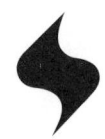

Stedman's
ORTHOPAEDIC
& REHAB
WORDS

INCLUDES
CHIROPRACTIC, OCCUPATIONAL THERAPY,
PHYSICAL THERAPY, PODIATRIC,
& SPORTS MEDICINE

FIFTH EDITION

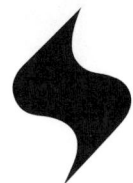

Stedman's

ORTHOPAEDIC & REHAB

WORDS

INCLUDES
CHIROPRACTIC, OCCUPATIONAL THERAPY,
PHYSICAL THERAPY, PODIATRIC, & SPORTS MEDICINE

FIFTH EDITION

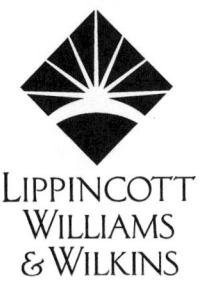

LIPPINCOTT
WILLIAMS
& WILKINS

Senior Publisher: Julie K. Stegman
Series Managing Editor: Eric Branger
Managing Editor: Steve Lichtenstein
Typesetter: Josephine Bergin
Printer & Binder: Malloy Litho, Inc.

Copyright © 2006 Lippincott Williams & Wilkins
351 West Camden Street
Baltimore, Maryland 21201-2436

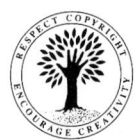

Printed in the United States of America

Fifth Edition, 2006

Library of Congress Cataloging-in-Publication Data
Stedman's orthopaedic & rehab words : includes chiropractic, occupational therapy, physical therapy, podiatric, & sportsmedicine. 5th ed.
    p. ; cm. -- (Stedman's word book series)
    Developed from the database of Stedman's medical dictionary, 27th ed., and supplemented by terminology found in current medical literature.
    Includes bibliographical references and index.
    ISBN 13: 978-0-7817-6182-6
    ISBN: 0-7817-6182-4 (alk. paper)
    1. Orthopedics—Terminology. 2. People with disabilities—Rehabilitation—Terminology. I. Stedman, Thomas Lathrop, 1853-1938. II. Stedman, Thomas Lathrop, 1853-1938. Stedman's medical dictionary. III. Title: Stedman's orthopaedic and rehab words.
    IV. Title: Orthopaedic & rehab words. V. Series: Stedman's word books.
    [DNLM: 1. Orthopedic Procedures—Terminology—English. 2. Athletic Injuries—Terminology—English. 3. Foot Diseases—Terminology—English. 4. Manipulation, Chiropractic—Terminology—English. 5. Physical Therapy Techniques—Terminology--English. 6. Rehabilitation--Terminology—English.   WE 15 S812 2006]
    RD723.S74 2006
    616.7'001'4--dc22

                                                                                    2005021543

06 07
2 3 4 5 6 7 8 9 10

Contents

Acknowledgements

An important part of our editorial process is the involvement of medical transcriptionists — as advisors, reviewers, and/or editors.

We extend special thanks to Nicole Peck, CMT, and Jeanne Bock, CSR, MT, for editing the manuscript, helping resolve many difficult questions, and contributing material for the appendix sections. We are grateful to our MT Editorial Advisory Board members, including Marty Cantu, CMT; Janice Deal, BSN, RN, ELS; Darcy Johnson; Beverly S. Oberline, CMT; and Jenifer Walker, MA, who were instrumental in the development of this reference. They recommended sources and shared their valuable judgment, insight, and perspective.

We also extend thanks to Jeanne Bock, CSR, MT, for working on the appendix. Additional thanks to Helen Littrell for performing the final pre-publication review. Other important contributors to this edition include Shemah Fletcher; Robin Koza; and Heather Little, CMT.

Special thanks to Lisa Fahnestock for her work in shaping and correcting the content.

As with all our Stedman's word references, this resource incorporates the suggestions and expertise of our many contacts in the medical transcriptionist community. Thanks to all of our advisory board participants, reviewers, and editors; AAMT meeting attendees; and others who have written us with requests and comments—keep talking, and we'll keep listening.

Editors' Preface

Life throws us many curves, often resulting in the unexpected. Stress can bring on headaches. Accidents can result in the fracture of any bone in our bodies. Repetitive movements can place a tremendous amount of strain on our muscles and joints. Our bodies are miracles—the network and teamwork of organs, bones, muscles, joints, blood, etc., that makes us function. Sadly, over time, with misuse and with diseases that invade, our bodies begin to wear down and need help to repair them. Even top athletes, who strive day after day to keep their bodies in top physical condition, suffer injuries and illnesses. The terminology of the myriad of problems related to muscles, bones, and joints under the umbrella of orthopaedic medicine are covered in this comprehensive 5th edition of *Stedman's Orthopaedic & Rehab Words*.

We anticipate the users of this reference will find much useful terminology related to orthopaedic injuries of the bones, joint, ligaments and spinal terminology related to such injuries.

We believe this edition will be especially helpful to the medical language specialist who has occasion to transcribe physical and/or occupational therapy dictation. This edition has an increased collection of terminology related to those two medical specialties that focus on rebuilding the strength, flexibility, and coordination of patients. Such therapy has the goal of returning patients to their original level of functionality or, alternatively, as high a level of functional independence as possible. Occupational and physical therapists work with patients who have lost these skills and abilities through deficits brought on by neurologic trauma, musculoskeletal trauma, or sometimes by the debilitation that can be seen from injury or other conditions found in a geriatric community.

Another advantageous feature of this edition is the inclusion of podiatric terms and images. Transcriptionists who need more specialized terminology relating to the foot and ankle will find the incorporation of these items into this edition of tremendous value.

Another edition of this book has come to fruition through the joint efforts of so many people. We'd like to take a moment to thank each of them for their hard work and dedication to this project: Lisa Fahnestock as the database editor; Steve Lichtenstein as the project manager; the Editorial Advisory Board; and all the medical transcriptionists who sent in suggestions and compiled new terms for inclusion in this book.

Nicole G. Peck, CMT

Jeanne Bock, CSR, MT

Publisher's Preface

Stedman's Orthopaedic & Rehab Words, Fifth Edition, offers an authoritative assurance of quality and exactness to the wordsmiths of the healthcare professions—medical transcriptionists, medical editors and copyeditors, health information management personnel, court reporters, and the many other users and producers of medical documentation.

We have received many requests to update this title. As a result, we have published this new edition that includes orthopaedic, rehabilitation, chiropractic, occupational therapy, physical therapy, and sports medicine terminology. In this new edition, we have expanded and revised all terminology, particularly in the areas of chiropractic and podiatric terminology. New to this edition is terminology relevant to kinesiology.

In *Stedman's Orthopaedic & Rehab Words, Fifth Edition*, users will nd protocols, diagnoses, and therapeutic procedures, new techniques, lab tests, clinical research terms, as well as abbreviations with their expansions pertinent to orthopaedics, rehabilitation, chiropractic, occupational therapy, physical therapy, and sports medicine. Users will also nd terms for protocols, diagnostic and therapeutic procedures, new techniques, lab tests, clinical research terms, as well as abbreviations with their expansions. The appendix sections provide anatomical illustrations with useful captions and labels; fracture illustrations; a table of muscles; a table of ligaments and tendons; style rules; professional organizations, associations, and titles; sample reports; common terms by procedure; and drugs by indication.

This compilation of more than 100,000 new and revised terms, fully cross-indexed for quick access, was built from a base vocabulary of approximately 66,000 medical words, phrases, abbreviations, and acronyms. The extensive A-Z list was developed from the database of Stedman's Medical Dictionary, 27th Edition, and supplemented by terminology found in current medical literature (see References on page xvii).

We at Lippincott Williams & Wilkins strive to provide you with the most up-to-date and accurate word references available. Your use of this word book will prompt new editions, which we will publish as often as updates and revisions justify. We welcome your suggestions for improvements, changes, corrections, and additions—whatever will make this Stedman's product more useful to you. Please complete the postpaid card in this book, and send your recommendations care of "Stedman's" at Lippincott Williams & Wilkins.

Explanatory Notes

Medical transcription is an art as well as a science. Both approaches are needed to correctly interpret the dictation of a physician, whose language is a product of education, training, and experience. This variety in medical language means that there are several acceptable ways to express certain terms, including jargon. *Stedman's Orthopaedic & Rehab Words, Fifth Edition*, provides variant spellings and phrasings for many terms. These elements, in addition to complete cross-indexing, make *Stedman's Orthopaedic & Rehab Words, Fifth Edition*, a valuable resource for determining the validity of terms as they are encountered.

Alphabetical Organization

Alphabetization of main entries is letter by letter as spelled, ignoring punctuation, spaces, prefixed numbers, or other characters. For example:

Nitalloy
2-nite
NiTi

Terms beginning or ending with Greek letters show the Greek letters spelled out and listed alphabetically. For example:

gamma, γ
  g. camera

In subentry alphabetization, the abbreviated singular form or the spelled-out plural form of the noun main entry word is ignored.

Format and Style

All main entries are in boldface to expedite locating a sought-after term, to enhance distinction between main entries and subentries, and to relieve the textual density of the pages.

Irregular plurals and variant spellings are shown on the same line as the singular or preferred form of the word. For example:

diaphysis, pl. **diaphyses**
orthopaedist, orthopedist

Hyphenation
As a rule of style, multiple eponyms (e.g., Mears-Rubash approach) are hyphenated. Also, hyphens have been added between a manufacturer and one or more eponyms (e.g., Vital-Metzenbaum dissecting scissors). Please note that in many cases, hyphenation is a question of style, not of accuracy, and thus is a matter of choice.

Possessives
Possessive forms have been dropped in this reference for the sake of consistency and conformance with the guidelines of the American Association for Medical Transcription (AAMT) and other groups. Please note, however, that in many cases, retaining the possessive, like hyphenating, is a question of style, not of accuracy, and thus is a matter of choice. To form the possessive of a word, simply add the apostrophe or apostrophe "s" to the end of the word.

Cross-indexing
The word list is in an index-like main entry-subentry format that contains two combined alphabetical listings:

(1) A noun main entry-subentry organization, which is typical of the A-Z section of medical dictionaries like *Stedman's*:

fixation	**shoe**
elastic f.	Canfield s.
graft f	cast s.
loop f.	Comed postoperative s.

(2) An *adjective* main entry-subentry organization, which lists words and phrases as you hear them. The main entries are the adjectives or modifiers in a multiword term. The subentries are the nouns around which the terms are constructed and to which the adjectives or modifiers pertain:

anterior
  a. cavus
  a. cervical approach
  a. cervical body fusion

bicipital
  b. muscle
  b. rib
  b. sulcus

This format provides the user with more than one way to locate and identify a multiword term. For example:

block
  Bier b.

Bier
  B. block

aquatic
  a. exercise

exercise
  aquatic e.

It also allows the user to see together all terms that contain a particular descriptor, as well as all types, kinds, or variations of a noun entity. For example:

magnetic
  m. resonance venography
  m. retriever
  m. sensor

patellar
  p. edge
  p. fat pad
  p. fossa

Wherever possible, abbreviations are separately defined and cross-referenced. For example:

IOM
　　interosseous membrane

interosseous
　　i. membrane (IOM)

membrane
　　interosseous m. (IOM)

References

In addition to the manufacturers' literature we gather at various medical meetings, scientific reports from hospitals, and the lists of our MT Editorial Advisory Board members (from their daily transcription work), we used the following sources for new terms in *Stedman's Orthopaedic & Rehab Words, Fifth Edition.*

Books

Adelaar RS. Complex Foot & Ankle Trauma. Philadelphia: Lippincott Williams & Wilkins, 1999.

Banks AS, Downey MS, Martin DE, Miller SJ. Foot and Ankle Surgery, 3rd Edition. Philadelphia: Lippincott Williams & Wilkins, 2001.

Banks AS, Downey MS, Martin DE, Miller SJ. McGlamry's Forefoot Surgery. Philadelphia: Lippincott Williams & Wilkins, 2004.

Blauvelt CT, Nelson FRT. A Manual of Orthopaedic Terminology, 6th Edition. Philadelphia: Mosby-Yearbook, 1998.

Bracker MD. The 5-Minute Sports Medicine Consult. Philadelphia: Lippincott Williams & Wilkins, 2001.

Brammer CM, Spires MC. Manual of Physical Medicine & Rehabilitation. Philadelphia: Hanley & Belfus, Inc., 2002.

Chang TJ, ed. Master Techniques in Podiatric Surgery: The Foot and Ankle. Baltimore: Lippincott Williams & Wilkins, 2005.

Crepeau EB, Cohn ES, Schell BAB, eds. Williard and Spackman's Occupational Therapy, 10th Edition. Philadelphia: Lippincott Williams & Wilkins, 2003.

Crim JR, Cracchiolo A, Hall RL. Imaging of the Foot and Ankle. Philadelphia: Lippincott Williams & Wilkins, 1996.

DeLisa JA, Gans BM, Walsh NE, eds. Physical Medicine and Rehabilitation, 4th Edition. Philadelphia: Lippincott Williams & Wilkins, 2004.

Dorland's Orthopedic Word Book for Medical Transcriptionists. Philadelphia: Saunders, 2002.

Drake E. Sloane's Medical Word Book, 4th Edition. Philadelphia: Saunders, 2001.

Garrison SJ, ed. Handbook of Physical Medicine and Rehabilitation Basics, 2nd Edition. Philadelphia: Lippincott Williams & Wilkins, 2003.

Gatterman M. Chiropractic Management of Spine Related Disorders, 2nd Edition. Baltimore: Lippincott Williams & Wilkins, 2003.

Greenspan A. Orthopedic Imaging: A Practical Approach, 4th Edition. Philadelphia: Lippincott Williams & Wilkins, 2004.

Herkowitz HN. The Lumbar Spine, 3rd Edition. Philadelphia: Lippincott Williams & Wilkins, 2004.

Hoppenfeld S, deBoer P. Surgical Exposures in Orthopaedics: The Anatomic Approach, 3rd Edition. Philadelphia: Lippincott Williams & Wilkins, 2003.

Karageanes SJ. Principles of Manual Sports Medicine. Philadelphia: Lippincott Williams & Wilkins, 2005.

Lance LL. Quick Look Drug Book. Baltimore: Lippincott Williams & Wilkins, 2002.

Leach RA. The Chiropractic Theories, 4th Edition. Philadelphia: Lippincott Williams & Wilkins, 2003.

Mow VC, Huskies R, eds. Basic Orthopaedic Biomechanics and Mechano-Biology, 3rd Edition. Philadelphia: Lippincott Williams & Wilkins, 2004.

Oatis CA. Kinesiology. Philadelphia: Lippincott Williams & Wilkins, 2004.

Olson T. A.D.A.M. Student Atlas of Anatomy. Philadelphia: Lippincott Williams & Wilkins,

1996.

Orthopedic/Neurology Words and Phrases, 2nd Edition. Modesto, CA: Health

Professions Institute, 2000.

Safran MR, McKeag DB, Van Camp SP. Manual of Sports Medicine. Philadelphia: Lippincott Williams & Wilkins, 1998.

Sponseller, PD, Frassica FJ, Wenz, JF. The 5-Minute Orthopaedic Consult. Philadelphia: Lippincott Williams & Wilkins, 2000.

Stedman's Medical Dictionary, 27th Edition. Baltimore: Lippincott Williams & Wilkins, 2000.

Stedman's Orthopaedic & Rehab Words, 4th Edition. Baltimore: Lippincott Williams & Wilkins, 2003.

Tessier C. The AAMT Book of Style. Modesto, CA: AAMT, 1995.

Thordarson DB, ed. Foot and Ankle. Philadelphia: Lippincott Williams & Wilkins, 2004.

Vera Pyle's Current Medical Terminology, 9th Edition. Modesto, CA: Health Professions Institute, 2003.

Images

Agur, AMR, Lee, MJ. Grant's Atlas of Anatomy, 10th Edition. Baltimore: Lippincott Williams & Wilkins, 1999.

Blackbourne LH, MD. Advanced Surgical Recall, 2nd Edition. Baltimore: Lippincott Williams & Wilkins, 2004.

Koval KJ, Zuckerman, JD. Atlas of Orthopaedic Surgery: A Multimeidal Reference. Philadelphia: Lippincott Williams & Wilkins, 2004.

LifeART Super Anatomy Collection 1-3, 5, 7 CD-ROM. Baltimore, Lippincott Williams & Wilkins.

MediClip Human Anatomy1-3, CD-ROM. Baltimore: Lippincott, Williams & Wilkins.

MediClip Manual Medicine II, CD-ROM. Baltimore: Lippincott Williams & Wilkins.

Neil O. Hardy. Westport, CT. From Stedman's Medical Dictionary, 27th Edition. Baltimore: Lippincott Williams & Wilkins, 2000.

Saurerland E, Saurerland W. Grant's Dissector, 12th Edition. Baltimore: Lippincott Williams & Wilkins, 1999.

Smeltzer SC, Bare BG. Textbook of Medical-Surgical Nursing, 9th Edition. Philadelphia: Lippincott Williams & Wilkins, 2000.

Stedman's Orthopedic & Rehab Words, 4th Edition. Baltimore: Lippincott Williams & Wilkins, 2003.

Journals

ACSM's Health & Fitness Journal. Baltimore: Lippincott Williams & Wilkins, 1999-2000.

Chiropractic Products. Los Angeles: Medical World Communications, Inc., 2000.

Clinical Journal of Sports Medicine. Philadelphia: Lippincott Williams & Wilkins, 2001-2002.

Current Opinion in Orthopaedics. Philadelphia: Lippincott Willaims & Wilkins, 2001-2002.

Foot & Ankle International. Philadelphia: Lippincott Willaims & Wilkins, 1999-2002.

Journal of the American Association for Medical Transcription. Modesto, CA: American Association for Medical Transcription, 2000-2001.

Journal of Bone & Joint Surgery. Needham, MA: The Journal of Bone & Joint Surgery, Inc. 1999-2005.

Journal of Foot & Ankle Surgery. Park Ridge, IL: American College of Foot and Ankle Surgeons, 1999-2005.

Latest Word. Philadelphia: Saunders, 1999-2005.

O & P Almanac. Alexandria, VA: American Orthotic and Prosthetic Association, 1999-2000.

OrthoKinetic Review. Los Angeles: MWC/Allied Healthcare Group, 2001.

Perspectives on the Medical Transcription Profession. Modesto, CA: Health Professions Institute, 2001.

Physical Therapy Products. Los Angeles: MWC/Allied Healthcare Group, 1998-1999.

Podiatric Products. Los Angeles: MWC/Allied Healthcare Group, 1999-2000.

Sports Medicine Digest. Philadelphia: Lippincott Williams & Wilkins, 2001-2002.

Websites

http://physicaltherapy.about.com

http://www.accessdata.fda.gov/scripts/cdrh/cfdocs/cfTopic/MDA/mda-list.cfm?list+1

http://www.aaos.org

http://www.aota.org

http://www.aotf.org

http://www.apma.org

http://www.askdrwalker.com/index/professional.organizations.htm

http://www.bonehome.com/Home/Topics/orthopedics/orthopedics.html

http://www.chiroweb.com

http://www.fda.gov

http://www.hpisum.com

http://www.mtdaily.com

http://www.mtdesk.com

http://www.mtmonthly.com

http://www.orthonurse.org/education/links.cfm

http://www.podiatrychannel.com

http://uwadmnweb.uwyo.edu/ATHTRN/Professional%20Organizations.htm

A
  A pin
  A wave
AA
  active-assistive
AAA
  autolyzed, antigen-extracted, allogenic
  diagnostic arthroscopy, operative
  arthroscopy, possible operative
  arthrotomy
    AAA bone
    AAA bone graft
AAD
  atlantoaxial dislocation
AAE
  active-assistive exercise
AAHS
  American Association for Hand Surgery
AAI
  activating adjusting instrument
  axial acetabular index
AAL
  anterior axillary line
Aalzet continuous infusion osmotic pump
AANA
  Arthroscopy Association of North
  America
AAOS
  American Academy of Orthopaedic
  Surgeons
    AAOS acetabular abnormality
    classification
    AAOS Knee Society Clinical
    Rating Score
AARF
  atlantoaxial rotatory fixation
AAROM
  active-assisted range of motion
Aarskog-Scott syndrome
AAS
  atlantoaxial subluxation
AAT
  animal-assisted therapy
AB/AD
  abduction/adduction
  abductor/adductor
  AB/AD ratio
Abaqus modeling program
abarthrosis
abarticular
abarticulation
abasia
    atactic a.
abasic

abatement
abatic
Abbe operation
Abbott
  A. brace
  A. gouge
  A. knee approach
  A. method
  A. operation
  A. posterior approach
  A. splint
Abbott-Carpenter posterior approach
Abbott-Fischer-Lucas hip arthrodesis
Abbott-Gill
  A.-G. epiphysial plate exposure
  A.-G. epiphysiodesis
  A.-G. osteotomy
Abbott-Lucas
  A.-L. arthrodesis
  A.-L. shoulder operation
Abbreviated Injury Scale (AIS)
ABC
  aneurysmal bone cyst
  Assessment Battery for Children
abdominal
  a. binder
  a. dressing
  a. flap
  a. lap pad
  a. muscle
  a. view
ABD pad
abduct
abducted thumb
abduction
  a. angle
  a. bolster
  a. brace
  a. contracture
  Cruiser hip a.
  a. cushion
  a. deformity
  a. and external rotation (ABER)
  a. external rotation test
  a. and external rotation view
  a. finger splint
  hinge a.
  hip a.
  a. hip orthosis
  a. humeral splint
  humerothoracic a.
  index finger a.
  a. knee separator
  a. load and shift test
  a. osteotomy

abduction *(continued)*
    a. pillow
    a. pillow cover splint
    a. sign
    a. stress test
    a. thumb splint
    a. traction technique
    a. wedge
abduction/adduction (AB/AD)
abduction-external
    a.-e. rotation (AER)
    a.-e. rotation fracture
abductor
    a. digiti minimi (ADM)
    a. digiti minimi muscle
    a. digiti minimi nerve
    a. digiti minimi opponensplasty
    a. digiti quinti (ADQ)
    a. digiti quinti muscle
    a. digiti quinti opponensplasty
    a. digiti quinti tendon
    a. hallucis longus flap
    a. hallucis muscle
    a. hallucis oblique head
    a. hallucis tendon
    a. hallucis transverse head
    a. insufficiency
    a. lever arm
    a. lurch
    a. lurch gait
    a. mechanism
    a. pollicis brevis
    a. pollicis brevis muscle
    a. pollicis brevis tendon
    a. pollicis longus (APL)
    a. pollicis longus muscle
    a. pollicis longus tendon
    side-lying hip a.
    a. slide technique
abductor/adductor (AB/AD)
    a./a. ratio
abductor-plasty
    flexor pollicis longus a.-p.
    Smith flexor pollicis longus a.-p.
abductory
    a. midfoot osteotomy
    a. wedge osteotomy
abductovalgus
    adolescent hallux a.
    hallux a. (HAV)
abductus
    digitus a.
    forefoot a.
    hallux a. (HA)
    interphalangeal a.
    metatarsus a.
    midfoot a.
    pes planovalgus a.
    pollex a.

ABER
    abduction and external rotation
    ABER view
Abernethy fascia
aberration
    hypokinetic a.
ABG cement-free hip system
ability, pl. **abilities**
    abstracting a.
    bathing and dressing a.
    conceptual a.
    constructional a.
    fluid absorption a.
    general a.
    McCarthy Scale of Children's
      Abilities
    positive a.
    self-help a.
    squatting a.
ablation
    cartilage a.
    cyst a.
    nerve rootlet a.
    radical nail bed a.
    surgical a.
    Zadik total nail bed a.
ablative
    a. arthroplasty
    a. laser therapy
    a. surgery
ablator
    Concept a.
Ableware Volumeter
abnormal
    a. fixation
    a. instantaneous axis of rotation
    A. Involuntary Movement Scale
      (AIMS)
    a. posterior talar process
    a. shoe wear
abnormality, pl. **abnormalities**
    alignment a.
    biochemical a.
    bony a.
    bulbar a.
    cranial nerve a.
    cytoarchitectonic a.
    dislocation contour a.
    engulfment a.
    fibropathic a.
    frontal plane growth a.
    sensorineural a.
    soft tissue a.
    sonographic a.
    spinal cord injury without
      radiographic a. (SCIWORA)
    tissue texture a. (TTA)
    torsional a.
Abouna splint

above
>a. elbow (AE)
>a. knee (AK)

above-elbow
>a.-e. amputation (AEA)
>a.-e. cast

above-knee
>a.-k. amputation (AKA)
>a.-k. prosthesis
>a.-k. suction enhancement system

abrader
>cartilage a.

Abramson catheter

abrasion
>a. arthroplasty
>a. chondroplasty
>graft-bony tunnel wall a.

Abrikossoff tumor

abscess
>arthrifluent a.
>bone a.
>Brodie a.
>bursal a.
>button a.
>cold a.
>collar-button a.
>growth plate a.
>gummatous a.
>horseshoe a.
>hypostatic a.
>intraosseous a.
>ischiorectal a.
>lumbar a.
>metaphysial a.
>midpalmar a.
>ossifluent a.
>paraspinal a.
>paravertebral a.
>pelvic a.
>periarticular a.
>posterior pharyngeal a.
>Pott a.
>psoas a.
>retropharyngeal a.
>retrosternal a.
>sacrococcygeal a.
>serous a.
>soft tissue a.
>spinal a.
>subaponeurotic a.
>subcutaneous a.
>subfascial a.
>subgaleal a.
>subperiosteal a.
>subphrenic a.
>subplatysmal a.
>subungual a.
>supralevator a.
>suture a.
>syphilitic a.
>thecal a.
>traumatic a.

abscessogram

absconsio

absence
>congenital intercalary limb a.
>congenital terminal limb a.
>limb a.

absent
>a. patella
>a. radius
>a. reflex
>a. spinous process
>a. tibia
>a. ulna

absolute
>A. absorbable screw
>a. refractory period
>a. scotoma

absorbable
>a. biomaterial
>a. collagen paste (ACP)
>a. polymeric pin
>a. polyparadioxanone pin
>a. suture anchor

Absorbine
>A. Antifungal Foot Powder
>A. Jr. Antifungal

absorptiometry
>dual-energy x-ray a. (DEXA, DXA)
>dual-photon a. (DPA, DPX)
>peripheral dual-energy x-ray a. (pDXA)

absorption
>bone a.
>bony a.
>a. cavity
>energy a.
>lysosomal a.
>shock a.

absorptive dressing

abstracting ability

Abumi technique

abut

NOTES

abutment
    calcaneofibular a.
    a. splint
    ulnocarpal a.
Abzorb cushioning
AC
    acromioclavicular
    AC joint
    AC joint separation
ACA
    augmentative communication aid
acampsia
acantha
acanthoma
    clear cell a.
    epidermolytic a.
acanthosis nigricans
acanthotic
Acapella chest physical therapy device
accelerated
    a. bone maturation
    a. chondral wear
acceleration
    angular a.
    swing-phase a.
    tibial a.
acceleration/deceleration injury
accelerator
    Bevatron a.
    linear a. (LINAC)
    Philips linear a.
    Siemens linear a.
accelerometer
    piezoelectric a.
Accell
    A. Connexus bone matrix
    A. DBM 100 bone matrix
    A. TBM bone matrix
    A. total bone matrix
acceptance
    weight a.
access
    eccentric a.
    A. Ostase
    southern a.
accessiflexor
accessory
    a. abductor hallucis
    a. atlantoaxial ligament
    Auto Glide walker a.
    a. bone
    a. cartilage
    a. communicating tendon
    a. digit
    a. epiphysis
    Isola spinal implant system a.
    a. lateral collateral ligament
    a. motion
    a. movement technique

    a. navicular
    a. navicular avulsion
    a. navicular cast
    a. navicular fracture
    a. nerve
    a. nerve injury
    a. ossicle
    a. ossicle fracture
    a. ossification center
    a. ossification center of calcaneus
    a. phalanx
    pneumatic drill a.
    portal a.
    a. portion
    a. sesamoid
    a. soleus
    a. soleus muscle
AccessTrainer exerciser
accident
    cerebrovascular a. (CVA)
    compensable a.
    motorcycle a. (MCA)
    motor vehicle a. (MVA)
    pedestrian a.
    vascular a.
acclimate
acclivity
Accolade hip prosthesis
accommodation
    a. curve
    a. reflex
accommodative
    a. brace
    a. equipment
    a. orthosis
    a. shoe
Accommodator arch support
accordion test
accoucheur hand
Accu-Back back support
Accucore II
Accu-Cut
    A.-C. osteotomy guide
    A.-C. osteotomy guide system
accuDEXA bone densitometer
Accuflate tourniquet
Accu-Flo
    A.-F. polyethylene bur hole cover
    A.-F. silicone rubber bur hole
      cover
    A.-F. ultrafiltration system
Accugraft
    A. allograft
    Puros A.
AccuGuide injection monitor
**Acculength arthroplasty measuring
system**
Accu-Line
    A.-L. dual pivot

A.-L. femoral resector
A.-L. guide
A.-L. knee instrument
A.-L. knee instrumentation
A.-L. tibial resector

accumulation
blood lactate a.
onset of blood lactate a. (OBLA)

AccuPressure heel cup

**Accurate Surgical and Scientific
Instruments Corporation (ASSI)**

**AccuSharp carpal tunnel release
instrument**

AccuSpan tissue expander

Accu-SPINA
A.-SPINA cervical decompression
machine
A.-SPINA system

AccuSway
A. balance measurement
A. balance measurement system

AccuTread shoe

Accu-Tron microcurrent machine

Accuvac smoke evacuation attachment

ACDF
anterior cervical discectomy and fusion

ace
A. adherent bandage
A. bandage reduction
A. brace
A. intramedullary (AIM)
A. intramedullary femoral nail
system
A. pin
A. screw
A. Unifix fixation
A. Unifix fixation apparatus
A. Unifix fixation device
A. wrap

Ace-Colles
A.-C. external fixator
A.-C. fixation
A.-C. fracture frame
A.-C. frame technique
A.-C. half ring

Ace-Fischer
A.-F. external fixator
A.-F. fixation
A.-F. fracture frame
A.-F. ring frame

Ace/Normed osteodistractor

ACET
aquatic cardiac evaluation and testing
ACET system

acetabula (*pl. of* acetabulum)

acetabular
a. allograft
a. angle
a. angle of Sharp
a. anteversion
a. augmentation graft
a. bone
a. branch
a. cap
a. cement compactor
a. component
a. component loosening
a. cup
a. cup arthroplasty
a. cup holder
a. cup peg drill guide
a. cup positioner
a. cup system
a. cup template
a. cyst
a. defect
a. deficiency
a. depth
a. depth to femoral head diameter
(AD/FHD)
a. dysplasia
a. endoprosthesis
a. expander
a. extensile approach
a. fossa
a. gauge
a. head index (AHI)
a. head quotient
a. index
a. knee
a. knife
a. labrum
a. libectomy
a. line
a. liner
a. notch
a. osteolysis
a. posterior wall fracture
a. pressurizer
a. prosthesis
a. prosthesis system
a. prosthetic interface
a. prosthetic liner
a. protrusio deformity

NOTES

acetabular *(continued)*
a. reamer
a. recess
a. reconstruction plate
a. reinforcement
a. reinforcement device
a. rim
a. rim fracture
a. rim syndrome
a. roof
a. round chisel
a. seating hole
a. shelf osteotomy
a. shell
a. slot
a. spacer
a. trial set
acetabulectomy
acetabuli
arteria a.
protrusio a.
acetabuloplasty
Albee a.
Lance a.
Pemberton a.
shelf a.
acetabulum, pl. **acetabula**
deep-shelled a.
dysplastic a.
false a.
floor of a.
lip of a.
malunited a.
true a.
acetate
compression-molded ethylene vinyl a. (CM EVA)
desmopressin a. (DDAVP)
ethylene vinyl a. (EVA)
mafenide a.
methylprednisolone a.
triamcinolone a.
acetic acid
acetylsalicylic acid
ACF
anterior cervical fusion
ACFS
anterior cervical plate fixation system
Dogbone ACFS
ache
a.'s and pains
theater a.
acheiria
acheiropodia
achieve
A. computer-assisted instruments
A. software
Achilles
A. bulge sign

A. heel pad
A. jerk
A. peritendinitis
A. squeeze test
A. tendinitis
A. tendinopathy
A. tendon (AT)
A. tendon advancement
A. tendon bursa
A. tendon bursitis
A. tendon contracture
A. tendon enthesis
A. tendon enthesis calcification
A. tendon lengthening
A. tendon pain
A. tendon reflex
A. tendon repair (ATR)
A. tendon resurfacing
A. tendon rupture (ATR)
A. tendon rupture repair comparison
A. tendon shortening
A. tendon taping technique
A. tendon test
A. tendon xanthoma
A. tendon Z-lengthening
A. tenotomy
A. triangle
A. + ultrasound bone densitometer
Achillis
tendo A.
achillobursitis
achillodynia
Albert a.
achillogram
Achillon instrument guide
achillorrhaphy
achillotenotomy
plastic a.
achillotomy
Achillotrain
A. active Achilles tendon support
Bauerfeind A.
achondrogenesis
achondroplasia
achondroplastic
a. dwarfism
a. pelvis
a. stenosis
achondroplasty
achromatopsia
Achromycin Topical
ACI
autologous chondrocyte implantation
acid
methylmalonic a.
peracetic a.
polyglycolic acid-polylactic a. (PGA-PLA)

poly-L-lactic a. (PLLA)
self-reinforcing polylevolactic a.
(SR-PLLA)
a. treatment
acid-citrate-dextrose solution
acidosis
lactic a.
acidosteophyte
Acinetobacter
A. *anitratus*
A. *wolffii*
ACIS
Assessment of Communication and
Interaction Skills
Ackerman
A. criteria for osteomyelitis
A. osteomyelitis criteria
ACL
Allen Cognitive Level
anterior cruciate ligament
ACL drill
ACL drill guide
ACL graft
ACL graft knife
ACL guide set
ACL Lite functional knee brace
ACL reconstruction
ACL repair
ACL Screen
Acland
A. clamp-applying forceps
A. clamp approximator
A. double-clamp approximator
A. microvascular clamp
aclasia
aclasis
diaphysial a.
metaphysial a.
tarsoepiphysial a.
aclastic
ACL-deficient knee
ACLR
anterior capsulolabral reconstruction
ACLS
Allen Cognitive Level Screen
acnemia, aknemia
Acoma scanner
acorn
Midas Rex a.
a. reamer
Acor Quikform I, II shoe
acoustical shadowing
acoustic myography

ACP
absorbable collagen paste
anterior cervical plate
AC-PC
anterior commissure-posterior
commissure
AC-PC line
AC-PC plane
ACPS
acrocephalopolysyndactyly
acquired
a. brain injury
a. clubfoot
a. digital fibrokeratoma
a. flatfoot
a. myopathy
a. tarsal coalition
a. thumb flexion contracture
a. torticollis
acquisita
myotonia a.
ACR
American College of Rheumatology
ACR classification
Acra-Cut wire pass drill
acral
a. digital fibrokeratoma
a. lentiginous melanoma
Acrel ganglion
acroarthritis
acroataxia
acrocephalopolysyndactyly (ACPS)
acrocephalosyndactylism
acrocephalosyndactyly
acrochordon
AcroContin drug delivery system
acrocontracture
acrocyanosis
acrodysesthesia
acrodysostosis
acrodysplasia
Acro-Flex artificial disc
acrokeratoelastoidosis
acrokinesia
acromacria
AcroMed
A. screw
A. VSP fixation system
A. VSP plate
acromegalic
a. arthralgia
a. arthritis
a. facies

NOTES

acromegalogigantism
acromegaloidism
acromegaly
acromelia
acromesomelic dysplasia
acrometagenesis
acromial
    a. angle
    a. bone
    a. profile
    a. spur
    a. spur index (ASI)
acromiale
    os a.
acromioclavicular (AC)
    a. arthroplasty
    a. articulation
    a. cyst
    a. disc
    a. immobilizer
    a. injury classification
    a. joint
    a. joint dislocation
    a. joint injury
    a. joint repair
    a. ligament
    a. separation
    a. sprain
acromiocoracoid ligament
acromiohumeral interval (AHI)
acromion
    hooked a.
    a. process
acromionectomy
    Armstrong a.
acromionizer tip
acromioplasty
    anterior a.
    arthroscopic a.
    decompressive a.
    McLaughlin a.
    McShane-Leinberry-Fenlin a.
    Neer a.
    Rockwood anterior a.
acromioscapular
acromyotonia
acromyotonus
acroosteolysis
    frostbite a.
acroosteosclerosis
acropachy
acropachyderma
acroparalysis
acroparesthesia
    Nothnagel a.
    Schultze a.
acropathology

acropathy
    amyotrophic a.
    ulcerative mutilating a.
acropectorovertebral dysplasia
acrosclerosis
acrostealgia
acrosyndactyly
    Apert a.
Acrotorque hand engine
acrylic
    a. bar prosthesis
    a. bone cement
    a. cap splint
    a. implant material
    a. orthotic device
    a. template splint
Acryl-X-II bone cement removal system
Acryl-X orthopaedic cement removal
    system
ACS
    anterior compartment syndrome
        ACS Gemini prosthesis
        ACS Profile prosthesis
        ACS Star prosthesis
ACSM
    American College of Sports Medicine
        ACSM Guidelines for Exercise
            Testing and Prescription
act
    A. joint support
    A. knee support
ACTH
    adrenocorticotropic hormone
actinic keratosis
actinomycosis
action
    concentric muscle a.
    a. current
    double-pendulum a.
    eccentric muscle a.
    A. elbow wrap
    A. Jr. wheelchair
    a. line
    Marshall Hall theory of reflex a.
    a. myoclonus
    a. potential (AP)
    reflex a.
    A. thumb sling
    A. ThumSling
    A. traction system
    a. tremor
    A. wrist wrap
activated partial thromboplastin time
    (APTT)
activating adjusting instrument (AAI)
activation
    antagonistic a.
    electromyographic a.
    a. force

latency of a.
order of a.
volitional a.

activator
tissue-type plasminogen a.

active
A. ankle brace
a. ankle joint complex range of motion
A. Ankle support
a. bending test
a. contraction
a. dorsiflexion
a. electrode
a. flexion
a. hip movement
a. insufficiency
a. integral range of motion (AIROM)
a. knee extension (AKE)
a. knee extension test
a. mobility
a. motion testing (AMT)
a. movement testing
a. muscle co-contraction
a. and passive range of motion
a. physiotherapy
a. range of motion (AROM)
a. range of motion exercise
a. restraint
a. sock
a. splint
A. support and brace
a. treatment

active-assisted
a.-a. range of motion (AAROM)
a.-a. range of motion exercise

active-assistive (AA)
a.-a. exercise (AAE)
a.-a. motion therapy

active-release technique (ART)

activity, pl. **activities**
a. adaptation
a. analysis
biphasic endplate a.
a. configuration
a. of daily living (ADL)
activities of daily living adjustment disorder agraphia
discrete a.
diversional a.
endplate a.
functional a.

a. grading
a. group
high-altitude a.
high-impact a.
A. Index and Meaningfulness of Activity Scale
involuntary a.
A. Loss Assessment (ALA)
mechanoreceptor a.
monophasic endplate a.
motion a.
motor a.
opsonic a.
physical a.
pivoting and cutting a.
pivot sport a.
purposeful a.
push-pull a.
spontaneous a.
sudomotor a.
a. synthesis
a. training (AT)
volitional a.
voluntary a.

Activity-Lite knee brace
activity-pattern analysis
Activ slideboard
actomyosin
actual leg length test
actuator
NYU-Hosmer prehension a.
ACU-derm wound dressing
AcuDriver osteotome
ACU-dyne antiseptic
Acufex
A. alignment guide
A. ankle distractor
A. arthroscopic instrument
A. arthroscopic instrumentation
A. bioabsorbable fixation device
A. bioabsorbable Suretac suture
A. bioabsorbable suture anchor
A. convex rasp
A. curette
A. curved basket forceps
A. distractor pin
A. double-lumen arthroscopic cannula
A. drill
A. drill-guide
A. Edge
A. gouge
A. grasper

NOTES

Acufex *(continued)*
- A. knee laxity arthrometer
- A. mallet
- A. meniscal basket
- A. meniscal stitcher
- A. microsurgical rear-entry to front-entry femoral guide system
- A. microsurgical tendon stripper
- A. MosaicPlasty instrument
- A. nerve hook
- A. osteotome
- A. probe
- A. rotary biting basket forceps
- A. rotary punch
- A. scissors
- A. tensiometer
- A. T-Fix suture anchor
- A. tibial guide

AcuFix anterior cervical plate system
Acuforce 7.0 therapy tool
Acu-Magnet therapy
AcuMatch
- A. A, L, M Series acetabular component
- A. integrated hip system
- A. L Series cemented femoral stem component
- A. M Series modular femoral hip prosthesis

Acumed
- A. congruent clavicle plate
- A. great toe system
- A. suture anchor

Acupoint stimulator
AcuPressor myotherapy tool
acupressure
- Neiguan point a.

Acu-Pressure slipper
acupuncture
- Korean hand a.
- laser a.
- a. needle
- a. point

Acuson imaging system
AcuSpark piezoelectric device
Acustar surgical navigation system
acute
- a. angular kyphosis
- a. avulsion fracture
- a. brachial radiculitis
- a. calcific tendinitis
- a. exertional compartment syndrome (AECS)
- a. foot strain
- a. gout
- a. hematogenous arthritis
- a. hematogenous osteomyelitis (AHO)

- a. inflammatory demyelinating polyradiculoneuropathy (AIDP)
- a. inflammatory polyradiculopathy
- a. inflammatory response
- a. ischemic contracture
- a. locked-back syndrome
- a. low back syndrome
- a. meniscal tear
- a. pain
- a. phase rehabilitation
- A. Physiology and Chronic Health Evaluation (APACHE)
- a. progressive myositis
- a. reflex bone atrophy
- a. repetitive seizure (ARS)
- a. spinal arthritis
- a. stretch injury
- a. transverse myelitis
- a. traumatic hemarthrosis
- a. traumatic lesion
- a. whiplash

AcuTENS transcutaneous nerve stimulator
Acutrak
- A. fusion system
- A. screw system
- A. small bone fixation system

Acu-Treat electroacupuncture
AcuVibe massager
adactylous
adactyly, adactylia
- partial a.

Adair-Dighton syndrome
Adair screw compressor
Adalat CC
Adam
- A. and Eve rib belt splint
- A. sign

Adamantiades-Behçet syndrome
adamantinoma
- a. of long bone
- tibial a.

Adamkiewicz artery
Adams
- A. forward-bending test
- A. hip operation
- A. position test
- A. procedure
- A. saw
- A. scoliosis test
- A. splint
- A. transmalleolar arthrodesis
- A. view

Adapta physical therapy table
adaptation
- activity a.
- high-altitude a.

adapted stroller

adapter, adaptor
    Christmas tree a.
    chuck a.
    Collet screwdriver a.
    French a.
    Grace plate 4-hole a.
    Hudson chuck a.
    Jacobs chuck a.
    Leksell a.
    Lloyd a.
    Mayfield a.
    SACH foot a.
    Smith-Petersen nail with Lloyd a.
    Trinkle brace and a.
    Trinkle chuck a.
Adapteur multifunctional drill guide
Adaptic
    A. crown
    A. dressing
    A. gauze
    A. pack
    A. packing
    A. sponge
adaptive equipment
adaptor (*var. of* adapter)
Adcon adhesive control gel
Adcon-L anti-adhesion barrier gel
Add-A-Clamp
    Hex-Fix A.-A-C.
adducent
adduct
adducta
    coxa a.
adducted thumb
adduction
    a. contracture
    a. deformity
    Edgarton-Grand thumb a.
    a. fracture
    a. load and shift test
    a. osteotomy
    a. sign
    a. stress to finger
    a. stress test
    a. traction technique
adduction-internal rotation deformity
adductocavus
    metatarsus a.
adductor
    a. aponeurosis
    a. hallucis longus
    a. hallucis muscle
    a. hallucis tendon
    a. hamstring tightness
    a. hiatus
    a. longus muscle rupture
    a. magnus
    a. magnus adductor flap
    a. muscle group
    a. origin
    a. pollicis brevis tendon
    a. pollicis muscle
    a. pollicis paralysis
    a. pollicus
    a. reflex
    a. sweep of thumb
    a. tendon and lateral capsular release
    a. tenotomy
    a. tenotomy and obturator neurectomy (ATON)
    a. tubercle
    a. tuberosity
adductovarus
    a. deformity
    forefoot a.
    metatarsus a.
adductus
    compensated metatarsus a.
    congenital metatarsus a.
    digitus a.
    dynamic metatarsus a.
    forefoot a.
    metatarsus a. (MTA)
    metatarsus primus a. (MPA)
    midfoot a.
    pes equinovarus a.
    simple metatarsus a.
    true metatarsus a. (TMA)
Adelaar-Williams-Gould 10-point scale
Adelmann operation
A-delta fiber
adenoma
    papillary a.
adenomyosis
adenosine thallium scan
AD/FHD
    acetabular depth to femoral head diameter
adherence
    skin a.
adherent
    a. profundus tendon
    Tuf-Skin tape a.
adhesion
    bandlike a.

NOTES

adhesion *(continued)*
    capsular a.
    fibrous a.
    filmy a.
    a. formation
    intraarticular a.
    subacromial bursal a.
    subdeltoid bursal a.
adhesion/cohesion mechanism
adhesive
    APR cement fixation a.
    a. arachnoiditis
    Aron Alpha a.
    benzoin a.
    Biobrane a.
    a. capsulitis
    Coe-pak paste a.
    Coverlet a.
    Cover-Roll gauze a.
    cyanoacrylate a.
    a. drape
    a. dressing
    fibrin glue a.
    Histoacryl glue a.
    hydroxyapatite a.
    Implast a.
    ligand a.
    LLPS hydroxyapatite a.
    Mastisol liquid a.
    medical a.
    methyl methacrylate a.
    a. neuralgia
    Orthomite II a.
    Palacos cement a.
    Simplex cement a.
    a. strapping
    Superglue a.
    Surfit a.
    Surgical Simplex P a.
    a. tenosynovitis
    T-Stick a.
    Zimmer low-viscosity a.
ADI
    atlantodens interval
adiabatic fast passage
adipofascial flap
adipose
    a. ligament
    a. tissue
adiposogenital dystrophy
adiposus
    panniculus a.
ADJ
    adjustable dynamic joint
adjoining pedicle
adjunct
    walking a.
adjunctive screw fixation
Adjustaback wheelchair backrest system

adjustability
    3D positional a.
adjustable
    A. Advanced Reciprocating Gait Orthosis (ARGO)
    a. aiming apparatus
    a. aiming device
    a. angle guide
    a. brace
    a. cane
    a. cane board
    a. dynamic joint (ADJ)
    A. Leg and Ankle Repositioning Mechanism (ALARM)
    a. nail
    a. pedicle connector
    a. 2-point caliper sensory assessment device
    a. postoperative protective prosthetic socket (APOPPS)
    a. splint
Adjusta-Wrist
    A.-W. hinge
    A.-W. splint
adjusting
    computer-assisted mechanical instrument a.
    mechanical instrument a.
    a. table
adjustive
    a. thrust
    a. treatment
adjustment
    atlas a.
    chiropractic spinal a.
    a. equipment
    figure-of-8 a.
    general a.
    level-specific chiropractic a.
    manual a.
    osseous a.
    psychological a.
    set-hold a.
    side-specific chiropractic a.
    specific a.
    a. of spine
    toggle-recoil a.
    vectored a.
    vertebral a.
adjuvant chemotherapy
adjuvant-induced arthritis (AIA)
ADK
    automated disposable keratome
Adkins
    A. spinal arthrodesis
    A. spinal fusion
ADL
    activity of daily living
    adrenoleukodystrophy

extended ADLs
hierarchial scales of ADLs
ADL index
indices of ADLs
instrumental ADLs
Northwick Park Index of
   Independence in ADL
Adlone Injection
ADM
   abductor digiti minimi
   Allen Diagnostic Module
admixed epinephrine
adolescent
   a. back pain
   a. condylar blade-plate
   a. hallux abductovalgus
   a. idiopathic scoliosis (AIS)
   a. kyphosis
   A. and Pediatric Pain Tool
      (APPT)
   A. and Pediatric Pain Tool Scale
   a. rigid foot
   A. Role Assessment (ARA)
   a. round back
   a. scoliosis
   a. tibia vara
adolescentium
   apophysitis tibialis a.
ADQ
   abductor digiti quinti
adrenal
   a. cortex
   a. disorder
adrenergic vagal function
adrenocorticotropic hormone (ACTH)
adrenoleukodystrophy (ADL)
Adriamycin
   A. PFS
   A. RDF
ADROM
   ankle dorsiflexion range of motion
adromia
Adson
   A. bur
   A. cerebellar retractor
   A. clip-introducing forceps
   A. conductor
   A. drill guide
   A. drill guide forceps
   A. enlarging bur
   A. hemilaminectomy retractor
   A. hypophysial forceps
   A. laminectomy chisel

A. maneuver
A. perforating bur
A. periosteal elevator
A. rongeur
A. saw guide
A. sign
A. spiral drill
A. suction tube
A. test
A. twist drill
A. wire saw
Adson-Rogers perforating drill
ADT
   anterior drawer test
adult
   a. acquired flatfoot
   a. flatfoot correction
   a. gait
   A. Nowicki Strickland Internal
      External Control Scale (ANSIE)
   A. Playfulness Scale
   a. rickets
   a. scoliosis
   a. scoliosis surgery
   Test of Visual-Motor Skills: Upper
      Level Adolescents and A.'s
      (TVMS:UL)
   Test of Visual-Perceptual Skills:
      Upper Level Adolescents
      and A.'s (TVPS:UL)
adult-acquired flatfoot deformity
advance
   A. PS total knee prosthesis
   A. PS total knee system
advanced
   A. mobile-bearing knee implant
   A. mobile-bearing prosthesis
advancement
   Achilles tendon a.
   Atasoy V-Y a.
   calcaneonavicular ligament-tibialis
      posterior tendon a.
   Chandler patellar a.
   en bloc a.
   a. flap
   a. flap graft
   frontoorbital a.
   heel cord a. (HCA)
   Johnson pronator a.
   Lloyd-Roberts-Swann trochanteric a.
   Maquet a.
   Murphy Achilles tendon a.
   Murphy heel cord a.

NOTES

advancement *(continued)*
    patellar a.
    plantar calcaneonavicular ligament-
      tibialis posterior tendon a.
    profundus a.
    tendon a.
    tongue-in-groove a.
    trochanteric a.
    vastus medialis a. (VMA)
    Wagner profundus a.
    Wagner trochanteric a.
advancer
advancing wedge appearance
Advanta Orthopaedics
Advantim
    A. revision knee system
    A. total knee prosthesis
    A. total knee system
    A. unconstrained prosthesis
adventitia
adventitial
    a. forceps
    a. scissors
adventitious
    a. bursa
    a. movement
adversive attack
advisor
    Schwinn Fitness A.
advocacy
    National Association for Rights,
      Protection, and A.
Advocate electric flexion distraction table
AE
  above elbow
    AE amputation
AE1, AE3 antibody
AEA
  above-elbow amputation
Aeby muscle
AECS
  acute exertional compartment syndrome
AEP
  auditory evoked potential
Aequalis
    A. head
    A. humeral prosthesis
    A. reamer
    A. reversed shoulder prosthesis
    A. stem
    A. system
AER
  abduction-external rotation
aerate
aeration
aerobic
    a. bacteria
    a. boxing

    a. capacity
    a. cellulitis
    a. conditioning
    a. conditioning functional
      assessment
    a. exercise
    a. infection
    a. walking
aerobics
    karate-inspired a.
AerobiCycle
    Universal A.
Aerodyn orthotic
Aeromonas hydrophilia
aeroplane splint
Aeroplast dressing
Aesculap
    A. ABC cervical plating system
    A. bipolar cautery
    A. bipolar cautery forceps
    A. clamp
    A. drill
    A. headholder
    A. saw
Aesculap-PM noncemented femoral prosthesis
aesthesiometer
AF
  antifungal
  arcuate fasciculus
affection
    patellar a.
afferent
    a. fiber
    a. nerve impulse
Affinity Anterior Cervical Cage System
AFG ankle/foot gauntlet
AFO
  ankle-foot orthosis
    articulated AFO
    AFO brace sock
    AFO molded
    AFO pediatric brace
    AFO posterior leaf-spring
    sliding AFO
    AFO standard shell
    Type C-50, C-90 AFO
A-Force dorsal night splint
A-frame
    A-f. notch
    A-f. orthosis
Aftate for Athlete's Foot
afterdrop
afterpotential
    negative a.
    positive a.
AG
  antigravity

AGC

anatomically graduated component
AGC Biomet total knee system
AGC femoral prosthesis
AGC knee prosthesis
AGC knee replacement system
AGC tibial prosthesis

AGE

angle of greatest extension

age

bone a.
Greulich-Pyle bone a.
skeletal a. (SA)

age-associated degenerative change

Agee

A. carpal tunnel release
A. carpal tunnel release system
A. endoscope
A. force-couple splint reduction
A. 4-pin fixation device
A. WristJack external fixator
A. WristJack fracture reduction
system

agency, pl. **agencies**

A. for Health Care Policy and
Research (AHCPR)
A. for Healthcare Research and
Quality (AHRQ)

agenesis

Bayne classification of radial a.
caudal spinal a.
lumbar a.
odontoid a.
radial a.
sacral a.

agenetic fracture

agent

Albunex ultrasound imaging a.
alpha-adrenergic blocking a.
anabolic a.
antifungal a.
antimicrobial a.
antiosteoclastic a.
antipyretic a.
cellulose hemostatic a.
chondroprotective a.
chymopapain blocking a.
contrast a.
enzymatic debriding a.
fibrinolytic a.
keratolytic a.
mechanical a.
nociceptor a.

phlogistic a.
physical a.
thermal a.
uricosuric a.
water-soluble contrast a.

AGF

angle of greatest flexion
autologous growth factor

aggressive

a. infantile fibromatosis
a. solitary plasmacytoma
a. tumor

agility

a. drill
A. total ankle system

agitans

paralysis a.

Agliette

A. measurement
A. supracondylar osteotomy

Agnew splint

agnosia

finger a.

agonist

gamma-aminobutyric acid a.
a. muscle

agonist-antagonist

agonistic muscle

agrammatism

agraphia

AHCPR

Agency for Health Care Policy and
Research
AHCPR guidelines
AHCPR guidelines for treatment of
acute low back pain

Ahern trochanteric débridement

AHI

acetabular head index
acromiohumeral interval
Arthritis Helplessness Index

Ahlback change

AHO

acute hematogenous osteomyelitis

AHP

American Hand Prosthetics
AHP digital prosthesis

AHRQ

Agency for Healthcare Research and
Quality

AHSC

Arizona Health Science Center
AHSC elbow prosthesis

NOTES

15

AHSC-Volz
> AHSC-V. elbow prosthesis
> AHSC-V. hinge

AIA
> adjuvant-induced arthritis

aid
> augmentative communication a.
> (ACA)
> Carex ambulatory a.
> erogenic a.
> extension a.
> mobility a.
> OrthoTurn standing transfer a.
> prosthetic speech a.
> seating a.
> sock a.
> speech a.
> StraddleSitter seating a.
> transfer a.
> Turn-Easy transfer a.
> ultrasonic mobility a.
> walking a.

AIDP
> acute inflammatory demyelinating
> polyradiculoneuropathy

AIIS
> anterior inferior iliac spine
> AIIS avulsion fracture

AIM
> Ace intramedullary
> AIM continuous passive motion
> AIM CPM
> AIM femoral nail system

aimer
> Arthrotek femoral a.
> tibial a.

aiming
> a. bow
> a. guide

AIMS
> Abnormal Involuntary Movement Scale
> Alberta Infant Motor Scales
> Arthritis Impact Measurement Scale

ainhum
Ainslie acrylic splint
Ainsworth
> A. modeling
> A. modification of Massie nail

air
> a. arthrography
> a. band
> a. bed
> a. bicycle
> a. compression osteotome
> a. contrast
> a. cylinder
> A. DonJoy patellofemoral brace
> a. drill
> a. embolism

> a. flow mat
> a. inflation system
> a. myelography
> a. plasma spray (APS)
> a. pressure splint
> a. sinus
> a. splint
> A. Townsend brace
> a. walker

Air-Back spinal system
airborne bacteria
Aircast
> A. ankle brace
> A. Cryo/Cuff
> A. Cryo/Cuff brace
> A. fracture brace
> A. Knee System
> A. leg brace
> A. pneumatic air stirrup
> A. Pneumatic Air Stirrup brace
> A. pneumatic walker
> A. Rolimeter
> A. Swivel-Strap
> A. Swivel-Strap brace
> A. walking brace

air-contrast study
air-driven
> a.-d. bur
> a.-d. oscillating saw

Air-Drop chiropractic table
Air-Dyne bicycle
Airex
> A. balance pad
> A. mat

AirFlex carpal tunnel splint
Air-Flex chiropractic table
air-flow enclosure
Airfoam splint
AirGEL ankle brace
Air-Limb amputation protector
Airlite
> A. alignable ankle block
> A. prosthesis

AirLITE support pad
AIROM
> active integral range of motion

airplane
> a. cast
> a. shears
> a. splint
> a. splint orthosis
> a. splint shoulder brace

air-powered cutting drill
Airprene
> A. Action knee brace
> A. hinged knee prosthesis

Air-Soft Splint
AirStance pylon
Air-Stirrup ankle training brace

A

Airtrac ambulatory cervical/lumbar traction system
airway management akathisia
AIS
Abbreviated Injury Scale
adolescent idiopathic scoliosis
Aitken
A. classification of epiphysial fracture
A. epiphysial fracture classification
A. femoral deficiency
AJ
ankle jerk
AJC
ankle joint complex
AK
above knee
applied kinesiology
AK prosthesis
AKA
above-knee amputation
akathisia
airway management a.
AKE
active knee extension
AKE test
Akin
A. bunionectomy
A. operation
A. procedure
A. proximal phalangeal osteotomy
akinesia amnestica
aknemia (*var. of* acnemia)
Akne-Mycin Topical
Akron midtarsal osteotomy
Akros
A. extended care mattress
A. pressure mattress
AkroTech mattress
ALA
Activity Loss Assessment
ala, pl. **alae**
a. ilii
sacral a.
AlamarBlue osteoblast proliferation assay
Alanson amputation
alar
a. bone
a. cartilage
a. chest
a. creaking
a. crease

a. dysgenesis
a. ligament
a. plate
a. rim
a. scapula
a. screw
a. spine
alaria
ALARM
Adjustable Leg and Ankle Repositioning Mechanism
alarm cushion
alata
scapula a.
ALB
Assessment of Ludic Behaviors
Albee
A. acetabuloplasty
A. bone graft
A. drill
A. hip arthrodesis
A. lumbar spinal fusion
A. olive-shaped bur
A. operation
A. orthopaedic table
A. osteotome
A. shelf procedure
Albee-Delbert operation
Albers-Schönberg
A.-S. disease
A.-S. marble bone
Albert
A. achillodynia
A. disease
A. knee operation
Alberta Infant Motor Scales (AIMS)
Albinus muscle
Albizzia
A. intramedullary nail
A. leg-lengthening procedure
A. technique
Albrecht bone
Albright
A. disease
A. dystrophy
A. hereditary osteodystrophy
A. syndrome
A. synovectomy
Albright-Chase arthroplasty
Albright-McCune-Sternberg syndrome
Albunex ultrasound imaging agent
Alcock canal

NOTES

alcohol
    a. cauterization
    a. fat embolism syndrome
    a. injection
    a. neurolysis
    A. Use Disorders Identification test
alcoholic neuropathy
Alcon
    A. Closure System
    A. Instrument Delivery System tray
Alden CDI orthotic
aldolase
aldose reductase inhibitor
Alexander
    A. chisel
    A. costal osteotome
    A. costal periosteotome
    A. gouge
    A. periosteal elevator
    A. rasp
    A. technique
    A. view
Alexander-Farabeuf
    A.-F. periosteotome
    A.-F. rasp
alexia
Alexian Brothers overhead frame
Alfenta Injection
alfentanil hydrochloride
algesimeter
    Aly a.
    Björnström a.
Alginate dressing
algiomotor
algiomuscular
AlgiSite Alginate wound dressing
algodystrophy syndrome
AlgoMed infusion system
algometer
    pressure a.
algometry
algoneurodystrophy
algorithm
    injury a.
    polytrauma a.
    Tile polytrauma a.
AliCool splint spray
AliCork Foot Orthosis
alien hand sign
aligner
    Charnley femoral inlay a.
    femoral a.
    patellar a.
    tibial a.
alignment
    a. abnormality
    anatomic a.
    angular a.
    atlantoaxial a.

    calcaneus a.
    colinear a.
    dynamic a.
    extramedullary a.
    foot a.
    a. of fracture fragment
    a. guide
    a. guide rod
    a. index
    integrity and a.
    a. measurement
    optimal a.
    patellar a.
    patellofemoral a.
    a. pin
    poor a.
    rotational a.
    static a.
    talocrural a.
    talus a.
    tibiofemoral a.
    toe a.
    torsional a.
    transfemoral a.
    a. of vertebral bodies
AliMed
    A. Conductive Patient Shifter
    A. diabetic night splint
    A. hemi arm sling
    A. insert
    A. orthosis
    A. putty
    A. sensor floor mat
    A. turnbuckle elbow splint
    A. wrist/thumb support
AliMed-Freedom arthritis support
alimentary osteopathy
Aliplast
    A. blank
    A. custom-molded foot orthosis
    A. insole
    A. pad
Alisoft splinting material
AliStrap Velcro-type strapping
Alivium
    A. implant metal
    A. implant metal prosthesis
alkaline phosphatase
alkaloid
alkaptonuria
Alkphase-B immunoassay
ALL
    anterior longitudinal ligament
all-alumina socket
Allen
    A. arthroscopic elbow positioner
    A. arthroscopic knee positioner
    A. arthroscopic wrist positioner
    A. Cognitive Battery

A. Cognitive Level (ACL)
A. Cognitive Level Screen (ACLS)
A. Diagnostic Module (ADM)
A. hand/arm surgery table
A. head screwdriver
A. maneuver
A. open reduction of calcaneal
fracture
A. reduction
A. Semantic Differential Scale
A. shoulder arthroscopy
A. shoulder/wrist arthroscopy
traction system
A. sign
A. stirrup
A. test
A. wrench
Allen-Brown prosthesis
Allender vertical laminar flow room
Allen-Ferguson Galveston pelvic fixation
Allen-Kocher clamp
allergenic arthritis
AllerMax Oral
Allevyn
A. Island dressing
A. wound dressing
Allgöwer
A. apparatus
A. stitch
A. suture technique
Allgöwer-Donati suture
Alliance rehabilitation system
alligator
a. bone-reduction forceps
a. grasping forceps
all-inside repair
Allis
A. clamp
A. maneuver
A. sign
A. test
A. tissue forceps
Allman
A. acromioclavicular injury
classification
A. modification of Evans ankle
reconstruction
all-median nerve hand
AlloAnchor
A. RC allograft
A. RC allograft device

AlloCraft
A. bone spacer substitute
A. PL allograft spacer
allodynia
heat a.
Allofit acetabular cup system
Allofix
A. freeze-dried bone
A. freeze-dried cortical bone pin
allogenic, allogeneic
autolyzed, antigen-extracted, a.
(AAA)
a. bone graft
a. lyophilized bone graft implant
material
allograft
Accugraft a.
acetabular a.
AlloAnchor RC a.
autologous bone-tissue a.
bone a.
a. bone graft
bone-tendon-bone a.
a. bone vise
a. coronary artery disease
a. cortical bone
femoral cortical ring a.
femoral diaphysial a.
freeze-dried cancellous a.
fresh-frozen nonirradiated bone-
patellar tendon-bone a.
HTO wedge human donor tissue a.
a. iliac bone
intercalary diaphysial a.
large composite a.
a. ligament replacement
MiCOR machine bone a.
MiCOR precision bone a.
napkin ring calcar a.
osteoarticular a.
osteochondral a.
a. paste
a. reconstruction
a. reconstruction of fibular
collateral ligament
Red Cross freeze-dried a.
shell a.
tendon-bone a.
a. transplantation
whole bone fresh-frozen a.
whole fresh-frozen calcaneal a.
allograft-host junction
AlloGrip bone vice

NOTES

AlloGro bone graft material
alloimplant
AlloMatrix
    A. bone graft putty
    A. injectable putty
    A. injectable putty bone graft
    substitute
allopathic medicine
alloplastic
    a. graft
    a. material
Allo-Pro hip system
all-or-none law
alloy
    cobalt-based a.
    cobalt-chromium a.
    Eligoy metal a.
    NiTi a.
    stainless steel a.
    titanium a.
All Poly Deltafit keel
all-polyethylene socket
Allport retractor
All-Pro ScanX-12 digital imaging
  system
all-purpose
Allstate view
All-Tronics scanner
all-ulnar nerve hand
Allurion foot prosthesis
Alm wound retractor
Aloe Grande creme
Alora Transdermal
Alouette
    A. amputation
    A. operation
ALP
  ankle ligament protector
    ALP Plus ankle brace
Alpers syndrome
alpha
    a. antagonist
    A. Chymar
    a. chymotrypsin
    A. cushion liner
    A. flat sheet
    a. index
    A. suction attachment block kit
alpha-adrenergic blocking agent
alpha-a_2-plasmin inhibitor
alphabet board
alpha-BSM
    a.-BSM bone repair material
    a.-BSM bone substitute material
alphaprodine
AlphaStar table
alpha-sympathomimetic

Alphatec
    A. mini lag-screw system
    A. small fragment system
ALPS
  anterior locking plate system
    Amset ALPS
    ALPS EasyLiner
ALPSA
  anterior labrum periosteal sleeve avulsion
    ALPSA lesion
Alps CustomPro custom liner
ALRI
  anterolateral rotary instability
    ALRI test
ALS
  amyotrophic lateral sclerosis
  anterolateral sclerosis
ALSAR
  Assessment of Living Skills and
  Resources
Alsberg
    A. angle
    A. triangle
alta
    A. advance tibial/humeral rod
    alteration architectural a.
    A. cancellous screw
    A. CFX reconstruction rod
    A. condylar buttress plate
    A. cortical screw
    A. cross-locking screw
    A. distal fracture plate
    A. lag screw
    A. modular trauma system
    patella a.
    A. supracondylar screw
    A. tibial-humeral rod
    A. tibial nail
    A. transverse screw
alteration architectural alta
altered
    a. intervertebral mechanics
    a. regional mechanics
    a. sensation
alternating
    a. pressure pad
    a. range of motion (ARM)
alternative
  graft material a.
    a. medicine
altitude syndrome
altitudinal anopsia
Alumafoam splint
alumina
    a. bioceramic joint replacement
    a. cemented total hip prosthesis
    a. ceramic
alumina-on-alumina total hip prosthesis

aluminum
- a. bridge splint
- a. contouring template set
- a. fence splint
- a. finger cot splint
- a. foam splint
- a. hand splint
- implant alloy a.
- a. master rod
- a. oxide arthroplasty material
- a. oxide ceramic coating
- a. toxicity
- a. wire splint

Alvarado
- A. collateral ligament protector
- A. knee holder
- A. legholder
- A. Orthopaedic Research

Alvar condylar bolt

alveolar
- a. bone fracture
- a. osteitis
- a. rhabdomyosarcoma
- a. soft-part sarcoma
- a. supporting bone

Aly algesimeter

Alzet continuous infusion osmotic pump

Alznner orthotic

amalgam

Ambi
- A. compression hip screw system
- A. fixation
- A. hip screw
- A. wrist brace

ambidextrous

AMBRI
- atraumatic, multidirectional, bilateral rehabilitation inferior
- AMBRI procedure

ambulate with assistance

ambulation
- assisted a.
- brace-free a.
- crutch a.
- functional a.
- a. index
- prosthetic a.
- a. skills
- a. training orthosis

ambulator
- Apex A.
- A. biomechanical footwear
- A. Bio-Rocker sole
- A. Chukka Boot
- A. conform footwear
- A. H1200 healing shoe

ambulatory
- a. function
- household a.
- A. shoe
- a. status
- a. traction

AMC total wrist prosthesis

AMD
- arthroscopic microdiscectomy
- articular motion device

AME
- American Medical Electronics
- Austin Medical Equipment
- AME bone growth stimulator
- AME microcurrent TENS unit
- AME pin site shield

amebiasis

amelanotic

amelia
- brachial a.
- complete a.

amenorrhea
- athletic a.
- exercise-induced a.

America
- Arthroscopy Association of North A. (AANA)
- Rehabilitation Engineering and Assistive Technology Society of North A. (RESNA)

American
- A. Academy of Orthopaedic Surgeons (AAOS)
- A. Academy of Orthopaedic Surgeons classification of acetabular deficiency
- A. Academy of Orthopaedic Surgeons/Hip Society Questionnaire
- A. Academy of Orthopaedic Surgeons Pediatrics Outcomes Instrument
- A. Association for Hand Surgery (AAHS)
- A. Board of Certification of Orthotics and Prosthetics
- A. Board of Physical Therapy Specialists
- A. Chiropractic College of Radiology adjusting table

NOTES

American *(continued)*
  A. College of Rheumatology
    (ACR)
  A. College of Sports Medicine
    (ACSM)
  A. Hand Prosthetics (AHP)
  A. Heyer-Schulte chin prosthesis
  A. Heyer-Schulte-Hinderer malar
    prosthesis
  A. Heyer-Schulte Radovan tissue
    expander prosthesis
  A. Joint Commission on Cancer
    staging systems
  A. Knee Society
  A. Knee Society score
  A. leech
  A. Medical Electronics (AME)
  A. Medical Society for Sports
    Medicine (AMSSM)
  A. Musculoskeletal Tumor Society
    rating scale
  A. Orthopaedic Association (AOA)
  A. Orthopaedic Foot and Ankle
    Society (AOFAS)
  A. Orthopaedic Foot and Ankle
    Society Ankle-Hindfoot Scale
  A. Orthopaedic Society for Sports
    Medicine (AOSSM)
  A. Rheumatism Association (ARA)
  A. Rheumatism Association
    classification
  A. Seating Access-O-Matic bed
  A. Shoulder and Elbow Surgeons
    rating
  A. Shoulder and Elbow Surgeons
    scale
  A. shoulder and elbow system
    (ASES)
  A. Society of Anesthesiologists
    physical status classification
    system
  A. Society for Surgery of the
    Hand (ASSH)
  A. Society for Testing and
    Materials (ASTM)
  A. Spinal Cord Injury Association
    classification
  A. Spinal Injury Association
    (ASIA)
  A. Spinal Injury Association
    impairment scale
A-methaPred Injection
AMFH
  angiomatoid malignant fibrous
    histiocytoma
Amfit
  A. custom orthosis
  A. digitizer
  A. orthotic

Amico drill
Amigo mechanical wheelchair
amikacin
aminoglycoside
**aminoglycoside-impregnated methyl
  methacrylate bead**
aminohydroxypropylidene diphosphonate
aminophylline
Amipaque contrast medium
amiprilose hydrochloride
AMIS
  anterior minimally invasive surgery
    AMIS extension table
AMK
  anatomic modular knee
    AMK fixed bearing knee system
    AMK total knee system
    AMK unconstrained prosthesis
AML
  anatomic medullary locking
    AML Plus prosthesis
    AML socket
    AML Tang femoral prosthesis
    AML total hip prosthesis
    AML total hip system
    AML trial hip component
AmLactin
  A. cream
  A. lotion
Ammens foot powder
AM-MI orthopaedic table
amnestica
  akinesia a.
amobarbital and secobarbital
amorphous eosinophilic material
Amoss sign
amphiarthrodial
  a. disc
  a. symphysis
amphiarthrosis
amphidiarthrodial joint
ampicillin and sulbactam
Amplatz anchor system
amplifier
  Omniace RT3200N
    electromyographic a.
amplitude
  high velocity, low a.
amplitude-summation
  a.-s. interferential current
  a.-s. interferential current therapy
    (ASICT)
Ampoxen sling
AMPS
  Assessment of Motor and Process Skills
amputation
  above-elbow a. (AEA)
  above-knee a. (AKA)
  AE a.

Alanson a.
Alouette a.
Anderson a.
ankle disarticulation a.
aperiosteal a.
BE a.
Béclard a.
below-elbow a. (BEA)
below-knee a. (BKA)
Berger interscapular a.
Bier a.
bilateral a.
bloodless a.
border ray a.
Boyd ankle a.
Bunge a.
Burgess below-knee a.
button toe a.
Callander a.
Carden a.
central ray a.
cervix a.
Chopart hindfoot a.
cinematic a.
cineplastic a.
circular open a.
circular supracondylar a.
closed flap a.
coat-sleeve a.
complete a.
consecutive a.
a. in contiguity
a. in continuity
corporectomy a.
cutaneous a.
diaclastic a.
Dieffenbach a.
digital a.
disarticular a.
disarticulation a.
distal thigh a.
double-flap a.
dry a.
Dupuytren a.
eccentric a.
elliptical a.
end-bearing a.
excentric a.
Farabeuf a.
femoral head a.
finger a.
fingertip a.
fishmouth a.

flap a.
flapless a.
forearm a.
forefoot digital a.
forequarter a.
Gordon-Taylor hindquarter a.
great toe a.
Gritti a.
Gritti-Stokes a.
guillotine a.
Guyon a.
Hancock a.
hand a.
Hey a.
hindfoot a.
hindquarter a.
immediate a.
incomplete a.
index ray a.
interilioabdominal a.
interinnominoabdominal a.
intermediary a.
intermediate a.
interpelviabdominal a.
interphalangeal a.
interscapular a.
interscapulothoracic forequarter a.
intrapyretic a.
Jaboulay a.
kineplastic a.
King-Steelquist hindquarter a.
Kirk distal thigh a.
knee disarticulation a.
a. knife
Krukenberg a.
Langenbeck a.
Larrey a.
Le Fort a.
linear a.
Lisfranc a.
lower extremity a. (LEA)
Mackenzie a.
Maisonneuve a.
major a.
Malgaigne a.
McKittrick transmetatarsal a.
mediotarsal a.
metacarpal a.
middle finger a.
midthigh a.
Mikulicz-Vladimiroff a.
minor a.
mixed a.

NOTES

amputation *(continued)*
>modified Boyd a.
>multiple ray a.
>musculocutaneous a.
>nonreplantable a.
>oblique a.
>open a.
>osteoplastic a.
>oval a.
>partial hand a.
>pathologic a.
>periosteoplastic a.
>phalangophalangeal a.
>Pirogoff a.
>primary a.
>provisional a.
>proximal level a.
>pulp a.
>quadruple a.
>racket a.
>ray a.
>rectangular a.
>replantable a.
>a. retractor
>Ricard a.
>a. saw
>secondary a.
>semicircular flap a.
>shoulder a.
>spontaneous a.
>1-stage a.
>Stokes a.
>a. stump
>a. stump neuroma
>subastragalar a.
>subperiosteal a.
>supracondylar a.
>supramalleolar open a.
>Syme ankle disarticulation a.
>tarsal a.
>tarsometatarsal a.
>tarsotibial a.
>Teale a.
>tertiary a.
>through-the-knee a.
>toe a.
>transcarpal a.
>transcondylar a.
>transfemoral a.
>transfixation a.
>transhumeral a.
>transiliac a.
>translumbar a.
>transmetacarpal a.
>transmetaphysial a.
>transmetatarsal a. (TMA)
>transpelvic a.
>transphalangeal a.
>transtibial a.

>transverse a.
>traumatic a.
>traverse a.
>Tripier a.
>Vladimiroff-Mikulicz a.
>Wagner modification of Syme a.
>Wagner 2-stage Syme a.

amputation-related bone pain

amputee
>a. athlete
>a. cushion
>transfemoral a.

Amrex
>A. muscle stimulator
>A. SynchroSonic muscle stimulation-ultrasound
>A. therapeutic ultrasound

AMS
>antimigration system
>AMS intramedullary fixation

Amset
>A. ALPS
>A. ALPS anterior locking plate system
>A. R-F fixation system
>A. R-F rod
>A. R-F screw

Amspacher-Messenbaugh closing wedge osteotomy

AMSSM
>American Medical Society for Sports Medicine

Amstutz
>A. cemented hip prosthesis
>A. femoral component
>A. reattachment
>A. resurfacing
>A. resurfacing operation
>A. resurfacing technique
>A. total hip replacement

Amstutz-Wilson osteotomy

AMT
>active motion testing

AMX knee brace

amyloid neuropathy

amyloidosis
>beta-2-microglobulin a.
>skeletal a.

amyoplasia congenita

amyostasia

amyostatic

amyosthenia

amyosthenic

amyotaxy

amyotonia
>a. congenita
>Oppenheim a.

amyotrophia

amyotrophic
    a. acropathy
    a. lateral sclerosis (ALS)
amyotrophy
    Aran-Duchenne a.
    diabetic a.
    hemiplegic a.
    neuralgic a.
    neuritic a.
    primary progressive a.
    progressive nuclear a.
    progressive spinal a.
    syphilitic a.
amyous
ANA
    antinuclear antibody
anabolic
    a. agent
    a. steroid
anaerobic
    a. bacteria
    a. cellulitis
    a. exercise
    a. infection
    a. osteomyelitis
    a. threshold (AT)
anal
    a. reflex
    a. triangle
    a. wink
analgesia
    patient-controlled a. (PCA)
analgesic
    nonnarcotic a.
analgia
analog, analogue
    a. neurotrophic factor
analogous signal detector
analysis, pl. **analyses**
    activity a.
    activity-pattern a.
    bioelectrical impedance a. (BIA)
    biomechanical a.
    cerebrospinal fluid a.
    chiropractic a.
    computerized gait a.
    computerized musculoskeletal a.
    deformity a.
    DeLee radiographic a.
    3-dimensional a.
    EMED gait a.
    fiber a.
    finite element a. (FEA)

    footprint a.
    force plate foot a.
    Fourier a.
    frequency a.
    F-Scan foot pressure a.
    gait a.
    high-resolution a.
    job task a. (JTA)
    Khan-Lewis phonological a.
    kinetic gait a.
    lateral flexion dynamic visual a.
    muscle a.
    musculoskeletal a.
    occipital-fiber a.
    peak-pressure a.
    pedobarographic a.
    phonological a.
    plumb line a.
    postural a.
    roentgen stereophotogrammetric a.
      (RSA)
    spinal a.
    trapezius fiber a.
    video-dimensional a. (VDA)
    video-gate a.
analyzer
    Arthrodial Protractor range of
      motion a.
    CA-6000 spine motion a.
    Elite Plus motion a.
    Futrex body fat a.
    Metrecom spinal a.
    NordicTrack Motion A.
    Pediatric Ultrasound Bone A.
    Sam Jr. posture a.
    Stride A.
    Tanita Professional Body
      Composition A.
Anametric
    A. total knee prosthesis
    A. total knee system
anaphylaxis
    exercise-induced a.
    latex a.
anapophysis
anarrhexis
anastomosis, pl. **anastomoses**
    extradural a.
    fishmouth a.
    flexor tendon a.
    gastrointestinal a. (GIA)
    intradural a.
    Martin-Gruber a.

NOTES

anastomosis *(continued)*
    microvascular surgical a.
    peroneus brevis to longus a.
    Riche-Cannieu a.
    surgical a.
anatomic
    a. alignment
    a. axis
    a. barrier
    a. fracture reduction principle
    a. hook
    a. insertion
    a. intermetatarsal angle
    a. landmark
    a. leg length inequality
    a. loading
    a. medullary locking (AML)
    a. medullary locking hip system
    a. modular knee (AMK)
    a. neck fracture
    a. nerve trunk
    a. plane
    porous-coated a. (PCA)
    a. porous replacement (APR)
    a. porous replacement hemispheric
      acetabular component
    a. position
    A. Precoat hip prosthesis
    a. reduction
    a. short leg
    a. snuffbox
    a. surface prosthesis
anatomical
    a. hip center of rotation
    a. vertical
anatomically
    a. based exercise system
    a. graduated component (AGC)
anatomopathological study
Anatomotor traction/massage table
anatomy
    cervicothoracic pedicle a.
    cross-sectional a.
    Daseler-Anson classification of
      plantaris muscle a.
    designed after natural a. (DANA)
    developmental a.
    dorsalis pedis artery a.
    neurovascular a.
    pedicle a.
anchor
    absorbable suture a.
    Acufex bioabsorbable suture a.
    Acufex T-Fix suture a.
    Acumed suture a.
    Anchorlok soft tissue a.
    Anspach suture a.
    Arthrex bone a.
    Arthrex TwistLoc suture a.

AxyaWeld bone a.
Bio-Anchor suture a.
Bio-FASTak a.
Biologically Quiet Mini-Screw
  suture a.
Biomet bone a.
Bio-Phase suture a.
BioROC a.
BioSphere suture a.
bone a.
Bone Bullet suture a.
Bone Button orthopaedic suture a.
buttress and button a.
Catera suture a.
compression locking a.
a. connector
Corkscrew suture a.
CurvTek drill bone a.
E-Z ROC a.
FASTak suture a.
Fastin suture a.
Fastin threaded a.
GII Snap-Pak a.
GLS suture a.
Harpoon suture a.
a. hole
Howmedica bone a.
implantable bone a.
Innovasive bone a.
intraosseous suture a.
Isola spinal implant system a.
ligament a.
Linvatec bone a.
MicroLite suture a.
Mini Bio-Phase suture a.
Mini GLS a.
Mini-Revo Screws suture a.
Mini-ROC a.
Mitek absorbable a.
Mitek bone a.
Mitek Fastin threaded a.
Mitek GII easy a.
Mitek GL a.
Mitek knotless a.
Mitek ligament a.
Mitek micro a.
Mitek Mini GLS a.
Mitek Panalok RC a.
Mitek rotator cuff a.
Mitek Tacit threaded a.
Ogden bone a.
Orthofix Ogden a.
PaBA a.
Panalok absorbable suture a.
PLA a.
a. plate
PLLA a.
Revo suture a.
ROC a.

A

RotorloC absorbable rotator cuff
  suture a.
a. screw
Sherlock threaded suture a.
a. splint
Stealth a.
suture a.
Tacit threaded a.
Therap-Loop door a.
threaded suture a.
traction a.
UltraFix MicroMite suture a.
UltraFix RC suture a.
UltraSorb suture a.
Wright Medical bone a.
Zimmer-Statak a.
anchorage-dependent growth
anchoring
  a. hole
  a. peg
  a. point
  a. tendon
Anchorlok
  A. soft tissue anchor
  A. soft tissue suture anchor system
ancient tuberculous arthritis
ancillary muscle group
anconeal
anconeus
  a. arthroplasty
  a. muscle
anconitis
anconoid
Anderson
  A. acetabular prosthesis
  A. amputation
  A. ankle fusion
  A. distractor
  A. fixation apparatus
  A. fixation device
  A. leg-lengthening apparatus
  A. leg-lengthening device
  A. medial-lateral grind test
  A. modeling
  A. modification of Berndt-Harty
  classification
  A. operation
  A. pin fixation
  A. screw placement technique
  A. splint
  A. system
  A. tibial lengthening

  A. tibial pseudarthrosis
  classification
  A. traction
Anderson-D'Alonzo odontoid fracture
  classification
Anderson-Fowler procedure
Anderson-Green growth prediction
Anderson-Hutchins unstable tibial shaft
  fracture
Anderson-Neivert osteotome
Andersson hip status system
Andren-von Rosen line
André Thomas sign
Andrews
  A. anterior instability test
  A. gouge
  A. iliotibial band reconstruction
  A. iliotibial band tenodesis
  A. lateral tenodesis
  A. osteotome
  A. spinal surgery frame
  A. SST-3000 spinal surgery table
  A. technique
androgenic-enhancing substance
  androstenediol
anemia
  blood loss a.
  Fanconi a.
  foot-strike hemolysis a.
  iron-deficiency a.
  sickle-cell a.
  sports a.
anergy
aneroid gauge
anesthesia
  ankle block a.
  Bier block a.
  bulbar a.
  compression a.
  continuous intravenous regional a.
  (CIVRA)
  crash induction of a.
  digital block a.
  dissociative a.
  epidural a.
  field block a.
  gauntlet a.
  general endotracheal a.
  glove a.
  glove-and-stocking a.
  graded spinal a.
  hypotensive a.
  inhalation a.

NOTES

anesthesia *(continued)*
 intrathecal a.
 intravenous block a.
 intravenous regional a. (IVRA)
 local standby a.
 lumbar a.
 Mayo block a.
 patient-controlled a. (PCA)
 peripheral nerve block a.
 regional a.
 ring block a.
 saddle block a.
 short-acting block a.
 spinal a.
 supraclavicular brachial block a.
 tactile a.
 thermal a.
 toe block a.
anesthetic
 foot a.
 Lido-Gel topical a.
aneurysm
 arterial a.
 benign bone a.
 brachial artery a.
 clavicular fracture a.
 false a.
 Park a.
aneurysmal bone cyst (ABC)
aneurysmorrhaphy
angel
 a. wing
 a. wing guide
Angell
 A. James dissector
 A. James hypophysectomy forceps
Anghelescu sign
angina cruris
angioblastoma
angiodysplasia
angioendotheliomatosis
angiofibroblastic
 a. hyperplasia tendinosis
 a. proliferation
angiofibroma
angiogram
 biplane a.
angiography
 digital subtraction a. (DSA)
 spinal cord a.
 vertebral a.
angiokeratoma
 diffuse a.
angioleiomyoma
angiolipoma
angioma
 cirsoid a.
angiomatoid malignant fibrous histiocytoma (AMFH)

angiomatosis
 skeletal-extraskeletal a.
angiosarcoma
angiosclerotica
 dysbasia a.
 myasthenia a.
angiospasm
angiotropic lymphoma
angle
 abduction a.
 acetabular a.
 acromial a.
 Alsberg a.
 anatomic intermetatarsal a.
 antegonial a.
 antetorsion a.
 a. of antetorsion
 a. of anteversion
 arch a.
 articular facet a.
 articular set a.
 Baumann a.
 Beatson combined ankle a.
 bimalleolar a.
 Böhler calcaneal a.
 Böhler lumbosacral a.
 Bowman a.
 Bragg a.
 C a.
 calcaneal inclination a.
 calcaneal pitch a. (CPA)
 calcaneal-second metatarsal a.
 calcaneoplantar a.
 calcaneotibial a.
 capital epiphysial a.
 capitolunate a.
 carrying a.
 CCD a.
 CE a.
 center-edge a.
 central collodiaphysial a.
 cervicothoracic pedicle a.
 Citelli a.
 Clarke arch a.
 Cobb scoliosis a.
 Codman a.
 collodiaphysial a.
 condylar a.
 condylar plateau a. (CPA)
 congruence a.
 a. of convergence
 costal a.
 costolumbar a.
 costophrenic a.
 costosternal a.
 costovertebral a. (CVA)
 craniofacial a.
 cuboid abduction a.
 cuboid declination a.

declination a.
a. of declination
distal articular set a. (DASA)
distal metatarsal articular a. (DMAA)
a. of divergence
dorsiflexion a. (DFA)
dorsoplantar talometatarsal a.
dorsoplantar talonavicular a.
Drennan metaphysial-epiphysial a.
elevation a.
Engel a.
epiphysial a.
Euler a.
eulerian a.
facet a.
femoral trunk a.
femorotibial a. (FTA)
Ferguson sacral base a.
a. finder
finger a.
first–fifth intermetatarsal a.
first–second intermetatarsal a.
flexion a.
foot a.
foot progression a. (FPA)
Fowler-Philip a.
functional intermetatarsal a.
a. of gait
Garden a.
gastrocnemius a.
Gissane a.
gonial a.
a. of greatest extension (AGE)
a. of greatest flexion (AGF)
hallux valgus a. (HVA)
hallux valgus interphalangeus a.
head-shaft a.
Hibbs metatarsocalcaneal a.
Hilgenreiner a.
hip joint a. (HJA)
hip-knee-ankle a.
HKA a.
humeroulnar a.
IM a.
inclination a.
a. of incongruity
increased carrying a.
inferior a.
intermetatarsal a. (IMA)
intrascaphoid a.
a. isometric testing
Kite a.

kyphotic a.
lateral patellofemoral a.
lateral slip a.
Laurin lateral patellofemoral a.
Levine Drennan a.
Lisfranc articular set a. (LASA)
Lovibond a.
Ludwig a.
lumbosacral joint a.
mandibular a.
manubriosternal a.
a. of Mary
Meary metatarsotalar a.
medial proximal tibial a.
mediolateral radiocarpal a.
Merchant congruence a.
metaphysial-diaphysial a.
metaphysial-epiphysial a.
metatarsal base a.
metatarsal phalangeal a.
metatarsocalcaneal a.
metatarsocuneiform a.
metatarsotalar a.
metatarsus adductus a.
metatarsus primus declination a.
Mikulicz a.
navicular to first metatarsal a.
neck-shaft a. (NSA)
negative congruence a.
neutral a.
occipitocervical a.
patellofemoral a.
Pauwels a.
pedicle axis a.
pelvic a.
pelvic-femoral a.
pennation a.
physial a.
plantar metatarsal a.
popliteal a.
proximal articular facet a.
proximal articular set a. (PASA)
Q a.
quadriceps a.
quadriceps neutral a. (QNA)
radiocarpal a.
resting forefoot supination a.
a. of retroversion
rib-vertebral a.
sacral base a.
sacrofemoral a.
sacrohorizontal a.
sacrovertebral a.

NOTES

angle *(continued)*
    sagittal pedicle a.
    salient a.
    scapholunate a.
    scoliosis a.
    set a.
    Sharp acetabular a.
    slip a.
    Southwick lateral slip a.
    spinographic a.
    a. splint
    sternoclavicular a.
    subscapular a.
    sulcus a.
    talar axis–first metatarsal base a.
      (TAMBA)
    talar declination a.
    talar tilt a.
    talocalcaneal a.
    talocrural a.
    talometatarsal a.
    talonavicular a.
    tarsometatarsal a.
    thigh-foot a. (TFA)
    a. of thoracic inclination
    tibiofemoral a. (TFA)
    tibiotalar a.
    toe-out a.
    a. of torsion
    Toygar a.
    transverse pedicle a.
    tuber a.
    tuber-joint a.
    tuberosity joint a.
    ulnohumeral a.
    valgus a.
    varus MTP a.
    a. of Wiberg
    Wiberg center-edge a.
    Wiberg fracture a.
    Wiltze a.
angled
    a. arthroscope
    a. awl
    a. bearing insert
    a. blade-plate fixation
    a. compression plate
    a. DeBakey clamp
    a. dissector
    a. jaw rongeur
    a. Lowman-type bone clamp
    a. pituitary rongeur
    a. probe
    a. rasp
angled-down forceps
angled-up forceps
angry backfiring C nociceptor
angular
    a. acceleration

    a. alignment
    a. bone rongeur
    a. curvature
    a. deviation
    a. displacement
    a. elevator
    a. hinge clamp
    a. momentum
    a. motion
    a. osteotomy
    a. parameter
    a. position
    a. process of orbit
    a. spine
    a. tilt
    a. velocity
angularity
angulated fracture
angulation
    anterior a.
    apex anterior a.
    apex dorsal a.
    apex posterior a.
    cephalic a.
    a. deformity
    degrees of valgus a.
    degrees of varus a.
    forefoot a.
    kyphotic a.
    limb length a.
    a. motion
    a. osteotomy
    plantar a.
    posttraumatic a.
    radius of a.
    screw a.
    spinal a.
    valgus a.
    varus-valgus a.
angulatory malunion
Angus-Cowell scale
anhidrosis, anidrosis
anhydrous ethanol
animal-assisted therapy (AAT)
animal beanbag exerciser
anion transport inhibitor
anisomelia
anisospondyly
anisotropy
Ank-L-Aid brace
ankle
    a. arthrodesis
    a. arthrography
    a. arthroplasty
    a. arthroscopy
    autologous reverse graft to a.
    a. block
    a. block anesthesia
    a. bone

Buechel-Pappas total a.
a. clonus
a. clonus test
a. contracture orthosis
C Stance a.
a. disarticulation
a. disarticulation amputation
disc of a.
a. disc device
a. disc training
a. dislocation
a. dorsiflexion range of motion (ADROM)
a. dorsiflexion test
a. effusion
a. equinus
a. eversion
a. exercise machine
footballer's a.
a. fracture classification
fused a.
a. fusion
a. guard
a. hitch
a. immobilizer
a. impingement
a. infectious arthritis
a. inferior transverse ligament
a. injury
a. instability
internal fixation compression arthrodesis of a.
a. inversion
a. inversion-eversion
a. inversion-eversion range of motion
Irvine a.
A. Isolator
A. Isolator ankle rehabilitator
A. Isolator foot and ankle exerciser
a. jerk (AJ)
a. jerk reflex
a. joint
a. joint complex (AJC)
a. joint leg-curl
a. laxity
a. ligament protector (ALP)
a. ligament protector brace
a. loose body
a. magnet
a. mortise
a. mortise diastasis

a. mortise fracture
a. mortise widening
multiaxis a.
neuropathic a.
New Jersey a.
a. orthosis (AO)
a. osteoarthritis
a. osteomyelitis
a. portal
a. prosthesis
a. reconstruction
a. rehabilitation pump
R-Hab lighter weight a.
a. rheumatoid arthritis
Rincoe human action bionic a.
a. scoring system of Baird and Jackson
snowboarder's a.
a. sprain
a. stability
a. stabilizer
a. stabilizing orthosis (ASO)
a. stabilizing orthosis support
a. stirrup brace
a. systolic pressure
tailor's a.
tendon Z-lengthening around knee and a.
a. traction bandage
transmalleolar a.
USMC multiaxis a.
a. weight
Wiltse osteotomy of a.
ankle-brachial pressure ratio
ankle-foot
a.-f. electrogoniometer
a.-f. orthosis (AFO)
a.-f. orthosis brace sock
a.-f. orthotic splint
a.-f. plastic orthosis
ankle-hindfoot scale
ankle-level arteriotomy
ankle-pump exercise
ankleRAP postsurgical wound wrap
AnkleTough rehabilitation system
ankylodactylia
ankylodactyly
ankylopoietic
ankylose
ankylosing
a. spinal hyperostosis
a. spinal stenosis
a. spondylitis

NOTES

ankylosis
>artificial a.
>bony a.
>capsular a.
>carpal bone fracture a.
>extraarticular a.
>extracapsular a.
>false a.
>fibrous a.
>intracapsular a.
>ligamentous a.
>operative a.
>partial a.
>shoulder a.
>spurious a.
>true a.
>unsound a.
>vertebral a.

ankylotic

anlage
>cartilaginous a.
>fibular a.
>radial head a.
>ulnar a.

Anna-Dote Positioning Support

Annandale operation

Ann Arbor double towel clamp

anneal

annular (*var. of* anular)

annulare
>limbus a.
>subcutaneous granuloma a.

annulotomy

annulus (*var. of* anulus)

anodal block

anomalous
>a. fibular nutrient artery
>a. insertion

anomaly, pl. **anomalies**
>congenital a.
>facet a.
>hand a.
>Kimerle a.
>Poland a.
>root a.
>vertebral abnormality, anal imperforation, tracheoesophageal fistula, and radial, ray, or renal anomalies (VATER)
>vertebral (defects), (imperforate) anus, tracheoesophageal (fistula), radial and renal (dysplasia) anomalies (VATER)
>vertebral segmentation a.

anonychia

anopsia
>altitudinal a.

anorgasmia

anoscope

anosteoplasia

anoxia

Ansaid Oral

anserine
>a. bursa
>a. bursitis

anserinus
>pes a.

ANSIE
>Adult Nowicki Strickland Internal External Control Scale

Anspach
>A. cementome
>A. 65K Universal instrument system
>A. power drill
>A. reamer
>A. suture anchor

antagonist
>alpha a.
>opiate receptor a.
>opioid a.
>reversal of a. (ROA)

antagonistic
>a. activation
>a. muscle
>a. reflex

antalgic
>a. gait
>a. lean
>a. limp

Ant-Cer dynamic cervical plate

anteater nose

antebrachial
>a. cutaneous nerve
>a. fascia
>a. fascial graft

antebrachium

antecedent sign

antecubital fossa

anteflex

anteflexion

antegonial angle

antegrade
>a. femoral nail
>a. method
>a. nailing

antegrade/retrograde compression nail

antenatal dislocation

antenna procedure

Antense antitension device

anterior
>a. acromioplasty
>a. acromioplasty approach
>a. acute flexion elbow splint
>a. angulation
>a. ankle impingement
>a. ankle shift operation
>a. apprehension test

a. aspiration
a. atlantooccipital membrane
a. atlantoodontoid interval
a. axillary approach
a. axillary line (AAL)
a. bending moment
a. calcaneal osteotomy
a. calcaneal process fracture
a. capsule
a. capsulectomy
a. capsulolabral reconstruction (ACLR)
a. capsulotomy
a. cavus
a. cervical approach
a. cervical body fusion
a. cervical cord syndrome
a. cervical discectomy
a. cervical discectomy and fusion (ACDF)
a. cervical fascia
a. cervical fixation
a. cervical fusion (ACF)
a. cervical plate (ACP)
a. cervical plate fixation system (ACFS)
a. cervicothoracic junction surgery
a. collateral ligament
a. column
a. column disruption
a. column fracture
a. column osteosynthesis
a. column of spine
a. commissure-posterior commissure (AC-PC)
a. compartment
a. compartment syndrome (ACS)
a. construct
a. cord compression
a. cord impingement
a. corpectomy
a. correction
a. cortex penetration
a. cruciate
a. cruciate deficit knee
a. cruciate ligament (ACL)
a. cruciate sprain
a. curvature
a. distraction instrumentation
a. drainage
a. drawer sign
a. drawer stress radiograph
a. drawer test (ADT)

a. epineurotomy
a. equinus
a. extensile approach
a. fiber-region
a. fibular ligament
a. foot draw sign
a. forceps
a. glenoid labrum
a. glide
a. heel
a. hiatal sign
a. hip dislocation
a. hip release
a. horn
a. horn cell
a. horn meniscal tear
a. horn of spinal cord
a. humeral line
a. iliofemoral technique
a. impingement spur
a. impingement syndrome
a. inferior iliac spine (AIIS)
a. innominate
a. innominate rotation
a. internal fixation
a. internal fixation device
a. interosseous nerve syndrome
a. joint impingement
a. jugular vein
a. Kostuik-Harrington distraction system
a. kyphosis
a. labrum periosteal sleeve avulsion (ALPSA)
a. locking plate system (ALPS)
a. longitudinal ligament (ALL)
a. long toe flexor
a. lower cervical spine surgery
a. lumbar vertebral interbody fusion
a. maxillary spine
a. medial ankle ligament
a. meniscofemoral ligament
a. metallic fixation
a. metatarsal arch
a. minimally invasive surgery (AMIS)
a. myocutaneous flap
a. neutralization
a. oblique bundle
a. oblique ligament (AOL)
a. oblique meniscal tear
a. occipitocervical arthrodesis

NOTES

anterior *(continued)*
a. occipitocervical spine
a. olisthesis
a. pelvic tilt
a. pes cavus
a. plate fixation
a. plate system (APS)
a. portal
a. and posterior (AP)
a. and posterior fusion
a. pronator teres
a. quadriceps musculocutaneous flap technique
a. quadrilateral triplane frame
a. radial collateral artery
a. recurrent tibial artery
a. retroperitoneal decompression
a. retroperitoneal flank approach
a. rotary drawer test
a. sacrococcygeal ligament
a. sacroiliac joint plate
a. sacroiliac ligament
a. scalene muscle
a. screw fixation
a. serratus muscle
a. shear
a. shin splint
a. short-segment stabilization
a. shoulder dislocation
a. shoulder instability
a. shoulder release
a. sliding tibial graft
a. slot graft arthrodesis
a. soft tissue impingement
a. spinal artery
a. spinal fixation
a. spinal fusion
a. spinal line
a. spinocerebellar tract
a. spinothalamic tract
a. spurring
a. stabilization procedure
a. sternoclavicular joint
a. sternomastoid approach
a. strap approach
a. superior iliac spine (ASIS)
a. surgical exposure
a. talar translation (ATT)
a. talofibular ligament (ATFL)
a. talofibular ligament rupture
a. talofibular sprain
a. talotibial ligament
a. talus shift
a. tarsal resection
a. tarsal tendinitis
a. tarsal tunnel syndrome
a. thoracic nerve
a. tibial artery
a. tibial compartment syndrome
a. tibial fasciocutaneous flap
tibialis a.
a. tibial margin
a. tibial muscle
a. tibial nerve
a. tibial nerve dermatome
a. tibial sign
a. tibial spine
a. tibial syndrome
a. tibial tendon
a. tibial tubercle
a. tibiofibular ligament
a. tibiotalar fascicle (ATTF)
a. tibiotalar ligament
a. transfer
a. translation
a. transthoracic approach
a. triangle
a. upper spine
a. view
a. Zielke instrumentation
anterior-draw stress view
anterior-inferior
a.-i. capsular ligament dysfunction
a.-i. compression
a.-i. dislocation
a.-i. fusion
a.-i. glide
a.-i. movement
a.-i. tibiofibular ligament
anterior-posterior
a.-p. compression (APC)
a.-p. fusion with SSI
a.-p. glide
a.-p. listhesis
a.-p. movement
anterior-screw fixation
anterocentral arthroscopic portal
anterodistal
anterograde AXT
anteroinferior
a. glenohumeral ligament
a. portal
a. spondylolisthesis
anterolateral
a. approach
a. capsule
a. compression fracture
a. decompression
a. dislocation
a. drainage
a. femorotibial ligament tenodesis
a. fragment
a. impingement syndrome
a. portal
a. raphe
a. release
a. rotary instability (ALRI)

a. rotary knee instability
a. sclerosis (ALS)
anterolateral-anteromedial rotary instability
anterolisthesis
anteromedial
a. bundle
a. capsule
a. drainage
a. glenohumeral ligament
a. humeral head defect
a. incision
a. portal
a. retropharyngeal approach
a. rotary instability
a. tubercle transfer
anteromedial-posteromedial rotary instability
anteroposterior (AP)
a. control orthosis
a. lateral sway
a. stress test
a. table (ATPC)
a. talocalcaneal
a. talocalcaneal divergence
a. tilt
a. translation
anteroproximal
anterosuperior (AS)
a. external ilium movement (ASEx)
a. glenohumeral ligament
a. iliac spine graft
a. ilium major
a. internal ilium movement (ASIn)
anteroventral
antetorsion
a. angle
femoral a.
anteversion
acetabular a.
a. determination
femoral a. (FA)
femoral head-neck a.
neutral a.
a. syndrome
anthropometric
a. caliper
a. measurement
a. measuring tape
a. method
a. total hip (ATH)
anthropometry
antibacterial pillow

antibiosis
antibiotic
a. bead
a. bead pouch
a. and saline solution
antibiotic-impregnated
a.-i. bead
a.-i. cement
a.-i. polymethyl methacrylate
antibiotic-loaded acrylic cement
antibody, pl. **antibodies**
AE1, AE3 a.
antihistocompatibility a.
antinuclear a. (ANA)
T-cell receptor a.
technetium-99m-labeled monoclonal antigranulocyte a.
anticavitation drill
anticentromere
anticoagulant
lupus a.
a. therapy
anticoagulation
prophylactic a.
anticonvulsant therapy
antidecubitus
a. mattress
a. pad
antidromic stimulation
antiembolic
a. position
a. stockings
antiemetic
antifungal (AF)
a. agent
antigen
antiproliferating cell nuclear a.
carcinoembryonic a. (CEA)
HLA-B27 blood a.
human leukocyte a. (HLA)
human lymphocyte a. (HLA)
transplantation a.
antigen-extracted, allogenic bone
antigenicity
antiglide plate
antigravity (AG)
antihistocompatibility antibody
antiinflammatory medication
antimicrobial
a. agent
a. benzalkonium chloride
antimigration system (AMS)

NOTES

antinuclear
    a. antibody (ANA)
    a. antibody test
antiosteoclastic agent
antiproliferating cell nuclear antigen
antiprotrusio cage
antipyretic agent
antirotation
    a. cable (ARC)
    a. device
antisense gene therapy
antiseptic
    ACU-dyne a.
    colored a.
    a. solution
Antishear gel sheet
antishock garment
Anti-Shox
    A.-S. foot cushion
    A.-S. gel insole
    A.-S. heel cup
    A.-S. orthosis
    A.-S. sports orthotic
antistreptolysin-O titer (ASOT)
antitension line
antithrombin III
antithrombotic therapy
antithrust seat
antitipper wheelchair
antitoxin
antituberculosis drug
antivibration glove
anular, annular
    a. cartilage
    a. constricting band syndrome
    a. fiber
    a. fibrosis
    a. groove
    a. injury
    a. ligament
    a. ligament entrapment
    a. ligament of radius
    a. periradial recess
    a. pulley (A1–A4)
anulospiral ending of muscle spindle
anulus, annulus
    a. fibrosus
anvil
    a. bone
    Bunnell a.
    a. sign
    a. test
any-angle splint
Anywear shoe
AO
    ankle orthosis
    atlantooccipital
    AO ankle fracture classification
    AO brace

    AO cancellous screw
    AO classification of ankle fracture
    AO compression
    AO compression apparatus
    AO condylar blade-plate
    AO contoured T plate
    AO contouring apparatus
    AO cortex screw
    AO drill bit
    AO dynamic compression plate
    AO dynamic compression plate
     construct
    AO external fixation
    AO femoral distractor
    AO fixateur interne
    AO fixateur interne instrumentation
    AO fracture pattern
    AO group
    AO group shoulder arthrodesis
    AO guidepin
    AO hook plate
    AO internal fixator
    AO lag screw
    AO minifragment set
    AO notched instrumentation
    AO plate bender
    AO procedure
    AO pseudoisochromatic color plate
     test
    AO reconstruction plate
    AO reduction forceps
    AO screw fixation
    AO semitubular plate
    AO slotted medullary nail
    AO small fragment plate
    AO spinal internal fixation
    AO spongiosa screw
    AO spoon plate
    AO surgical technique
    AO tap
    AO tension band
AOA
    American Orthopaedic Association
    AOA cervical immobilization brace
    AOA halo cervical traction
AO-ASIF
    AO-ASIF compression plate
    AO-ASIF compression technique
    AO-ASIF fixateur interne
    AO-ASIF orthopaedic implant
    AO-ASIF screw
AO-Danis-Weber ankle fracture
classification
AOF
    Assessment of Occupational Functioning
AOFAS
    American Orthopaedic Foot and Ankle
    Society

A

AOFAS hallux rating system
AOFAS score
AOL
anterior oblique ligament
AO-Morscher plate
A-ONE
Arnadottir Occupational Therapy
Activities of Daily Living
Neurobehavioral Evaluation
AOSSM
American Orthopaedic Society for Sports
Medicine
AP
action potential
anterior and posterior
anteroposterior
AP fusion
AP nail
AP supine view
AP translatory motion
APACHE
Acute Physiology and Chronic Health
Evaluation
aparthrosis
APB Hi all-purpose boot
APC
anterior-posterior compression
APC hip retractor
APC proximal femoral elevator
APD
automated percutaneous discectomy
ape
a. hand
a. thumb deformity
apelike hand
aperiosteal amputation
Apert
A. acrosyndactyly
A. disease
A. syndrome
aperta
spina bifida a.
aperture pad
apex, pl. **apices**
A. Ambulator
A. Ambulator shoe
a. anterior angulation
a. dorsal angulation
A. Energetics
a. of head of patella
A. insole
a. patellae
A. pin

a. plantar deformity
a. posterior angulation
A. Universal Drive and Irrigation
System
a. vertebra
Apfelbaum mirror
aphalangia
complete a.
congenital a.
partial a.
aphasia
Broca a.
Wernicke a.
apical
a. axis guide
a. corn
a. dental ligament
a. distraction
a. lordotic view
a. non-load-bearing bone fracture
a. segment
a. stitch
a. vertebra
apices (*pl. of* apex)
APL
abductor pollicis longus
APL Plus ankle brace
APLD
automated percutaneous lumbar
discectomy
Apley
A. compression test
A. distraction test
A. examination
A. grinding test
A. knee test
A. maneuver
A. scratch test
A. sign
A. traction
Apligraf
apocope
apodia
Apofix cervical instrumentation
Apollo
A. DXA bone densitometer
A. DXA bone densitometry system
A. hip prosthesis
A. hip system
A. hot/cold Pak
A. knee prosthesis system
A. TM electric flexion table
A. total knee system

NOTES

aponeurectomy
aponeurorrhaphy
aponeurosis
    adductor a.
    digital a.
    meniscal a.
    palmar a.
    plantar a.
    quadriceps a.
    a. of tendon
    woven gastrocnemius a.
aponeurositis
aponeurotic
    a. band
    a. fibroma
    a. lengthening
    a. reflex
    a. triangle
    a. troika
aponeurotome
aponeurotomy
apophysial, apophyseal
    a. complex
    a. fracture
    a. joint
    a. joint capsule
    a. joint osteophyte
apophysis, pl. **apophyses**
    calcaneus a.
    iliac a.
    medial epicondylar a.
    slipped vertebral a.
    spinal process a.
    vertebral ring a.
apophysitis
    calcaneal a.
    iliac a.
    a. tibialis
    a. tibialis adolescentium
apoplexy
    delayed a.
    posttraumatic a.
APOPPS
    adjustable postoperative protective
    prosthetic socket
apparatus
    Ace Unifix fixation a.
    adjustable aiming a.
    Allgöwer a.
    Anderson fixation a.
    Anderson leg-lengthening a.
    AO compression a.
    AO contouring a.
    Axer compression a.
    4-bar external fixation a.
    Bassett electrical stimulation a.
    Benedict-Roth a.
    Bovie electrocautery a.
    Buck convoluted traction a.

    Buck Redi-Traction a.
    Calandruccio triangular
      compression a.
    Cameron fracture a.
    Charnley centering a.
    Charnley compression a.
    compression a.
    coracoclavicular fixation a.
    coring a.
    CPM a.
    DeWald spinal a.
    Deyerle fixation a.
    driver tunnel locator a.
    electrocautery a.
    electronic bone stimulation a.
    a. extensor
    external skeletal fixation a.
    fixating a.
    Fox internal fixation a.
    Georgiade visor halo fixation a.
    Giliberty a.
    Golgi a.
    halo vest a.
    Hamilton a.
    Hare a.
    hinged-distraction a.
    Hoffmann-Vidal external fixation a.
    Ilizarov a.
    internal fixation a.
    isokinetic joint a.
    isokinetic resistance a.
    Kinetron muscle strengthening a.
    Kirschner a.
    Kronner external fixation a.
    Küntscher traction a.
    leg-holding a.
    McLaughlin osteosynthesis a.
    Mueller compression a.
    nail plate a.
    Nauth traction a.
    Neufeld a.
    optoelectric measuring a.
    optoelectric signal detection a.
    Orthofix a.
    Parham-Martin fracture a.
    Philips Angiodiagnostics 96 a.
    Quengel a.
    Rancho anklet foot control a.
    Redi-Trac traction a.
    Rezaian external fixation a.
    rod-mounted targeting a.
    Roger Anderson external fixation a.
    Sayre suspension a.
    snap-fit a.
    Southwick pin-holding a.
    spine a.
    subneural a.
    Sutter-CPM knee a.
    Taylor a.

Telectronics electrical stimulation a.
triplanar protractor a.
Vidal-Adrey modified Hoffman
  external fixation device a.
Volkov-Oganesian external
  fixation a.
Volkov-Oganesian-Povarov hinged
  distraction a.
Wagner external fixation a.
Wagner leg-lengthening a.
Wagner-Schanz screw a.
Zickel medullary a.
Zickel supracondylar fixation a.
Zimmer electrical stimulation a.

appearance
advancing wedge a.
bat-wing a.
blade of grass a.
bone-within-bone a.
candle flame a.
candle wax a.
cotton ball a.
crabmeat-like a.
horseshoe a.
mop-end a.
mouse-ear a.
picture frame a.
spongy a.

appendage clamp
appendiceal retractor
appendicular
a. bone mass measurement
a. skeletal muscle (ASM)
a. skeleton

Applause Super-Hemi wheelchair
apple-shape body
appliance (*See* device, orthosis)
DeWald spinal a.
Jobst a.
therapeutic a.

application
cast a.
cold a.
controlled force a.
diversified-type force a.
force a.
frame a.
Harrington rod instrumentation
  force a.
heat a.
ice a.
Isola spinal implant system a.
Kumar a.

paraffin wax therapeutic a.
paraspinal rod a.
traction a.
a. of traction device
transverse fixator a.

applicator
infrared a.

applied
a. kinesiology (AK)
a. load

applier
bayonet clip a.
bulldog clamp a.
clip a.
Ligaclip a.
Mayfield miniature clip a.
Mayfield temporary aneurysm
  clip a.
mini a.
surgical staple a.
Vari-Angle clip a.

apposing articular surface
apposition
axonal a.
bayonet a.
bone-to-bone a.
bony a.
facet a.

appositional growth
apprehension
a. shoulder
a. sign
a. test

apprentice kyphosis
approach
Abbott-Carpenter posterior a.
Abbott posterior a.
acetabular extensile a.
anterior acromioplasty a.
anterior axillary a.
anterior cervical a.
anterior extensile a.
anterior retroperitoneal flank a.
anterior sternomastoid a.
anterior strap a.
anterior transthoracic a.
anterolateral a.
anteromedial retropharyngeal a.
Aufranc lateral a.
Avila a.
axillary a.
Bailey-Badgley anterior cervical a.
Banks-Laufman a.

NOTES

approach *(continued)*
    Bennett posterior shoulder a.
    Berger-Bookwalter posterior a.
    Bosworth a.
    Boyd a.
    Boyd-Sisk a.
    Brackett-Osgood posterior a.
    Brodsky-Tullos-Gartsman a.
    Broomhead medial a.
    Brown lateral a.
    Bruser lateral a.
    Bryan-Morrey extensive posterior a.
    Callahan and Scuderi a.
    Campbell posterior shoulder a.
    Campbell posterolateral a.
    Carnesale acetabular extensile a.
    Carroll a.
    Cave hip a.
    Cave knee a.
    cervical a.
    Charnley-Müller lateral a.
    Cloward cervical disc a.
    Codman saber-cut shoulder a.
    Colonna-Ralston medial a.
    combined anterior and posterior a.
    combined low cervical and
      transthoracic a.
    Coonse-Adams knee a.
    costotransversectomy a.
    Cozen transverse a.
    Cubbins shoulder a.
    curved L a.
    de Andrade and MacNab
      anterior a.
    deBoer lateral a.
    deltoid-splitting shoulder a.
    deltopectoral a.
    Dickinson a.
    dorsal finger a.
    dorsal midline a.
    dorsalward a.
    dorsolateral a.
    dorsomedial a.
    dorsoplantar a.
    dorsoradial a.
    dorsorostral a.
    dorsoulnar a.
    Downey modification of Fowler-
      Philip a.
    Duran a.
    DuVries a.
    endoscopic a.
    extended iliofemoral a.
    extensile anterior a.
    extensile lateral a.
    extensive posterior a.
    extrabursal a.
    extraperitoneal a.
    extrapharyngeal a.

    Fahey a.
    femoral a.
    Fernandez extensile anterior a.
    Fowler-Philip a.
    Gallie a.
    Gibson a.
    Gordon a.
    Hardinge femoral a.
    Hardinge lateral a.
    Harmon cervical a.
    Harmon modified posterolateral a.
    Harris anterolateral a.
    Harris lateral a.
    Hay lateral a.
    Henderson posterolateral a.
    Henderson posteromedial a.
    Henry anterior strap a.
    Henry anterolateral a.
    Henry extensile a.
    Henry posterior interosseous
      nerve a.
    Henry radial a.
    Hirschhorn compression a.
    Hoffmann a.
    Hoppenfeld lateral a.
    Horwitz ankle fusion a.
    Howorth a.
    iliofemoral a.
    ilioinguinal acetabular a.
    inguinal a.
    Insall anterior a.
    intraforaminal a.
    ipsilateral a.
    Jones and Brackett anterior a.
    keyhole a.
    Kikuchi-MacNap-Moreau a.
    Kocher curved-L a.
    Kocher-Gibson posterolateral a.
    Kocher-Langenbeck a.
    Kocher lateral J a.
    Langenbeck anteromedial a.
    lateral deltoid-splitting a.
    lateral J a.
    lateral Kocher a.
    lateral Ollier a.
    lateral parapatellar a.
    Leslie-Ryan anterior axillary a.
    Letournel-Judet a.
    long deltopectoral a.
    low cervical a.
    Ludloff medial a.
    Mayo a.
    McConnell extensile a.
    McConnell median and ulnar
      nerve a.
    McLaughlin a.
    McWhorter posterior shoulder a.
    medial parapatellar capsular a.
    midlateral a.

midline medial a.
Mize-Bucholz-Grogan a.
modified posterolateral a.
Moore posterior a.
Moore-Southern a.
Murphy lateral a.
neurodevelopmental a.
Ollier arthrodesis a.
Ollier lateral a.
oropharyngeal a.
Osborne posterior a.
palmar a.
paramedian a.
parapatellar a.
pararectus a.
paraspinal a.
patella turndown a.
Perry extensile anterior a.
Phemister medial a.
Phemister posteromedial a.
plantar a.
Pogrund lateral a.
posterior costotransversectomy a.
posterior interosseous nerve a.
posterior inverted-U a.
posterior midline a.
posterior occipitocervical a.
posterior shoulder a.
posterior transolecranon a.
posterolateral a.
posteromedial a.
proprioceptive neuromuscular
  facilitation a.
proximal interphalangeal joint a.
proximal metatarsal a.
pulp a.
Putti posterior a.
radical a.
Radley-Liebig-Brown a.
Reinert acetabular extensile a.
retroperitoneal a.
retropharyngeal a.
Roberts a.
Robinson-Smith anterior cervical a.
Roos a.
Rowe posterior shoulder a.
saber-cut a.
sacral a.
sacroiliac a.
screw-plate a.
Senegas hip a.
sensorimotor stimulation a.
Shoemaker lateral a.

Sir Henry Platt transverse a.
Smith-Petersen a.
Smith-Robinson cervical disc a.
Somerville anterior a.
Southwick-Robinson anterior
  cervical a.
Spetzler anterior transoral a.
split heel a.
split patellar a.
stabilization a.
sternum-splitting a.
subclavicular a.
supraclavicular a.
surgical a.
Swedish a.
Thompson anterolateral a.
Thompson anteromedial a.
Thompson-Henry a.
Thompson posterior radial a.
thoracic a.
thoracoabdominal a.
thoracolumbar retroperitoneal a.
thoracotomy a.
thumb metacarpophalangeal joint a.
transacromial a.
transaxillary a.
transbrachioradialis a.
transcalcaneal a.
transclavicular a.
transfibular a.
transolecranon a.
transpedicular a.
transperitoneal a.
transsternal a.
transthoracic a.
transtrochanteric a.
transverse a.
triceps-splitting a.
triradiate acetabular extensile a.
triradiate transtrochanteric a.
trivector retaining a.
unilateral sacroiliac a.
Vermont Interdependent Services
  Team A. (VISTA)
volar a.
volarward a.
Wadsworth posterolateral a.
Wagner a.
Wagoner posterior a.
Watson-Jones anterior a.
Watson-Jones lateral a.
Wilson a.
Wiltberger anterior cervical a.

NOTES

approach *(continued)*
    Wiltse a.
    Yee posterior shoulder a.
    Young medial a.
    zigzag a.
    Z-plasty a.
approximator
    Acland clamp a.
    Acland double-clamp a.
    clamp a.
    double-clamp a.
    Henderson clamp a.
    hook a.
    Ikuta clamp a.
    Kleinert-Kutz clamp a.
    Lalonde tendon a.
    rib a.
    sternal a.
    Van Beek nerve a.
APPT
    Adolescent and Pediatric Pain Tool
APR
    anatomic porous replacement
    APR acetabular prosthesis
    APR cement fixation
    APR cement fixation adhesive
    APR femoral prosthesis
    APR hip stem
    APR I femoral stem
    APR II hip system
    APR II prosthesis
    APR total hip system
apraxia
    dressing a.
    Test of Oral and Limb A.
      (TOLA)
apraxic gait
ApriVera skin and hair cleanser
APRL
    Army Prosthetics Research Laboratory
    APRL hand prosthesis
    APRL prosthetic hook
apron
    quadriceps a.
apropulsive gait
APS
    air plasma spray
    anterior plate system
    APS Hi-Lo electric lift table
APTT
    activated partial thromboplastin time
APU brace
aqua
    a. PT dry physiotherapy
    a. PT water massage
    A. Spray
    A. Spray wet nail débridement
      system
    A. Thermassage

AquaBodyCiser aquatic mat
Aqua-Cel heating pad system
Aquachloral Supprettes
Aquaciser
    A. hydrodynamic measurement
      system
    A. pool
    A. 100R underwater treadmill
      system
    A. underwater treadmill
Aquaflex gel pad
AquaGaiter treadmill
AquaJogger buoyancy belt
AquaMED
    A. dry hydrotherapy
    A. dry hydrotherapy equipment
AquaMEPHYTON
AquaMotion pool
Aquanex hydrodynamic measurement
system
Aquaphor gauze dressing
Aquaplast
    A. splint
    A. splinting material
Aquarelle hydrogel nucleus viscoelastic
material
AquaRunners resistance footwear
AquaSens fluid monitoring system
AquaShield
    A. orthopaedic cast cover
    A. reusable cast cover
Aquasonic Transmission Gel
Aquasorb Hydrogel wound dressing
Aquatech cast pad
aquatherapy
Aquatherm bed pad
aquatic
    a. cardiac evaluation and testing
      (ACET)
    a. exercise
    a. exercise program
    a. map
    a. rehabilitation
    a. stabilization program
    a. therapy
    a. therapy pool
Aqua-Trainer
AquaTrek Wheelchair
Aquatrend water workout station
Aqua/Whirl bath
ARA
    Adolescent Role Assessment
    American Rheumatism Association
    ARA Test
arabinoside
arachidonate metabolism
arachidonic
arachnodactyly
arachnoid

arachnoiditis
  adhesive a.
arachnoid-shape Beaver blade
Arafiles
  A. elbow arthrodesis
  A. elbow prosthesis
Aralen Phosphate
Aran-Duchenne
  A.-D. amyotrophy
  A.-D. disease
Aravon footwear
ARC
  antirotation cable
arc
  carpal a.
  flexion-extension a.
  Leksell stereotactic a.
  monosynaptic reflex a.
  a. of motion
  painful a.
  reflex a.
  shoulder ROM a.
  stereotactic a.
arcade
  a. of Frohse
  Frohse ligamentous a.
  a. of Struthers
  superficialis a.
Arcelin view
arch, pl. **arches**
  a. angle
  anterior metatarsal a.
  axillary a.
  a. binder
  a. of bone
  carpal a.
  cervical a.
  a. cookie
  coracoacromial a.
  a. cushion
  deep a.
  dorsal venous a.
  fallen a.
  a. of foot
  a. fracture
  Hapad metatarsal a.
  Hapad scaphoid a.
  Hillock a.
  a. index
  ischiopubic a.
  Langer axillary a.
  a. loading
  longitudinal plantar a.

  medial longitudinal a.
  metatarsal a.
  palmar a.
  a. peak area
  plantar arterial a.
  posterior a.
  Roman a.
  scaphoid a.
  a. and slouch position
  a. stress
  superficial palmar a.
  a. support
  vertebral a.
archer's shoulder
arch-height
  a.-h. index
  a.-h. ratio
Archimedean drill
architectural alterations of bone
architecture
  bony a.
  foot a.
Arch-Lok
  Swede-O A.-L.
archplasty
arch-up test
Archxerciser foot exercise device
arciform
Arco classification
ArCom processed polyethylene
Arctic Blaze hot/cold pack
arcuate
  a. complex
  a. fasciculus (AF)
  a. foramen
  a. movement
  a. osteotomy
  a. popliteal ligament
arcuatus
  pes a.
arcus
ardeparin sodium
area
  arch peak a.
  Broca a.
  curvilinear a.
  dorsolumbar a.
  odontoid-axial a.
  Patrick trigger a.
  performance a.
  pressure-sensitive a.
  problem a.
  puboischial a.

NOTES

area *(continued)*
    pump bump a.
    a. scar
    thenar a.
    trapezial a.
    web a.
areflexia
    detrusor a.
areola of bone
Arglaes film dressing
ARGO
    Adjustable Advanced Reciprocating Gait
    Orthosis
Ariat shoe
Ariel computerized exercise system
Aristocort Forte
Arizona
    A. ankle brace
    A. Health Science Center (AHSC)
    A. Health Sciences Center-Volz
      hinge
    A. universal leg support
ARM
    alternating range of motion
    ARM method
    ARM method of physical
      examination
arm
    abductor lever a.
    articulating a.
    artificial a.
    a. band
    a. board
    a. cuff
    a. cylinder cast
    a. drift
    a. elevator sling
    flail a.
    a. flap
    a. fossa test
    2-a. goniometer
    grenade thrower's a.
    a. heel-strike synchrony
    a. holder
    lever a.
    Leyla a.
    linebacker's a.
    moment a.
    MonitorMate monitor a.
    outrigger a.
    Popeye a.
    a. positioner
    a. skate
    a. swathe
    tackler's a.
    Utah artificial a.
    wringer a.
    Yasargil Leyla retractor a.
armboard

armchair splint
Armistead
    A. technique
    A. ulnar lengthening
    A. ulnar lengthening operation
Armstrong
    A. acromionectomy
    A. plate
Army
    A. bone gouge
    A. osteotome
    A. Prosthetics Research Laboratory
      (APRL)
Army-Navy retractor
Arnadottir Occupational Therapy
    Activities of Daily Living
    Neurobehavioral Evaluation (A-ONE)
Arnold
    A. lumbar brace
    A. nerve
Arnold-Chiari
    A.-C. deformity
    A.-C. malformation
    A.-C. syndrome
AROM
    active range of motion
Aron Alpha adhesive
arrest
    epiphysial a.
    greater trochanteric apophysial a.
    growth a.
    mechanism of growth a.
    Shapiro classification of
      mechanisms of growth a.
arrow
    A. absorbable meniscal repair
      device
    Biofix meniscus a.
    Bionx a.
    meniscal a.
    A. pin clasp
ARS
    acute repetitive seizure
    ARS disorder
ART
    active-release technique
ArtAssist arterial assist device
arteria acetabuli
arterial
    a. aneurysm
    a. flap
    a. gas embolism
    a. occlusion sign
    a. oxygen saturation
    a. ring
    a. spasm
    a. trauma
arteries *(pl. of* artery)
arteriogram

arteriography
    femoral a.
    magnetic resonance a.
    peripheral a.
    spinal a.
    vertebral a.
arteriosclerosis obliterans
arteriotomy
    ankle-level a.
arteriovenous
    a. fistula (AVF)
    a. malformation
arteritis
artery, pl. **arteries**
    Adamkiewicz a.
    anomalous fibular nutrient a.
    anterior radial collateral a.
    anterior recurrent tibial a.
    anterior spinal a.
    anterior tibial a.
    ascending cervical a.
    axillary a.
    basilic a.
    brachial a.
    carotid a.
    cephalic a.
    cervical a.
    circumflex iliac a.
    circumflex scapular a.
    collateral a.
    common carotid a.
    common iliac a.
    deep circumflex iliac a.
    deltoid a.
    digital a.
    dorsal digital a. (DDA)
    dorsal metatarsal a.
    epiphysial a.
    facial a.
    femoral circumflex a.
    fibular plantar marginal a.
    first dorsal metacarpal a.
    first dorsal metatarsal a. (FDMA)
    first plantar metatarsal a. (FPMA)
    genicular a.
    geniculate a.
    gluteal a.
    hypogastric a.
    iliac a.
    iliofemoral flap a.
    iliolumbar a.
    inferior thyroid a.
    intercostal a.
    intermetatarsal a.
    internal carotid a.
    internal iliac a.
    interosseous a.
    lateral calcaneal a.
    lateral plantar a.
    lingual a.
    medial geniculate a.
    medial plantar a.
    metaphysial a.
    metatarsal a.
    middle sacral a.
    nutrient a.
    obturator a.
    paramalleolar a.
    perforating a.
    peripheral a.
    peroneal a.
    persistent sciatic a.
    plantar a.
    plantar digital a. (PDA)
    plantar metatarsal a.
    popliteal a.
    posterior inferior cerebellar a.
     (PICA)
    posterior radial collateral a.
    posterior tibial a.
    princeps pollicis a.
    profunda brachii a.
    pudendal a.
    radial a.
    radicular a.
    retinacular a.
    sacral a.
    saphenous a.
    second metatarsal a.
    spinal a.
    subclavian a.
    superficial circumflex iliac a.
    superficial femoral a. (SFA)
    superficial temporal a.
    superior laryngeal a.
    superior thyroid a.
    supraclavicular fossa a.
    tarsal canal a.
    tarsal sinus a.
    thoracoacromial a.
    thrombosis radial a.
    tibial a.
    ulnar a.
    vertebral a.
    volar digital a.
Arth-Aid Joint Formula

NOTES

arthralgia
> acromegalic a.
> intermittent a.
> migratory a.
> nonspecific a.
> periodic a.
> subtalar a.
> temporomandibular joint a.

arthrectomy

arthrempyesis

Arthrex
> A. arthroscopy instrument
> A. Bird-Beak device
> A. bone anchor
> A. coring reamer
> A. femoral guide
> A. instruments and systems
> A. meniscal dart
> A. meniscal dart gun
> A. Penetrator
> A. sheathed interference screw
> A. tibial guide
> A. TwistLoc suture anchor
> A. zebra pin

arthrifluent abscess

arthritic
> a. ankle joint narrowing
> a. atrophy
> a. destruction
> a. deterioration
> a. shoe
> a. talonavicular change

arthritides
> erosive a.

arthritis, pl. arthritides
> acromegalic a.
> acute hematogenous a.
> acute spinal a.
> adjuvant-induced a. (AIA)
> allergenic a.
> ancient tuberculous a.
> ankle infectious a.
> ankle rheumatoid a.
> assignment criteria for
>   rheumatoid a.
> atrophic a.
> bacterial a.
> base of thumb a.
> Bekhterev a.
> calcaneocuboid joint a.
> cervical a.
> Charcot a.
> chronic absorptive a.
> chronic villous a.
> chylous a.
> crystal-induced a.
> cystic rheumatoid a.
> a. deformans
> degenerative a. (DA)

enteropathic a.
filarial a.
A. Foundation
A. Foundation Pain Reliever
fungal a.
gonococcal septic a.
gouty a.
A. Helplessness Index (AHI)
hemophilic a.
hypertrophic a.
hypotrophic a.
A. Impact Measurement Scale
  (AIMS)
A. Impact Measurement Scale
  classification
infectious a.
inflammatory bowel disease
  associated a.
Jaccoud a.
juvenile chronic a.
juvenile-onset rheumatoid a.
juvenile rheumatoid a. (JRA)
Lyme disease a.
Marie-Strümpell a.
midfoot a.
migratory a.
monoarticular septic a.
a. mutilans
mutilans rheumatoid a.
mycobacterial a.
navicular a.
neonatal septic a.
neuropathic a.
New York diagnostic criteria for
  rheumatoid a.
a. nodosa
nonarticular a.
ochronotic a.
oligoarticular a.
pantalocrural a.
pantrapezial a.
patellofemoral a.
pauciarticular a.
periosteal a.
peritrapezial a.
pisotriquetral a.
polyarticular juvenile rheumatoid a.
postinfectious a.
postmenopausal a.
posttraumatic a.
primary degenerative a.
proliferative a.
psoriatic a.
pyogenic a.
a. Quality of Life Scale
radiocarpal a.
reactive a.
rheumatoid a. (RA)
robust rheumatoid a.

sarcoid a.
septic a.
seronegative rheumatoid a.
seropositive rheumatoid a.
silicone a.
a. sock
spinal a.
staphylococcal a.
subtalar joint a.
suppurative a.
tendon bowing in a.
tibiotalar a.
Tom Smith a.
traumatic a.
tuberculous a.
vertebral a.
viral-associated a.
WHO/LAR Response Criteria for
 Rheumatoid A.
arthritis-associated psoriasis
Arthro-7
ArthroCare
 A. arthroscopic system
 A. electrode
 A. wand
arthrocele
arthrocentesis
arthrochalasis
arthrochondritis
arthroclasia
arthrodesed digit
arthrodesis
 Abbott-Fischer-Lucas hip a.
 Abbott-Lucas a.
 Adams transmalleolar a.
 Adkins spinal a.
 Albee hip a.
 ankle a.
 anterior occipitocervical a.
 anterior slot graft a.
 AO group shoulder a.
 Arafiles elbow a.
 arthroscopic ankle a.
 arthroscopic subtalar a.
 atlantoaxial a.
 Baciu-Filibiu dowel ankle a.
 Baciu-Filibiu transmalleolar a.
 Badgley a.
 Barrasso-Wile-Gage a.
 Barr-Record ankle a.
 Batchelor-Brown extraarticular
  subtalar a.
 beak modification with triple a.

bimalleolar approach to ankle a.
Blair ankle a.
Blair anterior a.
Blair tibiotalar a.
Bosworth a.
Boyd ankle a.
Brett a.
Brewster triple a.
Brittain ischiofemoral a.
Brockman-Nissen a.
Brooks atlantoaxial a.
calcaneocuboid distraction a.
 (CCDA)
calcaneopelvic a.
calcaneotibial a.
Campbell-Akbarnia a.
Campbell posterior a.
Campbell-Rinehard-Kalenak
 anterior a.
Carceau-Brahms ankle a.
Carroll a.
cervical a.
Chandler a.
Chapchal knee a.
Charcot hip a.
Charnley ankle a.
Charnley compression a.
closing wedge a.
Cloward cervical a.
combined resection arthroplasty
 and a.
Compere-Thompson a.
compression a.
cone a.
coracoclavicular a.
cuneiform joint a.
Davis a.
Dennyson-Fulford extraarticular
 subtalar a.
distal fibulotalar a.
distraction bone block a.
distraction-compression bone
 graft a.
distraction subtalar a.
double a.
dowel a.
Dunn-Brittain triple a.
Dunn triple a.
elbow a.
Elmslie triple a.
Enneking knee a.
excisional a.

NOTES

arthrodesis *(continued)*
extension injury posterior
   atlantoaxial a.
extraarticular a.
failed triple a.
fibulotalar a.
first cuneiform joint a.
first cuneiform-navicular joint a.
first metatarsal-first cuneiform a.
flat-cut a.
flexion injury posterior
   atlantoaxial a.
fused a.
Gallie ankle a.
Gallie atlantoaxial a.
Gant hip a.
Garceau-Brahms a.
Gill a.
Gill-Stein a.
Gissane a.
glenohumeral a.
Goldner spinal a.
Graham ankle a.
Grice extraarticular subtalar a.
Grice-Green extraarticular
   subtalar a.
Guttmann subtalar a.
hallux interphalangeal joint a.
hallux rigidus a.
Harris-Beath a.
Heiple a.
Henderson a.
Hibbs a.
hindfoot a.
Hoke triple a.
Horwitz-Adams a.
Horwitz transmalleolar a.
Hunt-Thompson pantalar a.
Ilizarov ankle a.
interbody a.
intercarpal a.
internal fixation compression a.
interphalangeal a.
intertransverse process a.
intraarticular a.
John C. Wilson a.
joint a.
Kapandji-Sauvé a.
Key intraarticular knee a.
Kirkaldy-Willis a.
knee a.
Küntscher modified knee a.
Lambrinudi triple a.
Lapidus a.
Lapidus modified a.
lesser tarsal a.
limited intertarsal a.
Lipscomb metatarsophalangeal a.
Lipscomb modified McKeever a.

Lisfranc a.
Lord total hip a.
lunotriquetral a.
Mann modified McKeever a.
McKeever metatarsophalangeal a.
metatarsocuneiform a.
metatarsophalangeal joint a.
midcarpal a.
midfoot a.
Millender-Nalebuff wrist a.
Moberg a.
modified Boyd ankle a.
modified Lapidus a.
Mueller a.
Nalebuff a.
Naughton-Dunn triple a.
naviculocuneiform joint a.
nonfused a.
occipitocervical a.
panastragaloid a.
pantalar a.
paraarticular a.
Podiatry Institute procedures for
   ankle a.
Pontenza a.
posterior atlantoaxial a.
posterolateral a.
Potter a.
Pridie ankle a.
primary subtalar a.
Putti knee a.
radiocarpal a.
resection a.
Richards a.
Richardson subtalar a.
Robinson-Smith spinal a.
Robinson spinal a.
Ryerson triple a.
salvage ankle a.
scaphocapitolunate a. (SCL)
scaphotrapeziotrapezoid a.
scapulothoracic a.
Schneider hip a.
Scranton transmalleolar a.
a. screw
second metatarsophalangeal joint a.
Seoffert triple a.
shoulder a.
Simmons spinal a.
sliding a.
Smith-Robinson interbody a.
Soren a.
Spier elbow a.
spinal a.
Staples elbow a.
Stark a.
Steindler elbow a.
stone a.
subtalar a.

talar triple a.
talonavicular a.
tarsal a.
tarsometatarsal truncated-wedge a.
thoracoscapular a.
tibiocalcaneal a.
tibiotalar joint primary a.
tibiotalocalcaneal a.
transfibular a.
transmalleolar ankle a.
triple a.
triquetrum-lunate a.
triscaphe a.
Trumble a.
truncated tarsometatarsal wedge a.
Uematsu shoulder a.
ulnocarpal a.
Watson-Jones a.
Whitecloud-LaRocca cervical a.
White posterior a.
Wilson cone a.
Wolf blade plate ankle a.
arthrodial
    a. articulation
    a. cartilage
    a. protractor
    A. Protractor range of motion
      analyzer
arthrodiastasis
arthrodynia
arthrodysplasia
arthroempyesis
arthroendoscopy
arthroereisis
    Maxwell-Brancheau a. (MBA)
    peg-in-hole a.
    staple a.
    subtalar a.
arthrofibrosis
Arthrofile orthopaedic rasp
Arthro-Flo
    A.-F. arthroscopic irrigation system
    A.-F. irrigator
Arthroforce III hand instrument
arthrogenic gait
arthrogenous
arthrogram
    double-contrast a.
    Gordon-Broström single-contrast a.
    joint a.
    nuclear a.
    saline-enhanced MR a.
    single-contrast a.

arthrographic capsular distension and rupture technique
arthrography
    air a.
    ankle a.
    contrast a.
    coronal computed tomographic a.
    (CCTA)
    double-contrast a.
    joint a.
    magnetic resonance a.
    opaque a.
    osteochondral fracture a.
    saline-enhanced a.
arthrogryposis
    a. multiplex congenita
    myopathic a.
    neurogenic a.
arthrogrypotic clubfoot
arthrokatadysis
arthrokinematic
arthrokinetic reflex
arthrokleisis
arthrolith
arthrolithiasis
Arthro-Lock system
arthrology
    zygapophysial a.
Arthro-Lok system of Beaver blade
arthrolysis
arthromeningitis
arthrometer
    Acufex knee laxity a.
    Genucom a.
    joint a.
    knee laxity a.
    knee ligament a.
    KT-1000 joint a.
    KT-1000/Jr a.
    KT-1000 knee ligament a.
    KT-2000 knee ligament a.
    KT-1000/s surgical a.
    a. measurement
    Medmetric knee ligament a.
    Medmetric KT-1000 knee laxity a.
    Robinson a.
    stress-testing a.
    Stryker knee laxity a.
    a. test
    a. testing
arthrometric knee laxity measurement
arthrometry
arthroncus

NOTES

arthroneuralgia
arthronosos
arthroonychodysplasia syndrome
arthroophthalmopathy
    hereditary progressive a.
arthroosteoonychodysplasia
arthropathic
arthropathology
arthropathy
    Charcot a.
    crystal-induced a.
    crystal-related a.
    cuff tear a. (CTA)
    degenerative vertebral a.
    diabetic a.
    dislocating a.
    disuse a.
    gonococcal a.
    Heberden a.
    hemodialysis-related a.
    hemophilic a.
    inflammatory a.
    Jaccoud a.
    joint a.
    long leg a.
    midfoot a.
    neuropathic a. (NA)
    neuropathic spinal a.
    ochronotic a.
    palindromic a.
    pyrophosphate a.
    sacroiliac joint a.
    seronegative a.
    SLE a.
    static a.
    stationary a.
    tabetic a.
arthrophyte
arthroplasty
    ablative a.
    abrasion a.
    acetabular cup a.
    acromioclavicular a.
    Albright-Chase a.
    anconeus a.
    ankle a.
    Ashworth hand a.
    Ashworth implant a.
    Aufranc cup a.
    Aufranc-Turner a.
    Austin Moore a.
    autogenous interpositional
      shoulder a.
    Bankart a.
    Bechtol a.
    Bigliani/Flatow total shoulder a.
    bipolar hip a.
    Bosworth a.
    Bowers radial a.

Brain a.
Breslow a.
Bryan a.
a. bur
Campbell interpositional a.
Campbell resection a.
capitellocondylar total elbow a.
capsular interposition a.
carpometacarpal a.
Carroll and Taber a.
Castle-Schneider resection
  interposition a.
a. cement
cemented total hip a.
cementless surface replacement a.
  (CSRA)
cementless total hip a.
Charcot a.
Charnley low-friction a.
Charnley-Müller a.
Charnley total hip a.
Clayton forefoot a.
Clayton resection a.
Colonna trochanteric a.
condylar implant a.
constrained ankle a.
constrained shoulder a.
convex condylar-implant a.
Coonrad-Morrey total elbow a.
Coonrad total elbow a.
Cracchiolo forefoot a.
Cracchiolo-Sculco implant a.
Crawford-Adams acetabular cup a.
Cubbins a.
cuff tear a.
cup a.
Dewar-Barrington a.
distraction a.
DuVries a.
Eaton implant a.
Eaton volar plate a.
Eden-Hybbinette a.
elbow a.
Ewald capitellocondylar total
  elbow a.
Ewald-Walker kinematic knee a.
excision a.
extensor brevis a.
failed implant a.
fascial a.
finger joint a.
forefoot a.
Ganley modification of Keller a.
gap a.
Girdlestone resection a.
Global total shoulder a.
Gore-Tex interpositional a.
a. gouge
Green a.

Gristina-Webb total shoulder a.
Gunston a.
Gustilo-Kyle cementless total hip a.
Harrington total hip a.
Head hip a.
Helal flap a.
hemijoint a.
hemiresection interposition a.
hip a.
Hungerford-Krackow-Kenna knee a.
hydroxyapatite-coated ankle a.
ICLH double cup a.
implant a.
4-in-1 a.
Inclan-Ober a.
Inglis triaxial total elbow a.
Insall-Burstein-Freeman knee a.
interphalangeal a.
interpositional a.
ipsilateral total elbow a.
ipsilateral total shoulder a.
Irvine ankle a.
Jaccoud a.
Johnson resection a.
Jones resection a.
Kates forefoot a.
Keller a.
Keller-Brandes resection a.
Keller-Lelièvre a.
Keller-Mann resection a.
Keller-Mayo diabetic foot a.
Keller resection a.
knee a.
Koenig metatarsophalangeal joint a.
Lacey rotating hinge a.
Larmon forefoot a.
laser image custom a. (LICA)
Magnuson-Stack a.
Mann resection a.
Mark II Sorrells hip a.
Mayo ankle a.
Mayo resection a.
Mayo-Stone-Valenti hallux
  limitus/rigidus a.
Mayo total elbow a.
McKee-Farrar total hip a.
McLaughlin a.
metacarpophalangeal joint a.
metatarsophalangeal a.
Meuli a.
Millender a.
Miller-Galante knee a.
mobile-bearing knee a.

modified Keller resection a.
modified mold and surface
  replacement a.
mold acetabular a.
monospherical total shoulder a.
mosaic a.
Mould a.
Mueller hip a.
Mumford-Gurd a.
Nara a.
NEB a.
Neer unconstrained shoulder a.
Neviaser a.
New England Baptist hip a.
Nicola a.
Niebauer trapeziometacarpal a.
noncemented total hip a.
Post total shoulder a.
press-fit condylar knee a.
primary a.
A. Products Consultants foot and
  legholder
prosthetic a.
Putti-Platt a.
Regnauld modification of Keller a.
resection a.
revision hip a.
Robinson a.
rotator cuff tear a.
Sauvé-Kapandji a.
Schlein elbow a.
Schrock a.
Scott a.
semiconstrained total elbow a.
shoulder a.
silastic lunate a.
silicone implant a.
silicone rubber a.
silicone wrist a.
Smith-Petersen cup a.
Speed a.
Stanmore shoulder a.
Steffee thumb a.
surface replacement hip a.
Sutter silicone metacarpophalangeal
  joint a.
Swanson convex condylar a.
Swanson interpositional wrist a.
Swanson metatarsophalangeal
  joint a.
Swanson PIP joint a.
Swanson radial head implant a.
Swanson silicone wrist a.

NOTES

arthroplasty *(continued)*
    tendon interposition a.
    Thackray low friction a.
    Thompson a.
    total ankle a. (TAA)
    total articular replacement a.
        (TARA)
    total articular resurfacing a.
        (TARA)
    total elbow a.
    total hip a. (THA)
    total joint a. (TJA)
    total knee a. (TKA)
    total patellofemoral joint a.
    total shoulder a.
    total wrist a.
    triaxial total elbow a.
    Trillat a.
    Tupper a.
    UCLA anatomic shoulder a.
    ulnar hemiresection interposition a.
    unconstrained shoulder a.
    unicompartmental knee a. (UKA)
    Vainio a.
    Valenti a.
    Van Ness rotational a.
    vitallium cup a.
    volar plate a.
    Volz total wrist a.
    Woodward a.
arthropneumoradiography
arthropneumoroentgenography
arthropneumotography
Arthropor
    A. acetabular cup
    A. cup pad
    A. cup prosthesis
    A. II acetabular prosthesis
    A. II porous socket
    A. oblong cup for acetabular
        defect
ArthroProbe
    A. arthroscopic laser
    Contact A.
    A. laser system
arthropyosis
arthrorheumatism
arthrorisis
arthroscintigraphy
arthrosclerosis
arthroscope
    angled a.
    Baxter angled a.
    Citscope disposable a.
    disposable a.
    Dyonics a.
    Eagle straight-ahead a.
    fiberoptic a.
    GoldenEye a.

    O'Connor operating a.
    Panoview a.
    Sapphire View a.
    Storz oblique a.
    Stryker viewing a.
    triangulation technique for a.
    Trio a.
    Wolf a.
arthroscopic
    a. abrasion chondroplasty
    a. acromioplasty
    a. ankle arthrodesis
    a. augmentation
    a. Bankart repair
    a. cannula
    a. cheilectomy
    a. coplaning
    a. débridement
    a. drilling
    a. entry portal
    a. examination
    a. grabber
    a. knife
    a. knot
    a. laser instrument
    a. laser surgery
    a. leg holder
    a. legholder
    a. meniscectomy
    a. microdiscectomy (AMD)
    a. monopolar thermal stabilization
        forefoot compression sleeve
    a. mosaicplasty
    a. osteotome
    a. probe
    a. pump
    a. punch
    a. scissors
    a. screw fixation
    a. shaver
    a. shaving
    a. sheath
    a. shield
    a. subtalar arthrodesis
    a. synovectomy
    a. tourniquet
    a. transglenoid suture stabilization
        procedure
    a. transhumeral reconstruction
arthroscopically
    a. assisted anterior cruciate
        ligament reconstruction
    a. assisted synovectomy
arthroscopy
    Allen shoulder a.
    ankle a.
    A. Association of North America
        (AANA)
    a. basket forceps

calcaneonavicular joint a.
diagnostic and operative a. (DOA)
electrothermal a.
extraarticular a.
a. grasping forceps
Hawkeye suture needle for a.
knee a.
laser a.
lateral hip a.
metacarpophalangeal a.
midcarpal a.
operative a.
radiocarpal a.
Ringer a.
second-look a.
wrist a.

**arthroscopy-assisted patellar tendon
substitution**
ArthroSew arthroscopic suturing device
arthrosis
Charcot a.
crystal-induced a.
cystic a.
a. deformans
a. deformity
degenerative a.
Eaton CMC a. (stage I–IV)
end-stage a.
Malleoloc anatomic ankle a.
metatarsal-sesamoid a.
posttraumatic a.
primary cystic a.
subtalar a.
trapezial a.
uncovertebral a.

Arthrosol dressing
arthrosteitis
arthrostomy
arthrosynovitis
Arthrotek
A. calibrated cylinder
A. Ellipticut hand instrumentation
A. femoral aimer
A. meniscus staple
A. tibial fixation device

arthrotome
arthrotomography
double contrast shoulder a.

arthrotomy
diagnostic arthroscopy, operative
arthroscopy, possible operative a.
(AAA)
Magnuson-Stack shoulder a.

medial parapatellar a.
operative a.
parapatellar a.
subtalar a.

arthrotropic
ArthroWand
Caps A.
CAPSure A.
A. device
A. disposable surgical wand
Eliminator A.
Microblator A.
RazorVac A.
Saber Bisector A.
A. tool

arthroxerosis
arthroxesis
Arth-Support Formula
articular
a. block
a. blockage
a. bone lamella
a. bone tubercle
a. capsule
a. cartilage
a. cartilage autograft
a. cartilage autografting
a. cartilage lesion
a. cortex
a. crepitus
a. defect
a. disc
a. facet
a. facet angle
a. fragment
a. gout
a. insert
a. instability
a. labrum
a. mass separation
a. mass separation fracture
a. motion device (AMD)
a. nerve
a. pillar
a. pillar fracture
a. process
a. set angle
a. strain
a. structure
a. surface

articular-ligamentous system
articulated
a. AFO

NOTES

articulated *(continued)*
    a. chin implant
    a. external fixator
    a. skeleton
    a. tension device
articulate minifixator
articulating
    a. arm
    a. bone end
articulatio humeri
articulation
    acromioclavicular a.
    arthrodial a.
    atlantoaxial a.
    calcaneocuboid a.
    calcaneonavicular a.
    carpal a.
    carpometacarpal a.
    carporadial a.
    chondrosternal a.
    Chopart a.
    condylar a.
    congruent a.
    coracoclavicular a.
    costocentral a.
    costosternal a.
    costovertebral a.
    coxofemoral a.
    DIP a.
    a. disturbance
    ellipsoidal a.
    false a.
    a. of foot
    Goldman-Fristoe test of a.
    hinge a.
    humeroradial a.
    humeroulnar a.
    iliosacral a.
    immovable a.
    incongruent a.
    incudomalleolar a.
    intercarpal a.
    intermetacarpal a.
    interphalangeal a.
    Lisfranc joint a.
    manipulation of a.
    metacarpophalangeal a.
    metatarsocuneiform a.
    occipitocervical a.
    patellofemoral a.
    phalangeal a.
    PIP a.
    a. of pisiform bone
    plane-type acromioclavicular a.
    proximal radioulnar a.
    radiocapitellar a.
    radiocarpal a.
    radiohumeral a.
    radioscaphoid a.

    radioulnar a.
    sacrococcygeal a.
    sacroiliac a.
    scapuloclavicular a.
    slightly movable a.
    sternochondral a.
    sternoclavicular a.
    subtalar a.
    superior tibial a.
    talocalcaneonavicular ligament a.
    talofibular a.
    talonavicular a.
    tarsometatarsal a.
    tibiofemoral a.
    tibiofibular a.
    transverse tarsal a.
    trochoid a.
    ulnolunate a.
    ulnotriquetrum a.
    Vermont spinal fixator a.
    zygapophysial a.
articulatory
    a. procedure
    a. skill
    a. tic
Articulose-50 Injection
artifact
    electric a.
    friction a.
    movement a.
    a. on x-ray
    shock a.
    stimulus a.
artifactual
artificial
    a. ankylosis
    a. arm
    a. fat pad
    a. foot
    a. hand
    a. joint implant
    a. leech
    a. ligament
    a. limb
    a. vertebral body
Artisan cement system
Artscan
    A. 200 arthroscopic cartilage stiffness tester
    A. 200 arthroscopic cartilage stiffness testing device
arum fixation pin
arytenoid cartilage
arytenoidectomy
arytenoiditis
arytenoidopexy
AS
    anterosuperior

AS ilium
AS subluxation
ascending cervical artery
ascension
  A. MCP finger joint implant
  A. MCP total joint
  A. MCP total joint implant
  A. MCP total joint replacement
  A. PIP total joint
  A. PIP total joint replacement
Ascent total knee system
Asch
  A. forceps
  A. splint
ascites
  chylous a.
ASE
  axilla, shoulder, elbow
  ASE bandage
aseptic
  a. fashion
  a. felon
  a. loosening
  a. necrosis
ASES
  American shoulder and elbow system
  ASES shoulder score
ASEx
  anterosuperior external ilium movement
  ASEx ilium
  ASEx subluxation
Asher physical build assessment technique
Ashhurst
  A. fracture classification system
  A. leg splint
  A. sign
Ashhurst-Bromer ankle fracture classification
Ashworth
  A. hand arthroplasty
  A. implant arthroplasty
  A. muscle spasticity score
  A. scale
  A. score of muscle spasticity
ASI
  acromial spur index
ASIA
  American Spinal Injury Association
  ASIA impairment scale
  ASIA impairment scale for classification of spinal cord injury
Asics Gel-MC shoe

ASICT
  amplitude-summation interferential current therapy
ASIF
  Association for the Study of Internal Fixation
  ASIF broad dynamic compression bone plate
  ASIF cancellous screw
  ASIF chisel
  ASIF cortical screw
  ASIF malleolar screw
  ASIF right-angle blade-plate
  ASIF screw fixation operation
  ASIF screw fixation technique
  ASIF screw pin
  ASIF system
  ASIF T-plate
  ASIF twist drill
ASIn
  anterosuperior internal ilium movement
  ASIn ilium
  ASIn subluxation
ASIS
  anterior superior iliac spine
Asissto-Seat
  Maddapult A.-S.
Aslan endoscopic scissors
ASM
  appendicular skeletal muscle
Asnis
  A. 3 cannulated screw system
  A. 2 guided-screw system
  A. III cannulated screw
  A. pin
  A. pinning
  A. technique
ASO
  ankle stabilizing orthosis
  ASO ankle brace
  ASO support
ASOT
  antistreptolysin-O titer
aspect
  dorsal a.
  laminar cortex posterior a.
  medial a.
  posterolateral a.
  volar a.
aspen
  A. cervical collar
  A. CTO
  A. electrocautery

NOTES

Aspercin Extra
aspergillosis infection
Aspergillus
    A. fumigatus
    A. niger
aspirated fat
aspiration
    anterior a.
    bone marrow a.
    joint a.
    lateral a.
    medial a.
    a. needle biopsy
aspirator
    Cavitron ultrasonic surgical a.
    Sonocut ultrasonic a.
    ultrasonic a.
Aspirin Free Anacin Maximum Strength
assay
    AlamarBlue osteoblast
      proliferation a.
    cefazolin a.
    chemiluminescent microtiter protein
      kinase activity a.
    deoxypyridinoline crosslinks
      urine a.
    enzyme-linked immunosorbent a.
    microtiter protein kinase a.
    osteoblast proliferation
      fluorometric a.
    Pyrilinks-D urine a.
    radioisotope clearance a.
    vitamin D receptor gene serum a.
assembly
    foot-ankle a.
    Massie nail a.
    multiple hook a.
    nail a.
    nail-screw sideplate a.
    proximal drill-guide a.
assessment
    Activity Loss A. (ALA)
    Adolescent Role A. (ARA)
    aerobic conditioning functional a.
    A. Battery for Children (ABC)
    BFM arm impairment a.
    body composition a.
    Brief Test of Head Injury A.
    Brunnstrom-Fugl-Meyer
      impairment a.
    closed-chain functional a.
    A. of Communication and
      Interaction Skills (ACIS)
    environmental a.
    ergonomic a.
    Erhardt Developmental
      Prehension A. (EDPA)

    Erhardt Developmental Vision A.
      (EDVA)
    functional capacity a.
    gait a.
    home a.
    impairment a.
    injury a.
    isokinetic a.
    Jebsen a.
    joint a.
    a. for limiting condition
    A. of Living Skills and Resources
      (ALSAR)
    Löwenstein Occupational Therapy
      Cognitive A. (LOTCA)
    A. of Ludic Behaviors (ALB)
    Modified Dynamic Visual
      Processing A. (M-DVPA)
    Moire topographic scoliosis a.
    motor function a.
    A. of Motor and Process Skills
      (AMPS)
    Musculoskeletal Function A. (MFA)
    neurologic a.
    A. of Occupational Functioning
      (AOF)
    overuse injury a.
    palpatory technique for joint a.
    pressure ulcer a.
    rehabilitation a.
    return-to-play injury a.
    return-to-play musculoskeletal a.
    Rivermead Motor A.
    SCATBI A.
    Short Musculoskeletal Function A.
      (SMFA)
    sideline a.
    Tinetti gait a.
    Toglia Category A.
    vascular a.
    vocational a.
ASSH
    American Society for Surgery of the
    Hand
ASSI
    Accurate Surgical and Scientific
    Instruments Corporation
    ASSI coagulator
    ASSI wire-pass drill
assignment criteria for rheumatoid arthritis
assimilation
    atlantooccipital a.
    a. pelvis
assist
    Elite posterior spring a.
    first dorsal interosseous a.
    knee extension a.

Thera-Band a.
thumb interphalangeal extension a.
assistance
ambulate with a.
assistant
A. Free calibrated femoral tibial
spreader
A. Free foot/ankle support
A. Free hip surgery square frame
A. Free hip surgery standard
frame
A. Free long prong collateral
ligament retractor
A. Free orthopaedic needle holder
A. Free orthopaedic needle
holder/scissors
A. Free orthopaedic scissors
A. Free self-retaining hip surgery
retractor system
A. Free Shubbs short prong
collateral ligament retractor
A. Free Stulberg leg positioner
A. Free wide PCL retractor
assisted ambulation
assistive
a. device
a. movement
a. technology device (ATD)
Assmann disease
associated myofascial trigger point
association
American Orthopaedic A. (AOA)
American Rheumatism A. (ARA)
American Spinal Injury A. (ASIA)
Japanese Orthopaedic A. (JOA)
National Depressive and Manic-
Depressive A.
National Spinal Cord Injury A.
National Stroke A.
North American Riding for
Handicapped A.
A. Research Circulation Osseous
classification system
A. for the Study of Internal
Fixation (ASIF)
astasia
astasia-abasia gait
astereognosis
asterixis
asthenia
asthenic
asthma
exercise-induced a.

ASTM
American Society for Testing and
Materials
augmented soft tissue mobilization
ASTM augmented soft tissue
mobilization
ASTM designation of Biophase
Aston
A. cartilage reduction
A. patterning
astragalar bone
astragalectomy
astragalocalcaneal bone
astragalocalcanean
astragalocrural bone
astragaloid bone
astragaloscaphoid bone
astragalotibial bone
astragalus
aviator's a.
a. bone
Astramorph PF Injection
Astroturf toe
asymmetric
a. incurvatum reflex
a. skin fold
a. subtalar joint development
a. tonic neck reflex (ATNR)
a. wear
asymmetrical growth
asymmetry
interinnominate a.
pure limb apraxia limb a.
asyndesis
asyndetic communication
asynergia
asynergic
AT
Achilles tendon
activity training
anaerobic threshold
Atabrine
atactic abasia
Atak knee brace
Atasoy
A. triangular advancement flap
A. volar V-Y flap
A. V-Y advancement
A. V-Y technique
Atasoy-Kleinert flap
Atasoy-type flap for nail injury repair
Atavi
A. atraumatic spine fusion system

NOTES

Atavi *(continued)*
    A. atraumatic spine surgery system
    A. TiTLE rod fixation system
atavicus
    metatarsus primus a.
atavistic
    a. cuneiform
    a. epiphysial
    a. foot
ataxia
    Bruns a.
    cerebellar a.
    equilibratory a.
    Friedreich a.
    hereditary spinocerebellar a.
    limb a.
    locomotor a.
    spinocerebellar a.
    traumatic brain injury-related a.
    vestibulocerebellar a.
ataxiadynamia
ataxia-telangiectasia
ataxic
    a. cerebral palsy
    a. gait
ataxy
ATD
    assistive technology device
atelectasis
    platelike a.
    pulmonary a.
ateliotic dwarfism
atelocollagen gel
atelomyelia
atelopodia
atelorachidia
Aten olecranon screw
ATFL
    anterior talofibular ligament
ATH
    anthropometric total hip
atherectomy
atherosclerosis
atherostenosis
athetoid cerebral palsy
athetosis
athetotic
athlete
    amputee a.
    a. foot
    a. heart
    high-power a.
    a. pseudoanemia
    single-organ a.
    weekend a.
athletic
    a. amenorrhea
    a. brace
    a. heart syndrome

    a. injury
    a. pubalgia
    a. shoe carbon fiber plate
    a. trainer
Atkin epiphysial fracture
Atkinson endoprosthesis
Atlanta
    A. brace orthosis
    A. hip brace
atlantal transverse ligament
Atlanta-Scottish
    A.-S. Rite abduction orthosis
    A.-S. Rite brace
Atlantic
    A. overlap brace
    A. rim brace
Atlantis cervical plate system
atlantoaxial
    a. alignment
    a. arthrodesis
    a. articulation
    a. dislocation (AAD)
    a. fracture-dislocation
    a. fusion
    a. impaction
    a. instability
    a. interval
    a. joint
    a. lesion
    a. ligament
    a. luxation
    a. rotary displacement
    a. rotatory fixation (AARF)
    a. rotatory subluxation
    a. separation
    a. stabilization
    a. subluxation (AAS)
atlantodens interval (ADI)
atlantooccipital (AO)
    a. anterior membrane
    a. assimilation
    a. disability
    a. fusion
    a. joint
    a. joint dislocation
    a. junction
    a. ligament
    a. subluxation
atlantoodontoid
    a. interspace
    a. joint
atlas
    A. adjustable stand
    a. adjustment
    A. cable system
    a. fracture
    a. laterality
    A. modular humeral prosthesis

A. orthogonal percussion instrument
a. vertebral subluxation complex
atlas-axis
    a.-a. complex
    a.-a. movement
atlas-dens interval
ATNR
    asymmetric tonic neck reflex
ATODC
    atraumatic osteolysis of distal clavicle
ATON
    adductor tenotomy and obturator
    neurectomy
atonia
atony
atopic dermatitis
ATO walker
ATPC
    anteroposterior table
ATR
    Achilles tendon repair
    Achilles tendon rupture
    ATR brace
atracurium besylate
atraumatic
    a. forceps
    a. fracture
    a., multidirectional, bilateral
    rehabilitation inferior (AMBRI)
    a., multidirectional, bilateral
    rehabilitation inferior capsular
    shift
    a. multidirectional instability
    a. necrosis
    a. needle
    a. osteolysis
    a. osteolysis of distal clavicle
    (ATODC)
atretic
atrial natriuretic peptides
atrophic
    a. arthritis
    a. fracture
    a. muscular paralysis
    a. neuroarthropathy
    a. nonunion
atrophica
    myotonia a.
atrophy
    acute reflex bone a.
    arthritic a.
    Charcot-Marie a.
    Charcot-Marie-Tooth a.

cortical a.
Cruveilhier a.
disuse a.
Duchenne muscular a.
Erb a.
familial spinal muscular a.
fascioscapulohumeral muscular a.
fat pad a.
Fazio-Londe a.
gauntlet a.
Hoffmann muscular a.
inactivity a.
infantile progressive spinal
    muscular a.
juvenile muscular a.
Kienböck a.
Kugelberg-Welander juvenile spinal
    muscle a.
muscular a.
myopathic a.
neurogenic a.
neurotrophic a.
peroneal muscular a.
progressive muscular a. (PMA)
quadriceps a.
scapular peroneal a.
scapulohumeral a.
spinal cord a.
spinal muscular a. (type I–III)
    (SMA)
Sudeck a.
thenar a.
thigh a.
traction a.
Vulpian a.
Vulpian-Bernhardt spinal
    muscular a.
Werdnig-Hoffmann spinal
    muscular a.
Zimmerlin a.
A/T/S Topical
ATT
    anterior talar translation
ATT-300 LAT traction table
attachment
    Accuvac smoke evacuation a.
    capsular a.
    femoral a.
    fibrous a.
    ligamentous a.
    muscle-tendon a.
    muscular a.
    osseous a.

NOTES

attachment *(continued)*
 Pearson splint a.
 PRAFO PKA KAFO a.
 pyramid a.
 splint a.
 tendinous a.
 tendon-bone a.
 tendon-to-bone a.
 Thomas splint with Pearson a.
 a. versatility
attack
 adversive a.
 drop a.
Attenborough total knee prosthesis
attention
 Test of Everyday A. (TEA)
attenuate
attenuation
 bone ultrasound a. (BUA)
 a. of tendon
ATTF
 anterior tibiotalar fascicle
Atton disease
attrition
 ligamentous a.
 a. rupture of tendon
 a. of tendon
attritional perforation
atypical dislocation
auditory evoked potential (AEP)
Aufranc
 A. awl
 A. cobra hip prosthesis
 A. cobra retractor
 A. concentric hip mold
 A. cup arthroplasty
 A. gouge
 A. lateral approach
 A. modification
 A. modification of Smith-Petersen
 cup
 A. osteotome
 A. periosteal elevator
 A. reamer
Aufranc-Turner
 A.-T. acetabular cup
 A.-T. arthroplasty
 A.-T. cemented hip prosthesis
 A.-T. femoral component
 A.-T. operation
 A.-T. stem
Aufricht glabellar rasp
auger
augmentation
 arthroscopic a.
 bladder a.
 extraarticular a.
 fascial flap a.
 hamstring ligament a.

 iliotibial band graft a.
 Leach-Schepsis-Paul a.
 slotted acetabular a.
 synthetic a.
augmentative communication aid (ACA)
augmented
 a. reconstruction
 a. repair
 a. soft tissue mobilization (ASTM)
 a. Tinel sign
Augustine boat nail
AuRA cemented total hip system
aureus
 methicillin-resistant
 Staphylococcus a. (MRSA)
austenitic stainless steel
Austin
 A. bunionectomy
 A. chevron osteotomy fixation
 A. Medical Equipment (AME)
 A. Moore arthroplasty
 A. Moore chisel
 A. Moore extractor
 A. Moore femoral head prosthesis
 A. Moore hemiarthroplasty
 A. Moore hook
 A. Moore impactor
 A. Moore pin
 A. Moore rasp
 A. Moore reamer
 A. osteotomy
Austin-Akin bunionectomy
auto
 A. Glide walker accessory
 A. Suture stapler
autoamputation
autochthonous graft
autocinesis
autoclave
autocompression plate
autodistractor
autoerythrophagocytosis
Autoflex II, III CPM unit
autofusion
autogéné
 Soudre a.
Autogenesis
 A. automator
 A. automator for Ilizarov screw
autogenic
autogenous
 a. bone slurry
 a. cancellous bone graft
 a. cartilage transplantation
 a. fat
 a. fibular graft
 a. iliac bone
 a. interpositional shoulder
 arthroplasty

a. meniscal cartilage replantation
a. osteocartilage transfer
a. patellar ligament graft
a. patellar tendon reconstruction
a. quadrupled hamstring tendon graft
a. semitendinosus-gracilis graft

autograft
articular cartilage a.
bone-patellar tendon-bone a.
a. bridge
cartilage a.
free phalangeal bone a.
free revascularized a.
patellar bone-tendon-bone a.
Regnauld free phalangeal bone a.
Russell fibular head a.

autografting
articular cartilage a.
impaction cancellous a.

autoimmunization
surgical a.

Auto-Implant
A.-I. operation
A.-I. procedure

autologous
a. blood
a. blood transfusion
a. bone-tissue allograft
a. cancellous bone graft
a. chondrocyte implantation (ACI)
a. cultured chondrocyte
a. osteochondral transplantation
a. reverse graft
a. reverse graft to ankle
a. traction

autolyzed
a., antigen-extracted, allogenic (AAA)
a., antigen-extracted, allogenic bone

automated
a. disposable keratome (ADK)
a. percutaneous discectomy (APD)
a. percutaneous lumbar discectomy (APLD)
a. shaver

automatic
a. neonatal walking reflex
a. screwdriver
a. staple

automator
Autogenesis a.
A. device

autonomic
a. dysreflexia
a. nervous system
autonomous zone
Autophor
A. ceramic total hip prosthesis
A. femoral prosthesis
autoplastic graft
auto-reinforced polyglycolide rod
autosomal dominant mild short limb dwarfism
autotome drill
autotraction
autotransfusion suction
Autovac
A. autotransfusion canister
A. TC orthopaedic autotransfusion system
A-V
A-V Impulse foot pump
A-V Impulse system
A-V Impulse System foot pump DVT prophylaxis device
A-V Impulse System foot wrap DVT prophylaxis device
Avanta
A. MCP joint implant finger prosthesis
avascular
a. fragment
a. necrosis (AVN)
a. necrosis of femoral head (AVNFH)
a. nonunion
a. sequestrum
average evoked response
Averett hip prosthesis
Averill
A. press fit prosthesis
A. total hip replacement
AVF
arteriovenous fistula
aviator's astragalus
Avila
A. approach
A. operation
A. technique
Avitene
A. flour dressing
A. microfibrillar collagen
A. pack
AVN
avascular necrosis

NOTES

AVNFH
avascular necrosis of femoral head
avoidance gait
AVS spinal system
avulse
avulsed ligament
avulsion
accessory navicular a.
anterior labrum periosteal sleeve a.
(ALPSA)
bony humeral a.
chemical nail a.
a. chip fracture
coracoid tip a.
digitorum brevis a.
a. fragment
humeral a.
a. injury
isolated a.
labral a.
ligament a.
nail a.
a. of nail plate
posterior labrocapsular periosteal
sleeve a. (POLPSA)
a. stress fracture
syndesmotic a.
a. technique
tibial tubercle a.
tubercle a.
awakening trauma
awareness
body a.
kinesthetic a.
sensory a.
awl
angled a.
Aufranc a.
bone a.
Carter Rowe a.
curved a.
DePuy a.
Ender a.
Ferran a.
Küntscher a.
Mark II Kodros radiolucent a.
pointed a.
radiolucent a.
reaming a.
rectangular a.
Rush pin reamer a.
square-shaped a.
Stedman a.
Swanson lunate a.
Swanson scaphoid a.
T-handled a.
Zelicof orthopaedic a.
Zuelzer a.
Axel wire twister

Axer
A. compression apparatus
A. compression device
A. lateral opening wedge
osteotomy
A. operation
A. varus derotational osteotomy
Axer-Clark procedure
axes (*pl. of* axis)
axial
a. acetabular index (AAI)
a. calcaneal projection
a. calcaneus view
a. compression
a. compression injury
a. compression load
a. compression principle
a. compression screw
a. compression test
a. fat-suppressed turbo spin-echo
T2-weighted sequence
a. fixation
a. gripping strength
a. instability
a. loading
a. loading injury
a. loading of spine
a. load teardrop fracture
a. load test
a. manual traction test
a. musculature
a. neuritis
a. pattern flap
a. pin technique
a. plane
a. plane angular deformity
biomechanics
a. plate
a. resistance exerciser
a. rotation
a. sesamoid projection
a. sesamoid view
a. spinal system
a. stiffness
a. traction
axilla, pl. **axillae**
a., shoulder, elbow (ASE)
a., shoulder, elbow bandage
axillary
a. approach
a. arch
a. artery
a. block
a. contracture
a. crutch
a. flap
a. lateral view
a. nerve
a. nerve injury

a. region
a. vein

Axiom

A. modular knee system
A. total knee
A. total knee system

axis, pl. **axes**

anatomic a.
A. ankle brace
bimalleolar-foot a.
a. bone
cardinal axes (X, Y, Z)
deviation of atlas on a.
distal reference a. (DRA)
femoral shaft a.
A. fixation system
flexion a.
flexion-extension a.
foot-thigh a.
a. guide
hypothalamic-pituitary-adrenal a.
hypothalamoneurohypophysial a.
  (HNA)
interepicondylar a.
leg a.
long a.
longitudinal a.
longitudinal midtarsal joint a.
  (LMJA)
mechanical a.
metatarsal a.
middiaphysial a.
oblique midtarsal joint a. (OMJA)
proximal reference a. (PFA)
ray a.
a. of rib motion
a. of rotation
rotation a.
single a.

spinal a.
subtalar joint a. (SJA)
a. traction
transcondylar a. (TCA)
transepicondylar a.
transmalleolar a. (TMA)
transverse a.
vertical a.
weightbearing a.
X, Y, Z a.

axis-altering arthroereisis device
axle lock and bumper
axon

a. reflex
a. reflex test
a. response

axonal

a. apposition
a. degeneration
a. injury

axonopathy
axonotmesis
axoplasmic

a. aberration hypothesis
a. transport (AXT)

AXT

axoplasmic transport
anterograde AXT
retrograde AXT

AXT-blocking chemical
Axxess spinal cord stimulation lead
AxyaWeld

A. bone anchor
A. bone anchor system
A. instrument
A. J-tip suture welding system
A. product line

ayurvedic herb
azotemic osteodystrophy

NOTES

BA
bioactive
BA bone cement
Baastrup
B. disease
B. syndrome
Babcock
B. forceps
B. stainless steel wire
B. wire-cutting scissors
Babinski
B. percussion hammer
B. reflex
B. sign
B. test
Babinski-Fröhlich syndrome
Babinski-Nageotte syndrome
BacFix system
Baciguent Topical
bacille Calmette-Guérin (BCG)
bacitracin
b., neomycin, and polymyxin B
b. solution
Baciu-Filibiu
B.-F. dowel ankle arthrodesis
B.-F. transmalleolar arthrodesis
back
adolescent round b.
b. brace
B. Bubble gravity traction unit
B. Bull lumbar support cushion
B. Bull lumbar support system
b. creaking
b. crease
b. exercise
b. flexion
B. Hammer muscle stimulator
hollow b.
b. manipulation
old man's b.
b. pain
poker b.
b. range of motion (BROM)
b. range of motion device
b. range of motion instrument
B. Revolution Stick
B. Revolution Stick exercise
B. Revolution System
B. Revolution traction/exercise unit
rigid round b.
saddle b.
b. Seat torso-wrap brace
b. shu paraspinal point
B. Specialist chiropractic table
B. Specialist electric table

B. Specialist manual table
static b.
b. strain
b. support
sway b.
b. Trainer spinal exercise system
backache
Backbar device
backboard splint
backcutting osteotome
BackCycler continuous passive motion device
Back-Ease aromatherapy hot/cold pack
backfilling
bone substitute b.
b. reconstruction
backfire fracture
backfiring
Backhaus
B. towel clamp
B. towel forceps
Back-Huggar
Bodyline B.-H.
B.-H. lumbar support
B.-H. lumbar support cushion
Backjoy seat
back-knee deformity
Backnobber II massage tool
backout
screw b.
backpack
b. palsy
b. paralysis
backRAP postsurgical wound wrap
backside wear
backstroke
The B.
BackStrong lumbar extension machine
BackThing lumbar support
BackTracker
backward
b. bending
b. curvature
backward-cutting knife
bacon
B. bone rongeur
B. rasp
bacterial
b. arthritis
b. culture
b. flora
bacterium, pl. bacteria
aerobic bacteria
airborne bacteria
anaerobic bacteria

bacteruria
BactoShield Topical
Bac-Track
badger leg
Badgley
>B. arthrodesis
>B. combination procedure
>B. iliac wing resection
>B. laminectomy retractor
>B. operation
>B. plate
>B. resection of iliac wing
>B. technique

Bado classification
BADS
>Behavioral Assessment of the
>Dysexecutive syndrome

Bad Wildungen Metz spine system
BAEP
>brainstem auditory evoked potential

BAER
>brainstem auditory evoked response

Baer
>B. bone-cutting forceps
>B. bone rongeur
>B. rib shears

BaFPE
>Bay Area Functional Performance
>Evaluation

bag
>B. Bath
>containment b.
>Infusible pressure infusion b.
>Versi-Splint carry b.

Bagby angled compression plate
bag-of-bones technique
Bahler hinge
Bahnson appendage clamp
Bailey
>B. bur
>B. conductor
>B. drill
>B. rib contractor
>B. rib spreader
>B. saw guide
>B. wire saw

Bailey-Badgley
>B.-B. anterior cervical approach
>B.-B. cervical spine fusion
>B.-B. technique

Bailey-Dubow
>B.-D. nail
>B.-D. osteotomy
>B.-D. rod
>B.-D. technique

Bailey-Gibbon rib contractor
Bailey-Gigli saw guide
bail-lock
>b.-l. brace

>b.-l. knee joint
>b.-l. knee joint orthosis

baja
>patella b.

BAK
>BAK fusion cage
>BAK interbody fusion system
>BAK laparoscopic procedure

BAK/C Cervical Interbody Fusion System
Baker
>B. Achilles tendon lengthening
>procedure
>B. cyst
>B. lateral semitendinosus transfer
>B. patellar advancement operation
>B. technique
>B. trabecular traction
>B. translocation operation

Baker-Hill osteotomy
baker's leg
BAK Interbody Fusion System
BAK/Proximity interbody fusion implant
BAK/T thoracic interbody fusion system
Balacescu closing wedge osteotomy
balance
>b. beam scale
>b. board
>b. board training
>b. bridge
>Clinical Test of Sensory Integration
>and B. (CTSIB)
>column b.
>dynamic standing b.
>electrolyte b.
>fluid b.
>B. hip prosthesis
>B. Master
>B. Master rehabilitation evaluation
>B. Master training and assessment
>system
>nitrogen b.
>b. pad
>b. padding orthosis
>postural b.

balanced
>b. forearm
>b. forearm orthosis (BFO)
>b. hemivertebra
>b. skeletal traction
>b. splint
>b. suspension
>b. suspension traction

balancing
>Chopart amputation with tendon b.

Balcones Sensory Integration Screening Kit

Balfour
  B. clamp
  B. self-retaining retractor
Balkan
  B. beam
  B. femoral splint
  B. fracture frame
ball
  b. bearing
  Body B.
  Bouncewell medicine b.
  b. bur
  burst resistance fitness b.
  cold-weld femoral b.
  b. dissector
  Ex-Balls medicine b.
  ExerFlex b.
  b. extractor
  Finger Fitness Spring B.
  Fitness B.
  b. of foot
  Gertie b.
  Gripp squeeze b.
  b. guidepin
  gym b.
  Gymnastik b.
  Gymnic Plus exercise b.
  hand exercise b.
  Jurgan pin b.
  B. knee lock
  Ledraplastic exercise b.
  massage b.
  medicine b.
  New Versaback gym b.
  PhysioGymnic exercise b.
  Physio-Roll VisuaLiser exercise b.
  b. reamer
  R-Value exercise b.
  silastic b.
  Slo-Mo b.
  squeeze b.
  Swiss b.
  Thera-Band exercise b.
  Theragym b.
  Vari-Firm Medicine B.
  vestibular b.
ball-and-socket
  b.-a.-s. ankle prosthesis
  b.-a.-s. congruity
  b.-a.-s. giant pseudarthrosis
  b.-a.-s. giant pseudoarthritis
  b.-a.-s. joint
  b.-a.-s. trochanteric osteotomy

Ballantine
  B. clamp
  B. hemilaminectomy retractor
ball-catcherś view
Ballenger
  B. periosteotome
  B. swivel knife
Ballenger-Hajek chisel
ballismus
ballistic injury
balloon-assisted, endoscopic,
  retroperitoneal, gasless (BERG)
balloon cell nevus
ballottable
ballottement test
ball-peen splint
ball-point guidepin
ball-tip
  b.-t. guidepin
  b.-t. spike
ball-tipped Küntscher guide
ball-valve tumor
balmoral laced shoe
balneotherapy
Baló sclerosis
balsa wood filler block
Baltimore
  B. Therapeutic Equipment (BTE)
  B. Therapeutic Equipment Work
  Simulator
Bamberger-Marie
  B.-M. disease
  B.-M. syndrome
bamboo spine
Bamby clamp
banana
  b. finger extension splint
  b. knife
  B. Split Splint
Bancap HC
Bancroft sign
band
  air b.
  AO tension b.
  aponeurotic b.
  arm b.
  big b.
  Broca diagonal b.
  calf b.
  Can-Do exercise b.
  congenital anular b.
  congenital fibrous b.
  conjoined lateral b.

NOTES

band *(continued)*
    constriction b.
    deossification b.
    distal thigh b.
    exercise b.
    external b.
    fascial b.
    fibrous b.
    Fit-Lastic therapy b.
    GelBand arm b.
    Gennari b.
    iliopatellar b.
    iliotibial b. (ITB)
    internal b.
    Jobst air b.
    lateral b.
    M b.
    palpable b.
    Parham b.
    Parham-Martin b.
    Partridge b.
    patellar b.
    PDS b.
    pelvic b.
    periosteal b.
    pretendinous b.
    proximal thigh b.
    REP Bands exercise b.
    Resist-A-Band exercise b.
    Resist-A-Tube exercise b.
    rigid metal pelvic b.
    sagittal b.
    scar b.
    Simonart b.
    subsurface white b.
    taut b.
    tennis elbow arm b.
    b. tenodesis
    tension b.
    trochanteric b.
    True Blue exercise b.
    b. wire
    Xercise b.
    Z b.

bandage
    Ace adherent b.
    ankle traction b.
    ASE b.
    axilla, shoulder, elbow b.
    Barton b.
    capeline b.
    Champ elastic b.
    circular b.
    Comperm tubular elastic b.
    compression b.
    Conco elastic b.
    cotton elastic b.
    Cover-Roll stretch b.
    cravat b.

demigauntlet b.
Desault wrist b.
Dressinet netting b.
E Cotton b.
Elastic Foam b.
Elastomull elastic gauze b.
Elastoplast b.
Esmarch b.
Fabco gauze b.
fiberglass b.
figure-of-8 b.
Flex-Foam b.
flexible b.
Flexilite conforming elastic b.
Flex-Master b.
B. Gard cast protector
gauntlet b.
Gibney fixation b.
Gibson b.
gum rubber Martin b.
Hamilton b.
Helenca b.
Heliodorus b.
Hippocrates b.
Hueter b.
Hydron Burn B.
immobilizing b.
immovable b.
Kerlix b.
Kling elastic b.
Leukotape P stretch b.
Martin sheet rubber b.
Medi-Band b.
MPM b.
Nu Gauze b.
oblique b.
Orthoflex elastic plaster b.
Ortho-Trac adhesive skin
    traction b.
Ortho-Vent b.
Pavlik b.
plaster of Paris b.
Plast-O-Fit thermoplastic b.
polyurethane b.
Redigrip pressure b.
replantation b.
restrictive b.
Ribble b.
Richet b.
Robert Jones b.
roller b.
Sayre b.
scarf b.
Scultetus b.
Shur-Band self-closure elastic b.
Silesian b.
sling-and-swathe b.
spica b.
spiral b.

starch b.
stockinette b.
Thera-Boot b.
triangular b.
Tricodur compression support b.
Tricodur Epi compression b.
Tricodur Talus compression b.
Tru-Support EW b.
Tru-Support SA b.
TubeGauz b.
Tubigrip b.
tubular elastic b.
Velpeau b.
Webril b.

Bandi patellofemoral score
Band-It
    B.-I. magnetic elbow support
    B.-I. tennis elbow strap
bandlike
    b. adhesion
    b. pain
bandy-leg
Bane
    B. bone rongeur
    B. rongeur forceps
Bane-Hartmann bone rongeur
banjo
    b. cast
    b. splint
    b. traction
bank
    bone b.
Bankart
    B. arthroplasty
    B. fracture
    B. operation
    B. procedure
    B. reconstruction
    B. retractor
    B. shoulder dislocation
    B. shoulder lesion
    B. shoulder prosthesis
    B. shoulder repair
    B. shoulder repair set
    B. Tack implant
Bankart-Putti-Platt operation
banked bone
Bankhart procedure
Banks bone graft
Banks-Laufman
    B.-L. approach
    B.-L. incision
Banophen Oral

bantam
    B. CDH prosthesis
    B. wire-cutting scissors
BAP
    Behavioral Assessment of Pain
BAPS
    Biomechanical Ankle Platform System
    BAPS ankle system
    BAPS board
bar
    Bill b.
    b. bolt fixation
    bony b.
    broomstick b.
    calcaneonavicular b.
    cartilaginous b.
    congenital b.
    cross b.
    Denis Browne b.
    derotator b.
    distraction b.
    b. drill
    b. excision
    exercise grab b.
    1-b. external fixator
    Fillauer b.
    Gerster traction b.
    grab b.
    intramedullary b.
    Leyla b.
    Livingston intramedullary b.
    longitudinal spinal b.
    lumbrical b.
    medial talocalcaneal b.
    metatarsal flatfoot b.
    MT b.
    opponens b.
    patellar b.
    physial b.
    posterior thigh b.
    quad b.
    b. resection
    rigid b.
    rocker b.
    screw alignment b.
    b. section
    side-cutting Swanson b.
    spacer b.
    spondylotic b.
    Sports-Grip b.
    spreader b.
    stabilizing b.
    stall b.

B

NOTES

bar *(continued)*
    Stephen spreader b.
    tarsal b.
    Thera-P exercise b.
    Thornton b.
    Tommy trapeze b.
    torsion b.
    traction b.
    trapeze b.
    unsegmented vertebral b.
    valgus b.
    vertebral b.
    Zielke derotator b.

4-bar
    4-b. external fixation
    4-b. external fixation apparatus
    4-b. external fixation device
    4-b. link
    4-b. linkage on knee prosthesis
    4-b. linkage prosthetic knee
      mechanism
    4-b. polycentric knee prosthesis

bar-and-shoe orthosis
Bárány-Nylen maneuver
barbed
    b. broach
    b. staple
barbell
    Spring angled adjustable b.
barber chair position
barber-pole
    b.-p. fashion
    b.-p. vein graft
barbotage
Barbour
    B. cervical fixation
    B. technique
Bard clamp
Bardeen primitive disc
Bardeleben bone-holding forceps
Bardenheuer
    B. extension
    B. incision
Bard-Parker
    B.-P. blade
    B.-P. handle
    B.-P. knife
    B.-P. scalpel
Bareskin knee positioner
bariatric mat table
barked injury
Barker operation
Barkow ligament
barlike ventral defect
Barlow
    B. cruciform infant splint
    B. hip instability test
    B. maneuver

    B. provocative test
    B. sign
Barnes curve
barognosis
Baron suction tube
barotrauma
    middle ear b.
    pulmonary b.
Barouk
    B. button space
    B. cannulated bone screw
    B. microscrew with shortening
      osteotomy
    B. microstaple
    B. spacer
Barr
    B. anterior transfer
    B. bolt
    B. bolt nail
    B. hook
    B. open reduction and internal
      fixation
    B. pin
    B. tendon transfer operation
    B. tibial fracture fixation
Barraquer needle holder
Barrasso-Wile-Gage arthrodesis
barrel
    b. bur
    b. bur design
    b. chest
    b. crawl
    guide b.
    b. guide
    b. plate
    sideplate b.
barreled sideplate
Barre-Lieou syndrome
barrel-stave osteotomy
barrier
    anatomic b.
    blood-brain b. (BBB)
    calcium sulfate bone graft b.
    Capset calcium sulfate bone
     graft b.
    elastic b.
    B. lower extremity sheet
    motion b.
    pathologic b.
    physiologic b.
    side-bending b.
    b. technique
Barr-Record ankle arthrodesis
Barsky
    B. cleft closure
    B. macrodactyly reduction
    B. operation
    B. procedure
    B. technique

Barsony-Polgar syndrome
Barsony-Teschendorf syndrome
Barthel ADL index
Bartlett
    B. nail fold
    B. nail fold excision
    B. procedure
bar-to-bar clamp
Barton
    B. bandage
    B. fracture
    B. sling
    B. tongs
    B. traction handle
Barton-Cone tongs
Barwell operation
basal
    b. block cervical saddle
    b. bone
    b. chevron osteotomy
    b. closing wedge osteotomy
    b. extension
    b. joint
    b. metabolic rate (BMR)
    b. neck
    b. neck fracture
BASC
    Behavior Assessment Rating Scale
base
    Dycal b.
    b. of finger
    b. of fingernail
    b. of gait
    metacarpal b.
    b. of neck osteotomy
    plantar lateral b.
    Profix nonporous tibial b.
    b. of skull (BOS)
    b. of support
    b. of thumb arthritis
    b. wedge osteotomy
    b. wedge osteotomy/bunionectomy
baseball
    b. finger
    b. finger fracture
    b. finger splint
    b. fracture of hand
    b. pitcher's elbow
    b. shoulder
    b. stitch
    b. suture
baseline
    B. Bubble inclinometer

    b. capacity evaluation
    B. dynamometer
    b. view
basement membrane
basic
    b. calcium phosphate crystal deposition disease
    b. frame (type IV)
    b. hand splint
    B. I, II cranial adjusting procedure
    b. lamella
    b. multicellular remodeling unit
    b. technique
basicervical fracture
basilar
    b. bone
    b. cartilage
    b. closing wedge metatarsal osteotomy
    b. crescentic osteotomy
    b. femoral neck fracture
    b. impression
    b. invagination
    b. plantarflexory metatarsal osteotomy
    b. region
    b. vertebra
Basile hip screw
basilic artery
basioccipital
basivertebral
basket
    Acufex meniscal b.
    b. forceps
    b. rongeur
    rotary b.
    b. stockinette
    walker b.
basketball foot
basket-weave ankle taping
Basmajian technique
basograph
Basser syndrome
Bassett
    B. electrical stimulation apparatus
    B. electrical stimulation device
    B. electrical stimulation system
    B. sign
Basswood splint
Batchelor
    B. plaster
    B. plaster hip spica cast
    B. plate

NOTES

B

Batchelor-Brown extraarticular subtalar arthrodesis
Batch-Spittler-McFaddin
 B.-S.-M. knee disarticulation
 B.-S.-M. technique
Bateman
 B. femoral neck prosthesis
 B. finger prosthesis
 B. hemiarthroplasty
 B. shoulder operation
 B. UPF II bipolar knee system
 B. UPF II bipolar prosthesis
 B. UPF II shoulder prosthesis
bath
 Aqua/Whirl b.
 Bag B.
 contrast b. (CB)
 Dickson paraffin b.
 galvanic b.
 hot and cold contrast b.
 hot water b.
 mud pack b.
 Para-Care paraffin therapy b.
 paraffin b. (PB)
 whirlpool b. (WPB)
Bathe Away cleanser
bathing and dressing ability
Bathlifter
 Leo B.
batrachian
 b. gait
 b. posture
Batson
 vein of B.
 B. vertebral brain system
battery
 Allen Cognitive B.
 Rand Functional Limitations B.
 Rand Physical Capacities B.
battery-driven hand drill
battery-pack Osteo-Stim bone stimulator
battery-powered instrument
batting
 Dacron b.
battledore incision
Battle sign
bat-wing appearance
Batzdorf
 B. cervical wire passer
 B. cervical wire twister
Bauerfeind
 B. Achillotrain
 B. ankle brace
 B. Comprifix knee brace
 B. Malleolic Ankle Orthosis
 B. silicone heel pad
 B. SofSpot Heel Cup
 B. support
Bauer-Jackson classification

Baumann angle
Baumgaertel and Gotzen calcaneal fracture reduction technique
Baumgard-Schwartz tennis elbow technique
Baumrucker clamp irrigator
Bavarian splint
Baxter
 B. angled arthroscope
 B. nerve release
 B. personal Von-Loc ice pack
Baxter-D'Astous procedure
Bay Area Functional Performance Evaluation (BaFPE)
Bayer
 B. Buffered Aspirin
 B. Low Adult Strength
 B. Select Pain Relief Formula
Bayley Scales of Infant Development
Baylor
 B. adjustable cross splint
 B. metatarsal splint
Bayne
 B. classification of radial agenesis
 B. radial agenesis classification
 B. ulnar ray deficiency classification
Bayne-Klug centralization
bayonet
 b. apposition
 b. clip applier
 b. dislocation
 b. fracture position
 b. knife
 b. leg
 b. nonunion
 b. osteotome
 b. position of fracture
 b. rongeur
 b. saw
 b. sign
 b. spacer
bayonet-point wire
Bazooka support surface
BB
 BB marker
 BB to MM examination
BBB
 blood-brain barrier
BBC
 biceps, brachialis, coracobrachialis
 BBC muscles
BB to MM
 bellybutton to medial malleolus
BCG
 bacille Calmette-Guérin
BDD
 blistering distal dactylitis

B

BDH
    biologically designed hip
    BDH prosthesis
BE
    below elbow
    BE amputation
BEA
    below-elbow amputation
beach chair position
beachcomber
    The B. prosthetic foot
    B. waterproof prosthesis
bead
    aminoglycoside-impregnated methyl
      methacrylate b.
    antibiotic b.
    antibiotic-impregnated b.
    copolymer starch copolymer b.
    gentamicin b.
    metallic b.
    methyl methacrylate b.
    b. pouch
    Septobal b.
    targeting b.
bead-blasted prosthesis
beaded
    b. guidewire
    b. hip pin
    b. reamer guidepin
    b. transfixion wire
beaded-pin wrench
bead-loaded wire
beak
    b. fingernail
    b. fracture
    b. ligament
    metacarpal b.
    b. modification with triple
      arthrodesis
    b. nail
    talar b.
beaked
    b. cervicomedullary junction
    b. pelvis
beaking
    b. of head of talus
    b. joint
    talar b.
beaklike osteophyte formation
Beals
    B. syndrome
    B. test

beam
    Balkan b.
    load b.
    primary x-ray b.
    b. theory
beanbag
bearing
    ball b.
    ceramic b.
    pretibial b. (PTB)
    radial b.
    spinal load b.
    Steinmann pin with ball b.
    ulnar b.
    unipolar b.
bearing-seating forceps
bear's paw hand
Beasley-Babcock forceps
3-beat clonus
Beath
    B. bone intramedullary peg
    B. needle
    B. pin
    B. view
Beatson combined ankle angle
Beaty lateral release
Beaufort seating orthosis
Beau line
beaver
    B. blade
    B. blade handle
    B. cataract knife
    B. discission blade
    B. keratome blade
    B. saw
Beaver-DeBakey
    B.-D. blade
    B.-D. knife
Bebax
    B. Bootie
    B. orthosis
    B. shoe
Bechterew (*var. of* Bekhterev)
Bechtol
    B. acetabular component
    B. arthroplasty
    B. hip prosthesis
    B. screw
    B. shoulder prosthesis
    B. system prosthesis
Beckenbaugh
    B. correction
    B. technique

NOTES

Becker
- B. brace
- B. hand prosthesis
- B. 655 motion control limiter
- B. muscular dystrophy (BMD)
- B. orthopaedic spinal system (BOSS)
- B. orthopaedic spinal system orthotic device
- B. orthopaedic thermoformable ankle system
- B. screwdriver
- B. technique
- B. tendon repair
- B. variant
- B. variant of Duchenne dystrophy

Becker-type tardive muscular dystrophy
Beckhterev test
Beckman retractor
Beck-Steffee total ankle prosthesis
Béclard amputation
Becton
- B. Colles fracture plate
- B. open reduction
- B. technique

bed
- air b.
- American Seating Access-O-Matic b.
- BioDyne b.
- bone graft b.
- Borg-Warner orthopaedic b.
- Burke Bariatric b.
- Chick-Foster orthopaedic b.
- circle b.
- CircOlectric b.
- Clinitron air b.
- b. cradle
- DMI orthopaedic b.
- Flexicair b.
- FluidAir b.
- Foster b.
- fracture b.
- fusion b.
- Gatch b.
- Goodman orthopaedic b.
- Hausted orthopaedic b.
- high-air-loss b.
- high muscular resistance b.
- Hill-Rom orthopaedic b.
- Hollywood b.
- Inland Super Multi-Hite orthopaedic b.
- Joerns orthopaedic b.
- Keane mobility b.
- KinAir b.
- Lapidus b.
- low-air-loss b.
- Magnum 800 b.

- Medicus b.
- Mega-Air b.
- Mega Tilt and Turn b.
- b. mobility skill
- nail b.
- obese b.
- orthopaedic b.
- Plastazote foot b.
- b. rest
- Restcue b.
- b. rest-related deconditioning
- b. of rib
- Roho b.
- Roto-Rest b.
- Simmons Multi-Matic orthopaedic b.
- Simmons Vari-Hite orthopaedic b.
- skeletal b.
- Skytron b.
- SMI 3000, 5000 b.
- Smith-Davis Converta-Hite orthopaedic b.
- Spa B.
- Stryker b.
- Superior Sleeprite Hi-Lo orthopaedic b.
- Swinger car b.
- TheraPulse b.
- Tilt and Turn Paragon b.
- Ultraflex orthopaedic b.
- b. wedge

Bed-Bar support rail
Bednar tumor
bedroom fracture
bed-to-chair transfer
Beebe wire-cutting scissors
beefburger procedure
Beery-Buktenica Developmental Test of Visual-Motor Integration
Beery Visual Motor Integration Test
Beeson
- B. cast spreader
- B. plaster spreader

bee venom therapy
Beevor sign
behavior
- Assessment of Ludic B.'s (ALB)
- B. Assessment Rating Scale (BASC)
- compensatory b.
- occupational b.

behavioral
- B. Assessment of the Dysexecutive syndrome (BADS)
- B. Assessment of Pain (BAP)
- B. Assessment of Pain Questionnaire
- B. Inattention Test (BIT)
- b. mapping

Behçet syndrome
Behr syndrome
Beighton hypermobility syndrome
  criteria
Bekhterev, Bechterew
    B. arthritis
    B. deep reflex
    B. disease
    B. rheumatoid spondylitis
    B. sitting test
Bekhterev-Mendel reflex
Bekhterev-Strümpell spondylitis
Belix Oral
bell
    Hydro-Tone B.
    B. palsy
    b. rasp
    B. suture
    B. table
Bell-Dally cervical dislocation
Bellemore-Barrett closing wedge
  osteotomy
Bell-Tawse
    B.-T. open reduction
    B.-T. open reduction technique
    B.-T. procedure
Bellucci alligator scissors
belly
    bellybutton to medial malleolus
    (BB to MM)
    muscle b.
bellybutton
    b. to medial malleolus (BB to MM)
    b. to medial malleolus examination
belly-press test
Belos compression pin
below
    b. elbow (BE)
    b. knee (BK)
below-elbow
    b.-e. amputation (BEA)
    b.-e. prosthesis
below-knee
    b.-k. amputation (BKA)
    b.-k. prosthesis
    b.-k. suspension
    b.-k. walking cast
belt
    AquaJogger buoyancy b.
    Carabelt therapeutic b.
    cast b.
    Cool-Flex A/K suspension b.
    gait b.

    Meek pelvic traction b.
    pelvic traction b.
    Posey b.
    Reed cast b.
    rib b.
    sacroiliac b.
    Schiek B.
    Serola sacroiliac b.
    SI b.
    Silesian b.
    Soma sacroiliac stabilization b.
    Spine Power pelvic stabilizer b.
    S'port Max sacroiliac b.
    Sports Plus II back b.
    TES b.
    Thera-Band Aqua B.
    Tri-Flex auxiliary suspension b.
    waist suspension b.
Benadryl Oral
Ben-Allergin-50 Injection
bench
    Ensolite padded transfer b.
    b. examination
    Invacare vinyl transfer b.
    Paramount 3-way press b.
    pelvic b.
    b. test
    Winco adjusting b.
bend
    deep knee b. (DKB)
    sitting side b.
    standing side b.
Bend-A-Boot foot splint
bender
    AO plate b.
    Bunnell knuckle b.
    cast b.
    DePuy rod b.
    French rod b.
    Luque rod b.
    plate b.
    rod b.
    Rush b.
bending
    backward b.
    cantilever b.
    forward b.
    b. fracture
    ipsilateral side b.
    lateral b.
    b. load
    rod b.
    side b.

NOTES

bending (*continued*)
    b. strength
    b. stress
    b. toward the side of injury
benediction
    b. attitude sign
    b. posture
Benedict-Roth apparatus
BeneFin clinical shark cartilage
benefit
    pedal disability b.
    Viscolas heel pain and
      disability b.
BeneFix
Benefoot & Birkenstock orthotic sandal
BeneJoint analgesic cream
benign
    b. bone aneurysm
    b. chondroblastoma
    b. congenital myopathy
    b. cortical defect
    b. fasciculation
    b. hypermobile joint syndrome
    b. joint hypermobility syndrome
      (BJHS)
    b. subsidence
    b. tumor
Benink tarsal index
Bennett
    B. basic hand dislocation
    B. basic hand fracture
    B. basic hand splint
    B. bone retractor
    B. comminuted fracture
    B. elevator
    B. fracture-dislocation
    B. fracture of thumb
    B. Hand Tool Dexterity Test
    B. lesion
    B. nail biopsy
    B. orthosis
    B. pain model
    B. posterior shoulder approach
    B. quadriceps plastic operation
    B. quadriceps plastic procedure
    B. thumb fracture classification
    B. tibial retractor
bent
    b. Hohman retractor-narrow
    b. Hohman retractor-wide
    b. nail
    B. operation
bent-knee
    b.-k. cast
    b.-k. syndrome
Benton Constructional Praxis Test
Bentson procedure
benzalkonium chloride
benzoic acid and salicylic acid

benzoin
    b. adherent tape
    b. adhesive
    tincture of b.
benztropine mesylate
BeOK hand exercise putty
Berens
    B. muscle clamp
    B. muscle clamp forceps
    B. osteotomy
BERG
    balloon-assisted, endoscopic,
      retroperitoneal, gasless
    BERG lumbar interbody fusion
Berg
    B. Balance Scale
    B. balance test
Berger
    B. capsulodesis
    B. exercise
    B. interscapular amputation
    B. operation
    B. paresthesia
Berger-Bookwalter posterior approach
Bergman mallet
Bergstrom
    B. cannula
    B. needle
Berke clamp
Berliner percussion hammer
Berman-Gartland
    B.-G. metatarsal osteotomy
    B.-G. procedure
Berman-Moorhead metal locator
Bermuda spica cast
Berndt
    B. classification
    B. hip ruler
Berndt-Harty
    B.-H. classification
    B.-H. classification of transchondral
      fracture
Berndt-Harty classification
Bernese periacetabular osteotomy
Bernhard clamp
Berstein cast table
Bertin
    B. bone
    B. hip retractor
    B. ligament
Bertolotti syndrome
Besnier rheumatism
Bestfoam insole
besylate
    atracurium b.
Betadine
    B. dressing
    B. First Aid Antibiotics +
      Moisturizer

B. paint
B. scrub
B. scrub solution
B. soak
B. soap
Betadine-soaked pledget
beta-endorphin
plasma b.-e.
beta-2-microglobulin
b.-2-m. amyloidosis
b.-2-m. deposition
Beta Pile II, III splint strap
beta-sympathomimetic
Bethesda bone
Bethune
B. periosteal elevator
B. rib shears
Bethune-Coryllos rib shears
Bevatron accelerator
bevel
beveled chisel
Bevin shoe
Beyer rongeur
BF+ bone void filler
BFM
Brunnstrom-Fugl-Meyer
BFM arm impairment assessment
BFM impairment
BFO
balanced forearm orthosis
BFO Kit
BFO Orthosis
BGS
bone graft substitute
BHAGL
bony humeral avulsion of glenohumeral
ligament
BHAGL lesion
B.H. Moore procedure
BIA
bioelectrical impedance analysis
Bi-Angular shoulder prosthesis
biarticular
b. bone-cutting forceps
b. bone shears
biarticulate
bias-cut
b.-c. stockinette
b.-c. tape
biaxial
b. flap
b. joint
B. Weave composite prosthesis

BICAP
Bipolar Circumactive Probe
BICAP cautery
bicapsular
bicentric prosthesis
biceps
b., brachialis, coracobrachialis
(BBC)
b. brachialis muscle transfer
b. brachialis tendon
b. brachii muscle
b. brachii tendon
b. elevator
b. femoris
b. femoris muscle
b. femoris tendon
b. interval
b. interval lesion (BIL)
b. jerk (BJ)
b. jerk reflex test
b. reflex
b. tendinitis
b. tenodesis
Bichat ligament
bichloracetic acid
Bicillin C-R 900/300 Injection
bicipital
b. bursitis
b. groove
b. muscle
b. rib
b. sulcus
b. syndrome
b. tendinitis
b. tendon
b. tenosynovitis
b. tuberosity
b. tuberosity view
Bickel
B. intramedullary nail
B. intramedullary rod
B. legholder
bicolumn fracture
bicompartmental
b. implant
b. knee implant prosthesis
b. replacement
b. replacement of knee
b. soft tissue sarcoma
biconcave
b. deformity
b. vertebra

NOTES

B

bicondylar
 b. ankle prosthesis
 b. graft
 b. knee prosthesis
 b. tibial plateau
 b. T-shaped fracture
 b. Y-shaped fracture
Bicon-Plus Cup
bicortical
 b. iliac bone
 b. iliac bone graft
 b. ilial strip graft
 b. screw
 b. screw fixation
bicycle, bike
 air b.
 Air-Dyne b.
 b. brace
 b. ergometer
 b. ergometry
 b. exerciser
 FES exercise b.
 b. injury
 Monark b.
 New Schwinn 900 b.
 New Schwinn elliptical b.
 recumbent b.
 Schwinn Air-Dyne b.
 Schwinn Spinner b.
 Schwinn 900 stationary b.
 b. spoke fracture
BID
 bilateral interfacetal dislocation
bidirectional traction
Bielschowsky head tilt test
Bielschowsky-Jansky disease
Bier
 B. amputation
 B. amputation saw
 B. block
 B. block anesthesia
 B. lumbar puncture needle
 B. operation
bifid
 b. condyle
 b. foot
 b. graft
 b. hook
 b. spinous process
 b. thumb
 b. thumb deformity
bifida
 spina b.
bifilar needle recording electrode
biflanged drill
Bi-Flex
bifocal manipulative with distraction jing
biframed distraction technique

bifrontal incision
bifurcate
 b. ligament
 b. navicular
bifurcated
 b. blade-plate
 b. vein graft for vascular reconstruction
bifurcation osteotomy
bifurcatum
 ligamentum b.
big
 b. band
 b. toe test
Bigelow
 B. crural
 B. iliopectineal
 B. ligament
 B. maneuver
 B. septum
Bigliani/Flatow
 B./F. complete shoulder
 B./F. shoulder system
 B./F. total shoulder arthroplasty
biglycan
bike (*var. of* bicycle)
Bike ankle brace
BIL
 biceps interval lesion
bilateral
 b. acute radicular syndrome
 b. amputation
 b. arm raise back exercise technique
 b. chronic radicular syndrome
 b. frame
 b. hemiplegia
 b. heterotopic ossification
 b. interfacetal dislocation (BID)
 b. lateral fusion
 strength test eccentric b.
 b. talocalcaneal coalition
 b. variable screw placement system
Bilhaut-Cloquet procedure
Bill bar
bilobed
 b. digital neurovascular island flap
 b. flap reconstruction
 b. skin flap
bilocular joint
Bilos
 B. pin
 B. pin extractor
bimalleolar
 b. angle
 b. ankle fracture
 b. approach to ankle arthrodesis
bimalleolar-foot axis

Bi-Metric
  B.-M. hip prosthesis
  B.-M. Interlok femoral prosthesis
  B.-M. porous primary femoral
    prosthesis
Bindegewebsmassage
binder
  abdominal b.
  arch b.
  cloth b.
  Dale abdominal b.
  Helenca b.
  sacroiliac b.
  Scultetus b.
binding
  biologic b.
bind wire
Bing-Horton syndrome
binocular loupe
Bio-1000 knee brace system
bioabsorbable
  b. material
  b. mesh scaffold
  b. tack repair
Bio-Absorbable interference screw
BioAction great toe implant
bioactive (BA)
  b. bone cement
  b. implant
Bio-Anchor suture anchor
Bio-Boot
Biobrane
  B. adhesive
  B. glove
  B. synthetic skin substitute
BioCast wrist/hand orthosis
bioceramic implant material
biochemical
  b. abnormality
  b. integrity
  b. marker
  b. response
Bio-Chromatic hand prosthesis
Bioclad with pegs reinforced acetabular
  prosthesis
BioCleanse tissue sterilization process
Bioclusive select transparent film
  dressing
biocompatibility
  b. characteristic
  implant b.
biocompatible
BioCompression Pneumatic Sleeve

Biocoral bone graft substitute
Bio-Corkscrew
  headed B.-C.
biocorrosion
BioCuff
  B. bioresorbable screw and spiked
    washer implant
  B. C bioresorbable cannulated
    screw
  B. C bioresorbable cannulated
    screw and spike washer implant
  B. C bioresorbable spike washer
    implant
biodegradable
  b. calcium phosphate cement
  b. fixation device
  b. fixation instrumentation
  b. implant
  b. plate
  b. surgical tack
  b. synthetic polymer
Biodel implant
Bio-Dermal Hydrogel kit
Biodex
  B. Balance System
  B. cycle ergometer
  B. Gait Trainer
  B. isokinetic dynamometer
  B. isokinetic testing machine
  B. Multi-Joint System 3 MVP
  B. target balance trainer
  B. test
  B. Unweighing Support System
  B. Unweighing System partial
    weight therapy
Biodynamic Molding System
BioDyne bed
bioelectric
  b. phenomenon
  b. potential
bioelectrical
  b. impedance
  b. impedance analysis (BIA)
  b. repair
  b. repair of delayed union or
    nonunion
bioenergy imbalance syndrome (BIS)
Bio-FASTak
  B.-F. anchor
  B.-F. suture
biofeedback-assisted method
Biofeedback 5DX
BioFit Press-Fit acetabular prosthesis

NOTES

Biofix
>B. absorbable fixation
>B. absorbable fixation system
>B. arrow gun
>B. biodegradable implant
>B. meniscus arrow
>B. system pin

BIOflex
>B. Magnet Back Support
>B. magnetic counterforce brace
>B. medical magnet
>B. orthotic

Bio Flote air flotation system
Biofoot orthotic
Bio-Form glove
Bio-Gel decubitus pillow
Bioglass prosthesis
Bio-Groove
>B.-G. acetabular prosthesis
>B.-G. Macrobond HA femoral prosthesis

bioimplant
>OrthoBlast osteoinductive b.

Bio-Interference
>B.-I. screwdriver
>B.-I. tibial screw

biokinetic remediation
Biokinetics pedobarograph
BioKnit garment electrode
Biolectron bone growth stimulator
biologic
>b. binding
>b. dressing
>b. fixation
>b. fracture management

biologically
>b. designed hip (BDH)
>B. Quiet interference screw
>B. Quiet Mini-Screw suture anchor
>B. quiet stapler

Biolox ceramic coating
biomagnet
biomaterial
>absorbable b.
>carbon-based b.
>ceramic b.
>collagen-based b.
>PGA-PLA b.
>polymethylmethacrylate b.

biomechanical
>b. analysis
>B. Ankle Platform System (BAPS)
>b. control
>b. deficiency
>b. evaluation of foot function during stance phase of gait
>b. factor
>b. failure of implant
>b. frame of reference
>b. integrity
>b. principle
>b. stress
>b. testing

biomechanics
>axial plane angular deformity b.
>bone b.
>distraction instrumentation b.
>Dwyer instrumentation b.
>gait b.
>impact b.
>posterior fixation system b.
>propulsion b.
>soft tissue b.
>walking b.

biomedium
>Dynafill graft b.

BioMed TENS unit
Biomet
>B. acetabular cup
>B. AGC knee prosthesis
>B. ankle arthrodesis nail
>B. Ascent total knee
>B. bone anchor
>B. button
>B. cement-removal hand chisel
>B. custom implant
>B. fracture brace
>B. hip prosthesis
>B. M2A metal-on-metal articulation for hip replacement system
>B. MARS acetabular component
>B. Maxim knee system
>B. revision acetabular component
>B. revision hip stem
>B. revision knee system
>B. Second Assistant knee positioner
>B. shoulder component
>B. staple
>B. total toe prosthesis
>B. Ultra-Drive cement remover
>B. Ultra-Drive ultrasonic revision system

biometal
Biometric prosthesis
Bio-Modular
>B.-M. shoulder prosthesis
>B.-M. total shoulder system

Bio-Moore endoprosthesis
bionic
>Rincoe human action b.

Bionicare 1000 stimulator system
Bionx
>B. absorbable cannulated screw
>B. arrow
>B. self-reinforced PLLA smart screw
>B. servohydraulic testing machine

Bio-Oss
    B.-O. collagen
    B.-O. synthetic bone
Biophase
    ASTM designation of B.
    B. implant metal
    B. implant metal prosthesis
Bio-Phase suture anchor
biophysics
    chiropractic b. (CBP)
bioplastic
biopolymeric graft
BioPro ceramic TARA head
bioprosthesis
    bovine collagen b.
biopsy, pl. biopsies (Bx)
    aspiration needle b.
    Bennett nail b.
    bone marrow b.
    b. cannula
    channel-and-core b.
    closed core needle b.
    cone bone b.
    core needle b.
    Dunn b.
    excisional b.
    forage core b.
    b. forceps
    Fosnaugh nail b.
    freehand CT-guided b.
    incisional b.
    lumbar spine b.
    Michele vertebral b.
    needle b.
    open b.
    percutaneous core bone b.
    punch b.
    Scher nail b.
    spinal infection b.
    synovial b.
    thoracic spine b.
    trephine needle b.
    Turkel bone b.
    ultrasound-guided echo b.
    ultrasound-guided stereotactic b.
    Valls-Ottolenghim-Schajowicz
    needle b.
    Zaias nail b.
BioRCI bioabsorbable screw
bioresorbable
    b. drug delivery system
    b. implant

    b. pin
    b. screw
BioROC anchor
Bio-R-Sorb resorbable poly-L-lactic acid
    ministaple
BioScrew absorbable interference screw
Biosensor biomechanical testing system
BioSkin
    B. DP wrist support
    B. Q knee brace
BioSole-GEL orthotic
BioSorbFX SR self-reinforced plate and
    screw
BioSorb suture
BioSphere
    B. suture anchor
    B. suture anchor implant
BioStim Digital NMS muscle stimulator
BioStinger low-profile fixation device
BioStop G bone cement restrictor
Biosyn synthetic monofilament suture
Biotens neurostimulator
Biotex
    B. implant metal
    B. implant metal prosthesis
biothesiometer testing
Biothotic
    B. foot orthosis
    B. orthotic
    B. orthotic mold
Biotone Polar lotion
biotribology
Bio-Wick sock
BioWrap lumbosacral/sacral support
BioZone nutrition system
bipartita
    patella b.
bipartite
    b. fracture
    b. ossification
    b. patella
    b. scaphoid
    b. tibial sesamoid
bipedal walking
bipedicle dorsal flap
biphasic
    b. action potential
    b. endplate activity
    b. waveform
bipivotal hinge knee brace
biplanar
    b. fixator
    b. radiography

B

NOTES

biplane
- b. angiogram
- b. Dwyer osteotomy
- b. padding
- b. roentgenogram
- b. trochanteric osteotomy

biplaning of osteotomy

bipolar
- b. acetabular cup
- b. cauterization
- b. cautery
- B. Circumactive Probe (BICAP)
- b. coagulator
- b. femoral component
- b. femoral head prosthesis
- b. forceps
- b. hip arthroplasty
- b. hip arthroplasty component
- b. hip replacement prosthesis
- b. IF waveform
- b. needle recording electrode
- b. prosthetic cup
- b. release
- b. stimulating electrode
- b. vertebral traction

Bircher
- B. bone-holding clamp
- B. cartilage clamp
- B. meniscotome
- B. meniscus knife

Bircher-Ganske cartilage forceps
birdcage splint
Bird & Cronin wrist brace
birefringent lipid crystals in tendinitis
Birkenstock
- B. Blue Footbed arch support
- B. high-flange arch support
- B. shoe

birth
- b. fracture
- b. injury
- b. trauma

BIS
- bioenergy imbalance syndrome

bisacromial
Bischof myelotomy
bisector line
Bishop
- B. bone clamp
- B. chisel
- B. classification
- B. gouge
- B. saw

BIT
- Behavioral Inattention Test

bit
- AO drill b.
- cannulated drill b.
- b. drill

drill b.
- femoral drill b.
- Gore b.
- hip fracture compaction drill b.
- Howmedica Microfixation System drill b.
- Leibinger Micro System drill b.
- Luhr Microfixation System drill b.
- Storz Microsystems drill b.
- Synthes Microsystems drill b.

biter
- Stille bone b.
- suction b.

bite sign
bivalved
- b. cylinder cast
- b. overlap brace
- b. pancake plaster hand cast

bizarre
- b. high-frequency discharge
- b. parosteal osteochondromatous proliferation (BPOP)
- b. repetitive discharge
- b. repetitive potential

BJ
- biceps jerk

BJHS
- benign joint hypermobility syndrome

Björk
- B. prosthesis
- B. rib drill

Björnström algesimeter
BK
- below knee
- BK mole syndrome
- BK prosthesis

BKA
- below-knee amputation

black
- B. heel syndrome
- B. Max mid size knee component
- B. peroneal tendon sheath injection
- B. rasp
- B. repair
- B. technique

Blackburn
- B. technique
- B. traction

Blackburne ratio
Blackburn-Peel
- B.-P. measurement
- B.-P. ratio

black-dot heel
bladder
- b. augmentation
- b. dysfunction
- b. injury
- neurogenic b.

blade
>
> arachnoid-shape Beaver b.
> Arthro-Lok system of Beaver b.
> Bard-Parker b.
> Beaver b.
> Beaver-DeBakey b.
> Beaver discission b.
> Beaver keratome b.
> cartilage shaver b.
> Caspar b.
> cast b.
> chisel b.
> Curdy b.
> curved meniscotome b.
> Dynagrip handle of b.
> Dyonics arthroscopic b.
> Field b.
> Gigli saw b.
> b. of grass appearance
> Hebra b.
> Hibbs b.
> hook b.
> Incisor arthroscopic b.
> K b.
> keratome Beaver b.
> knife b.
> Magnum Tiger b.
> Merlin arthroscopy b.
> mini-meniscus b.
> 3M Maxi Driver b.
> narrow Assistant Free retractor b.
> notchplasty b.
> Paufique b.
> PowerCut drill b.
> resector b.
> retrograde Beaver b.
> retrograde meniscal b.
> rosette Beaver b.
> shoulder b.
> sickle-shape Beaver b.
> side-cutting b.
> Smillie-Beaver b.
> Superblade b.
> Swann-Morton surgical b.
> Synovator arthroscopic b.
> synovectomy b.
> Taylor spinal retractor b.
> Temperlite saw b.
> Tiger b.
> triradial resector b.
> Zimmer-Gigli saw b.

blade-plate
>
> adolescent condylar b.-p.
> AO condylar b.-p.
> ASIF right-angle b.-p.
> bifurcated b.-p.
> Blair talar body fusion b.-p.
> Blair tibiotalar arthrodesis b.-p.
> Blanchard traction device b.-p.
> b.-p. construct
> b.-p. driver
> b.-p. fixation
> fixed-angle AO b.-p.
> Giebel b.-p.
> Mueller compression b.-p.
> pediatric b.-p.
> semitubular b.-p.
> Zimmer femoral condyle b.-p.

blade-point retractor
blade-spike retractor
Blair
>
> B. ankle arthrodesis
> B. ankle fusion
> B. anterior arthrodesis
> B. chisel
> B. elevator
> B. knife
> B. procedure
> B. saw guide
> B. talar body fusion blade-plate
> B. technique
> B. tibiotalar arthrodesis
> B. tibiotalar arthrodesis blade-plate

Blair-Brown skin graft
Blair-Omer rerouting
Blake inverted orthotics
Blalock clamp
Blanchard
>
> B. traction device
> B. traction device blade-plate

blank
>
> Aliplast b.
> implant b.
> Nickelplast b.
> Plastazote b.

Blanke inverted tibialis posterior tendon orthotic
blanket
>
> Hollister Hot/Ice knee b.
> Rowe b.

Blastomyces dermatitidis
blastomycosis
>
> North American b.

blastomycotic osteomyelitis

NOTES

Blatt
 B. capsulodesis
 B. procedure
Blauth knee prosthesis
Blazina
 B. prosthesis
 B. tendinopathy
BLE
 both lower extremities
bleb capsulodesis
Bleck
 B. iliopsoas recession
 B. metatarsus adductus classification
 B. method
 B. recession technique
Bledsoe
 B. cast brace
 B. fracture brace
 B. knee brace
 B. leg brace
 B. Ultimate brace
bleeding
 b. bone
 b. point
blennorrhagica
 keratoderma b.
blind
 b. anchorage hole
 b. medullary nail
 b. medullary nailing
blink
 b. reflex
 b. response
Bliskunov implantable femoral distractor
blister
 bone b.
 b. of bone
 B. Film dressing
 fracture b.
blistering distal dactylitis (BDD)
Blix contractile force curve
bloc
 en b.
Bloch equation
block
 Airlite alignable ankle b.
 ankle b.
 anodal b.
 articular b.
 axillary b.
 balsa wood filler b.
 Bier b.
 bone b.
 Boyd posterior bone b.
 brachial plexus b.
 Campbell posterior bone b.
 common peroneal nerve b.
 conduction b.
 condyle b.

cutting b.
4-in-1 cutting b.
depolarization b.
differential spinal b.
digital nerve b.
facet joint b.
femoral nerve b.
field b.
filler b.
B. fixator
forefoot nerve b.
functional grip pushup b.
ganglion b.
ganglionic b.
Gill posterior bone b.
graduated-height b.
graduated spinal b. (GSB)
hand b.
Hara infiltration b.
Howard bone b.
HyProCure sinus tarsi implant b.
iliac crest bone b.
Inclan posterior bone b.
intercostal nerve b.
interscalene b.
joint b.
Kohs b.
lumbar sympathetic b.
Mayo nerve b.
median nerve b.
metacarpal b.
metatarsal b.
Mikhail bone b.
motor point b.
musculocutaneous nerve b.
nerve root b.
neurolytic b.
neuromuscular b.
b. osteotomy
parasacral b.
paravertebral b.
patellar tendon bone b.
PED b.
pelvic b.
perineural b.
peripheral nerve b.
plantar V infiltration b.
plexus b.
2-point nerve b.
popliteal sciatic nerve b.
posterior bone b.
presacral b.
pudendal b.
push-up b.
Putti posterior bone b.
recurrent median nerve b.
regional b.
sacral b.
sacroiliac b.

scalene b.
sciatic leg b.
sciatic nerve b.
S-cutting b.
sphenopalatine ganglion b.
spinal cord b.
Steinberg infiltration b.
stellate sympathetic ganglion b.
Styrofoam filler b.
subarachnoid b.
sympathetic b.
b. test
tibial cutting b.
transsacral b.
ulnar nerve b.
b. vertebra
vertebral b.
blockade
central neural b.
popliteal fossa neural b.
sympathetic b.
blockage
articular b.
extensor tendon b.
blocker
b. exostosis
hook b.
blood
autologous b.
b. cast
b. culture
b. flow
b. lactate
b. lactate accumulation
b. loss
b. loss anemia
b. pool phase
b. pressure
b. pressure monitor (BPM)
b. pressure monitoring
b. supply
b. transfusion
b. vessel tumor
b. viscosity
b. volume pulse (BVP)
blood-borne infection
blood-brain barrier (BBB)
bloodless
b. amputation
b. field
bloody effusion

bloom
B. splint
B. syndrome
Bloomberg sign
Bloom-Raney modification
blot test
Blount
B. anvil retractor
B. blade plate
B. bone spreader
B. brace
B. disease
B. displacement osteotomy
B. epiphysiodesis
B. fracture staple
B. knee retractor
B. knife
B. laminar spreader
B. osteotome
B. splint
B. stapling
B. technique for osteoclasis
B. tracing technique
Blount-Barber disease
Blount-Schmidt Milwaukee brace
blow-in fracture
blow-out fracture
B&L pinch gauge
Blucher
B. design
B. laced shoe
blue
B. Brand Therapy Putty
b. foot syndrome
B. Line orthotic
B. Line ThumbStay splint
B. Line UNO splint
B. Line Wrist Control splint
methylene b.
b. nevus
b. toe syndrome
Blumensaat line
Blumenthal bone rongeur
Blumer shelf
Blundell-Jones
B.-J. hip osteotomy
B.-J. operation
B.-J. varus osteotomy
blunt
b. arthroscopic cannula
b. caliper
b. dissection
b. forceps

NOTES

blunt (*continued*)
    b. hook
    b. hook dissector
    b. nose hemostat
    b. obturator
    b. pressure testing
    b. stylet
    b. tapered T-handled reamer
    b. trocar
blunt-tip
    b.-t. iris scissors
    b.-t. probe
BMC
    bone mineral content
BMD
    Becker muscular dystrophy
    bone mineral density
BME
    brief maximal effort
BMI
    body mass index
BMP
    bone marrow pressure
    bone morphogenetic protein
    BMP cabling and plating system
BMR
    basal metabolic rate
BNP
    brain natriuretic peptide
Bo
    Tae B.
board
    adjustable cane b.
    alphabet b.
    arm b.
    balance b.
    BAPS b.
    broad-based cane b.
    English cane b.
    Euroglide MKII slide b.
    exercise b.
    Flexisplint flexed arm b.
    glider cane b.
    grid maze b.
    Hadfield hand b.
    hand b.
    J b.
    Lowman balance b.
    manipulation b.
    memory b.
    powder b.
    quad b.
    Rock ankle exercise b.
    rocker b.
    Rock & Roller exercise b.
    spine b.
    b. splint
    Spri Xercise b.
    string drawing b.

    transfer b.
    vertical foot b.
    wobble b.
BoarderAnkle brace
boat nail
Bobath technique
Bobechko
    B. sliding barrel hook
    B. spreader
bob and weave
Bock
    B. knee prosthesis
    B. nerve
Bodenstab tourniquet
Bodnar retractor
body, pl. **bodies**
    alignment of vertebral bodies
    ankle loose b.
    apple-shape b.
    B. Armor short leg walker
    B. Armor walker cast
    artificial vertebral b.
    b. awareness
    B. Ball
    b. building
    cartilaginous loose b.
    b. cast syndrome
    b. composition
    b. composition assessment
    fibrous loose b.
    foreign b. (FB)
    B. Gard neoprene support
    B. Glove orthopaedic product
    intraarticular loose b.
    b. jacket
    b. jacket cast
    Kelvin b.
    b. logic rehabilitation system
    loose joint b.
    b. mass index (BMI)
    B. Master
    B. Masters MD 510 hi-lo pulley system
    Maxwell b.
    b. mechanics
    B. Mechanics Evaluation Checklist
    b. mechanics examination chart
    melon-seed b.
    navicular b.
    newtonian b.
    Ortho-Mold lumbar b.
    B. Oscillation Integrates Neuromuscular Gain (BOING)
    osteocartilaginous loose b.
    osteochondrotic loose b.
    pear-shaped b.
    B. Pedestal
    pedunculated loose b.
    Renaut b.

B. Response system
rice b.
b. righting reflex
rigid b.
b. of scapula
b. side integration
B. Sport ankle brace
B. Sticks massager
b. sway
talar b.
Verocay b.
b. of vertebra
vertebral b.
3-b. wear
b. weight
b. weight/composition
winterize b.
BodyBilt chair
Bodyblade
bodyCushion
SwimEx aquatic therapy b.
body-exhaust suit
BodyIce
B. cold pack
B. cold pack wrap
Bodyline
B. Back-Huggar
B. sleeper mattress overlay
B. Sports Brace
Bodynapper Comfort Pillow
body-powered prosthetic device
Body-Solid exercise equipment
bodywork
Boeck sarcoid
bogginess
boggy
b. consistency
b. swelling
b. synovitis
Böhler
B. brace
B. calcaneal angle
B. calcaneal fracture reduction
technique
B. calcaneal view
B. cast breaker
B. clamp
B. extension bow
B. fracture frame
B. guideline
B. lumbosacral angle
B. lumbosacral view
B. nail

B. pin
B. reducing frame
B. skintight cast
B. stirrup
B. tongs
B. tong traction
B. wire splint
Böhler-Braun
B.-B. frame
B.-B. leg sling
B.-B. splint
Böhler-Knowles hip pin
Böhler-Steinmann
B.-S. pin
B.-S. pin holder
Bohlman
B. anterior cervical vertebrectomy
B. cervical fusion technique
B. pin
B. triple-wire fusion
B. triple-wire technique
Boies forceps
BOING
Body Oscillation Integrates
Neuromuscular Gain
Bold compression screw
Boldrey brace
Bolero lift bath trolley
Bolin wedge filter system
bollard device
Bollinger knee brace
Boloxie OT Prehension Game
bolster
abduction b.
cotton b.
finger b.
knee b.
padded b.
roll control b.
rubber b.
Telfa b.
tie-over b.
bolt
Alvar condylar b.
Barr b.
bone lock b.
cannulated b.
condylar b.
connecting b.
b. cutter
DePuy b.
expansion b.
Fenton tibial b.

NOTES

B

87

bolt *(continued)*
    b. fixation
    fixation b.
    Hardinge expansion b.
    Harris b.
    Herzenberg b.
    hexhead b.
    Holt b.
    Hubbard b.
    Norman tibial b.
    Recon proximal drill guide b.
    Richmond b.
    slotted b.
    solid hex b.
    tibial b.
    transfixion b.
    trochanteric b.
    Webb stove b.
    Wilson b.
    wire fixation b.
    Zimmer tibial b.
Boltzmann distribution
bolus
bombardment by nociceptor
Bombelli-Mathys-Morscher hip prosthesis
Bombelli-Morscher femoral component
Bond arm splint
Bondek suture
bonding
    bone b.
    Poly-Lock b.
bone
    AAA b.
    b. abscess
    b. absorption
    accessory b.
    acetabular b.
    acromial b.
    adamantinoma of long b.
    b. age
    b. age according to Greulich and
     Pyle
    b. age ratio
    alar b.
    Albers-Schönberg marble b.
    Albrecht b.
    Allofix freeze-dried b.
    b. allograft
    allograft cortical b.
    allograft iliac b.
    alveolar supporting b.
    b. anchor
    ankle b.
    antigen-extracted, allogenic b.
    anvil b.
    arch of b.
    architectural alterations of b.
    areola of b.
    articulation of pisiform b.

astragalar b.
astragalocalcaneal b.
astragalocrural b.
astragaloid b.
astragaloscaphoid b.
astragalotibial b.
astragalus b.
b. autogenous graft
autogenous iliac b.
autolyzed, antigen-extracted,
  allogenic b.
b. awl
axis b.
b. bank
banked b.
basal b.
basilar b.
Bertin b.
Bethesda b.
bicortical iliac b.
b. biomechanics
Bio-Oss synthetic b.
b. biopsy needle
bleeding b.
b. blister
blister of b.
b. block
b. block fusion
b. block graft
b. block procedure
b. bonding
bone in b.
b. in bone finding
Bonfiglio b.
b. borer
b. bowing
bregmatic b.
Breschet b.
bridging b.
brittle b.
b. bruise
b. bruise sign
B. Bullet suture anchor
bundle b.
b. bur
B. Button orthopaedic suture
  anchor
cadaver b.
calcaneal b.
calcaneocuboid b.
b. callus
calvarial free b.
cancellated b.
cancellous versus cortical b.
candle wax appearance of b.
cannon b.
capitate b.
carpal b.
cavalry b.

b. cavity
b. cement
central b.
cervical vertebral b.
chalky b.
chevron b.
b. chip
b. chip graft
b. chisel
coalition of b.
coccygeal b.
coffin b.
collar b.
compact b.
b. conduction threshold
cone and socket b.
continuity of b.
convoluted b.
b. core
3-cornered b.
coronary b.
cortical b.
corticocancellous b.
costal b.
coxal b.
cranial b.
crazy b.
b. crisis
cuboid b.
cuneiform b.
b. curette
b. cyst
b. cyst excision
b. cyst fracture probability
b. cyst treatment
dead b.
b. debris
b. defect
demineralized b.
dense b.
b. densitometer
b. densitometry
b. density
b. density and arthritis testing
  system
b. density measurement
b. density study
b. deposition
b. depression
dermal b.
b. destructive process
detritus b.
b. development

dimple the b.
b. disease
disorganized b.
b. dissection
b. dollop
b. dowel
b. drill set
Durapatite b.
b. dysplasia
eburnated b.
ectocuneiform b.
ectopic b.
elbow b.
b. elevator
enchondral b.
enchondroma of b.
b. end
endochondral b.
entocuneiform b.
entrapped plantar b.
eosinophilic granuloma of b.
epactal b.
epipteric b.
exercise b.
exoccipital b.
b. extension clamp
femoral b.
b. femoral plug
fibular b.
b. file
b. fixation kit
b. fixation surface coating
flank b.
b. flap fixation plate
flat b.
1-b. forearm
3-b. forearm
b. formation
fourth turbinated b.
fovea centralis b.
fractured b.
b. fragment
fragmental b.
freeze-dried b.
freshening of b.
frontal b.
funny b.
fusiform periosteal new b.
Goethe b.
b. gouge
b. graft bed
b. graft collapse
b. graft decompression

NOTES

bone *(continued)*
  grafted b.
  b. graft extrusion
  b. graft incorporation
  b. graft placement
  b. graft punch
  b. graft putty
  b. graft repair
  b. graft shoe horn
  b. graft substitute (BGS)
  greater multangular b.
  great toe b.
  b. growth
  growth center of b.
  b. growth stimulator
  hamate b.
  b. hand drill
  b. harvesting
  b. healing
  heterotopic b.
  highest turbinated b.
  b. holder
  b. hole punch
  hollow b.
  b. hook
  hooked b.
  hook of hamate b.
  b. hook with cable/wire hole
  host b.
  human cancellous b.
  human cortical b.
  humeral b.
  hydroxyapatite b.
  hyoid b.
  hyperplastic b.
  b. hypertrophy
  iliac b.
  immature b.
  b. impactor
  b. implant
  b. implant material
  incarial b.
  incisive b.
  incomplete fracture of b.
  b. infarct
  b. infarction
  infected b.
  b. infection
  b. ingrowth
  innominate b.
  intermaxillary b.
  interparietal b.
  Interpore b.
  b. interstice
  intrachondrial b.
  irregular b.
  ischial b.
  b. island
  b. isograft

  ivory b.
  jugal b.
  Kiel b.
  knuckle b.
  Krause b.
  lacrimal b.
  b. lacuna
  lamellar b.
  lamellated b.
  laminar b.
  b. lavage
  lenticular b.
  lesser multangular b.
  b. and limb growth velocity ratios
  b. liner
  b. lip
  b. lock bolt
  long axis of b.
  b. loss
  lunate b.
  lunocapitate b.
  luxated b.
  lyophilization of b.
  malar b.
  b. mallet
  marble b.
  b. marrow
  b. marrow aspiration
  b. marrow biopsy
  b. marrow edema
  b. marrow embolism
  b. marrow graft
  b. marrow pressure (BMP)
  b. marrow stimulating technique
  b. marrow tumor
  b. mass
  b. matrix
  b. maturation
  b. maturity
  b. meal
  medial metacarpal b.
  membranous b.
  mesocuneiform b.
  b. metabolic unit
  metacarpal b.
  metaphysial b.
  b. metastasis
  metatarsal b.
  b. mill
  b. mineral content (BMC)
  b. mineral density (BMD)
  b. mineralization isotope
  morcellized b.
  b. morphogenetic protein (BMP)
  b. mortise
  B. Mulch screw
  multangular b.
  navicular b.
  b. necrosis

necrotic b.
b. neoplasm
new b.
newly woven b.
Nicoll b.
nonlamellar b.
nonlamellated b.
nonloadbearing fractured b.
occipital b.
omovertebral b.
orbitosphenoidal b.
osteoclast-mediated b.
osteonal lamellar b.
osteopenic b.
osteoporotic b.
osteotomized b.
pagetoid b.
palatine b.
parietal b.
particle of b.
b. paste
b. pathology
b. peg
b. peg epiphysiodesis
b. pegging
b. peg graft
perilesional b.
periosteal new b.
petrosal b.
petrous temporal b.
phalangeal b.
ping-pong b.
Pirie b.
pisiform b.
plantar b.
B. Plast bone replacement material
b. plate integrity
b. plate selection
b. plombage
b. plug cutter
b. plug extractor
b. plug setter
porotic b.
postulnar b.
preinterparietal b.
primary lymphoma of b. (PLB)
primitive b.
b. production
b. prosthesis
pterotic b.
pterygoid b.
pubic b.
b. punch forceps

b. punch rongeur
quadripartite b.
radial b.
raw b.
b. reamer
b. remodeling
b. remodeling transient
b. remodeling unit
replacement b.
b. replacement graft
b. resection
b. resorption
b. resurfacing
resurrection b.
rider's b.
Riolan b.
rudimentary b.
sacral b.
b. saw
b. scan
scaphoid b.
b. scintigraphy
b. sclerosis
sclerotic b.
b. screw depth gauge
b. screw ruler gauge
b. screw targeter
scroll b.
semilunar b.
b. sequestrum
sesamoid b.
b. setting
b. shaft
b. shaft fracture
shank b.
shin b.
short b.
shoulder b.
b. sialoprotein
b. skid
sliver of b.
b. slurry
soft b.
b. spacer
b. spicule
spike of b.
splint b.
spongy b.
b. spreader
b. spur
squamooccipital b.
squamous-type b.
b. staple system

B

NOTES

bone *(continued)*
   b. stock
   b. strength
   structured b.
   stump of b.
   subchondral b.
   subcoracoid b.
   subperiosteal new b.
   b. substance
   b. substitute
   b. substitute backfilling
   supernumerary b.
   supporting b.
   supraoccipital b.
   suprasternal b.
   b. surface lesion
   b. survey
   sutural b.
   b. suture fixation
   b. suturing wire chisel-tip wire
   synthetic cortical b.
   talonavicular b.
   b. tamp
   tarsal b.
   temporal b.
   thoracic b.
   tibia b.
   trabecular b.
   b. transfer
   trapezium b.
   trapezoid b.
   b. trephine
   triangular wrist b.
   tripartite b.
   triquetrum b.
   b. trough
   b. tuberculoma
   tumor-bearing b.
   b. tunnel
   turbinated b.
   b. turnover
   tympanic b.
   ulna b.
   ulnar sesamoid b.
   ulnar styloid b.
   b. ultrasound attenuation (BUA)
   unciform b.
   uncinate b.
   vascular bundle implantation
    into b.
   vascular metaphysial b.
   vertebral b.
   vesalian b.
   Vesalius b.
   Vitoss synthetic b.
   vomer b.
   b. wax
   b. wax gelatin sponge
   b. wedge

   whettle b.
   b. wire guide
   wormian b.
   woven b.
   wrist b.
   xiphoid b.
   zygomatic b.
bone-biting forceps
bone-breaking forceps
bone-cement interface
bone-cutting forceps
bone-forming
   b.-f. sarcoma bone imaging
   b.-f. tumor
bone-graft plug
bone-grasping forceps
bone-holding
   b.-h. clamp
   b.-h. forceps
   b.-h. instrumentation
bone-implant interface
bone-ingrowth fixation
bonelet
Boneloc cement
Bone-Lok device
bonemeal tablet
bone-nibbling rongeur
bone-patellar
   b.-p. ligament-bone (BPB)
   b.-p. tendon-bone (BPB, BPTB)
   b.-p. tendon-bone autograft
   b.-p. tendon-bone preparation
bone-peg interface
BonePlast bone void filler
bone-remodeling
bone-screw interface strength
BoneSource hydroxyapatite cement
bone-specific alkaline phosphatase
   (BSAP)
bone-splitting forceps
bone-tendon
   b.-t. exposure
   b.-t. graft
   b.-t. graft material
bone-tendon-bone
   b.-t.-b. allograft
   b.-t.-b. graft
bone-to-bone
   b.-t.-b. apposition
   b.-t.-b. graft
bone-within-bone appearance
Bonferroni correction
Bonfiglio
   B. bone
   B. bone graft
   B. bone replacement material
   B. modification
   B. modification of Phemister
    technique

Bonner position
bonnet
    gluteal b.
Bonney clamp
Bonney-Kessel dorsiflexionary tilt-up
   osteotomy
Bonola technique
bony
    b. abnormality
    b. absorption
    b. ankylosis
    b. apposition
    b. architecture
    b. bar
    b. bridge
    b. bridge resection
    b. consolidation
    b. crepitus
    b. deformity
    b. demineralization
    b. distal end
    b. eburnation
    b. element destruction
    b. encroachment
    b. erosion
    b. excrescence
    b. exostosis
    b. fossa
    b. hallux limitus
    b. humeral avulsion
    b. humeral avulsion of
      glenohumeral ligament (BHAGL)
    b. interface
    b. landmark
    b. lesion
    b. mass
    b. metastasis
    b. necrosis
    b. necrosis and destruction
    b. osteophyte
    b. overgrowth
    b. pelvis
    b. procedure
    b. process
    b. purchase
    b. reabsorption
    b. semicircular canal
    b. sequestrum
    b. skeleton
    b. slurry leakage
    b. spurring
    b. tenderness
    b. union

Boo-Boo Pacs
Book Butler book-grip device
boomerang wrist support
boot
    Ambulator Chukka B.
    APB Hi all-purpose b.
    b. brace
    Bunny b.
    cast b.
    Chukka b.
    clamshell AFO b.
    compression b.
    Conformer diabetic b.
    Cryo/Cuff b.
    De Lorme b.
    derotation b.
    external sequential pneumatic
      compression b.
    fluid barrier b.
    fracture b.
    gelatin compression b.
    Gibney b.
    Hang Ups gravity b.
    Heelift suspension b.
    Heelift traction b.
    Heel-Up Boot suspension b.
    In-Bed AFO b.
    Jobst b.
    Junod b.
    L'Nard b.
    Markell brace b.
    Markell open-toe b.
    Moon b.
    Multi Podus b.
    Ongoing Ambulating AFO b.
    pneumatic compression b.
    Primer modified Unna b.
    quadriceps De Lorme b.
    Rik FootHugger fluid heel b.
    rocker b.
    sequential pneumatic compression b.
    SlimLine cast b.
    Sorrel-type snowboard b.
    Spenco b.
    Unna paste b.
    Venodyne b.
    weight b.
    Wilke b.
    b. wrap
booth
    B. test
    B. wire osteotomy

NOTES

B

bootie
> Bebax B.

boot-top
> b.-t. fracture
> b.-t. laceration

Boplant
> B. Surgibone
> B. Surgibone bovine bone
> substitute

Bora
> B. centralization
> B. operation
> B. technique

borazone blade cutting machine
Borchardt olive-shaped bur
Borchgrevin traction
border
> brush b.
> coast of California b.
> coast of Maine b.
> cryptotic medial b.
> lateral acromial b.
> medial b.
> b. ray
> b. ray amputation
> scapular b.
> scapulovertebral b.
> superior b.
> vertebral b.
> web b.

bore needle
borer
> bone b.
> cork b.

Borg
> B. Numerical Pain Scale
> B. Scale of Rating Perceived
> Exertion

Borggreve
> B. limb rotation
> B. method

Borggreve-Hall technique
Borg-Warner orthopaedic bed
boring pain
Boropak astringent solution
borotannic complex
Borrelia burgdorferi
BOS
> base of skull

Bose
> B. nail fold excision
> B. procedure

BOSS
> Becker orthopaedic spinal system

boss
> carpal b.
> carpometacarpal b.

bosselated
bosselation

bossing
> frontal b.

Bostick staple
Boston
> B. bivalve cast
> B. brace thoracolumbosacral
> orthosis
> B. Classification System
> B. Diagnostic Aphasia examination
> B. elbow system
> B. LINAC
> B. overlap brace
> B. postoperative hip orthosis
> B. scoliosis brace
> B. soft body jacket
> B. soft corset
> B. thoracic brace
> B. thoracic splint

B&O Supprettes
Bosworth
> B. approach
> B. arthrodesis
> B. arthroplasty
> B. bone peg insertion
> B. coracoclavicular screw
> B. crown drill
> B. femoroischial transplant
> B. femoroischial transplantation
> B. fracture
> B. lumbar spinal fusion
> B. screwdriver
> B. shelf operation
> B. shelf procedure
> B. spine plate
> B. splint
> B. technique
> B. tendo calcaneus repair

Bosworth-type reverse plasty
botfly
> human b.

both
> b. lower extremities (BLE)
> b. upper extremities (BUE)

both-bone fracture
both-column fracture
Botox injection
botryoid sarcoma
bottleneck femoral tunnel
bottle sign
bottom
> hoof b.
> weaver's b.

Bottoms-Up posture system
Bouchard
> B. node
> B. nodule
> B. sign

bouche de tapir
bougie needle

bounce home test
Bouncewell medicine ball
bouncing
    ligamentous b.
Bourgery ligament
Bourneville disease
boutonnière
    b. deformity
    b. hand dislocation
    b. splint
Bouvier maneuver
Bovie
    B. cauterization
    B. cautery
    B. coagulating unit
    B. electrocautery apparatus
    B. electrocautery device
    B. knife
    underwater B.
bovine
    b. collagen
    b. collagen bioprosthesis
    b. collagen graft
    b. collagen implant
    b. collagen material prosthesis
bow
    aiming b.
    B. & Arrow cannulated drill guide
    Böhler extension b.
    cupid's b.
    extension b.
    finger extension b.
    Framer finger extension b.
    Kirschner wire traction b.
    maximum radial b.
    posterior b.
    posteromedial b.
    Schwarz finger extension b.
    traction b.
    wire traction b.
Bowden cable suspension system
bowed leg
bowel
    neurogenic b.
    b. training
Bowen
    B. chisel
    B. disease
    B. osteotome
    B. periosteal elevator
    B. suture drill

Bowers
    B. radial arthroplasty
    B. technique
bowing
    bone b.
    congenital posteromedial b.
    b. deformity
    b. fracture
    lateral b.
    tendon b.
    tibial b.
Bowlby arm splint
bowl curette
bowleg
    b. brace
    b. deformity
bowler's thumb
Bowman
    B. angle
    B. disc
    B. muscle
bowstring
    b. sign
    b. tear
    b. test
bowstringing
bow-tie sign
box
    b. and block test of arm disability
    BTE Bolt B.
    b. chisel
    b. curette
    fracture b.
    high toe b.
    ligamentous b.
    b. osteotome
    sit-and-reach b.
    toe b.
    wide toe b.
box-end wrench
boxer's
    b. elbow
    b. fracture
    b. knuckle
    b. punch
boxwood mallet
Boyd
    B. ankle amputation
    B. ankle arthrodesis
    B. approach
    B. classification
    B. communicating perforation vein
    B. dual-onlay bone graft

B

NOTES

Boyd (*continued*)
    B. formula
    B. hip disarticulation
    B. modification of Tardieu spastic
       measurement scale
    B. operation
    B. perforator
    B. podiatry chair
    B. posterior bone block
    B. side plate
    B. type II fracture
Boyd-Anderson
    B.-A. biceps tendon repair
    B.-A. technique
Boyd-Griffin trochanteric fracture classification
Boyd-Ingram-Bourkhard treatment
Boyd-McLeod
    B.-M. procedure
    B.-M. tennis elbow technique
Boyd-Sisk
    B.-S. approach
    B.-S. posterior capsulorrhaphy
Boyer degenerative joint disease grading system
Boyes
    B. brachioradialis transfer technique
    B. test
    B. transfer
Boyes-Goodfellow hook
Boyle-Davis retractor
Boytchev procedure
Bozzini light conductor
BPB
    bone-patellar ligament-bone
    bone-patellar tendon-bone
       BPB autologous graft
BPM
    blood pressure monitor
       Laserflo BPM
BPOP
    bizarre parosteal osteochondromatous
       proliferation
BPTB
    bone-patellar tendon-bone
       BPTB graft
BPTI
    brachial plexus traction injury
brace
    Abbott b.
    abduction b.
    accommodative b.
    Ace b.
    ACL Lite functional knee b.
    Active ankle b.
    Active support and b.
    Activity-Lite knee b.
    adjustable b.
    AFO pediatric b.

Aircast ankle b.
Aircast Cryo/Cuff b.
Aircast fracture b.
Aircast leg b.
Aircast Pneumatic Air Stirrup b.
Aircast Swivel-Strap b.
Aircast walking b.
Air DonJoy patellofemoral b.
AirGEL ankle b.
airplane splint shoulder b.
Airprene Action knee b.
Air-Stirrup ankle training b.
Air Townsend b.
ALP Plus ankle b.
Ambi wrist b.
AMX knee b.
Ank-L-Aid b.
ankle ligament protector b.
ankle stirrup b.
AO b.
AOA cervical immobilization b.
APL Plus ankle b.
APU b.
Arizona ankle b.
Arnold lumbar b.
ASO ankle b.
Atak knee b.
athletic b.
Atlanta hip b.
Atlanta-Scottish Rite b.
Atlantic overlap b.
Atlantic rim b.
ATR b.
Axis ankle b.
back b.
Back Seat torso-wrap b.
bail-lock b.
Bauerfeind ankle b.
Bauerfeind Comprifix knee b.
Becker b.
bicycle b.
Bike ankle b.
BIOflex magnetic counterforce b.
Biomet fracture b.
BioSkin Q knee b.
bipivotal hinge knee b.
Bird & Cronin wrist b.
bivalved overlap b.
Bledsoe cast b.
Bledsoe fracture b.
Bledsoe knee b.
Bledsoe leg b.
Bledsoe Ultimate b.
Blount b.
Blount-Schmidt Milwaukee b.
BoarderAnkle b.
Bodyline Sports B.
Body Sport ankle b.
Böhler b.

Boldrey b.
Bollinger knee b.
boot b.
Boston overlap b.
Boston scoliosis b.
Boston thoracic b.
bowleg b.
Brite-Life wrist b.
Buck knee b.
cable-twister b.
cage-back b.
Caligamed b.
caliper b.
Callender derotational b.
Camp b.
CAM Walker ankle b.
CAM Walker leg b.
Can Am b.
canvas b.
Capener b.
Carpal Lock CTS b.
Carpal Lock wrist b.
carpenter's b.
CASH b.
Castaway leg b.
Cast Boot polypropylene hip
  abduction b.
Castiglia ankle b.
Centec Formfit ankle b.
cervical collar b.
chairback b.
Charleston nighttime bending b.
Charleston scoliosis b.
Charnley b.
Cheetah ankle b.
CHH cervical b.
Chopart b.
CI functional knee b.
Cinch Lock CTS b.
Cincinnati ACL b.
clamshell b.
Clinch Lock CTS wrist b.
CM-Band 505N b.
CM-Band silicone rubber b.
Cole hyperextension b.
collar b.
Combined Instabilities functional
  knee b.
contraflexion b.
controlled-motion b.
controlled position b. (CPB)
Cook walking b.
cool CPB b.

Cooper ankle b.
Counter Rotation System b.
Count'R-Force arch b.
cowhorn b.
CRM rehab b.
CRS b.
Cruiser hip abduction b.
Cruiser OA b.
CTi b.
CTi2 knee b.
Cunningham b.
custom-fitted b.
cutout patellar b.
Dalco Astro ankle b.
Darco back b.
DarcoGel ankle b.
Defiance functional knee b.
Dennison cervical b.
DePuy fracture b.
derotation b.
derotational b.
3D fracture walker b.
dial-lock b.
DonJoy ALP b.
DonJoy Gold Point knee b.
DonJoy Opal knee b.
DonJoy 4-point Super Sport
  knee b.
DonJoy Quadrant shoulder b.
DonJoy Universal ankle b.
dorsiflexion stop b.
double-upright short leg b.
doughnut support b.
b. drill
dropfoot b.
drop-lock knee b.
Drytex RocketSoc ankle b.
dual-lock ankle b.
Duncan shoulder b.
Dura-Flex back b.
dynamic abduction b.
dynamic hinge elbow fracture b.
Easy Lok ankle b.
Easy-On elbow b.
Eclipse Gel ankle b.
economy ROM b.
EconoSoc ankle b.
Edge knee b.
elastic-hinge knee b.
elastic knee sleeve b.
Elite knee b.
English b.
Equalizer cast b.

NOTES

brace *(continued)*
    Exotec b.
    EZ ROM postoperative knee b.
    felt b.
    figure-of-8 b.
    Fisher b.
    Flagg fiberglass knee b.
    Flex Foam b.
    flexor hinge hand-splint b.
    FlexTech knee b.
    Floam ankle stirrup b.
    Florida back b.
    Florida cervical b.
    Florida contraflexion b.
    Florida extension b.
    Florida hyperextension b.
    Florida J-24, J-35, J-45, J-55 b.
    Florida post-fusion b.
    Florida spinal b.
    foot-ankle b.
    footdrop b.
    Forrester cervical collar b.
    Frazer wrist b.
    Friedman b.
    functional fracture b.
    functional knee b.
    furniture b.
    Futuro wrist b.
    Galveston metacarpal b.
    Generation II 3DX b.
    Generation II Unloader ADJ
      knee b.
    Generation II Unloader Select
      knee b.
    Genutrain knee b.
    GII Unloader ADJ knee b.
    GII Unloader OA b.
    Gillette b.
    GLS b.
    GoldPoint ACL functional knee b.
    GoldPoint hinged knee b.
    GoldPoint PCL functional knee b.
    Goldthwait b.
    Guilford cervical b.
    halo b.
    hand b.
    H buttress support
      patellofemoral b.
    head b.
    Hennessy knee b.
    Hessing b.
    high-tide walking b.
    Hilgenreiner b.
    hinged knee b.
    Hi-Top foot/ankle b.
    Hoke lumbar b.
    horseshoe patellofemoral b.
    Hudson-Jones knee-cage b.
    Hudson TLSO b.

    humeral b.
    hyperextension b.
    Ilfeld b.
    InCare b.
    Inner Lok ankle b.
    internal tibial torsion b.
    Intrepid functional knee b.
    I-Plus system humeral fracture b.
    I-Plus system ulnar fracture b.
    ischial weightbearing leg b.
    IsoDyn knee b.
    Jewett-Benjamin cervical b.
    Jones b.
    Juzo b.
    Juzo Patellaligner b.
    Kallassy b.
    Key wrist b.
    Kicker Pavlik harness hip
      abduction b.
    King cervical b.
    Kleinert postoperative traction b.
    Klengall b.
    Klenzak spring b.
    Kling cervical b.
    knee cage b.
    knee MD b.
    KneeRanger hinged knee b.
    Knight back b.
    Knight-Taylor thoracic b.
    knock-knee b.
    KS 5 ACL b.
    KSO b.
    Küntscher-Hudson b.
    Kydex b.
    kyphosis b.
    lace-on b.
    lace-up RocketSoc ankle b.
    lacing ankle b.
    lateral buttress support J
      patellofemoral b.
    leaf-spring b.
    LeCocq b.
    leg b.
    Legend ACL functional knee b.
    Legend PCL functional knee b.
    Lenox Hill derotational knee b.
    Lenox Hill Spectralite knee b.
    Lerman hinge b.
    Liberty CMC thumb b.
    ligamentous control b.
    limb b.
    long arm b.
    long leg hinged b.
    Lorenz b.
    low-tide walking b.
    LSU reciprocation-gait orthosis b.
    lumbar b.
    lumbosacral b.
    MacAusland lumbar b.

Magnetic Support b.
M-Brace knee b.
McClintoch b.
McCollough internal tibial torsion b.
McDavid knee b.
McKee b.
MCL b.
MC walker b.
MD b.
Medical Design b.
Medipedic Multicentric knee b.
Metcalf spring drop b.
Miami fracture b.
Miami TLSO scoliosis b.
b. migration
Milwaukee scoliosis b.
Minerva cervical b.
MKS II knee b.
Monarch knee b.
Moon Boot b.
Mooney b.
MTA b.
Mueller ATF ankle b.
Mueller hinged knee b.
Mueller Lite ankle b.
Mueller orthopaedic shoulder b.
Mueller Ultralite b.
Mueller wrap-around knee b.
Multi-Lig knee b.
Multi-Lock knee b.
Murphy b.
Nakamura b.
neck b.
neoprene wrist b.
Nevin ankle b.
New England scoliosis b.
Newington b.
Newport MC hip orthosis b.
Nextep knee b.
night b.
nonweightbearing b.
Northville b.
no-stretch RocketSoc b.
OAdjuster knee b.
OA knee b.
OAsys knee b.
offloading knee b.
Omni knee b.
Opiela b.
Oppenheim b.
Orbital shoulder stabilizer b.
Orthomedics b.

Ortho-Mold spinal b.
Orthoplast fracture b.
Orthotech Controller knee b.
Osgood-Schlatter knee b.
OS-5/Plus 2 knee b.
OsteoArthritic knee b.
osteoarthritis padded night sleeve b.
out-of-cast ankle b.
outside-the-boot b.
oyster-shell b.
Palumbo dynamic patellar b.
Palumbo stabilizing b.
pantaloon b.
parachutist ankle b.
Patellaligner knee b.
patellar stabilizing b. (PSB)
patellar tendon-bearing b.
patellofemoral b.
Patten-Bottom-Perthes b.
pediatric PRAFO b.
pelvic b.
performer ultralight knee b.
Perlstein b.
PFT traction b.
Phelps b.
Philadelphia Plastizote cervical b.
piano-wire dorsiflexion b.
Playmaker functional knee b.
PlayTuf knee b.
PMT halo system b.
PneuGel ankle b.
Pneu Knee b.
Pneu-trac neck b.
4-point IROM b.
6-point knee b.
4-point SuperSport functional knee b.
Polaris knee rehab b.
2-poster b.
4-poster cervical b.
postfusion b.
Power Play knee b.
PPG-AFO b.
PPG-TLSO b.
Pro-8 ankle b.
Procase Ankle-Lock b.
progressive resistance b.
Proline Stomatex shoulder b.
Protonic b.
PTB b.
PTS knee b.
Push medical b.

NOTES

brace *(continued)*
Quadrant advanced shoulder b.
QualCare knee b.
Raney flexion jacket b.
range of motion b.
ratchet-type b.
reamer b.
Rebel knee b.
Rehab TROM b.
Rhino Triangle polypropylene hip
  abduction b.
Richie b.
rigid postoperative b.
Ritchie b.
RocketSoc ankle b.
Rolyan TakeOff Sprint b.
Rolyan tibial fracture b.
ROM knee b.
ROM walker b.
Saltiel b.
Sarmiento fracture b.
SAS II b.
Sawa shoulder b.
Schanz collar b.
SCOI shoulder b.
scoliosis overlap b.
Scottish Rite b.
Selectively Lockable knee b.
semirigid ankle b.
Seton hip b.
short arm b.
short leg caliper b.
short leg double-upright b.
short leg walking b.
shoulder subluxation inhibitor b.
SmartBrace b.
SmartWrap elbow b.
Smedberg b.
snap-lock b.
SofTec rigid b.
SOMI b.
Speed b.
Spinal Technology bivalve
  TLSO b.
SpineCor nonrigid b.
Sports-Caster I, II knee b.
SSI b.
Stardox wrist b.
Stealth knee b.
Stille b.
Stimprene electrotherapy b.
stirrup b.
stop action b.
straight walker b.
Strap Lok ankle b.
Stromgren ankle b.
Stubbs 4-way clavicle b.
Sully shoulder stabilizer b.
Sure Step ankle b.

Swede-O Ankle Loc b.
Swede-O-Universal b.
Swivel-Strap ankle b.
Taylor back b.
Taylor-Knight b.
Taylor spine b.
telescoping b.
Teufel cervical b.
Teurlings wrist b.
Thermoskin b.
Thomas cervical collar b.
Thomas walking b.
thoracolumbar standing orthosis b.
TLSO b.
toe-drop b.
Tomasini b.
Toronto b.
total anatomical hinge knee b.
Townsend Rebel convertible b.
Tracker knee b.
Tri-angle shoulder abduction b.
Trinkle b.
TROM knee b.
Tru-Fit b.
turnbuckle ankle b.
turnbuckle knee b.
UBC b.
UCLA functional long leg b.
ulnar b.
Ultrabrace b.
underarm b.
unilateral calcaneal b. (UCB)
University of British Columbia b.
Unloader ADJ Unloader b.
Unloader Bi-ComPF knee b.
Unloader Express Unloader b.
Unloader Select Unloader b.
Unloader Spirit knee b.
Value Walker b.
Varney acromioclavicular b.
Verlow b.
Victorian b.
von Lackum transection shift
  jacket b.
walking b.
Warm Springs b.
Watco b.
weightbearing b.
Wheaton Pavlik Harness b.
Wilke boot b.
Williams b.
Wilmington scoliosis b.
Wright Universal b.
wrist b.
Yale b.
Zimmer reamer b.
Zinco Air Cam b.
Zinco Airprene b.
Zinco Cam Walker b.

B

Zinco Castaway D b.
Zinco Hi-Top b.
Zinco Minerva cervical b.
Zinco Multi-Lig knee b.
Zinco Pin Cam Walker b.
brace/corset
Hoke lumbar b./c.
brace-free ambulation
bracelet
Nussbaum b.
Q-Ray b.
b. test
brace-type reamer
brachia (*pl. of* brachium)
brachial
b. amelia
b. artery
b. artery aneurysm
b. artery injury
b. neuralgia
b. neuritis
b. plexopathy
b. plexus
b. plexus block
b. plexus injury
b. plexus neuropathy
b. plexus palsy
b. plexus paralysis
b. plexus repair
b. plexus tendon
b. plexus tension test
b. plexus traction injury (BPTI)
brachialgia
brachialis
b. muscle
b. tendon
brachiocephalic vein
brachiocrural
brachiocubital
brachiocyllosis
brachiocyrtosis
brachiogram
brachioradialis
b. flap
b. muscle
b. reflex
b. tendon
b. transfer
b. transfer for wrist extension
brachium, pl. **brachia**
brachybasia
brachybasocamptodactyly
brachybasophalangia

brachycnemic
brachydactylia
brachydactyly
brachykerkic
brachymelia
brachymesophalangia
brachymetacarpalia
brachymetacarpia
brachymetapody
brachymetatarsia
brachyphalangia
brachypodous
brachyskelic
brachyskelous
brachystasis
brachytelephalangia
bracing
cast b.
fracture b.
postoperative b.
bracket
longitudinal epiphysial b.
bracketed splint
Brackett-Osgood
B.-O. knee approach
B.-O. posterior approach
Brackett osteotomy
Braden risk assessment scale
Bradford
B. fracture frame
B. fusion
Bradley femoral canal preparation scraper
Brady
B. balanced-suspension splint
B. leg splint
bradycinesia
Brady-Jewett technique
bradykinesia
bradykinin
bradymetatarsalgia
Bragard
B. reinforcement
B. sign
B. test
Bragg angle
Bragg-peak photon-beam therapy
Brahms
B. foot operation
B. procedure
braid
carbon fiber lamination b. (CFLB)
braided suture

NOTES

Brailsford disease
brain
    B. arthroplasty
    b. natriuretic peptide (BNP)
    B. reflex
brainstem
    b. auditory evoked potential
    (BAEP)
    b. auditory evoked response
    (BAER)
    transtentorial b.
brake
    b. lever extension
    b. phenomenon
branch
    acetabular b.
    calcaneal b.
    digital b.
    distal communicating b. (DCB)
    dorsal ulnar cutaneous b.
    interosseous b.
    motor b.
    posterior interosseous b.
    proper digital nerve b.
    proximal communicating b. (PCB)
    superior laryngeal nerve external b.
    thenar b.
branched calculus
brand
    B. tendon-holding forceps
    B. tendon passer
    B. tendon-passing forceps
    B. tendon stripper
    B. tendon transfer technique
Branhamella catarrhalis
Brannock
    B. Device shoe sizer
    B. foot measuring device
Brant aluminum splint
Brantigan interbody fusion cage
brassiere
    Jobst b.
Brattström condylar height ratio
Braun
    B. frame
    B. procedure
    B. shoulder tenotomy
    B. skin graft
breach
    cortical b.
    naviculocuneiform b.
break
    b. point
    b. screw extractor
    b. test
breakable screw breaker
breakage
    pedicle screw b.

    screw b.
    tack b.
breakaway
    b. lap cushion
    b. pin
    b. weakness
breakdancer's thumb
breakdown
    skin b.
breaker
    Böhler cast b.
    breakable screw b.
    cast b.
    Wolfe-Böhler cast b.
breast
    chicken b.
    funnel b.
    pigeon b.
breastbone
breaststroker's knee
breathing
    paradoxical b.
Breck
    B. pin
    B. pin cutter
Breezee Mist Antifungal
bregma
bregmatic
    b. bone
    b. bone Brissaud scoliosis
bregmatomastoid suture
Bremer
    B. AirFlo halo vest
    B. halo cervical traction
    B. Halo Crown cervical collar
    B. halo system
Breschet bone
Breslow
    B. arthroplasty
    B. classification
    B. classification of melanoma
Breslow classification
Brett
    B. arthrodesis
    B. osteotomy
Breuerton view
breve
    vinculum b.
brevicollis
breviflexor
Brevio nerve conduction monitor
brevis
    abductor pollicis b.
    extensor carpi radialis b. (ECRB)
    extensor digitorum b. (EDB)
    extensor pollicis b. (EPB)
    flexor digitorum b. (FDB)
    flexor digitorum quinti b. (FDQB)
    flexor hallucis b. (FHB)

flexor pollicis b. (FPB)
peroneus b. (PB)
b. release
Brewster triple arthrodesis
Brickner position
bridge
    autograft b.
    b. back exercise technique
    balance b.
    bony b.
    fascial b.
    b. graft
    B. Hip system
    iliac crest b.
    b. of meniscus
    osseous b.
    physial b.
    b. plate
    b. plate fixation
    skin b.
    tarsal b.
    tendon-bone b.
bridging
    b. bone
    b. callus
    b. of defect
    myocardial b.
    b. osteophyte
bridle
    b. posterior tibial tendon transfer operation
    B. procedure
brief
    b. maximal effort (BME)
    B. Pain Inventory
    b., small, abundant, polyphasic potential (BSAPP)
    b., small, abundant potential (BSAP)
    B. Test of Head Injury (BTHI)
    B. Test of Head Injury Assessment
Brigham prosthesis
Brighton electrical stimulation system
brim
    pelvic b.
    proximal medial b.
    quadrilateral b.
brisement
    b. forcé
    b. therapy

Brissaud
    B. scoliosis
    B. syndrome
Bristow
    B. operation
    B. periosteal elevator
    B. procedure
    B. rasp
    B. shoulder reconstruction
Bristow-Helfet procedure
Bristow-Latarjet procedure
Bristow-May procedure
Brite-Life wrist brace
British test
Brittain
    B. chisel
    B. ischiofemoral arthrodesis
    B. operation
brittle
    b. bone
    b. bone disease
    b. bone failure
    b. nail
broach
    barbed b.
    cemented b.
    cementless b.
    Charnley femoral b.
    chipped-tooth b.
    drilling b.
    b. extractor
    femoral prosthesis b.
    Harris b.
    Koenig metatarsal b.
    orthopaedic b.
    root canal b.
    smooth b.
    square-hole b.
    Swanson metatarsal b.
    Zimmer femoral canal b.
broad
    b. AO dynamic compression plate
    b. foot
    b. thumb–big toe syndrome
broad-based
    b.-b. cane
    b.-b. cane board
    b.-b. gait
Broadbent-Woolf 4-limb Z-plasty
broad-spectrum antibiotic
broad-toed shoe

NOTES

Broberg-Morrey
> B.-M. elbow function scale
> B.-M. fracture

Broca
> B. aphasia
> B. area
> B. convolution
> B. diagonal band

Brockman
> B. foot operation
> B. incision
> B. procedure

Brockman-Nissen arthrodesis

Broden
> B. stress examination
> B. stress radiography
> B. view

Brodie
> B. abscess
> B. bursa
> B. disease
> B. knee
> B. ligament

Brodsky-Tullos-Gartsman approach

BROM
> back range of motion

bromelain powder

bromfenac sodium

bromidrosis, bromhidrosis
> plantar b.

Bromi-Lotion antiperspirant lotion

Bromi-Talc Plus antiperspirant powder

Brooke Army Hospital splint

Brooker
> B. classification of heterotopic ossification (I–IV)
> B. double-locking unreamed tibial nail
> B. femoral nail
> B. frame
> B. heterotopic bone formation classification (I-IV)
> B. wire

Brooker-Wills nail

Brooks
> B. atlantoaxial arthrodesis
> B. cervical fusion
> B. cervical fusion operation
> B. shoe
> B. technique

Brooks-Gallie cervical fusion

Brooks-Jenkins
> B.-J. atlantoaxial fusion
> B.-J. atlantoaxial fusion technique
> B.-J. cervical fusion

Brooks-type fusion

Broomhead medial approach

broomstick
> b. bar
> b. cast
> b. curl-up

Brophy periosteal elevator

Broström
> B. injection technique
> B. lateral ankle ligament repair
> B. ligament reconstruction
> B. procedure

Broström-Evans procedure

Broström-Gould ankle instability operation

Browlift bone bridge system

brown
> B. dermatome
> b. fat tumor
> B. fibular transfer
> B. knee approach
> B. knee approach operation
> B. knee joint reconstruction
> B. lateral approach
> B. periosteotome
> B. 2-portal carpal tunnel release
> B. rasp
> B. technique
> B. tissue forceps
> b. tumor of hyperparathyroidism

Brown-Adson forceps

Brown-Cushing forceps

Browne splint

Brown-Mueller T-fastener set

Brown-Roberts-Wells (BRW)
> B.-R.-W. stereotactic frame

Brown-Séquard
> B.-S. lesion
> B.-S. syndrome (BSS)

Brucella **osteomyelitis**

brucellosis
> spinal b.

Bruce protocol

Bruck disease

Brudzinski
> B. reflex
> B. sign

Bruening chisel

Bruening-Citelli rongeur

Bruininks-Oseretsky Test of Motor Proficiency

bruisability

bruise
> bone b.
> reticular bone b.

Brunhilde strain

Brunner
> B. modified incision
> B. palmar incision
> B. rib shears

Brunn plaster shears

Brunnstrom-Fugl-Meyer (BFM)
> B.-F.-M. impairment assessment

Bruns
- B. ataxia
- B. bone curette
- B. gait apraxia Bruns syndrome

Brunswick-Mack rotating drill

Bruser
- B. knee approach
- B. lateral approach
- B. skin incision
- B. technique

brush
- b. border
- Cohort bone b.
- delta b.
- Plak-Vac oral suction b.
- b. test

brush-evoked pain testing

bruxism

BRW
- Brown-Roberts-Wells
- BRW head ring halo

Bryan
- B. arthroplasty
- B. procedure
- B. total knee implant prosthesis

Bryan-Morrey
- B.-M. elbow approach
- B.-M. extensive posterior approach
- B.-M. technique

Bryant
- B. line
- B. sign
- B. traction
- B. triangle

BSAP
- bone-specific alkaline phosphatase
- brief, small, abundant potential

BSAPP
- brief, small, abundant, polyphasic potential

BSS
- Brown-Séquard syndrome

BST-CarGel

BTE
- Baltimore Therapeutic Equipment
- BTE Assembly Tree
- BTE Bolt Box
- BTE dynamic lift

BTHI
- Brief Test of Head Injury

BUA
- bone ultrasound attenuation

bubbly bone lesion

buccinator
- b. muscle
- b. myomucosal flap

Buchanan disease

Buchholz
- B. acetabular cup
- B. prosthesis

buck
- B. bone curette
- B. convoluted traction apparatus
- B. convoluted traction device
- B. extension
- B. extension splint
- B. fascia
- B. femoral cement restrictor inserter
- B. knee brace
- B. method
- B. neurological hammer
- B. operation
- B. percussion hammer
- B. periosteal elevator
- B. plug
- B. Redi-Traction apparatus
- B. traction
- B. traction splint
- B. traction stockinette

bucket
- Denis Browne b.
- kick b.
- Lenox b.

bucket-handle
- b.-h. fracture
- b.-h. fragment
- b.-h. plica
- b.-h. rib
- b.-h. rib motion
- b.-h. tear

Buck-Gramcko
- B.-G. gouge
- B.-G. pollicization
- B.-G. technique

buckle
- b. fracture
- wire-fixation b.

Buckley chisel

buckling
- plantar b.
- reverse b.

Bucky
- B. diaphragm
- B. view
- B. x-ray tray

NOTES

B

Bucy-Frazier suction cannula
bud
>limb b.

buddy
>b. splint
>b. strap
>b. taping

BuddyWrap
>FoamWrap B.

Budge
>ciliospinal center of B.

Budin
>B. hammertoe splint
>B. joint
>B. toe splint

Budin-Chandler
>B.-C. anteversion determination
>B.-C. method

BUE
>both upper extremities
>BUE strength

Buechel-Pappas
>B.-P. total ankle
>B.-P. total ankle prosthesis
>B.-P. total ankle replacement
>B.-P. total ankle replacement system

Buerger-Allen exercise
buffalo hump
buffing sponge
Buffinol Extra
Buford complex
Bugg-Boyd technique
buggy
>cruiser b.
>Maclaren mobile b.

Buhl spirometer
Builder Grip hand exerciser
buildup
>Elevations shoe b.

bulb
>b. dynamometer
>irrigation b.
>b. neuroma
>b. suture
>b. and thumb screw valve

bulbar
>b. abnormality
>b. anesthesia
>b. necrosis

bulbocavernosus reflex
bulge
>disc b.

bulging disc
bulk
>b. flow axoplasmic transport
>b. graft

bulky hand dressing
bulla, pl. **bullae**
>hemorrhagic b.

bulldog
>b. clamp
>b. clamp applier
>b. clamp-applying forceps

bullet
>b. driver
>b. stretching

bullosa
>epidermolysis b.

Bullseye femoral guide
bull's eye shoulder
BuMelTT
>busulfan, melphalan, thiotepa

bump
>Haglund b.
>hip b.
>inion b.
>pump b.
>runner's b.

bumper
>axle lock and b.
>b. cast
>dorsiflexion b.
>flexion b.
>b. fracture
>b. wedge

Buncke
>B. technique
>B. transfer

bundle
>anterior oblique b.
>anteromedial b.
>b. bone
>cleidoepitrochlear b.
>b. dressing
>b. function
>interdigital nerve b.
>intermediate b.
>medial neurovascular b.
>b. nailing
>neurovascular b.
>posterolateral b.
>posteromedial b.
>superior gluteal neurovascular b.
>b. suture

bundle-nailing method
Bunge amputation
bungee effect
bunion
>b. complex
>b. deformity
>b. dissector
>dorsal b.
>b. formation
>juvenile b.

b. shield
tailor's b.
bunionectomy
Akin b.
Austin b.
Austin-Akin b.
b. capsular closure
chevron b.
closing wedge osteotomy b.
DuVries-Mann modified b.
Hauser b.
Hohmann b.
Joplin b.
Juvara b.
juvenile b.
Kalish b.
Kelikian modified Z b.
Keller b.
Kreuscher b.
Lapidus b.
Ludloff b.
Mann b.
Mau b.
Mayo b.
McBride b.
McKeever b.
Mitchell b.
modified Hohmann b.
modified Mau b.
modified McBride b.
modified Z b.
osteotomy b.
Reverdin b.
Reverdin-Green b.
Reverdin-Laird b.
Reverdin-McBride b.
scarf osteotomy b.
short Z b.
Silver b.
Stone b.
supratubercular wedge osteotomy b.
tailor's b.
tricorrectional b.
Wilson b.
Wu b.
Z b.
bunionette
b. deformity
b. excision
tailor's b.
bunionette-hallux valgus-splayfoot complex
bunion-hallux valgus complex

bunk
b. bed fracture
b. bed injury
Bunker footpiece
Bunnell
B. active hand and finger splint
B. anvil
B. atraumatic technique
B. bone drill
B. crisscross suture
B. digital exertion measurer
B. dissecting probe
B. dressing
B. figure-of-8 suture
B. finger extension splint
B. finger loop
B. forwarding probe
B. gutter splint
B. hand drill
B. knuckle bender
B. modification
B. modification of Steindler flexorplasty
B. opponensplasty
B. outrigger splint
B. posterior tibial tendon transfer
B. posterior tibial tendon transfer operation
B. pullout wire
B. reverse knuckle-bender splint
B. safety-pin splint
B. solution
B. stitch
B. technique of pulley reconstruction
B. tendon needle
B. tendon passer
B. tendon repair
B. tendon stripper
B. tendon suturing technique
B. tendon transfer technique
B. test
B. wire pull-out suture
B. zigzag fashion
Bunnell-Littler test
bunny
B. boot
B. boot foot splint
bur, burr
Adson enlarging b.
Adson perforating b.
air-driven b.
Albee olive-shaped b.

NOTES

bur *(continued)*
   arthroplasty b.
   Bailey b.
   ball b.
   barrel b.
   bone b.
   Borchardt olive-shaped b.
   carbide b.
   coarse carbide cone b.
   coarse-olive b.
   cone b.
   conical b.
   crosscut b.
   Cushing b.
   cutting b.
   cylindrical b.
   decortication b.
   dental b.
   D'Errico enlarging drill b.
   D'Errico perforating drill b.
   diamond b.
   3-in-1 diamond b.
   Doyen cylindrical b.
   Doyen spherical b.
   b. drill
   Dyonics arthroplasty b.
   enlarging b.
   Fantastic Burr nail b.
   fine olive b.
   finish b.
   fissure b.
   flame-tip b.
   Hall b.
   Happy podiatric b.
   high-speed b.
   high-torque b.
   b. hole
   Hudson bone b.
   Hudson brace with b.
   large-nail spicule b.
   Lindemann b.
   long coarse b.
   long-stemmed powered b.
   McKenzie enlarging b.
   medium carbide cone b.
   medium fine b.
   Midas Rex b.
   motorized b.
   nail b.
   new happy b.
   old smoothie b.
   olive-shaped b.
   orthopaedic b.
   paronychia b.
   pear b.
   perforating b.
   pilot b.
   podiatric b.
   Podi-Burr nail b.

   power b.
   right ankle b.
   Rosen b.
   Rotablator rotating b.
   rotary b.
   rotating b.
   round b.
   short coarse b.
   short fine b.
   side-cutting b.
   small nail spicule b.
   smoothie junior b.
   spherical b.
   Stille b.
   water-cooled power b.
   Zimmer rotary b.
Burch-Schneider antiprotrusio cage
bur-down technique
Burford-Finochietto rib spreader
Burford rib spreader
Burgess
   B. below-knee amputation
   B. technique
buried
   b. K-wire fixation
   b. K-wire fixation in digital fusion
Burke
   B. Bariatric bed
   B. test
Burkhalter
   B. modification of Stiles-Bunnell
     technique
   B. transfer technique
Burkhalter-Reyes
   B.-R. method
   B.-R. method phalangeal fracture
burn
   B. bench test
   b. boutonnière deformity
   b. contracture
   b. dressing
   irrigation b.
   mafenide acetate for b.
   plaster cast application b.
   b. syndactyly
burner
   b. injury
   B. phenomenon
Burnet clonal selection theory
Burnham
   B. finger splint
   B. thumb splint
   B. view
burning
   b. foot
   b. pain
   paroxysmal b.
burning-feet syndrome
burn-related pigmentation change

Burns
  B. disease
  B. ligament
  B. plate
Burns-Haney incision
Burow
  B. skin flap technique
  B. triangle
burr (*var. of* bur)
Burroughs solution
Burrows technique
bursa, pl. **bursae**
  Achilles tendon b.
  adventitious b.
  anserine b.
  Brodie b.
  calcaneal b.
  deltoid b.
  Fleischmann b.
  infrapatellar b.
  intermetatarsal b.
  intermetatarsophalangeal b.
  ischiogluteal b.
  Luschka b.
  Monro b.
  no-name, no-fame b.
  olecranon b.
  patellar b.
  pisiform b.
  pre-Achilles b.
  prepatellar b.
  radial b.
  radiohumeral b.
  retro-Achilles b.
  retrocalcaneal b.
  rider's b.
  sacral b.
  scapulohumeral b.
  subacromial b.
  subacromiodeltoid b.
  subdeltoid b.
  subtendinous iliac b.
  subtendinous prepatellar b.
  synovial b.
  trochanteric b.
  ulnar b.
  Voshell b.
bursal
  b. abscess
  b. cyst
  b. débridement
  b. flap
  b. fluid

  b. inflammation
  b. projection
  b. sac
  b. synovitis
  b. tissue
bursata
  exostosis b.
bursectomy
bursitis
  Achilles tendon b.
  anserine b.
  bicipital b.
  calcaneal b.
  calcific b.
  cubital b.
  Duplay b.
  gastrocnemius b.
  hip b.
  iliopectineal b.
  iliopsoas b.
  infracalcaneal b.
  infrapatellar b.
  intermetatarsal b.
  intermetatarsophalangeal b.
  intertubercular b.
  ischial b.
  ischiogluteal b.
  lateral premalleolar b.
  medial gastrocnemius b.
  olecranon b.
  patellar b.
  pelvic region b.
  pigmented villonodular b.
  postcalcaneal b.
  pre-Achilles b.
  premalleolar b.
  prepatellar b.
  pyogenic b.
  radiohumeral b.
  retrocalcaneal b.
  scapulothoracic b.
  semimembranosus b.
  septic b.
  subacromial b.
  subcalcaneal b.
  subdeltoid b.
  subgluteal b.
  subscapularis b.
  tarsal navicular b.
  tibial collateral ligament b.
  Tornwaldt b.
  trochanteric b.
  tuberculous trochanteric b.

B

NOTES

bursocentesis
bursography
    Mikasa subacromial b.
    subacromial b.
bursolith
bursopathy
bursotomy
burst
    b. fracture
    b. injury
    b. resistance fitness ball
bursting dislocation
burst-type laceration
Burton-Pelligrini excising trapezium
Burton sign
Burwell-Scott
    B.-S. modification
    B.-S. modification of Watson-Jones
      incision
Busenkell posterior hip retractor
bushing
    guide b.
    Uniflex drill b.
Busquet disease
busulfan, melphalan, thiotepa
  (BuMelTT)
butabarbital sodium
Butisol Sodium
Butler
    B. fifth toe operation
    B. procedure to correct overlapping
      toes
butterfly
    B. cushion
    B. cushion with strap
    b. flap
    b. fracture
    b. fracture fragment
    b. vertebra
butterfly-shaped monoblock vertebral
  plate
buttocks
    heart-shaped b.
    b. pad
button
    b. abscess
    Biomet b.
    Charnley suture b.

    collared b.
    Drummond b.
    Hewson ligament b.
    b. hook
    ligament b.
    padded b.
    patellar b.
    periosteal b.
    polyethylene b.
    pull-out b.
    b. sequestrum
    silastic b.
    B. Spacer
    subdural b.
    b. suture
    b. toe amputation
    Wisconsin b.
buttonhole
    b. deformity
    b. fracture
    b. rupture
buttress
    b. and button anchor
    b. pad
    b. pie plate
    b. pin
    pretibial b. (PTB)
    rotator cuff b. (RCB)
    b. thread screw
buttressed hook
buttressing
    b. in internal fixation
    b. procedure
buttress-type plate
butyrophenone
BVP
    blood volume pulse
Bx
    biopsy
Byars mandibular prosthesis
bypass
    dorsal pedal b.
    extended tibial in situ b.
    femoral above-knee popliteal b.
    femorodistal b.
    popliteus b.
    b. surgery

C

C angle
C knife
C sign
C Stance ankle
C washer
CA-5000 drill-guide isometer
CA-6000 spine motion analyzer
cable

antirotation c. (ARC)
cerclage c.
c. cerclage method
chrome-cobalt c.
Dall-Miles c.
Dwyer scoliosis c.
fiberoptic c.
Flex Ranger stretch c.
FlexStrand c.
Gallie fusion-using c.
Howmedica cerclage c.
interspinous c.
liquid c.
c. nerve graft
scoliosis correction with Dwyer c.
Songer c.
stretch c.
c. suspension system
c. tensioner
titanium c.
twister c.
cable-hook compression instrumentation
Cable-Ready cable grip system
cable-twister

c.-t. brace
c.-t. orthosis
cable/wire hole
Cabot

C. leg splint
C. posterior splint
Cacchione syndrome
cacomelia
CAD

coronary artery disease
CAD femoral stem prosthesis
cadaver

c. bone
c. bone graft
cadaveric

c. knee
c. specimen
CAD/CAM

computer-aided design/computer-aided
manufacturing
CAD/CAM prosthesis

caddy

SwingAlong walker c.
cadence of gait
Cadenza

C. girdle
C. panty
CAECS

chronic anterior exertional compartment
syndrome
café-au-lait spot
Caffey

C. disease
C. hyperostosis
C. syndrome
Caffey-Kenny disease
Caffey-Silverman syndrome
Caffinière trapeziometacarpal prosthesis
cage

antiprotrusio c.
BAK fusion c.
Brantigan interbody fusion c.
Burch-Schneider antiprotrusio c.
carbon-fiber-composite c.
carbon-fiber-reinforced c.
elastic knee c.
fusion c.
Harms c.
InterFix RP threaded spinal
fusion c.
InterFix titanium threaded spinal
fusion c.
Link acetabular c.
lumbar intersomatic fusion
expandable c. (LIFEC)
Moss c.
Novus LC threaded interbody
fusion c.
Novus LT titanium threaded
interbody fusion c.
osseocartilaginous thoracic c.
protrusio c.
Pyramesh c.
Ray TFC threaded fusion c.
rib c.
SL c.
stereolithography c.
Swedish knee c.
threaded fusion c. (TFC)
threaded spinal fusion c.
cage-back brace
CAH

Camber axis hinge
Cairns hemostatic forceps
Calandriello procedure

Calandruccio
- C. cemented hip prosthesis
- C. clamp
- C. external fixation system
- C. fixation
- C. II compression device
- C. impaction screw-plate
- C. nail
- C. side plate
- C. technique
- C. triangular compression apparatus
- C. triangular compression fixation device

Calcanea fracture plate
calcaneal
- c. apophysitis
- c. avulsion fracture
- c. axial view
- c. bone
- c. bone graft
- c. bone plug
- c. branch
- c. bursa
- c. bursitis
- c. compartment pressure measurement
- c. displaced fracture
- c. distraction
- c. facet
- c. fat pad
- c. fracture reduction
- c. fracture (type I–III)
- c. gait
- c. gait pattern
- c. inclination angle
- c. L osteotomy
- c. malunion
- c. neck lengthening
- c. nerve
- c. pin
- c. pin traction
- c. pitch
- c. pitch angle (CPA)
- c. pseudocyst
- c. region
- c. resection
- c. sliding corrective osteotomy
- c. spreader
- c. spur
- c. spur cookie orthosis
- c. spur pad in shoe
- c. spur syndrome
- c. stance
- c. sulcus
- c. tendon
- c. tenodesis
- c. tuberosity
- c. valgus

- c. varus
- c. Y plate

calcaneal-second metatarsal angle
calcanectomy
calcanei (*pl. of* calcaneus)
calcaneoapophysitis
calcaneoastragaloid ligament
calcaneocavovarus deformity
calcaneocavus
- c. deformity
- c. foot
- talipes c.

calcaneoclavicular ligament
calcaneocuboid (CC)
- c. articulation
- c. bone
- c. coalition
- c. distraction arthrodesis (CCDA)
- dorsal c. (DCC)
- c. joint
- c. joint arthritis
- c. joint nutcracker injury
- c. ligament
- long c. (LCC)
- short c. (SCC)
- c. subluxation

calcaneocuboideum
- ligamentum c.

calcaneodynia
calcaneofibular
- c. abutment
- c. ligament (CFL)
- c. sprain

calcaneonavicular
- c. articulation
- c. bar
- c. bar resection
- c. bar section
- c. coalition
- c. joint
- c. joint arthroscopy
- c. ligament
- c. ligament-tibialis posterior tendon advancement

calcaneopelvic arthrodesis
calcaneoplantar angle
calcaneoscaphoid
calcaneotibial
- c. angle
- c. arthrodesis
- c. fusion
- c. ligament

calcaneovalgocavus
calcaneovalgus
- c. deformity
- c. flatfoot
- c. foot
- talipes c.

calcaneovarus
    c. deformity
    talipes c.
calcaneus, pl. **calcanei**
    accessory ossification center of c.
    c. alignment
    c. apophysis
    c. deformity
    displaced intraarticular c.
    distal c.
    c. excursion
    pes c.
    sulcus calcanei
    talipes c.
    tendo c.
    c. tongue fracture
    tuberosity of c.
calcanodynia
calcar
    c. collar
    c. femorale development
    c. pedis
    pivot of c.
    c. pivot
    c. planer
    c. reamer
    c. replacement
    c. replacement femoral prosthesis
    c. replacement stem
Cal Carb-HD
calcareous deposit
calcidiol test
Calciferol
    C. Injection
    C. Oral
calcific
    c. bursitis
    c. density
    c. deposit
    c. spur
    c. tendinitis
    c. tendinosis
calcificans
    chondrodystrophia c.
calcification
    Achilles tendon enthesis c.
    central c.
    eggshell-like c.
    falx c.
    c. of falx
    flocculent focus of c.
    focal c.
    heterotopic c.

    juvenile intervertebral disc c.
    (JIDC)
    paraarticular c.
    periarticular c.
    provisional c.
    soft tissue c.
    supraspinatus c.
calcified
    c. cartilage
    c. osteoid
calcify
calcifying aponeurotic fibroma
Calcimar Injection
calcinosis
    c. circumscripta
    c., Raynaud, esophageal motility
    disorders, sclerodactyly,
    telangiectasia (CREST)
    tumoral c.
calciphylaxis
Calcitite
    C. graft
    C. graft material
calcitriol
calcium
    c. alginate dressing
    c. carbonate
    c. carbonate bone replacement graft
    c. carbonate graft material
    c. channel blocker
    c. deposit
    c. glubionate
    c. gout
    c. hydroxyapatite (CHA)
    c. hydroxyapatite crystal
    c. hydroxyapatite crystal deposition
    disease
    c. hydroxyapatite pellet
    c. lactate
    c. oxalate deposition
    c. phosphate
    c. phosphate ceramic
    c. phosphate, dibasic
    c. pyrophosphate dihydrate
    deposition (CPPD)
    c. pyrophosphate dihydrate
    deposition disease
    serum c.
    c. sulfate bone graft barrier
    c. sulfate ceramic
calcodynia
calculus, pl. **calculi**
    branched c.

C

NOTES

calculus *(continued)*
    hemic c.
    staghorn c.
Caldani ligament
Caldesene Topical
Caldwell hanging cast
calf, pl. **calves**
    c. band
    c. bone dowel
    c. circumference
    football c.
    gnome's c.
    c. hypertension
    c. raise back exercise
    c. shell
    c. squeeze test
calibrated
    c. clubfoot splint
    c. guidepin
    c. guide wire
    c. monofilament
    c. pin
    c. pin guide
    c. probe
calibration curve
calibrator
    screw depth c.
California
    C. soft spinal system (CASS)
    C. welt construction
Caligamed
    C. ankle orthosis
    C. brace
caliper
    anthropometric c.
    blunt c.
    c. brace
    Digimatic c.
    digital c.
    Harpenden c.
    Lafayette skinfold c.
    Lange skinfold c.
    Mitutoyo digital c.
    c. orthosis
    c. rib movement
    skinfold c.
    Thomas walking c.
    Townley femur c.
    Vernier c.
    weight-relieving c.
Callahan
    C. extension
    C. extension of cervical injury
    C. fusion technique
    C. method
    C. and Scuderi approach
Callander amputation
Callaway test
Calleja exercise

Callender
    C. derotational brace
    C. technique hip prosthesis
callosal lesion
callosity
    metatarsal c.
    plantar c.
    shearing c.
callotasis
callous
    c. bone union
    c. formation
callus
    bone c.
    bridging c.
    central c.
    definitive c.
    c. distraction
    c. distraction procedure
    elephant-foot c.
    ensheathing c.
    florid c.
    fracture c.
    horse's foot c.
    intermediate c.
    irritation c.
    c. massage
    medullary c.
    myelogenous c.
    nail groove c.
    permanent c.
    pinch c.
    provisional c.
    shearing c.
    temporary c.
    c. weld
Calmette-Guérin
    bacille C.-G. (BCG)
Calnan-Nicolle
    C.-N. finger implant
    C.-N. finger prosthesis
    C.-N. metatarsophalangeal prosthesis
    C.-N. synthetic joint prosthesis
calor
calvarial
    c. free bone
    c. free bone graft
Calvé disease
Calvé-Legg-Perthes syndrome
Calvé-Perthes disease
calves (*pl. of* calf)
Calypso lift
CAM
    Cognitive Assessment of Minnesota
    complimentary and alternative medicine
    computer-assisted myelography
    controlled ankle motion
    CAM Lock knee joint
    CAM Walker ankle brace

CAM Walker ankle walker
CAM Walker II
CAM Walker leg brace
Cama Arthritis Pain Reliever
Camber axis hinge (CAH)
cambium layer
camelback sign
camera
DyoCam 550 arthroscopic video c.
DyoCam arthroscopic view c.
Endius spinal endoscopic c.
gamma c.
Saticon tube c.
Sony CCD/RGB DXC-151 color video c.
Stryker c.
Vidicon vacuum chamber pickup tube for video c.
Cameron
C. femoral component removal
C. fracture apparatus
C. fracture device
Camino catheter technique
Camitz
C. opponensplasty
C. technique
C. tendon transfer
camouflage prosthesis
camp
C. brace
C. corset
C. Diversity arthritis program
Campbell
C. ankle operation
C. ankle procedure
C. cannulated screw
C. corset
C. elbow approach
C. gouge
C. interpositional arthroplasty
C. ligament
C. nerve root retractor
C. onlay bone graft
C. osteotome
C. periosteal elevator
C. posterior arthrodesis
C. posterior bone block
C. posterior shoulder approach
C. posterolateral approach
C. reamer
C. resection arthroplasty
C. rongeur
C. screw fixation

C. technique
C. tibial osteotomy
C. traction splint
C. transfer
C. triceps reflection
Campbell-Akbarnia arthrodesis
Campbell-Rinehard-Kalenak anterior arthrodesis
camper
C. chiasma
C. fascia
camphor and phenol
camplodactyly
camptocormia
camptodactyly
camptomelia
camptomelic dwarfism
camptospasm
CamStar
C. exercise machine
C. power leg press
Camurati-Engelmann disease
Canadian
C. Academy of Sports Medicine emergency kit
C. crutch
C. hip disarticulation prosthesis
C. Knee Orthosis
C. Occupational Performance Measure (COPM)
Canakis beaded hip pin
canal
Alcock c.
bony semicircular c.
carpal c.
cartilage c.
central c.
cerebrospinal c.
cervical c.
Civinini c.
cortical bone primary c.
Dorello c.
Dupuytren c.
femoral medullary c.
c. finder
Guyon c.
haversian c.
humeral c.
Hunter c.
hydrops c.
iliac c.
c. innominate osteotomy
intersacral c.

NOTES

canal *(continued)*
intramedullary c.
lumbar c.
marrow c.
medullary c.
narrowing of spinal c.
Richet tibial-astragalocalcaneal c.
sacral c.
spinal cord c.
talar c.
tarsal c.
tibial medullary c.
tight spinal canal trefoil c.
vertebral c.
Volkmann c.

Canale
C. osteotomy
C. technique
C. view

Canale-Kelly
C.-K. talar neck fracture
C.-K. talar neck fracture
classification
C.-K. view

canaliculus, pl. **canaliculi**
canal-to-calcar isthmus ratio
Can Am brace
Canavan disease
Canavan-van Bogaert-Bertrand disease
cancellated bone
cancellectomy
cancellous
c. bone carrier
c. bone screw
c. bone surface
c. chip
c. chip bone graft
c. insert
c. insert graft
c. morselized bone graft
c. non-load-bearing bone fracture
c. pin
c. screw thread
c. versus cortical bone

cancer treatment-related lymphedema
Candela SPTL laser
Candida onychomycosis
candle
c. flame appearance
c. wax appearance
c. wax appearance of bone

Can-Do exercise band
cane
adjustable c.
broad-based c.
Double Duty c.
English c.
glider c.
MAFO c.

offset c.
quad c.
single-point c.
small-base quad c.
Thera c.
tripod c.

Canfield shoe
canister
Autovac autotransfusion c.

cannon
c. bone
C. Law of Denervation
Supersensitivity

cannula
Acufex double-lumen
arthroscopic c.
arthroscopic c.
Bergstrom c.
biopsy c.
blunt arthroscopic c.
Bucy-Frazier suction c.
Concept c.
Dyonics c.
Endotrac c.
Eriksson muscle biopsy c.
inflow c.
large-bore inflow c.
large egress c.
McCain TMJ c.
microirrigating c.
outflow c.
self-sealing c.
small egress c.
suction c.
suprapatellar c.
c. system
Teflon c.
zone-specific c.

cannulated
c. bolt
c. bone screw
c. cancellous lag screw
c. cortical step drill
c. drill
c. drill bit
c. drill point
c. expulsion piston
c. guided hip screw system
c. hip screw
c. nail
C. Plus screw system
c. reaming technique
c. screwdriver
c. wrench

cannulation
unilateral pedicle c.

canted finger hook
Cantharone

cantilever
    c. bending
    c. external fixator
canvas brace
CAOS
    computer-assisted orthopaedic surgery
caoutchouc pelvis
cap
    acetabular c.
    C.'s ArthroWand
    C.'s ArthroWand device
    Carnation corn c.'s
    cartilaginous c.
    Cloward drill guard c.
    digit c.
    egg-shaped c.
    flexor c.
    nerve c.
    offset c.
    plaster toe c.
    plastic end c.
    Silipos mesh c.
    c. splint
    toe c.
    Zang metatarsal c.
    Zimmer tibial nail c.
capacitive
    c. coupling
    c. sensor
capacity
    aerobic c.
    exercise c.
    forced vital c.
    physical work c. (PWC)
cap-and-anchor plate
Caparosa wire crimper
CAPE
    Children's Assessment of Participation
    and Enjoyment
    Clifton Assessment Procedures for the
    Elderly
    continuous anatomical passive exerciser
capeline bandage
Capello
    C. press-fit prosthesis
    C. slim-line abduction pillow
    C. technique
    C. total hip replacement
Capener
    C. brace
    C. coil splint
    C. finger splint

    C. gouge
    C. lateral rhachotomy
capillary
    c. filling time (CFT)
    c. fracture
    c. hemangioma
    c. ischemia
    c. refill
    c. refill, sensation, motor function,
    temperature (CSMT)
    c. refill time
capital
    C. and Codeine
    c. crescentic shelf osteotomy
    c. epiphysial angle
    c. epiphysis (CE)
    c. femoral epiphysis
    c. fragment
    c. ligament
capitate bone
capitate-hamate joint
capitate-lunate
    c.-l. instability
    c.-l. joint
capitellar
    c. fracture
    c. osteochondritis
capitellocondylar
    c. total elbow arthroplasty
    c. unconstrained elbow prosthesis
capitellum
    Hahn-Steinthal fracture of c.
    Kocher-Lorenz fracture of c.
capitolunate angle
capitular
    c. epiphysis
    c. process
capitulum fracture
Caplan
    C. Indented Paragraph Test
    C. syndrome
Capner gouge
capped elbow
caprolactam suture
Caprosyn suture
**Capset calcium sulfate bone graft
barrier**
capsular
    c. adhesion
    c. ankylosis
    c. attachment
    c. deficiency
    c. flap

C

NOTES

capsular *(continued)*
 c. imbrication
 c. imbrication procedure
 c. incision
 c. interposition arthroplasty
 c. layer
 c. length insufficiency
 c. ligament
 c. plication
 c. reconstruction
 c. reefing
 c. release
 c. shift
 c. shift procedure
 c. strap
 c. support tissue
capsular-ligamentous tension
capsular-shift reconstruction
capsule
 anterior c.
 anterolateral c.
 anteromedial c.
 apophysial joint c.
 articular c.
 dorsal c.
 elbow c.
 facet c.
 fibrous c.
 c. formation
 Gerota c.
 joint c.
 medial talonavicular c.
 meniscofemoral c.
 meniscotibial c.
 metatarsophalangeal joint c.
 midlateral c.
 midmedial c.
 peripheral c.
 plantar c.
 posterior c.
 posterolateral c.
 posteromedial c.
 c. repair
 suprasellar c.
 talonavicular c.
 trapeziometacarpal c.
 volar c.
 wrist c.
capsulectomy
 anterior c.
 circumferential c.
 silhouette c.
capsulitis
 adhesive c.
 dorsal carpal c.
 glenohumeral adhesive c.
capsulodesis
 Berger c.
 Blatt c.

 bleb c.
 dorsal c.
 intercarpal ligament c.
 Zancolli flexion c.
capsulolabral
 c. complex
 c. repair
capsuloligamentous
 c. complex
 c. mechanism
 c. system
 c. tissue
capsuloperiosteal
 c. envelope
 c. flap
capsuloplasty
 Zancolli c.
capsuloputaminal infarction
capsuloputaminocaudate infarction
capsulorrhaphy
 Boyd-Sisk posterior c.
 electrothermally assisted c. (ETAC)
 laser-assisted c.
 medial c.
 open-staple c.
 pants-over-vest c.
 posterior c.
 Rockwood posterior c.
 Roux-duToit staple c.
 staple c.
 c. staple
 thermal c.
 Tibone posterior c.
capsulotomy
 anterior c.
 Curtis PIP joint c.
 dorsal transverse c.
 dorsolateral and medial c.
 dorsoplantar c.
 hourglass c.
 linear c.
 L-shaped c.
 medial V-Y c.
 metatarsophalangeal c.
 posterior c.
 stereotaxic anterior c.
 subtalar c.
 talonavicular c.
 transmetatarsal c.
 transverse c.
 T-shaped c.
 V c.
 vertical c.
CAPSure ArthroWand
CAQ
 Clinical Analysis Questionnaire
Carabelt
 C. lower back support
 C. therapeutic belt

Cara Klenz cleansing agent
carbide bur
CarboFlex odor-control dressing
carbohydrate oxidation
CarboJet lavage
carbol-fuchsin solution
carbolic acid
carbon
    C. Copy high performance foot
      prosthesis
    C. Copy HP foot prosthesis
    C. Copy II foot prosthesis
    C. Copy II Light Foot
    C. Copy II Light prosthesis
    c. dioxide laser
    c. fiber fixator
    c. fiber graft
    c. fiber half ring
    c. fiber lamination braid (CFLB)
    c. fiber-reinforced plate
    c. fiber-reinforced polyethylene
    c. implant
    c. Monotube long bone fracture
      external fixation system
    pyrolytic c. (PyC)
    c. steel drill point
carbon-based biomaterial
carbon-fiber-composite cage
carbon-fiber-reinforced cage
carbon-tungsten rasp
CarbonX active heel
Carboplast
    C. II composite
    C. II sheeting
    C. II sheet orthotic material
Carborundum grinding wheel
Carceau-Brahms ankle arthrodesis
carcinoembryonic antigen (CEA)
carcinogen
    chemical c.
carcinoma
    clear cell c.
    joint verrucous c.
carcinomatous myopathy
Carcon stent
Carden amputation
cardiac
    c. output
    c. precautions
cardinal axes (X, Y, Z)
cardioboxing
CardioKarate
CardioKickboxing

cardiomyopathy
    dilated c.
    hypertrophic c.
    nonspecific c.
    right ventricular c.
Cardona keratoprosthesis prosthesis
care
    corrective spinal c.
    Miami Acute C. (MAC)
    palliative c.
    postoperative wound c.
    rehabilitation c.
Caregiver Strain Index (CSI)
Carex ambulatory aid
car hand control
caries sicca
carinatum
    pectus c.
carisoprodol, aspirin, and codeine
Carleton spot
Carl P. Jones traction splint
C-arm
    C-a. fluoroscope
    C-a. fluoroscopy
    C-a. fluoroscopy unit
    C-a. image intensifier
Carman meniscus sign
Carmody perforator drill
Carnation corn caps
Carnesale
    C. acetabular extensile approach
    C. hip approach
    C. hip approach operation
    C. technique
Carnesale-Stewart-Barnes classification of
  hip dislocation
Carolina rocker
Carolon AFO sock
carotid
    c. artery
    c. artery compression
    c. sheath
    c. vein
carpal
    c. arc
    c. arch
    c. articulation
    c. bone
    c. bone fracture ankylosis
    c. bone stress fracture
    c. boss
    c. canal
    C. Care carpal tunnel exerciser

C

NOTES

carpal *(continued)*
- C. Care exercise
- C. Care rehabilitative program
- c. coalition
- c. compression test
- c. dislocation
- c. height ratio
- c. instability
- c. instability, dissociative (CID)
- c. instability, nondissociative (CIND)
- c. ligament
- C. Lock cock-up splint
- C. Lock CTS brace
- C. Lock wrist brace
- C. Lock wrist splint
- c. lunate implant prosthesis
- c. navicular fracture
- c. pedal spasm
- c. row
- c. scaphoid
- c. scaphoid bone fracture
- c. scaphoid implant prosthesis
- c. scaphoid screw
- c. sulcus
- c. synovectomy
- C. Trac traction
- C. Trac traction device
- c. tunnel (CT)
- c. tunnel decompression (CTD)
- c. tunnel glove
- c. tunnel release (CTR)
- c. tunnel stretch
- C. Tunnel Stretch exerciser
- c. tunnel surgery relief kit
- c. tunnel syndrome (CTS)
- c. tunnel syndrome injection therapy
- c. tunnel view

carpal-intercarpal joint
Carpal-Lock wrist support
carpal-metacarpal
carpectomy
- distal row c.
- Omer-Capen c.
- proximal row c.

carpenter
- c. brace
- c. knee
- C. syndrome

carpet layer's knee
carpi *(pl. of carpus)*
carpometacarpal (CMC)
- c. arthroplasty
- c. articulation
- c. boss
- c. fracture-dislocation
- c. joint
- c. joint dislocation
- c. joint fracture
- c. joint radiography
- c. ligament

carpophalangeal joint
carporadial articulation
carposcope
carprofen
carpus, pl. **carpi**
- complex instability of c. (CIC)
- c. curvus
- carpi radialis brevis tendon
- carpi radialis longus tendon

Carrel
- C. method
- C. patch
- C. suture
- C. treatment

Carrell
- C. fibular substitution
- C. fibular substitution technique
- C. resection

Carrell-Girard screw
Carrie car seat
carrier
- cancellous bone c.
- clamp c.
- double-headed stereotactic c.
- Finochietto clamp c.
- ligature c.
- Miya hook ligature c.
- Yasargil ligature c.

Carrington Dermal wound gel
Carroll
- C. approach
- C. arthrodesis
- C. bone-holding forceps
- C. dressing forceps
- C. hand retractor
- C. periosteal elevator
- C. skin hook
- C. and Taber arthroplasty
- C. tendon-pulling forceps
- C. tendon retriever
- C. test
- C. tissue forceps

Carroll-Bennett retractor
Carroll-Bunnell drill
Carroll-Legg periosteal elevator
Carr-Purcell-Meiboom-Gill sequence
Carr-Purcell sequence
carrying
- c. angle
- c. angle of forearm

Carstan reverse wedge osteotomy
cart
- Harloff c.

Cartam-Treander reverse wedge osteotomy

Carter
- C. elevation pillow
- C. foam pillow
- C. immobilization cushion
- C. mycetoma
- C. Rowe awl
- C. splint

Carter-Rowe
- C.-R. shoulder score
- C.-R. view

Carter-Wilkinson criteria for hypermobility syndrome

cartilage
- c. ablation
- c. abrader
- accessory c.
- alar c.
- anular c.
- arthrodial c.
- articular c.
- arytenoid c.
- c. autograft
- basilar c.
- calcified c.
- c. canal
- c. cell
- circumferential c.
- c. clamp
- condylar c.
- connecting c.
- costal c.
- cricoid c.
- cryopreserved c.
- degenerated c.
- diarthrodial c.
- eburnation of c.
- elastic c.
- c. elastic pullover kneecap splint
- ensiform c.
- falciform c.
- fibroelastic c.
- fibrous c.
- floating c.
- c. forceps
- free flap of c.
- glenoid c.
- c. graft
- c. healing
- hyaline c.
- c. hypertrophy
- c. implant
- interarticular c.
- interosseous c.
- intervertebral c.
- c. knife
- c. lacuna
- loose c.
- nonossified tarsal navicular c.
- c. oligomeric matrix protein (COMP)
- patellofemoral groove c.
- physial c.
- pitted c.
- quadrangular c.
- roughened c.
- c. scissors
- scored c.
- semilunar c.
- c. shaver blade
- shelling off of c.
- slipping rib c.
- c. space
- c. stripper
- c. synovium
- tendon c.
- thyroid c.
- triradial c.
- triradiate c.
- c. volume
- yellow c.

cartilage-hair hypoplasia (CHH)

cartilaginous
- c. anlage
- c. bar
- c. cap
- c. cap of phalangeal head
- c. coalition
- c. degeneration
- c. disc
- c. fragment
- c. glenoid labrum
- c. growth plate
- c. hallux limitus
- c. hamartoma
- c. hypertrophy
- c. joint
- c. lesion
- c. loose body
- c. metaplasia
- c. navicular
- c. ossification
- c. ring
- c. spur
- c. tissue
- c. tumor

cartwheel fracture

NOTES

Cartwright implant
cascade
    clotting c.
    C. Up and About system
Cascading Tower Technology
Casey pelvic clamp
CASH
    cruciform anterior spinal hyperextension
    CASH brace
    CASH thoracolumbosacral orthosis
CASP
    Child and Adolescent Social Perception
      Measure
    contoured anterior spinal plate
Caspar
    C. alligator forceps
    C. anterior cervical plating
      technique
    C. anterior instrumentation
    C. blade
    C. cervical plate
    C. cervical screw
    C. retractor
Caspari
    C. arthroscopic portal
    C. repair
    C. shuttle
    C. suture punch
CASS
    California soft spinal system
Casselberry suture punch
casserian muscle
Casser perforated muscle
cast
    above-elbow c.
    accessory navicular c.
    airplane c.
    c. application
    arm cylinder c.
    banjo c.
    Batchelor plaster hip spica c.
    below-knee walking c.
    c. belt
    c. bender
    bent-knee c.
    Bermuda spica c.
    bivalved cylinder c.
    bivalved pancake plaster hand c.
    c. blade
    blood c.
    Body Armor walker c.
    body jacket c.
    Böhler skintight c.
    c. boot
    C. Boot polypropylene hip
      abduction brace
    Boston bivalve c.
    c. bracing
    c. breaker

broomstick c.
bumper c.
Caldwell hanging c.
circular c.
Comfort C.
corrective c.
Cotrel scoliosis c.
cotton c.
c. cover
C. Cozy
C. Cozy toe covering
c. cushion
Cutter c.
c. cutter
cylinder walking c.
double hip spica c.
EDF scoliosis c.
elbow c.
Equalizer short leg walking c.
c. equipped with rubber pedestal
extension body c.
fiberglass c.
figure-of-8 c.
3-finger spica c.
flexion body c.
full thumb spica c.
gaiter c.
C. Gard cast protector
gauntlet c.
gel c.
Gelocast c.
gravity equinus c.
groin-to-ankle c.
gutter c.
Gypsona c.
halo c.
handshake c.
hanging arm c.
Hexcelite c.
hinged cylinder c.
hip spica c.
hyperextension c.
c. immobilization
c. immobilizer
inhibitive c.
intermediate c.
intern's triangle in hip spica c.
Jones compression c.
Kite clubfoot c.
Kite metatarsal c.
c. knife
leg walking c.
light c.
c. liner
localizer c.
long arm c. (LAC)
long arm finger c.
long bent-knee leg c.
long leg c. (LLC)

long leg walking c. (LLWC)
long leg weightbearing c.
  (LLWBC)
Lorenz c.
Lovell clubfoot c.
medial malleolus c.
3M fiberglass c.
Minerva c.
modified Cotrel c.
Moe modified Cotrel c.
Mooney c.
Munster c.
negative impression c.
Neufeld c.
nonwalking c.
O'Donoghue cotton c.
one-half spica c.
one and one-half spica c.
onlay bone graft c.
Orfizip knee c.
Orfizip wrist c.
Orthoplast slipper c.
outrigger c.
c. padding
pantaloon spica c.
pantaloon walking c.
patellar dislocation c.
patellar tendon weightbearing c.
petaling the c.
Petrie spica c.
plaster of Paris c.
plastic c.
3-point pressure c.
polyurethane c.
pontoon spica c.
POP c.
PTB c.
quadriceps femoris muscle c.
Quengel c.
removable c.
c. removal
rigid below-knee c.
Risser localizer scoliosis c.
Risser turnbuckle c.
Sarmiento short leg patellar
  tendon-bearing c.
Sbarbaro spica c.
Schmeisser spica c.
scoliosis c.
semirigid fiberglass c. (SRF)
serial wedge c.
c. shoe
short arm c. (SAC)

short arm fiberglass c.
short arm gauntlet c.
short arm navicular c. (SANC)
short leg c. (SLC)
short leg plaster c.
short leg walking c. (SLWC)
short walking c.
shoulder spica c.
single-leg spica c.
skin-tight c.
slipper c.
c. sock
spica c.
SP Walker c.
sugar-tong c.
c. syndrome
c. table
c. tape
thumb spica c.
toe spica c.
toe-to-groin c.
toe-to-midthigh c.
tone-inhibiting leg c.
total contact c.
traction c.
turnbuckle c.
underarm c.
univalve c.
Unna boot c.
Velpeau c.
c. walker
walking boot c.
warm-and-form c.
c. wedge
wedging c.
well-leg c.
c. window
windowed c.
c. with dorsal toe plate extension
c. with volar toe plate extension
zipper c.
castaway
  C. ankle walker
  C. leg brace
  C. leg walker
Castech extremity support
Castellani paint
Castiglia ankle brace
casting
  foam c.
  intermittent c.
  negative c.
  postoperative c.

NOTES

123

casting *(continued)*
    c. process
    serial c.
    total contact c. (TCC)
Castle procedure
Castle-Schneider resection interposition arthroplasty
Castroviejo
    C. bladebreaker knife
    C. needle holder
    C. trephine
CAT
    computerized axial tomography
Cataflam Oral
Catagni criteria
Catalyn vitamin
Catalyst anterior instrument set
catapophysis
catastrophic deterioration
cat-back
    rachitic c.-b.
CAT-CAM
    contoured adduction trochanteric-controlled alignment method
catch and clunk test
catching sensation
catch-up clunk
category
    functional ambulation c. (FAC)
    Rehabilitation Impairment C. (RIC)
    Risser c.
    Westin-Turco c.
Catera suture anchor
Cateye
    C. Ergociser
    C. T220 treadmill
Cathcart Orthocentric hip prosthesis
cathepsin
catheter
    Abramson c.
    condom c.
    c. entrapment
    c. kinking
    Mentor Self-Cath soft c.
    Simpson arthrectomy c.
    tracer c.
    wicking c.
cathode
Catlin amputating knife
Caton method
Cat's Paw exerciser
Catterall
    C. classification
    C. hip score
cauda
    c. equina
    c. equina compression
    c. equina syndrome
caudad anterior mold

caudal
    c. lamina resection
    c. retinaculum
    c. spinal agenesis
    c. translation
    c. vertebra
caudalward
caudocephalad
caudocranial
causalgia
causalgic pain
cauterization
    alcohol c.
    bipolar c.
    Bovie c.
    phenol c.
    unipolar c.
cautery
    Aesculap bipolar c.
    BICAP c.
    bipolar c.
    Bovie c.
    chemical c.
    Concept handheld c.
    Hotsy C.
    intraarticular c.
    Mira c.
    monopolar c.
    slow c.
    unipolar c.
cavalry bone
cavalryman's osteoma
cave
    C. hip approach
    C. knee approach
    C. operation
cavern chordoma
cavernous
    c. hemangioma
    c. lymphangioma
Cavin osteotome
cavitary
    c. defect
    c. deficiency
    glenoid c.
cavitation
    joint c.
    manual c.
Cavitron ultrasonic surgical aspirator
cavity
    absorption c.
    bone c.
    c. cavity
    cotyloid c.
    glenoid c.
    idiopathic bone c.
    joint c.
    marrow c.
    Meckel c.

medullary c.
saclike c.
synovial c.
cavoequinovarus
cavovalgus
pes c.
talipes c.
cavovarus
c. deformity
c. foot
pes c.
talipes c.
cavus
anterior c.
combined c.
c. foot
c. foot deformity
c. foot support
forefoot c.
global c.
hindfoot c.
lesser tarsus c.
local c.
metatarsus c.
midfoot c.
pes c.
posttraumatic c.
c. posture
pronated pes c.
rigid foot c.
talipes c.
CAWO
closing abductory-wedge osteotomy
CB
contrast bath
C-bar orthosis
CBCL
Child Behavior Checklist
CBI
Child Behaviors Inventory of Playfulness
CBP
chiropractic biophysics
CBP technique
CBWO
closed base wedge osteotomy
CC
calcaneocuboid
coracoclavicular
CC joint
CC ligament
CC Rider closed-chain rehabilitation
system

CCD
central collodiaphysial
CCD angle
CCDA
calcaneocuboid distraction arthrodesis
CCF
compound comminuted fracture
C-clamp
Fukushima C-c.
CCN
cervical cord neurapraxia
CCPQ
Children's Comprehensive Pain
Questionnaire
CCS
chronic compartment syndrome
CCTA
coronal computed tomographic
arthrography
C-D
Cotrel-Dubousset
C-D fixation device
C-D hook
C-D instrumentation
C-D instrumentation device
C-D instrumentation fixation
strength
C-D instrumentation rigidity
C-D rod insertion
C-D screw modification
CD
CD Horizon M8 multiaxial screw
CD Horizon Sextant System
CDH
congenital dislocation of hip
congenital dysplasia of hip
CDH cup inserter
CDH Precoat Plus hip prosthesis
CDP
computerized dynamic posturography
CE
capital epiphysis
CE angle
CEA
carcinoembryonic antigen
Cebotome
C. bone cement drill
C. osteotome
Cedell fracture
**Cedell-Magnusson classification of
arthritis on x-ray**
cefamandole
Ceftin Oral

NOTES

Celestone Soluspan
cell
  anterior horn c.
  cartilage c.
  chondrosarcoma c.
  c. cushion
  dorsal horn c.
  endothelial c.
  mesenchymal c.
  osteoclastic giant c.
  osteogenic c.
  osteoprogenitor c.
  Schwann c.
  squamous c.
  synovial stromal c.
  c. therapy
cell-mediated immunity
cellular
  c. immunity
  c. level response
  c. periosteal osteocartilaginous mass
  c. response to implant material
  c. schwannoma
cellulitis
  aerobic c.
  anaerobic c.
celluloid implant material
cellulose
  c. hemostatic agent
  Oxycel oxidized c.
CEM
  central extensor mechanism
cement
  acrylic bone c.
  antibiotic-loaded acrylic c.
  arthroplasty c.
  BA bone c.
  bioactive bone c.
  biodegradable calcium phosphate c.
  bone c.
  Boneloc c.
  BoneSource hydroxyapatite c.
  c. centralizer
  centrifugation of c.
  CMW bone c.
  c. compactor
  c. curette
  DePuy CMW 1 bone c.
  c. disease
  doughy c.
  Duall 88 c.
  c. eater
  Endurance bone c.
  excess c.
  Howmedica c.
  hydroxyapatite-coated porous
    alumni c.
  Implast bone c.
  c. injection gun

  c. interface
  Ketac c.
  key the c.
  KyphX HV-R bone c.
  c. line
  low-viscosity bone c.
  c. mantle
  c. mantle grade classification
  master c.
  medium-viscosity c.
  methyl methacrylate c.
  Norian SRS c.
  Orthocomp c.
  orthopaedic c.
  Orthoset radiopaque bone c.
  Osteobond copolymer bone c.
  Palacos radiopaque bone c.
  Palacos R bone c.
  c. patty
  c. plug
  PMMA bone c.
  polymerization of bone c.
  polymethyl methacrylate bone c.
  pressurized c.
  Pronto c.
  prosthetic antibiotic-loaded
    acrylic c. (PROSTALAC)
  Protoplast c.
  c. pump
  radiopaque bone c.
  c. removal
  removal of excess c.
  residual c.
  c. restrictor
  c. restrictor inserter
  Simplex P bone c.
  c. spacer inserter
  c. spatula
  SRS injectable c.
  surface c.
  Surgical Simplex P radiopaque
    bone c.
  c. syringe
  VersaBond medium-viscosity
    bone c.
  Zimmer bone c.
  Zimmer low-viscosity c.
cemental fracture
cementation
cement-bone interface
cemented
  c. broach
  c. component
  c. hip prosthesis
  c. total hip arthroplasty
cementing fibroma
cementless
  c. broach
  c. disease

c. femoral component
c. fixation
c. prosthesis
c. Sportono (CLS)
c. surface replacement arthroplasty (CSRA)
c. technique
c. total hip arthroplasty
c. total hip replacement

cementome
Anspach c.

cementophyte
cement-removal hand chisel
cement-wedge sign
Cemex system
cenesthopathy
Centec Formfit ankle brace
center
accessory ossification c.
Arizona Health Science C. (AHSC)
c. of axial rotation
central micturition c.
c. of gravity (CG, COG)
growth c.
C. for Independent Living (CIL)
Louisiana State University Medical C. (LSUMC)
c. of mass
Midwest Regional Spinal Cord Injury C.
National Aging Information C.
National Consumer Supporter Technical Assistance C.
National Empowerment C.
National Rehabilitation Information C.
ossification primary c.
ossification secondary c.
pontine micturition c.
primary c.
secondary c.
Veterans Administration Prosthetic C. (VAPC)

center-edge
c.-e. angle
c.-e. angle of Wiberg

centering
c. drill
c. hole

Centinela supraspinatus test
central
c. bone
c. calcification

c. callus
c. canal
c. canal stenosis
c. collodiaphysial (CCD)
c. collodiaphysial angle
c. column
c. cord
c. cord syndrome
c. core disease
c. deficiency
c. disc protrusion
c. dislocation
c. electromyography
c. extensor mechanism (CEM)
c. fiber-region
c. heel pad syndrome
c. herniation
c. herniation syndrome
c. horn
c. meniscal flap
c. micturition center
c. modulation
c. necrosis
c. nervous system (CNS)
c. neural blockade
c. physiolysis
c. polydactyly
c. posterior-anterior pressure
c. ray
c. ray amputation
c. segment
c. semi suture-loop meniscal repair technique
c. slip
c. slip sparing technique
c. spine spondylosis
c. splitting technique
c. talus fracture
c. transpatellar tendon portal

Centralign precoat hip prosthesis
centralization
Bayne-Klug c.
Bora c.
Manske-McCarroll-Swanson c.
c. of radius operation
tendon c.

centralizer
cement c.
PMMA c.

centralizing rod
centrifugation of cement
centrifuged methyl methacrylate

NOTES

centromedullary
   c. nail
   c. nailing
centronuclear myopathy
centrosclerosis
cephalad
   c. anterior mold
   c. translation
cephalic
   c. angulation
   c. artery
   c. vein
cephalocaudad
cephalocaudal
cephalomedullary nail fracture
cephaloscapular projection
Cephalosporium **nail infection**
ceramic
   c. acetabular cup
   alumina c.
   c. bearing
   c. biomaterial
   calcium phosphate c.
   calcium sulfate c.
   c. femoral head prosthesis
   c. implant
   c. ossicular prosthesis
   resorbable c.
   c. vertebral spacer
ceramic-on-ceramic
   c.-o.-c. bearing surface
   c.-o.-c. coupling
Ceramion prosthesis
Cerasorb resorbable synthetic bone void filler
cerclage
   c. cable
   Dall-Miles cable c.
   c. fibreux
   Howmedica c.
   c. technique
   c. wire
   c. wire fixation
   c. wire inserter
   c. wire twister
cerclaged component
cerebella (*pl. of* cerebellum)
cerebellar
   c. ataxia
   c. function test
   c. gait
   c. retractor
cerebellopontine angle tumor
cerebellum, pl. **cerebella**
cerebral
   c. palsy (CP)
   c. palsy-related dystonia
cerebroside reticulocytosis

cerebrospinal
   c. canal
   c. fluid
   c. fluid analysis
cerebrovascular accident (CVA)
Ceres' Secret aloe vera gel
cervical
   c. acceleration/deceleration syndrome
   c. AOA halo traction
   c. approach
   c. arch
   c. artery
   c. arthritis
   c. arthrodesis
   c. canal
   c. chair
   c. collar
   c. collar brace
   c. compaction test
   c. cord neurapraxia (CCN)
   c. corpectomy
   c. cushion
   c. Derifield procedure electromyocardiography
   c. disc
   c. disc disease
   c. discectomy
   c. disc excision
   c. discography
   c. discopathy
   c. disc surgery
   c. dorsal glide
   c. dorsal outlet syndrome
   c. drill
   c. extension strength
   c. fascia
   c. fracture tongs
   c. general rotation
   c. halter traction
   c. hypolordosis
   c. interbody fusion
   c. joint
   c. laminectomy punch
   c. ligament of tarsal sinus
   c. lordosis
   c. mallet
   c. manual traction
   c. microtrauma
   c. midline disc herniation
   c. mover ligament
   c. myofascial pain
   c. nerve root encroachment
   c. nerve root injection
   c. nerve root injury
   c. oblique facet wiring
   c. orthosis (CO)
   c. outlet
   c. plate
   c. plexus

c. punch forceps
c. radiculitis
c. radiculopathy
c. range of motion (CROM)
c. range of motion device
c. region
c. rib
c. rib syndrome
c. roll
c. rongeur
c. root
c. rotation in extension
c. saddle
c. screw insertion technique
c. sidegliding test
c. sleep pillow
c. specific rotation
c. specific rotation in flexion
c. spinal cord
c. spinal injury
c. spine (C-spine)
c. spine decompression
c. spine extension injury
c. spine internal fixation
c. spine kyphotic deformity
c. spine laminectomy
c. spine posterior fusion
c. spine posterior ligament
   disruption
c. spine screw-plate fixation
c. spine stabilization
c. spine trauma
c. spondylolysis
c. spondylosis
c. spondylotic myelopathy
c. spondylotic myelopathy fusion
   technique
c. spondylotic myelopathy
   vertebrectomy
c. stairstep
c. stenosis
c. stress line
c. support
c. support pillow
c. sympathectomy
c. sympathetic chain
c. sympathetic chain location
c. synostosis
c. tension myositis (CTM)
c. thoracic orthosis
c. traction pillow
c. triangle
c. trochanteric displaced fracture
c. trochanteric fracture
c. vertebra
c. vertebral bone
c. vertebrectomy

cervicalgia
cervical/lumbar hammer
cervicitis
cervicoaxillary
cervicobrachial
cervicobrachialgia
cervicocranial
cervicodorsal
cervicoencephalic syndrome
cervicogenic
   c. dorsalgia
   c. headache
   c. syndrome
cervicomedullary junction
cervicooccipital fusion
cervicoplasty
cervicoscapular
cervicothoracic
   c. curve
   c. jacket
   c. junction
   c. junction stabilization
   c. junction surgery
   c. orthosis (CTO)
   c. pedicle anatomy
   c. pedicle angle
   c. transition
**cervicothoracolumbosacral orthosis
   (CTLSO)**
cervicotrochanteric
Cervifix system
Cervitrak device
cervix amputation
CES
   cranial electrical stimulation
Cestan-Chenais syndrome
CFL
   calcaneofibular ligament
CFLB
   carbon fiber lamination braid
C-Flex supine cervical traction
CFS
   contoured femoral stem
      CFS hip prosthesis
CFT
   capillary filling time
CG
   center of gravity

NOTES

C

C-guide
> screw placement C-g.

CH
> coracohumeral
> CH ligament

CHA
> calcium hydroxyapatite
> CHA crystal
> CHA crystal deposition disease

Chaddock
> C. reflex
> C. sign
> C. test

CHAG
> coralline hydroxyapatite Goniopora
> CHAG bone graft substitute
>   material

chain
> cervical sympathetic c.
> closed kinematic c.
> closed kinetic c. (CKC)
> kinematic c.
> kinetic c.
> open kinematic c.
> paravertebral sympathetic c.
> pelvic kinematic c.
> c. reaction exercise
> sympathetic c.
> wheelchair c.

chair
> BodyBilt c.
> Boyd podiatry c.
> cervical c.
> dynamic integrated stabilization c.
>   (DISC)
> ergonomically correct c.
> EZ Rider support c.
> Gardner c.
> Hogg c.
> Invacare padded shower c.
> Kaleidoscope c.
> Orthokinetics travel c.
> Pogon c.
> Portal Pro 2 treatment c.
> sit/stand c.
> STC 900-series travel c.
> Vess c.

chairback
> c. brace
> c. lumbosacral orthosis

ChairCiser adjustable exerciser
Chalet frame
chalk-stick fracture
chalky bone
chamber
> monoplace hyperbaric c.
> multiplace hyperbaric c.

Portable Topical Hyperbaric
>   Oxygen Extremity C.
> Pudenz flushing c.

Chamberlain
> C. line
> C. method

Chambers
> C. osteotomy
> C. procedure

chamfer
> c. cut
> c. cut jig
> c. reamer

chamfered cylinder acetabular
> **component**
champ
> C. CTS cold therapy wrap
> C. elastic bandage
> C. Insulated Propac II

champagne bottle leg
champion
> C. Power Sox
> C. Trauma Score (CTS)

Championnière bone drill
chance
> C. fracture thoracolumbar spine
> C. vertebral fracture

Chandler
> C. arthrodesis
> C. bone elevator
> C. disease
> C. felt collar splint
> C. hip fusion
> C. knee retractor
> C. patellar advancement
> C. procedure
> C. spinal perforating forceps
> C. tendon transfer
> C. unreamed interlocking tibial nail

change
> age-associated degenerative c.
> Ahlback c.
> arthritic talonavicular c.
> burn-related pigmentation c.
> Charcot c.
> degenerative arthritic c.
> diurnal c.
> Fairbanks c.
> Iowa degenerative c.
> kinematic gait pattern c.
> neuromuscular gait pattern c.
> sarcomatous c.
> therapeutic lifestyle c. (TLC)
> trophic c.

Chang-Miltner incision
Chang pin clamp
channel
> interosseous anastomosing c.
> tibial c.

channel-and-core biopsy
Chapchal knee arthrodesis
Chapman point treatment
Chaput
  C. fracture
  C. fragment
  C. method
  C. tubercle
characteristic
  biocompatibility c.
  electrooptical c. (EOC)
  receiver operating c.
Charcot
  C. arthritis
  C. arthropathy
  C. arthroplasty
  C. arthrosis
  C. change
  C. chondroma
  C. collapse
  C. deformity
  C. degeneration
  C. disruption
  C. foot
  C. gait
  C. hip arthrodesis
  C. joint
  C. joint disease
  C. neuroarthropathy
  C. restraint orthotic walker
  (CROW)
  C. spine
  C. syndrome
  C. triad
Charcot-Marie atrophy
Charcot-Marie-Tooth (CMT)
  C.-M.-T. atrophy
  C.-M.-T. disease
  C.-M.-T. Evaluation
charger view
Charles Bonnet syndrome
Charleston
  C. nighttime bending brace
  C. scoliosis brace
charley horse
Charlie Chaplin gait
Charnley
  C. acetabular cup
  C. acetabular cup prosthesis
  C. ankle arthrodesis
  C. ankle fusion procedure
  C. arthrodesis clamp
  C. bone clamp

  C. bone curette
  C. brace
  C. brace handle
  C. cemented prosthesis
  C. centering apparatus
  C. centering drill
  C. centering ring
  C. classification of function
  C. compression
  C. compression apparatus
  C. compression arthrodesis
  C. compression clamp
  C. compression-type knee fusion
  C. deepening reamer
  C. expanding reamer
  C. external fixation clamp
  C. external fixation device
  C. femoral broach
  C. femoral condyle drill
  C. femoral condyle radius gauge
  C. femoral inlay aligner
  C. femoral inlay guillotine
  C. femoral prosthesis neck punch
  C. femoral prosthesis pusher
  C. flat-back femoral component
  C. foam suture pad
  C. functional classification
  C. hip score
  C. horizontal retractor
  C. implant
  C. incision
  C. initial incision retractor
  C. introducer
  C. knee retractor
  C. laminar flow room
  C. low-friction arthroplasty
  C. low-friction hip prosthesis
  C. narrow-stem component
  C. offset-bore cup
  C. pain and function grading scale
  C. pilot drill
  C. pin
  C. pin clamp
  C. pin retractor
  C. rasp
  C. self-retaining retractor
  C. socket gauge
  C. standard-stem component
  C. starting drill
  C. suction drain
  C. suture button
  C. taper reamer
  C. template

NOTES

Charnley *(continued)*
>C. tibial onlay jig
>C. total hip arthroplasty
>C. total hip prosthesis
>C. total hip replacement
>C. total hip system
>C. towel
>C. trochanter holder
>C. trochanter reamer
>C. wire-holding forceps
>C. wire passer
>C. wire tightener

Charnley-Hastings prosthesis
Charnley-Howorth Exflow system
Charnley-Merle
>C.-M. d'Aubigné disability grading scale
>C.-M. d'Aubigné disability grading system

Charnley-Müller
>C.-M. arthroplasty
>C.-M. hip prosthesis
>C.-M. lateral approach

Charpy impact test
Charriere
>C. amputation saw
>C. bone saw

CHART
>Craig Handicap Assessment and Reporting Technique

chart
>body mechanics examination c.
>Reality Orientation C.
>sclerotome pain c.

Chassaignac
>C. axillary muscle
>C. tubercle

Chattanooga
>C. balance system Checkrein deformity
>C. traction
>C. traction device

Chatzidakis hinged Vitallium implant prosthesis
chauffeur's fracture
Chaves muscle transfer
Chaves-Rapp paralysis
CHD
>congenital hip dysplasia
>CHD prosthesis

check
>Derifield pelvic leg c.
>head c.
>shoulder-to-head c.
>c. socket

Checkerboard wheelchair cushion
checklist
>Body Mechanics Evaluation C.
>Child Behavior C. (CBCL)

>Feasibility Evaluation C. (FEC)
>Low Back Pain Symptom C.
>McGill pain c.
>Mother-Child Interaction c.
>Role c. (RC)
>Ways of Coping c.

checkrein
>c. deformity
>c. ligament
>c. procedure

cheese-grater hemispherical reamer
Cheetah ankle brace
cheilectomy
>arthroscopic c.
>dorsal c.
>first MTP c.
>Garceau c.
>Mann-Coughlin-DuVries c.
>Sage c.
>Sage-Clark c.

cheilotomy
cheiralgia paresthetica
cheirarthritis
cheiroarthropathy
cheirobrachialgia
cheirognostic
cheiromegaly
cheiroplasty
cheiropodalgia
cheirospasm
chelation therapy
chemical
>AXT-blocking c.
>c. carcinogen
>c. cautery
>c. matricectomy
>c. nail avulsion
>c. neurolysis
>c. selective suppression (CHESS)
>c. sympathectomy

chemiluminescent microtiter protein kinase activity assay
chemocautery
chemonucleolysis
>chymopapain c.
>double-needle c.

chemosterilized graft
chemosurgery
>phenol c.

chemotactic peptide
chemotherapy
>adjuvant c.
>neoadjuvant c.

chemotherapy-related neuropathy
Cherf
>C. cast stand
>C. legholder

cherry
>C. drill

C. osteotome
C. screw extractor
C. tong traction
C. traction tongs
Cherry-Austin drill
CHES
Children's Handwriting Evaluation Scale
CHES-M
Children's Handwriting Evaluation Scale
for Manuscript Writing
CHESS
chemical selective suppression
chest
alar c.
barrel c.
cobbler c.
c. contusion
c. expansion test
flat c.
foveated c.
funnel c.
keeled c.
paralytic c.
phthinoid c.
pigeon c.
pterygoid c.
c. roll
c. tube
chest-band transmitter
Chester-Erdheim disease
chevron
c. bone
c. bunionectomy
c. fusion
c. hallux valgus correction
c. incision
c. laceration
c. modification
c. modification of Mitchell
osteotomy
c. osteotomy
c. osteotomy with rigid screw
fixation
c. procedure
c. technique
chevron-Akin double osteotomy
CHF
congestive heart failure
CHH
cartilage-hair hypoplasia
CHH cervical brace
chi
tai c.

Chiari
C. formation
C. innominate osteotomy
C. malformation
C. shelf procedure
C. technique
chiasma
Camper c.
Chiba spinal system
chick
C. CLT operating frame
C. CLT operating table
C. fracture table
C. nail
chicken breast
Chick-Foster orthopaedic bed
Chick-Langren orthopaedic table
Chiene test
chilblain
child
C. and Adolescent Social
Perception Measure (CASP)
C. Behavior Checklist (CBCL)
C. Behaviors Inventory of
Playfulness (CBI)
C. Development Inventory
c. flatfoot correction
children
Assessment Battery for C. (ABC)
C.'s Assessment of Participation
and Enjoyment (CAPE)
Choosing Outcomes and
Accommodations for C. (COACH)
C.'s Comprehensive Pain
Questionnaire (CCPQ)
C.'s Dynafed Jr.
Functional Independence Measure
for C. (WeeFIM)
C.'s Handwriting Evaluation Scale
(CHES)
C.'s Handwriting Evaluation Scale
for Manuscript Writing (CHES-M)
C.'s Hospital hand drill
C.'s Hospital screwdriver
c. mat
C.'s Motrin Oral Suspension
Movement Assessment Battery
for C.
C.'s Paced Auditory Serial
Addition Test (CHIPASAT)
C.'s Silapap
sized orthotics for c. (SOCS)

NOTES

children *(continued)*
    Test of Everyday Attention for C. (TEA-Ch)
    Total Knee for C.
Childress
    C. ankle fixation
    C. ankle fixation technique
    C. duck waddle test
Chinese
    C. fingertrap suture
    C. fingertrap tube
    C. flap
    C. medicine
    C. red line sign
chin-to-chest test
ChinUpps cervicofacial support
chip
    bone c.
    cancellous c.
    c. fracture
    c. graft
CHIPASAT
    Children's Paced Auditory Serial Addition Test
Chippaux-Smirak arch index
chipped-tooth broach
C-2 hip system
chirarthritis
Chiroflow
    C. adjustable back support
    C. back rest
Chiro-Klenz tea
Chiro-Manis chiropractic table
chiropodalgia
chiropodical
chiropodist
chiropody
chiropractic
    c. adjustment procedure
    c. analysis
    c. biophysics (CBP)
    c. joint manipulation
    c. laser nonsurgical facelift
    c. lesion
    c. management
    c. manipulative reflex technique (CMRT)
    c. manipulative therapy (CMT)
    c. manual manipulation
    c. manual manipulation of spine
    c. mattress
    c. spinal adjustment
    sports c.
    c. thermography
    c. x-ray film
chiropractor
chiropraxis
Chiroslide Jamar Hand Dynamometer
chirospasm

Chirotech x-ray system
chirurgicum mallei
chisel
    acetabular round c.
    Adson laminectomy c.
    Alexander c.
    ASIF c.
    Austin Moore c.
    Ballenger-Hajek c.
    beveled c.
    Biomet cement-removal hand c.
    Bishop c.
    c. blade
    Blair c.
    bone c.
    Bowen c.
    box c.
    Brittain c.
    Bruening c.
    Buckley c.
    cement-removal hand c.
    Cloward spinal fusion c.
    cold c.
    Converse c.
    Cottle c.
    Dautrey c.
    D'Errico lamina c.
    c. elevator
    Fomon c.
    c. fracture
    Freer c.
    gold-paneled c.
    Hajek c.
    Harmon c.
    Hibbs c.
    hollow c.
    Kerrison c.
    Lambert-Lowman c.
    laminectomy c.
    Lexer c.
    Lowman c.
    Lowman-Hoglund c.
    Lucas c.
    Magnum c.
    Martin cartilage c.
    meniscotomy c.
    Metzenbaum c.
    Meyerding c.
    Miles bone c.
    Moore prosthesis-mortising c.
    mortising c.
    Oratec c.
    orthopaedic c.
    Partsch c.
    Passow c.
    Pick c.
    Puka c.
    Schwartze c.
    seating c.

Sheehan c.
Simmons c.
Smillie cartilage c.
Smillie meniscectomy c.
Smith-Petersen c.
square-hollow c.
Stille bone c.
straight c.
swan-neck c.
Trautmann c.
U.S. Army bone c.
West bone c.
White c.
chisel-edge elevator
chisel-tip wire
chloral hydrate
chloramphenicol osteomyelitis
chlorhexidine gluconate
chloride
polyvinyl c. (PVC)
chloroquine phosphate
Cho
C. anterior cruciate ligament
reconstruction
C. tendon technique
choke
c. hold
c. syndrome
choked disc
choline
c. magnesium trisalicylate
c. salicylate
cholinergic vagal function
cholinesterase inhibitor
chondral fragment
chondralgia
chondrectomy
chondrification
chondritis
chondroblast
chondroblastic sarcoma
chondroblastoma
benign c.
humeral c.
chondrocalcinosis
chondroclast
chondrocyte
autologous cultured c.
Carticel autologous cultured c.
hypertrophic c.
chondrodiastasis
chondrodynia

chondrodysplasia
genotypic c.
hereditary deforming c.
hyperplastic c.
McKusick-type metaphysial c.
metaphysial c.
c. punctata
rhizomelic-type c.
chondrodystrophia calcificans
chondrodystrophy
chondroepiphysis
chondroepiphysitis
chondrofibroma
chondrogenesis
chondrography
chondroid syringoma
chondroitin
chondroitin/glucosamine sulfate complex
chondrolipoma
chondrolysis
chondroma
Charcot c.
extraskeletal c.
joint c.
juxtacortical c.
periosteal c.
synovial c.
chondromalacia
c. patellae
patellar c.
chondromalacic
chondromatosis
Henderson-Jones c.
synovial c.
chondromatous hamartoma
chondrometaplasia
chondromyofibroma
chondromyoma
chondromyxofibroma
chondromyxoid fibroma
chondromyxoma
chondromyxosarcoma
chondronecrosis
chondroosseous
c. growth
c. spur
chondroosteodystrophy
chondropathology
chondropathy
chondrophyte
chondroplastic
c. dwarfism
c. myotonia

C

NOTES

chondroplasty
    abrasion c.
    arthroscopic abrasion c.
    c. knife
chondroporosis
chondroprotective agent
chondrosarcoma
    c. cell
    clear cell c.
    dedifferentiated c.
    differentiated c.
    extracortical c.
    extraskeletal c.
    juxtacortical c.
    mesenchymal c.
    myxoid c.
    parosteal c.
    periosteal c.
    pseudocapsule c.
chondrosarcomatosis
chondrosis
chondrosteoma
chondrosternal articulation
chondrosternoplasty
chondrotomy
chondrotrophic
chondroxiphoid
chonechondrosternon
Chonstruct
    C. chondral repair
    C. chondral repair system
Choosing Outcomes and
  Accommodations for Children
  (COACH)
Chopart
    C. amputation with tendon
      balancing
    C. ankle dislocation
    C. articulation
    C. brace
    C. hindfoot amputation
    C. joint line
    C. midtarsal joint
    C. operation
    C. osseous joint injury
    C. partial foot prosthesis
Cho-pat
    C.-p. Achilles tendon strap
    C.-p. Dual Action Knee Strap
    C.-p. elbow strap
    C.-p. ITB Strap
    C.-p. knitted compression support
choppy sea sign
chordoblastoma
chordocarcinoma
chordoma
    cavern c.
    sacrococcygeal c.
chordosarcoma

chordotomy
choreatic gait
choreiform
choristoma
chow
    C. endoscopic carpal tunnel release
    C. transbursal carpal tunnel release
      technique
Choyce MK II keratoprosthesis
  prosthesis
CHPS
    chronic heel pain syndrome
Chrisman-Snook
    C.-S. ankle technique
    C.-S. correction
    C.-S. correction of ankle instability
    C.-S. reconstruction
    C.-S. reconstruction of ankle
      ligament
    C.-S. technique modification
    C.-S. tenodesis
    C.-S. weave procedure
Christensen interlocking nail
Christiani maneuver
Christiansen hip prosthesis
Christmas
    C. tree adapter
    C. tree reamer
chromatography
    high-performance liquid c. (HPLC)
    high-pressure liquid c. (HPLC)
chromatolysis
chrome
    cobalt c.
chrome-cobalt
    c.-c. cable
    c.-c. screw
chromium-cobalt-alloy implant
chromium-cobalt mesh
chromomycosis
chronaxie, chronaxy
chronic
    c. absorptive arthritis
    c. Achilles tendinitis
    c. ankle sprain
    c. anterior exertional compartment
      syndrome (CAECS)
    c. compartment syndrome (CCS)
    c. foot sprain
    c. functional instability
    c. heel pain syndrome (CHPS)
    c. heel wound
    c. hemorrhagic villous synovitis
    c. intractable benign pain syndrome
      (CIBPS)
    c. lateral ankle instability
    c. low back pain (CLBP)
    c. microtraumatic soft tissue injury

c. musculoskeletal pain syndrome (CMPS)
c. periostalgia
c. purulent synovitis
c. recurrent ankle joint dislocation
c. retrocalcaneal bursitis
c. rheumatism
c. sclerosing osteomyelitis of Garré
c. subtalar joint pain
c. tophaceous disease
c. tophaceous gout
c. traumatic encephalopathy (CTE)
c. villous arthritis
c. whiplash

chronotropic impairment
CHSD
congenital hyperphosphatasemic skeletal dysplasia

chuck
c. adapter
c. drill
gold-handled c.
hand c.
Jacobs c.
3-jaw c.
pin c.
Steinmann pin with pin c.
T-handle Zimmer c.
Zimmer c.

Chuinard autogenous bone graft
Chukka boot
chylothorax
chylous
c. arthritis
c. ascites
c. leakage

Chymar
Alpha C.

CI
confidence interval
CI functional knee brace

Cibacalcin Injection
CIBPS
chronic intractable benign pain syndrome

CIC
complex instability of carpus

Cica-Care wound dressing
cicatricial scoliosis
cicatrix, pl. **cicatrices**
cicatrization
Cicherelli bone rongeur
ciclopirox

CID
carpal instability, dissociative

Cierny-Mader technique
ciguatera
CIL
Center for Independent Living

ciliospinal center of Budge
cinch
C. instant suction B.K. prosthesis
joint c.
C. Lock CTS brace

Cincinnati
C. ACL brace
C. incision
C. Knee Rating System
C. knee scoring questionnaire
C. technique

CIND
carpal instability, nondissociative

cine
c. memory
c. view

cinearthrography
triple-injection c.

cinefluoroscopy
Cinelli osteotome
cine-magnetic resonance imaging (cine-MRI)
cinematic amputation
cinematographic gait study
cine-MRI
cine-magnetic resonance imaging

cineplastic amputation
cineplastics
cineradiography
cineroentgenography
cingulotomy, cingulumotomy
Cintor
C. bone rongeur
C. knee prosthesis

Cipro
C. Injection
C. Oral

CIQ
Community Integration Questionnaire

CircAid elastic stockings
circle
c. bed
c. draw test

CircOlectric
C. bed
C. frame

CircPlus bandage/wrap system

NOTES

Circul'Air shoe process system
circular
- c. bandage
- c. cast
- c. fine-wire external fixator
- c. fixation
- c. fixation device
- c. laminar hook with offset top
- c. open amputation
- c. saw
- c. supracondylar amputation
- c. wire
- c. wire fixator

circulation
- collateral c.
- extraosseous c.
- femoral c.
- intraosseous c.
- perichondral c.

Circulator boot system
circulatory embarrassment
Circulon
- C. dressing
- C. wrap

circumduction maneuver
circumductor table
circumference
- calf c.
- pelvic c.

circumferential
- c. capsulectomy
- c. cartilage
- c. dedicated knee coil
- c. dressing
- c. fracture
- c. grommet
- c. lamella
- c. ligamentous sleeve
- c. release
- c. release of clubfoot
- c. wire
- c. wire-loop fixation
- c. wiring

circumflex
- c. iliac artery
- c. scapular artery

circumscribed
circumscribing incision
circumscripta
- calcinosis c.
- Dubreuilh melanosis c.

Cirrus
- C. composite prosthetic foot
- C. foot prosthesis
- C. foot prosthetic

cirsoid angioma
citalopram hydrobromide

Citanest
- C. Forte
- C. Plain

Citelli
- C. angle
- C. punch forceps

Citscope disposable arthroscope
Civinini
- C. canal
- C. ligament
- C. process
- C. spine

CIVRA
- continuous intravenous regional anesthesia

CKC
- closed kinetic chain

CKCE
- closed kinetic chain exercise

CKS
- Continuum knee system
- CKS implant
- CKS knee system

Claiborne external fixator
clamp
- Acland microvascular c.
- Aesculap c.
- Allen-Kocher c.
- Allis c.
- angled DeBakey c.
- angled Lowman-type bone c.
- angular hinge c.
- Ann Arbor double towel c.
- appendage c.
- c. approximator
- Backhaus towel c.
- Bahnson appendage c.
- Balfour c.
- Ballantine c.
- Bamby c.
- Bard c.
- bar-to-bar c.
- Berens muscle c.
- Berke c.
- Bernhard c.
- Bircher bone-holding c.
- Bircher cartilage c.
- Bishop bone c.
- Blalock c.
- Böhler c.
- bone extension c.
- bone-holding c.
- Bonney c.
- bulldog c.
- Calandruccio c.
- c. carrier
- cartilage c.
- Casey pelvic c.
- Chang pin c.

Charnley arthrodesis c.
Charnley bone c.
Charnley compression c.
Charnley external fixation c.
Charnley pin c.
Cooley graft c.
Cooley iliac c.
Cooley multipurpose angled c.
Cooley multipurpose curved c.
Dandy c.
Davidson muscle c.
Diethrich bulldog c.
Dingman bone and cartilage c.
disposable muscle biopsy c.
dissecting c.
distraction c.
Doctor Collins fracture c.
double c.
Edna towel c.
exclusion c.
extension bone c.
femoral c.
Ferguson bone c.
c. fixator
c. forceps
Freeman c.
full-curved c.
Gerster bone c.
Goodwin bone c.
Greenberg c.
Halifax interlaminar c.
Harrington hook c.
Harrington rod c.
hemostat c.
hemostatic thoracic c.
Hex-Fix Universal swivel c.
Hey Groves c.
Hoen c.
Hoffmann ligament c.
c. holder
hook c.
iliac c.
c. insert
interlaminar c.
Jackson bone c.
Jackson bone-extension c.
Jackson bone-holding c.
Jacobson bulldog c.
Jameson muscle c.
Jarit anterior resection c.
Jarit cartilage c.
Jarit meniscal c.
Jarit small bone-holding c.

Johns Hopkins bulldog c.
Jones thoracic c.
Jones towel c.
Kantrowitz thoracic c.
Kelly c.
Kern bone-holding c.
Kocher c.
Lahey c.
Lalonde oblique fracture large
  bone c.
Lalonde oblique fracture medium
  bone c.
Lalonde oblique metacarpal fracture
  bone c.
Lalonde small bone c.
Lambert-Lowman bone c.
Lambotte bone-holding c.
Lamis patellar c.
Lane bone-holding c.
Lewin bone-holding c.
ligament c.
lobster-type c.
Locke bone c.
locking c.
Lowman bone-holding c.
Lowman-Gerster bone c.
Lowman-Hoglund c.
Malis hinge c.
Martin cartilage c.
Martin meniscal c.
Martin muscular c.
Masterson curved c.
Masterson pelvic c.
Masterson straight c.
Mastin muscular c.
Matthew cross-leg c.
Mayo c.
medial malleolar/small bone
  fragment c.
meniscal c.
metal c.
microvascular c.
miniature multipurpose c.
mini-Ullrich bone c.
Mixter ligature-carrier c.
Mixter right-angle c.
mosquito c.
Moynihan towel c.
multipurpose angled c.
multipurpose curved c.
muscle biopsy c.
muscular c.
Naraghi-DeCoster reduction c.

NOTES

139

clamp (continued)
OBrien bone c.
osteoplastic flap c.
padded c.
Parham-Martin bone-holding c.
patellar cement c.
patellar reduction c.
Pean c.
pedicle c.
pelvic C c.
Pemberton spur-crushing c.
phalangeal c.
pin c.
pin-to-bar c.
point-of-reduction c.
Price muscular biopsy c.
ratchet c.
Rayport muscular biopsy c.
reamer c.
Richards bone c.
rod c.
rubber shod c.
Rumel myocardial c.
Rumel rubber c.
Rumel thoracic c.
Rush bone c.
saddle c.
Satinsky c.
Schlein c.
Seidel bone-holding c.
self-retaining c.
Semb bone-holding c.
sesamoid c.
single c.
Slocum meniscal c.
Smith bone c.
Southwick c.
speed-lock c.
sponge c.
spur-crushing c.
stainless steel c.
Steinhauser bone c.
Steri-Clamp c.
swivel c.
towel c.
trochanter-holding c.
Ulrich bone-holding c.
Universal wire c.
Verbrugge bone c.
Vermont spinal fixator c.
vessel c.
VSF c.
Walton cartilage c.
Walton meniscal c.
Wells pedicle c.
Wester meniscal c.
wire-tightening c.
Wylie lumbar bulldog c.

X c.
Zimmer cartilage c.
clamping mechanism
clamshell
c. AFO boot
c. brace
c. prosthesis
Clancy
C. cruciate ligament reconstruction
C. lateral compartment
C. ligament technique
C. patellar tendon graft
Clancy-Andrews reconstruction
Clanton
C. turf toe
C. turf toe grading system
Clark
C. classification
C. classification of melanoma
C. pectoralis major transfer
C. sign
C. transfer technique
Clarke
C. arch angle
C. patellar compression test
Clarus SpineScope
CLASP
compression locking anchor with
secondary purchase
clasp
Arrow pin c.
Epi-Sport epicondylitis c.
clasped
c. thumb
c. thumb deformity
classification
AAOS acetabular abnormality c.
ACR c.
acromioclavicular injury c.
Aitken epiphysial fracture c.
Allman acromioclavicular injury c.
American Rheumatism
Association c.
American Spinal Cord Injury
Association c.
Anderson-D'Alonzo odontoid
fracture c.
Anderson modification of Berndt-
Harty c.
Anderson tibial pseudarthrosis c.
ankle fracture c.
AO ankle fracture c.
AO-Danis-Weber ankle fracture c.
Arco c.
Arthritis Impact Measurement
Scale c.
Ashhurst-Bromer ankle fracture c.
Bado c.
Bauer-Jackson c.

Bayne radial agenesis c.
Bayne ulnar ray deficiency c.
Bennett thumb fracture c.
Berndt c.
Berndt-Harty c.
Bishop c.
Bleck metatarsus adductus c.
Boyd c.
Boyd-Griffin trochanteric fracture c.
Breslow c.
Brooker heterotopic bone
  formation c. (I-IV)
Canale-Kelly talar neck fracture c.
Catterall c.
cement mantle grade c.
Charnley functional c.
Clark c.
Clatter c.
Codman c.
Colonna hip fracture c.
Colton c.
Crowe congenital hip dysplasia c.
Danis-Weber fracture c.
d'Antonio acetabular c.
Darrow pain c.
Deknatel suture c.
DeLee c.
Denis Browne sacral fracture c.
Denis Browne spinal fracture c.
Denis compression fracture c.
Denis seat-belt injury c.
Devas stress fracture c.
Dorr bone c.
Durie-Salmon c.
Dyck-Lambert c.
Edwards and Lee tibiofibular
  diastasis and syndesmotic
  injury c.
Ellis c.
Enneking c.
Epstein hip dislocation c.
Essex-Lopresti calcaneal fracture c.
Evans intertrochanteric fracture c.
femoral fracture following total hip
  replacement c.
Ficat femoral head osteonecrosis c.
Ficat stage of avascular necrosis c.
Fielding femoral fracture c.
Flatt c.
floating knee fracture c.
Foucher c.
fracture c.
Fränkel neurologic deficit c.

Freeman calcaneal fracture c.
Fries score for rheumatoid
  arthritis c.
Frykman distal radius fracture c.
Garden femoral neck fracture c.
Gartland humeral supracondylar
  fracture c.
Gartland Universal radial
  fracture c.
Gertzbein seat-belt injury c.
Graf c.
Grantham femur fracture c.
Greenfield spinocerebellar ataxia c.
Gumley seat beat injury c.
Gustilo-Anderson open fracture c.
Gustilo-Anderson tibial plafond
  fracture c.
Gustilo puncture wound c.
Gustilo tibial fracture c.
Hahn-Steinthal capitellum
  fracture c.
Hannover c.
Hansen fracture c.
Hardcastle c.
Hawkins talar fracture c.
Henderson c.
Herbert scaphoid bone fracture c.
Herndon hip c.
Herring lateral pillar c.
Heyman hip c.
hip dislocation c.
Hohl-Luck tibial plateau fracture c.
Hohl tibial condylar fracture c.
Holdsworth spinal fracture c.
Hughston Clinic injury c.
Ideberg glenoid fracture c.
Insall patellar injury c.
Jahss ankle dislocation c.
Jahss metatarsophalangeal joint
  dislocation c.
Janis tibialis posterior tendon
  dysfunction c.
Jeffery radial fracture c.
Johansson fracture c.
Johnson and Strom tibialis
  posterior tendon dysfunction c.
Jones congenital tibial deficiency c.
Jones diaphysial fracture c.
Judet epiphysial fracture c.
Kalamchi c.
Kelikian nail deformity c.
Kilfoyle humeral medial condylar
  fracture c.

C

NOTES

classification *(continued)*
King thoracic scoliosis c.
Kocher c.
Kocher-Lorenz capitellum
fracture c.
Kostuik-Errico spinal stability c.
Kuwada Achilles tendon injury c.
Kyle fracture c.
Langenskiöld c. (stage I–VI)
lateral condylar fracture c.
Lauge-Hansen ankle fracture c.
Lenke c.
Letournel-Judet acetabular
fracture c.
Leung thumb loss c.
Lichtman aseptic necrosis c.
Lichtman radiographic c.
Lindell c.
load-sharing c.
LSUMC c.
Macewen c.
MacNichol-Voutsinas c.
Mason radial head fracture c.
Mathews olecranon fracture c.
Mayo carpal instability c.
Mayo elbow fracture c.
Mazur ankle elevation c.
McDermott radiological c.
Melone distal radius fracture c.
Merland perimedullary arteriovenous
fistula c.
Meyers-McKeever tibial fracture c.
Milch condylar fracture c.
Milch elbow fracture c.
modified Fränkel c.
modified Sillence c.
modified Stahl c. (stage I-V)
Moore tibial plateau fracture c.
MRC muscle function c.
Mueller femoral supracondylar
fracture c.
Mueller humerus fracture c.
Mueller tibial fracture c.
Neer femur fracture c.
Neer-Horowitz humerus fracture c.
Neer humerus fracture c.
Neer shoulder fracture c.
Neviaser frozen shoulder c.
Newman radial neck and head
fracture c.
New York diagnostic criteria c.
Nicoll c.
Nurick spondylosis c.
O'Brien radial fracture c.
Oden peroneal tendon
subluxation c.
Ogden epiphysial fracture c.
Ogden knee dislocation c.
Olerud and Molander fracture c.

O'Rahilly limb deficiency c.
ordinal c.
Orthopaedic Trauma Association c.
osteoarthritis grading c.
Outerbridge c.
Ovadia-Beals tibial plafond
fracture c.
Paley c.
Palmer triangular fibrocartilage
complex lesion c.
Papavasiliou olecranon fracture c.
Pauwels femoral neck fracture c.
Pennal c.
peripheral nerve tumor c.
pilon fracture c.
Pipkin posterior hip dislocation c.
Pipkin subclassification of Epstein-
Thomas c.
Poland epiphysial fracture c.
pressure ulcer c.
Pritsch talar osteochondroma c.
Prosthetic Problem Inventory
Scale c.
Quénu-Küss tarsometatarsal
injury c.
Quinby pelvic fracture c.
Ranawat c.
Ratliff avascular necrosis c.
Regnauld hallux rigidus c.
Riordan club hand c.
Riseborough-Radin intercondylar
fracture c.
Risser c.
Rockwood c.
Rosenthal c.
Rowe calcaneal fracture c.
Ruedi-Allgower c.
Russe c.
Russell-Taylor c.
Rüter c.
Saha shoulder muscle c.
Sakellarides calcaneal fracture c.
Salter epiphysial fracture c.
Salter-Harris-Rang epiphysial
fracture c.
Salter-Harris tibial-fibular injury c.
Salter-Thompson c.
Sanders CT C.
Sanders intraarticular calcaneal
fracture c.
scalar c.
Schatzker tibial plateau fracture c.
Seddon c.
Seinsheimer femoral fracture c.
Severin c.
Shapiro c.
Shelton femoral fracture c.
Sillence osteogenesis imperfecta c.
Singh osteoporosis c.

Sorbie calcaneal fracture c.
Speed radial head fracture c.
5 c.'s of spondylolisthesis
Stahl Kienbock disease c.
Stahl c. (stage I-V)
Steinbrocker rheumatoid arthritis c.
Steinert epiphysial fracture c.
Stelling and Tucker polydactyly c.
Steward-Milford fracture c.
Stulberg hip c.
Sunderland nerve injury c.
Swanson c.
Tachdjian c.
talocalcaneal index c.
Thomas c.
Thompson-Epstein c.
Three Color Concept of Wound c.
tibial tuberosity fractures in
  children c.
Tile c.
Torg c.
Toronto pelvic fracture c.
Tronzo intertrochanteric fracture c.
Trunkey fracture c.
Tscherne c.
Universal distal radius fracture c.
Universal spine c. (type A-C)
Venn-Watson c.
Vostal radial fracture c.
Wagner c.
Waldenström c.
walking footprints c.
Wassel thumb duplication c.
Watanabe discoid meniscus c.
Watson-Jones navicular fracture c.
Watson-Jones spinal fracture c.
Watson-Jones tibial fracture c.
Weber-Danis ankle injury c.
Weber fracture c.
Weiland c.
Weissman c.
Wiberg patellar c.
Wiley-Galey c.
Winquist femoral shaft fracture c.
Winquist-Hansen femoral fracture c.
Winquist-Hansen fracture
  comminution c.
Woofry-Chandler c.
Young pelvic fracture c.
Zickel c.
Zwipp c.
Clatter classification
Claude syndrome

claudication
  intermittent c. (IC)
  jaw c.
  neurogenic c. (NC)
claudicatory
clavicectomy
clavicle
  atraumatic osteolysis of distal c.
    (ATODC)
  distal c.
  c. excision
  floating c.
  intraarticular c.
  c. orthosis
  c. pin
  tuberosity of c.
  weightlifter's c.
clavicotomy
clavicular
  c. birth fracture
  c. cross splint
  c. epiphysis
  c. fracture aneurysm
  c. notch
claviculectomy
clavipectoral
  c. fascia
  c. triangle
clavulanic acid
clavus
  c. foot
  c. formation
claw
  c. finger
  c. foot
  c. hand
  c. toe
  c. toe deformity
clawed
  c. hallux
  c. pedicle hook
clawfoot
  c. contracture
  c. deformity
clawhand
  c. deformity
  c. sign
clawing
  toe c.
claw-type basic frame
clay shoveler's fracture
Clayton
  C. forefoot arthroplasty

NOTES

Clayton *(continued)*
C. greenstick splint
C. osteotome
C. procedure
C. procedure with panmetatarsal head resection
C. prosthesis
C. resection arthroplasty
CLBP
chronic low back pain
cleanser
ApriVera skin and hair c.
wound c.
cleansing
pressure ulcer c.
Cleanwheel
C. disposable neurological pinwheel
C. presterilized disposable device
clear
c. cell acanthoma
c. cell carcinoma
c. cell chondrosarcoma
c. cell sarcoma
c. space measurement
Clearfix screw
clearinghouse
National Accessible Apartment C.
National Maternal and Child Health C.
National Mental Health Consumers' Self-Help C.
Clearpro suction socket
cleavage
c. fracture
horizontal c.
c. lesion
c. line
c. tear
Cleeman sign
cleft
c. closure
c. foot
c. foot deformity
gluteal c.
Hahn c.
c. hand
c. hand deformity
intergluteal c.
interinnominoabdominal c.
retropharyngeal fascial c.
c. spine
c. spinous process
venous c.
c. vertebra
vertebral column c.
clefting of meniscus
C-Leg
C.-L. lower limb prosthesis
C.-L. System artificial leg

cleidagra
cleidal
cleidarthritis
cleidocostal
cleidocranial
c. dysostosis
c. dysplasia
cleidoepitrochlear bundle
cleidomastoid
Cleland ligament
clenched
c. fist syndrome
c. fist view
Cleocin
C. HCl
C. Pediatric
C. Phosphate
Cleveland
C. bone-cutting forceps
C. bone rongeur
Clevisphere ankle joint
CLI
critical limb ischemia
click
hip c.
Mulder c.
Ortolani c.
c. sign
clicker
compression c.
Clifton Assessment Procedures for the Elderly (CAPE)
Climara Transdermal
climber
Fitstep II stair c.
Sprint C.
clinarthrosis
Clinch Lock CTS wrist brace
clinical
C. Analysis Questionnaire (CAQ)
c. bone sonometer
c. diagnosis
c. examination
c. parameter
C. Test of Sensory Integration and Balance (CTSIB)
c. trial
Clinisert mattress
Clinitron air bed
clinodactyly
clinoid process
clinotherapy
ClinsWound wound cleanser
clip
c. applier
c. gauge
Indiana tome c.
Michel c.
palmar c.

towel c.
Weck c.
clip-applying forceps
clip-bending forceps
clip-cutting forceps
clip-introducing forceps
clivus
clock
    c. balance test
    shoulder c.
clog
    Hollander c.
    Markell Mobility Health C.'s
    wooden postoperative c.'s
clonus
    ankle c.
    3-beat c.
    drawn ankle c.
    patellar c.
    persistent c.
    sustained ankle c.
    transient c.
    unsustained c.
clorazepate dipotassium
Clorpactin WCS-90
closed
    c. ankle fracture
    c. base wedge osteotomy (CBWO)
    c. core needle biopsy
    c. Cotrel-Dubousset hook
    c. dislocation
    c. drainage system
    c. femoral diaphysial shortening
    c. flap amputation
    c. indirect fracture
    c. intramedullary osteotomy
    c. irrigation
    c. kinematic chain
    c. kinetic chain (CKC)
    c. kinetic chain exercise (CKCE)
    c. kinetic chain injury
    c. kinetic chain progressive-resistance exercise
    c. Küntscher nail
    c. Küntscher nailing
    c. loop EndoButton
    c. manipulative maneuver
    c. medullary nailing
    c. pinning
    c. pseudarthrosis
    c. reduction (CR)
    c. reduction of fracture
    c. rupture

c. soft tissue injury
c. suction irrigation
c. surgery
c. transverse process TSRH hook
c. treatment
c. unlocked nail
c. wedge osteotomy/bunionectomy
c. wound
closed-chain
    c.-c. exercise
    c.-c. functional assessment
closed-form bar theory
Close Encounter nut
Closer stapler
closing
    c. abductory-wedge osteotomy (CAWO)
    c. base wedge
    c. base-wedge osteotomy
    voluntary c. (VC)
    c. wedge arthrodesis
    c. wedge greenstick dorsal proximal metatarsal osteotomy
    c. wedge high tibial osteotomy (CWHTO)
    c. wedge manipulation
    c. wedge manipulation and reapplication of plaster
    c. wedge osteotomy bunionectomy
clostridial
    c. infection
    c. myonecrosis
    c. myositis
Clostridium
    C. difficile
    C. perfringens
closure
    Barsky cleft c.
    bunionectomy capsular c.
    cleft c.
    delayed primary c. (DPC)
    epiphysial c.
    lace c.
    myofascial c.
    physial c.
    premature c.
    primary c.
    secondary c.
    skin c.
    Steri-Strip skin c.
    SureClosure c.
    tissue c.
    vacuum-assisted c. (VAC)

C

NOTES

closure *(continued)*
    Velcro c.
    visual c.
    wound c.
clot
    exogenous fibrin c.
    fibrin c.
cloth
    c. binder
    c. tape occlusion method of Litt
clotheslining
clothespin spinal fusion graft
clotting
    c. cascade
    c. disorder
Cloutier unconstrained knee prosthesis
cloven-hoof
    c.-h. fracture
    c.-h. fracture of finger
cloverleaf
    c. condylar plate fixation
    c. deformity
    c. Küntscher nail
    c. met foot pad
    c. pattern
    c. pin
    c. pin extractor
    c. plate
Cloward
    C. anterior spinal fusion
    C. back fusion
    C. blade retractor
    C. bone graft impactor
    C. cervical arthrodesis
    C. cervical disc approach
    C. cervical drill
    C. cervical drill guard
    C. cervical drill tip
    C. depth gauge
    C. dowel cutter
    C. dowel ejector
    C. drill guard cap
    C. drill guide
    C. drill shaft
    C. fusion discography
    C. hammer
    C. intervertebral disc rongeur
    C. operation
    C. osteophyte elevator
    C. periosteal elevator
    C. spinal fusion chisel
    C. spinal fusion osteotome
    C. spreader
    C. surgical saddle
    C. technique
cloxacillin
CLS
    cementless Sportono
    CLS hip system

clubbed
    c. finger
    c. nail
    c. toe
clubfoot
    acquired c.
    arthrogrypotic c.
    circumferential release of c.
    c. deformity
    extrinsic c.
    intrinsic c.
    posteromedial release of c.
    c. release
    resistant c.
    c. splint
clubhand
    c. deformity
    radial c.
    ulnar c.
clumsy
    c. gait
    c. hand dysarthria
    c. hand syndrome
cluneal nerve
clunk
    catch-up c.
    spontaneous wrist c.
    c. test
Clutton joint
Clyburn
    C. Colles fracture fixator
    C. external fixator
Clyde Mood scale
CM
    combined mechanical
CMAP
    compound muscle action potential
    compound muscle-motor action potential
CM-Band
    CM-B. 505N brace
    CM-B. silicone rubber brace
CMC
    carpometacarpal
    CMC fusion
    CMC joint
    CMC splint
CME-MRI
    contrast medium-enhanced magnetic
     resonance imaging
CM EVA
    compression-molded ethylene vinyl
     acetate
CMPS
    chronic musculoskeletal pain syndrome
CMRT
    chiropractic manipulative reflex
     technique
CMT
    Charcot-Marie-Tooth

chiropractic manipulative therapy
Contextual Memory Test
   CMT disease
   CMT Evaluation
CMW
   CMW bone cement
   CMW cement gun
cnemial
cnemis
cnemitis
CNS
   central nervous system
CO
   cervical orthosis
COACH
   Choosing Outcomes and
   Accommodations for Children
coach's finger
coagulated plasma
coagulating forceps
coagulation
   c. disorder
   disseminated intravascular c. (DIC)
   c. factor
   c. necrosis
coagulative necrosis
coagulator
   ASSI c.
   bipolar c.
   Concept bipolar c.
   Malis CMC-II bipolar c.
   Polar-Mate c.
coalescence
coalition
   acquired tarsal c.
   bilateral talocalcaneal c.
   c. of bone
   calcaneocuboid c.
   calcaneonavicular c.
   carpal c.
   cartilaginous c.
   complete c.
   congenital complete subtalar c.
   cubonavicular c.
   fibrous talocalcaneal c.
   c. formation
   incomplete c.
   interphalangeal c.
   lunatotriquetral c.
   Minaar classification of c.
   multiple tarsal c.'s

   naviculocuneiform c.
   nonosseous tarsal c.
   osseous c.
   subtalar c.
   talocalcaneal c.
   tarsal c.
   c. view
coapt
coaptation
   c. plate
   c. splint
coarse carbide cone bur
coarse-olive bur
coast
   c. of California border
   c. of Maine border
coated
   c. implant
   c. prosthesis
coating
   aluminum oxide ceramic c.
   Biolox ceramic c.
   bone fixation surface c.
   cobalt-chrome powder c.
   DePuy total hip system with
     porous c.
   Porocoat porous c.
   porous c.
   sintering of cobalt-chrome
     powder c.
coat-sleeve amputation
coaxial needle electrode
Coballoy
   C. implant metal
   C. implant metal prosthesis
   C. twist drill
cobalt
   c. chrome
   c. implant
cobalt-based alloy
cobalt-chrome
   c.-c. alloy and polyethylene
     implant
   c.-c. powder coating
   c.-c. power sintering
cobalt-chromium
   c.-c. alloy
   c.-c. head
   c.-c. implant
   ion-bombarded c.-c.
   smooth c.-c.

C

NOTES

cobalt-chromium-alloy prosthesis
cobalt-chromium-molybdenum (Co-Cr-Mo)
cobalt-chromium-tungsten-nickel (Co-Cr-W-Ni)
Coban
    C. elastic dressing
    C. elastic wrap
Cobb
    C. attachment for Albee-Compere fracture table
    C. curette
    C. gauge
    C. method
    C. method for measuring scoliosis
    C. osteotome
    C. periosteal elevator
    C. scoliosis angle
    C. scoliosis measuring technique
    C. spinal gouge
    C. syndrome
    technique of C.
    C. tibialis posterior tendon dysfunction procedure
cobbler chest
Coblation spinal surgery system
cobra
    C. Master
    c. retractor
cobra-design femoral component
cobra-head plate
Coccidioides immitis
coccidioidomycosis
coccyalgia
coccydynia
coccygalgia
coccygeal
    c. bone
    c. joint
    c. sinus
    c. spine
    c. vertebra
coccygectomy
coccygerector
coccygodynia
coccygotomy
coccyodynia
coccyx fracture
cockade image
Cockayne syndrome
cocked-half flap
Cocke maxillectomy
Cockett communicating perforating veins
cocking injury
Cocklin toe operation
cock-robin head tilt
cock-up
    c.-u. arm splint

    c.-u. deformity
    c.-u. deformity of toe
    c.-u. hand splint
    c.-u. splint orthosis
    c.-u. wrist splint
    c.-u. wrist support
co-contraction
    active muscle c.-c.
    c.-c. exercise
Co-Cr-Mo
    cobalt-chromium-molybdenum
    Co-Cr-Mo alloy implant metal
    Co-Cr-Mo alloy prosthesis
    Co-Cr-Mo pin
Co-Cr-W-Ni
    cobalt-chromium-tungsten-nickel
    Co-Cr-W-Ni alloy implant metal
    Co-Cr-W-Ni alloy prosthesis
codfish
    c. deformity
    c. vertebra
Codivilla
    C. extension
    C. operation
    C. tendon lengthening
    C. tendon lengthening technique
Codman
    C. ACP system
    C. angle
    C. anterior cervical plating system
    C. classification
    C. exercise
    C. saber-cut shoulder approach
    C. sign
    C. Ti-frame posterior fixation system
    C. triangle
    C. tumor
    C. wire-passing drill
Codman-Kerrison laminectomy rongeur
coefficient of friction
Coe-pak
    C.-p. paste
    C.-p. paste adhesive
coffin bone
Coffin-Lowry syndrome
Cofield
    C. shoulder prosthesis
    C. technique
    C. total shoulder system
CoFilm dressing
Co-Flex
    C.-F. adherent wrap
    C.-F. dressing
COG
    center of gravity
cogent
    C. light

C. LightWear headlight
C. XL illuminator

cognitive

C. Assessment of Minnesota (CAM)
C. Performance Test (CPT)

cogwheel

c. gait
c. rigidity
c. sign

Cohen

C. periosteal elevator
C. rongeur

cohesion

glenohumeral joint c.

cohort

C. anterior plate system
C. bone brush
C. bone screw
C. spinal impactor
c. study

COI

combination of isotonics

coil

circumferential dedicated knee c.

coin

fracture en c.

Coker-Arnold collar
ColBenemid
colchicine and probenecid
Colclough laminectomy rongeur
cold

c. abscess
c. application
c. chisel
c. compressive dressing
c. injury
c. intolerance
c. laser
c. laser treatment
c. pack
c. pad
c. pressor test
c. rolled rod
c. therapy
c. weld

cold-curing polymer
Coldflo

C. cold therapy
C. cold therapy and sequential compression

Coldhot pack
cold-mold prosthesis

cold-weld

c.-w. femoral ball
c.-w. femoral prosthesis

Cole

C. fracture frame
C. hyperextension brace
C. hyperextension frame
C. operation
C. osteotomy
C. osteotomy for midfoot deformity
C. procedure
C. technique
C. tendon fixation

Coleman

C. flatfoot technique
C. lateral block test
C. plasty

colinear alignment
colistin
collagen

Avitene microfibrillar c.
Bio-Oss c.
bovine c.
c. fiber
microcrystalline c.
c. scaffold
c. skin dressing
c. vascular disease (CVD)

collagen-based biomaterial
collagenous schwannoma
Collagraft bone graft matrix
collapse

bone graft c.
Charcot c.
exercise-associated c.
exercise-induced c.
foot c.
hindfoot-midfoot c.
hyperthermic exercise-associated c.
neuropathic c.
scapholunate advanced c. (SLAC)
scapholunate arthritis c. (SLAC)
vertebral body c.

collapsible

c. internal fixation device
c. pin

collapsing pes valgo planus
collar

Aspen cervical c.
c. bone
c. brace
Bremer Halo Crown cervical c.
calcar c.

C

NOTES

149

collar *(continued)*
cervical c.
Coker-Arnold c.
Cowboy C.
c. and crown scissors
c. and cuff
dynamization c.
Exo-Static cervical c.
Exo-Static neck c.
foam c.
Forrester-Brown c.
Georgiade visor cervical c.
hard c.
Headmaster c.
Houston halo traction cervical c.
implant c.
Lerman-Minerva c.
Lewin c.
MAC cervical c.
Marlin cervical c.
Mayo rigid cervical c.
Mayo-Thomas c.
Miami Acute cervical c.
Miami J cervical c.
molded Thomas c.
myocervical c.
periosteal bone c.
Philadelphia cervical c.
Philadelphia rigid c.
pillow c.
Plastazote cervical c.
plastic c.
Pneu-trac cervical c.
2+2 Rehab C.
rigid c.
Schanz c.
serpentine foam c.
soft c.
Thomas rigid c.
Tuxedo c.
wire frame c.
collar-and-cuff sling
collar-button abscess
collar-calcar support femoral prosthesis
collared
c. button
c. femoral head
c. press-fit femoral stem
implantation
collarless
c., polished, tapered (CPT)
c. stem
collateral
c. artery
c. circulation
c. fibular ligament
c. ligament instability
c. ligament laxity
c. ligament rupture

c. radial ligament
c. tibial ligament
c. ulnar ligament
collection
epidural fluid c.
multiloculated fluid c.
collectomy
shortening c.
college
C. Park TruStep foot
C. Park TruStep foot prosthesis
Colles
C. fascia
C. fracture
C. ligament
C. splint
Collet
C. screwdriver adapter
tibial C.
colli
fibromatosis c.
pterygium c.
collicular fracture
colliculus, pl. **colliculi**
posterior c.
Collier sign
collimation
collimator
Multileaf C.
Collimator plugging pattern
Collin
C. amputating knife
C. osteoclast
Collins
C. dynamometer
C. rib shears
Collis
C. broken femoral stem technique
C. retractor
C. TDR instrument
Collis-Dubrul femoral stem removal
Collison
C. body drill
C. cannulated hand drill
C. plate
C. screw
C. screwdriver
C. tap drill
Collis-Taylor retractor
collodiaphysial
c. angle
central c. (CCD)
collodion dressing
colloid solution
colocutaneous fistula
Colonna
C. hip fracture classification
C. shelf operation
C. trochanteric arthroplasty

Colonna-Ralston
    C.-R. ankle approach
    C.-R. incision
    C.-R. medial approach
color
    digital c.
    c. duplex imaging
color-coded therapy putty
colored antiseptic
Colpacs pack
Coltart
    C. calcaneotibial fusion
    C. fracture
    C. fracture technique
Colton classification
Columbus
    C. McKinnon assist for lifting or transfer
    C. McKinnon Hugger device
column
    anterior c.
    c. balance
    central c.
    2-c. cervical spine injury
    contrast c.
    radial c.
    resistive weighed c.
    spinal c.
    ulnar c.
    vertebral c.
3-column
    3-c. cervical spine injury
    3-c. concept
    3-c. spine
    3-c. spine theory
comb
    toe c.
Combat Task Test
CombiDERM nonadhesive absorbent dressing
Combi Multi-Traction System
combination
    film-screen c.
    Grafton bone matrix/marrow c.
    Isola spinal implant system plate-rod c.
    c. of isotonics (COI)
    c. of isotonics technique
    jab and hook punch c.
combined
    c. ankle and knee motion gait determinant
    c. anterior cavus

    c. anterior and posterior approach
    c. cavus
    c. cavus deformity
    c. curve
    c. fixation device
    c. flexion-distraction injury and burst fracture
    c. flexion phenomenon
    C. Instabilities functional knee brace
    c. instability
    c. low cervical and transthoracic approach
    c. magnetic field system
    c. mechanical (CM)
    c. nerve palsy
    c. radial-ulnar-humeral fracture
    c. resection arthroplasty and arthrodesis
    c. scintigraphy
    c. stenosis
Combunox
Comed postoperative shoe
Comet fragment
Comfeel Ulcus occlusive dressing
Comforfoam splint
comfort
    C. Ag prosthetic sock
    C. Cast
    C. Cast stirrup
    C. Club tub pillow
    C. Cool neoprene support
    c. level
    C. n' Care Seamfree socks
    C. Rite footwear
    C. Take-Along wheelchair cushion
    C. wrist immobilizer
comforter
    C. Splint
    Thermo hand c.
    Thermo knee c.
Comf-Orthotic
    C.-O. 3/4-length insole
    C.-O. sports replacement insole
    C.-O. wool felt insole
Comfortseat
    Flo-Fit C.
Comfort-U total body pillow
ComfortWalk
    C. foot system
    C. prosthetic foot
comfy
    C. Elbow Orthosis

C

NOTES

comfy *(continued)*
    C. elbow splint
    C. Knee Orthosis
    C. toilet lift seat
    C. walker
command
    C. hip instrumentation system
    C. instrument system surgical
        instrument
    C. joint replacement instrument
        system
comma sign
commemorative sign
comminuted
    c. bursting fracture
    c. intraarticular fracture
    c. pilon fracture
    c. teardrop fracture
comminution
    interposed c.
commissural myelorrhaphy
commissure
    anterior commissure-posterior c.
        (AC-PC)
committee
    Fitness Safety Standards C.
    International Knee
        Documentation C. (IKDC)
common
    c. carotid artery
    c. digital nerve
    c. dural sac
    c. extensor tendon
    c. iliac artery
    c. iliac vein
    c. peroneal nerve
    c. peroneal nerve block
    c. peroneal nerve paralysis
    c. peroneal nerve syndrome
communicans
    Gray ramus c.
communicating hydrosyringomyelia
communication
    asyndetic c.
communis
    extensor digitorum c. (EDC)
    flexor digitorum c. (FDC)
community
    C. Integration Questionnaire (CIQ)
    c. rehabilitation
Comolli sign
COMP
    cartilage oligomeric matrix protein
compact
    c. bone
    c. osteoma
compaction
    C. pliers
    vertical sacral c.

compactor
    acetabular cement c.
    cement c.
company
    United States Manufacturing C.
        (USMC)
    U.S. Manufacturing C.
comparative radiographic examination
comparison
    Achilles tendon rupture repair c.
compartment
    anterior c.
    Clancy lateral c.
    deep posterior c.
    dorsal c.
    fascial c.
    c. fasciotomy
    4-c. fasciotomy
    interosseous c.
    lateral c.
    medial c.
    Mueller lateral c.
    osteofascial c.
    patellofemoral c.
    plantar c.
    posterior c.
    posterolateral c.
    posteromedial c.
    superficial posterior c.
    c. syndrome
compartmental
    c. II knee prosthesis
    c. pressure
compass
    C. hinge
    C. Hinge external fixator
    C. stereotactic system
Compeed protective dressing
compensable accident
compensated
    c. metatarsus adductus
    c. talipes equinus
compensation reaction
compensatory
    c. basilar osteotomy
    c. behavior
    c. curve
    c. deformity
    c. hypermobility
    c. lordosis
    c. movement
    c. scoliosis
    c. structural subluxation
    c. wedge
Compere
    C. fixation wire
    C. lengthening
    C. operation

C. osteotome
C. threaded pin
Compere-Thompson arthrodesis
Comperm tubular elastic bandage
competence
    mechanism of reflex
      immunologic c.
    reflex immunologic c.
complement
complete
    c. amelia
    c. amputation
    c. aphalangia
    c. coalition
    c. dislocation
    c. fracture
    c. paraxial hemimelia
    c. phocomelia
    c. subtalar release (CSR)
    c. syndactyly
complex
    c. acetabular reconstruction
    ankle joint c. (AJC)
    apophysial c.
    arcuate c.
    atlas-axis c.
    atlas vertebral subluxation c.
    borotannic c.
    Buford c.
    bunion c.
    bunionette-hallux valgus-splayfoot c.
    bunion-hallux valgus c.
    capsulolabral c.
    capsuloligamentous c.
    Edinger-Westphal c.
    Eisenmenger c.
    epiphysial c.
    fabellofibular c.
    femur button graft c.
    femur-fibular-ulna c.
    fibrocartilage c.
    foot-ankle c.
    forearm c.
    c. fracture
    c. fracture dislocation
    gastrocnemius-soleus c.
    Ghon-Sachs c.
    hallux valgus-metatarsus primus
      varus c.
    hindfoot joint c.
    c. instability of carpus (CIC)
    3-joint c.
    knee c.

    lateral quadruple c.
    ligament-bone c.
    ligamentous c.
    Lisfranc joint c.
    lumbopelvic c.
    lymphedema c.
    medial quadruple c.
    c. meniscal tear
    c. motor unit action potential
    occipital-atlantoaxial c.
    occipitoatlantoaxial joint c.
    plantar capsuloligamentous c.
    postural c.
    quadruple c.
    radial collateral ligament c.
      (RCLC)
    Ranke c.
    c. regional pain syndrome (CRPS)
    c. regional pain syndrome type 2
      (CRPS-2)
    Remimembranosus c.
    c. repetitive discharge
    shoulder c.
    c. skewfoot
    SNARE c.
    soleus c.
    spinal cord-meningeal c.
    spring ligament c.
    c. syndactyly
    talocalcaneonavicular c.
    tibiocalcaneal joint c.
    trialkylphosphine gold c.
    triangular fibrocartilage c. (TFC,
      TFCC)
    ulnar collateral ligament c. (UCLC)
    vertebral subluxation c. (VSC)
    zygomatic-malar c. (ZMC)
compliant prestress system (CPS)
complicated
    c. complex syndactyly
    c. dislocation
    c. fracture
complication
    iatrogenic c.
    intraoperative c.
    neurologic c.
    neurovascular c.
    postoperative c.
    pulmonary c.
    urologic c.
complimentary and alternative medicine
(CAM)

NOTES

C

component

acetabular c.
AcuMatch A, L, M Series
   acetabular c.
AcuMatch L Series cemented
   femoral stem c.
AML trial hip c.
Amstutz femoral c.
anatomically graduated c. (AGC)
anatomic porous replacement
   hemispheric acetabular c.
Aufranc-Turner femoral c.
Bechtol acetabular c.
Biomet MARS acetabular c.
Biomet revision acetabular c.
Biomet shoulder c.
bipolar femoral c.
bipolar hip arthroplasty c.
Black Max mid size knee c.
Bombelli-Morscher femoral c.
cemented c.
cementless femoral c.
cerclaged c.
chamfered cylinder acetabular c.
Charnley flat-back femoral c.
Charnley narrow-stem c.
Charnley standard-stem c.
cobra-design femoral c.
custom-designed swan-neck
   femoral c.
Definition PM femoral implant c.
DePuy trispiked acetabular c.
dorsi stop c.
Duramer polyethylene c.
Durasul prosthetic c.
energy conservation walking c.
failed acetabular c.
femoral c.
fluid controlled   c.
c. of gait
glenoid c.
Gustilo-Kyle femoral c.
Harris-Galante hip replacement
   acetabular c.
Harris-Galante I porous-coated
   acetabular c.
head-neck c.
Healey revision acetabular c.
Hoffmann II compact external
   fixation c.
humeral c.
hybrid fixation of hip
   replacement c.
Infinity femoral c.
internal rotary component of
   force c.
keel of glenoid c.
kinesiopathologic c.
large-head humeral c.

Lubinus acetabular c.
MARS revision acetabular c.
Meridian ST femoral implant c.
metal-backed acetabular c.
Metasul hip joint c.
modular hip implant c.
modular large-head
monoblock femoral c.
Morse taper lock of modular hip
   implant c.
neck c.
Neer II humeral c.
neuromuscular c.
NexGen c.
OEC lag screw c.
Ogee acetabular c.
Osteolock acetabular c.
Osteolock HA femoral c.
Osteonics Omnifit-HA c.
performance c.
polyethylene liner implant c.
porous cementless c.
porous-coated c.
posterior c.
postural c.
press-fit femoral c.
Profix porous femoral c.
progression walking c.
prosthesis c.
quadrant sparing acetabular c.
   (QSAC)
Reliance CM femoral implant c.
roof-reinforcement ring hip
   arthroplasty c.
sensory c.
Smith & Nephew reflection
   acetabular cup implant c.
Springlite II foot c.
Springlite G foot c.
S-ROM modular femoral c.
standing stability walking c.
stem c.
sternal attachment c.
straight stem femoral c.
structural c.
c. subsidence
sympathetic c.
Taperloc femoral c.
Tharies femoral resurfacing c.
Tharies hip c.
thoracic extension c.
Ti-Bac acetabular c.
tibial c.
c. trial
trial femoral c.
Tri-Con c.
Tricon-M c.
Ultima C femoral c.
uncemented femoral c.

Universal radial c.
V40 femoral head implant c.
Vitalock cluster acetabular c.
Vitalock solid-back acetabular c.
wheel chair seating c.
Zimmer NexGen LPS knee
  femoral c.

composite
Carboplast II c.
c. defect
E-A-R specialty c.
c. fracture
c. free tissue transfer
c. groin fascial free flap
c. joint
c. knee score
c. material
c. prosthetic foot
c. rib graft
c. skin graft
c. spring elastic splint
void metal c. (VMC)

composition
body c.

compound
c. comminuted fracture (CCF)
c. dislocation
Hurler-Scheie c.
c. joint
c. mixed nerve action potential
c. motor nerve action potential
c. muscle action potential (CMAP)
c. muscle-motor action potential
  (CMAP)
c. nevus
OCT c.
photoactive naphthalimide c.
c. sensory nerve action potential
c. shattered elbow

Compoz
C. Gel Caps
C. Nighttime Sleep Aid

compression
c. anesthesia
anterior cord c.
anterior-inferior c.
anterior-posterior c. (APC)
AO c.
c. apparatus
c. arthrodesis
axial c.
c. bandage
c. boot

carotid artery c.
cauda equina c.
Charnley c.
c. clicker
Coldflo cold therapy and
  sequential c.
cord c.
disc c.
c. dressing
duodenal c.
dynamic c. (DC)
elastic c.
c. fracture
c. garment
c. glove
Harrington rod instrumentation c.
c. hip screw
c. hook
c. inserter-extractor
c. instrumentation posterior
  construct
interfragmentary c.
intermittent impulse c.
intermittent pneumatic c.
ischemic c.
c. lag screw
lateral c. (LC)
c. load
c. loading
c. locking anchor
c. locking anchor with secondary
  purchase (CLASP)
lower nerve root c.
lower sacral nerve root c.
  (LSNRC)
median nerve c.
c. molding
napkin ring c.
nerve root c.
neuraxial c.
c. overload
c. paralysis
c. pattern
c. phenomenon
c. plate
c. plate fixation
c. plating
pneumatic pedal c.
c. pump
c. rod
c. rod treatment
c. screw-plate device
sequential c.

C

NOTES

compression *(continued)*
 c. sideplate
 c. sleeve shin splint
 snap-off c. (SOC)
 spinal cord c.
 c. spring
 static c.
 c. stockings
 c. strain
 c. syndrome
 c. technique
 c. test
 c. testing
 c. therapy
 c. ultrasonography
 c. ultrasound
 c. U-rod instrumentation
 vasopneumatic intermittent c.
 venous c.
 vertebral c.
 vertical c.
 c. wire
 c. wiring
compression-molded
 c.-m. ethylene vinyl acetate (CM
  EVA)
 c.-m. prosthesis
compression-plus-torque cervical injury
compressive
 c. centripetal wrapping
 c. extension
 c. flexion
 c. flexion injury
 c. hyperextension injury
 c. internal fixating device
 c. neuropathy
compressor
 Adair screw c.
 screw c.
Comprifix
 C. active ankle support
 C. ankle splint
compromise
 c. osteotomy
 soft tissue c.
Compro Plus Knee support
Compton clavicle pin
Compudriver digital torque-meter
computed tomography (CT)
**computer-aided design/computer-aided
 manufacturing (CAD/CAM)**
computer-assisted
 c.-a. carpal tunnel syndrome
 c.-a. design
 c.-a. design/computer-assisted
  manufacturing prosthesis
 c.-a. mechanical instrument
  adjusting

 c.-a. myelography (CAM)
 c.-a. orthopaedic surgery (CAOS)
 c.-a. percutaneous internal fixation
computerized
 c. axial tomography (CAT)
 c. dynamic posturography (CDP)
 c. gait analysis
 c. isokinetic dynamometer
 c. musculoskeletal analysis
Conaxial ankle prosthesis
concave
 c. articular surface
 c. loading socket
 c. rod
concave-surface reamer
concavity
 flexural c.
 glenoid c.
concavity-compression effect
concavoconcave
concavoconvex
concealed straight leg raising test
concentrate
 platelet c.
concentric
 c. bilateral isokinetic
 c. contraction
 c. function
 c. hip cup
 c. isokinetic leg press exercise
 c. lamella
 c. loading
 c. muscle action
 c. needle electrode
 c. plantar flexion peak torque
  newton-meter
 c. reduction
 c. work
concept
 c ablator
 c arthroscopy power system
 c beach chair shoulder positioning
  system
 c bipolar coagulator
 c cannula
 3-column c
 c CTS Relief Kit
 Eftekhar c
 c handheld cautery
 hinge axis c
 c II rowing ergometer
 juvenile hinge axis c
 Klein-Vogelbach functional
  movement c
 one wound-one scar c
 c 2-pin passer
 c Precise ACL guide system
 c rotator cuff repair system

c self-compressing cannulated screw
system
c Sterling arthroscopy blade system
conceptual ability
concetric hip cup
concise
    C. cementing sculp
    C. compression hip screw
    C. compression hip screw system
    C. side plate
Conco elastic bandage
concomitant
concretion
concurrent force system
concussion
    sideline assessment of c. (SAC)
concussor
condensing osteitis
condition
    assessment for limiting c.
    degenerative spine c.
    diabetic foot ulcerative c.
    dysvascular c.
    limiting c.
    postsurgical heel c.
    sterile c.
    tumorous c.
conditioned stimulus (CS)
conditioner
    Shuttle cardiomuscular c.
conditioning
    aerobic c.
    musculoskeletal evaluation,
      rehabilitation and c. (MERAC)
    work c.
condom catheter
conduction
    c. block
    c. time
    c. velocity
    c. velocity test
    volume c.
conductive Hydrogel wound dressing
conductor
    Adson c.
    Bailey c.
    Bozzini light c.
    light c.
conduit
    Neurotube bioabsorbable nerve c.
condylar
    c. angle
    c. articulation

c. bolt
c. cartilage
c. compression fracture
c. cuff
c. defect
c. femoral fracture
c. implant
c. implant arthroplasty
c. plate
c. plateau angle (CPA)
c. screw fixation
c. split fracture
condyle
    bifid c.
    c. block
    femoral c.
    flare of c.
    humeral c.
    lateral femoral c.
    lateral tibial c.
    medial femoral c.
    medial humeral c.
    medial/lateral femoral c.
    occipital c.
    odontoid c.
    tibial c.
    volar c.
condylectomy
    DuVries phalangeal c.
    DuVries plantar c.
    phalangeal c.
    plantar c.
condylocephalic
    c. nail
    c. nailing
condyloid
    c. joint
    c. process
condylotomy
cone
    c. arthrodesis
    c. bone biopsy
    c. bur
    C. checkers game
    cutting c.
    hand c.
    Posey Palm C.
    prosthetic c.
    C. ring curette
    c. and socket bone
    C. splint
    stacking c.
    C. suction biopsy curette

NOTES

cone
coned-down view
confidence interval (CI)
configuration
  activity c.
  Cotrel-Dubousset hook claw c.
  double cruciate c.
  spoke-wheel c.
  triangular base transverse bar c.
confinement
  wheelchair c.
confirmatory testing
confluent
confocal microscopy
Conform dressing
Conformer diabetic boot
confrontational test
congenita
  amyoplasia c.
  amyotonia c.
  arthrogryposis multiplex c.
  dyskeratosis c.
  fragilitas ossium c.
  luxatio coxae c.
  myotonia c.
  osteogenesis imperfecta c. (OIC)
  pachyonychia c.
  paramyotonia c.
congenital
  c. above-elbow amputation
  c. anomaly
  c. anular band
  c. aphalangia
  c. atlantoaxial instability
  c. atonic pseudoparalysis
  c. band syndrome
  c. bar
  c. below-elbow amputation
  c. clasped thumb
  c. complete subtalar coalition
  c. convex pes plano valgus
  c. dislocation of hip (CDH)
  c. dysplasia of hip (CDH)
  c. dystrophy
  c. fibrous band
  c. fracture
  c. general fibromatosis
  c. hemivertebra
  c. hip dislocation
  c. hip dysplasia (CHD)
  c. hip subluxation
  c. hyperphosphatasemic skeletal
    dysplasia (CHSD)
  c. hypotonia
  c. intercalary limb absence
  c. kyphosis (type I, II)
  c. laxity
  c. laxity of ligament
  c. limb deficiency

c. limb disorder
c. lymphedema
c. metatarsus adductus
c. myopathy
c. myotonia
c. nevus
c. osteochondroma
c. patella dislocation
c. plexopathy
c. posteromedial bowing
c. predisposition
c. pseudoarthritis
c. radioulnar synostosis
c. ring
c. rocker-bottom flatfoot
c. scapular elevation
c. scoliosis
c. spondylolisthesis
c. stenosis
c. talipes equinovarus
c. terminal limb absence
c. tibial deficiency
c. tibial pseudarthrosis
c. torticollis
c. trigger digit
c. trigger finger
c. ulnar drift
c. vertical talus (CVT)
c. vertical talus foot deformity
c. wry neck
congenitally short limb
congestion
  flap c.
  intraosseous vascular c.
congestive heart failure (CHF)
congruence
  c. angle
  joint c.
  patellofemoral c.
congruent
  c. articulation
  c. metatarsophalangeal joint
  c. reduction
congruity
  ball-and-socket c.
congruous cup-shaped reamer
conical
  c. bur
  c. nut wrench
  c. obturator
  c. reamer
conical-point wire
conjoined
  c. gastrocnemius soleus fascial slip
  c. lateral band
  c. tendon
conjugated
  c. estrogens
  c. linoleic acid (CLA)

Conley pin
connecting
  c. bolt
  c. cartilage
  c. plate
connection
  Martin-Gruber c.
  neuroendocrine-immune c.
  Riche-Cannieu c.
  vincula longa c.
connective
  c. tissue
  c. tissue disease
  c. tissue massage (CTM)
  c. tissue plasticity
connector
  adjustable pedicle c.
  anchor c.
  domino spinal instrumentation c.
  intrinsic transverse c.
  longitudinal member to anchor c.
  longitudinal member to longitudinal
    member c.
  pedicle c.
  tandem c.
  transverse c.
Con-Nex reamer
Connolly
  C. procedure
  C. technique
Conn operation
conoid
  c. ligament
  c. process
  c. tubercle
conoidal ankle prosthesis
conoideum
Conrad-Bugg
  C.-B. trapping
  C.-B. trapping of soft tissue
Conradi
  C. disease
  C. syndrome
consecutive
  c. amputation
  c. dislocation
conservatism
  therapeutic c.
conservative
  c. management
  c. therapy
Conserve hip system

consideration
  return-to-play c.
consistency
  boggy c.
  doughy c.
console compression garment
consolidated graft
consolidation
  bony c.
  delayed c.
  fracture line c.
  premature c.
constancy
  form c.
constant
  c. direct current stimulator
  c. massive motion
  C. and Murley shoulder scoring
    system
  c. tension splint
constant-friction knee
constant-touch perception
ConstaVac
  C. autoreinfusion system
  C. drainage
constellation of clinical findings
constitutional stenosis
constrained
  c. ankle arthroplasty
  c. condylar knee
  c. hinged knee prosthesis
  c. nonhinged knee prosthesis
  c. shoulder arthroplasty
constriction
  c. band
  c. band syndrome
  hourglass c.
  c. ring
constrictive edema
construct
  anterior c.
  AO dynamic compression plate c.
  blade-plate c.
  compression instrumentation
    posterior c.
  disease c.
  double-rod c.
  Edwards modular system bridging
    sleeve c.
  Edwards modular system
    compression c.
  Edwards modular system
    distraction-lordosis c.

C

NOTES

construct *(continued)*
Edwards modular system kyphoreduction c.
Edwards modular system neutralization c.
Edwards modular system rod sleeve c.
Edwards modular system scoliosis c.
Edwards modular system spondylar c.
Edwards modular system standard sleeve c.
hook-to-screw L4-S1 compression c.
iliosacral and iliac fixation c.
pedicle screw c.
c. pedicle screw-laminar claw c.
posterior c.
rod-hook c.
screw-to-screw compression c.
segmental compression c.
single-rod c.
triplane c.
TSRH double-rod c.
upper cervical spine anterior c.
upper cervical spine posterior c.
Wiltse system double-rod c.
Wiltse system H c.
Wiltse system single-rod c.

construction
California welt c.
corticocancellous c.

constructional ability

contact
C. ArthroProbe
c. force
c. healing
c. laser delivery system
c. manipulation
manual c.
c. point
Richards maximum c. (RMC)
c. shield
C. SPH cups system
standing knee bend PSIS-sacrum c.
c. stress

contained
c. disc herniation
c. herniated disc

container
Quickbox c.

containment bag

content
bone mineral c. (BMC)

context
performance c.

Contextual Memory Test (CMT)

contiguity
amputation in c.

contiguous
c. articular surface
c. vertebral structure

continuity
amputation in c.
c. of bone
neuroma in c.
synthesis of c.

continuous
c. anatomical passive exerciser (CAPE)
c. cryotherapy
c. intravenous regional anesthesia (CIVRA)
c. LVG
c. passive motion (CPM)
c. passive motion machine
c. stimulation
c. wave arthroscopy pump

continuum
C. bipolar acetabular head
C. elliptical acetabular cup
C. hip stem
C. knee system (CKS)
C. knee system implant
C. polyethylene acetabular cup
C. P/S total knee
C. total knee base plate
C. unconstrained prosthesis

contour
C. DF-80 total hip operation
double hump c.
C. internal prosthesis
C. Meniscus Arrow bioresorbable repair system
patellar c.
polyethylene proximal brim in quadrilateral c.
spinal c.
Wiberg type II patellar c.

contoured
c. adduction trochanteric-controlled alignment method (CAT-CAM)
c. anterior spinal plate (CASP)
c. anterior spinal plate drill guide
c. anterior spinal plate technique
c. felt padding
c. femoral stem (CFS)
c. T-plate plate
c. washer

contract

contractile force curve

contractility
muscle c.

contraction
active c.
concentric c.
detrusor c.
direct c.

eccentric c.
extrafusal fiber c.
c. fasciculation
isometric c.
isotonic c.
lengthening c.
maintained c.
maximal voluntary c. (MVC)
muscular c.
reflex muscular c.
repeated quick stretch superimposed
  upon an existing c. (RQS-SEC)
shortening c.
tetanic c.
c. tremor
c. type
volitional c.
contractor
Bailey-Gibbon rib c.
Bailey rib c.
Lemmon rib c.
rib c.
Sellors rib c.
contract-relax technique
contracture
abduction c.
Achilles tendon c.
acquired thumb flexion c.
acute ischemic c.
adduction c.
axillary c.
burn c.
clawfoot c.
c. deformity
digital c.
Dupuytren c.
equinus c.
established c.
c. exercise
extension c.
external rotation c.
fixed flexion c. (FFC)
flexion, abduction, external
  rotation c.
flexor digitorum longus tendon c.
flexor hallucis tendon c.
forearm c.
gastrocnemius-soleus c.
hip flexor c.
intrinsic c.
ischemic c.
knee c.
lumbrical intrinsic c.

metacarpophysial joint extension c.
muscle c.
opposition c.
paralytic c.
pelvic flexion c. (PFC)
postpoliomyelitic c.
pronation c.
quadriceps c.
rectus femoris c.
retropatellar fat pad c.
rotational c.
shoulder c.
Skoog procedure for release of
  Dupuytren c.
soft tissue c.
spastic intrinsic c.
supination c.
valgus c.
varus c.
Volkmann c.
web c.
wrist c.
contraflexion brace
contraindication
stretching c.
contralateral
c. double vertical fracture
c. foot
c. hypoplastic/agenetic pedicle
c. pain
c. sign
c. spondylolysis
c. straight leg raising
c. straight leg raising test
contrast
c. agent
air c.
c. arthrography
c. bath (CB)
c. column
c. medium-enhanced magnetic
  resonance imaging (CME-MRI)
contrecoup
c. contusion
fracture by c.
c. fracture
c. injury
control
biomechanical c.
car hand c.
3D positional c.
Dupaco knee c.

C

NOTES

control *(continued)*
 evaluation, prediction,
  intervention, c. (EPIC)
 exsanguination tourniquet c.
 fluoroscopic c.
 habitual c.
 hip joint aspiration under
  fluoroscopic c.
 maximum c. (MC)
 monitored anesthesia c. (MAC)
 motion c.
 nudge c.
 postural c.
 pronation c.
 pronation/spring c. (PSC)
 rotary c.
 swing-phase c.
 Total Environment C. (TEC)
 tourniquet c.
 trunk c.
 verticality c.
 voluntary c. (VC)
controlled
 c. ankle motion (CAM)
 c. ankle walker
 c. comminuted fracture
 c. force application
 c. position brace (CPB)
 c. range of motion (CRM)
 c. rotational osteotomy
controlled-motion brace
controller
 shoulder c.
 C. shoulder orthosis
contusion
 chest c.
 contrecoup c.
 coup c.
 cuff c.
 hip pointer c.
 muscle c.
 osteochondral c.
 pelvic region c.
 quadriceps c.
 rib c.
 rotator cuff c.
conus medullaris syndrome
ConvaDERM Plus dressing
conventional
 c. cutting needle
 c. osteosarcoma
 c. silicone elastomer (CSE)
 c. single-axis knee prosthesis
 c. technique
 c. tomography
convergence
 angle of c.
 c. facilitation
 c. projection

converse
 C. chisel
 C. periosteal elevator
 C. splint
conversion
 Tilt-In-Space wheelchair c.
Convery polyarticular disability index
convex
 c. condylar-implant arthroplasty
 c. fusion
 c. pes valgus
 c. rasp
 c. rod
convexity
 distal ulnar c.
 left lumbar c.
 c. of spine
 ulnar c.
convoluted bone
convolution
 Broca c.
Conyers technique
cookbook
 c. stimulation
 c. stimulation of acupuncture points
Cook-Gordon mechanism
cookie
 arch c.
 c. cutter
 Gelfoam c.
 metatarsal c.
 navicular shoe c.
 scaphoid shoe c.
 shoe c.
Cooksey-Cawthorne exercise
Cook walking brace
cool
 c. CPB brace
 c. Irom splint
 c. pack
 c. pack cryotherapy
Cool-Aid continuous controlled cold
 therapy
Cooley
 C. graft clamp
 C. iliac clamp
 C. multipurpose angled clamp
 C. multipurpose curved clamp
 C. rib retractor
 C. rib shears
Cooley-Baumgarten wire twister
Cool-Flex A/K suspension belt
cooling machine
CoolSorb absorbent cold transfer
 dressing
Coombs bone biopsy system
Coonrad
 C. hinged prosthesis

C. semiconstrained elbow prosthesis
C. total elbow arthroplasty
Coonrad-II prosthesis
Coonrad-Morrey
C.-M. elbow prosthesis
C.-M. implant
C.-M. total elbow arthroplasty
Coonse-Adams
C.-A. knee approach
C.-A. quadricepsplasty
C.-A. technique
Cooper
C. ankle brace
C. reduction
Coopercare Lastrap support wrap
Coopernail sign
Coopervision irrigation/aspiration handpiece
coordinate
C. complete revision knee system
c. system (X, Y, Z)
coordinated mobility
coordination
muscular c.
Copeland-Howard
C.-H. scapulothoracic fusion
C.-H. shoulder procedure
Copeland humeral resurfacing head
Copeland-Kavat classification of metatarsophalangeal dislocation
Copenhagen Stroke study
Coping Strategies Questionnaire (CSQ)
coplaning
arthroscopic c.
COPM
Canadian Occupational Performance Measure
copolymer
c. ankle-foot orthosis
c. foam
LactoSorb resorbable c.
c. orthotic material
c. starch copolymer bead
CO_2 powered gun system
copper
c. deficiency syndrome
c. mallet
copropraxia
coracoacromial
c. arch
c. ligament
c. ligament transfer
c. process

coracobrachialis
biceps, brachialis, c. (BBC)
coracobrachial muscle
coracoclavicular (CC)
c. arthrodesis
c. articulation
c. distance
c. fixation apparatus
c. joint
c. ligament
c. screw
c. screw fixation
c. suture fixation
c. technique
coracohumeral (CH)
c. ligament
coracoid
c. fracture
c. impingement syndrome
c. notch
c. process
c. tip avulsion
c. tuberosity
coracoiditis
coracoradialis
coracoulnaris
Coraderm dressing
Corail
C. HA-coated stem
C. HA-coated stem hip implant
C. hip system
C. press-fit prosthesis
coral
madreporic c.
Corbett bone rongeur
cord
anterior horn of spinal c.
central c.
cervical spinal c.
c. compression
digital c.
heel c.
lateral c.
MGHL c.
natatory c.
c. portion
pretendinous c.
retrovascular c.
space available for c. (SAC)
spinal c.
Sport C.
tenodesis of heel c.

C

NOTES

cord *(continued)*
    tethered spinal c.
    vocal c.
Cordase injectable collagenase
cordate pelvis
cordiform pelvis
Cordis implantable drug reservoir device
cordlike structure
Cordon-Colles fracture splint
cordotomy
cord-traction syndrome
corduroy cloth pattern
core
    c. biopsy obturator
    bone c.
    c. decompression
    c. decompression of femoral head
    c. drilling procedure
    C. Hibak Rest
    C. Lobak Rest
    C. Max-Relax Cushion
    c. needle biopsy
    C. Reflex wrist support
    C. Sitback Rest
    C. Slimrest
    c. suture
    C. Universal elastic knee support
    C. Universal elbow support
    C. Universal rib support
Corfit System 7000 Series Lumbosacral Support
coring
    c. apparatus
    c. device
Corin hip arthroplasty system
cork
    c. borer
    sheet c.
corkscrew
    c. femoral head extractor
    C. Parachute
    C. rotator cuff repair system
    C. suture anchor
corn
    apical c.
    end c.
    hard c.
    interdigital c.
    Lister c.
    neurovascular c.
    plantar c.
    soft c.
    web c.
Cornelia de Lange syndrome
corner
    c. fracture
    c. fragment
    c. of knee

    4-c. midcarpal fusion
    posteromedial c.
3-cornered bone
corneum
    stratum c.
cornuate navicular
cornuradicular zone
Cornwall hip fracture study
Coromega dietary supplement
coronal
    c. computed tomographic arthrography (CCTA)
    c. plane
    c. plane correction
    c. plane deformity
    c. plane deformity sagittal translation
    c. split fracture
    c. tilting
    c. T1-weighted sequence
coronary
    c. artery disease (CAD)
    c. bone
    c. ligament
coronoid
    c. fragment
    c. line
    c. process
    c. process fracture
corpectomy
    anterior c.
    cervical c.
    c. model
    vertebral body c.
corporation
    Accurate Surgical and Scientific Instruments C. (ASSI)
corporectomy amputation
corporotransverse
    c. inferior ligament
    c. superior ligament
correction
    adult flatfoot c.
    anterior c.
    Beckenbaugh c.
    Bonferroni c.
    chevron hallux valgus c.
    child flatfoot c.
    Chrisman-Snook c.
    coronal plane c.
    cubitus varus c.
    curvature c.
    frontal plane c.
    hallux varus c.
    hammertoe c.
    King curve posterior c. (type IV)
    kyphosis c.
    Lapidus-type c.
    loss of c.

mechanism of c.
neuromechanical c.
phalangeal malunion c.
rotational c.
Ruiz-Mora c.
scoliosis c.
somatovisceral c.
Steel c.
V-Y plasty c.

corrective
c. cast
c. lengthening osteotomy
c. orthosis
c. shoe
c. soft dressing
c. spinal care
c. therapy

corrosion
crevice c.
fretting c.
metal implant c.

corrugated reamer
corrugator muscle
corset
Boston soft c.
Camp c.
Campbell c.
dorsal lumbar c.
elastic ankle c.
c. front
Hoke lumbar c.
Kampe c.
leather ankle c.
lumbodorsal support c.
lumbosacral c.
soft c.
surgical c.
c. suspension
thigh c.
thoracolumbar c.
Warm 'n' Form lumbosacral c.

cortex, pl. **cortices**
adrenal c.
articular c.
femoral c.
lateral c.
c. screw
vertebral body anterior c.

cortical
c. ASIF screw
c. atrophy
c. bone

c. bone graft
c. bone modeling
c. bone primary canal
c. bone remodeling
c. bone screw
c. breach
c. cancellous screw
c. débridement
c. defect
c. desmoid
c. desmoid tumor
c. destruction
c. fibrous dysplasia
c. fracture
c. fragment
c. index
c. lucency
c. perforation
c. pin
c. plasticity
c. plate
c. step drill
c. strut graft
c. thickening
c. thickness
c. thumb
c. window
c. windowing

corticalization
cortices (*pl. of* cortex)
corticocancellous
c. bone
c. bone graft
c. bone strip
c. chip graft
c. construction

corticospinal tract
corticosteroid (CS)
depot c.
c. injection
postoperative c.
c. therapy

corticosteroid-induced avascular necrosis
corticotomy
DeBastiani c.
Ilizarov c.
percutaneous c.
c. of proximal tibia

COR/T implant
cortisone
c. acetate
c. injection

C

NOTES

165

Cortisporin
>   C. Topical Cream
>   C. Topical Ointment

Cortone Acetate
Cortoss bone void filler
corundum ceramic implant material
Coryllos rasp
cosmesis
>   foot c.
>   poor c.
>   scarring c.

cosmetically acceptable foot
Cosmolon closure for splint
costal
>   c. angle
>   c. bone
>   c. cartilage
>   c. notch
>   c. periosteotome

costalgia
costectomy
Costen syndrome
costocentral articulation
costochondral
>   c. joint
>   c. junction of ribs

costochondritis
costoclavicular
>   c. ligament
>   c. maneuver
>   c. space
>   c. syndrome
>   c. syndrome test

costocoracoid
costogenic
costoinferior
costolumbar angle
costophrenic angle
costopleural
costoscapular
costoscapularis
costosternal
>   c. angle
>   c. articulation

costosternoplasty
costotransversarium
costotransverse
>   c. joint
>   c. ligament

costotransversectomy
>   c. approach
>   Seddon dorsal spine c.
>   c. technique

costovertebral
>   c. angle (CVA)
>   c. angle tenderness (CVAT)
>   c. articulation
>   c. joint

costoxiphoid

cot
>   finger c.

Cotrel
>   C. pedicle screw
>   C. pedicle screw fixation strength
>   C. pedicle screw rigidity
>   C. scoliosis
>   C. scoliosis cast
>   C. traction

Cotrel-Dubousset (C-D)
>   C.-D. derotation operation
>   C.-D. dynamic transverse traction device
>   C.-D. hook claw configuration
>   C.-D. hook-rod
>   C.-D. pedicle screw instrumentation
>   C.-D. rod
>   C.-D. rod flexibility
>   C.-D. spinal instrument

Cotting ingrown nail procedure
Cottle
>   C. chisel
>   C. mallet
>   C. osteotome
>   C. rasp
>   C. saw

cotton
>   C. ankle fracture
>   C. ankle instability test
>   c. ball appearance
>   c. bolster
>   c. cast
>   c. cast padding
>   c. dressing
>   c. elastic bandage
>   c. elbow reduction
>   C. fibular bone hook test
>   C. procedure
>   C. reduction of elbow dislocation
>   c. roll
>   c. sheet wadding
>   c. suture

Cotton-Berg syndrome
cottonloader position
cottonoid patty
cotyloid
>   c. cavity
>   c. notch

cotyloplasty technique
cotylosacral
cough
>   c. fracture
>   c. test

Coulter counter
council
>   Medical Research C. (MRC)

counseling
>   rehabilitation c. (RC)

count
  instrument, sponge, needle c.
  lymphocyte c.
  platelet c.
  potassium-40 c.
  white blood cell c.
counter
  Coulter c.
  extended medial shoe c.
  heel c.
  c. nutation
  c. rotating saw
  C. Rotation System (CRS)
  C. Rotation System brace
  c. sink
counterbalance
counterclockwise
counterextension
counterforce strap
counterrotational splint
countersinking osteotomy
countersink screw head
counterstrain technique
countersunk
countertraction splint
counterweight
Count'R-Force arch brace
coup contusion
coupled
  c. discharge
  c. motion
coupler
  Ferrier c.
coupling
  capacitive c.
  ceramic-on-ceramic c.
Couvelaire incision
Covaderm Plus adhesive barrier dressing
Coventry
  C. distal femoral osteotomy
  C. proximal tibial osteotomy
  C. screw
  C. staple
  C. vagal osteotomy
cover
  Accu-Flo polyethylene bur hole c.
  Accu-Flo silicone rubber bur hole c.
  AquaShield orthopaedic cast c.
  AquaShield reusable cast c.
  cast c.
  Overcast cast c.
  ShowerSafe waterproof cast and bandage c.
  soft cosmetic c.
  Springlite polyolefin BK c.
  Springlite polyurethane AK, BK conical c.
coverage
  skin c.
  soft tissue c.
covering
  Cast Cozy toe c.
  epineural c.
  fascial sheath c.
Coverlet
  C. adhesive
  C. adhesive surgical dressing
  C. Strips wound dressing
Cover-Roll
  C.-R. adhesive gauze dressing
  C.-R. gauze
  C.-R. gauze adhesive
  C.-R. stretch bandage
Covertell composite secondary dressing
Cowboy Collar
Cowden syndrome
cowhorn brace
Co-Wrap dressing
coxa, pl. **coxae**
  c. adducta
  c. plana
  c. senilis
  c. valga
  c. vara
  c. vara deformity pelvic radiotherapy
coxal bone
coxalgia
coxalgic pelvis
coxankylometer
coxarthria
coxarthritis
coxarthrocace
coxarthropathy
  Postel c.
coxarthrosis
  end-stage c.
Cox flexion-distraction technique
coxitic scoliosis
coxitis
coxodynia
coxofemoral
  c. articulation
  c. joint

C

NOTES

coxotomy
coxotuberculosis
Cozen
    C. test
    C. transverse approach
Cozen-Brockway Z-plasty
cozy
    Cast C.
CP
    cerebral palsy
CP2 inflatable cold pack
CPA
    calcaneal pitch angle
    condylar plateau angle
CPB
    controlled position brace
CPM
    continuous passive motion
        AIM CPM
        CPM apparatus
        CPM device
        CPM exerciser machine
CPPD
    calcium pyrophosphate dihydrate
    deposition
CPS
    compliant prestress system
cps, c/sec
    cycle per second
CPT
    Cognitive Performance Test
    collarless, polished, tapered
        CPT hip system
        CPT prosthesis
CR
    closed reduction
crab gait
crabmeat-like appearance
Cracchiolo
    C. forefoot arthroplasty
    C. procedure
Cracchiolo-Sculco implant arthroplasty
crack
    c. fracture
    hairline c.
cracking
    environmental stress c.
    c. of joint
    stress-corrosion c.
cradle
    c. arm sling
    bed c.
    Posey bed c.
Crafoord thoracic scissors
Craig
    C. abduction splint
    C. Handicap Assessment and
      Reporting Technique (CHART)
    C. pin

    C. pin remover
    C. vertebral biopsy set
Craig-Scott orthosis
Cramer wire splint
cramp
    c. discharge
    heat c.
    muscle c.
    muscular c.
cramping
    heat c.
Cram test
crane
    C. mallet
    C. osteotome
    C. shoulder exercise
cranial
    c. bone
    c. defect
    c. electrical stimulation (CES)
    c. helmet
    c. nerve abnormality
    c. tongs
cranial-sacral respiratory mechanism
(CRSM)
cranioacromial
craniocaudal glide
craniocervical plate
craniofacial
    c. angle
    c. dysjunction fracture
craniomandibular dysfunction
craniosacral
    c. table
    c. theory
    c. therapy (CST)
    c. therapy technique
craniospinal trauma
craniotabes
craniovertebral
crank
    c. frame retractor
    c. table
    c. test
crankshaft phenomenon
crash induction of anesthesia
craterization
cravat bandage
Crawford
    C. head frame
    C. incision
    C. low lithotomy crutch
    C. L-shaped osteotomy
Crawford-Adams
    C.-A. acetabular cup
    C.-A. acetabular cup arthroplasty
crawl
    barrel c.

crazy
> c. bone
> c. bone of elbow

C-reactive protein

creaking
> alar c.
> back c.
> distal medial c.
> flexion c.
> infragluteal c.
> metatarsophalangeal c.
> palmar c.
> PIP flexion c.
> popliteal flexion c.
> skin c.
> thenar c.
> ulnar c.
> wrist c.

cream (*See also* creme)
> AmLactin c.
> Diapedic foot c.
> Free-Up massage c.
> massage c.
> Naftin c.
> Thera-Gesic c.

crease
> alar c.
> back c.
> distal palmar c. (DPC)
> flexor skin c.
> infragluteal c.
> metatarsophalangeal c.
> palmar c.
> popliteal c.
> skin c.
> thenar palmar c. (TPC)

creatine phosphokinase

creation
> kyphosis c.
> lordosis c.

Creative diabetic socks

Credé maneuver

Credo operation

Creed dissector

creep
> transient compressive c.
> viscoelastic c.
> webspace c.

creeping substitution

Crego
> C. elevator
> C. femoral osteotomy
> C. hip reduction

> C. periosteal elevator
> C. retractor
> C. tendon transfer technique

cremasteric reflex

creme (*See also* cream)

crepitans
> peritendinitis c.
> tenalgia c.
> tenosynovitis c.

crepitant

crepitation
> patellofemoral c.
> "Rice Krispie" c.

crepitus
> articular c.
> bony c.

crescent
> C. Complete Sleeper pillow
> C. memory pillow
> c. sign

crescentic
> c. base wedge osteotomy
> c. base wedge
> osteotomy/bunionectomy
> c. basilar first metatarsal osteotomy
> c. calcaneal osteotomy
> c. rupture
> c. saw
> c. shelf osteotomy (CSO)

Crescent-Pillo pillow

crescent-shaped
> c.-s. fibrocartilaginous disc
> c.-s. osteotomy

CREST
> calcinosis, Raynaud, esophageal motility
> disorders, sclerodactyly, telangiectasia
> CREST syndrome

crest
> c. buttress pad
> iliac c.
> Maquet elevation of tibial c.
> neural c.
> palpation of iliac c.
> c. sign
> c. sign side
> tibial c.
> toe c.

cretinism

crevice corrosion

crick in the neck

cricoid
> c. cartilage
> c. ring

C

NOTES

cricopharyngeal sphincter muscle
cricothyroid membrane
Crile
    C. forceps
    C. gasserian ganglion knife and
    dissector
    C. head traction
    C. hemostat
    C. knife
Crile-Wood needle holder
crimped Dacron prosthesis
crimper
    Caparosa wire c.
    pin c.
    Simmons c.
    washer c.
    wire c.
crisis, pl. crises
    bone c.
crispation
crista
criterion, pl. criteria
    Ackerman osteomyelitis c.
    Beighton hypermobility syndrome
    criteria
    Catagni criteria
    Garcia wrist laxity criteria
    Harris criteria
    Hodgkinson acetabular component
    loosening criteria
    Insall criteria
    Kellgren degenerative disc disease
    criteria
    Mulholland and Gunn criteria
    New York diagnostic criteria
    Rome criteria
    Salter criteria
    Severin hip criteria
    White and Panjabi cervical spine
    criteria
    WHO/LAR Response C.
Criticaid lotion
critical
    c. limb ischemia (CLI)
    c. load
CRM
    controlled range of motion
    CRM cup
    CRM rehab brace
    CRM stem
    CRM system
crochet
    main en c.
CROM
    cervical range of motion
Crosby reduction
cross
    c. bar

    c. friction
    c. leg pain
cross-arm flap
cross-bracing
    spinal rod c.-b.
    Wiltse system c.-b.
crosscut
    c. bur
    c. saw
crossed
    c. adductor reflex
    c. extensor reflex
    c. flexor reflex
    c. intrinsic transfer
    c. Kirschner wire
    c. straight leg raise
    c. straight leg raise test
    c. straight leg raising (CSLR)
crossed-leg pike down stretch
cross-extremity flap
cross-finger flap
cross-friction massage
crosshead displacement
crossing
    nerve c.
    c. screws
cross-leg
    c.-l. flap
    c.-l. Patrick maneuver
cross-legged gait
crosslink
    Edwards modular system rod c.
    free pyridinium c.
    Galveston fixation with TSRH c.
    c. plate
    c. plate size
    pyridinium collagen c. (PYD)
    pyridinoline collagen c. (PYD)
    TSRH c.
crosslinked EVA copolymer foam
cross-locking screw
crossover
    femoral-femoral c.
    c. second toe
    c. syndrome
    c. test
crossover-toe deformity
cross-screw fixation
cross-sectional anatomy
cross-slot screwdriver
cross-table
    c.-t. lateral radiograph
    c.-t. lateral view (CTLV)
crossunion
crotch strap
crouch gait
Crouzon syndrome
CROW
    Charcot restraint orthotic walker

Crowe
 C. congenital hip dysplasia classification
 C. congenital hip dysplasia classification system
 C. congenital hip dysplasia (type I-IV)
 C. hip scale
 C. pilot point
 C. pilot point on Steinmann pin
 C. subluxation
 C. tip pin
crown
 Adaptic c.
 c. and collar scissors
 c. drill
 c. drill screw
 Unitek steel c.
CRPS
 complex regional pain syndrome
CRPS-2
 complex regional pain syndrome type 2
CRS
 Counter Rotation System
 CRS brace
 CRS Tibial Torsion System
CRSM
 cranial-sacral respiratory mechanism
crucial angle of Gissane
cruciate
 anterior c.
 c. condylar knee system
 c. condylar unconstrained prosthesis
 c. pulley (C1–C3)
 c. fashion
 c. head bone screw
 c. incision
 c. ligament
 c. ligament laxity
 c. ligament reconstruction
 c. ligament rupture
 c. paralysis
 posterior c.
 c. punch
cruciate-retaining prosthesis
cruciate-sacrificing prosthesis
cruciform
 c. anterior spinal hyperextension (CASH)
 c. anterior spinal hyperextension orthosis
 c. head bone screw

 c. screwdriver
 c. tibial base plate
cruiser
 c. buggy
 C. hip abduction
 C. hip abduction brace
 C. OA brace
crural
 Bigelow c.
 c. fascia
cruris
 angina c.
 tinea c.
crush
 c. fracture
 c. injury
 c. syndrome
crushed eggshell fracture
crushing osteochondritis
crutch
 c. ambulation
 axillary c.
 c. and belt femoral closed nail
 c. and belt femoral closed nailing
 Canadian c.
 Crawford low lithotomy c.
 EuroCuff forearm c.
 hands-free c.
 Hardy aluminum c.
 iWALKfree hands-free c.
 Lofstrand c.
 c. palsy
 c. paralysis
 platform c.
 c. walking
 weightbearing c.
Crutchfield
 C. bone drill
 C. drill point
 C. hand drill
 C. operation
 C. pin
 C. skeletal tong traction
Crutchfield-Raney
 C.-R. drill
 C.-R. tongs
Cruveilhier
 C. atrophy
 C. disease
 C. joint
 C. ligament
 C. paralysis
cryoanalgesia

C

NOTES

Cryo/Cuff
> Aircast C./C.
> C./C. ankle dressing
> C./C. boot
> C./C. compression support
> C./C. Knee Compression Dressing System

Cryocup ice massager
cryogenic
> c. denervation
> c. neuroablation

cryohypophysectomy
cryoprecipitate
cryopreserved cartilage
cryosurgery
cryotherapy
> continuous c.
> cool pack c.
> liquid nitrogen c.
> c. rehabilitation
> verruca c.

cryptococcal infection
cryptococcosis
Cryptococcus neoformans
cryptopodia
cryptotic medial border
cry reflex
crystal
> C. adjusting table
> calcium hydroxyapatite c.
> CHA c.
> c. deposition
> monosodium urate c.
> C. polymer gel
> uric acid c.

crystal-induced
> c.-i. arthritis
> c.-i. arthropathy
> c.-i. arthrosis
> c.-i. synovitis

crystalloid solution
crystal-related
> c.-r. arthropathy
> c.-r. joint disease

CS
> conditioned stimulus
> corticosteroid

CSE
> conventional silicone elastomer

c/sec (*var. of* cps)
> cycle per second

C-shaped
> C-s. foot
> C-s. plate

CSI
> Caregiver Strain Index

CSLR
> crossed straight leg raising

CSMT
> capillary refill, sensation, motor function, temperature

CSO
> crescentic shelf osteotomy

CSQ
> Coping Strategies Questionnaire

CSR
> complete subtalar release
> McKay-Simons CSR

CSRA
> cementless surface replacement arthroplasty

CST
> craniosacral therapy

CT
> carpal tunnel
> computed tomography
> > CT bone densitometer
> > CT scan

CTA
> cuff tear arthropathy

CT-based CAD/CAM revision femoral implant
CTD
> carpal tunnel decompression
> cumulative trauma disorder

CTE
> chronic traumatic encephalopathy

C-Tek anterior cervical plate system
CTi2 knee brace
CTi brace
CTLSO
> cervicothoracolumbosacral orthosis
> > CTLSO orthosis

CTLV
> cross-table lateral view

CTM
> cervical tension myositis
> connective tissue massage

CTO
> cervicothoracic orthosis
> > Aspen CTO

CTR
> carpal tunnel release

CTS
> carpal tunnel syndrome
> Champion Trauma Score
> > CTS gauge
> > CTS Gripfit splint

CTSIB
> Clinical Test of Sensory Integration and Balance

Cubbins
> C. arthroplasty
> C. bone screwdriver
> C. incision
> C. open reduction
> C. operation

C. screw
C. shoulder approach
C. shoulder dislocation technique
cube
Temper Foam c.
CUBEx multifunctional step
cubital
c. bursitis
c. joint
c. nerve
c. process
c. tunnel
c. tunnel splint
c. tunnel syndrome
cubitocarpal
cubitoradial
cubitus
patella c.'s
c. pseudovarus
c. recurvatum
c. valgus
c. varus
c. varus correction
cuboid
c. abduction angle
c. bone
c. decancellation
c. declination angle
c. fracture
c. fusion
c. notch
c. sulcus
c. syndrome
c. wedge osteotomy
cuboidal tuberosity
cuboid-calcaneal osteotomy
cuboideonavicular ligament
cubonavicular
c. coalition
c. joint
cucullaris muscle
cucumber heel
Cuda shaver
cuff
arm c.
collar and c.
condylar c.
c. contusion
c. of fascia
hand c.
joint distraction c.
leather c.
C. Link orthopaedic device

musculotendinous c.
pneumatic tourniquet c.
push c.
Push-Ease Quad C.
c. resection
rotator c. (RC)
shoulder c.
Steri-Cuff disposable tourniquet c.
supracondylar c.
suprapatellar c. (SPC)
c. suspension
c. tear arthropathy (CTA)
c. tear arthroplasty
thigh c.
Western Ontario Rotator C.
(WORC)
cuing strategy
Culler hook
Culley ulnar splint
culture
bacterial c.
blood c.
DTM c.
urine c.
wound c.
Cummins procedure
cumulative trauma disorder (CTD)
cuneiform
atavistic c.
c. bone
c. fracture
c. injury
c. joint
c. joint arthrodesis
c. mortise
c. osteotomy
cuneiform-first metatarsal exostosis
cuneocuboid
cuneometatarsal joint
cuneonavicular
c. joint
c. ligament
cuneoscaphoid
Cuniard and Campell technique
cuniculatum
epithelioma c.
Cunningham brace
cup
AccuPressure heel c.
acetabular c.
Anti-Shox heel c.
c. arthroplasty
Arthropor acetabular c.

C

NOTES

cup *(continued)*

Aufranc modification of Smith-Petersen c.
Aufranc-Turner acetabular c.
Bauerfeind SofSpot Heel C.
Bicon-Plus C.
Biomet acetabular c.
bipolar acetabular c.
bipolar prosthetic c.
Buchholz acetabular c.
ceramic acetabular c.
Charnley acetabular c.
Charnley offset-bore c.
concentric hip c.
c. and cone method
Continuum elliptical acetabular c.
Continuum polyethylene acetabular c.
Crawford-Adams acetabular c.
CRM c.
custom-made acetabular c.
DePuy bipolar c.
DePuy Tri-Lock interlocking acetabular c.
Essential Energy C.
Flo-Trol drinking c.
Ganz c.
Gap c.
Gemini c.
Harris-Galante acetabular c.
Hedrocel c.
heel c.
hip c.
c. holder
c. holder handle
Integrity acetabular c.
interlocking acetabular c.
Interseal acetabular c.
jumbo acetabular c.
Kennedy spillproof c.
Laing concentric hip c.
Lineage acetabular c.
Lord c.
low-profile c.
Luck hip c.
McKee-Farrar acetabular c.
metal-backed acetabular c.
migration of acetabular c.
monolithic A1203 c.
Mueller c.
multipolar bipolar c.
NEB acetabular c.
New England Baptist acetabular c.
oblong polyethylene acetabular c.
Opti-Fix II acetabular c.
Osteonics acetabular c.
patella c.
plastic heel c.
Polysorb heel c.

porous-coated acetabular c.
c. positioner
PQ premium heel c.
press-fit c.
prosthesis c.
c. reamer
Reflection I, V, FSO acetabular c.
Restoration GAP acetabular c.
retroversion of acetabular c.
Riecken PQ premium heel c.
rubber held c.
screw-in ceramic acetabular c.
Silipos Silicone Wonder C.
Smith-Petersen c.
Sorbothane II heel c.
S-ROM acetabular c.
S-ROM Super C.
trial acetabular c.
TuliGel heel c.
Tuli Pro Heel C.
Tuli rubber heel c.
University of California Biomechanics Laboratory heel c.
Wonder-Cup heel c.
Wonder-Spur heel c.
ZTT I, II c.
ZTT acetabular c.

cup-and-ball osteotomy
cup-cement interface
cupid's

c. bow
c. bow contour sign

cup-on-cup arthroplasty of hip
cupped

c. curette
c. grasping forceps

curative soft tissue procedure
curb tenotomy
Curdy blade
curettage

excision and c.

curette, curet

Acufex c.
bone c.
bowl c.
box c.
Bruns bone c.
Buck bone c.
cement c.
Charnley bone c.
Cobb c.
Cone ring c.
Cone suction biopsy c.
cupped c.
curved c.
Daubenspeck bone c.
Epstein c.
Faulkner c.
fine-angled c.

fine bone c.
Gillquist suction c.
Halle bone c.
Hardy hypophysial c.
Hatfield bone c.
hex handle c.
Hibbs c.
hypophysial c.
Innomed bone c.
Jansen bone c.
Kerpel bone c.
Kerrison c.
Kevorkian c.
Latitude c.
Lempert bone c.
long c.
Magnum c.
Malis c.
Martini bone c.
mastoid c.
McCain TMJ c.
McElroy c.
meniscal c.
Meyhoeffer bone c.
Microsect c.
Moe bone c.
orthopaedic c.
oval curved-cup c.
Piffard c.
ring c.
Schede bone c.
Scoville c.
short c.
Spratt bone c.
Spratt mastoid c.
Statak c.
stout-neck c.
straight c.
T-handle c.
Volkmann bone c.
Walker ruptured disc c.
Whitney single-use plastic c.
Williger bone c.

curl

dynamic trunk c.
neutral wrist c.
preacher c.
reverse wrist c.
seated hamstring c.
trunk c.
wrist c.

curl-up

broomstick c.-u.

curly

c. toe
c. toe deformity

current

action c.
amplitude-summation interferential c.
cutting c.
direct c.
interferential c.
low-frequency alternating c. (LFAC)

Currey model
Curry

C. hip nail
C. walking splint

Curschmann-Steinert disease
Curtin

C. incision
C. plantar fibromatosis excision

Curtis

C. PIP joint capsulotomy
C. technique

curvature

angular c.
anterior c.
backward c.
c. correction
dorsal kyphotic c.
humpbacked spinal c.
lateral c.
posterior c.
Pott spinal c.
spinal c.

curve

accommodation c.
Barnes c.
Blix contractile force c.
calibration c.
cervicothoracic c.
combined c.
compensatory c.
contractile force c.
displacement c.
double major spinal c.
double thoracic c.
flattening of normal lordotic c.
fractional c.
full c.
Hadley S-c.
King thoracic and lumbar c. (type I–IV)
kyphotic c.
length-tension c.
load-deflection c.

NOTES

curve *(continued)*
    load-deformation c.
    load-displacement c.
    lordotic c.
    low single thoracic c.
    lumbar lordotic c.
    major c.
    c. measurement
    minor c.
    nonstructural c.
    normal lordotic c.
    c. pattern (type I, II)
    primary c.
    c. progression
    c. progression in scoliosis
    right thoracic c.
    rigid c.
    scoliotic c.
    severe rigid thoracic c.
    specific c.
    standardized growth c.
    strain-stress c.
    strength c.
    strength-duration c.
    stress-strain c.
    structural c.
    tension c.
    thoracic c.
    thoracolumbar c.
    torque c.
curved
    c. awl
    c. basket forceps
    c. bone rongeur
    c. curette
    c. gouge
    c. incision
    c. Küntscher nail system
    c. L approach
    c. Mayo scissors
    c. meniscotome
    c. meniscotome blade
    c. osteotome
    c. osteotomy
    c. passer
    c. periosteal elevator
    c. retractor
curvilinear
    c. area
    c. chin implant
    c. incision
CurvTek
    C. drill bone anchor
    C. TSR bone drill
Cushing
    C. bur
    C. disc rongeur
    C. dural hook
    C. flat drill

    C. Little Joker elevator
    C. perforator drill
    C. periosteal elevator
    C. retractor
    C. saw guide
    C. syndrome
Cushing-Gigli saw guide
Cushing-Hopkins periosteal elevator
cushion
    abduction c.
    alarm c.
    amputee c.
    Anti-Shox foot c.
    arch c.
    Back Bull lumbar support c.
    Back-Huggar lumbar support c.
    breakaway lap c.
    Butterfly c.
    Carter immobilization c.
    cast c.
    cell c.
    cervical c.
    Checkerboard wheelchair c.
    Comfort Take-Along wheelchair c.
    Core Max-Relax C.
    Disc-O-Sit Jr. c.
    Dry Flotation wheelchair c.
    Easy Up c.
    EcstaSeat seat c.
    enhancer c.
    FB cast c.
    foam c.
    foot c.
    gel c.
    Gel-Foam Ultra-Wedge c.
    Geo-Matt contour c.
    C. Grip Flatware
    Healthier seating c.
    heel c.
    c. heel
    Hudson Hydrofloat C.
    hydrofloat c.
    Invacare Comfort-Mate extra c.
    invalid c.
    Isch-Dish Plus c.
    J2 c.
    Jay basic c.
    Jay Combi c.
    Jay Rave c.
    Jay Triad c.
    Jay Xtreme c.
    laptop c.
    latex c.
    lumbar support c.
    MaxiFloat wheelchair c.
    Pediplast c.
    pommel c.
    Postura wheelchair c.
    Posture Curve lumbar c.

Posture Wedge seat c.
pressure c.
pressure-relief c.
Prop'R Toes hammertoe c.
Quadtro c.
ring c.
Roho Pack-It c.
saddle c.
Sat-A-Lite contoured wedge seat c.
seat c.
seating c.
Shockmaster heel c.
c. shoe liner
Sit-Straight wheelchair c.
Skil-Care c.
Sorbothane heel c.
Temper Foam c.
T-Foam c.
T-Gel c.
trilaminate c.
Vac-Lok immobilization c.
Viscoheel K heel c.
Viscoheel N c.
Viscoheel SofSpot viscoelastic
   heel c.
Viscolas heel c.
ViscoSpot heel c.
wheelchair c.
cushioned shoe insert
cushioning
Abzorb c.
cushion-throat wire cutter
Custodis implant
custom
c. implant
c. prosthesis
c. rasp
custom-designed swan-neck femoral
   component
custom-fitted brace
custom-made
c.-m. acetabular cup
c.-m. insert
c.-m. shoe
custom-molded
c.-m. orthotics
c.-m. shoe
custom-threaded prosthesis
cut
chamfer c.
freehand c.
horizontal gantry c.
jack upper c.

notch c.
Z-step c.
cutaneous
c. amputation
c. axon reflex
c. distribution
c. flap
c. fold
c. graft
c. horn
c. icing
c. maceration
c. nerve
c. neuroma
c. pressure threshold
cut-back zone
Cutinova
C. cavity dressing
C. foam dressing
C. thin dressing
cutout
c. knee support
c. patellar brace
c. shoe
c. table
cutter
bolt c.
bone plug c.
Breck pin c.
cast c.
C. cast
Cloward dowel c.
cookie c.
cushion-throat wire c.
diamond pin c.
diamond wire c.
double-action c.
dowel c.
end c.
c. guide
Hefty-bite pin c.
Horsley bone c.
C. implant
Jarit pin c.
Kalish Duredge wire c.
Kirschner wire c.
Kleinert-Kutz bone c.
Leibinger Micro System plate c.
Luhr Microfixation System plate c.
Martin diamond wire c.
meniscal c.
Midas Rex bone c.
milling c.

NOTES

cutter *(continued)*
  motorized meniscal c.
  M-Pact cast c.
  multiaction pin c.
  multiple action c.
  pin c.
  plate c.
  plug c.
  Redi-Vac cast c.
  rib c.
  Rochester harvest bone c.
  Rochester recipient bone c.
  Roos rib c.
  side c.
  side-cut pin c.
  Sklar pin c.
  Spartan jaw wire c.
  Storz Microsystems plate c.
  Synthes Microsystems plate c.
  toothed c.
  wire c.
  Wister wire/pin c.
cutting
  c. block
  c. bur
  c. cone
  c. current
  c. current knife
  c. forceps
  c. jig
  c. needle
  c. shaver
  c. weight
CVA
  cerebrovascular accident
  costovertebral angle
    CVA Sling
    CVA tenderness
CVAT
  costovertebral angle tenderness
CVD
  collagen vascular disease
CVT
  congenital vertical talus
C-Walk foot 1C40 prosthetic foot
CWHTO
  closing wedge high tibial osteotomy
C-wire inserter
cyanoacrylate
  c. adhesive
  c. glue
cyanocobalamin
cyanosis
cybernetics
Cybertech 1000 back support
Cybex
  C. back rehabilitation equipment
  C. cycle ergometer
  C. device

C. I, II+ exercise system
C. II, II+ isokinetic exerciser
C. II isokinetic dynamometer
C. 340 isokinetic rehabilitation and
  testing system
C. isokinetic test
C. machine
C. tester
C. testing
C. Torso Rotation Testing and
  Rehabilitation Unit
C. training system
C. Trunk Extension Flexion unit
cycle
  Ergociser exercise c.
  c. ergometer
  Exer-Pedic c.
  gait c.
  c. per second (cps, c/sec)
  Power Trainer c.
  recumbent c.
  Saratoga c.
  Schwinn bi-directional Windjammer
    upper body c.
  c. time
  upper body c.
  walking c.
cycled stimulation
cyclic loading
cycling
  studio c.
cyclobenzaprine HCl
cyclooxygenase product
cyclops
  c. formation
  c. lesion
  c. syndrome
cyclosporin A
cyclothymia
cylinder
  air c.
  Arthrotek calibrated c.
  Feldenkrais c.
  c. walking cast
cylindrical
  c. autologous dowel graft
  c. bur
  c. dowel
  c. osteotomy
  c. sleeve
cyma line
Cyriax
  C. evaluation
  C. technique
cyst
  c. ablation
  acetabular c.
  acromioclavicular c.
  aneurysmal bone c. (ABC)

Baker c.
bone c.
bursal c.
digital mucoid c.
expansile c.
ganglion c.
giant popliteal synovial c.
inclusion c.
c. index
juxtaarticular bone c.
lipid inclusion c.
meniscal c.
mucous c.
myxoid c.
perimeniscal c.
porencephalic c.
postfracture c.
rheumatoid c.
sacral c.
simple bone c.
solitary bone c.

subarticular c.
subchondral bone c.
synovial c.
Tarlov c.
tibiofibular c.
traumatic bone c.
unicameral bone c.
cystic
    c. arthrosis
    c. bone lesion
    c. defect
    c. disease
    c. hygroma
    c. osteomyelitis
    c. rheumatoid arthritis
    c. tumor
cytoarchitectonic abnormality
cytotoxic drug
Cytoxan
    C. Injection
    C. Oral

C

NOTES

3D

3-dimensional
3D fracture walker brace
3D plate
3D positional adjustability
3D positional control

D/3

distal third

DA

degenerative arthritis

d'accoucheur

main d.

Dacron

D. batting
D. graft
D. polyester
D. prosthesis
D. stent
D. suture
D. synthetic ligament material

Dacron-impregnated silicone rod
dactylalgia
dactylitis

blistering distal d. (BDD)
tuberculous d.

dactylocampsis
dactylocampsodynia
dactylodynia
dactylogryposis
dactylospasm
DAF

dynamic axial fixator

Dafilon suture
Dagrofil suture
DAI

diffuse axonal injury

Daily Adjusted Progressive Resistance Exercise (DAPRE)
Dakin

D. solution
D. tubing

Dalco Astro ankle brace
Dale

D. abdominal binder
D. first rib rongeur

Dallas grading system
Dall-Miles

D.-M. cable
D.-M. cable cerclage
D.-M. cable/crimp cerclage system
D.-M. cable grip system
D.-M. cerclage wire

DALY

disability adjusted life year

damage

physial d.

damage-control orthopaedics
d'Ambrosia test
damp heat
DANA

designed after natural anatomy
DANA shoulder prosthesis

dance

high-impact aerobic d. (HIAD)
low-impact aerobic d. (LIAD)
d. medicine

dancer's

d. foot
d. fracture
d. pad

dancing

d. bear gait
d. bear syndrome

dandy

D. clamp
D. maneuver

Dandy-Walker deformity
dangling foot
Daniel iliac bone graft
Danis-Weber

D.-W. classification of ankle injury
D.-W. classification of malleolar fracture
D.-W. fracture classification

Danniflex CPM exerciser
Dansko shoe
d'Antonio acetabular classification
DAPRE

Daily Adjusted Progressive Resistance Exercise
DAPRE strength training

Darco

D. back brace
D. Body Armor Hi
D. Body Armor Lo
D. Body Armor short leg walker
D. foot splint
D. Medical-Surgical shoe
D. Medical-Surgical shoe and toe alignment splint
D. moldable insole
D. OrthoWedge healing shoe
D. Podospray
D. Softie shoe
D. surgical shoe
D. Wedge shoe

DarcoGel ankle brace
Darier-White disease

Darrach
D. periosteal elevator
D. procedure
D. resection
D. retractor
D. ulnar tenodesis
Darrow pain classification
dart
Arthrex meniscal d.
Darvon Compound-65 Pulvules
Das
D. Gupta procedure
D. Gupta scapular excision
D. Gupta scapulectomy
DASA
distal articular set angle
Dasco Pro angle finder
Daseler-Anson classification of plantaris muscle anatomy
DASH
Disabilities of Arm, Shoulder, and Hand
DASH questionnaire
DASH scale
dashboard
d. dislocation
d. fracture
d. knee injury
dashpot
DataHand system
DATT
deep anterior tibiotalar
DATT ligament
Daubenspeck bone curette
d'Aubigné
d. femoral prosthesis
d. femoral reconstruction
d. hip status system
d. patellar transplant
d. resection reconstruction
d'Aubigné-Postel postoperative function score
Dautrey
D. chisel
D. osteotome
David drainage
Davidson muscle clamp
Davidson-Sauerbruch-Doyen periosteal elevator
Davies-Colley operation
Davis
D. arthrodesis
D. drainage technique
D. dura dissector
D. fusion
D. law
D. metacarpal splint
D. muscle-pedicle graft
D. percussion hammer
D. pin

D. saw guide
D. series
Dawbarn sign
Dawson-Yuhl
D.-Y. impactor
D.-Y. periosteal elevator
D.-Y. rongeur forceps
D.-Y. suction tube
Dawson-Yuhl-Kerrison rongeur forceps
Dawson-Yuhl-Key elevator
Dawson-Yuhl-Leksell rongeur forceps
day
D. fixation device
D. fixation pin
D. fixation staple
d. treatment rehabilitation
DayTimer carpal tunnel support
Daytona cervical orthosis
DBM
demineralized bone matrix
DBS
deep bonding system
Denis Browne splint
DC
dynamic compression
DC-101 chiropractic table
DCB
distal communicating branch
DCC
dorsal calcaneocuboid
DCC ligament
D-Core support pillow
DCP
dynamic compression plate
DCS
dorsal column stimulator
Dynamic condylar screw
DCS pin
DDA
dorsal digital artery
DDAVP
desmopressin acetate
DDD
degenerative disc disease
DDH
developmental dislocation of hip
developmental dysplasia of hip
DDH orthosis
DDP
dual drop pelvis
DDP table
de
de Andrade and MacNab anterior approach
de Barsy syndrome
de Kleyn position
de Kleyn test
de La Caffinière trapeziometacarpal prosthesis

de Lange syndrome
De Lorme boot
De Mayo hip positioner
de Morgan spot
de Quervain disease
de Quervain fracture
de Quervain stenosing tenosynovitis
de Quervain syndrome
de Quervain tendinitis

dead
d. arm syndrome
d. ball exercises
d. bone
d. lift
d. space

deafferentation pain
deafness
lentigines, electrocardiographic
abnormalities, ocular hypertelorism,
pulmonary stenosis, abnormalities
of genitalia, retardation of
growth, d. (sensorineural)
(LEOPARD)
d., onychoosteodystrophy, mental
retardation (DOOR)

Dean
D. bone rongeur
D. scissors

Deane unconstrained knee prosthesis
death
exercise-induced sudden d.
quadrant of d.

Deaver retractor
DeBakey prosthesis
DeBastiani
D. corticotomy
D. distractor
D. external fixator
D. femoral lengthening
D. fixation
D. technique

deBoer lateral approach
debonded femoral stem prosthesis
debonding
débridement
Ahern trochanteric d.
arthroscopic d.
bursal d.
cortical d.
diagnostic arthroscopy and d.
enzymatic d.
exploration and d.
irrigation and d. (I&D)

Magnuson d.
d. patella

debris
bone d.
fibrin d.
fibrofatty d.
joint d.
loose d.
metallic d.
particulate wear d.
polyethylene d.
polymeric d.
pulvinar fibrofatty d.
tissue d.
wear d.

debris-incited osteolysis
debris-induced osteolysis
debris-retaining reamer
Debrunner kyphometer
debulking
d. procedure
Tsuge d.

deburring
Decadron Phosphate
decalcification
decancellation
cuboid d.

decerebrate posture
dechondrification
deciduous
Decker rongeur
deck plate
declination
angle of d.
d. angle

decompression
anterior retroperitoneal d.
anterolateral d.
bone graft d.
carpal tunnel d. (CTD)
cervical spine d.
core d.
d. equipment
extensive posterior d.
d. fasciotomy
foot d.
foramen magnum d.
fracture d.
lateral d.
leg d.
lumbar spine d.
nerve root d.
posterior nerve d.

NOTES

D

decompression *(continued)*
    posterolateral d.
    retroperitoneal d.
    d. rhachotomy
    sacral spine d.
    spinal d.
    subacromial d.
    d. technique
    thoracic spine d.
    thoracolumbar spine d.
    vertebral body d.
decompressive
    d. acromioplasty
    d. laminectomy
    d. osteotomy
deconditioned foot
deconditioning
    bed rest-related d.
    stroke-related d.
    d. syndrome
decorticate posture
decortication
    d. bur
    d. technique
decremental response
DeCube mattress
Decubitene oxygenated oil
decubitus
    d. position
    d. ulcer
decussation
dedifferentiated chondrosarcoma
Dee
    D. elbow hinge
    D. totally constrained elbow
      prosthesis
deep
    d. anterior tibiotalar (DATT)
    d. anterior tibiotalar ligament
    d. arch
    d. bonding system (DBS)
    d. circumflex iliac artery
    d. collateral ligament
    d. delayed infection
    d. fascia
    d. friction massage
    d. heat modality
    d. iliac dissection
    d. intracompartmental soft tissue
      sarcoma
    d. knee bend (DKB)
    d. lateral femoral notch sign
    d. muscle therapy
    d. peroneal nerve
    d. posterior compartment
    d. posterior sacrococcygeal ligament
    d. posterior tibiotalar (DPTT)
    d. posterior tibiotalar ligament
    D. Relief

    d. retractor
    d. stroking
    d. stroking and kneading massage
    d. tendon reflex (DTR)
    d. transverse carpal ligament
    d. transverse intermetatarsal
      ligament
    d. transverse metacarpal ligament
    d. transverse metatarsal ligament
    d. TV metatarsal ligament
    d. venous thrombosis (DVT)
    d. venous thrombosis prophylaxis
    d. wound infection
deepening reamer
deepithelialized rectus abdominis muscle (DRAM)
deep-shelled acetabulum
Deerfield test
deer tick disease
defect
    acetabular d.
    anteromedial humeral head d.
    Arthropor oblong cup for
      acetabular d.
    articular d.
    barlike ventral d.
    benign cortical d.
    bone d.
    bridging of d.
    cavitary d.
    composite d.
    condylar d.
    cortical d.
    cranial d.
    cystic d.
    developmental d.
    diaphysial d.
    femoral condylar d.
    fibrous cortical d.
    fibrous metaphysial d.
    fusiform d.
    impression d.
    Klippel-Feil segmentation d.
    mapping the d.
    metaphysial fibrous cortical d.
    neural tube d.
    nonsubperiosteal cortical d.
    d. nonunion
    osseous d.
    osteoarticular d.
    osteochondral d.
    pars d.
    posterior superior humeral head d.
    radial ray d.
    reverse Hill-Sachs d.
    segmental bone d.
    segmentation d.
    skeletal d.
    step d.

subcortical d.
subperiosteal cortical d.
tibial d.
triangular d.
trochlear d.
unremodeled d.

defervesce
Defiance functional knee brace
deficiency, pl. **deficiencies**
    acetabular d.
    Aitken femoral d.
    American Academy of Orthopaedic
      Surgeons classification of
      acetabular d.
    biomechanical d.
    capsular d.
    cavitary d.
    central d.
    congenital limb d.
    congenital tibial d.
    factor VIII, IX d.
    focal d.
    Jones classification of congenital
      tibial d.
    long bone d.
    longitudinal d.
    magnesium d.
    proximal femoral focal d.
    proximal focal femoral d. (PFFD)
    radial d.
    segmental d.
    skeletal limb d.
    tibial longitudinal d.
    transverse d.
    vitamin C, D, K d.
deficient
    d. knee
    d. spinous process
deficit
    executive function d.
    motor d.
    motor function d.
    neurologic d.
    perception d.
    proprioceptive d.
    sensorimotor d.
    sensory d.
    somatosensory d.
Definition PM femoral implant
  component
definitive
    d. callus

d. cerclage wire
d. stabilization
deformability
deformans
    arthritis d.
    arthrosis d.
    malum d.
    osteitis d.
    osteoarthritis d.
    osteochondrodystrophia d.
    Paget osteitis d.
    spondylitis d.
    spondylosis d.
deformation
    elastic d.
    plastic d.
    stem d.
deformity, pl. **deformities**
    abduction d.
    acetabular protrusio d.
    adduction d.
    adduction-internal rotation d.
    adductovarus d.
    adult-acquired flatfoot d.
    d. analysis
    angulation d.
    ape thumb d.
    apex plantar d.
    Arnold-Chiari d.
    arthrosis d.
    back-knee d.
    biconcave d.
    bifid thumb d.
    bony d.
    boutonnière d.
    bowing d.
    bowleg d.
    bunion d.
    bunionette d.
    burn boutonnière d.
    buttonhole d.
    calcaneocavovarus d.
    calcaneocavus d.
    calcaneovalgus d.
    calcaneovarus d.
    calcaneus d.
    cavovarus d.
    cavus foot d.
    cervical spine kyphotic d.
    Charcot d.
    Chattanooga balance system
      Checkrein d.
    checkrein d.

D

NOTES

deformity *(continued)*
    clasped thumb d.
    clawfoot d.
    clawhand d.
    claw toe d.
    cleft foot d.
    cleft hand d.
    cloverleaf d.
    clubfoot d.
    clubhand d.
    cock-up d.
    codfish d.
    Cole osteotomy for midfoot d.
    combined cavus d.
    compensatory d.
    congenital vertical talus foot d.
    contracture d.
    coronal plane d.
    crossover-toe d.
    curly toe d.
    Dandy-Walker d.
    digital d.
    digitus flexus d.
    dinner fork d.
    DISI d.
    double corn d.
    dynamic digital d.
    elevatus d.
    equinocavovarus d.
    equinovalgus d.
    equinovarus hindfoot d.
    equinus d.
    Erlenmeyer flask d.
    eversion-external rotation d.
    extension d.
    femoral head d.
    finger d.
    fishtail d.
    fixed d.
    flat back d.
    flatfoot d.
    flexible clawtoe d.
    flexible hammertoe d.
    flexion-internal rotational d.
    flexion valgus d.
    foot d.
    forefoot abduction d.
    fracture d.
    garden spade d.
    genu valgum d.
    genu varum d.
    gibbus d.
    gull-wing d.
    gunstock d.
    Haglund foot d.
    hallux limitus d.
    hallux valgus d.
    hallux varus d.
    hammertoe d.

    hatchet-head d.
    Hibbs extensor tendon transfer cavus d.
    Hill-Sachs d.
    hindfoot d.
    hollow foot clawfoot d.
    hook-nail d.
    hourglass d.
    humpback d.
    hyperextension d.
    Ilfeld-Holder d.
    internal rotation d.
    intrinsic minus d.
    intrinsic plus d.
    J-hook d.
    joint d.
    Kelikian classification of nail d.
    Kirner d.
    knock-knee d.
    kyphotic d.
    lobster-claw d.
    lumbar spine kyphotic d.
    Madelung d.
    mallet finger d.
    mallet toe d.
    medial ray adduction d.
    metatarsus adductus d.
    metatarsus primus varus d.
    metatarsus varus d.
    midfoot d.
    multiplanar d.
    nail d.
    neuropathic foot d.
    oblique osteotomy for tibial d.
    pannus d.
    pencil and cup d.
    pes arcuatus clawfoot d.
    pes cavus clawfoot d.
    pes planovalgus d.
    pes planus d.
    pes valgo planus d.
    1-plane d.
    2-plane d.
    3-plane d.
    planovalgus d.
    plantarflexion-inversion d.
    posttraumatic spinal d.
    procurvatum d.
    protrusio d.
    pseudoboutonnière d.
    pseudo-Hurler d.
    pump bump d.
    rearfoot d.
    recurvatum angulation d.
    reduction d.
    rheumatoid d.
    rigid equinovarus d.
    rigid flatfoot d.
    rockerbottom flatfoot d.

rotational d.
round shoulder d.
saber shin d.
sagittal d.
scaphoid humpback d.
seal-fin d.
shepherd's crook d.
shoulder d.
silver-fork d.
skeletal d.
skewfoot d.
spastic hindfoot valgus d.
spastic thumb-in-palm d.
spinal coronal plane d.
spine d.
splayfoot d.
split-hand d.
split-nail d.
Sprengel d.
S-shaped d.
static foot d.
subcondylar d.
supination d.
swan-neck finger d.
talipes cavus d.
talus foot d.
thoracic spine kyphotic d.
thoracic spine scoliotic d.
thumb d.
thumb-in-palm d.
tibial d.
torsional d.
triphalangeal thumb d.
turned-up pulp d.
ulnar deviation d.
ulnar drift d.
valgus heel d.
varus hindfoot d.
Velpeau d.
vertical talus foot d.
volar angulation d.
Volkmann clawhand d.
windblown d.
windswept d.
wrist d.
Zancolli procedure for clawhand d.
Z foot d.
zigzag compensatory d.
deformity/instability
spinal d./i.
Defourmentel bone rongeur
DeGangi-Berk Test of Sensory Integration

Dega pelvic osteotomy
degenerated cartilage
degeneration
axonal d.
cartilaginous d.
Charcot d.
disc d.
endoneurium d.
fascicular d.
fibrinoid d.
immobilization d.
joint d.
Kirkaldy-Willis 3 phases of d.
mucoid d.
Regnauld-type great toe d.
retrograde d.
rotator cuff d.
Sandoz 4-phase model of spinal d.
spinal d.
spinocerebellar d.
wallerian d.
wear-and-tear d.
Zenker d.
degenerative
d. arthritic change
d. arthritis (DA)
d. arthrosis
d. disc disease (DDD)
d. disorder
d. joint disease (DJD)
d. lumbar scoliosis
d. lumbar spine fusion
d. meniscal tear
d. meniscus
d. olisthesis
d. osteoarthritis
d. spine condition
d. spondylolisthesis
d. spondylosis
d. spondylosis decompression and fusion
d. spur
d. spurring
d. stenosis
d. vertebral arthropathy
degloving
d. injury
phalangeal d.
d. procedure
degradable polyglycolide rod
degree
d.'s of freedom (DOF)

D

NOTES

degree *(continued)*
    6 d.'s of freedom
    electrogoniometer
    d. of separation
    d.'s of valgus angulation
    d.'s of varus angulation
degrees-of-freedom joint motion
dehiscence
    prosthesis d.
    wound d.
    Zuckerkandl d.
Dejerine
    D. disease
    D. percussion hammer
    D. sign
Dejerine-Davis percussion hammer
Dejerine-Sottas
    D.-S. disease
    D.-S. syndrome
Deknatel
    D. orthopaedic autotransfusion
    system
    D. suture classification
delamination
DeLaura knee prosthesis
DeLaura-Verner knee prosthesis
delay
    electromechanical d. (EMD)
    sensory d.
delayed
    d. apoplexy
    d. bone imaging
    d. bone maturation
    d. closure
    d. consolidation
    d. femoral osteotomy
    d. fracture union
    d. graft
    d. healing bone fracture
    d. onset
    d. open reduction
    d. primary closure (DPC)
    d. primary repair
    d. reflex
    d. response
delayed-onset muscle soreness
Delbet splint
DeLee
    D. classification
    D. radiographic analysis
Delitala
    D. T-nail nail
    D. T-pin
Dellon ulnar nerve transposition
Del-Mycin Topical
Delore method
DeLorme exercise
Delrin-handle bone saw
Delrin joint

delta
    d. brush
    d. femoral nail
    d. frame
    d. phalanx
    d. receptor
    D. Recon nail
    D. Recon proximal drill guide
    d. rod
    d. tibial nail
    D. walker
Delta-Cortef Oral
Deltafit Keel
Delta-Lite
    D.-L. casting tape
    D.-L. FlashCast
Delta-Rol cast padding
deltoid
    d. artery
    d. bursa
    d. fascia
    d. flap
    d. insertion
    d. ligament
    d. ligament tear
    d. muscle
    d. origin
    d. reflex
    d. region
    d. sprain
Deltoid-Aid arm support
deltoid-splitting
    d.-s. incision
    d.-s. shoulder approach
deltopectoral
    d. approach
    d. flap
    d. groove
    d. interval
deltotrapezius fascial ligament
deluxe
    d. FIN pin
    d. FIN pin inserter
demand
    motion d.
    specific adaptation to imposed d.
    (SAID)
demarcation
    line of d.
DeMartel wire saw
DeMartel-Wolfson clamp holder
DeMay hip positioner
DeMayo suture passer
dementia
Demianoff sign
demigauntlet bandage
demineralization
    bony d.

demineralized
    d. bone
    d. bone graft
    d. bone matrix (DBM)
demyelination
denatured alcohol
dendritic synovitis
denervation
    cryogenic d.
    d. disease
    d. potential
    d. procedure
    d. supersensitivity
Denham
    D. external fixation
    D. external fixation device
    D. pin
Denis
    D. Browne bar
    D. Browne bar foot orthosis
    D. Browne bucket
    D. Browne clubfoot splint
    D. Browne 3-column model
    D. Browne 3-column spine theory
    D. Browne hip splint
    D. Browne sacral fracture
      classification
    D. Browne spinal fracture
      classification
    D. Browne splint (DBS)
    D. Browne talipes hobble splint
    D. Browne tray
    D. compression fracture
      classification
    D. seat-belt injury classification
    D. spinal fracture
Dennison cervical brace
Dennyson-Fulford extraarticular subtalar arthrodesis
DENS
    direct electrical nerve stimulation
dens
    d. anterior screw fixation
    d. fracture
    d. x-ray view
dense bone
densitometer
    Discovery bone d.
densitometry
    bone d.
    dual photon d. (DPD)
    fracture site nonunion Norland
      bone d.

    Norland bone d.
    photon d.
    scanning d.
    video d. (VD)
density
    bone d.
    bone mineral d. (BMD)
    calcific d.
    fiber d.
    lumbosacral junction bone d.
    proton d.
dental
    d. bur
    d. drill
    d. mirror
    d. pick
dentate
    d. fracture
    d. ligament
dentinogenesis imperfecta
Denuce
    quadrate ligament of D.
denudation
denude
deodorant
    Deoshoes d.
Deoshoes deodorant
deossification band
deoxypyridinoline crosslinks urine assay
DEPA
    depth of ulcer, extent of bacterial
    colonization, phase of ulcer, associated
    etiology
    DEPA system
DePalma
    D. hip prosthesis
    D. modified patellar technique
    D. staple
    D. staple procedure
dependent edema
depGynogen Injection
depletion
    T-cell d.
depMedalone Injection
DepoDur
Depo-Estradiol injection
Depogen Injection
Depoject Injection
depolarization block
depolymerization
    increased d.
    unbalanced d.
Depo-Medrol Injection

D

NOTES

Depopred Injection
deposit
> calcareous d.
> calcific d.
> calcium d.
> gouty tophaceous d.
> rotator cuff calcified d.
> tophaceous d.

deposition
> beta-2-microglobulin d.
> bone d.
> calcium oxalate d.
> calcium pyrophosphate dihydrate d. (CPPD)
> crystal d.
> hemosiderin d.
> pseudotumorous mucin d.

depot corticosteroid
depressed
> d. fracture
> d. reflex

depression
> bone d.
> d. of fragment
> Hamilton Rating Scale for D.
> Nation Alliance for Research on Schizophrenia and D.
> postactivation d.

depth
> acetabular d.
> d. caliper-meter stick method
> d. gauge
> d. inlay shoe
> D. orthopaedic shoe
> d. of ulcer, extent of bacterial colonization, phase of ulcer, associated etiology (DEPA)
> wire penetration d.

depth-check drill
DePuy
> D. acetabular liner
> D. acetabular lining
> D. aeroplane splint
> D. AML hip
> D. AML Porocoat stem prosthesis
> D. any-angle splint
> D. awl
> D. bipolar cup
> D. bolt
> D. calcar grinder
> D. CMW 1 bone cement
> D. coaptation splint
> D. drill
> D. femoral acetabular overlay guide
> D. fracture brace
> D. Global Advantage shoulder eccentric humeral head
> D. Global shoulder glenoid component with fin
> D. graft preparation table
> D. halter
> D. hip prosthesis
> D. hip prosthesis with Scuderi head
> D. interference screw
> D. LCS mobile-bearing knee
> D. open-spindle splint
> D. open-thimble splint
> D. orthopaedic implant
> D. pin
> D. plate
> D. rainbow frame
> D. rasp
> D. reamer
> D. reducing frame
> D. rocking leg splint
> D. rod bender
> D. rolled Colles splint
> D. screwdriver
> D. support
> D. total hip system with porous coating
> D. Tri-Lock interlocking acetabular cup
> D. trispiked acetabular component

DePuy-Pott splint
derangement
> Hey internal d.
> internal d.
> joint internal d.
> structural d.
> d. syndrome
> vertebral d.

derby
> d. hat fracture
> D. nail

Derifield pelvic leg check
Derifield-Thompson test
dermabrader
Dermacentor
> *D. andersoni*
> *D. variabilis*

DermaFlex Gel
DermaFreeze topical anesthetic
Dermagraft
Dermagran
> D. hydrophilic gauze dressing
> D. ointment
> D. ointment wound dressing
> D. spray
> D. wound cleanser with zinc

dermal
> d. bone
> d. fasciectomy
> d. fibromatosis
> d. interposition splint

d. sinus
d. substitute
DermaMend
D. foam wound dressing
D. Hydrogel dressing
DermaSite dressing
DermAssist wound-filling material
Dermatell hydrocolloid dressing material
DermaTemp infrared thermographic sensor
dermatitis, pl. **dermatitides**
atopic d.
shoe d.
venous stasis d.
dermatoarthritis
Dermatobia hominis
dermatocele
dermatofibroma
dermatofibrosarcoma protuberans
dermatogenic torticollis
dermatolymphangitis
dermatomal
d. pain
d. pattern
dermatome
anterior tibial nerve d.
Brown d.
electric d.
d. mapping
mechanical d.
Padgett electric d.
Reese d.
sacral d.
Stryker d.
Zimmer d.
dermatomyositis
dermatophyte test medium (DTM)
dermatosensory evoked potential
dermatosis, pl. **dermatoses**
juvenile plantar d.
plantar d.
Derma-Wand germicidal lamp
Dermiflex dressing
dermodesis
resection d.
dermographia
dermometer
dermomyotome
derotate
derotation
d. boot
d. brace
oblique osteotomy with d.

derotational
d. brace
d. osteotomy
d. pin
d. reflex
derotator
d. bar
d. splint
DeRoyal LMB finger splint
D'Errico
D. enlarging drill bur
D. lamina chisel
D. perforating drill
D. perforating drill bur
D. retractor
Desault
D. fracture
D. sign
D. wrist bandage
D. wrist dislocation
descending lymphedema
Deschamps needle
Descot fracture
designed after natural anatomy (DANA)
DesignLine orthotic
desirudin
desk
Posture-Rite lap d.
Desk-rest arm support
desktop therapy portal
desmalgia
desmectasis
desmitis
desmocytoma
desmodynia
desmoid
cortical d.
d. fibroma
d. lesion
periosteal d.
d. tumor
desmoma
desmopathy
desmoplasia
desmoplastic fibroma
desmopressin acetate (DDAVP)
desmorrhexis
desmosis
desmotomy
despotic nevus
desquamation
Destot sign

D

NOTES

destruction
    arthritic d.
    bony element d.
    bony necrosis and d.
    cortical d.
    geographic d.
    localized bone d.
    moth-eaten d.
    pantalocrural arthritic d.

destructive
    d. articular lesion
    d. bone disease
    d. joint disease

desyndactylization
    Weinstock d.

detector
    analogous signal d.
    Isometer bone graft placement
      site d.

deterioration
    arthritic d.
    catastrophic d.

determinant
    combined ankle and knee motion
      gait d.
    knee flexion during stance phase
      motion gait d.
    pelvic rotation motion gait d.
    pelvic shift motion gait d.
    pelvic tilt motion gait d.

determination
    anteversion d.
    Budin-Chandler anteversion d.
    fusion limit d.
    leg length d.
    skin blood flow d.
    transcutaneous oxygen tension d.
    Whitesides tissue pressure d.

detritus
    d. bone
    hyaline cartilage d.

detrusor
    d. areflexia
    d. contraction
    d. hyperreflexia

detrusor-sphincter synergia
Deune knee prosthesis
Deutschländer disease
Devas stress fracture classification
development
    asymmetric subtalar joint d.
    Bayley Scales of Infant D.
    bone d.
    calcar femorale d.
    motor d.
    National Institute for Child Health
      and Human D.
    postural d.
    reflex d.

    D. Test of Visual Perception, 2nd
      Edition (DTVP-2)

developmental
    d. anatomy
    d. coxa vara
    d. defect
    d. dislocated hip orthosis
    d. dislocation of hip (DDH)
    d. dyscalculia
    d. dysplasia of hip (DDH)
    d. hip dysplasia

Deverle fixation
deviation
    angular d.
    d. of atlas on axis
    gait d.
    lateral d.
    medial d.
    proximal set angle d.
    radial d.
    rotary d.
    standard d.
    ulnar d.

device
    Acapella chest physical therapy d.
    acetabular reinforcement d.
    Ace Unifix fixation d.
    acrylic orthotic d.
    Acufex bioabsorbable fixation d.
    AcuSpark piezoelectric d.
    adjustable aiming d.
    adjustable 2-point caliper sensory
      assessment d.
    Agee 4-pin fixation d.
    AlloAnchor RC allograft d.
    Anderson fixation d.
    Anderson leg-lengthening d.
    ankle disc d.
    Antense antitension d.
    anterior internal fixation d.
    antirotation d.
    application of traction d.
    Archxerciser foot exercise d.
    Arrow absorbable meniscal
      repair d.
    ArtAssist arterial assist d.
    Arthrex Bird-Beak d.
    ArthroSew arthroscopic suturing d.
    Arthrotek tibial fixation d.
    ArthroWand d.
    articular motion d. (AMD)
    articulated tension d.
    Artscan 200 arthroscopic cartilage
      stiffness testing d.
    assistive technology d. (ATD)
    Automator d.
    A-V Impulse System foot pump
      DVT prophylaxis d.

A-V Impulse System foot wrap
DVT prophylaxis d.
Axer compression d.
axis-altering arthroereisis d.
Backbar d.
BackCycler continuous passive
motion d.
back range of motion d.
4-bar external fixation d.
Bassett electrical stimulation d.
Becker orthopaedic spinal system
orthotic d.
biodegradable fixation d.
BioStinger low-profile fixation d.
Blanchard traction d.
body-powered prosthetic d.
bollard d.
Bone-Lok d.
Book Butler book-grip d.
Bovie electrocautery d.
Brannock foot measuring d.
Buck convoluted traction d.
Calandruccio II compression d.
Calandruccio triangular compression
fixation d.
Cameron fracture d.
Caps ArthroWand d.
Carpal Trac traction d.
C-D fixation d.
C-D instrumentation d.
cervical range of motion d.
Cervitrak d.
Charnley external fixation d.
Chattanooga traction d.
circular fixation d.
Cleanwheel presterilized
disposable d.
collapsible internal fixation d.
Columbus McKinnon Hugger d.
combined fixation d.
compression screw-plate d.
compressive internal fixating d.
Cordis implantable drug
reservoir d.
coring d.
Cotrel-Dubousset dynamic transverse
traction d.
CPM d.
Cuff Link orthopaedic d.
Cybex d.
Day fixation d.
Denham external fixation d.
Deyerle fixation d.

Deyo d.
Disk-Criminator nerve stimulation
measuring d.
distal targeting d.
DressFlex orthotic d.
Dr. Grip writing d.
Dunn fracture d.
Dwyer d.
dynamic transverse traction d.
Easy-Pull sock aide d.
EBI d.
Econo-Cerv traction d.
Edwards modular system sacral
fixation d.
Elbow-Up Protector elbow
suspension d.
Electronics electrical stimulation d.
electrotherapy d.
Encore Orthopedics d.
EndoPearl bioabsorbable d.
EndoPearl fixation d.
Endoskeleton TA structural d.
Epos Ultra extracorporeal shock
wave therapy d.
Epos Ultra orthopaedic shock wave
therapy d.
Evershears surgical instrument d.
Exeter intramedullary bone plug d.
EX-FI-RE external fixation d.
Exogen 2000 noninvasive, low-
intensity, pulsed ultrasound d.
E-Z Flex jaw exercising d.
EZ-Trac orthopaedic suspension d.
FastOut d.
fixation d.
FootFlex performance stretching d.
forearm lift assist adjustable
spring-loaded d.
Fox internal fixation d.
fracture fixation d.
Fromm triangle orthopaedic d.
geometric d.
Georgiade fixation d.
Giliberty d.
Golgi d.
Graftmaster d.
Grip-Ease d.
halo-gravity traction d.
halo vest d.
Hare splint d.
Harrington fixation d.
Harrington-Kostuik distraction d.

D

NOTES

device *(continued)*

Harrington rod instrumentation distraction outrigger d.
Harris-Aufranc d.
Heyer-Schulte antisiphon d.
hipGRIP body positioning d.
Hoffmann mini-lengthening fixation d.
Hoffmann-Vidal external fixation d.
hot/ice cold therapy cooler therapy d.
humeral d.
Ikuta fixation d.
Ilizarov d.
implantable bone anchor d.
inductive coupling d.
InFuse bone graft/LT-Cage lumbar tapered fusion d.
Innovasive d.
Insta-Nerve d.
Intelect laser system d.
Inter Fix RP threaded spinal fusion cage d.
Inter Fix threaded spinal fusion cage d.
intraarticular cautery d.
Intracell mechanical muscle d.
Intracell myofascial trigger-point d.
InvertaChair traction d.
isometric d.
Jace W550 CPM d.
JAS elbow motion d.
Kaneda distraction d.
Kendrick extrication d. (KED)
Kennedy ligament augmenting d.
Kerboull acetabular reinforcement d.
Kessler fixation d.
Kin-Con d.
kinetic rehab d. (KRD)
Kirschner d.
Knott rod distraction d.
KRD L2000 rehab d.
Kronner external fixation d.
Kuhlman cervical traction d.
Küntscher traction d.
Lawrence d.
Legasus support CPM d.
legGRIP body positioning d.
leg-holding d.
leg-lengthening d.
Leinbach d.
Leksell adapter to Mayfield d.
LifeGait partial weightbearing therapy d.
ligament augmentation d. (LAD)
Link Orthopaedics d.
LiteGait partial weightbearing gait therapy d.
LT-Cage lumbar tapered fusion d.

lumbar tapered-cage lumbar tapered fusion d.
Luque fixation d.
Mayfield d.
Mayo elbow distraction d.
McAtee compression screw d.
McKeever patellar resurfacing d.
McLaughlin osteosynthesis d.
MediRule II measuring d.
Merry Walker ambulation d.
MicroFET2 muscle testing d.
Mobilimb CPM d.
Mueller fixation d.
muscle and neurological stimulation electrotherapy d.
MyoTrac d.
nail-bending d.
nail-mounted compression d.
nail plate d.
Nauth traction d.
Necktrac traction d.
Nervoscope d.
Neufeld d.
Neuro-Aide testing d.
newer-generation d.
notcher d.
NuPulse d.
Ogden Anchor soft tissue d.
Ommaya reservoir d.
Omni-Flexor d.
Oppociser exercise d.
Orateck d.
Original Jacknobber II muscle-massage d.
Orthofix external fixation d.
Orthofix ISKD d.
Ortholav irrigation and suction d.
orthotic d.
OssaTron noninvasive extracorporeal shock wave therapy d.
OssaTron Orthotripter d.
OsteoAnalyzer d.
OsteoView x-ray d.
Oxford uncompartmental d.
Parham-Martin fracture d.
passive motion d.
passive positioning d.
PDN d.
peg d.
pegboard lateral positioning d.
Percuss-O-Matic jackhammer d.
Pivot Pole walking d.
Plastazote orthotic d.
PlexiPulse intermittent pneumatic compression d.
PLM d.
pneumatic external compression d.
pneumatic peripheral circulation improvement d. (PPCID)

PodoFlex reflexology d.
Polar Care 500 cryotherapy d.
posterior reduction d. (PORD)
PPT orthotic d.
Pressure-Specified Sensory D.
pronation spring-control d.
Pronex patient controlled pneumatic traction d.
prosthetic disc nucleus d.
ProTrac measurement d.
pulsatile pneumatic plantar-compression d.
pyrolytic carbon d.
Quartzo d.
Quengel d.
Rancho ankle foot control d.
Redi-Trac traction d.
Reichert-Mundinger stereotactic d.
Rezaian external fixation d.
Rezaian interbody d.
Richards lag screw d.
RMC knee replacement d.
Rochester bone trephine d.
rod distraction d.
rod-mounted targeting d.
Roeder manipulative aptitude test d.
Roger Anderson compression d.
Roger Anderson external fixation d.
Roger Anderson stabilization d.
RollerBack self-massage d.
Rolz d.
rope stretching d.
rotation d.
Safe-T mate anti-rollback d.
SAFHS ultrasound d.
Scully Hip S'port hip d.
sequential compression d. (SCD)
sequential foot compression d. (SFCD)
Servox d.
Sgarlato d.
shear-off d.
sighting d.
single-use d.
Sleeper Gripper prosthetic d.
sliding fixation d.
sliding nail d.
Slot distraction d.
snap-fit d.
Sock-Assist d.
Sofamor spinal d.

SofPulse d.
SOLEutions custom orthotic d.
SOLEutions Prefab orthotic d.
Sorbothane orthotic d.
Southwick pin-holding d.
Spenco orthotic d.
spinal fusion d.
Sport-Rite Olympian d.
Sport-Rite Runner d.
sports terminal d.
SporTX stimulation d.
StairClimber assist d.
Statak soft tissue attachment d.
Stellbrink fixation d.
Stone clamp-locking d.
Stress-Ray varus-valgus d.
Stryker knee joint laxity d.
STx lumbar traction d.
STx Saunders lumbar disc d.
Sukhtian-Hughes fixation d.
SuperQuad assistive d.
SureClosure d.
Suretac bioabsorbable shoulder fixation d.
Sutter d.
Sutter-CPM knee d.
Tacticon peripheral neuropathy screening d.
Tekscan in-shoe monitoring d.
Telectronics electrical stimulation d.
telescoping tubular d.
Tenderlett d.
terminal d. (TD)
T-Fix absorbable meniscal repair d.
ThermaStim muscle warming d.
thermocouple skin temperature d.
The Rope stretch-and-traction d.
The Rope stretching d.
Thumper d.
titanium geometric d.
toe-straight d.
totally implantable lengthening d.
traction d.
transpedicularly implanted anterior spinal support d.
transverse loading d.
d. for transverse traction (DTT)
triangular compression d.
TriggerWheel d.
TSRH corkscrew d.
TSRH mini-corkscrew d.
Valenti arthroereisis d.
Vapr coagulation and cautery d.

D

NOTES

device *(continued)*
>VariFix spinal implant d.
>VariGrip spinal implant d.
>Vectra Genisys laser system d.
>Vidal-Adrey modified Hoffmann external fixation d.
>Viladot arthroereisis d.
>visor halo fixation d.
>Volkov-Oganesian elbow distraction d.
>Volkov-Oganesian external fixation d.
>voluntary closing terminal d.
>voluntary opening terminal d.
>Wagner distraction d.
>Wagner external fixation d.
>Wagner-Schanz screw d.
>Walk-Rite d.
>Wanger leg lengthening d.
>WasherLoc d.
>Wasserstein fixation d.
>wood probe reflexology d.
>Wrist Pro wrist support d.
>Xercise Band exercise d.
>Xercise tube resistive d.
>XTB knee extension d.
>Zickel supracondylar d.
>Zielke distraction d.
>Zimmer electrical stimulation d.
>Zimmer orthopaedic d.
>Zipper antidisconnect d.

devitalized
>d. bone graft
>d. portion
>d. tissue

DeWald
>D. spinal apparatus
>D. spinal appliance

Dewar
>D. posterior cervical fixation procedure
>D. posterior cervical fusion
>D. posterior cervical fusion technique

Dewar-Barrington
>D.-B. arthroplasty
>D.-B. clavicular dislocation technique

Dewar-Harris
>D.-H. paralysis
>D.-H. shoulder technique

DEXA
>dual-energy x-ray absorptiometry
>DEXA scan

Dexasone L.A.
Dexone LA
Dexon suture
dexterity
>finger d.

dextran prophylaxis
dextrorotary scoliosis
dextrorotoscoliosis
dextroscoliosis scoliosis
Deyerle
>D. drill
>D. femoral fracture technique
>D. fixation apparatus
>D. fixation device
>D. II pin
>D. interlocking screw
>D. plate
>D. punch
>D. sciatic tension test

Deyo device
DFA
>dorsiflexion angle

D-Foam
DFS
>distraction-flexion stage

DHC Plus
DH pressure relief walker
DHS
>dynamic hip screw

Diab-A-Foot
>D.-A-F. protection system
>D.-A-F. rocker insole

Diab-A-Pad insole
Diab-A-Sheet
Diab-A-Sole
>D.-A-S. flat insole
>D.-A-S. molded insole

Diab-A-Thotics orthotic
diabetes mellitus
diabetic
>d. amyotrophy
>d. arthropathy
>d. Charcot foot
>D. Diagnostic insole
>D. D-Sole foot orthosis
>d. femoral mononeuropathy
>d. foot
>d. foot ulcerative condition
>d. limb salvage
>d. neuropathy
>d. neurotrophic ulcer
>d. orthosis kit
>d. plantar hallux ulcer
>d. polyradiculopathy
>d. pressure relief shoe
>D. Quality of Life
>d. sock

diaclasis
diaclastic amputation
diacondylar fracture
diadochokinesia

diagnosed
>National Association for Dually D. (NADD)

diagnosis, pl. **diagnoses**
>clinical d.
>differential d.
>palpatory d.

diagnostic
>d. arthroscopy
>d. arthroscopy and débridement
>d. arthroscopy, operative arthroscopy, possible operative arthrotomy (AAA)
>d. imaging
>d. and operative arthroscopy (DOA)
>d. strategy

diagonal stretch

diagram
>free body d.

dial
>d. pelvic osteotomy
>d. periacetabular osteotomy
>d. test

dial-lock
>d.-l. brace
>d.-l. orthosis

diameter
>acetabular depth to femoral head d. (AD/FHD)
>horizontal pedicle d.
>lumbar spine pedicle d.
>neck d.
>orthonormal d.
>pedicle d.
>sagittal pedicle d.
>sagittal spinal canal d.
>thoracic spine pedicle d.
>transpedicular fixation effective pedicle d.
>transverse pedicle d.
>vertical pedicle d.

diametral

diametric pelvic fracture

diamond
>D. biomechanical table
>d. bur
>d. fraise
>d. high-speed drill
>d. inlay bone graft
>D. nail
>d. pin cutter
>d. point needle

>d. rasp
>d. tip wire
>d. wire cutter

Diamondback
>D. 1100 recumbent stepper
>D. 1100 self-generated stepper
>D. 100 upright stepper

3-in-1 diamond bur
Diamond-Gould syndactyly operation
diamond-point wire double-strand wire
diamond-shaped medullary nail
diapedesis
Diapedic foot cream
diaphragm
>Bucky d.
>urogenital d.

diaphysectomy
diaphyses (*pl. of* diaphysis)
diaphysial, diaphyseal
>d. aclasis
>d. defect
>d. dysplasia
>d. fracture
>d. osteotomy
>d. plating
>d. region
>d. sclerosis
>d. tuberculosis

diaphysial-epiphysial fusion
diaphysis, pl. **diaphyses**
>femoral d.

diaplasis
diaplastic
diarthrodial
>d. cartilage
>d. joint

diarthrosis
diastasis
>ankle mortise d.
>d. fibula
>frank d.
>interosseous d.
>latent d.
>pubic d.
>symphysis pubis d.
>syndesmotic d.
>tibiofibular d.
>tibiotalar d.

diastatic fracture
diastematomyelia
diastrophic
>d. dwarfism
>d. dysplasia

D

NOTES

diathermy
>Magnatherm SSP pulse shortwave d.
>microwave d. (MWD)
>pulsed d.
>shortwave d. (SWD)

diathesis
>Dupuytren d.

Diaz disease

DIC
>disseminated intravascular coagulation

dichlorodifluoromethane and trichloromonofluoromethane

Dick AO fixateur interne

Dickinson
>D. approach
>D. calcaneal bursitis technique

Dickson
>D. geometric osteotomy
>D. muscle transfer
>D. operation
>D. paraffin bath
>D. paralysis
>D. transplant technique

Dickson-Diveley
>D.-D. foot operation
>D.-D. procedure

dicondylar fracture

Didiee view

Dieffenbach
>D. amputation
>D. operation

die punch fracture

diet
>Gerson d.
>gouty d.
>tea-and-toast d.
>d. therapy
>training d.
>very low calorie d. (VLCD)

dietary
>d. modification
>d. protein
>d. reference intake (DRI)

Diethrich bulldog clamp

difference

differential
>d. diagnosis
>d. spinal block
>temperature d. (TD)
>d. variable reluctance transducer (DVRT)

differentiated chondrosarcoma

differentiation failure

diffuse
>d. angiokeratoma
>d. axonal injury (DAI)
>d. fasciitis
>d. idiopathic skeletal hyperostosis (DISH)
>d. idiopathic skeletal hyperostosis syndrome
>d. infantile fibromatosis
>d. pigmented villonodular synovitis (DPVNS)

digastric muscle

DiGeorge syndrome

Digi-Flex
>D.-F. finger exerciser
>D.-F. hand exerciser

Digikit finger tourniquet

Digimatic caliper

Digi Sleeve stockinette dressing

digit
>accessory d.
>arthrodesed d.
>d. cap
>congenital trigger d.
>flail d.
>infantile trigger d.
>multiple d.'s
>replantation of amputated d.
>sausage d.
>d. splint
>supernumerary d.
>trigger d.
>d. tube
>d. wrap

Digit-Aide fifth toe splint

digital
>d. amputation
>d. aponeurosis
>d. artery
>d. artery of foot
>d. artery protection
>D. Biofeedback System
>d. block anesthesia
>d. blood perfusion
>d. branch
>d. branch of plantar nerve
>d. caliper
>D. Care kit
>d. color
>d. contracture
>d. cord
>d. deformity
>d. edge-detection
>d. extensor mechanism
>d. extensor tendon
>d. flexor tendinitis
>d. flexor tendon
>d. flexor tendon sheath
>d. formula
>d. fusion
>d. impaction
>d. implant
>d. inclinometry

d. joint
d. mucoid cyst
d. nail
d. nerve block
d. pad
d. palpation
d. photoplethysmography
d. plethysmography
d. prosthesis
d. reflex
d. response test
d. self-retaining retractor
d. shortening
d. subtraction angiography (DSA)
d. theca
d. tourniquet
d. vibrogram
Digitalis lanata
Digit-grip device
digiti quinti proprius tendon
digitizer
Amfit d.
Metrecom d.
digitorum
d. brevis avulsion
d. communis tendon
extensor d. (ED)
flexor d. (FD)
digitus
d. abductus
d. adductus
d. annularis
d. flexus deformity
d. medius
d. minimus
d. primus
d. valgus
d. varus
Di Guglielmo disease
dihydrocodeine compound
dilated cardiomyopathy
dilator
Eder-Puestow metal olive d.
lacrimal duct d.
vessel d.
Dillwyn-Evans
D.-E. osteotomy
D.-E. resection
dilutional pseudoanemia
dimelia
ulnar d.

dimension
D. hip prosthesis
D. hip system
3-dimensional (3D)
3-d. analysis
Dimension-C femoral stem prosthesis
diminished sensation
Dimon-Hughston
D.-H. fracture fixation
D.-H. intertrochanteric osteotomy
D.-H. technique
Dimon osteotomy
dimple
d. the bone
pilonidal d.
d. sign
ding foot
Dingman
D. bone and cartilage clamp
D. bone-holding forceps
D. mouth gag
D. osteotome
dinner fork deformity
diode
infrared light-emitting d.
d. laser
diorthosis
Dioval Injection
DIP
distal interphalangeal
DIP articulation
DIP fusion
DIP joint
dipalmitoyl phosphatidylcholine (DPPC)
diparesis
spastic d.
diphasic
diphosphonate
methylene d. (MPD)
DIPJ
distal interphalangeal joint
diplegia
spastic d.
diplegic foot
Diplococcus pneumoniae
diplomyelia
diploscope
dipropionate
dipyridamole
d. handgrip test
d. thallium imaging
direct
d. contraction

NOTES

199

direct (*continued*)
    d. current
    d. current electrotherapy
    d. electrical nerve stimulation (DENS)
    d. fracture
    d. injury elbow dislocation
    d. lateral portal
    d. vertex impact
direct-impact prosthesis
director
    grooved d.
direct-vision carpal tunnel release
disability, pl. **disabilities**
    d. adjusted life year (DALY)
    Disabilities of Arm, Shoulder, and Hand (DASH)
    Disabilities of Arm, Shoulder, and Hand questionnaire
    Disabilities of Arm, Shoulder, and Hand scale
    atlantooccipital d.
    box and block test of arm d.
    functional d.
    Models of Media Representation of D.
    National Council on D.
    National Information Center for Children and Youth with Disabilities
    Oswestry Low Back Pain D.
    permanent d.
    permanent partial d. (PPD)
    permanent and total d. (PTD)
    reversible ischemic neurologic d. (RIND)
    d. scale
    d. screening questionnaire
    secondary d.
    tapping test of arm d.
disappearing bone disease
disarticular amputation
disarticulation
    d. amputation
    ankle d.
    Batch-Spittler-McFaddin knee d.
    Boyd hip d.
    elbow d. (ED)
    joint d.
    Lisfranc d.
    Mazet knee d.
    metatarsophalangeal joint d.
    sacroiliac d.
    shoulder d. (SD)
    wrist d. (WD)
DISC
    dynamic integrated stabilization chair
disc, disk
    Acro-Flex artificial d.

    acromioclavicular d.
    amphiarthrodial d.
    d. of ankle
    articular d.
    Bardeen primitive d.
    Bowman d.
    d. bulge
    bulging d.
    cartilaginous d.
    cervical d.
    choked d.
    d. compression
    contained herniated d.
    crescent-shaped fibrocartilaginous d.
    d. degeneration
    d. diffusion method
    d. diffusion test
    d. electrode
    Engelmann d.
    d. excision
    excision of intervertebral d.
    extruded d.
    d. extrusion
    fibrocartilaginous d.
    fixation d.
    d. forceps
    d. fragment
    frayed d.
    d. grabber
    hard d.
    herniated d.
    herniated intervertebral d. (HID)
    d. herniation
    I d.
    interarticular d.
    intermediate d.
    interpubic d.
    intervertebral d.
    intraarticular d.
    isotropic d.
    J d.
    d. lesion
    locking d.
    lumbar d.
    massive herniated d.
    noncontained d.
    d. plication
    d. pressure
    d. prolapse
    protruding d.
    d. protrusion
    Q d.
    d. rongeur
    ruptured d.
    sequestered d.
    sequestrated d.
    slipped d.
    d. space
    d. space saline acceptance test

sternoclavicular d.
swollen d.
d. syndrome
thin d.
transverse d.
vacuum d.
Z d.
discectomy, diskectomy
anterior cervical d.
automated percutaneous lumbar d.
(APLD)
cervical d.
fluoroscopic d.
laminotomy and d.
lumbar d.
microlumbar d. (MLD)
microsurgical d. (MSD)
partial d.
PercScope percutaneous d.
percutaneous lumbar d.
Robinson anterior cervical d.
SMALL fluoroscopic d.
Smith-Robinson anterior cervical d.
Williams d.
Wiltse d.
d. with Cloward fusion
discharge
bizarre high-frequency d.
bizarre repetitive d.
complex repetitive d.
coupled d.
cramp d.
double d.
d. frequency
grouped d.
high-frequency d.
multiple d.
myokymic d.
myotonic d.
neuromyotonic d.
paired d.
pseudomyotonic d.
repetitive d.
triple d.
waning d.
disci (*pl. of* discus)
discission knife
discitis, diskitis
juvenile d.
discogenic, diskogenic
d. neck pain
discogram, diskogram
d. needle

discography, diskography
cervical d.
Cloward fusion d.
lumbar d.
microlumbar d.
Williams d.
discoid
d. lateral meniscus
d. meniscus saucerization
discoligamentous injury
discometry, diskometry
discontinuity
pelvic d.
discopathogenic
discopathy
cervical d.
traumatic cervical d.
Disc-O-Sit Jr. cushion
discotome, diskotome
Pheasant d.
discovery
D. bone densitometer
D. elbow system
discrepancy
leg length d. (LLD)
limb length d.
discrete activity
discrimination
2-point d.
right/left d.
sharp/dull d.
tactile d.
Weber static 2-point d.
discus, pl. **disci**
disease
Albers-Schönberg d.
Albert d.
Albright d.
allograft coronary artery d.
Apert d.
Aran-Duchenne d.
Assmann d.
Atton d.
Baastrup d.
Bamberger-Marie d.
basic calcium phosphate crystal
deposition d.
Bekhterev d.
Bielschowsky-Jansky d.
Blount d.
Blount-Barber d.
bone d.
Bourneville d.

D

NOTES

disease *(continued)*

Bowen d.
Brailsford d.
brittle bone d.
Brodie d.
Bruck d.
Buchanan d.
Burns d.
Busquet d.
Caffey d.
Caffey-Kenny d.
calcium hydroxyapatite crystal
  deposition d.
calcium pyrophosphate dihydrate
  deposition d.
Calvé d.
Calvé-Perthes d.
Camurati-Engelmann d.
Canavan d.
Canavan-van Bogaert-Bertrand d.
cement d.
cementless d.
central core d.
cervical disc d.
CHA crystal deposition d.
Chandler d.
Charcot joint d.
Charcot-Marie-Tooth d.
Chester-Erdheim d.
chronic tophaceous d.
CMT d.
collagen vascular d. (CVD)
connective tissue d.
Conradi d.
d. construct
coronary artery d. (CAD)
Cruveilhier d.
crystal-related joint d.
Curschmann-Steinert d.
cystic d.
Darier-White d.
deer tick d.
degenerative disc d. (DDD)
degenerative joint d. (DJD)
Dejerine d.
Dejerine-Sottas d.
denervation d.
de Quervain d.
destructive bone d.
destructive joint d.
Deutschländer d.
Diaz d.
Di Guglielmo d.
disappearing bone d.
double Charcot d.
Duchenne d.
Duchenne-Aran d.
Duplay d.
Dupuytren d.

Eddowes d.
Ehlers-Danlos d.
Ehrenfeld d.
Emery-Dreifuss d.
Engelmann d.
Engel-Recklinghausen d.
Erb-Landouzy d.
Erdheim-Chester d.
Erichsen d.
facet joint d. (FJD)
fascioscapulohumeral muscle
  atrophy d.
Felix d.
fibromuscular d.
Forestier d.
Freiberg d.
Freiberg-Kohler d.
Friedreich d.
Garré d.
Garrod d.
Gaucher d.
glenohumeral joint d.
Gorham d.
Grisel d.
Gumboro d.
Haas d.
Haglund d.
handcuff d.
Hand-Schüller-Christian d.
Hansen d.
Heberden d.
Henderson-Jones d.
hereditary neuropathic d.
Hoffa d.
Hoffa-Kastert d.
Hospital for Joint D. (HJD)
Hurler d.
hydroxyapatite deposition d.
hypophosphatemic bone d.
ischemic leg d.
ischemic limb d. (ILD)
Iselin d.
Jaffe d.
Jansen d.
joint d.
Jüngling d.
Kashin-Bek d.
Kienböck d.
Koehler d.
Köhler d.
Köhler-Pellegrini-Stieda d.
König d.
Kugelberg-Welander d.
Kümmell d.
Kümmell-Verneuil d.
Lance d.
Larsen d.
Larsen-Johansson d.
Ledderhose d.

Legg-Calvé-Perthes d. (LCPD)
Legg-Calvé-Waldenström d.
Legg-Perthes d.
Leri d.
Leri-Weill d.
Letterer-Siwe d.
Lichtman d.
Lichtman radiographic classification
of Kienböck d. (stages I, II,
IIIa, IIIb, IV)
Lobstein d.
Lyme d.
MacLean-Maxwell d.
Maffucci d.
Marie-Bamberger d.
Marie-Charcot-Tooth d.
Marie-Strümpell d.
Maroteaux-Lamy d.
marrow d.
Martin d.
Mauclaire d.
McArdle d.
metabolic bone d.
metastatic d.
Meyer-Betz d.
milk-alkali d.
mini-core d.
mixed connective tissue d.
modified Kienböck d.
modified Stahl classification of
Kienböck d. (stage I-V)
Moeller-Barlow d.
Morquio d.
Morquio-Ullrich d.
Morton d.
motor neuron d.
Mouchet d.
Munchmeyer d.
Nakamura d.
National Institute of Arthritis and
Musculoskeletal and Skin D.'s
(NIAMS)
neurogenic d.
neuromuscular d.
neuropathic joint d.
Niemann-Pick d.
noninflammatory degenerative
joint d. (NIDJD)
oligoarticular d.
Ollier d.
Oppenheim d.
Osgood-Schlatter d.
Otto d.

Paas d.
Paget d.
Panner d.
Parkinson d.
Pauzat d.
Pellegrini d.
Pellegrini-Stieda d.
peripheral arterial occlusive d.
(PAOD)
peripheral vascular d. (PVD)
peripheral vascular obstructive d.
Perrin-Ferraton d.
Perthes d.
Poncet d.
posttraumatic degenerative d.
Pott d.
Poulet d.
Preiser d.
pseudo-Pott d.
Pyle d.
Quervain d.
quiet hip d.
Raynaud d.
Recklinghausen d.
Reiter d.
rheumatoid d.
Ribbing d.
Roussy-Lévy d.
Rust d.
sacroiliac joint d.
Schanz d.
Scheuermann d.
Schlatter d.
Schlatter-Osgood d.
Schmid d.
Schmorl d.
senile hip d.
Sever d.
Silfverskiöld d.
Sinding-Larsen-Johansson d.
skeletal hypoplasia d.
spotted bone d.
Steinert d.
steroid-induced bone d.
Still d.
Strümpell d.
Strümpell-Marie d.
Sudeck d.
Swediauer d.
synovial d.
Talma d.
Taratynov d.
Thiemann d.

D

NOTES

disease *(continued)*
    Thomsen d.
    thromboembolic d. (TED)
    tophaceous d.
    Trevor d.
    Trevor-Fairbank d.
    Truswell-Hansen d.
    upper motor neuron d.
    van Buchem d.
    Van der Hoeve d.
    Van Neck d.
    venous thromboembolic d. (VTED)
    Volkmann d.
    von Recklinghausen d.
    Voorhoeve d.
    Vrolik d.
    Wagner d.
    Waldenström d.
    Wegner d.
    Werdnig-Hoffmann d.
    Wilson d.
    Wohlfart-Kugelberg-Welander d.
    Woringer-Kolopp d.
    Worth d.
    Ziehen-Oppenheim d.
disease-modifying antirheumatologic drug (DMARD)
disfigured foot
DISH
    diffuse idiopathic skeletal hyperostosis
    DISH syndrome
dishpan fracture
DISI
    distal intercalated segment instability
    dorsal intercalated segment instability
    dorsiflexed intercalated segment instability
    DISI collapse pattern
    DISI deformity
disinfectant
    high-level d.
    intermediate d.
disk *(var. of* disc)
Diskard head halter
Disk-Criminator
    D.-C. nerve stimulation measuring device
    D.-C. sensory testing
diskectomy *(var. of* discectomy)
diskitis *(var. of* discitis)
diskogenic *(var. of* discogenic)
diskogram *(var. of* discogram)
diskography *(var. of* discography)
diskometry *(var. of* discometry)
diskotome *(var. of* discotome)
dislocated
    d. knee
    d. patella
dislocating arthropathy

dislocatio erecta
dislocation
    acromioclavicular joint d.
    ankle d.
    antenatal d.
    anterior hip d.
    anterior-inferior d.
    anterior shoulder d.
    anterolateral d.
    d. of articular process
    atlantoaxial d. (AAD)
    atlantooccipital joint d.
    atypical d.
    Bankart shoulder d.
    bayonet d.
    Bell-Dally cervical d.
    Bennett basic hand d.
    bilateral interfacetal d. (BID)
    boutonnière hand d.
    bursting d.
    Carnesale-Stewart-Barnes classification of hip d.
    carpal d.
    carpometacarpal joint d.
    central d.
    Chopart ankle d.
    chronic recurrent ankle joint d.
    closed d.
    complete d.
    complex fracture d.
    complicated d.
    compound d.
    congenital hip d.
    congenital patella d.
    consecutive d.
    d. contour abnormality
    Copeland-Kavat classification of metatarsophalangeal d.
    Cotton reduction of elbow d.
    dashboard d.
    Desault wrist d.
    direct injury elbow d.
    divergent elbow d.
    dorsal perilunate d.
    dorsal transscaphoid perilunar d.
    elbow d.
    facet d.
    d. factor
    fracture d.
    frank d.
    gamekeeper's thumb d.
    glenohumeral joint d.
    habitual d.
    Hill-Sachs shoulder d.
    hip d.
    incomplete d.
    interfacetal d.
    interphalangeal joint d.
    intraarticular d.

irreducible fracture d.
isolated d.
Jahss classification of ankle d.
joint d.
Kienböck d.
knee d.
Kocher reduction of shoulder d.
ligamentous anterior d. (LAD)
Lisfranc d.
lumbosacral d.
lunate d.
luxatio erecta shoulder d.
medial swivel d.
metacarpophalangeal d.
metatarsophalangeal joint d.
Meyn reduction of elbow d.
milkmaid's elbow d.
Monteggia d.
Nélaton ankle d.
neuropathic joint d.
occipitoatlantal d.
old unreduced d.
open d.
Osborne-Cotterill elbow d.
Otto pelvis d.
Palmer transscaphoid perilunar d.
panclavicular d.
parachute jumper's d.
partial d.
patellar intraarticular d.
pathologic d.
perilunar transscaphoid d.
perilunate carpal d.
peroneal d.
phalangeal d.
posterior facet d.
posterior hip d.
posterior shoulder d.
posteromedial d.
prenatal d.
primitive d.
proximal tibiofibular joint d.
radial head d.
radiocarpal d.
radioulnar d.
recent d.
recurrent patellar d.
retrosternal d.
sacroiliac d.
shoulder d.
simple d.
Smith d.
spontaneous hyperemic d.

sternoclavicular joint d.
subastragalar d.
subcoracoid shoulder d.
subglenoid shoulder d.
subspinous d.
subtalar joint d.
superior d.
swivel d.
talar d.
talonavicular d.
tarsal d.
tarsometatarsal d.
temporomandibular joint d.
teratologic d.
tibialis posterior d.
tibiofibular joint d.
transscaphoid perilunate d.
traumatic d.
triquetrolunate d.
unilateral interfacetal d. (UID)
unreduced d.
volar semilunar wrist d.

dislodgment
hook d.

disorder
adrenal d.
ARS d.
clotting d.
coagulation d.
congenital limb d.
cumulative trauma d. (CTD)
degenerative d.
gait d.
mixed connective tissue d.
motor speech d.
movement d.
muscle d.
myeloproliferative d.
National Organization for
  Rare D.'s
neurocompressive d.
neurogenic d.
neurologic d.
neuromuscular junction d.
nontotal-contact d.
occupation-related d.
patellofemoral d.
peripheral neurocompressive d.
progressive neurologic d.
recurrent d.
repetitive strain d.
repetitive stress d.
repetitive trauma d. (RTD)

D

NOTES

disorder *(continued)*
    retrocalcaneal d.
    rheumatoid d.
    rheumatologic d.
    spastic d.
    tendon d.
    trophic joint d.
    vasomotor d.
disorganized bone
disparity
    limb length d.
dispenser
    Jet Vac cement d.
dispersion
    temporal d.
displaced
    d. intraarticular calcaneus
    d. intraarticular fracture
    d. pilon fracture
    d. vertebra
displacement
    angular d.
    d. anterior cavus V osteotomy
    atlantoaxial rotary d.
    crosshead d.
    d. curve
    Ellis-Jones peroneal tendon d.
    fracture fragment d.
    interregional d.
    lateral patella d.
    lateral rotary d.
    Laurin lateral patella d.
    left-right leg d.
    load-to-grip d.
    medial d.
    oblique d.
    patella d.
    peroneal tendon d.
    posterior facet d.
    rotary d.
    sagittal plane d.
    tendon d.
    translational d.
    traumatic d.
    Y-axis translatory d.
display
    head-mounted d. (HMD)
    high-definition video d.
disposable
    d. arthroscope
    d. muscle biopsy clamp
    d. 1-piece osteotome
Disposatrode disposable electrode
disproportionate dwarfism
disrelationship
    persistent occiput/atlas d.
disruption
    anterior column d.
    cervical spine posterior ligament d.

Charcot d.
end-stage d.
facet capsule d.
fibular joint d.
forefoot d.
glenolabral articular d. (GLAD)
interosseous ligament d.
joint d.
lateral compartment d.
ligamentous d.
medial compartment d.
pedicle cortex d.
physial d.
sesamoid d.
skeletal d.
talocalcaneal ligament d.
dissecans
    osteochondritis d. (OCD, OD)
dissecting
    d. clamp
    d. probe
    d. scissors
dissection
    blunt d.
    bone d.
    deep iliac d.
    extracapsular d.
    field of d.
    fingertip d.
    Pack-Ehrlich deep iliac d.
    sharp d.
    subligamentous d.
    subperiosteal d.
dissector
    Angell James d.
    angled d.
    ball d.
    blunt hook d.
    bunion d.
    Creed d.
    Crile gasserian ganglion knife
      and d.
    Davis dura d.
    dura d.
    Freer d.
    golf-stick d.
    grooved d.
    Hajek-Ballenger d.
    hand d.
    hockey-stick d.
    joker d.
    Kidner d.
    Kocher d.
    Lewin bunion d.
    McDonald d.
    Penfield 4 d.
    sesamoidectomy d.
    transsphenoidal d.
    West hand d.

disseminated
    d. intravascular coagulation (DIC)
    d. pigmented villonodular synovitis
dissociation
    hypnotic d.
    lunotriquetral d.
    d. movement
    radioulnar d.
    scapholunate d.
    scapulothoracic d.
dissociative
    d. anesthesia
    carpal instability, d. (CID)
distal
    d. Akin phalangeal osteotomy
    d. articular set angle (DASA)
    d. biceps brachii tendon rupture
    d. bone end
    d. calcaneus
    d. clavicle
    d. clavicular excision
    d. communicating branch (DCB)
    d. compression test
    d. concave articular surface
    d. dystrophy
    d. femoral cutting guide
    d. femoral epiphysial fracture
    d. femoral resection
    d. femur
    d. fibula
    d. fibulotalar arthrodesis
    d. first metatarsal osteotomy
    d. forearm
    d. fragment
    d. humeral epiphysis
    d. humeral fracture
    d. humerus
    d. intercalated segment instability (DISI)
    d. interlocking
    d. interphalangeal (DIP)
    d. interphalangeal joint (DIPJ)
    d. interphalangeal joint approach
    d. intrinsic release
    d. latency
    d. locking
    d. locking screw
    d. L osteotomy
    d. medial creaking
    d. metaphysis
    d. metatarsal articular angle (DMAA)
    d. neurolysis

    d. oblique sliding osteotomy
    d. palmar crease (DPC)
    d. parabola toe length
    d. phalanx (DP)
    d. phocomelia
    d. radial fracture
    d. radioulnar joint (DRUJ)
    d. radioulnar joint prosthesis
    d. radioulnar joint stabilization
    d. radius
    d. realignment
    d. reference axis (DRA)
    d. row carpectomy
    d. segment weight
    d. soft tissue release (DSTR)
    d. star pad
    d. targeting
    d. targeting device
    d. thigh amputation
    d. thigh band
    d. third (D/3, distal/3)
    d. third of shaft
    d. tibia
    d. tibial epiphysial injury
    d. tibial physis
    d. tibiofibular fusion
    d. tibiofibular joint
    d. transfer
    d. tuberosity
    d. tuberosity of finger
    d. tuberosity of toe
    d. tuft
    d. ulna
    d. ulnar convexity
    d. Wagner femoral metaphysial shortening
distal/3
    distal third
distalward
distance
    coracoclavicular d.
    focal film d.
    fulcrum d.
    interpedicular d.
    protrusion d.
distention, distension
distolateral
distoocclusal
distortion
    multisegmental spinal d.
    sacral base d.
    structural intersegmental d.

NOTES

D

distraction
    apical d.
    d. arthroplasty
    d. bar
    d. bone block arthrodesis
    calcaneal d.
    callus d.
    d. clamp
    fixed d.
    flexion d.
    d. force
    d. of fracture
    fracture fragment d.
    Guhl d.
    halo-cast d.
    halo-femoral d.
    halo-pelvic d.
    d. histogenesis
    d. hook
    d. injury
    d. instrumentation
    d. instrumentation biomechanics
    joint d.
    d. laminoplasty
    d. lengthening
    longitudinal d.
    manipulation with d.
    Monticelli-Spinelli d.
    d. osteogenesis
    d. osteogenesis technique
    physial d.
    d. pin
    d. rod
    d. screw
    slow d.
    small step d.
    spinal d.
    d. subtalar arthrodesis
    d. technique
    d. test
distraction-compression
    d.-c. bone graft arthrodesis
    d.-c. scoliosis treatment
distraction-flexion stage (DFS)
distractive
    d. extension
    d. flexion
    d. motion
distractor
    Acufex ankle d.
    Anderson d.
    AO femoral d.
    Bliskunov implantable femoral d.
    DeBastiani d.
    femoral d.
    hook d.
    Ilizarov d.
    intramedullary skeletal kinetic d.
      (ISKD)

    joint d.
    Kessler metacarpal d.
    Mark II distal femur d.
    McCarthy hip d.
    Monticelli-Spinelli d.
    Mueller d.
    Orthofix M-100 d.
    Pinto d.
    Santa Casa d.
    turnbuckle d.
    Wagner d.
distribution
    Boltzmann d.
    cutaneous d.
    Moe-Kettleson d.
    stocking-glove d.
    stress d.
disturbance
    articulation d.
    gait d.
    pain-related sleep d.
disuse
    d. arthropathy
    d. atrophy
    d. osteoporosis
diurnal
    d. change
    d. variation in straight leg raising
divergence
    angle of d.
    anteroposterior talocalcaneal d.
divergent elbow dislocation
diversified
    D. chiropractic manipulative therapy
    d. manipulation
diversified-type force application
diversional activity
divided navicular
division
    Swafford-Lichtman d.
divisionary line
divot sign
Dix-Hallpike maneuver
DJD
    degenerative joint disease
DKB
    deep knee bend
DK 201 cryotherapy wrap
D-L internal fixator
DMAA
    distal metatarsal articular angle
DMARD
    disease-modifying antirheumatologic
    drug
D-Med Injection
DMI
    Duro-Med Industries
    DMI orthopaedic bed
DMP wire twister

DOA
    diagnostic and operative arthroscopy
Doane knee retractor
dobutamine echocardiography
doctor (Dr, Dr.)
    D. Collins fracture clamp
    d. of podiatric medicine (DPM)
documented pseudarthrosis
Dodd perforator
DOF
    degrees of freedom
doffing
    donning and d.
    d. prosthesis
Dogbone ACFS
dog-ear repair
dogleg fracture
dolichostenomelia
doll
    D. trochanteric reattachment
    D. trochanteric reattachment
    technique
dollar
    d. sign
    d. sign side
dollop
    bone d.
doll's eye sign
dolorimeter
dolorosus
    hallux d.
dome
    d. fracture
    d. plunger
    d. proximal tibial osteotomy
    shoulder d.
    talar d.
    weightbearing acetabular d.
Domeboro
dome-shaped osteotomy
dominance
    hand d.
    left-hand d.
    right-hand d.
domino spinal instrumentation connector
Donaghy angled suture needle holder
Donati suture
DonJoy
    D. ALP brace
    D. Gold Point knee brace
    D. knee splint
    D. Opal knee brace
    D. 4-point Super Sport knee brace

    D. Quadrant shoulder brace
    D. Ultrasling shoulder immobilizer
    D. Universal ankle brace
    D. wrist splint
donning
    d. and doffing
    d. prosthesis
donning-doffing skill
donor
    d. site
    d. team
DOOR
    deafness, onychoosteodystrophy, mental
    retardation
    DOOR syndrome
Doppler
    D. ankle systolic pressure
    D. pulse evaluation
    D. scope
    D. study
    D. technique
    D. ultrasound
    D. ultrasound flowmeter
Dorello canal
Dormarex 2 Oral
Dormin Oral
Dorr
    D. bone classification
    D. ratio
Dorrance
    D. hand prosthesis
    D. hook
    D. procedure
dorsal
    d. arch of wrist
    d. aspect
    d. bunion
    d. calcaneocuboid (DCC)
    d. calcaneocuboid ligament
    d. calcaneonavicular ligament
    d. capsule
    d. capsulodesis
    d. carpal capsulitis
    d. carpal ligament
    d. carpometacarpal ligament
    d. cheilectomy
    d. closing wedge osteotomy
    d. closing wedge proximal
    phalangeal osteotomy
    d. columella implant
    d. column stimulator (DCS)
    d. column stimulator implant
    d. compartment

NOTES

dorsal *(continued)*
  d. cross-finger flap
  d. cuboideonavicular ligament
  d. cuneocuboid ligament
  d. cuneonavicular ligament
  d. cutaneous nerve
  d. digital artery (DDA)
  d. drainage
  d. drawer test
  d. extension block splint
  d. finger approach
  d. glide
  d. hood
  d. horn cell
  d. intercalated segment instability
    (DISI)
  d. intercarpal ligament
  d. intercuneiform ligament
  d. interosseous muscle
  d. kyphotic curvature
  d. linear incision
  d. lithotomy position
  d. longitudinal incision
  d. lordosis
  d. lumbar corset
  d. malalignment
  d. metacarpal ligament
  d. metatarsal artery
  d. metatarsal ligament
  d. midline approach
  d. neuroma
  d. pedal bypass
  d. pedal pulse
  d. perilunate dislocation
  d. planar x-ray
  d. plate
  d. plate extender
  d. point
  d. proximal metatarsal osteotomy
  d. radial slope
  d. radiocarpal ligament
  d. ramus
  d. recumbent position
  d. reflex
  d. ridge
  d. root entry zone (DREZ)
  d. root ganglion (DRG)
  d. root ganglionectomy
  d. scapular nerve
  d. skin
  d. subcutaneous nerve transposition
  d. synovectomy
  d. talonavicular ligament
  d. tarsometatarsal ligament
  d. tenosynovectomy
  d. toe plate extension
  d. T-plate
  d. translation

  d. transscaphoid perilunar
    dislocation
  d. transverse capsulotomy
  d. transverse incision
  d. ulnar cutaneous branch
  d. venous arch
  d. venous arch of hand
  d. vertebra
  d. V osteotomy
  d. wing
  d. wing fracture
  d. wire-loop fixation
  d. wrist splint
  d. wrist splint with outrigger
dorsalgia
  cervicogenic d.
dorsalia
  ligamenta carpometacarpaliad d.
dorsalis
  d. pedis artery anatomy
  d. pedis fasciocutaneous flap
  d. pedis pulse
  tabes d.
dorsalward approach
Dorsey screw-holding screwdriver
dorsi
  elastofibroma d.
  d. jam syndrome
  latissimus d.
  osteochondritis deformans
    juvenilis d.
  d. stop component
dorsiflexed
  d. intercalated segment instability
    (DISI)
  d. metatarsal
dorsiflexion
  active d.
  d. angle (DFA)
  d. assist ankle joint ankle-foot
    orthosis
  d. bumper
  d. flexion
  d. foot splint
  d. metatarsal osteotomy
  passive d.
  resisted d.
  d. stop brace
  d. stress ankle x-ray
  d. view
dorsiflexion-eversion test
dorsiflexion-plantar flexion position
dorsiflexor gait
dorsiflexory wedge osteotomy
Dorsiwedge night splint
dorsodynia
dorsolateral
  d. approach
  d. and medial capsulotomy

dorsolumbar area
dorsomedial
 d. approach
 d. cutaneous nerve
 d. incision
dorsoplantar
 d. approach
 d. capsulotomy
 d. projection
 d. radiograph
 d. radiographic view
 d. talometatarsal angle
 d. talonavicular angle
dorsoradial
 d. approach
 d. ligament (DRL)
dorsorostral approach
dorsoulnar approach
dorsovolar
dorsum of hand
double
 d. arthrodesis
 d. bent Hohmann acetabular
  retractor
 d. binocular operating microscope
 d. camelback sign
 d. Charcot disease
 d. clamp
 d. Cobra plate
 d. contrast arthrotomography of
  shoulder
 d. contrast shoulder
  arthrotomography
 d. corn deformity
 d. cruciate configuration
 d. crush syndrome
 d. discharge
 d. drape
 D. Duty cane
 D. Duty cane reacher
 d. flexion wave
 d. fracture
 d. hemiplegia
 d. hip spica cast
 d. hump contour
 d. incision
 d. inflow cannula system
 d. jointed
 d. leg raise test
 d. major curve pattern
 d. major curve scoliosis
 d. major spinal curve

 d. osteotomy
 d. PCL sign
 d. pearl-face hip joint
 d. portal technique
 d. right-angle suture
 d. simultaneous sensory stimulation
 d. sugar-tong splint
 d. support time
 d. tendon transfer
 d. thoracic curve
 d. thoracic curve scoliosis
 d. tourniquet
 d. Zielke instrumentation
double-action
 d.-a. ankle joint
 d.-a. bone-cutting forceps
 d.-a. cutter
 d.-a. rongeur
double-arc sign
double-cannula system
double-clamp approximator
double-contrast
 d.-c. arthrogram
 d.-c. arthrography
 d.-c. study
double-ended
 d.-e. nail
 d.-e. right-angle retractor
double-flap amputation
double-flexion knee motion
double-headed stereotactic carrier
double-hollow nail
double-H plate
double-incision fasciotomy
double-leg
 d.-l. stance
 d.-l. stance phase
 d.-l. stance phase of gait
double-looped
 d.-l. cerclage wire
 d.-l. gracilis graft
 d.-l. semitendinous and gracilis
  hamstring graft knee
  reconstruction technique
double-L spinal rod
double-needle chemonucleolysis
double-occlusal splint
double-open hook
double-opposing Z-plasty
double-pendulum action
double-pronged skin hook
double-ring frame

D

NOTES

211

double-rod
    d.-r. construct
    d.-r. technique
double-sharp forceps
double-slot screwdriver
double-stem
    d.-s. silicone implant
    d.-s. silicone lesser MP joint
double-step gait
double-stranded wire double-twisted wire
doublet
double-tap gait
double-threaded Herbert screw
double-thumb thrust
double-upright short leg brace
double-Z rhombic skin flap
doughnut
    d. headrest
    d. ring
    d. support brace
doughy
    d. cement
    d. consistency
Douglas skin graft
Dow
    D. Corning titanium hemi-implant
    D. Corning Wright finger joint prosthesis
dowager's hump
dowel
    d. arthrodesis
    bone d.
    d. bone graft
    calf bone d.
    d. cutter
    cylindrical d.
    graft d.
    Graftech structural allograft cervical d.
    d. graft technique
    d. grip
    iliac crest d.
    d. spinal fusion
    threaded cortical d.
doweled
doweling
    d. spondylolisthesis
    d. spondylolisthesis technique
down
    D. epiphysial knife
    D. syndrome
down-angle hook
downbiting rongeur
Downey
    D. hemilaminectomy retractor
    D. modification

    D. modification of Fowler-Philip approach
    D. texture discrimination test
Downey-McGlamery procedure
Downey-Rubin overlapping toe repair procedure
downgoing toes
Downing
    D. cartilage knife
    D. staple
downsized circular laminar hook
Doyan periosteal elevator
Doyen
    D. bone mallet
    D. costal rasp
    D. cylindrical bur
    D. cylindrical drill
    D. rib elevator
    D. rib rasp
    D. spherical bur
Dozier radiolucent Bennett retractor
DP
    distal phalanx
    DP pulse
    Springlite Advantage DP
DPA
    dual-photon absorptiometry
DPB
    dynamic pedobarography
DPC
    delayed primary closure
    distal palmar crease
DPD
    dual photon densitometry
DPM
    doctor of podiatric medicine
DPPC
    dipalmitoyl phosphatidylcholine
DPTT
    deep posterior tibiotalar
    DPTT ligament
DPVNS
    diffuse pigmented villonodular synovitis
DPX
    dual-photon absorptiometry
Dr
    doctor
    Dr Scholl's Athlete's Foot
    Dr Scholl's Maximum Strength Tritin
Dr.
    doctor
    Dr. Grip writing device
    Dr. Joseph's diabetic foot kit
    Dr. Joseph's Original Footbrush
DRA
    distal reference axis
drafting
    overlay d.

Dragstedt skin graft
drag-to gait
drain
Charnley suction d.
fishmouth d.
Hemovac Hydrocoat d.
Heyer-Schulte wound d.
Jackson-Pratt d.
Nélaton rubber tube d.
open fracture wound d.
Penrose d.
polyethylene d.
PVC d.
rubber d.
Shirley d.
silastic d.
subcutaneous d.
Surgivac d.
Wound-Evac d.
drainage
anterior d.
anterolateral d.
anteromedial d.
ConstaVac d.
David d.
dorsal d.
ilium d.
incision and d. (I&D)
infusion-aspiration d.
Klein d.
lateral d.
medial d.
Ober posterior d.
open d.
pelvic d.
posterior d.
posterolateral d.
posteromedial d.
suction d.
draining infected nonunion
DRAM
deepithelialized rectus abdominis muscle
DRAM flap
drape
adhesive d.
double d.
fenestrated d.
foot d.
incise d.
isolation d.
lint-free d.
Loban adhesive d.
3M skin d.

NeuroDrape surgical d.
Opmi microscopic d.
Opraflex d.
draped out
drawer
flexion-rotation-d. (FRD)
d. sign
d. test
drawing
pain d.
preoperative d.
Ransford Pain D.
drawn ankle clonus
dream
D. Pillow
D. Ride car seat
Dremel Moto-tool
Drennan
D. metaphysial-epiphysial angle
D. posterior transfer
DressFlex
D. orthotic
D. orthotic device
Dressinet netting bandage
dressing
abdominal d.
absorptive d.
ACU-derm wound d.
Adaptic d.
adhesive d.
Aeroplast d.
Alginate d.
AlgiSite Alginate wound d.
Allevyn Island d.
Allevyn wound d.
d. apraxia
Aquaphor gauze d.
Aquasorb Hydrogel wound d.
Arglaes film d.
Arthrosol d.
Avitene flour d.
Betadine d.
Bioclusive select transparent film d.
biologic d.
Blister Film d.
bulky hand d.
bundle d.
Bunnell d.
burn d.
calcium alginate d.
CarboFlex odor-control d.
Cica-Care wound d.

NOTES

213

dressing *(continued)*
    Circulon d.
    circumferential d.
    Coban elastic d.
    CoFilm d.
    Co-Flex d.
    cold compressive d.
    collagen skin d.
    collodion d.
    CombiDERM nonadhesive
      absorbent d.
    Comfeel Ulcus occlusive d.
    Compeed protective d.
    compression d.
    conductive Hydrogel wound d.
    Conform d.
    CoolSorb absorbent cold transfer d.
    Coraderm d.
    corrective soft d.
    cotton d.
    Covaderm Plus adhesive barrier d.
    Coverlet adhesive surgical d.
    Coverlet Strips wound d.
    Cover-Roll adhesive gauze d.
    Covertell composite secondary d.
    Co-Wrap d.
    Cryo/Cuff ankle d.
    Cutinova cavity d.
    Cutinova foam d.
    Cutinova thin d.
    Dermagran hydrophilic gauze d.
    Dermagran ointment wound d.
    DermaMend foam wound d.
    DermaMend Hydrogel d.
    DermaSite d.
    Dermiflex d.
    Digi Sleeve stockinette d.
    dry sterile d. (DSD)
    DuoDerm d.
    Eakin cohesive seal d.
    elastic d.
    Elastikon d.
    Elastomull d.
    Elastoplast d.
    Ensure-It d.
    Epigard d.
    Esmarch d.
    Exu-Dry wound d.
    Fabco gauze d.
    felt d.
    figure-of-8 d.
    fixed d.
    Flexderm wound d.
    flexible burn d.
    Flexigrid d.
    Flexinet d.
    Flexzan foam wound d.
    fluff d.
    foam wound d.

    Fuller shield d.
    Furacin gauze d.
    FyBron d.
    gauze d.
    Geliperm d.
    Gelocast Unna boot compression d.
    Glasscock ear d.
    Granuflex d.
    hydrocolloid occlusive d.
    Hydrocol wound d.
    Hydrogel wound d.
    hydrophilic d.
    Inerpan flexible burn d.
    Intact d.
    IntraSite d.
    J&J ulcer d.
    Jones d.
    Kaltostat d.
    Kelikian foot d.
    Kerlix d.
    Kling adhesive d.
    Koch-Mason d.
    Kollagen d.
    LYOfoam C d.
    LYOfoam wound d.
    Medi-Rip d.
    Microfoam d.
    Mills d.
    modified Robert Jones d.
    moleskin strip d.
    Mother Jones d.
    neoprene d.
    nonadherent gauze d.
    N-Terface d.
    Nu Gauze d.
    NutraFill hydrophilic d.
    NutraStat wound d.
    Oasis wound d.
    occlusive d.
    O'Donoghue d.
    Omniderm d.
    Opraflex d.
    OpSite wound d.
    Orthoflex d.
    Orthoplast d.
    OsmoCyte island wound-care d.
    Owen gauze d.
    palm-to-axilla d.
    Panogauze Hydrogel wound d.
    patch d.
    petroleum gauze d.
    pledget d.
    Polyderm hydrophilic polyurethane
      foam d.
    PolyMem wound care d.
    polymeric d.
    Polyskin d.
    polyurethane foam d. (PFD)
    PolyWic d.

postoperative d.
pressure ulcer d.
Primaderm d.
Primapore wound d.
ProCyte transparent d.
Profore wound d.
Promogran matrix wound d.
PVD d.
RepliCare wound d.
Reston d.
Restore CalciCare d.
rigid d.
Robert Jones d.
Schanz d.
Scherisorb d.
semirigid postoperative d.
Setopress d.
SignaDRESS hydrocolloid d.
silastic gel d.
silk mesh gauze d.
SkinTemp collagen skin d.
sling d.
Sof-Rol d.
soft bulky d.
Sof-Wick d.
Spenco Second Skin d.
stent d.
sterile dry d. (SDD)
d. stick
Stimson d.
SuperSkin thin film d.
Surgilast tubular elastic d.
Suture-Self d.
Synthaderm d.
Tegaderm d.
Telfa gauze d.
THINSite d.
Toe-Aid d.
toe-to-groin modified Jones d.
transparent adhesive d.
Tricodur Epi compression d.
Tricodur Talus compression d.
Tubex gauze d.
Tubigrip d.
ulcer d.
Ultec thin d.
Uniflex d.
VAC GranuFoam heel d.
Velpeau d.
Vi-Drape d.
Vigilon d.
Webril d.
wet-to-dry d.

wide-mesh petroleum gauze d.
wound d.
Xeroform gauze d.
Dreyer formula
Dreyfus
    D. prosthesis forceps
    D. prosthesis placement instrument
DREZ
    dorsal root entry zone
    DREZ lesion
    DREZ modification of Eriksson
      technique
    DREZ procedure
DRG
    dorsal root ganglion
DRI
    dietary reference intake
Driessen hinged plate
drift
    arm d.
    congenital ulnar d.
    leg d.
    osseous d.
    pronator d.
    radial d.
    ulnar d.
drill
    ACL d.
    Acra-Cut wire pass d.
    Acufex d.
    Adson-Rogers perforating d.
    Adson spiral d.
    Adson twist d.
    Aesculap d.
    agility d.
    air d.
    air-powered cutting d.
    Albee d.
    Amico d.
    Anspach power d.
    anticavitation d.
    Archimedean d.
    ASIF twist d.
    ASSI wire-pass d.
    autotome d.
    Bailey d.
    bar d.
    battery-driven hand d.
    biflanged d.
    bit d.
    d. bit
    d. bit fracture
    Björk rib d.

D

NOTES

drill *(continued)*

bone hand d.
Bosworth crown d.
Bowen suture d.
brace d.
Brunswick-Mack rotating d.
Bunnell bone d.
Bunnell hand d.
bur d.
cannulated d.
cannulated cortical step d.
Carmody perforator d.
Carroll-Bunnell d.
Cebotome bone cement d.
centering d.
cervical d.
Championnière bone d.
Charnley centering d.
Charnley femoral condyle d.
Charnley pilot d.
Charnley starting d.
Cherry d.
Cherry-Austin d.
Children's Hospital hand d.
chuck d.
Cloward cervical d.
Coballoy twist d.
Codman wire-passing d.
Collison body d.
Collison cannulated hand d.
Collison tap d.
cortical step d.
crown d.
Crutchfield bone d.
Crutchfield hand d.
Crutchfield-Raney d.
CurvTek TSR bone d.
Cushing flat d.
Cushing perforator d.
dental d.
depth-check d.
DePuy d.
D'Errico perforating d.
Deyerle d.
diamond high-speed d.
Doyen cylindrical d.
driver nail d.
Elan d.
Elan-E power d.
extractor nail d.
fingernail d.
Fisch d.
flat d.
Galt hand d.
Gates-Glidden d.
glenoid d.
Gray bone d.
d. guard
d. guide

d. guide forceps
Hall air d.
Hall-Dundar d.
Hall Micro-Aire d.
Hall power d.
Hall stepdown d.
Hall Versipower d.
hand d.
hand-operated d.
Harold Crowe d.
Harris-Smith anterior interbody d.
Hewson d.
high-speed twist d.
hip fraction compaction d.
d. hole
hollow mill d.
Hudson bone d.
Hudson brace d.
initiator d.
intramedullary d.
Jacobs chuck d.
Kerr electro-torque d.
Kerr hand d.
Kirschner bone d.
Kirschner wire d.
Kodex d.
Küntscher d.
Loth-Kirschner d.
Luck bone d.
Lusskin bone d.
Macewen d.
Magnuson twist d.
Mathews hand d.
Mathews load d.
McKenzie bone d.
McKenzie perforating twist d.
Michelson-Sequoia air d.
Micro-Aire d.
Midas Rex d.
mini-Stryker power d.
Minos air d.
Mira d.
Moore bone d.
nail d.
Neurain d.
Neurairtome d.
nippers nail d.
Orthairtome II d.
Osseodent surgical d.
Osteone air d.
Patrick d.
pencil-tip d.
penetrating d.
Penn finger d.
perforating twist d.
perforator d.
pilot d.
d. pin
pistol-grip hand d.

Podospray podiatry d.
d. point
Portmann d.
power d.
pronator d.
Ralks bone d.
Ralks fingernail d.
Raney bone d.
Raney perforator d.
retention d.
rib d.
Rica bone d.
Richards Lovejoy bone d.
Richards pistol-grip d.
Richmond subarachnoid twist d.
Richter bone d.
right-angle dental d.
rotating d.
scissors nail d.
Shea d.
Sherman-Stille d.
Sklar bone d.
d. sleeve
Smedberg hand d.
Smedberg twist d.
Smith automatic perforated d.
spiral d.
Spirec d.
step d.
step-down d.
Stille bone d.
Stille hand d.
Stille-Sherman bone d.
Stiwer hand d.
Stryker d.
Suretac d.
Surgairtome air d.
surgical orthopaedic d.
suture hole d.
Synthes d.
tap d.
Toti trephine d.
Treace stapes d.
trephine d.
Trinkle bone d.
Trinkle power d.
Trinkle Super-Cut twist d.
Trowbridge-Campau bone d.
Trow Bridge triple-speed d.
twist d.
Ullrich d.
Uniflex calibrated step d.
union broach retention d.

Universal 2-speed hand d.
Warren-Mack rotating d.
wire d.
Wolferman d.
Xomed d.
Zimmer Cebotome bone cement d.
Zimmer hand d.
Zimmer-Kirschner hand d.
Zimmer Universal d.

drill-guide
Acufex d.-g.

drilling
arthroscopic d.
d. broach
excision, curettage, d. (ECD)
d. jig
percutaneous transmalleolar d.
retrograde d.
d. technique
transmalleolar d.

drill-tipped guidewire
D-ring strap
drip-suck irrigation
Drisdol Oral
drive
Jacobs chuck d.
worm d.

driver
blade-plate d.
bullet d.
femoral head d.
Flatt d.
graft d.
Hall d.
Harrington hook d.
Jewett d.
Ken d.
Kirschner wire d.
Küntscher nail d.
K-wire d.
Linvatec d.
Lloyd nail d.
Massie d.
Maxi-Driver d.
McReynolds d.
Micro Series wire d.
Moore d.
nail d.
d. nail drill
Orthairtome wire d.
ParaMax angled d.
plate d.
polyethylene-faced d.

D

NOTES

driver *(continued)*
    prosthesis d.
    Pugh d.
    Rush d.
    Sage d.
    Schneider nail d.
    staple d.
    supine position d.
    surgical pin d.
    Teflon-coated d.
    tibial d.
    trial d.
    d. tunnel locator apparatus
    wire d.
    Zimmer Orthair ream d.
driver-bender-extractor
    Rush d.-b.-e.
driver-extractor
    Hansen-Street d.-e.
    Ken d.-e.
    McReynolds d.-e.
    Sage d.-e.
    Schneider d.-e.
drivethrough sign
DRL
    dorsoradial ligament
dromedary gait
droopy shoulder syndrome
drop
    d. attack
    d. finger
    d. shoulder
    wrist d.
    d. wrist splint
drop-arm
    d.-a. sign
    d.-a. test
drop-entry (closed body) hook
droperidol and fentanyl
dropfoot
    d. brace
    d. gait
    d. redression stockings
    d. splint
drop-lock
    d.-l. knee brace
    d.-l. ring
dropped
    d. foot
    d. hallux
drug
    antituberculosis d.
    cytotoxic d.
    disease-modifying
      antirheumatologic d. (DMARD)
    National Collegiate Athletic
      Association prohibited d.
    nonsteroidal antiinflammatory d.
      (NSAID)

    slow-acting antirheumatic d.
      (SAARD)
drug-induced myotonia
drug-infusion fever
drug-related hydantoin syndrome
DRUJ
    distal radioulnar joint
    DRUJ instability
    DRUJ prosthesis
drummer-boy palsy
Drummond
    D. button
    D. and Hastings cuboid extrusion
    injury
    D. hook
    D. hook holder
    D. spinal instrumentation
    D. spinous wiring technique
    D. wire
drumstick finger
drunken sailor gait
dry
    d. amputation
    D. Flotation wheelchair cushion
    d. gangrene
    d. heat therapy
    d. hydrotherapy
    d. infected nonunion
    d. joint
    d. necrosis
    d. sterile dressing (DSD)
    d. synovitis
Drytex RocketSoc ankle brace
DSA
    digital subtraction angiography
DSD
    dry sterile dressing
DSIS
    dynamic stabilizing innersole system
    DSIS orthotic
D-Soles
    D-S. insole
    D-S. orthotic
DSTR
    distal soft tissue release
DTM
    dermatophyte test medium
DTM culture
DTR
    deep tendon reflex
DTT
    device for transverse traction
    DTT implant
    DTT system
DTVP-2
    Development Test of Visual Perception,
    2nd Edition
dual
    D. AFO Boot orthotic

d. compression scoliosis treatment
d. drop pelvis (DDP)
d. nerve root suction retractor
d. onlay cortical bone graft
d. photon densitometry (DPD)
d. photon densitometry test
d. photon densitometry test for osteoporosis
d. pin redresser
d. plate
D. Range Limiter System
dual-energy x-ray absorptiometry (DEXA, DXA)
Dualer Plus inclinometer
Duall 88 cement
dual-lock
d.-l. ankle brace
d.-l. total hip prosthesis
d.-l. total hip replacement system
dual-photon
d.-p. absorptiometry (DPA, DPX)
d.-p. electrospinal orthosis
dual-threaded screw
Dubreuilh
D. melanosis circumscripta
melanosis circumscripta preblastomatosis of D.
Duchenne
D. disease
D. muscular atrophy
D. muscular dystrophy
Duchenne-Aran disease
Duchenne-Erb palsy
duckbill
d. elevator
d. rongeur
duck-waddle
d.-w. gait
d.-w. test
duck waddle
duct
thoracic d.
ductile failure
ductility
Dugas test
Duhot line
dull aching pain
dumbbell
d. tumor
d. wagon
Dumon-Gilliard prosthesis introducer
Duncan
D. loop

D. prone rectus test
D. shoulder brace
Dunlop traction
Dunn
D. biopsy
D. fracture device
D. hip operation
D. multiple comparison test
D. osteotomy
D. technique
D. triple arthrodesis
Dunn-Brittain triple arthrodesis
Duocentric prosthesis
Duo-Cline Dual Support contoured bed wedge
Duocondylar knee prosthesis
duodenal compression
DuoDerm dressing
Duo-Drive screw
Duofilm Solution
Duo-Lock hip prosthesis
duopatellar unconstrained prosthesis
Dupaco
D. knee control
D. knee prosthesis
Dupel blue iontophoresis electrode
Duplay
D. bursitis
D. disease
D. syndrome
duplex
d. Doppler ultrasonography
d. ultrasound
duplicate
d. sternum
d. thumb
duplicated metacarpal
duplication
Marks-Bayne technique for thumb d.
symmetric thumb d.
thumb d.
Wassel thumb d. (type IV)
duPont Bunion Rating Score
Dupont distal humeral plate system
Dupré muscle
Dupuytren
D. amputation
D. canal
D. contracture
D. contracture release
D. diathesis
D. disease

D

NOTES

Dupuytren *(continued)*
- D. exostosis
- D. fascia
- D. fasciitis
- D. fibromatosis
- D. fracture
- D. hydrocele
- D. operation
- D. sign
- D. splint
- D. suture

dura
- d. dissector
- d. hook
- d. mater
- d. mater graft

DuraBoot orthosis

Duracon
- D. knee implant
- D. prosthesis

Dura-Flex back brace

Duragesic Transdermal

Dura-Kold reusable compression ice wrap

dural
- d. ectasia
- d. elevator
- d. ligament
- d. repair

Duraleve custom molded foot orthotic

Durallium implant

Duraloc
- D. acetabular cup system
- D. acetabular liner
- D. prosthesis

Duralone Injection

duralumin

Duramer polyethylene component

Duramorph Injection

Duran
- D. approach
- D. passive mobilization

Duran-Houser wrist splint

Durapatite
- D. bone
- D. bone replacement material
- D. implant

DuraPrep

Dura-Soft soft-compression reusable ice or heat wrap

Dura-Stick adhesive electrode

Durasul
- D. head system
- D. polyethylene
- D. polyethylene, high wear resistant acetabular insert
- D. prosthetic component

Duraval Hook & Loop strap material

Durham
- D. flatfoot operation
- D. plasty
- D. procedure
- D. procedure for flatfoot

Durie-Salmon classification

Durkan
- D. carpal compression test
- D. CTS gauge

Duro-Med Industries (DMI)

durometer

durum
- heloma d. (HD)
- osteoma d.

dust
- nail d.

Dutchman's roll

duToit shoulder staple

Duval elevator

Duverney fracture

DuVries
- D. approach
- D. arthroplasty
- D. deltoid ligament reconstruction technique
- D. hammertoe repair
- D. incision
- D. modified McBride hallux valgus operation
- D. phalangeal condylectomy
- D. plantar condylectomy
- D. procedure
- D. resection
- D. technique for overlapping toe

DuVries-Mann modified bunionectomy

Dvorak test

DVRT
- differential variable reluctance transducer

DVT
- deep venous thrombosis
- Flowtron DVT
- DVT prophylaxis

dwarfism
- achondroplastic d.
- ateliotic d.
- autosomal dominant mild short limb d.
- camptomelic d.
- chondroplastic d.
- diastrophic d.
- disproportionate d.
- Langer mesomelic d.
- Laron d.
- metatropic d.
- micromelic d.
- phocomelic d.
- Pott d.
- proportionate d.

Russell-Silver d.
short-limb d.
dwarf pelvis
Dwyer
D. calcaneal osteotomy
D. clawfoot operation
D. correction of scoliosis
D. device
D. incision
D. instrumentation biomechanics
D. osteotomy
D. procedure
D. scoliosis cable
D. spinal instrumentation
D. spinal mechanical stapler
D. spinal screw
D. tensioner
Dwyer-Hall plate
Dwyer-Wickham electrical stimulation system
DXA
dual-energy x-ray absorptiometry
DXA scan
Dycal base
Dycem roll matting
Dyck-Lambert classification
Dycor
D. Geriatric ADL single axis foot prosthesis
D. prosthetic foot
dye
d. extravasation
methylene blue d.
d. punch fracture
d. punch injury
Dyggve-Melchior-Clausen syndrome
dying bug exercise
Dyke-Davidoff-Masson syndrome
Dyna-Disc
Exertools D.-D.
D.-D. gymball
DYNAfabric material
Dynafed IB
Dynafill graft biomedium
DynaFix external fixation system
DynaFlex
D. Gyro exerciser
D. multilayer compression system
DynaGraft implant
Dynagrip
D. blade handle
D. handle of blade
DynaHeat hot pack

Dyna-Hex Topical
Dyna knee splint
Dyna-Lok
D.-L. pedicle screw system
D.-L. plating system
dynametric testing
dynamic
d. abduction brace
d. alignment
d. axial fixator (DAF)
d. balance
d. canal glide
d. compression (DC)
d. compression plate (DCP)
d. compression plate fixation
d. compression plate instrumentation
D. condylar screw (DCS)
d. condylar screw fixation
d. condylar screw tap
d. digital deformity
D. digit extensor tube
d. double tendon replacement
D. Edge rehabilitation equipment
D. elbow orthosis
d. electromyography
d. external fixation
d. fault
d. footprint
D. foot stabilizer
d. friction
d. gait
d. hallux varus
d. hammertoe
d. hinge elbow fracture brace
d. hip screw (DHS)
d. integrated stabilization chair (DISC)
d. joint force
D. knee orthosis
d. listing
d. listing nomenclature
d. loading
d. locking nail
d. lumbar stabilization
d. magnetic resonance imaging
d. metatarsus adductus
D. Motion Foot 1D35
d. motion x-ray
d. movement
d. MRI
d. muscle transfer
d. pedobarography (DPB)
d. pedodynographic finding

NOTES

dynamic *(continued)*
    d. repair
    d. splint
    d. splinting
    d. stability index
    d. stabilization trainer
    d. stabilizing innersole system
      (DSIS)
    d. standing balance
    d. stress x-ray view
    d. stump exercise
    d. traction method
    d. transverse traction device
    d. trunk curl
    D. wrist orthosis
dynamics
    foot d.
dynamization collar
dynamometer
    Baseline d.
    Biodex isokinetic d.
    bulb d.
    Chiroslide Jamar Hand D.
    Collins d.
    computerized isokinetic d.
    Cybex II isokinetic d.
    electromechanical d.
    hand grip d.
    handheld d. (HHD)
    Harpenden d.
    isokinetic d.
    Jamar hydraulic hand d.
    Lido isokinetic d.
    orthopaedic d.
    Smedley d.
    Spark handheld d.
    squeeze d.
dynamometry
    isokinetic d.
    tip-pinch d.
DynaPak electrode kit
Dynaphor iontophoresis
Dynaplex knee prosthesis
DynaPrene splinting thermoplastic
Dynaslipper night shoe
Dynasplint
    D. knee extension
    D. knee extension unit
    D. shoulder system
DynaSport athletic tape
Dynatron
    D. 50, 125, 525 electrotherapy
    D. Mini 2000 electrotherapy
    D. 2000 muscle test
    D. TX 900 electrotherapy
DyoCam
    D. 550 arthroscopic video camera
    D. arthroscopic view camera

Dyonics
    D. arthroplasty bur
    D. arthroscope
    D. arthroscopic blade
    D. cannula
    D. Golden Retriever magnet
    D. shaver
dysarthria
    clumsy hand d.
    spinal d.
dysarthrosis
    patellofemoral d.
dysbaric
    d. osteonecrosis
    d. oxygen
dysbasia
    d. angiosclerotica
    d. lordotica progressiva
dyscalculia
    developmental d.
dyschondroplasia
    Ollier d.
dyschondrosteosis
dyscollagenosis
dyscrasia
    plasma cell d.
dyscrasic fracture
dysdiadochokinesia
dysesthesia
dysfunction
    anterior-inferior capsular ligament d.
    bladder d.
    craniomandibular d.
    endothelial d.
    extensor mechanism d.
    facet joint d.
    fixation d.
    flexor hallucis longus d. (FHLD)
    iliacus d.
    intervertebral d.
    joint d.
    mechanical d.
    motor d.
    neuroarticular d.
    organic d.
    painful minor intervertebral d.
      (PMID)
    patellofemoral d. (PFD)
    pelvic pain and organic d.
    pelvic ring d.
    pilomotor d.
    posterior tibial tendon d. (PTTD)
    posttraumatic sacroiliac d.
    sacroiliac d.
    sacroiliac-iliosacral d.
    scapular d.
    segmental d.
    somatic d.

sympathetic d.
d. syndrome
dysgenesis
alar d.
epiphysial d.
dyshidrosis, dyshydrosis
dyskeratosis congenita
dyskinesia
d. intermittens
positional d.
poststatic d. (PSDK)
retrolisthesis positional d.
dyskinetic cerebral palsy
dysmetria
lower limb d.
truncal d.
dysnomia
dysostosis
cleidocranial d.
Jansen metaphysial d.
metaphysial d.
Schmid metaphysial d.
Spahr metaphysial d.
dysplasia
acetabular d.
acromesomelic d.
acropectorovertebral d.
bone d.
cleidocranial d.
congenital hip d. (CHD)
congenital hyperphosphatasemic
skeletal d. (CHSD)
cortical fibrous d.
Crowe congenital hip d. (type I-
IV)
developmental hip d.
diaphysial d.
diastrophic d.
dyssegmental d.
epiarticular osteochondromatous d.
d. epiphysealis
epiphysial d.
faciodigitogenital d.
femoral head d.
fibrous d.
focal fibrocartilaginous d.
foot d.
d. of hip
hip d.
Holt-Oram d.
hyperphosphatasemic skeletal d.
intracortical fibrous d.
Meyer d.

Mondini d.
monostotic fibrous d.
multiple epiphysial d.
Namaqualand hip d.
oculoauriculovertebral d.
osteochondromatous d.
osteofibrous d.
patellofemoral d.
polyostotic fibrous d.
progressive diaphysial d.
rhizomesomelic bone d.
skeletal d.
Sponastrine d.
spondyloepiphysial d.
Streeter d.
dysplastic
d. acetabulum
d. fibula
d. nevus syndrome
d. spondylolisthesis
d. tibia
dysponetic
dysraphism
spinal d.
dysreflexia
autonomic d.
dyssegmental dysplasia
dysstasia
dysstatic
dyssynergia
dystaxia
dystelephalangy
dystonia
cerebral palsy-related d.
focal d.
d. lenticularis
d. musculorum
d. musculorum deformans
torsion d.
dystopia
shoulder d.
dystrophic
d. gait
d. nail
d. spondylosis
d. toenail
dystrophica
myotonia d.
dystrophinopathy
dystrophy
adiposogenital d.
Albright d.
Becker muscular d. (BMD)

NOTES

D

dystrophy *(continued)*
    Becker-type tardive muscular d.
    Becker variant of Duchenne d.
    congenital d.
    distal d.
    Duchenne muscular d.
    Emery-Dreifuss d.
    Erb muscular d.
    fascioscapulohumeral muscular d.
    Fröhlich adiposogenital d.
    Gowers muscular d.
    humeroperoneal muscular d.
    juvenile muscular d.
    Kiloh-Nevin ocular form of
      progressive muscular d.
    Landouzy-Dejerine d.

    Leyden-Möbius muscular d.
    limb-girdle muscular d.
    muscular d. (MD)
    myotonic muscular d.
    neurovascular d.
    osseous d.
    pelvofemoral muscular d.
    posttraumatic d.
    progressive muscular d. (PMD)
    pseudohypertrophic d.
    reflex neurovascular d.
    reflex sympathetic d. (RSD)
    sex-linked muscular d.
    sympathetic reflex d.
    tardive muscular d.

dysvascular condition

E-2
    E-2 foot prosthesis
    E-2 hydrocollator heating unit
EACS
  exertional anterior compartment
  syndrome
EADL
  electronic aid for daily living
  extended activities of daily living
eagle
    E. arthroscope
    e. beak bone-cutting forceps
    E. straight-ahead arthroscope
Eagle-Barrett syndrome
Eakin cohesive seal dressing
Earle sign
EARLY
  ergonomic assessment of risk and
  liability
Early Fit night splint
E-A-R specialty composite
earth electrode
EAS
  endoskeletal alignment system
EAST
  external rotation-abduction stress test
Easton cock-up splint
East-West retractor
Eastwood technique
easy
    E. Access foot splint
    E. Lok ankle brace
    E. Up cushion
EasyAnchor
    GII E.
EasyLiner
    ALPS E.
Easy-On elbow brace
Easy-Pull sock aide device
Easyslide sliding mat
Easyspine pedicle screw and rod
system
EasyStand 6000 glider
EasyStep pressure relief walker
eater
  cement e.
  Zimmer Cibatome cement e.
Eaton
    E. closed reduction
    E. CMC arthrosis (stage I–IV)
    E. implant arthroplasty
    E. splint
    E. trapezium finger joint
    replacement prosthesis
    E. volar plate arthroplasty

Eaton-Lambert syndrome
Eaton-Littler
    E.-L. ligament reconstruction
    E.-L. technique
Eberle
    E. contracture release
    E. contracture release technique
EBGS
  electrical bone-growth stimulation
  electrical bone-growth stimulator
EBI
  electronic bone stimulation
    EBI device
    EBI external fixator
    EBI Medical OsteoGen bone
    growth stimulator
    EBI Medical Systems bone healing
    system
    EBI Medical Systems Orthofix
    fixation system
    EBI SpF-2 implantable bone
    stimulator
    EBI SpF-T implantable bone
    stimulator
    EBI XFix DynaFix System
EBL
  estimated blood loss
ebonation
eburnate
eburnated
    e. bone
    e. bone surface
eburnation
  bony e.
  e. of cartilage
eburneum
  osteoma e.
eccentric
    e. access
    e. amputation
    e. axis of ankle rotation
    e. axis of rotation of the ankle
    e. contraction
    e. drill guide
    e. dynamic compression plate
    (EDCP)
    e. exercise
    e. function
    e. loading
    e. muscle action
    e. muscle training
    e. wear
    e. work
eccentro-osteochondrodysplasia
ecchondroma, pl. **ecchondromata**

E

ecchondrotome
ecchymosis
eccrine
    e. poroma
    e. sweat gland
ECD
    excision, curettage, drilling
echinococcosis
Echlin
    E. bone rongeur
    E. duckbill rongeur
    E. rongeur forceps
Echlin-Luer rongeur
echo
    e. time
    e. train length (ETL)
echocardiography
echography
eclipse
    E. Gel ankle brace
    E. Gel elbow strap
    E. TENS unit
EcoNail nail lacquer
Econo
    E. 90 lumbar home traction
    E. 90 traction unit
Econo-Cerv
    E.-C. supine cervical traction
    E.-C. traction device
economic self-sufficiency WHO Handicap Scale
economy ROM brace
EconoSoc ankle brace
Econo-Strap
E Cotton bandage
ECRB
    extensor carpi radialis brevis
    ECRB muscle
    ECRB tendon
ECRL
    extensor carpi radialis longus
    ECRL muscle
    ECRL tendon
EcstaSeat seat cushion
ECT
    European compression technique
    extended code therapy
    ECT bone screw
    ECT internal fracture fixation
    ECT internal fracture fixation
      system
ectasia
    dural e.
ectocuneiform bone
ectomesomorphic physique
ectomorph
ectomorphic physique
ectopic
    e. bone

    e. bone growth
    e. ossification
ECTR
    endoscopic carpal tunnel release
ectrodactyly
ectromelia
ECU
    extensor carpi ulnaris
    ECU muscle
    ECU tendon
ED
    elbow disarticulation
    extensor digitorum
EDB
    extensor digitorum brevis
    EDB muscle
    EDB tendon
EDC
    extensor digitorum communis
EDCP
    eccentric dynamic compression plate
Eddowes
    E. disease
    E. syndrome
edema
    bone marrow e.
    constrictive e.
    dependent e.
    endoneurial e.
    goose-egg e.
    e. heat therapy
    intracompartmental e.
    leg e.
    marrow e.
    mushy e.
    nonpitting e.
    pitting e.
    posttraumatic e.
    pretibial e.
    rheumatismal e.
    e. sock
    stump e.
    transient bone marrow e.
edematous
Eden-Hybbinette
    E.-H. arthroplasty
    E.-H. operation
    E.-H. procedure
Eden-Lange procedure
Eden test
Eder-Puestow metal olive dilator
EDF
    elongation, derotation, flexion
    elongation, derotation, lateral flexion
    EDF scoliosis cast
EDG
    electrodynogram
    EDG system
Edgarton-Grand thumb adduction

edge
> Acufex E.
> 3-e. cutting forceps
> E. knee brace
> patellar e.

edge-detection
> digital e.-d.

Edinburgh
> E. method
> E. Rehabilitation Status Scale
> (ERSS)

Edinger-Westphal complex

Edintrak II system

EDit
> electric differential therapy

edition
> Development Test of Visual
> Perception, 2nd E. (DTVP-2)

EDL
> extensor digitorum longus

EDM
> extensor digiti minimi

Edna towel clamp

EDPA
> Erhardt Developmental Prehension
> Assessment

EDPCS
> exertional deep posterior compartment
> syndrome

EDQ
> extensor digiti quinti

EDS
> Ehlers-Danlos syndrome

EDSS
> Expanded Disability Status Scale

education
> lifestyle e. (LSE)
> posture e.

EDVA
> Erhardt Developmental Vision
> Assessment

Edwards
> E. D-L modular fixator
> E. D-L modular screw rod
> E. hook
> E. instrumentation
> E. and Lee tibiofibular diastasis
> and syndesmotic injury
> classification
> E. modular system
> E. modular system bridging sleeve
> construct

E. modular system compression
construct
E. modular system construct
selection
E. modular system distraction-
lordosis construct
E. modular system dynamic
loading
E. modular system kyphoreduction
construct
E. modular system load sharing
E. modular system neutralization
construct
E. modular system rod crosslink
E. modular system rod sleeve
construct
E. modular system sacral fixation
device
E. modular system scoliosis
construct
E. modular system spinal/sacral
screw
E. modular system spinal sleeve
E. modular system spondylar
construct
E. modular system standard sleeve
construct
E. modular system Universal rod
E. polyethylene sleeve
E. procedure
E. seamless prosthesis
E. syndrome

Edwards-Levine
> E.-L. hook
> E.-L. rod
> E.-L. sleeve

Edwin Smith papyrus

EDX, EDx
> electrodiagnosis

effect
> bungee e.
> concavity-compression e.
> Hick e.
> Ilizarov tension-stress e.
> magic angle e.
> neurophysiologic e.
> rake-handle e.
> scarring e.
> spindle e.
> steal e.
> Steindler e.
> tenodesis e.
> tethering e.

E

NOTES

effect *(continued)*
  vasodilatory e.
  windshield wiper e.
efferent nerve impulse
Effler-Groves hook
effleurage massage
effluent
  pelvic e.
effort
  brief maximal e. (BME)
  maximum voluntary e. (MVE)
  e. thrombosis
effort-induced thrombosis
effusion
  ankle e.
  bloody e.
  joint e.
  knee joint e.
  shoulder joint e.
Eftekhar
  E. broken femoral stem technique
  E. concept
  E. long-stem prosthesis
Eftekhar-Charnley hip prosthesis
Egawa sign
eggcrate mattress
Eggers
  E. bone plate
  E. contact splint
  E. neurectomy
  E. operation
  E. screw
  E. tendon transfer technique
  E. tenodesis
  E. transfer
Eggsercizer
  E. CTS exerciser
  E. resistive hand exerciser
egg-shaped cap
eggshell
  e. fracture
  e. procedure
eggshell-like calcification
egress of arthroscopic fluid
Egyptian foot
EHL
  extensor hallucis longus
  EHL tendon
Ehlers-Danlos
  E.-D. disease
  E.-D. syndrome (EDS)
Ehrenfeld disease
EI
  external ilium
Eichenholz stage
Eicher
  E. femoral prosthesis
  E. hip prosthesis
Eikenella corrodens

Eilers-Armstrong unicompartmental knee prosthesis
EIP
  extensor indicis proprius
  EIP muscle
  EIP tendon
Eisenmenger complex
EJ
  elbow jerk
ejector
  Cloward dowel e.
Ekbom restless leg syndrome
Elan drill
Elan-E power drill
Elase-Chloromycetin
  E.-C. ointment
  E.-C. Topical
Elase Topical
Elastafit tubing kit
ElastaTrac
  E. home lumbar traction system
  E. home lumbar traction unit
  E. lumbar traction
elastic
  e. ankle corset
  e. barrier
  e. cartilage
  e. compression
  e. deformation
  e. dressing
  e. fixation
  E. Foam bandage
  e. knee cage
  e. knee cage orthosis
  e. knee cage with medial and lateral contoured knee joints
  e. knee sleeve brace
  e. limit
  e. plaster of Paris
  e. property
  e. recoil
  e. stable intramedullary nailing (ESIN)
  e. stockings
  e. strain
  e. strap
  e. stretch
  e. traction
  e. tubing
  e. twister orthosis
  e. wristlet
  e. zone
elastic-hinge knee brace
Elastichrome stain
elasticity
  modulus of e.
Elastikon
  E. dressing
  E. elastic tape

elastofibroma dorsi
Elasto-Gel
    E.-G. hot/cold wrap
    E.-G. shoulder therapy wrap
elastoidosis
Elasto-Link joint wrap
elastoma
elastomer
    conventional silicone e. (CSE)
    high performance silicone e.
    medical e. X7-2320
    polyolefin e.
    e. skin molding
    thermoplastic e. (TPE)
Elastomull
    E. dressing
    E. elastic gauze bandage
    E. splint
Elastoplast
    E. bandage
    E. dressing
elastosis
elbow
    above e. (AE)
    e. arthrodesis
    e. arthroplasty
    axilla, shoulder, e. (ASE)
    baseball pitcher's e.
    e. bone
    boxer's e.
    capped e.
    e. capsule
    e. cast
    compound shattered e.
    crazy bone of e.
    e. disarticulation (ED)
    e. dislocation
    epicondylitis of e.
    e. extension splint
    e. extensor tendon
    fat pad of e.
    e. flexion splint
    e. flexion test
    floating e.
    e. fracture
    Frohse arcade of e.
    golfer's e.
    e. hinge
    e. injury
    E. Injury Management Kit
    javelin thrower's e.
    e. jerk (EJ)
    e. jerk reflex test

    e. joint
    Little Leaguer's e.
    e. magnet
    milkmaid's e.
    miner's e.
    nursemaid's e.
    NYU-Hosmer electric e.
    e. orthosis (EO)
    e. pad
    e. prosthesis
    pulled e.
    e. radiography
    e. reflex
    e. region
    e. replacement
    reverse tennis e.
    e. sleeve
    slipped e.
    Sorbie-Questor e.
    e. stability
    student's e.
    supermarket e.
    temper tantrum e.
    tennis e.
    thrower's e.
    varus-valgus stress of e.
    Wilson procedure for extraarticular
      fusion of e.
    wrestler's e.
Elbow-Up Protector elbow suspension
  device
elbow-wrist-hand orthosis (EWHO)
Elderberry Sambu Internal Cleansing
  Program
elderly
    Clifton Assessment Procedures for
      the E. (CAPE)
electric
    e. artifact
    e. cast saw
    e. dermatome
    e. differential therapy (EDit)
    e. joint fluoroscopy
    e. wheelchair
electrical
    e. bone-growth stimulation (EBGS)
    e. bone-growth stimulator (EBGS)
    e. implant
    e. inactivity
    e. injury
    e. modality
    e. nerve stimulation
    e. potential

E

NOTES

electrical *(continued)*
    e. silence
    e. stimulation rehabilitation
    e. stimulation therapy
    e. stimulator waveform
    e. surface stimulation
    e. surface stimulation treatment for
      scoliosis
Electri-Cool
    E.-C. cold therapy system
    E.-C. continuous controlled cold
      therapy
electroacupuncture
    Acu-Treat e.
    Electro-Acuscope e.
Electro-Acuscope
    E.-A. electroacupuncture
    E.-A. 85 stimulator
electrocardiography
electrocautery
    e. apparatus
    Aspen e.
electrocoagulation
electrode
    active e.
    ArthroCare e.
    bifilar needle recording e.
    BioKnit garment e.
    bipolar needle recording e.
    bipolar stimulating e.
    coaxial needle e.
    concentric needle e.
    disc e.
    Disposatrode disposable e.
    Dupel blue iontophoresis e.
    Dura-Stick adhesive e.
    earth e.
    Electro-Mesh e.
    Excel Plus e.
    exploring e.
    e. glove
    e. grid
    ground e.
    indifferent e.
    LSI Easy Stims self-adhesive e.
    LSI silver self-adhesive
      disposable e.
    macro-EMG needle e.
    microcurrent e.
    monopolar needle recording e.
    multilead e.
    needle e.
    e. paste
    e. placement
    Polystim e.
    prizm Electro-Mesh Sock e.
    recording e.
    reference e.
    Silver-Thera stocking e.

    single-fiber needle e.
    e. sock
    Sportstim muscle stimulation e.
    stigmatic e.
    stimulating e.
    surface e.
    Teq-Trode e.
    Ultra Stim silver e.
    unipolar needle e.
    Versa-Stim self-adhering e.
electrodesiccated bleeding point
electrodesiccation
electrodiagnosis (EDX, EDx)
    mononeuropathy e.
**Electro-Diagnostic Instruments Model
720 Bilateral Tetrapolar**
electrodiagnostic medicine
electrodynogram (EDG)
electrogoniometer (elgon)
    ankle-foot e.
    6 degrees of freedom e.
    parallelogram e.
electrokinetic potential
Electro-Link joint wrap
electrolyte
    e. balance
    e. replacement
electromagnet
    spring-mounted e.
electromagnetic field
electromassage
electromechanical
    e. delay (EMD)
    e. dynamometer
Electro-Mesh
    E.-M. electrode
    E.-M. sleeve
electromyocardiography
    cervical Derifield procedure e.
electromyogram (EMG)
    ulnar nerve motor/sensory e.
electromyographic activation
electromyography (EMG)
    central e.
    dynamic e.
    integrated e.
    single-fiber e. (SFEMG)
    surface e. (sEMG)
electron beam therapy
electroneuromyography (ENMG)
electroneurophysiologic
electronic
    e. aid for daily living (EADL)
    e. bone stimulation (EBI)
    e. bone stimulation apparatus
    e. goniometer
electronics
    American Medical E. (AME)
    E. electrical stimulation device

electronystagmography
electrooptical characteristic (EOC)
electrophysiologic study
electrosurgical
 e. generator
 e. instrument
 e. pencil
electrotherapeutic point stimulation (ETPS)
electrotherapy
 e. device
 direct current e.
 Dynatron 50, 125, 525 e.
 Dynatron Mini 2000 e.
 Dynatron TX 900 e.
 Mettler e.
 PET e.
 e. system (ES)
 ultrasound e.
electrothermal arthroscopy
electrothermally assisted capsulorrhaphy (ETAC)
Elekta stereotactic head frame
element
 neural e.
 posterior e.
elementary fracture
elephant-ear clavicular splint
elephant-foot
 e.-f. callus
 e.-f. fracture
 e.-f. fracture nonunion
elevata
 scapula e.
elevated
 e. rim acetabular liner
 e. scapula
elevating osteotomy
elevation
 e. angle
 congenital scapular e.
 e. exercise
 e. of extremity
 ice, compression, e. (ICE)
 Maquet e.
 periosteal e.
 e. pillow
 protection, restricted activity, ice, compression, e. (PRICE)
 rest, ice, compression, e. (RICE)
 scapular e.
 E.'s shoe buildup

elevator
 Adson periosteal e.
 Alexander periosteal e.
 angular e.
 APC proximal femoral e.
 Aufranc periosteal e.
 Bennett e.
 Bethune periosteal e.
 biceps e.
 Blair e.
 bone e.
 Bowen periosteal e.
 Bristow periosteal e.
 Brophy periosteal e.
 Buck periosteal e.
 Campbell periosteal e.
 Carroll-Legg periosteal e.
 Carroll periosteal e.
 Chandler bone e.
 chisel e.
 chisel-edge e.
 Cloward osteophyte e.
 Cloward periosteal e.
 Cobb periosteal e.
 Cohen periosteal e.
 Converse periosteal e.
 Crego periosteal e.
 curved periosteal e.
 Cushing-Hopkins periosteal e.
 Cushing Little Joker e.
 Cushing periosteal e.
 Darrach periosteal e.
 Davidson-Sauerbruch-Doyen periosteal e.
 Dawson-Yuhl-Key e.
 Dawson-Yuhl periosteal e.
 Doyan periosteal e.
 Doyen rib e.
 duckbill e.
 dural e.
 Duval e.
 Endotrac e.
 extra-leverage proximal femoral e.
 Farabeuf periosteal e.
 Fomon periosteal e.
 fracture reducing e.
 Frazier e.
 Freer periosteal e.
 Freer septal e.
 Gardner e.
 hand e.
 Harrington spinal e.
 Heel Minder foot e.

E

NOTES

elevator *(continued)*
> Herczel rib e.
> Hibbs chisel e.
> Hoen periosteal e.
> Iowa University periosteal e.
> Jannetta duckbill e.
> joker periosteal e.
> Joseph periosteal e.
> J-periosteal e.
> Kennerdell-Maroon e.
> Key periosteal e.
> Kleinert-Kutz periosteal e.
> Kocher e.
> Lambotte e.
> lamina e.
> Lane periosteal e.
> Langenbeck periosteal e.
> Lempert periosteal e.
> Lewis periosteal e.
> liberator e.
> Locke e.
> Love-Adson periosteal e.
> lumbosacral fusion e.
> Malis e.
> Matson-Alexander rib e.
> Matson periosteal e.
> Matson rib e.
> McGlamry e.
> Mead periosteal e.
> modified Darrach-type e.
> Molt periosteal e.
> Moore bone e.
> e. muscle
> narrow proximal femoral e.
> nasal e.
> orthopaedic shoulder e.
> OSI extremity e.
> osteophyte e.
> Penfield periosteal e.
> periosteal e.
> e. periosteotome
> Phemister e.
> posterior glenoid e.
> proximal femoral e.
> Rhoton e.
> rib e.
> Rochester lamina e.
> Rochester spinal e.
> Rolyan arm e.
> Rosen e.
> round-tapped e.
> Sauerbruch rib e.
> Sayre e.
> Sebileau periosteal e.
> Sedillot periosteal e.
> Sheffield hand e.
> Sisson fracture reducing e.
> spiked Darrach-type e.
> staphylorrhaphy e.

> straight periosteal e.
> Sunday staphylorrhaphy e.
> Swanson e.
> Tenzel e.
> T-handle e.
> Tronzo e.
> von Langenbeck periosteal e.
> Ward periosteal e.
> Wiberg periosteal e.
> wide periosteal e.
> Williger periosteal e.
> Woodson e.
> Yankauer periosteal e.
> Yasargil e.

elevator-dissector
> Freer e.-d.

elevator-periosteotome

elevatus
> e. deformity
> extrinsic metatarsus primus e.
> hallux e.
> iatrogenic e.
> intrinsic metatarsus primus e.
> metatarsus primus e.

elgon
> electrogoniometer

Eligoy metal alloy

Eliminator ArthroWand

elite
> E. Farley retractor
> E. hip system
> E. knee brace
> E. Plus motion analyzer
> e. posterior adjustable stop
> E. posterior spring assist
> E. Power Station gym

Elithorn Maze Test

Elizabethtown osteotomy

Elliott femoral condyle blade plate

ellipsoidal articulation

ellipsoid joint

elliptical
> e. amputation
> e. incision
> e. machine
> e. overlap shadow

Ellis
> E. classification
> E. Jones peroneal tendon operation
> E. skin traction technique
> E. technique for Barton fracture

Ellis-Jones
> E.-J. peroneal tendon displacement
> E.-J. peroneal tendon technique

Ellison
> E. fixation staple
> E. iliotibial band tenodesis
> E. lateral knee reconstruction
> E. technique

Ellis-van Creveld syndrome
Elmslie
    E. peroneal tendon operation
    E. peroneal tendon procedure
    E. reconstruction
    E. triple arthrodesis
    E. weave procedure
Elmslie-Cholmeley
    E.-C. foot operation
    E.-C. procedure
Elmslie-Trillat
    E.-T. osteotomy
    E.-T. patellar operation
    E.-T. patellar procedure
    E.-T. patellar realignment method
    E.-T. realignment
    E.-T. transplant
elongation
    e., derotation, flexion (EDF)
    e., derotation, lateral flexion (EDF)
    ligament e.
    peroneus brevis e.
    e. property
    repeated quick stretch from e.
    (RQS-E)
    tissue e.
Elson middle slip test
Elvarex
    E. compression garment
    E. support garment
Ely heel-to-buttock test
emanate
Embarc bone repair material
embarrassment
    circulatory e.
emboli (*pl. of* embolus)
embolic mononeuropathy
embolism (*See also* embolus)
    air e.
    arterial gas e.
    bone marrow e.
    fat e.
    pulmonary e.
embolization
embolotherapy
embolus, pl. **emboli** (*See also* embolism)
embryonal rhabdomyosarcoma
EMD
    electromechanical delay
EMED
    EMED gait analysis
    EMED insole
EMED-F foot-force measurement

EMED-SF
    EMED-SF pedobarograph
    EMED-SF sensor mat
emedullate
Emerald implantation system
emergency
    e. closed manipulative measure
    e. muscle
Emery-Dreifuss
    E.-D. disease
    E.-D. dystrophy
EMG
    electromyogram
    electromyography
    EMG biofeedback system
    fine wire EMG
    integrated rectified EMG (IEMG)
    EMG retrainer biofeedback unit
    scanning EMG
    single-channel surface EMG
    single-fiber EMG
Emgel Topical
eminence
    hypothenar e.
    medial e.
    thenar e.
    tibial e.
eminentia
emission
    otoacoustic e. (OAE)
    e. tomography
Emmon osteotomy
emollient
    vitamin E e.
Empirin With Codeine
empty
    e. can exercise
    e. can position
    e. can syndrome
    e. can test
empyema
empyemic scoliosis
EMS 2000 neuromuscular stimulator
en
    en bloc
    en bloc advancement
    en bloc laminectomy
    en bloc resection
enarthrodial joint
encapsulation
encased screw
encephalitis
encephalocele

E

NOTES

encephalopathy
    chronic traumatic e. (CTE)
encerclage
enchondral
    e. bone
    e. ossification
enchondroma
    e. of bone
    e. of hand
    multiple e.
    e. protuberans
    solitary e.
enchondromatosis
    multiple e.
enchondromatous myxoma
encircling wire
enclavement
    Regnauld e.
enclosure
    air-flow e.
encore
    E. Orthopedics
    E. Orthopedics device
encroachment
    bony e.
    cervical nerve root e.
    foraminal osteophyte e.
    osseous foraminal e.
end
    articulating bone e.
    bone e.
    bony distal e.
    e. corn
    e. cutter
    distal bone e.
    e. feel
    lateral e.
    medial e.
    e. plate
    e. play
    e. point
    e. range of motion
    e. vertebra
endarteritis obliterans
end-bearing amputation
end-biting forceps
end-cutting
    e.-c. reamer
    e.-c. reciprocating saw
endemic
    e. hypertrophy
    e. osteoarthritis
endemica
    osteoarthritis deformans e.
Ender
    E. awl
    E. femoral fracture technique
    E. flexible medullary nail
    E. nail fixation

    E. nailing
    E. pin
    E. rod
    E. rod fixation
    E. rod fixation of fracture
Endermologie cellulite treatment
end-feel palpation
ending
    flower-spray e.
    nerve e.
Endius
    E. bipolar sheath
    E. endoscopic access system
    E. spinal endoscope/camera
    E. spinal endoscopic camera
    E. TriFix thoracolumbar pedicle
       screw system
Endless Pool physical therapy pool
Endo
    E. Multi-Mode stimulator
    E. rotating knee joint prosthesis
endoabdominal fascia
EndoAvitene
EndoButton
    closed loop E.
    E. FM
endochondral
    e. bone
    e. ossification
    e. osteogenesis
endochondromatosis
endocrine fracture
EndoFix bioabsorbable interference
  screw
Endo-FixL screw
Endoflex endoscopic lumbar discectomy
  scope
endogenous pain
Endolite
    E. prosthesis
    E. transtibial system
Endo-Model
    E.-M. hinged knee prosthesis
    E.-M. rotating knee joint prosthesis
    E.-M. sled prosthesis
endomorph
endomysial
endomysium
endoneural
    e. fibrosis
    e. tube
endoneurial edema
endoneurium degeneration
endoneurolysis
EndoPearl
    E. bioabsorbable device
    E. fixation device
endoplasmic reticulum

endoprosthesis
    acetabular e.
    Atkinson e.
    Bio-Moore e.
    femoral e.
    F.R. Thompson e.
    nonporous-coated e.
    smooth e.
    tibial e.
    TPP hip e.
    tumor-replacement e.

endoprosthetic flange
end-organ
endorthesis
endorthosis
endoscope
    Agee e.

endoscope/camera
    Endius spinal e./c.

endoscopic
    e. anterior cruciate ligament
      reconstruction
    e. approach
    e. carpal tunnel instrumentation
    e. carpal tunnel release (ECTR)
    e. carpal tunnel release system
    e. correction of scoliosis
    e. gastrocnemius recession
    e. plantar fasciotomy (EPF)

endoscopy
    fiberoptic intraosseous e.
    laser-assisted spinal e. (LASE)
    lumbar epidural e.
    percutaneous transcaudal epidural e.
    tendon sheath e.

endoskeletal
    e. alignment system (EAS)
    e. socket
    solid ankle flexible e. (SAFE)
    stationary attachment flexible e.
      (SAFE)

Endoskeleton TA structural device
endosteal
    e. hypertrophy
    e. lamella
    e. revascularization
    e. scalloping
    e. surface
    e. vessel

endosteum
endotenon

endothelial
    e. cell
    e. dysfunction

endothelium
    vascular e.

endothoracic fascia
Endotrac
    E. blade system
    E. cannula
    E. carpal tunnel release system
    E. elevator
    E. endoscopic carpal tunnel release
    E. rasp

endotracheal intubation
endovaginal lipoma
endplate
    e. activity
    e. fragmentation
    e. invagination
    e. noise
    e. ossification
    posterior e.
    e. potential (EPP)
    e. sclerosis
    e. spike
    superior e.
    vertebral body e.
    e. zone

endpoint of orthopaedic test
end-stage
    e.-s. arthrosis
    e.-s. coxarthrosis
    e.-s. disruption

end-to-end
    e.-t.-e. suture
    e.-t.-e. tendon repair

end-to-side repair
EnduraFIX tape
endurance
    E. bone cement
    e. event
    e. exercise
    e. limit
    e. training

EnduraSPORTS tape
EnduraTape tape
Enduron acetabular liner
energetics
    Apex E.

energy
    e. absorption
    e. conservation walking component
    e. expenditure

E

NOTES

energy *(continued)*
    e. intake
    kinetic e.
    e. metabolism
    muscle e.
    E. Plus shoe insert
    e. storing foot prosthesis
    strain e.
    thermal e.
Engebretsen procedure
Engel
    E. angle
    E. plaster saw
Engelmann
    E. disc
    E. disease
    E. thigh splint
Engel-Recklinghausen disease
Engen
    E. extension orthosis
    E. palmar finger orthosis
    E. palmar wrist splint
Engh
    E. porous metal hip prosthesis
    E. total hip replacement
Engh-Glassman femoral stem
engine
    Acrotorque hand e.
engineering
    functional tissue e. (FTE)
Englehardt femoral prosthesis
English
    E. anvil nail nipper
    E. brace
    E. cane
    E. cane board
English-McNab shoulder prosthesis
engulfment abnormality
enhancer cushion
enjoyment
    Children's Assessment of
        Participation and E. (CAPE)
enlarged frontal horn
enlargement
    tibial tunnel e.
enlarging bur
ENMG
    electroneuromyography
Enneking
    E. classification
    E. disease stage
    E. knee arthrodesis
    E. principle
    E. question
    E. resection-arthrodesis
    E. rod
    E. staging
    E. staging of malignant soft tissue
    tumor

enostosis
ensheathing callus
ensiform cartilage
Ensolite padded transfer bench
Ensure-It dressing
Entegra prosthesis
Enterobacter
    E. agglomerans
    E. cloacae
enterocutaneous fistula
enteropathic arthritis
enthesis
    Achilles tendon e.
enthesitis
enthesopathy
entocuneiform bone
entrapment
    anular ligament e.
    catheter e.
    lateral canal e.
    median nerve e.
    meniscoid e.
    nerve root e.
    e. neuropathy
    peripheral nerve e.
    peroneal nerve e.
    popliteal fossa e.
    posterior interosseous nerve e.
    posterior tibial nerve e.
    e. syndrome
    ulnar nerve e.
entrapped plantar bone
Entrex small joint arthroscopy
  instrument set
entry point
entubulation
    nerve e.
enucleate
enucleation
enucleator
    Rhoton e.
envelope
    e. arm sling
    capsuloperiosteal e.
    soft tissue e.
environment
    Home Observation and
        Measurement of the E. (HOME)
environmental
    e. assessment
    e. stress cracking
Envision anterior cervical plate system
enzymatic
    e. débridement
    e. debriding agent
enzyme-based lactic acid blood testing
enzyme-linked immunosorbent assay
EO
    elbow orthosis

EOC
    electrooptical characteristic
      EOC goniometer
eosinophilia-myalgia syndrome
eosinophilic
    e. granuloma
    e. granuloma of bone
epactal bone
EPB
    extensor pollicis brevis
ependymoma
EPF
    endoscopic plantar fasciotomy
epiarticular osteochondromatous
  dysplasia
EPIC
    evaluation, prediction, intervention,
      control
      EPIC functional evaluation system
epicondylalgia
    e. externa
    radial e.
epicondylar
    e. avulsion fracture
    e. ridge
epicondyle
    femoral e.
    humeral e.
    lateral e.
    medial e.
epicondylectomy
    medial e.
epicondylitis
    e. of elbow
    external humeral e.
    humeral e.
    lateral humeral e.
    medial e.
    radiohumeral e.
epicritic
    e. pain
    e. receptor
    e. sensation
    e. sensation erythrasma
Epic wheelchair
epidermal cell tumor
epidermis, pl. **epidermides**
epidermodysplasia verruciformis
epidermolysis bullosa
epidermolytic acanthoma
epidermophytid reaction
Epidermophyton floccosum

epidural
    e. abscess evacuation
    e. anesthesia
    e. fluid collection
    e. neurolysis
    e. space
    e. space infection
    e. steroid
    e. steroid injection (ESI)
    e. tumor evacuation
    e. venography
epidurography
epifascicular epineurotomy
Epigard dressing
epilepsy
    jacksonian e.
    myoclonic e.
    posttraumatic e.
epileptic myoclonus
Epi-Lock elbow support
epiloia
epimeric muscle
epimysiotomy
epimysium
epineural
    e. covering
    e. repair
    e. scarring
epineurectomy
    interfascicular e.
epineurial
    e. neuropathy
    e. neurorrhaphy
epineurial-perineurial neuropathy
epineurium
epineurolysis
    volar e.
epineurotomy
    anterior e.
    epifascicular e.
    interfascicular e.
    local e.
epiphyses (*pl. of* epiphysis)
epiphysial, epiphyseal
    e. angle
    e. arrest
    e. artery
    e. aseptic necrosis
    atavistic e.
    e. bar resection
    e. chondromatous giant cell tumor
    e. closure
    e. complex

E

NOTES

epiphysial *(continued)*
  e. dysgenesis
  e. dysplasia
  e. exostosis
  e. growth plate
  e. growth plate fracture
  e. hyperplasia
  e. injury
  e. ischemic necrosis
  e. line
  e. osteochondritis
  e. osteochondroma
  e. oxygen
  e. ring
  e. slip fracture
  e. staple
  e. stapling
  e. tibial fracture
epiphysial-metaphysial osteotomy
epiphysiodesis
  Abbott-Gill e.
  Blount e.
  bone peg e.
  Heyman-Herndon e.
  medial tibial e.
  open bone graft e.
  percutaneous e.
  proximal phalangeal e.
  screw e.
  spontaneous postfracture e.
  White e.
epiphysiolysis
  femoral e.
  proximal femoral e.
epiphysiopathy
epiphysis, pl. epiphyses
  accessory e.
  capital e. (CE)
  capital femoral e.
  capitular e.
  clavicular e.
  distal humeral e.
  femoral e.
  humeral e.
  iliac e.
  Morrissy percutaneous fixation of
    slipped e.
  Perthes e.
  pressure e.
  slipped capital femoral e. (SCFE)
  slipped under femoral e. (SUFE)
  stippled e.
  tibial e.
  traction e.
epiphysitis
  traction e.
  transient e.
Epipoint elbow support
epipteric bone

Epi-Sport epicondylitis clasp
epitendineum
epitenon suture
epithelialization
epithelioid
  e. hemangioepithelioma
  e. sarcoma
epithelioma cuniculatum
epithesis
Epitrain
  E. active elbow support
  E. knitted elbow support
  E. Viscoped support
epitrochlea
epitrochlear
epitrochleoanconeus muscle
Epker osteotome
EPL
  extensor pollicis longus
epoetin alfa
eponychia
eponychium
Epos
  E. Ultra extracorporeal shock wave
    therapy device
  E. Ultra orthopaedic shock wave
  E. Ultra orthopaedic shock wave
    therapy device
EPP
  endplate potential
Eppright dial osteotomy
epsilon receptor
Epsom salts soak
Epstein
  E. bone rasp
  E. curette
  E. hip dislocation classification
  E. neurological hammer
EPTFE
  expanded polytetrafluoroethylene
  EPTFE graft prosthesis
epX suspension sleeve
Equagesic
equalizer
  E. air walker
  E. cast brace
  E. Pro massager
  E. short leg walking cast
equation
  Bloch e.
  Jackson-Pollock skinfold e.
equilibratory ataxia
equilibrium
  intrinsic e.
  e. reaction
  e. reflex
equina
  cauda e.
equine gait

equinocavovarus deformity
equinocavus foot
equinovalgus
    e. deformity
    e. foot
    pes e.
    spastic e.
    talipes e.
equinovarus
    congenital talipes e.
    e. foot
    e. hindfoot deformity
    pes e.
    e. posturing
    psychogenic e.
    talipes e. (TEV)
    Turco repair of talipes e.
equinus
    ankle e.
    anterior e.
    compensated talipes e.
    e. contracture
    e. deformity
    e. foot
    forefoot e.
    gastrocnemius e.
    gastrosoleal e.
    global metatarsus e.
    heel e.
    metatarsus primus e.
    osseous e.
    pes e.
    e. position
    residual heel e.
    residual hindfoot e.
    spastic e.
    e. step
    talipes e.
equipment
    accommodative e.
    adaptive e.
    adjustment e.
    AquaMED dry hydrotherapy e.
    Austin Medical E. (AME)
    Baltimore Therapeutic E. (BTE)
    Body-Solid exercise e.
    Cybex back rehabilitation e.
    decompression e.
    Dynamic Edge rehabilitation e.
    home medical e.
    insertion e.
    Invertrac e.

    National Operating Committee on
      Standards for Athletic E.
      (NOCSAE)
    OsteoStat single-use power
      surgical e.
    Reflex exercise and
      rehabilitation e.
    Response rehabilitation and
      fitness e.
    stainless steel e.
equivalent
    human skin e.
Erb
    E. atrophy
    E. muscular dystrophy
    E. palsy
    E. point
Erb-Duchenne palsy
Erb-Landouzy disease
Erdheim-Chester disease
Erdheim syndrome
ERE
    external rotation in extension
erect
    e. position
    e. view
erecta
    dislocatio e.
    luxatio e.
erector spinae
ERF
    external rotation in flexion
Ergo
    E. Cush back support
    E. style flexion table
Ergociser
    Cateye E.
    E. exercise cycle
Ergoflex Premiere back support
ergogenic aid
ergograph
    Mosso e.
ErgoLogic keyboard
ergolytic
ergometer
    bicycle e.
    Biodex cycle e.
    Concept II rowing e.
    Cybex cycle e.
    cycle e.
    handgrip e.
    upper body e. (UBE)

E

NOTES

ergometry
    bicycle e.
ergonomic
    e. assessment
    e. assessment of risk and liability
      (EARLY)
    e. chair
    e. factor
    e. injury
    e. risk
    e. safety
ergonomically
    e. correct chair
    e. designed transducer
ergoreceptor
ergostat
Ergos work simulator
ergotherapy
Erhardt
    E. Developmental Prehension
      Assessment (EDPA)
    E. Developmental Vision
      Assessment (EDVA)
Erichsen
    E. disease
    E. sign
Erich splint
erigentes
    nervi e.
Eriksson
    E. brachial block technique
    E. cruciate ligament reconstruction
    E. knee prosthesis
    E. ligament technique
    E. muscle biopsy cannula
ER/IR
    external rotation/internal rotation
    ER/IR ratio
Erlenmeyer
    E. flask deformity
    E. flask shape
erogenic aid
erosion
    e. of articular surface
    bony e.
    osteoclastic e.
    pedicle e.
erosive
    e. arthritides
    e. osteoarthritis
EROS therapy
ERSS
    Edinburgh Rehabilitation Status Scale
EryDerm Topical
Erygel Topical
Erymax Topical
erythema of joint

erythematosus
    lupus e. (LE)
    systemic lupus e. (SLE)
erythralgia
erythrasma
    epicritic sensation e.
erythrocyte sedimentation rate (ESR)
erythromelalgia
    idiopathic e.
    secondary e.
erythromycin
erythromycin, topical
erythropoietin
ES
    electrotherapy system
eschar
escharotic
escharotomy
Escherichia coli
Esclim Transdermal
E-Series hip system
ESI
    epidural steroid injection
ESIN
    elastic stable intramedullary nailing
Eska modular hip system
Esmarch
    E. bandage
    E. dressing
    E. plaster knife
    E. plaster shears
    E. tourniquet
    E. tube
E-Solve-2 Topical
ESR
    erythrocyte sedimentation rate
essential
    E. Energy Cup
    E. Energy Water
    E. Energy Whole House Wand
    e. fatty acid
    e. tremor
Esser skin graft
Essex-Lopresti
    E.-L. axial fixation technique
    E.-L. calcaneal fracture
      classification
    E.-L. calcaneal fracture technique
    E.-L. fixation
    E.-L. fixation of calcaneal fracture
    E.-L. injury
    E.-L. joint depression fracture
    E.-L. lesion
    E.-L. method
    E.-L. open reduction
    E.-L. tongue-type fracture
ESSF
    external spinal skeletal fixator
established contracture

esterified estrogens
Esterom solution
Estersohn
    E. osteotomy
    E. osteotomy for tailor's bunion
esthesia
esthesiometry
    Semmes-Weinstein monofilament
    pressure e.
estimated blood loss (EBL)
estimation
    Simple Calculated Osteoporosis
    Risk E. (SCORE)
Estrace Oral
Estraderm Transdermal
Estra-L Injection
Estratest H.S.
Estro-Cyp Injection
estrogen
    conjugated e.'s
    e.'s and medroxyprogesterone
    e.'s and methyltestosterone
ETAC
    electrothermally assisted capsulorrhaphy
ethanol
    anhydrous e.
Ethibond suture
Ethicon suture
Ethiflex suture
Ethilon suture
ethinyl estradiol
ethmoid forceps
Ethrone implant material
ethyl
    e. chloride
    e. chloride and
    dichlorotetrafluoroethane
ethylene
    e. oxide
    e. oxide sterilization
    e. vinyl acetate (EVA)
etidronate
    e. disodium
    sodium e.
etiology
    depth of ulcer, extent of bacterial
    colonization, phase of ulcer,
    associated e. (DEPA)
    e. undetermined
    e. unknown
ETL
    echo train length

ETPS
    electrotherapeutic point stimulation
    ETPS therapy
ETS-2% Topical
Eucalyptamint arthritis pain ointment
eukinesia
Euler
    E. angle
    E. angle of wrist motion
    E. load
eulerian angle
eumelanin
eumycetoma
EuroCuff forearm crutch
Euroglide MKII slide board
European
    E. Chiropractic Union
    E. compression technique (ECT)
European-style screwdriver
Eurotaper 12/14 taper
Eurotech
    E. Diamond table
    E. Emerald table
    E. Platinum table
    E. Sapphire table
EVA
    ethylene vinyl acetate
evacuation
    epidural abscess e.
    epidural tumor e.
    nail bed hematoma e.
evaluation
    Acute Physiology and Chronic
    Health E. (APACHE)
    Arnadottir Occupational Therapy
    Activities of Daily Living
    Neurobehavioral E. (A-ONE)
    Balance Master rehabilitation e.
    baseline capacity e.
    Bay Area Functional
    Performance E. (BaFPE)
    Charcot-Marie-Tooth E.
    CMT E.
    Cyriax e.
    Doppler pulse e.
    Evans tenodesis e.
    Evolution hip prosthesis e.
    Fugl-Meyer e.
    functional capacity e. (FCE)
    Hughston knee e.
    isokinetic e.
    job capacity e. (JCE)
    Mazur ankle e.

E

NOTES

evaluation *(continued)*
orthopaedic e.
physical capacity e. (PCE)
e., prediction, intervention, control
(EPIC)
preoperative e.
Smith physical capacities e.
static e.
Toddler and Infant Motor E.
(TIME)
E. Tool of Children's Handwriting
Touch-Test sensory e.
uniaxial balance e. (UBE)
vocational e. (VE)
evaluator
Touch-Test sensory e.
Evans
E. ankle joint instability operation
E. ankle reconstruction technique
E. anterior opening wedge
calcaneal osteotomy
E. calcaneal lengthening
E. calcaneal lengthening osteotomy
site
E. calcaneal reconstruction
E. fracture classification system
E. intertrochanteric fracture
classification
E. lateral ankle reconstruction
E. procedure
E. tenodesis
E. tenodesis evaluation
Evans-Burkhalter protocol
Evazote
E. cushioning material
E. foam
event
endurance e.
eventration
Eve reconstructive procedure
Ever-Flex insole
Evershears surgical instrument device
eversion
ankle e.
heel e.
e. injury
e. osteotomy
e. stress test
eversion-external rotation deformity
evertor
e. force
e. tendon
evidence-based orthopaedics
evoked
e. compound muscle action
potential
e. potential study
e. response
Evolis femoral cutting guide

evolution
E. hip prosthesis
E. hip prosthesis evaluation
Ewald
E. capitellocondylar total elbow
arthroplasty
E. elbow arthroplasty rating system
E. total elbow replacement
E. unconstrained elbow prosthesis
Ewald-Walker
E.-W. kinematic knee arthroplasty
E.-W. knee implant
EWHO
elbow-wrist-hand orthosis
Ewing
E. sarcoma
E. tumor
exacerbation
Exact-Fit ATH hip replacement system
exaggeration reaction
examination, exam
Apley e.
ARM method of physical e.
arthroscopic e.
BB to MM e.
bellybutton to medial malleolus e.
bench e.
Boston Diagnostic Aphasia e.
Broden stress e.
clinical e.
comparative radiographic e.
full spine radiographic e.
lateral full-spine radiographic e.
Mini Mental State E. (MMSE)
motor e.
neurologic e.
neurological nerve conduction
velocity e.
palpatory e.
pedodynographic e.
physical e.
radiographic e.
reflex e.
sensory e.
stress e.
tender point e.
thermographic e.
exarticulation
Ex-Balls medicine ball
excavatum
pectus e.
Excel Plus electrode
excentric amputation
·**excess cement**
excessive
e. joint play
e. laxity test
e. sweating

exchange
    isolated modular tibial insert e.
    e. nailing
excision
    e. arthroplasty
    bar e.
    Bartlett nail fold e.
    bone cyst e.
    Bose nail fold e.
    bunionette e.
    cervical disc e.
    clavicle e.
    e. and curettage
    e., curettage, drilling (ECD)
    Curtin plantar fibromatosis e.
    Das Gupta scapular e.
    disc e.
    distal clavicular e.
    Ferciot e.
    Ferciot-Thomson e.
    Flatt e.
    funicular e.
    hemivertebral e.
    e. and implantation
    e. of intervertebral disc
    intracapsular e.
    intralesional e.
    marginal e.
    McKeever-Buck fragment e.
    meniscal e.
    microlumbar disc e.
    e. of osteochondroma
    radical compartmental e.
    retropulsed bone e.
    ruptured disc e.
    split-thickness skin e. (STSE)
    Stewart distal clavicular e.
    Thompson e.
    ulnar head e.
    wide e.
    William microlumbar disc e.
excisional
    e. arthrodesis
    e. biopsy
excision-curettage technique
excitatory postsynaptic potential
exclusion clamp
excochleation
excoriation
excrescence
    bony e.
excursion
    e. amplifier sleeve

    calcaneus e.
    hindfoot e.
    insertional e.
    range of e.
    tendon e.
executive function deficit
Exelderm Topical
Exerball kit
Exerband
    E. Pak bilateral tube
    E. Pak unilateral tube
    E. tubing
Exerboard
    Velcro Hand E.
exercise
    active-assisted range of motion e.
    active-assistive e. (AAE)
    active range of motion e.
    aerobic e.
    anaerobic e.
    ankle-pump e.
    aquatic e.
    back e.
    Back Revolution Stick e.
    e. band
    Berger e.
    e. board
    e. bone
    Buerger-Allen e.
    calf raise back e.
    Calleja e.
    e. capacity
    Carpal Care e.
    chain reaction e.
    closed-chain e.
    closed kinetic chain e. (CKCE)
    closed kinetic chain progressive-resistance e.
    co-contraction e.
    Codman e.
    concentric isokinetic leg press e.
    contracture e.
    Cooksey-Cawthorne e.
    Crane shoulder e.
    Daily Adjusted Progressive Resistance E. (DAPRE)
    dead ball e.'s
    DeLorme e.
    dying bug e.
    dynamic stump e.
    eccentric e.
    elevation e.
    empty can e.

E

NOTES

exercise *(continued)*
 endurance e.
 explosive e.
 external rotation e.
 FITT e.
 flexibility e.
 flexion-extension e.
 forearm ischemic e.
 Frenkel e.'s
 gastrocnemius resistive e.
 e. grab bar
 gripping e.'s
 hamstring-setting e.
 handgrip e.
 heel cord stretching e.
 heel raise e.
 heel rock e.
 hip abductor strengthening e.
 hip extension e.
 hook-lying pectoral stretch e.
 horizontal shoulder abduction e.
 increment after e.
 internal rotation e.
 e. intolerance
 inversion-eversion e.
 e. ischemia
 isokinetic e.
 isometric e.
 isotonic e.
 kinesthetic e.
 knee extension e.
 knee pump e.
 e. log
 low-stress aerobic e.
 McKenzie extension e.
 muscle-setting e.
 muscle-strengthening e.
 e. myopathy
 open-chain e.
 open kinetic chain e. (OKCE)
 orthokinetic e.
 6-pack hand e.
 parallel squat e.
 passive assistance e.
 passive range of motion e.
 passive resistive e.
 passive stretch e.
 pelvic floor e.
 pendulum e.
 peroneal strengthening e.
 e. physiology
 Pilates method e.
 plyometric e.
 pneumatic resistance e.
 PNF e.
 e. program
 progressive-resistance e.
 progressive-resistive e. (PR, PRE)
 prone scapular retraction e.

 proprioceptive e.
 pulley e.
 e. putty
 quadriceps-setting e.
 quadriceps strengthening e.
 race-pace e.
 range of motion e.
 Regen flexion e.
 rehabilitation flexibility e.
 remedial e.
 repetitive e.
 resistive e.
 rotation e.
 E. Sandal
 e. science
 seated scapular retraction e.
 e. self-efficacy
 E. Self-Efficacy Scale
 Seradge hand e.'s
 single-row e.
 sports anemia e.
 stair-climbing e.
 step e.
 straight leg raising e.
 Super-Seven e.
 supinator fossa supraclavicular fossa
  Frenkel e.'s
 supported extension e.
 tai chi chuan e.
 e. testing
 Thera-Band Max resistive e.
 therapeutic e.
 toe gripping e.
 toe raise e.
 towel e.
 unrestricted closed and open chain
  knee extension e.
 VMO e.
 volitional e.
 wall-slide e.
 Williams flexion e. (WFE)
 work hardening e.
 wrist stretch e.
exercise-associated collapse
exercise-induced
 e.-i. amenorrhea
 e.-i. anaphylaxis
 e.-i. asthma
 e.-i. breast pain
 e.-i. collapse
 e.-i. compartment syndrome
 e.-i. myokymia
 e.-i. sudden death
exerciser
 AccessTrainer e.
 animal beanbag e.
 Ankle Isolator foot and ankle e.
 axial resistance e.
 bicycle e.

Builder Grip hand e.
Carpal Care carpal tunnel e.
Carpal Tunnel Stretch e.
Cat's Paw e.
ChairCiser adjustable e.
continuous anatomical passive e.
  (CAPE)
Cybex II, II+ isokinetic e.
Danniflex CPM e.
Digi-Flex finger e.
Digi-Flex hand e.
DynaFlex Gyro e.
Eggsercizer CTS e.
Eggsercizer resistive hand e.
Exer-Cor e.
ExtendaFLEX e.
finger e.
Finger Helper hand e.
Finger Platter hand e.
Flextender Plus hand e.
Grahamizer I e.
Gripp squeeze ball hand e.
Gyro-Flex upper extremity e.
hand e.
Hand Helper hand e.
isokinetic Unex III e.
Iso-Quadron e.
Jace shoulder e.
jaw e.
Jux-A-Cisor e.
Knead-A-Ball e.
microcomputer upper limb e.
  (MULE)
MiniMedBall hand e.
Morpho E.
Motivator FTR2000 e.
MULE upper limb e.
Nelson finger e.
NordiCare Enabler e.
NordiCare Strider e.
NordicTrack ski e.
NuStep e.
Omni-Flexor wrist e.
Oppociser hand e.
Orthotron e.
pedal e.
Plyo-Sled e.
Powerflex CMP e.
Power Pogo stationary e.
Power Web hand e.
Power Web Jr. e.
Preston Traveler CPM e.
ProStretch e.

Pul-Ez e.
resistive e.
rickshaw rehabilitation e.
rocky boat e.
Rotaflex e.
Roylan ergonomic hand e.
Seated Cable Row e.
soft touch hand e.
squeeze e.
strengthening e.
Stronghands hand e.
Stryker CPM e.
Stryker leg e.
Swanson Grip-X hand e.
Thera-Band ASSIST e.
Thera-Band hand e.
Thera-Band resistive e.
Thera Cane shoulder e.
Theraflex wrist e.
Ther-A-Hoop e.
Thera-Loop e.
Thera-Putty CTS e.
Toronto Medical CPM e.
Tuf Nex neck e.
Tunturi hand e.
Versa-Trainer e.
Walk-'n-Tone e.
Wilco ankle e.
Wristiciser e.
Zimmer continuous anatomical
  passive e.
exercise-related headache
Exer-Cor exerciser
Exercycle
ExerFlex ball
Exer-Pedic cycle
Exerstrider walking pole
exertion
  Borg Scale of Rating Perceived E.
  rated perceived e. (RPE)
  rating of perceived e. (RPE)
exertional
  e. anterior compartment syndrome
    (EACS)
  e. deep posterior compartment
    syndrome (EDPCS)
  e. hypotension
  e. rhabdomyolysis
Exertools
  E. Dyna-Disc
  E. gymball
Exeter
  E. cemented hip prosthesis

E

NOTES

Exeter *(continued)*
    E. intramedullary bone plug
    E. intramedullary bone plug device
    E. stem
    E. total hip system
Exeter-Femora press fit prosthesis
EX-FI-RE
    external fixation reduction
    EX-FI-RE external fixation
    EX-FI-RE external fixation device
    EX-FI-RE external fixation system
exhaustion
    postactivation e.
    posttetanic e.
Exidine Scrub
Exo-Bed traction unit
exoccipital bone
Exogen
    E. bone healing system
    E. 2000 noninvasive, low-intensity, pulsed ultrasound device
    E. 2000+ noninvasive ultrasound
    E. 2000+ noninvasive ultrasound therapy
    E. 2000 sonic accelerated fracture healing system
exogenous
    e. fibrin clot
    e. reconstruction
Exo-Overhead traction unit
Exo-Static
    E.-S. cervical collar
    E.-S. neck collar
    E.-S. traction
exostectomy
    lateral e.
    medial e.
exostosectomy
exostosis, pl. **exostoses**
    blocker's e.
    bony e.
    e. bursata
    cuneiform-first metatarsal e.
    Dupuytren e.
    epiphysial e.
    Haglund e.
    hereditary multiple e.
    hypertrophic e.
    impinging e.
    marginal e.
    metatarsal cuneiform e.
    metatarsocuneiform joint e.
    multiple hereditary osteochondral e. (MHOCE)
    osteocartilaginous e.
    pump bump e.
    retrocalcaneal e.
    subungual e.
    tackler's e.

    talar neck e.
    talotibial e.
    traction e.
    turret e.
Exotec brace
expanded
    E. Disability Status Scale (EDSS)
    e. polytetrafluoroethylene (EPTFE)
expander
    AccuSpan tissue e.
    acetabular e.
    Mentor tissue e.
    tissue e.
expanding reamer
Expandover athletic tape
expansile
    e. cyst
    e. lesion
expansion
    e. bolt
    lateral extensor e.
    medial extensor e.
    e. screw
expansive laminaplasty
expenditure
    energy e.
experimental threshold
exploration
    e. and débridement
    e. and revision
exploratory incision
exploring electrode
explosion
    e. fracture
    front kick e.
    e. injury
explosive exercise
exposure
    Abbott-Gill epiphysial plate e.
    anterior surgical e.
    bone-tendon e.
    extrapharyngeal e.
    Henry posterior interosseous nerve e.
    Kocher-Langenbeck e.
    subperiosteal e.
    surgical e.
    thoracolumbar junction surgical e.
    thoracolumbar spine anterior e.
    transperitoneal e.
    upper cervical spine anterior e.
    vertebral e.
expulsion
    graft e.
exsanguinate
exsanguination tourniquet control
extend
    E. stem
    E. total hip system

ExtendaFLEX exerciser
extended
    e. activities of daily living
      (EADL)
    e. ADLs
    e. code therapy (ECT)
    e. iliofemoral approach
    e. maxillotomy
    e. medial shoe counter
    e. slide trochanteric osteotomy
    e. steel shank
    e. steel-shank shoe
    e. tibial in situ bypass
extended-counter shoe
extender
    dorsal plate e.
    nail e.
    Rousek e.
    Rush e.
    Superstabilizer cemented stem e.
    Superstabilizer press-fit stem e.
Extend-It finger splint
extensibility
extensible
extensile
    e. anterior approach
    e. lateral approach
extension
    active knee e. (AKE)
    e. aid
    angle of greatest e. (AGE)
    Bardenheuer e.
    basal e.
    e. block splint
    e. block splinting method
    e. body cast
    e. bone clamp
    e. bow
    brachioradialis transfer for wrist e.
    brake lever e.
    Buck e.
    Callahan e.
    cast with dorsal toe plate e.
    cast with volar toe plate e.
    cervical rotation in e.
    Codivilla e.
    compressive e.
    e. contracture
    e. deformity
    distractive e.
    dorsal toe plate e.
    Dynasplint knee e.
    external rotation in e. (ERE)

    femoral trunk e.
    flexion and e.
    flexion, abduction, external
      rotation, e. (FABERE)
    flexion, adduction, internal
      rotation, e. (FADIR, FADIRE)
    e. gap
    headrest e.
    hip e.
    Hittenberger halo e.
    e. injury posterior atlantoaxial
      arthrodesis
    e. instability
    internal rotation in e. (IRE)
    isokinetic knee e.
    Legg-Perthes shoe e.
    lumbar e.
    e. malposition
    e. maneuver
    Maquet table e.
    e. nail
    nail e.
    NexGen offset stem e.
    e. osteotomy
    range of e.
    e. restriction
    shoe e.
    sitting knee e.
    skeletal e.
    terminal knee e.
    toe plate e.
    volitional resisted flexion and e.
    wrist e.
extensive
    e. neoplasm
    e. posterior approach
    e. posterior decompression
extensometer
    strain-gauge e.
extensor
    apparatus e.
    e. brevis arthroplasty
    e. carpi radialis brevis (ECRB)
    e. carpi radialis brevis muscle
    e. carpi radialis brevis tendon
    e. carpi radialis longus (ECRL)
    e. carpi radialis longus muscle
    e. carpi radialis longus tendon
    e. carpi ulnaris (ECU)
    e. carpi ulnaris muscle
    e. carpi ulnaris tendon
    e. communis muscle
    e. digiti minimi (EDM)

E

NOTES

extensor *(continued)*
  e. digiti minimi muscle
  e. digiti minimi tendon
  e. digiti quinti (EDQ)
  e. digiti quinti muscle
  e. digiti quinti tendon
  e. digitorum (ED)
  e. digitorum brevis (EDB)
  e. digitorum brevis flap
  e. digitorum brevis muscle
  e. digitorum brevis tendon
  e. digitorum communis (EDC)
  e. digitorum communis muscle
  e. digitorum communis tendon
  e. digitorum longus (EDL)
  e. digitorum longus muscle
  e. digitorum longus tendon
  e. digitorum transfer
  e. hallucis
  e. hallucis brevis muscle
  e. hallucis longus (EHL)
  e. hallucis longus muscle
  e. hallucis longus strength
  e. hallucis longus tendon
  e. hallucis longus tenodesis
  e. hallucis longus transfer
  e. hood
  e. hood mechanism
  e. hood release
  e. indicis proprius (EIP)
  e. indicis proprius muscle
  e. indicis proprius tendon
  knee e.
  long e.
  e. mechanism dysfunction
  e. pollicis brevis (EPB)
  e. pollicis brevis muscle
  e. pollicis brevis tendon
  e. pollicis longus (EPL)
  e. pollicis longus muscle
  e. pollicis longus tendon
  e. quinti tendon
  radial wrist e.
  e. retinaculum
  e. substitution
  e. tendon blockage
  e. tendon injury
  e. tendon lengthening
  e. tendon repair
  e. tendon transfer
  e. tenotomy
  e. thrust reflex
  toe e.
  ulnar e.
  e. wad of 3 muscles
  e. wand
  wrist e.
extensus
  hallux e.

exteriorization
externa
  epicondylalgia e.
external
  e. band
  e. elastic strap
  e. fixation reduction (EX-FI-RE)
  e. fixator
  e. fixator frame
  e. hamstring reflex
  e. humeral epicondylitis
  e. ilium (EI)
  e. ilium movement
  e. immobilization
  e. immobilizer
  e. intercostal muscle
  e. malleolus
  e. neurolysis
  e. oblique muscle
  e. oblique reflex
  posteroinferior e. (PIEx)
  e. prehallux
  e. ring fixation
  e. rotation
  e. rotation-abduction stress test (EAST)
  e. rotation contracture
  e. rotation exercise
  e. rotation in extension (ERE)
  e. rotation in flexion (ERF)
  e. rotation/internal rotation (ER/IR)
  e. rotation/internal rotation ratio
  e. rotation stress test
  e. rotator
  e. sequential pneumatic compression boot
  e. skeletal fixation apparatus
  e. spinal fixation
  e. spinal skeletal fixator (ESSF)
  e. support
  e. tibial torsion
  e. traction
  e. version
external-alignment compression jig
external-coil electrical stimulation
externally
  e. powered tenodesis orthosis
  e. rotated
externum
externus
  malleolus e.
exteroceptive sensation
exteroceptor
  postural e.
extirpation
extraabdominal desmoid tumor
extraarticular
  e. ankylosis
  e. arthrodesis

e. arthroscopy
e. augmentation
e. fracture
e. graft
e. Grice procedure
e. hip fusion
e. knee ligament
e. pain syndrome
e. pigmented villonodular synovitis
e. pseudarthrosis
e. reconstruction
e. resection
e. structure
e. subtalar fusion
e. subtalar joint
e. technique
e. tuberculosis
extrabursal approach
extracapsular
e. ankylosis
e. arterial ring
e. dissection
e. fracture
e. ligament
e. rupture
extracompartmental soft tissue sarcoma
extracorporeal
e. shock wave therapy
e. shock wave treatment
extracortical chondrosarcoma
extracting forceps
extraction pliers
extractor
Austin Moore e.
ball e.
Bilos pin e.
bone plug e.
break screw e.
broach e.
Cherry screw e.
cloverleaf pin e.
corkscrew femoral head e.
femoral head e.
femoral trial e.
FIN e.
Jewett e.
Kalish Duredge wire e.
Küntscher e.
Mark II femoral component e.
Mark II tibial component e.
Massie e.
metatarsal head e.
Moore prosthesis e.

Moreland femoral component e.
e. nail drill
Nicoll e.
Rousek e.
Sage e.
Schneider e.
Snap Lock wire/pin e.
Southwick screw e.
staple e.
stem e.
Sven-Johansson e.
Take-Out E.
Universal modular femoral hip
component e.
Zimmer e.
extractor-driver
Schneider e.-d.
extractor-impactor
Fox e.-i.
extra-depth
e.-d. posterior acetabular retractor
e.-d. shoe
extradural
e. anastomosis
e. granulation
extrafascial nerve injection
extrafusal fiber contraction
extra-large hip retractor
extra-leverage proximal femoral elevator
extramedullary
e. alignment
e. alignment guide
e. fixation
e. plasmacytoma
e. tibial alignment jig
extraoctave fracture
extraosseous
e. circulation
e. factor
extraperitoneal approach
extrapharyngeal
e. approach
e. exposure
extrapyramidal gait
extraskeletal
e. chondroma
e. chondrosarcoma
e. osteosarcoma
extravasation
dye e.
e. extremity
e. extrusion

E

NOTES

extravasation *(continued)*
    e. injury
    e. irrigation solution
Extreme foot orthotic
extremity, pl. **extremities**
    both lower extremities (BLE)
    both upper extremities (BUE)
    elevation of e.
    extravasation e.
    left lower e. (LLE)
    left upper e. (LUE)
    lower e. (LE)
    e. mobilization strap
    e. mobilization technique
    e. pump
    right lower e. (RLE)
    right upper e. (RUE)
    scanogram of lower e.
    upper e. (UE)
extrinsic
    e. clubfoot
    e. entrapment test
    finger e.'s
    e. ligament
    e. metatarsus primus elevatus
    e. muscle
    e. muscle strength
    e. rearfoot post
    e. tightness test
    e. toe flexor
extruded
    e. bar polyethylene
    e. disc

extrusion
    bone graft e.
    disc e.
    extravasation e.
extubation
    postoperative e.
exuberant
    e. granulation tissue
    e. synovium
exudate
exude
Exu-Dry wound dressing
eye sign
Eyler flexorplasty
Eyre-Brook epiphysial index
EZ
    EZ Bend sponge
    EZ hand pump
    EZ Rider support chair
    EZ ROM postoperative knee brace
    EZ "T" orthopaedic shirt
E-Z
    E-Z arm abduction orthosis
    E-Z Flex jaw exercising device
    E-Z Reacher
    E-Z ROC anchor
Ezeform splint
EZ-Trac orthopaedic suspension device
EZ-Up inversion table
Ezy
    E. Wrap lumbosacral support
    E. Wrap shoulder immobilizer

F
>F latency
>F wave

F2L Multineck femoral stem

FA
>femoral anteversion

Fabco
>F. gauze bandage
>F. gauze dressing

fabella syndrome

fabellofibular
>f. complex
>f. ligament

FABER
>flexion, abduction, external rotation
>FABER test

FABERE
>flexion, abduction, external rotation, extension
>FABERE sign
>FABERE test

Fabian screw

fabric
>neoprene f.
>Staph-Chek Synergy f.

FAC
>functional ambulation category

facebow
>Ortho-Yomy f.

facelift
>chiropractic laser nonsurgical f.

facet
>f. angle
>f. anomaly
>f. apposition
>articular f.
>calcaneal f.
>f. capsule
>f. capsule disruption
>f. dislocation
>f. excision technique
>fibular f.
>f. fracture stabilization wiring
>fusion f.
>f. fusion
>inferior f.
>f. injection
>f. joint
>f. joint block
>f. joint disease (FJD)
>f. joint dysfunction
>f. joint irritation
>f. joint preparation
>f. joint syndrome
>f. joint vacuum

>lateral patellar f.
>locked f.
>malleolar f.
>oblique wiring f.
>f. plane
>posterior f.
>proximal fibular f.
>f. replacement
>f. screw system
>f. subluxation
>f. subluxation stabilization wiring
>f. surface
>f. synovial impingement
>f. tropism

facetectomy
>O'Donoghue f.

face validity of rehabilitation testing

facial artery

facies
>acromegalic f.
>swan-neck f.

facilitated
>f. spinal system
>f. subluxation

facilitation
>convergence f.
>Law of F.
>neuromuscular f.
>f. pattern
>postactivation f.
>posttetanic f.
>proprioceptive neuromuscular f. (PNF)

facilitatory technique

facioauriculovertebral (FAV)

faciodigitogenital dysplasia

facioscapulohumeral (FSH)

factitious
>f. injury
>f. lymphedema

factor
>analog neurotrophic f.
>biomechanical f.
>coagulation f.
>dislocation f.
>ergonomic f.
>extraosseous f.
>high-risk f.
>insulin-like growth f. (IGF)
>leg protection f. (LPF)
>nerve growth f.
>neurotrophic f.
>platelet-derived growth f. (PDGF)
>RA f.
>rheumatoid arthritis f.

F

factor *(continued)*
skeletal growth f.
transforming growth f. (TGF)
f. VIII, IX deficiency
FADIR
flexion, adduction, internal rotation
flexion, adduction, internal rotation, extension
FADIR sign
FADIR test
FADIRE
flexion, adduction, internal rotation, extension
fad therapy
Fahey
F. approach
F. pin
F. retractor
F. technique
failed
f. acetabular component
f. back surgery syndrome (FBSS)
f. back syndrome (FBS)
f. back syndrome with documented pseudarthrosis
f. femoral osteotomy
f. flatfoot surgery
f. implant arthroplasty
f. joint replacement
f. procedure
f. surgery syndrome
f. triple arthrodesis
fail-safe mechanism
failure
brittle bone f.
congestive heart f. (CHF)
f. of conservative management
differentiation f.
ductile f.
fatigue f.
Harrington rod instrumentation f.
heart f.
implant f.
metal f.
spinal implant load to f.
stem f.
Fairbanks
F. change
F. sign
F. technique
F. technique with Sever modification
Fairbanks-Sever procedure
Fajersztajn crossed sciatic sign
FAL
functional and anatomic loading
falces (*pl. of* falx)

falciform
f. cartilage
f. ligament
Fallat-Buckholz method
fallen arch
fallen-fragment sign
fallen-leaf sign
false
f. acetabulum
f. aneurysm
f. ankylosis
f. articulation
f. coxa vara
f. joint
f. ligament
f. neuroma
f. pelvis
f. profile view
f. rib
f. vertebra
false-negative result
falx, pl. **falces**
calcification of f.
f. calcification
FAM
functional assessment measure
familial
f. expansile osteolysis
f. lymphedema
f. myoglobinuria
f. osteoectasia
f. periodic paralysis
f. shape
f. spinal muscular atrophy
family management model
fan
Schmitt f.
f. sign
Fanconi
F. anemia
F. syndrome
Fanconi-Albertini-Zellweger syndrome
Fantastic Burr nail bur
Farabeuf
F. amputation
F. bone-holding forceps
F. bone rasp
F. periosteal elevator
Farabeuf-Lambotte
F.-L. bone-holding forceps
F.-L. rasp
far fashion
far-field potential
farmer
F. operation
F. technique
far-out syndrome
Farrior wire-crimping forceps

Fartlek training
fascia, pl. **fascias, fasciae**
Abernethy f.
antebrachial f.
anterior cervical f.
Buck f.
Camper f.
cervical f.
clavipectoral f.
Colles f.
crural f.
cuff of f.
deep f.
deltoid f.
Dupuytren f.
endoabdominal f.
endothoracic f.
gluteal f.
hypothenar f.
infraspinous f.
investing f.
f. lata
f. lata femoris
f. lata freeze-thawed graft
lumbar f.
lumbodorsal f. (LDF)
medial geniculate f.
Osborne f.
palmar f.
plantar f.
popliteal f.
pubic f.
quadratus femoris f.
f. of quadratus lumborum muscle
retrosacral f.
Scarpa f.
f. sheath
Sibson f.
thenar f.
transversalis f.
vertebral f.
fascial
f. arthroplasty
f. band
f. bridge
f. compartment
f. fibromatosis
f. flap augmentation
f. graft
f. plane
f. plexus
f. release
f. sarcoma

f. septum
f. sheath covering
f. space
f. space infection
f. subcutaneous turn-down flap
f. suture
fascial-muscle interface
fasciaplasty, fascioplasty
fascias (*pl. of* fascia)
fascia-splitting incision
fascicle
anterior tibiotalar f. (ATTF)
motor f.
muscle f.
popliteomeniscal f.
sensory f.
silent f.
fascicular
f. degeneration
f. neuropathy
f. repair
fasciculation
benign f.
contraction f.
malignant f.
f. potential
proprioceptive neuromuscular f. (PNF)
fasciculus, pl. **fasciculi**
arcuate f. (AF)
fasciectomy
dermal f.
limited f.
partial f.
radical palmar f.
subtotal plantar f.
fasciitis, fascitis
diffuse f.
Dupuytren f.
iliotibial band f.
ITB f.
necrotizing f.
nodular f.
plantar f.
proliferative f.
pseudosarcomatous f.
recalcitrant plantar f.
fasciocutaneous
f. axial pattern flap
f. island flap
fasciodesis
fascio-fat graft
fasciogram

F

NOTES

fascioplasty (*var. of* fasciaplasty)
fasciorrhaphy
fascioscapulohumeral
    f. dystrophy
    f. muscle atrophy disease
    f. muscular atrophy
    f. muscular dystrophy
fasciotome
    intercompartment f.
    Masson f.
    Moseley f.
fasciotomy
    compartment f.
    4-compartment f.
    decompression f.
    double-incision f.
    endoscopic plantar f. (EPF)
    minimal incision plantar f.
    palmar f.
    percutaneous plantar f. (PPF)
    plantar f.
    prophylactic f.
    single-incision f.
    subcutaneous palmar f.
    uniportal plantar f.
    Yount f.
fascitis (*var. of* fasciitis)
fashion
    aseptic f.
    barber-pole f.
    Bunnell zigzag f.
    cruciate f.
    far f.
    near-far f.
FASS
    foot and ankle severity scale
FAST
    Functional Assessment Staging
    FAST 1 intraosseous infusion
      system
fast
    f. axoplasmic transport (FAXT)
    f. imaging with steady procession
      (FISP)
    F. Lanex rare earth screen
    f. low-angle shot (FLASH)
    f. muscle
FASTak
    F. suture anchor
    F. suture anchor system
fastener
    Intrafix ACL tibial f.
Fastex proprioceptive and agility test
Fastin
    F. suture anchor
    F. threaded anchor
Fastlok implantable staple
FastOut device
Fas-Trac strip

fast-twitch muscle fiber
fat
    aspirated f.
    autogenous f.
    f. embolism
    f. embolism syndrome
    f. and fat-free mass (FFM)
    f. graft
    f. loading
    f. oxidation
    f. pad
    f. pad atrophy
    f. pad of elbow
    f. pad retractor
    f. pad sign
    f. pad syndrome
    f. saturation
fat-blood
    f.-b. interface (FBI)
    f.-b. interface sign
fat-fluid level
fatigue
    f. bone graft
    f. failure
    f. fracture
    implant f.
    metal f.
    static f.
    f. strength
    f. stress
    f. tolerance
    volitional f.
fat-suppressed turbo spin-echo T2-
weighted sequence
fatty
    f. tissue
    f. tissue tumor
Faulkner curette
fault
    dynamic f.
faulty union
FAV
    facioauriculovertebral
    FAV syndrome
FAXT
    fast axoplasmic transport
Fazio-Londe
    F.-L. atrophy
    F.-L. syndrome
FB
    foreign body
    FB cast cushion
FBI
    fat-blood interface
    FBI sign
FBS
    failed back syndrome
FBSS
    failed back surgery syndrome

FCE
functional capacity evaluation
FCER
Foundation for Chiropractic Education
and Research
FCL
fibular collateral ligament
FCR
flexor carpi radialis
FCS
full cervical spine
FCS view
FCS x-ray
FCU
flexor carpi ulnaris
FD
flexor digitorum
FDB
flexor digitorum brevis
FDC
flexor digitorum communis
FDICT
frequency-difference interferential current
therapy
FDL
flexor digitorum longus
FDMA
first dorsal metatarsal artery
FDP
flexor digitorum profundus
FDQB
flexor digitorum quinti brevis
FDS
flexor digitorum sublimis
flexor digitorum superficialis
FEA
finite element analysis
Feagin shoulder dislocation test
fear-near
f.-n., near-far suture
f.-n., near-far suture technique
feasibility
F. Evaluation Checklist (FEC)
vocational f.
febricitans
pes f.
FEC
Feasibility Evaluation Checklist
feeder
offset suspension f.
suspension f.
Tumble Forms f.

feel
end f.
initiation f.
through-range f.
feet (*pl. of* foot)
Feiss line
Feldenkrais
F. cylinder
F. foam roll
F. method
Felix disease
fell on outstretched hand (FOOSH)
felon
aseptic f.
f. infection
felt
f. apron Bowden cable suspension
system
f. brace
f. collar splint
f. dressing
orthopaedic f.
f. padding
f. patch
rolled f.
F. shears
female
f. athletic triad
f. reamer
f. washer
femora (*pl. of* femur)
femoral
f. above-knee popliteal bypass
f. aligner
f. alignment jig
f. antetorsion
f. anteversion (FA)
f. approach
f. arteriography
f. attachment
f. bone
f. Buck plug procedure
f. canal
f. canal restrictor
f. circulation
f. circumflex artery
f. clamp
f. component
f. component pusher
f. component removal
f. condylar defect
f. condylar shaving
f. condylar template

F

NOTES

femoral *(continued)*
    f. condyle
    f. cortex
    f. cortical index
    f. cortical perforation
    f. cortical ring allograft
    f. cortical window
    f. cutaneous nerve
    f. derotation osteotomy
    f. diaphysial allograft
    f. diaphysis
    f. distractor
    f. drill bit
    f. drill tunnel
    f. endoprosthesis
    f. epicondyle
    f. epiphysiolysis
    f. epiphysis
    f. footprint
    f. fossa
    f. fracture following total hip
    replacement classification
    f. groove
    f. guide pin
    f. guidepin
    f. head
    f. head amputation
    f. head bone removal reamer
    f. head cork screw
    f. head deformity
    f. head driver
    f. head dysplasia
    f. head extractor
    f. head line (FHL)
    f. head and neck
    f. head-neck anteversion
    f. head-neck junction
    f. head-neck ratio
    f. head osteonecrosis
    f. head vascularity
    f. impactor
    f. intramedullary guide
    f. intratrochanteric fracture
    f. lengthening
    f. medullary canal
    f. metaphysial shortening
    f. metaphysis
    f. muscle
    f. nailing
    f. neck fracture
    f. neck fracture reduction
    f. neck nail
    f. neck prosthesis
    f. neck version
    f. nerve block
    f. nerve paralysis
    f. nerve stretch test
    f. nerve traction test
    f. notch guide

    f. offset
    f. osteolysis
    f. osteomyelitis
    f. osteoporosis
    f. plate
    f. plug
    f. prosthesis broach
    f. prosthesis fixation
    f. rasp
    f. reflex
    f. region
    f. resection
    f. resector
    f. retrotorsion
    f. retroversion
    f. rollback
    f. sarcoma
    self-articulating f. (SAF)
    f. shaft
    f. shaft axis
    f. shaft fracture
    f. shaft malunion
    f. sheath
    f. stem removal
    f. supracondylar fracture
    f. torsion
    f. trial extractor
    f. trunk angle
    f. trunk extension
    f. trunk flexion
    f. tuberosity
    f. tunnel
    f. vein injury
femoral-femoral
    f.-f. bypass graft
    f.-f. crossover
femoris
    biceps f.
    fascia lata f.
    fovea capitis f.
    linea aspera f.
    profunda f.
    quadratus f. (QF)
    rectus f.
femorocrural graft
femorodistal
    f. bypass
    f. bypass procedure
femoroiliac thrombophlebitis
femoroischial transplantation
femoropatellar joint
femorotibial
    f. angle (FTA)
    f. joint (FTJ)
    f. ligament tenodesis
    f. torsion
femur, pl. **femora**
    f. button graft complex
    distal f.

F. Finder instrument
f. graft
f. length (FL)
f. length to abdominal
circumference ratio (FL/AC)
proximal f.
spiral line of f.
femur-fibular-ulna complex
fenamic acid
fence splint
fender fracture
fenestrated
f. drape
f. reamer
f. stem
f. tenotomy
fenestration
Fenlin total shoulder system
Fentanyl Oralet
Fenton tibial bolt
Ferciot
F. excision
F. tiptoe splint
Ferciot-Thomson excision
Ferguson
F. bone clamp
F. bone holder
F. bone-holding forceps
F. hip reduction
F. sacral base angle
F. scoliosis measuring method
F. view
Ferguson-Frazier suction tube
Fergusson
F. forceps
F. method for measuring scoliosis
Ferkel
F. bipolar release
F. C guide
F. torticollis technique
Fernandez
F. extensile anterior approach
F. osteotomy
F. point-score wrist assessment
system
F. scale posttraumatic wrist
assessment system
Ferno
F. AquaCiser underwater treadmill
system
F. custom therapy pool
Ferran awl
ferric subsulfate

Ferrier coupler
Ferris-Smith
F.-S. bone-biting forceps
F.-S. rongeur
F.-S. rongeur forceps
F.-S. tissue forceps
Ferris-Smith-Kerrison
F.-S.-K. forceps
F.-S.-K. laminectomy rongeur
Ferris-Smith-Spurling disc rongeur
ferromagnetic
f. metal plate
f. relaxation
ferumoxide injectable solution
FES
functional electrical stimulation
FES exercise bicycle
festinating gait
festination
fetal
f. alcohol syndrome
f. substantia nigra graft
fetalis
myodystrophia f.
fever
drug-infusion f.
fracture f.
rheumatic f.
f. of undetermined origin (FUO)
feverfew extract
FF
further flexion
FFC
fixed flexion contracture
FFI
Foot Function Index
FFM
fat and fat-free mass
FGS
FHB
flexor hallucis brevis
FHL
femoral head line
flexor hallucis longus
FHL release technique
FHL tendon transfer/augmentation
FHLD
flexor hallucis longus dysfunction
FI
Functional Integration
fiber
A-delta f.
afferent f.

F

NOTES

fiber *(continued)*
    f. analysis
    anular f.
    collagen f.
    f. density
    fast-twitch muscle f.
    intrafusal f.
    f. metal taper
    ragged-red f.
    Sharpey f.
    skeletal muscle f.
    tendinous f.
    X-Static silver fiber shoe lining f.
fiberglass
    f. bandage
    f. cast
    f. splint
fiberglass-free cast tape
fiber-metal peg
fiberoptic
    f. arthroscope
    f. cable
    f. intraosseous endoscopy
    f. light source
fiber-region
    anterior f.-r.
    central f.-r.
fiber-splitting incision
fibreux
    cerclage f.
fibrillar absorbable hemostat material
fibrillation
    f. potential
    synchronized f.
fibrin
    f. clot
    f. debris
    f. glue adhesive
    f. island
fibrinoid degeneration
fibrinolysin and desoxyribonuclease
fibrinolysis
fibrinolytic agent
fibroadipose tissue
fibroblast
    regenerated f.
fibroblastic
    f. phase
    f. proliferation
    f. sarcoma
    f. tumor
fibrocartilage
    f. complex
    triangular f.
fibrocartilaginous
    f. disc
    f. joint
    f. pad

    f. plate
    f. tissue
fibrochondrocyte
fibroconnective tissue
fibrodysplasia ossificans progressiva
fibroelastic cartilage
fibroepithelial polyp
fibroepithelioma of Pinkus
fibroepitheliomatous
fibrofatty
    f. debris
    f. infiltrate
    f. tissue
fibroid tumor
fibrokeratoma
    acquired digital f.
    acral digital f.
fibrolipoma
    massive f.
fibrolipomatosis
    macrodactylia f.
fibroma
    aponeurotic f.
    calcifying aponeurotic f.
    cementing f.
    chondromyxoid f.
    desmoid f.
    desmoplastic f.
    juvenile aponeurotic f.
    Koenen periungual f.
    f. molle
    nonossifying f. (NOF)
    nonosteogenic f.
    ossifying f.
    osteogenic f.
    perineural f. (PNR)
    periosteal f.
    periungual f.
    soft f.
    subungual f.
fibromatosis
    aggressive infantile f.
    f. colli
    congenital general f.
    dermal f.
    diffuse infantile f.
    Dupuytren f.
    fascial f.
    Garrod f.
    generalized f.
    infantile dermal f.
    irradiation f.
    juvenile hyaline f.
    palmar f.
    plantar f.
    pseudosarcomatous f.
    solitary f.
    sternocleidomastoid muscle f.
    subcutaneous pseudosarcomatous f.

fibromuscular disease
fibromyalgia syndrome (FMS)
fibromyalgic pain
fibromyositis
fibromyxoma
fibronectin
fibroosseous
    f. pulley
    f. ring
    f. ring of Lacroix
    f. sheath
    f. tunnel
fibropathic abnormality
fibroplasia
fibrosa
    myositis f.
    progressive myositis f.
fibrosarcoma
fibrosis
    anular f.
    endoneural f.
    intraneural f.
    perineural f.
    retroperitoneal f.
fibrositis
    f. ossificans progressiva
    periarticular f.
fibrosus
    anulus f.
    lacertus f.
fibrotic strut
fibrous
    f. adhesion
    f. ankylosis
    f. attachment
    f. band
    f. capsule
    f. cartilage
    f. cortical defect
    f. dysplasia
    f. dysplasia ossificans progressiva
    f. hamartoma
    f. histiocytoma
    f. hyperplasia
    f. joint
    f. lesion
    f. loose body
    f. metaphysial defect
    f. metaplasia
    f. scar tissue
    f. spur
    f. talocalcaneal coalition
    f. tissue implant

    f. tumor
    f. union
    f. xanthoma
fibrovascular connective tissue stroma
fibroxanthoma
fibula, pl. **fibulae, fibulas**
    diastasis f.
    distal f.
    dysplastic f.
    f. protibial synostosis
    proximal f.
    short f.
    f. shortening
fibular
    f. anlage
    f. bone
    f. bone hook test
    f. collateral ligament (FCL)
    f. collateral sprain
    f. compression test
    f. diaphysial fracture
    f. facet
    f. groove
    f. head
    f. head resection
    f. hemimelia
    f. joint disruption
    f. malleolus
    f. margin
    f. metaphysis
    f. muscle
    f. neck
    f. onlay-inlay graft
    f. ostectomy
    f. osteotomy
    f. peg
    f. plantar marginal artery
    f. pseudarthrosis
    f. sesamoid
    f. sesamoidal ligament
    f. sesamoidectomy
    f. shortening
    f. strut graft
    f. transfer
    f. transplant
fibulectomy
    partial f.
fibulocalcaneal ligament
fibulotalar
    f. arthrodesis
    f. ligament
fibulotalocalcaneal (FTC)
    f. ligament

F

NOTES

Ficat

F. and Arlet disease stage
F. classification of femoral head osteonecrosis
F. femoral head osteonecrosis classification
F. procedure
F. stage of avascular necrosis classification
F. view

Fick method
fiducial
field

F. blade
f. block
f. block anesthesia
bloodless f.
f. of dissection
electromagnetic f.
f. focused nuclear magnetic resonance (FONAR)
ionized gas f.
peripheral nerve cutaneous f. (PEMF)
pulsating electromagnetic f. (PEMF)
pulsed electromagnetic f. (PEMF)
QRS Quantronic Resonance pulsating magnetic f.

Fielding

F. femoral fracture classification
F. modification of Gallie technique

fifth

f. finger
f. metacarpal

fighter's fracture
figure-of-4

f.-o.-4 position
f.-o.-4 test

figure-of-8

f.-o.-8 adjustment
f.-o.-8 bandage
f.-o.-8 brace
f.-o.-8 cast
f.-o.-8 dressing
f.-o.-8 harness
f.-o.-8 suture
f.-o.-8 taping
f.-o.-8 test
f.-o.-8 thoracic orthosis
f.-o.-8 wire
f.-o.-8 wire loop
f.-o.-8 wiring

filarial

f. arthritis
f. synovitis

file

bone f.
orthopaedic bone f.
orthopaedic surgical f.

filiform
fill

fit and f.

Fillauer

F. bar
F. bar foot orthosis
F. dorsiflexion assist ankle joint
F. endoskeletal alignment system
F. modular shuttle lock system
F. night splint
F. PDC ankle joint
F. prosthesis liner
F. Scottish Rite orthosis kit
F. silicone suction liner
F. silicone suspension liner

filler

BF+ bone void f.
f. block
BonePlast bone void f.
Cerasorb resorbable synthetic bone void f.
Cortoss bone void f.
nonosteoconductive bone-void f.
OsteoSet bone f.
ProOsteon implant 500 coralline hydroxyapatite bone void f.
shoe f.
Springlite toe f.
synthetic cancellous bone void f.
synthetic cortical bone void f.
TheriLok bone void f.
Vitoss Scaffold synthetic cancellous bone void f.

filleted graft
fillet local flap graft
film

chiropractic x-ray f.
lateral cervical spine f.
scout f.
spot f.
stress f.
working orthopaedic surgery f.

film-screen combination
filmy adhesion
filtration system
filum terminale syndrome
FIM

functional independence measure

FIN

flexible intramedullary nail
FIN extractor
FIN pin guide
FIN system

fin

DePuy Global shoulder glenoid component with f.
F. & Flipper exercise log
f. of the implant
prosthetic stem lateral f.

finder
> angle f.
> canal f.
> Dasco Pro angle f.
> gravity-driven angle f.
> Leisure Activities F. (LAF)
> pedicle f.

finding
> bone in bone f.
> constellation of clinical f.'s
> dynamic pedodynographic f.
> thermographic f.

fine
> f. bone curette
> f. manipulation
> f. olive bur
> f. osteotome
> f. wire EMG

fine-angled curette
fine-tooth electric saw
finger
> adduction stress to f.
> f. agnosia
> f. amputation
> f. angle
> f. in balloon sign
> base of f.
> baseball f.
> F. Blocking Tree
> f. bolster
> claw f.
> cloven-hoof fracture of f.
> clubbed f.
> coach's f.
> congenital trigger f.
> f. cot
> f. cot splint
> f. deformity
> f. dexterity
> distal tuberosity of f.
> drop f.
> drumstick f.
> f. exerciser
> f. extension bow
> f. extension clockspring splint
> f. extrinsics
> fifth f.
> F. Fitness Spring Ball
> f. flap
> f. flexion glove
> f. flexion splint
> f. flexor muscle
> football f.

> f. gauge
> f. goniometer
> hammer f.
> F. Helper hand exerciser
> hippocratic f.
> f. hook
> HP-100 prosthetic f.
> hypoplastic f.
> index f.
> f. intrinsic
> jammed f.
> jerk f.
> jersey f.
> f. joint
> f. joint arthroplasty
> f. joint implant
> f. joint implant prosthesis
> f. ladder
> little f.
> lock f.
> long f.
> f. loop
> lumbrical-plus f.
> lumbrical syndrome f.
> mallet f.
> middle f.
> multiple f.
> f. opposition
> f. pad
> paradoxical lumbrical-plus f.
> F. Platter hand exerciser
> prosthetic f.
> f. pulp
> f. ray
> replantation of f.
> ring f.
> rugby jersey f.
> sausage f.
> f. separator
> f. sled splint
> f. sling
> snap f.
> spade f.
> 3-f. spica cast
> spider f.
> spring f.
> stuck f.
> syndactylized f.
> f. technique
> f. tourniquet
> trigger f.
> f. tuft

F

NOTES

finger *(continued)*
    f. web
    webbed f.
fingerbreadth
Finger-Hugger splint
fingernail
    base of f.
    beak f.
    f. drill
finger-thumb reflex
fingertip
    f. amputation
    f. cold intolerance
    f. dissection
    f. guard
    f. pad
fingertips-to-floor test
finger-to-finger test
finger-to-nose test
fingertrap
    f. suspension
    f. suture
    f. traction
    f. tube
finish bur
finisher
    Küntscher f.
finite element analysis (FEA)
Finkelstein
    F. maneuver
    F. sign
    F. test
    F. test for synovitis
Finn
    F. hinged knee prosthesis
    F. knee system
Finney-Flexirod prosthesis
Finney prosthesis
Finochietto
    F. clamp carrier
    F. rib retractor
Fiorinal with Codeine
firearm injury
Fired-Hendel procedure
firing
    f. pattern
    f. rate
Firm D-Ring wrist support splint
FirmFlex
    F. custom orthosis
    F. custom orthotic
first
    f. carpometacarpal joint fracture
    f. cervical vertebra
    f. cuneiform joint arthrodesis
    f. cuneiform-navicular joint
      arthrodesis
    f. dorsal interosseous assist
    f. dorsal metacarpal artery

    f. dorsal metatarsal artery (FDMA)
    f. intention
    f. intermetacarpal ligament
    f. metacarpal
    f. metatarsal-first cuneiform
      arthrodesis
    f. metatarsal head (FMH)
    f. metatarsus rise test
    f. MTP cheilectomy
    f. plantar metatarsal artery (FPMA)
    f. ray surgery
    f. rib rasp
    f. rib resection
    f. toe Jones repair
    f. web space
    wrist f.
first–fifth intermetatarsal angle
first–second intermetatarsal angle
FirstSTEP Developmental Screening
  Test
Fisch
    F. bone drill irrigator
    F. bone rongeur
    F. drill
Fischer
    F. pressure threshold meter
    F. ring
    F. tendon stripper
    F. transfixing pin
fish
    F. cuneiform osteotomy
    F. cuneiform osteotomy technique
    f. vertebra
Fisher
    F. advancement flap
    F. brace
    F. guide
    F. half pin
    F. Protected Least Significant
      Difference test
    F. rasp
fishmouth
    f. amputation
    f. anastomosis
    f. drain
    f. end-to-end suture
    f. incision
fishtail
    f. deformity
    f. sign
Fiskars scissors
Fisk-Fernandez volar wedge bone graft
FISP
    fast imaging with steady procession
fissure bur
fissured
    f. fracture
    f. nail
Fist-Palm-Side Test

fist position
Fist-Ring Test
fistula, pl. **fistulas, fistulae**
    arteriovenous f. (AVF)
    colocutaneous f.
    enterocutaneous f.
    perilymphatic f. (PLF)
    synovial f.
    vesicocutaneous f.
fistulography
FIT
    Footwear Integration Technology
    Fracture Intervention Trial
fit
    f. and fill
    interference f.
    press f.
    snap f.
    trial f.
Fit-Lastic
    F.-L. therapy band
    F.-L. therapy tubing
fitness
    F. Ball
    F. Safety Standards Committee
Fitnet joint testing system
Fits-All
    F.-A. sling
    F.-A. support
Fitstep
    F. II stair climber
    Universal F.
FITT
    frequency, intensity, time, type
    FITT exercise
fitting
    immediate postsurgical f. (IPSF)
    prosthetic f.
    temporary prosthetic f.
    Velcro f.
Fitzgerald rating
Fixateur
    F. Interne fixation system
    F. Interne rod
    F. Interne screw
fixating apparatus
fixation
    abnormal f.
    Ace-Colles f.
    Ace-Fischer f.
    Ace Unifix f.
    adjunctive screw f.
    Allen-Ferguson Galveston pelvic f.

Ambi f.
AMS intramedullary f.
Anderson pin f.
angled blade-plate f.
anterior cervical f.
anterior internal f.
anterior metallic f.
anterior plate f.
anterior-screw f.
anterior screw f.
anterior spinal f.
AO external f.
AO screw f.
AO spinal internal f.
APR cement f.
arthroscopic screw f.
Association for the Study of
   Internal F. (ASIF)
atlantoaxial rotatory f. (AARF)
Austin chevron osteotomy f.
axial f.
bar bolt f.
Barbour cervical f.
4-bar external f.
Barr open reduction and internal f.
Barr tibial fracture f.
bicortical screw f.
Biofix absorbable f.
biologic f.
blade-plate f.
bolt f.
f. bolt
bone-ingrowth f.
bone suture f.
bridge plate f.
buried K-wire f.
buttressing in internal f.
Calandruccio f.
Campbell screw f.
cementless f.
cerclage wire f.
cervical spine internal f.
cervical spine screw-plate f.
chevron osteotomy with rigid
   screw f.
Childress ankle f.
circular f.
circumferential wire-loop f.
cloverleaf condylar plate f.
Cole tendon f.
compression plate f.
computer-assisted percutaneous
   internal f.

NOTES

F

fixation *(continued)*
condylar screw f.
coracoclavicular screw f.
coracoclavicular suture f.
cross-screw f.
DeBastiani f.
Denham external f.
dens anterior screw f.
Deverle f.
f. device
Dimon-Hughston fracture f.
f. disc
dorsal wire-loop f.
dynamic compression plate f.
dynamic condylar screw f.
dynamic external f.
f. dysfunction
f. dysfunction of lumbar spine
ECT internal fracture f.
elastic f.
Ender nail f.
Ender rod f.
Essex-Lopresti f.
EX-FI-RE external f.
external ring f.
external spinal f.
extramedullary f.
femoral prosthesis f.
fracture f.
Gallie subtalar f.
Galveston pelvic f.
Ganz f.
Georgiade visor halo f.
Gouffon pin f.
graft f.
greenstick f.
Hackethal intramedullary bouquet f.
half-pin f.
Halifax clamp posterior cervical f.
Hammer external f.
Harrington rod f.
Herbert bone screw f.
Hex-Fix external f.
Hoffmann external f.
3-hole suture tendon f.
hook-pin f.
hook-plate f.
Hughes f.
hybrid f.
Ikuta f.
iliac f.
Ilizarov external f.
f. imaging
ingrowth f.
Innovasive f.
interference fit f.
internal fracture f.
internal spinal f.
interosseous wire f.

intersegmental f.
Intrafix f.
intramedullary bouquet f.
intramedullary rod f.
intraosseous f.
intrapedicular f.
f. jig
Kavanaugh-Brower-Mann f.
Kempf internal screw f.
Kirschner pin f.
Kirschner wire f.
Kristiansen-Kofoed external f.
Kronner external f.
Kronner ring f.
K-wire f.
Kyle internal f.
lag screw f.
long-bone f.
loop f.
LPPS hydroxyapatite f.
lumbar pedicle f.
lumbar spine segmental f.
lumbar spine transpedicular f.
Luque-Galveston f.
Luque loop f.
Luque rod f.
Luque segmental f.
Magerl posterior cervical screw f.
Magerl transarticular screw f.
Matta-Saucedo f.
McKeever medullary clavicle f.
mechanical f.
medial malleolus f.
medullary nail f.
Meniscus Arrow f.
Minerva f.
minifragment plate f.
Modulock posterior spinal f.
monofilament wire f.
Monticelli-Spinelli leg f.
Morrissy percutaneous slipped
  epiphysis f.
multiple-point sacral f.
Murray f.
nail plate f.
neutralization plate f.
nonloop f.
Obwegeser-Dalpont internal screw f.
occipitocervical f.
odontoid fracture internal f.
Olerud transpedicular f.
open reduction and internal f.
  (ORIF)
OrthoSorb pin f.
os calcis pin f.
pedicle screw f.
pedicular f.
f. peg
pelvic f.

percutaneous f.
phalangeal fracture f.
Phemister acromioclavicular pin f.
pin f.
f. pin
pin-and-plaster f.
plate f.
plate-screw f.
4-point f.
porous ingrowth f.
posterior cervical f.
posterior screw f.
posterior segmental f.
Precision Osteolock f.
press-fit f.
prophylactic skeletal f.
provisional f.
reduction f.
ReUnite hand f.
Rezaian external f.
rib f.
rigid internal f.
rod sleeve f.
Roger Anderson f.
Rogozinski spinal f.
Roy-Camille posterior screw
plate f.
sacral fusion screw f.
sacral pedicle screw f.
sacral spine f.
sacroiliac extension f.
sacroiliac flexion f.
Sangeorzan internal f.
Schneider f.
Schuind external f.
scoliosis f.
scoliotic curve f.
f. screw
screw f.
screw-and-keel f.
screw-and-plate f.
screw-and-wire f.
screw-plate f.
segmental f.
Seidel intramedullary f.
Shepherd internal screw f.
Slatis f.
SmartTack f.
Spiessel internal screw f.
spinal f.
spinopelvic transiliac f. (STIF)
spondylolisthesis reduction f.
spring f.

Stableloc II external f.
staple f.
static f.
Steinmann pin f.
f. strength
strut plate f.
sublaminar f.
f. subluxation
Sukhtian-Hughes f.
suprasyndesmotic screw f.
Suretac shoulder f.
surgical f.
suture f.
f. technique
tendon f.
tension band f.
thin pin f.
TiMesh implantable hardware f.
transarticular screw f.
transarticular wire f.
transcapitellar wire f.
TransFix ACL system f.
transiliac rod f.
transpedicular f.
transsyndesmotic screw f.
transverse f.
triangular external ankle f.
True-Lok external f.
TSRH rod f.
tunnel-and-sling f.
Turvy internal screw f.
Versa-Fx femoral f.
Vidal-Adrey modified Hoffmann f.
Volkov-Oganesian external f.
VSP f.
Wagner f.
Wasserstein f.
Webb f.
wedge f.
white f.
Wilson-Jacobs tibial f.
wire loop f.
Wisconsin wire f.
Wolvek sternal approximation f.
Zickel nail f.
Zickel subtrochanteric fracture f.

fixator
Ace-Colles external f.
Ace-Fischer external f.
Agee WristJack external f.
AO internal f.
articulated external f.
1-bar external f.

F

NOTES

fixator *(continued)*
 biplanar f.
 Block f.
 cantilever external f.
 carbon fiber f.
 circular fine-wire external f.
 circular wire f.
 Claiborne external f.
 clamp f.
 Clyburn Colles fracture f.
 Clyburn external f.
 Compass Hinge external f.
 DeBastiani external f.
 D-L internal f.
 dynamic axial f. (DAF)
 EBI external f.
 Edwards D-L modular f.
 external f.
 external spinal skeletal f. (ESSF)
 f. frame
 Ganz antishock pelvic f.
 half-pin external f.
 Herbert screw f.
 Hex-Fix monolateral external f.
 hinged articulated f.
 Hoffmann C-series external f.
 Hoffmann dynamic external f.
 Hoffmann-Vidal external f.
 HTO f.
 hybrid external f.
 Ilizarov circular external f.
 Ilizarov external ring f.
 Ilizarov hybrid f.
 Jacquet f.
 Kessler external f.
 L-frame f.
 Lima external f.
 Manuflex external f.
 mini-Hoffmann external f.
 mini-Kessler external f.
 mini-Orthofix f.
 modified Hoffmann quadrilateral external f.
 Monofixateur external f.
 Monticelli-Spinelli f.
 f. muscle
 Olerud internal f.
 Orthofix monolateral femoral external f.
 Oxford f.
 Pennig dynamic wrist f.
 pin external f.
 1-plane bilateral external f.
 2-plane bilateral external f.
 1-plane unilateral external f.
 2-plane unilateral external f.
 Rezaian spinal f.
 Richards Colles external f.
 ring external f.

 Roger Anderson external f.
 spanning external f.
 Stableloc Colles fracture external f.
 temporary external f.
 thin-wire Ilizarov f.
 Thomas f.
 Vermont spinal f. (VSF)
 Wagner device external f.
 Wiltse f.

fixator-augmented nailing
fixed
 f. anatomic patellar implant
 f. bearing knee implant
 f. deformity
 f. distraction
 f. dressing
 f. femoral head prosthesis
 f. flexion contracture (FFC)
 f. hammertoe
 f. hammertoe deformity repair
 f. inversion
 f. sagittal imbalance
 f. torticollis

fixed-angle AO blade-plate
fixed-offset guide
fixer
 Wagner f.

Fixion intramedullary humeral nail
Fix-Sil silicone adhesive
FJD
 facet joint disease
FL
 femur length
FL/AC
 femur length to abdominal circumference ratio
  FL/AC ratio
flaccid
 f. cerebral palsy
 f. flatfoot
 f. gait
 f. leg
 f. paralysis
flaccidity
flag
 f. flap
 f. sign
Flagg fiberglass knee brace
flail
 f. arm
 f. digit
 f. foot
 f. implant
 f. joint
 f. knee
 f. shoulder
 f. toe
flail-elbow hinge

FLAIR
   fluid attenuation inversion recovery
flake hamate fracture
flame-tip bur
Flanagan-Burem apposing hemicylindric
  graft
flange
   endoprosthetic f.
4-flanged nail
flanged revision prosthesis
flank bone
flap
   abdominal f.
   abductor hallucis longus f.
   adductor magnus adductor f.
   adipofascial f.
   advancement f.
   f. amputation
   anterior myocutaneous f.
   anterior tibial fasciocutaneous f.
   arm f.
   arterial f.
   Atasoy-Kleinert f.
   Atasoy triangular advancement f.
   Atasoy volar V-Y f.
   axial pattern f.
   axillary f.
   biaxial f.
   bilobed digital neurovascular
    island f.
   bilobed skin f.
   bipedicle dorsal f.
   brachioradialis f.
   buccinator myomucosal f.
   bursal f.
   butterfly f.
   capsular f.
   capsuloperiosteal f.
   central meniscal f.
   Chinese f.
   cocked-half f.
   composite groin fascial free f.
   f. congestion
   cross-arm f.
   cross-extremity f.
   cross-finger f.
   cross-leg f.
   cutaneous f.
   deltoid f.
   deltopectoral f.
   dorsal cross-finger f.
   dorsalis pedis fasciocutaneous f.
   double-Z rhombic skin f.

DRAM f.
extensor digitorum brevis f.
fascial subcutaneous turn-down f.
fasciocutaneous axial pattern f.
fasciocutaneous island f.
finger f.
Fisher advancement f.
flag f.
flexor hallucis brevis f.
foot first-web f.
forearm f.
free fasciocutaneous f.
free latissimus dorsi f.
free microsurgical f.
free scapular f.
free skin f.
gastrocnemius f.
Gilbert scapular f.
gluteus maximus f.
gracilis f.
f. graft
groin f.
hemipulp f.
horseshoe-shaped f.
hypogastric f.
iliac osteocutaneous f.
iliofemoral pedicle f.
intercostal f.
inverted skin f.
island adipofascial f.
island skin f.
Kutler double lateral
  advancement f.
Kutler lateral V-Y f.
Kutler V-Y f.
lateral arm f.
lateral thigh f.
lateral thoracic f.
latissimus dorsi f.
lazy-V deepithelialized turn-over
  fasciocutaneous f.
Limberg f.
local f.
long posterior f.
medialis pedis f.
medial plantar fasciocutaneous f.
f. meniscal tear
microvascular free muscle f.
Moberg advancement f.
Morrison neurovascular free f.
multistaged carrier f.
muscle f.
musculocutaneous free f.

F

NOTES

flap *(continued)*
    musculotendinous f.
    myocutaneous f.
    neurocutaneous hand f.
    neurovascular free f.
    nutrient f.
    omental f.
    f. operation
    osteocutaneous free f.
    osteomusculocutaneous f.
    osteoperiosteal f.
    palmar advancement f.
    palmar cross-finger f.
    parascapular f.
    pectoralis major f.
    pedicle groin f.
    peroneal island f.
    plantar artery f.
    plantar V-Y advancement f.
    f. plasty
    posterior f.
    pulp f.
    radial-based f.
    radial forearm f.
    random pattern f.
    rectus abdominis f.
    rectus femoris f.
    remote pedicle f.
    reverse cross-finger f.
    reverse-flow f.
    reverse forearm island f.
    rhomboid f.
    rotational f.
    saphenous f.
    scapular f.
    Schrudde rotational f.
    serratus anterior f.
    single-lobed skin f.
    skew f.
    skin f.
    sliding f.
    soft tissue f.
    Steichen neurovascular free f.
    supramalleolar f.
    sural island f.
    temporalis fascia f.
    tensor fascia femoris f.
    tensor fascia lata muscle f.
    thenar f.
    thoracoepigastric f.
    TRAM f.
    transposition f.
    triangular advancement f.
    turn-down tendon f.
    Urbaniak neurovascular free f.
    Urbaniak scapular f.
    vascularized free f.
    V-Y advancement f.
    V-Y Kutler f.

    webspace f.
    wraparound neurovascular free f.
    4-f. Z-plasty
flapless amputation
flare
    f. of condyle
    foot f.
    medial tibial f.
flared spinal rod
FLASH
    fast low-angle shot
FlashCast
    Delta-Lite F.
flat
    f. back deformity
    f. back syndrome
    f. bone
    f. bone graft
    f. chest
    f. drill
    f. flexible foot
    F. Foot insole
    f. hand
    f. metatarsal head
    f. palpation
    f. plate
    f. plate radiography
    f. retractor
    f. splint
flat-bottomed Kerrison rongeur
flat-cut
    f.-c. arthrodesis
    f.-c. technique
flatfoot
    acquired f.
    adult acquired f.
    calcaneovalgus f.
    congenital rocker-bottom f.
    f. deformity
    Durham procedure for f.
    flaccid f.
    f. gait
    hypermobile f.
    Kidner f.
    neonatal f.
    pediatric f.
    peroneal spastic f.
    physiologic f.
    posttraumatic f.
    pronated straight f.
    rigid f.
    rockerbottom f.
    spastic f.
flat-hand test
Flatt
    F. classification
    F. driver
    F. excision
    F. finger-joint prosthesis

F. finger-thumb prosthesis
F. implant
F. recess
F. self-retaining screwdriver
F. technique
F. tendon transfer

flattening of normal lordotic curve
F&L attenuating glove
flattop talus
flatware

Cushion Grip F.
Melaware f.

flava (*pl. of* flavum)
flaval ligament
flavectomy
flavum, pl. **flava**

hypertrophied ligamentum f.

fleck

F. fracture
f. fracture
F. sign

Fleischmann bursa
flesh

proud f.

Fletching femoral hernia implant material
Flex

F. Foam brace
F. Foam orthosis
F. Ranger stretch cable
F. Ranger stretch cable with pulley

flex

f. against gravity
F. H/A total ossicular prosthesis

Flexall gel
Flexderm wound dressing
flexed position
Flex-Foam bandage
Flex-Foot Modular III prosthesis
flexibility

f. conditioning program
Cotrel-Dubousset rod f.
f. exercise
f. training

flexible

f. bandage
f. burn dressing
f. clawtoe deformity
f. digital implant
f. hammertoe
f. hammertoe deformity
f. hinge implant

f. hinge suspension
f. intramedullary nail (FIN)
f. medullary nail
f. medullary reamer
f. orthosis
f. pes planus
f. pes valgus
f. socket
f. sound
f. talipes

Flexicair bed
Flexigrid dressing
Flexi-Grip exercise putty
Flexilite conforming elastic bandage
fleximeter
Flexinet dressing
flexing
flexion

f., abduction, external rotation (FABER)
f., abduction, external rotation (FABER)
f., abduction, external rotation contracture
f., abduction, external rotation, extension (FABERE)
active f.
f., adduction, internal rotation (FADIR)
f., adduction, internal rotation, extension (FADIR, FADIRE)
f. angle
angle of greatest f. (AGF)
f. axis
back f.
f. body cast
f. body jacket
f. bumper
cervical specific rotation in f.
f. compression spine injury stabilization
compressive f.
f. creaking
f. distraction
distractive f.
dorsiflexion f.
elongation, derotation, f. (EDF)
elongation, derotation, lateral f. (EDF)
f. and extension
external rotation in f. (ERF)
femoral trunk f.
forced passive full forward f.

NOTES

flexion *(continued)*
>>forced plantar f.
>>forward f.
>>full fist f.
>>further f. (FF)
>>f. gap
>>f. glove
>>hip f.
>>f. injury posterior atlantoaxial
>>>arthrodesis
>>f. instability
>>internal rotation in f. (IRF)
>>knee f.
>>lateral f.
>>left lateral f.
>>lumbar lateral f.
>>lumbosacral f.
>>f. malposition
>>f. osteotomy
>>palmar f.
>>passive f.
>>resisted active f.
>>f. restriction
>>right lateral f.
>>Riordan finger f.
>>Schober test of lumbar f.
>>shelf f.
>>sitting f.
>>f. spinal radiography test
>>spine f.
>>standing f.
>>f. teardrop fracture
>>toe f.
>>transverse axis knee f.
>>uninhibited f.
>>f. valgus deformity
>>volitional resisted f.

flexion-adduction

flexion-burst fracture

flexion-compression fracture

flexion-distraction
>>f.-d. chiropractic table
>>f.-d. fracture
>>f.-d. injury
>>f.-d. therapy

flexion-extension
>>f.-e. arc
>>f.-e. axis
>>f.-e. control cervical orthosis
>>f.-e. exercise
>>f.-e. gap
>>hip f.-e.
>>f.-e. injury
>>knee f.-e.
>>f.-e. maneuver
>>f.-e. MRI
>>f.-e. plane
>>f.-e. radiography

flexion-internal rotational deformity

flexion-rotation-compression maneuver

flexion-rotation-drawer knee instability test

Flexisplint flexed arm board

FlexiSport orthotic

FlexiTherm
>>F. diabetic diagnostic insole
>>F. Thermographic System

FlexLite hinged knee support

Flex-Master bandage

flexometer
>>Moeltgen f.

flexor
>>anterior long toe f.
>>f. cap
>>f. carpi radialis (FCR)
>>f. carpi radialis muscle
>>f. carpi radialis tendon
>>f. carpi ulnaris (FCU)
>>f. carpi ulnaris muscle
>>f. carpi ulnaris syndrome
>>f. carpi ulnaris tendon
>>f. digiti quinti muscle
>>f. digitorum (FD)
>>f. digitorum brevis (FDB)
>>f. digitorum communis (FDC)
>>f. digitorum communis tendon
>>f. digitorum longus (FDL)
>>f. digitorum longus muscle
>>f. digitorum longus tendon
>>f. digitorum longus tendon
>>>contracture
>>f. digitorum longus tendon transfer
>>f. digitorum profundus (FDP)
>>f. digitorum profundus muscle
>>f. digitorum profundus tendon
>>f. digitorum quinti brevis (FDQB)
>>f. digitorum slip
>>f. digitorum sublimis (FDS)
>>f. digitorum sublimis muscle
>>f. digitorum sublimis tendon
>>f. digitorum superficialis (FDS)
>>f. digitorum superficialis muscle
>>f. digitorum superficialis tendon
>>f. to extensor tendon transfer
>>extrinsic toe f.
>>f. glove
>>f. groove
>>f. hallucis brevis (FHB)
>>f. hallucis brevis flap
>>f. hallucis brevis muscle
>>f. hallucis brevis tendon
>>f. hallucis longus (FHL)
>>f. hallucis longus dysfunction
>>>(FHLD)
>>f. hallucis longus muscle
>>f. hallucis longus release technique
>>f. hallucis longus tendon
>>f. hallucis longus tendon release

f. hallucis longus tenosynovitis
f. hallucis tendon contracture
f. hinge hand-splint brace
f. hinge orthosis
f. hinge splint
long toe f.
f. mechanism
f. origin syndrome
f. phase
f. plate
f. plate release
f. pollicis brevis (FPB)
f. pollicis brevis muscle
f. pollicis brevis tendon
f. pollicis longus (FPL)
f. pollicis longus abductor-plasty
f. pollicis longus muscle
f. pollicis longus tendon
f. profundus tendon
f. pronator slide
f. retinaculum
f. retinaculum of hand
f. skin crease
snapping thumb f.
f. sublimis tendon
f. tendon anastomosis
f. tendon graft
f. tendon laceration
f. tendon repair
f. tendon rupture
f. tendon sheath
f. tenolysis
f. tenosynovectomy
f. tenotomy
toe f.
f. wad
f. wad of 5 muscles
f. withdrawal reflex
flexorplasty
Bunnell modification of Steindler f.
Eyler f.
Steindler f.
flexor-pronator
f.-p. origin
f.-p. origin release
flexor-to-extensor tendon transfer
FlexPosure endoscopic retractor
Flex-Sprint prosthesis
FlexStrand cable
FlexTech knee brace
Flextender Plus hand exerciser
flexural concavity

flexure
perineal f.
Flexzan foam wound dressing
Flip-Flop pillow
flipped meniscus sign
flipper hand
flip test
Floam ankle stirrup brace
floating
f. arch fracture
f. cartilage
f. clavicle
f. elbow
f. gait
f. knee
f. knee fracture classification
f. ligament
f. patella
f. rib
f. shoulder
f. thumb
f. time
f. toe
f. traction
flocculent
f. foci
f. focus of calcification
Flo-Fit Comfortseat
floor
f. of acetabulum
f. mat
f. sitter
floor-reaction ankle-foot orthosis
floppy
f. infant
f. infant syndrome
f. toe
flora
bacterial f.
florid
f. callus
f. reactive periostitis
f. rickets
f. synovitis
Florida
F. back brace
F. cervical brace
F. contraflexion brace
F. extension brace
F. hyperextension brace
F. J-24, J-35, J-45, J-55 brace
F. post-fusion brace
F. spinal brace

F

NOTES

Flotan thumb
Flo-Tech prosthetic socket
Flo-Trol drinking cup
flottant
flounce
    meniscal f.
flow
    blood f.
Flower index
flower-spray ending
flowing hyperostosis
flow-mediated vasodilation (FMD)
flowmeter
    Doppler ultrasound f.
flowmetry
    laser Doppler f.
Flowtron
    F. DVT
    F. pneumatic compression system
      BioCryo system
FLP
    Functional Limitation Profile
fluctuation test
fluff dressing
Fluftex gauze roll
fluid
    f. absorption ability
    f. attenuation inversion recovery (FLAIR)
    f. balance
    f. barrier boot
    bursal f.
    cerebrospinal f.
    f. controlled component
    egress of arthroscopic f.
    f. homeostasis
    hypotonic f.
    interstitial f.
    f. overhydration
    f. prosthesis
    f. sign
    synovial f.
FluidAir bed
fluid-fluid level
fluidotherapy
Fluidotherapy sterile dry heat modality
fluocinolone acetonide
fluorescein
    f. perfusion monitoring
    f. study
Fluori-Methane Topical Spray
FluoroNav virtual fluoroscopy system
fluoroquinolone-associated Achilles tendon disorder
FluoroScan imaging system
fluoroscopic
    f. control
    f. discectomy
    f. table

fluoroscopy
    C-arm f.
    electric joint f.
    intraoperative f.
    2-plane f.
    portable C-arm image intensifier f.
    XiScan f.
flush
    heparinized saline f.
    peroxide f.
flute of cannulated screw
fluted
    f. medullary rod
    f. reamer
    f. Sampson nail
    f. titanium nail
Flynn
    F. femoral neck fracture reduction
    F. technique
FM
    EndoButton FM
FMD
    flow-mediated vasodilation
FMH
    first metatarsal head
FMP acetabular system
fMRI
    functional magnetic resonance imaging
FMS
    fibromyalgia syndrome
    FMS Intracell stick
FO
    foot orthosis
foam
    f. casting
    f. collar
    copolymer f.
    crosslinked EVA copolymer f.
    f. cushion
    Evazote f.
    foam compression molded ethylene vinyl acetate f.
    gelatin f.
    high-density f.
    Neoplush f.
    f. pad
    Pedilen polyurethane f.
    f. pillow
    Plastazote f.
    polyethylene f.
    prosthetic f.
    f. ring
    f. slant
    soft copolymer f.
    f. tape
    Temper F.
    tube f.
    f. tubing
    f. wound dressing

Foamart foot impression system
FoamWrap
- F. BuddyWrap
- F. Final Flexion wrap
- F. finger sling
- F. finger trapper
- F. ThumDuction strap
- F. ThumWrap

focal
- f. calcification
- f. deficiency
- f. dystonia
- f. fibrocartilaginous dysplasia
- f. film distance
- f. nodular myositis
- f. pigmented villonodular synovitis
- f. scleroderma

focus, pl. **foci**
- flocculent foci

Foerster forceps
fold
- asymmetric skin f.
- Bartlett nail f.
- cutaneous f.
- nail f.
- synovial f.

folding
- f. fracture
- f. frame wheelchair

fold-over finger splint
Folex PFS
folic acid
Folius muscle
folliculitis
fomentation therapy
Fomon
- F. chisel
- F. periosteal elevator
- F. periosteotome
- F. rasp

FONAR
- field focused nuclear magnetic resonance
- FONAR Stand-Up MRI

fondaparinux sodium
FOOSH
- fell on outstretched hand
- FOOSH injury

foot, pl. **feet**
- adolescent rigid f.
- f. alignment
- f. anesthetic
- f. angle
- f. and ankle severity scale (FASS)

- arch of f.
- f. architecture
- articulation of f.
- artificial f.
- atavistic f.
- athlete's f.
- ball of f.
- basketball f.
- bifid f.
- broad f.
- burning f.
- calcaneocavus f.
- calcaneovalgus f.
- Carbon Copy II Light F.
- cavovarus f.
- cavus f.
- f. central compartment pressure measurement
- Charcot f.
- Cirrus composite prosthetic f.
- clavus f.
- claw f.
- cleft f.
- f. collapse
- College Park TruStep f.
- ComfortWalk prosthetic f.
- composite prosthetic f.
- contralateral f.
- f. cosmesis
- cosmetically acceptable f.
- C-shaped f.
- f. cushion
- C-Walk foot 1C40 prosthetic f.
- dancer's f.
- dangling f.
- f. decompression
- deconditioned f.
- f. deformity
- diabetic f.
- diabetic Charcot f.
- digital artery of f.
- ding f.
- diplegic f.
- disfigured f.
- f. drape
- dropped f.
- f. drop strap
- Dycor prosthetic f.
- Dynamic Motion F. 1D35
- f. dynamics
- f. dysplasia
- Egyptian f.
- equinocavus f.

F

NOTES

foot (*continued*)
    equinovalgus f.
    equinovarus f.
    equinus f.
    f. first-web flap
    flail f.
    f. flare
    flat flexible f.
    Flex-Walk II prosthetic f.
    forced f.
    Friedreich f.
    functional disability of f.
    F. Function Index (FFI)
    F. Function Index questionnaire
    Greek f.
    Hardy-Clapham classification of
      sesamoid bones of f.
    F. Health Status Questionnaire
    hemiplegic f.
    hollow f.
    hooked f.
    F. Hugger foot support
    hypermobile f.
    hypoflexibility of f.
    immersion f.
    f. imprinter
    inferior extensor of f.
    insensate f.
    f. ischemia
    ischemic f.
    Kingsley Steplite f.
    lateral spring ligament of f.
    F. Levelers custom orthotic
    F. Levelers orthosis
    F. Levelers sandalthotics
    f. lift-off
    lobster-claw f.
    Lo Rider prosthetic f.
    low-arch f.
    Madura f.
    f. magnet
    malodorous f.
    march f.
    f. model
    Morand f.
    Morton f.
    mossy f.
    multiaxis f.
    neuroarthropathic f.
    neuropathic f.
    f. orthosis (FO)
    f. orthotic management
    Otto Bock 1A30 Greissinger
      Plus f.
    Otto Bock 1D25 Dynamic Plus f.
    paralytic f.
    parrot f.
    Pathfinder prosthetic f.
    Persian slipper f.

    f. pillow
    f. placement test
    planovalgus f.
    plantar f.
    plantigrade f.
    f. plate
    polydactylous cleft f.
    f. progression angle (FPA)
    pronated f.
    pronation of f.
    f. prosthesis
    prosthetic f.
    f. puncture wound
    Quantum f.
    reel f.
    Re-Flex VSP artificial f.
    f. rest
    rheumatoid f.
    rigid f.
    rockerbottom f.
    f. rotation
    SACH f.
    SAFE f.
    F. screw system
    serpentine f.
    shortened f.
    single-axis Syme DYCOR f.
    skew f.
    f. slap
    f. sling
    sole of f.
    solid ankle, cushioned heel f.
    spatula f.
    split f.
    f. sprain
    spread f.
    S-shaped f.
    f. stabilization
    f. stabilizer
    f. stagnation
    stairclimber's f.
    f. stool
    f. strain
    f. stump
    superior extensor retinaculum of f.
    supination of f.
    Sure-Flex III prosthetic f.
    Syme Dycor prosthetic f.
    tabetic f.
    taut f.
    The Beachcomber prosthetic f.
    trench f.
    tripod f.
    Trow Bridge TerraRound f.
    f. type
    valgus f.
    Vari-Flex prosthetic f.
    f. volumeter

weak f.
Z f.
foot-ankle
  f.-a. assembly
  f.-a. brace
  f.-a. complex
football
  f. calf
  f. finger
  f. player shoulders
footballer's
  f. ankle
  f. groin
  f. hernia
footbed
  Velocor f.
Footbrush
  Dr. Joseph's Original F.
footdrop
  f. brace
  f. gait
  f. night splint
Foot-Fitter
FootFlex performance stretching device
footgear
Footmaster orthotic
footpiece
  Bunker f.
  traction f.
footplate (*var. of* foot plate)
footprint
  f. analysis
  dynamic f.
  femoral f.
  Harris-Beath f.
  f. index
  f. mat
  static f.
  tibial f.
footrest
Foot-Station 3-D foot imaging system
foot-strike
  f.-s. hemolysis
  f.-s. hemolysis anemia
  f.-s. phase
  f.-s. phase of gait
foot-thigh axis
footwear
  Ambulator biomechanical f.
  Ambulator conform f.
  AquaRunners resistance f.
  Aravon f.
  Comfort Rite f.

F. Integration Technology (FIT)
Milano Shoethotic f.
Mobils Professionals pedorthic f.
forage
  f. core biopsy
  f. procedure
foramen, pl. **foramina**
  arcuate f.
  Hartigan f.
  intravertebral f. (IVF)
  ischiopubic f.
  f. magnum
  f. magnum decompression
  neural f.
  open exit f.
  sciatic f.
  f. transversarium
  Weitbrecht f.
foraminal
  f. compression test
  f. encroachment subluxation
  f. osteophyte encroachment
  f. stenosis
foraminoplasty
  laminaplasty with extended f.
foraminotomy
  neural f.
Forbes
  F. modification of Phemister graft technique
  F. onlay bone graft
force
  activation f.
  f. application
  contact f.
  distraction f.
  dynamic joint f.
  evertor f.
  forefoot f.
  f. gauge
  gravity ground reaction f.
  ground reaction f.
  hamstring f.
  invertor f.
  isometric f.
  joint f.
  knee f.
  lateral compression f.
  moment of f.
  Newton f.
  f. nucleus
  patellofemoral joint reaction f.
  f. plate

NOTES

F

force *(continued)*
    f. plate foot analysis
    prehension f.
    reaction f.
    shearing f.
    subthreshold f.
    tensile f.
    tension f.
    torque f.
    f. transducer
    translatory f.
    weightbearing ground reaction f.
forcé
    brisement f.
    redressement f.
force-couple splint reduction
forced
    f. adduction test
    f. flexion injury
    f. foot
    f. passive full forward flexion
    f. passive internal rotation
    f. plantar flexion
    f. vital capacity
forceps
    Acland clamp-applying f.
    Acufex curved basket f.
    Acufex rotary biting basket f.
    Adson clip-introducing f.
    Adson drill guide f.
    Adson hypophysial f.
    adventitial f.
    Aesculap bipolar cautery f.
    alligator bone-reduction f.
    alligator grasping f.
    Allis tissue f.
    Angell James hypophysectomy f.
    angled-down f.
    angled-up f.
    anterior f.
    AO reduction f.
    arthroscopy basket f.
    arthroscopy grasping f.
    Asch f.
    atraumatic f.
    Babcock f.
    Backhaus towel f.
    Baer bone-cutting f.
    Bane rongeur f.
    Bardeleben bone-holding f.
    basket f.
    bearing-seating f.
    Beasley-Babcock f.
    Berens muscle clamp f.
    biarticular bone-cutting f.
    biopsy f.
    bipolar f.
    Bircher-Ganske cartilage f.
    blunt f.

Boies f.
bone-biting f.
bone-breaking f.
bone-cutting f.
bone-grasping f.
bone-holding f.
bone punch f.
bone-splitting f.
Brand tendon-holding f.
Brand tendon-passing f.
Brown-Adson f.
Brown-Cushing f.
Brown tissue f.
bulldog clamp-applying f.
Cairns hemostatic f.
Carroll bone-holding f.
Carroll dressing f.
Carroll tendon-pulling f.
Carroll tissue f.
cartilage f.
Caspar alligator f.
cervical punch f.
Chandler spinal perforating f.
Charnley wire-holding f.
Citelli punch f.
clamp f.
Cleveland bone-cutting f.
clip-applying f.
clip-bending f.
clip-cutting f.
clip-introducing f.
coagulating f.
Crile f.
cupped grasping f.
curved basket f.
cutting f.
Dawson-Yuhl-Kerrison rongeur f.
Dawson-Yuhl-Leksell rongeur f.
Dawson-Yuhl rongeur f.
Dingman bone-holding f.
disc f.
double-action bone-cutting f.
double-sharp f.
Dreyfus prosthesis f.
drill guide f.
eagle beak bone-cutting f.
Echlin rongeur f.
3-edge cutting f.
end-biting f.
ethmoid f.
extracting f.
Farabeuf bone-holding f.
Farabeuf-Lambotte bone-holding f.
Farrior wire-crimping f.
Ferguson bone-holding f.
Fergusson f.
Ferris-Smith bone-biting f.
Ferris-Smith-Kerrison f.
Ferris-Smith rongeur f.

Ferris-Smith tissue f.
Foerster f.
Friedman rongeur f.
gall duct f.
Gardner bone f.
glenoid-reaming f.
grasping f.
Greene f.
Gunderson bone f.
Gunderson muscle f.
Hajek-Koffler bone punch f.
Halsted f.
Harrington clamp f.
Harrison bone-holding f.
Hartmann mosquito f.
Heermann alligator f.
hemostatic f.
Hibbs bone-cutting f.
Hinderer cartilage f.
Hirsch hypophysis punch f.
Hoen f.
Horsley bone-cutting f.
Horsley-Stille bone-cutting f.
Horsley-Stille rib shears f.
Howmedica Microfixation System f.
Hudson f.
Hurd bone-cutting f.
implant f.
Jackson broad-blade staple f.
Jackson dressing f.
Jackson tendon-seizing f.
Jacobson mosquito f.
James wound f.
Jansen monopolar f.
Jarell f.
Jarit tendon-pulling f.
jeweler's f.
Juers-Lempert rongeur f.
Kelly f.
Kern bone-holding f.
Kern-Lane bone f.
King wound f.
Kleinert-Kutz bone-cutting f.
Kleinert-Kutz rongeur f.
Kleinert-Kutz tendon f.
Knight bone-cutting f.
knotting f.
Kocher f.
Lalonde hook f.
Lambotte bone-holding f.
Landolt spreading f.
Lane bone-holding f.
Lane screw-holding f.

Lane self-retaining bone-holding f.
Langenbeck bone-holding f.
Larsen tendon-holding f.
Leibinger Micro System plate-
  holding f.
Leksell rongeur f.
Lempert rongeur f.
LeRoy clip-applying f.
Lester muscle f.
Lewin bone-holding f.
Lewin spinal perforating f.
lion f.
lion-jaw f.
Liston bone-cutting f.
Liston-Key bone-cutting f.
Liston-Littauer bone-cutting f.
Liston-Stille bone-cutting f.
Littauer-Liston bone-cutting f.
Llorente dissecting f.
long-jaw basket f.
Lore suction tube and tip-
  holding f.
Love-Gruenwald alligator f.
Love-Kerrison rongeur f.
Lowman bone-holding f.
Luer rongeur f.
Luer-Whiting rongeur f.
Luhr Microfixation System plate-
  holding f.
Malis-Jensen microbipolar f.
Malis jeweler bipolar f.
Mantis retrograde f.
Markwalder rib f.
Martin cartilage f.
Mayfield f.
McGee-Priest wire f.
McGee wire-crimping f.
McIndoe rongeur f.
meniscus f.
MicroBite f.
Micro-One dissecting f.
Micro-Two f.
Mixter f.
mosquito f.
mosquito-tip grasping f.
nail-pulling f.
Nicola f.
Niro bone-cutting f.
Niro wire-twisting f.
Olivecrona clip-applying and
  removing f.
orthopaedic f.
Overholt clip-applying f.

F

NOTES

forceps *(continued)*
  perforating f.
  Perman cartilage f.
  pick-up f.
  pin-seating f.
  plain tissue f.
  plate-holding f.
  Poppen f.
  Potts-Smith dressing f.
  Preston ligamentum flavum f.
  punch f.
  Raimondi hemostatic f.
  rat-tooth f.
  reduction f.
  rib f.
  Riches artery f.
  ring f.
  Rochester-Carmalt f.
  Rochester-Ochsner f.
  Rochester-Pean f.
  rongeur f.
  rotary basket f.
  Rowe disimpaction f.
  Rowe glenoid-reaming f.
  Rowe-Harrison bone-holding f.
  Rowe modified-Harrison f.
  Ruskin bone-cutting f.
  Ruskin bone-splitting f.
  Ruskin-Liston bone-cutting f.
  Ruskin rongeur f.
  Ruskin-Rowland bone-cutting f.
  Russian f.
  Samuels f.
  Sauerbruch rib f.
  Schlesinger cervical punch f.
  Schlesinger rongeur f.
  Schwartz clip-applying f.
  Schwartz temporary clamp-
   applying f.
  screw-holding f.
  Seaber f.
  seizing f.
  self-centering bone-holding f.
  self-retaining bone-holding f.
  Selverstone rongeur f.
  Semb bone f.
  Semb rib f.
  septal f.
  sequestrum f.
  Shutt Mantis retrograde f.
  side-cutting basket f.
  small plate f.
  Smithwick clip-applying f.
  smooth-tipped jeweler's f.
  spatula f.
  Spence rongeur f.
  sponge-holding f.
  spreading f.
  Spurling-Kerrison rongeur f.

  Steinmann tendon f.
  Stille-Horsley bone f.
  Stille-Horsley rib f.
  Stille-Liston bone-cutting f.
  Stille-Luer rongeur f.
  Stiwer bone-holding f.
  straight basket f.
  Synthes Microsystems plate-
   holding f.
  tack-and-pin f.
  Take-apart f.
  taper-jaw f.
  tenaculum-reducing f.
  tendon f.
  tendon-braiding f.
  tendon-holding f.
  tendon-passing f.
  tendon-pulling f.
  tendon-retrieving f.
  tendon-seizing f.
  tendon-tunneling f.
  Thompson hip prosthesis f.
  thumb f.
  tissue f.
  titanium microsurgical bipolar f.
  Toennis tumor f.
  toothed tissue f.
  Tudor-Edwards bone-cutting f.
  tumor-grasping f.
  tying f.
  Ulrich bone-holding f.
  Ulrich-St. Gallen f.
  Universal bone grafting/impacting f.
  upbiting basket f.
  upcurved punch f.
  Utrata f.
  Van Buren sequestrum f.
  vascular f.
  Verbrugge bone-holding f.
  Walter-Liston f.
  Walton-Ruskin f.
  Walton wire-pulling f.
  Weller cartilage f.
  Wiet cup f.
  Wilde ethmoid f.
  Wilde rongeur f.
  wire-cutting f.
  wire-extracting f.
  wire-holding f.
  wire prosthesis-crimping f.
  wire-pulling f.
  wire-tightening f.
  wire-twisting f.
  X-long cement f.
  Zimmer-Hoen f.
  Zimmer-Schlesinger f.

force-time integral (FTI)
Ford triangulation technique

forearm
  f. amputation
  balanced f.
  1-bone f.
  3-bone f.
  carrying angle of f.
  f. compartment syndrome
  f. complex
  f. contracture
  distal f.
  f. flap
  f. fracture
  f. ischemic exercise
  f. lift assist adjustable spring-
    loaded device
  f. lift-assist prosthesis
  f. splint
  f. stabilizer
  f. supination test
  f. tourniquet
forefoot
  f. abduction deformity
  f. abductus
  f. adduction correction test
  f. adductovarus
  f. adductus
  f. angulation
  f. arthroplasty
  f. block test
  f. cavus
  f. compression sleeve
  f. digital amputation
  f. disruption
  f. equinus
  f. force
  f. FPA
  hooked f.
  Larmon f.
  narrowing of f.
  f. nerve block
  f. peak pressure
  f. splaying
  f. striker
  f. valgus
  f. varus
forefoot-to-rearfoot striker
foreign
  f. body (FB)
  f. body granuloma
  f. body reaction
  f. body response
  f. body screw
forequarter amputation

Forestier
  F. bowstring sign
  F. disease
forged cobalt-chromium alloy prosthesis
fork
  f. strap
  f. strap prosthetic support
form
  f. constancy
  IKDC f.
  International Knee Documentation
    Committee f.
  International Knee Documentation
    Committee Subjective Knee F.
  Jettmobile positioning and
    tumble f.
  Vestibulator positioning tumble f.
formal hemipelvectomy
formation
  adhesion f.
  beaklike osteophyte f.
  bone f.
  bunion f.
  callous f.
  capsule f.
  Chiari f.
  clavus f.
  coalition f.
  cyclops f.
  gouty tophus f.
  intramembranous f.
  lappet f.
  new bone f.
  osteomyelitic cloaca f.
  osteophyte f.
  periosteal new bone f.
  Pfitzner theory of coalition f.
  pincer nail f.
  procallus f.
  reactive bone f.
  rouleaux f.
  scar f.
  spur f.
  subperiosteal new bone f.
  tophus f.
  trellis f.
Formatray mandibular splint
forme, pl. **formes**
  f. fruste
  formes frustes neurofibromatosis
formula, pl. **formulae, formulas**
  Arth-Aid Joint F.
  Boyd f.

F

NOTES

formula *(continued)*
    digital f.
    Dreyer f.
    pediatric nutritional f.
    vertebral f.
Forrester
    F. cervical collar brace
    F. splint
Forrester-Brown collar
Forte
    F. ES
    F. harness
Fortin finger test
fortitude
    F. Ti titanium spinal fixation
    product
    F. Vue titanium spinal fixation
    product
forward
    f. bending
    f. flexion
    f. flexion posture
    f. head posture
forward-cutting knife
FOS
    fructooligosaccharides
Fosnaugh nail biopsy
fossa, pl. **fossae**
    acetabular f.
    antecubital f.
    bony f.
    femoral f.
    glenoid f.
    intercondylar f.
    ischiorectal f.
    Jobert f.
    lower f. active, lateral knee pain,
    long leg on the side ipsilateral
    to the weak f. (LLL)
    Mohrenheim f.
    olecranon f.
    patellar f.
    popliteal f.
    sphenoidal f.
    supinator f.
    supraclavicular f.
    upper f. active, medial knee pain,
    and short leg on the side
    ipsilateral to the weak f. (UMS)
Foster
    F. bed
    F. splint
    F. turning frame
Foster-Kennedy maneuver
Foucher
    F. classification
    F. classification of epiphysial
    injury
Foucher classification

foulage
foundation
    Arthritis F.
    F. for Chiropractic Education and
    Research (FCER)
    level f.
    Musculoskeletal Transplant F.
    (MTF)
    National Headache F.
    National Osteoporosis F.
    Osteogenesis Imperfecta F. (OIF)
    F. total knee and hip system
fourchée
    main f.
Fourier
    F. analysis
    F. transform infrared spectroscopy
Fournier test
fourth
    f. metacarpal
    f. metatarsophalangeal joint
    f. turbinated bone
fovea, pl. **foveae**
    f. capitis femoris
    f. centralis bone
foveal fat pad
foveate
foveated chest
foveation
Fowler
    F. central slip tenotomy
    F. knee system
    F. maneuver
    F. osteotomy
    F. position
    F. procedure
    F. spread
    F. technique
    F. tendon transfer
    F. tenodesis
    F. test
Fowler-Philip
    F.-P. angle
    F.-P. approach
    F.-P. incision
Fowles
    F. dislocation technique
    F. open reduction
Fox
    F. clavicular splint
    F. extractor-impactor
    F. impactor-extractor
    F. internal fixation apparatus
    F. internal fixation device
    F. wrench
FP5000 pump system
FPA
    foot progression angle

forefoot FPA
hindfoot FPA
FPB
flexor pollicis brevis
FPL
flexor pollicis longus
FPMA
first plantar metatarsal artery
F.R.
F.R. Thompson endoprosthesis
F.R. Thompson femoral prosthesis
fraction
linear f.
motor unit f.
fractional
f. curve
f. lengthening
fractionation
Fractomed splint
fracture
abduction-external rotation f.
accessory navicular f.
accessory ossicle f.
acetabular posterior wall f.
acetabular rim f.
acute avulsion f.
adduction f.
agenetic f.
AIIS avulsion f.
Aitken classification of
epiphysial f.
Allen open reduction of
calcaneal f.
alveolar bone f.
anatomic neck f.
Anderson-Hutchins unstable tibial
shaft f.
angulated f.
ankle mortise f.
anterior calcaneal process f.
anterior column f.
anterolateral compression f.
AO classification of ankle f.
apical non-load-bearing bone f.
apophysial f.
arch f.
articular mass separation f.
articular pillar f.
Atkin epiphysial f.
atlas f.
atraumatic f.
atrophic f.
avulsion chip f.

avulsion stress f.
axial load teardrop f.
backfire f.
Bankart f.
Barton f.
basal neck f.
baseball finger f.
basicervical f.
basilar femoral neck f.
bayonet position of f.
beak f.
f. bed
bedroom f.
bending f.
Bennett basic hand f.
Bennett comminuted f.
Berndt-Harty classification of
transchondral f.
bicolumn f.
bicondylar T-shaped f.
bicondylar Y-shaped f.
bicycle spoke f.
bimalleolar ankle f.
bipartite f.
birth f.
f. blister
blow-in f.
blow-out f.
bone shaft f.
f. boot
boot-top f.
Bosworth f.
both-bone f.
both-column f.
bowing f.
f. box
boxer's f.
Boyd type II f.
f. bracing
Broberg-Morrey f.
bucket-handle f.
buckle f.
bumper f.
bunk bed f.
Burkhalter-Reyes method
phalangeal f.
burst f.
butterfly f.
buttonhole f.
calcaneal avulsion f.
calcaneal displaced f.
calcaneal f. (type I–III)
calcaneus tongue f.

F

NOTES

fracture *(continued)*
    f. callus
    f. callus loading
    Canale-Kelly talar neck f.
    cancellous non-load-bearing bone f.
    capillary f.
    capitellar f.
    capitulum f.
    carpal bone stress f.
    carpal navicular f.
    carpal scaphoid bone f.
    carpometacarpal joint f.
    cartwheel f.
    Cedell f.
    cemental f.
    central talus f.
    cephalomedullary nail f.
    cervical trochanteric f.
    cervical trochanteric displaced f.
    chalk-stick f.
    Chance vertebral f.
    Chaput f.
    chauffeur's f.
    chip f.
    chisel f.
    circumferential f.
    f. classification
    clavicular birth f.
    clay shoveler's f.
    cleavage f.
    closed ankle f.
    closed indirect f.
    closed reduction of f.
    cloven-hoof f.
    coccyx f.
    Colles f.
    collicular f.
    Coltart f.
    combined flexion-distraction injury and burst f.
    combined radial-ulnar-humeral f.
    comminuted bursting f.
    comminuted intraarticular f.
    comminuted pilon f.
    comminuted teardrop f.
    complete f.
    complex f.
    complicated f.
    composite f.
    compound comminuted f. (CCF)
    compression f.
    condylar compression f.
    condylar femoral f.
    condylar split f.
    congenital f.
    contralateral double vertical f.
    contrecoup f.
    f. by contrecoup
    controlled comminuted f.

coracoid f.
corner f.
coronal split f.
coronoid process f.
cortical f.
Cotton ankle f.
cough f.
crack f.
craniofacial dysjunction f.
crush f.
crushed eggshell f.
cuboid f.
cuneiform f.
dancer's f.
Danis-Weber classification of malleolar f.
dashboard f.
f. decompression
f. deformity
delayed healing bone f.
Denis spinal f.
dens f.
dentate f.
depressed f.
de Quervain f.
derby hat f.
Desault f.
Descot f.
diacondylar f.
diametric pelvic f.
diaphysial f.
diastatic f.
dicondylar f.
die punch f.
direct f.
dishpan f.
f. dislocation
displaced intraarticular f.
displaced pilon f.
distal femoral epiphysial f.
distal humeral f.
distal radial f.
distraction of f.
dogleg f.
dome f.
dorsal wing f.
double f.
drill bit f.
Dupuytren f.
Duverney f.
dye punch f.
dyscrasic f.
eggshell f.
elbow f.
elementary f.
elephant-foot f.
Ellis technique for Barton f.
f. en coin
Ender rod fixation of f.

endocrine f.
f. en rave
epicondylar avulsion f.
epiphysial growth plate f.
epiphysial slip f.
epiphysial tibial f.
Essex-Lopresti fixation of
  calcaneal f.
Essex-Lopresti joint depression f.
Essex-Lopresti tongue-type f.
explosion f.
extraarticular f.
extracapsular f.
extraoctave f.
fatigue f.
femoral intratrochanteric f.
femoral neck f.
femoral shaft f.
femoral supracondylar f.
fender f.
f. fever
fibular diaphysial f.
fighter's f.
first carpometacarpal joint f.
fissured f.
f. fixation
f. fixation device
flake hamate f.
Fleck f.
fleck f.
flexion-burst f.
flexion-compression f.
flexion-distraction f.
flexion teardrop f.
floating arch f.
folding f.
forearm f.
fragility f.
f. fragment
f. fragment displacement
f. fragment distraction
f. fragment nonunion
f. fragment separation
f. frame
Freiberg f.
fresh f.
Frykman radial f.
fulcrum f.
Gaenslen f.
Galeazzi f.
f. gap
Garden femoral neck f.
glenoid rim f.

Gosselin f.
graft f.
greater trochanteric femoral f.
greenstick f.
grenade thrower's f.
gross f.
growth plate f.
Guérin f.
gunshot f.
Gustilo-Anderson open clavicular f.
Gustilo tibial f.
Hahn-Steinthal f.
hairline f.
hamate tail f.
hangman's f.
Hawkins talus f. (type 1)
head f.
head-splitting humeral f.
healed f.
f. healing
heat f.
hemicondylar f.
Henderson f.
Herbert scaphoid bone f.
Hermodsson f.
hickory-stick f.
high-energy f.
Hill-Sachs f.
hip avulsion f.
hockey-stick f.
Hoffa f.
Holstein-Lewis f.
hoop stress f.
horizontal f.
humeral head-splitting f.
humeral physial f.
humeral shaft f.
humeral supracondylar f.
Hutchinson f.
hyperextension teardrop f.
hyperflexion teardrop f.
ice skater's f.
idiopathic f.
impacted articular f.
impacted valgus f.
impaction f.
implant f.
impression f.
incomplete f.
indirect f.
inflammatory f.
infraction f.
insufficiency f.

F

NOTES

fracture (*continued*)
    interarticular f.
    intercondylar femoral f.
    intercondylar humeral f.
    intercondylar tibial f.
    internally fixed f.
    interperiosteal f.
    intertrochanteric femoral f.
    intertrochanteric 4-part f.
    F. Intervention Trial (FIT)
    intraarticular calcaneal f.
    intraarticular proximal tibial f.
    intracapsular f.
    intraoperative f.
    intraperiosteal f.
    inverted-Y f.
    ipsilateral femoral neck f.
    ipsilateral femoral shaft f.
    irreducible f.
    ischioacetabular f.
    Jefferson cervical burst f.
    joint depression f.
    Jones f.
    junctional f.
    juvenile Tillaux f.
    juxtaarticular f.
    juxtacortical f.
    Kapandji f.
    knee f.
    Kocher f.
    Kocher-Lorenz f.
    Köhler f.
    laminar f.
    lap seatbelt f.
    lateral column calcaneal f.
    lateral humeral condyle f.
    laterally displaced f.
    lateral malleolus f.
    lateral mass f.
    lateral talar process f.
    lateral tibial plateau f.
    lateral wedge f.
    Lauge-Hansen stage II supination-
      eversion f.
    Laugier f.
    lead pipe f.
    Le Fort fibular f.
    Le Fort II f.
    Le Fort mandible f.
    Le Fort-Wagstaffe f.
    lesser trochanter f.
    f. line
    linear f.
    f. line consolidation
    Lisfranc f.
    Lloyd-Roberts f.
    local compression f.
    local decompression f.
    long bone f.

    longitudinal f.
    long oblique f.
    loose f.
    Looser zone in insufficiency f.
    lorry driver's f.
    low-energy f.
    low lumbar spine f.
    low T humerus f.
    lumbar spine burst f.
    lumbosacral junction f.
    lunate f.
    Maisonneuve fibular f.
    malar f.
    Malgaigne pelvic f.
    malleolar chip f.
    mallet f.
    f. malreduction
    malunited calcaneus f.
    malunited forearm f.
    malunited radial f.
    f. management
    mandibular f.
    march f.
    marginal f.
    Marmor-Lynn f.
    Mason f.
    maxillary f.
    medial column calcaneal f.
    medial epicondyle humeral f.
    medial malleolar f.
    metacarpal neck f.
    metaphysial tibial f.
    metatarsal f.
    middle tibial shaft f.
    midfacial f.
    midfoot f.
    midnight f.
    midshaft f.
    minimally displaced f.
    mini-pilon f.
    missed f.
    monomalleolar ankle f.
    Monteggia forearm f.
    Montercaux f.
    Moore f.
    Mouchet f.
    multangular ridge f.
    multilevel f.
    multipartite f.
    multiple f.
    multiray f.
    navicular dorsal lip f.
    navicular tuberosity f.
    naviculocapitate f.
    f. of necessity
    neck f.
    Neer-Horowitz classification of
      humeral f.
    neoplastic f.

neurogenic f.
neuropathic f.
neurotrophic f.
Newman radial f.
nightstick f.
night-walker f.
nonarticular distal radial f.
noncontiguous f.
nondisplaced f.
nonloadbearing bone f.
nonphysial f.
nonrotational burst f.
nonunion horse-hoof f.
nonunion long-bone f.
nonunion torsion wedge f.
nonunited f.
nutcracker f.
oblique f.
obliquity f.
obturator avulsion f.
occipital condyle f.
occult f.
odontoid condyle f.
old f.
olecranon tip f.
open-book f.
open-break f.
open reduction of f.
open f. (type I, II, III, IIIA, IIIB, IIIC)
ossification-associated f.
osteochondral non-load-bearing bone f.
osteochrondral slice f.
osteoporotic ankle f.
os trigonum f.
Palmer primary f.
paratrooper f.
parry f.
pars interarticularis f.
1-part f.
2-part f.
3-part f.
4-part f.
patellar sleeve f.
pathologic f.
f. pattern
Pauwels f.
pedicle f.
pelvic avulsion f.
pelvic rim f.
pelvic ring f.
pelvic straddle f.

penetrating f.
percutaneous pinning of f.
perforating f.
periarticular f.
periprosthetic f.
peritrochanteric f.
PER-IV f.
pertrochanteric f.
phalangeal diaphysial f.
physial plate f.
physis f.
Piedmont f.
pillow f.
pilon f.
ping-pong f.
Pipkin-type femoral head f.
plafond f.
plastic bowing f.
plateau f.
pond f.
Posada f.
posterior arch f.
posterior column f.
posterior element f.
posterior process f.
posterior talar process f.
posterior wall f.
postirradiation f.
postmortem f.
postoperative f.
Pott ankle f.
Pouteau f.
pressure f.
Prevent Recurrence of Osteoporotic F.'s (PROOF)
profundus artery f.
pronation-abduction f.
pronation-eversion f.
pronation-eversion-external rotation f.
proximal end tibia f.
proximal femoral f.
proximal humeral f.
proximal tibial metaphysial f.
pseudo-Jones f.
puncture f.
pyramidal f.
radial head f.
radial neck f.
radial styloid f.
f. reducing elevator
reduction of f.
f. reduction

F

NOTES

fracture (*continued*)

f. repair
resecting f.
retrodisplaced f.
reverse Barton f.
reverse Colles f.
reverse Monteggia f.
reverse obliquity f.
rib f.
ring f.
f. risk
Rolando f.
rotational burst f.
Ruedi f.
Ruedi-Allgower tibial plafond f.
sacral f.
sacroiliac f.
Salter f.
Salter-Harris f. (type I–VI)
sandbagging long bone f.
Sanders f.
Sangeorzan navicular f.
scaphoid f.
scapular f.
Schatzker f.
secondary f.
segmental f.
Segond tibial avulsion f.
Séguin f.
senile subcapital f.
sentinel f.
SER IV f.
sesamoid f.
shaft f.
shear f.
Shepherd f.
short oblique f.
sideswipe elbow f.
silver-fork f.
simple f.
single-column f.
f. site
f. site nonunion Norland bone
    densitometry
skier's f.
Skillern f.
sleeve f.
small f.
Smith ankle f.
Sneppen talar f.
snowboarder's f.
sourcil f.
spinal f.
spinous process f.
spiral oblique f.
f. splint
splintered f.
split f.
split-depression f.

split heel f.
spontaneous f.
sprain f.
Springer f.
sprinter's f.
f. stabilization
stable burst f.
stairstep f.
Steida f.
stellate f.
step-off of f.
sternum f.
Stieda f.
straddle f.
strain f.
stress f.
styloid f.
subcapital f.
subcutaneous f.
subperiosteal f.
subtrochanteric femoral f.
supination-adduction f.
supination-eversion f.
supination-external rotation IV f.
supracondylar humeral f.
supracondylar Y-shaped f.
suprasyndesmotic f.
supratectal transverse f.
surgical neck f.
sustentaculum tali f.
synchondritic f.
T f.
f. table
talar avulsion f.
talar neck f.
talar osteochondral f.
talus body f.
tarsal bone f.
T condylar f.
teacup f.
teardrop f.
teardrop-shaped flexion-
    compression f.
temporal bone f.
tennis f.
tension f.
thalamic f.
thoracic spine f.
thoracolumbar burst f.
through-and-through f.
thrower's f.
Thurston-Holland f.
tibial plafond f.
tibial plateau f.
tibiofibular f.
Tillaux f.
Tillaux-Chaput f.
toddler's f.
tongue f.

torsional f.
torus f.
total talus f.
traction f.
transcapitate f.
transcervical femoral f.
transchondral f.
transcondylar f.
transepiphysial f.
transhamate f.
transiliac f.
transsacral f.
transscaphoid dislocation f.
transtriquetral f.
transverse process f.
trapezium f.
trimalleolar ankle f.
triplane tibial f.
triquetral f.
trophic f.
T-shaped f.
tuberosity avulsion f.
tuft f.
ulnar styloid f.
unciform f.
uncinate process f.
undisplaced f.
unicondylar f.
unstable f.
ununited f.
vertebral body f.
vertebral plana f.
vertebral stable burst f.
vertebral wedge compression f.
vertical shear f.
volar shear f.
Volkmann f.
Vostal classification of radial f.
V-shaped f.
wagon wheel f.
Wagstaffe f.
Wagstaffe-Le Fort f.
waist f.
Walther f.
Watson-Jones navicular f.
Weber B, C f.
wedge compression f.
wedge flexion-compression f.
wedge-shaped uncomminuted tibial
  plateau f.
willow f.
Wilson f.

Winquist-Hansen classification of
  femoral f.
f. with scoliosis
Y f.
Y-T f.
Zickel f.
ZMC f.
f. zone

fractured
f. bone
f. bone mobility
f. vertebra

fracture-dislocation
atlantoaxial f.-d.
Bennett f.-d.
carpometacarpal f.-d.
Galeazzi f.-d.
intermediate cuneiform f.-d.
Lisfranc f.-d.
Monteggia f.-d.
perilunate f.-d. (PLFD)
posterior f.-d.
f.-d. reduction
tarsometatarsal f.-d.
thoracolumbar spine f.-d.
tibial plateau f.-d.
transcapitate f.-d.
transhamate f.-d.
transtriquetral f.-d.
unstable f.-d.
f.-d. with anterior ligament

fragile X syndrome
fragilitas ossium congenita
fragility fracture
Fragmatome tip
fragment
alignment of fracture f.
anterolateral f.
articular f.
avascular f.
avulsion f.
bone f.
bucket-handle f.
butterfly fracture f.
capital f.
cartilaginous f.
Chaput f.
chondral f.
Comet f.
corner f.
coronoid f.
cortical f.
depression of f.

NOTES

F

fragment *(continued)*
    disc f.
    distal f.
    fracture f.
    free f.
    free-floating cartilaginous f.
    hinged f.
    hypervascular f.
    intraarticular f.
    loose f.
    major fracture f.
    osteochondral f.
    retrolisthesed f.
    retropulsed bony f.
    step-off between bone fracture f.'s
    superomedial f.
    sustentacular f.
    thalamic f.
    Thurston-Holland f.
    tuberosity f.
    wedge-shaped uncomminuted f.
fragmental bone
fragmentation
    endplate f.
    graft f.
fraise
    diamond f.
frame
    Ace-Colles fracture f.
    Ace-Fischer fracture f.
    Ace-Fischer ring f.
    Alexian Brothers overhead f.
    Andrews spinal surgery f.
    anterior quadrilateral triplane f.
    f. application
    Assistant Free hip surgery
      square f.
    Assistant Free hip surgery
      standard f.
    Balkan fracture f.
    basic f. (type **IV**)
    bilateral f.
    Böhler-Braun f.
    Böhler fracture f.
    Böhler reducing f.
    Bradford fracture f.
    Braun f.
    Brooker f.
    Brown-Roberts-Wells stereotactic f.
    Chalet f.
    Chick CLT operating f.
    CircOlectric f.
    claw-type basic f.
    Cole fracture f.
    Cole hyperextension f.
    Crawford head f.
    delta f.
    DePuy rainbow f.
    DePuy reducing f.

    double-ring f.
    Elekta stereotactic head f.
    external fixator f.
    fixator f.
    Foster turning f.
    fracture f.
    fusion f.
    GaitMaster low-profile f.
    Gardner-Wells fixation f.
    Goldthwait f.
    Granberry f.
    Hastings f.
    Herzmark f.
    Hibbs f.
    Hitchcock stereotactic
      immobilization f.
    Hoffmann f.
    Hoffmann-Vidal double f.
    Ilizarov f.
    Jones abduction f.
    Jordan f.
    Kessler traction f.
    laminectomy f.
    Malcolm-Lynn C-RXF cervical
      retractor f.
    Mayfield fixation f.
    Monticelli-Spinelli f.
    pelvic fracture f.
    phantom f.
    Pittsburgh pelvic f.
    1-plane bilateral f.
    2-plane bilateral f.
    1-plane unilateral f.
    2-plane unilateral f.
    4-poster f.
    quadrilateral f.
    rectangular f.
    f. of reduction
    f. of reference
    Relton-Hall f.
    Risser f.
    scoliosis operating f.
    Slatis pelvic fracture f.
    sling f.
    spinal turning f.
    spine f.
    Stealth f.
    Stryker fracture f.
    Stryker turning f.
    Taylor spinal f.
    tent f.
    Thomas f.
    Thompson f.
    triangular ankle fusion f.
    triangulate triple f.
    triple f.
    Wagner f.
    Watson-Jones f.
    Weber f.

Whitman f.
Wilson convex f.
Wolfson f.
Zimmer fracture f.
Zimmer laminectomy f.

Framer
F. finger extension bow
F. splint
F. tendon passer
F. tendon-passing needle

frank
f. diastasis
f. dislocation
F. and Johnson modification
F. and Johnson modification of Heyman procedure

Fränkel
F. neurologic deficit classification
F. sign
F. white line

Frankfort horizontal plane
frayed
f. disc
f. meniscus

fraying of meniscus
Frazer wrist brace
Frazier
F. elevator
F. suction tip

FRD
flexion-rotation-drawer
FRD test

free
f. body diagram
f. fasciocutaneous flap
f. fat graft
f. flap of cartilage
f. flap transfer
f. fragment
f. gracilis muscle transfer
f. latissimus dorsi flap
f. microsurgical flap
f. phalangeal bone autograft
f. pyridinium crosslink
f. revascularized autograft
f. scapular flap
f. skin flap
f. skin graft
f. tie
f. tissue transfer
f. toe transfer
f. vascularized bone transplant
f. weight rehabilitation

Freebody
F. pin
F. stay-retractor

freedom
F. accommodator arch support
F. arthritis support
F. back support
degrees of f. (DOF)
F. elastic long wrist support
F. Micro Pro stimulator
f. of movement
F. neutral position splint
F. omni progressive splint
F. Palm Guard
F. Progressive Resting splint
F. sportsfit splint
F. thumbkeeper
F. thumb spica
F. thumb stabilizer
F. ultimate grip splint
F. USA wristlet

free-floating
f.-f. cartilaginous fragment
f.-f. osteotomy

Free-Flow system prosthesis
freehand
f. CT-guided biopsy
f. cut
F. prosthesis system
f. suturing technique

freely movable joint
Freeman
F. calcaneal fracture classification
F. clamp
F. modular total hip prosthesis

Freeman-high neck press fit prosthesis
Freeman-Samuelson knee prosthesis
Freeman-Sheldon syndrome
Freeman-Swanson
F.-S. knee prosthesis
F.-S. knee system

Freer
F. chisel
F. dissector
F. elevator-dissector
F. periosteal elevator
F. septal elevator

free-spinning probe
free-swinging knee gait
Free-Up massage cream
free-walking velocity
freeze-dried
f.-d. bone

NOTES

F

freeze-dried *(continued)*
    f.-d. bone pin
    f.-d. cancellous allograft
    f.-d. cortical bone
    f.-d. graft
freeze-thawed graft
Freiberg
    F. cartilage knife
    F. disease
    F. fracture
    F. meniscectomy knife
    F. traction
Freiberg-Kohler disease
Frejka
    F. jacket
    F. pillow
    F. pillow orthosis
    F. pillow splint
    F. traction
fremitus
French
    F. adapter
    F. fracture technique
    F. lateral closing-wedge osteotomy
    F. rod bender
    F. scale
    F. supracondylar fracture operation
frenectomy
Frenkel
    F. exercises
    F. movement
    F. track
frenulum, pl. **frenula**
frequency
    f. analysis
    discharge f.
    f., intensity, time, type (FITT)
    onset f.
    recruitment f.
frequency-difference interferential current therapy (FDICT)
freshening of bone
freshen the surface
fresh fracture
fresh-frozen
    f.-f. graft
    f.-f. nonirradiated bone-patellar tendon-bone allograft
Fresnel prism
fretting corrosion
friable
Friatec manual arthroscopy instrument
fricative
friction
    f. artifact
    coefficient of f.
    cross f.
    dynamic f.
    f. lock pin

    f. massage
    patient-on-table f.
    f. rub
frictional torque
friction-reduced
    f.-r. examination table
    f.-r. segmented table
Friedman
    F. bone rongeur
    F. brace
    F. rongeur forceps
    F. splint
    F. support
Friedreich
    F. ataxia
    F. disease
    F. foot
Fries
    F. rheumatoid arthritis score
    F. score for rheumatoid arthritis classification
fringe
    f. joint
    f. of osteophyte
    synovial f.
frog-leg
    f.-l. lateral radiograph
    f.-l. lateral view
    f.-l. position
    f.-l. splint
Fröhlich adiposogenital dystrophy
Frohse
    arcade of F.
    F. arcade of elbow
    F. ligamentous arcade
Froimson
    F. procedure
    F. splint
    F. technique
Froimson-Oh
    F.-O. arm procedure
    F.-O. repair
frôlement
FROM
    full range of motion
Froment
    F. paper sign
    F. ulnar nerve function test
Fromm triangle orthopaedic device
frond
    synovial f.
front
    corset f.
    f. kick explosion
frontal
    f. bone
    f. bossing
    f. motion
    f. plane

f. plane correction
f. plane growth abnormality
f. plane XY
f. plane Z-plasty
f. plate
front-entry guide
fronting of velar
frontoorbital advancement
front-opening orthosis
frontside snowboard stance
frost
F. foot operation
F. foot procedure
F. H-block
F. partial matricectomy
F. posterior tibialis technique
F. posterior tibialis tendon
lengthening
F. stitch
frostbite
f. acroosteolysis
f. of hand
f. injury
frozen
f. pelvis
f. shoulder
f. shoulder syndrome
FRS
fusion and reconstruction system
FRS screw
fructooligosaccharides (FOS)
fruste
forme f.
Frykman
F. distal radius fracture
classification
F. radial fracture
F. wrist fracture classification
F-Scan
F-S. foot force and gait analysis
system
F-S. foot pressure analysis
F-S. in-shoe system
F-S. pressure measurement system
FSH
facioscapulohumeral
FSI
Functional Status Index
FSQ
Functional Status Questionnaire
FSU
functional spinal unit
FT03C transducer

FTA
femorotibial angle
FTC
fibulotalocalcaneal
FTC ligament
FTE
functional tissue engineering
FTI
force-time integral
FTJ
femorotibial joint
FTSG
full-thickness skin graft
Fugl-Meyer
F.-M. evaluation
F.-M. Evaluation of Physical
Performance
Fukuda humeral head retractor
Fukushima C-clamp
fulcrum, pl. **fulcra, fulcrums**
f. distance
f. fracture
joint f.
f. test
fulcruming
Fulford procedure
fulgurate
Fulkerson
F. functional knee score
F. oblique tibial tubercle osteotomy
full
f. cervical spine (FCS)
f. curve
f. fist flexion
f. interference pattern
f. lateral position
f. range of motion (FROM)
f. spine radiographic examination
f. thumb spica cast
f. weightbearing (FWB)
full-circle goniometer
full-curved clamp
Fuller shield dressing
full-hand splint
full-occlusal splint
full-radius
f.-r. resector
f.-r. resector knife
full-thickness
f.-t. cuff tear
f.-t. skin graft (FTSG)
fully constrained tricompartmental knee
prosthesis

F

NOTES

fulminans
>purpura f.

fulminate

function
>adrenergic vagal f.
>ambulatory f.
>bundle f.
>Charnley classification of f.
>cholinergic vagal f.
>concentric f.
>eccentric f.
>hand f.
>intrinsic f.
>Jebsen assessment of hand f.
>LSUMC classification of motor and sensory f.
>motor f.
>neurologic f.
>perverted f.
>physical condition, upper limb function, lower limb function, sensory component, excretory function, support f. (PULSES)
>position of f.
>Quadriplegia Index of F. (QIF)
>reflex f.
>rotator cuff f.
>sensory f.
>splinted in position of f.
>subtalar joint f. (SJF)
>sudomotor f.
>throwing f.
>tibialis posterior f.

functional
>f. activity
>f. ambulation
>f. ambulation category (FAC)
>f. and anatomic loading (FAL)
>f. assessment measure (FAM)
>F. Assessment Staging (FAST)
>f. axial rotation
>f. back pain
>f. capacity assessment
>f. capacity evaluation (FCE)
>f. capacity measurement
>f. disability
>f. disability of foot
>f. electrical stimulation (FES)
>f. fracture brace
>f. grip pushup block
>f. independence measure (FIM)
>F. Independence Measure for Children (WeeFIM)
>f. instability
>F. Integration (FI)
>f. intermetatarsal angle
>f. knee brace
>f. leg length inequality
>F. Limitation Profile (FLP)

>f. loss
>f. magnetic resonance imaging (fMRI)
>f. neuromuscular stimulation
>f. orthotic
>f. performance
>f. phase rehabilitation
>F. Rating Score
>f. recovery
>f. refractory period
>f. restoration
>f. scoliosis
>f. short leg
>f. spinal unit (FSU)
>f. splint
>f. squats back exercise technique
>F. Status Index (FSI)
>F. Status Questionnaire (FSQ)
>f. subluxation
>f. tissue engineering (FTE)
>f. training

functionally debilitating symptom

functioning
>Assessment of Occupational F. (AOF)
>Self-Assessment of Occupational F. (SAOF)

fungal
>f. arthritis
>f. infection

Fungi-Nail antifungal solution

fungoid
>F. AF Topical Solution
>F. Creme

fungous synovitis

funicular excision

funiculitis

funiculus

Funk tibialis posterior tendon dysfunction classification syndrome

funnel
>f. breast
>f. chest
>f. technique

funnelization of metaphysis

funny bone

Funsten supination splint

Funston syndrome

FUO
>fever of undetermined origin

Furacin gauze dressing

furniture brace

furrowing
>scarring and f.

further flexion (FF)

furunculosis

Fusarium solani

fused
>f. ankle

fusiform
f. arthrodesis
f. hip
f. vertebra

fusiform
f. defect
f. periosteal new bone
f. soft tissue swelling

fusimotor
f. neuron
f. system

fusion
Adkins spinal f.
Albee lumbar spinal f.
Anderson ankle f.
ankle f.
anterior cervical f. (ACF)
anterior cervical body f.
anterior cervical discectomy and f.
  (ACDF)
anterior-inferior f.
anterior lumbar vertebral
  interbody f.
anterior and posterior f.
anterior spinal f.
AP f.
atlantoaxial f.
atlantooccipital f.
Bailey-Badgley cervical spine f.
f. bed
BERG lumbar interbody f.
bilateral lateral f.
Blair ankle f.
Bohlman triple-wire f.
bone block f.
Bosworth lumbar spinal f.
Bradford f.
Brooks cervical f.
Brooks-Gallie cervical f.
Brooks-Jenkins atlantoaxial f.
Brooks-Jenkins cervical f.
Brooks-type f.
buried K-wire fixation in digital f.
f. cage
calcaneotibial f.
cervical interbody f.
cervical spine posterior f.
cervicooccipital f.
Chandler hip f.
Charnley compression-type knee f.
chevron f.
Cloward anterior spinal f.
Cloward back f.
CMC f.

Coltart calcaneotibial f.
convex f.
Copeland-Howard scapulothoracic f.
4-corner midcarpal f.
cuboid f.
Davis f.
degenerative lumbar spine f.
degenerative spondylosis
  decompression and f.
Dewar posterior cervical f.
diaphysial-epiphysial f.
digital f.
DIP f.
discectomy with Cloward f.
distal tibiofibular f.
dowel spinal f.
extraarticular hip f.
extraarticular subtalar f.
facet f.
f. facet
f. frame
Gallie atlantoaxial f.
Gallie cervical f.
Gallie subtalar ankle f.
Gallie wire f.
Gissane ankle f.
Goldstein spinal f.
f. graft
Hall facet f.
hammertoe correction with
  interphalangeal f.
H-graft f.
Hibbs spinal f.
Horwitz-Adams ankle f.
Horwitz ankle f.
hyperostotic bony f.
interbody spinal f.
interdigital bone f.
interfacet wiring and f.
interphalangeal f.
interspinous process f.
intertransverse f.
intraarticular hip f.
intraarticular knee f.
joint f.
Kellogg-Speed lumbar spinal f.
Kennedy modification of Gallie
  ankle f.
King intraarticular hip f.
knee f.
Langenskiöld f.
lateral f.
f. limit determination

NOTES

F

293

fusion (*continued*)
long segment spinal f.
lower cervical spine f.
lumbar spine f.
lumbar vertebral interbody f.
lumbosacral f.
lunotriquetral f.
McKeever metatarsophalangeal f.
metatarsocuneiform joint f.
metatarsophalangeal joint f.
minimally invasive lumbar
   interbody f. (MiLIF)
Müller intraarticular shoulder f.
multilevel f.
naviculocuneiform f.
f. nonunion rate
occipitoatlantoaxial f.
occipitocervical f.
pantalar ankle f.
f. plate
posterior cervical f.
posterior lumbar interbody f.
   (PLIF)
posterior spinal f.
posterolateral interbody f. (PLIF)
posterolateral lumbosacral f.
posterolateral spine f.
radiolunate f.
radioscaphoid f.
f. and reconstruction system (FRS)
Robinson anterior cervical f.
Robinson cervical spine f.
Robinson-Southwick f.
Robins-Riley spinal f.
Rowe f.
sacral spine f.
sacroiliac joint f.
salvage f.
scaphocapitate f.
scapulothoracic f.
scoliosis spinal f.
screw f.
selective thoracic spine f.
short segment spinal f.
Simmons cervical spine f.
single-level spinal f.
Smith-Petersen sacroiliac joint f.
Smith-Robinson anterior f.
Smith-Robinson cervical
   interbody f.
Soren ankle f.
spinal f.

2-stage hip f.
Stamm procedure for intraarticular
   hip f.
f. stiffness
subastragalar f.
subaxial posterior cervical spinal f.
subtalar distraction bone block f.
symmetric vertebral f.
talar body f.
talocalcaneal f.
talocrural f.
talonavicular f.
f. technique
thoracic facet f.
thoracic spinal f.
tibiocalcaneal f.
tibiofibular f.
tibiotalar f.
tibiotalocalcaneal ankle f.
transfibular f.
transpedal multiplanar wedge f.
trapeziometacarpal f.
triple tarsal f.
triple-wire f.
triscaphe f.
upper cervical spine f.
vertebral f.
Watkins f.
Watson scaphotrapeziotrapezoidal f.
White posterior ankle f.
Wilson ankle f.
Wiltse bilateral lateral f.
Winter convex f.
Zielke instrumentation for scoliosis
   spinal f.
Fusobacterium nucleatum
fustigation
Futrex body fat analyzer
Futura
   F. conical subtalar implant
   F. flexible digital implant
   F. metal hemi-toe implant
Future implant
Futuro
   F. splint
   F. wrist brace
   F. wrist support
F-wave response
FWB
   full weightbearing
FyBron dressing

G5

G5 Fleximatic massage/percussion
unit
G5 Fleximatic massager/percussor
massager
G5 Porta-Plus muscle stimulator
G5 Vibracare massager/percussor
G5 Vibramatic massage/percussion
unit

**gadolinium-diethylenetriamine pentaacetic
acid**

**gadolinium-labeled diethylenetriamine
pentaacetic acid**

**gadopentetate-dimeglumine-enhanced
magnetic resonance imaging**

GADS

gas atomized dispersion strengthened
GADS technology

Gaenslen

G. fracture
G. osteomyelitis
G. sign
G. spike
G. split-heel incision
G. split-heel technique
G. test

Gaffney

G. ankle prosthesis
G. joint

gag

Dingman mouth g.

Gage

G. distal transfer
G. sign

gain

Body Oscillation Integrates
Neuromuscular G. (BOING)
heat g.

GAIT

great toe arthroplasty implant technique

gait

abductor lurch g.
G. Abnormality Rating Scale
(GARS)
G. Abnormality Rating Scale
Modified Version (GARS-M)
adult g.
g. analysis
angle of g.
antalgic g.
apraxic g.
apropulsive g.
G., Arms, Legs, and Spine
(GALS)

G., Arms, Legs, and Spine
screening
arthrogenic g.
g. assessment
astasia-abasia g.
ataxic g.
avoidance g.
base of g.
batrachian g.
g. belt
g. biomechanics
broad-based g.
cadence of g.
calcaneal g.
cerebellar g.
Charcot g.
Charlie Chaplin g.
choreatic g.
clumsy g.
cogwheel g.
component of g.
crab g.
cross-legged g.
crouch g.
g. cycle
dancing bear g.
g. deviation
g. disorder
g. disorder, autoantibody, late-age
onset, polyneuropathy (GALOP)
g. disturbance
dorsiflexor g.
double-leg stance phase of g.
double-step g.
double-tap g.
drag-to g.
dromedary g.
dropfoot g.
drunken sailor g.
duck-waddle g.
dynamic g.
dystrophic g.
equine g.
extrapyramidal g.
festinating g.
flaccid g.
flatfoot g.
floating g.
footdrop g.
foot-strike phase of g.
free-swinging knee g.
gastrocnemius-soleus g.
glue-footed g.
gluteal g.
gluteus maximus g.

G

gait *(continued)*
    gluteus medius g.
    heel-and-toe g.
    heel-contact phase of g.
    heel-off phase of g.
    heel-strike phase of g.
    heel-toe g.
    helicopod g.
    hemiparetic g.
    hemiplegic g.
    high-steppage g.
    hip extensor g.
    hobbling g.
    hyperextended knee g.
    hysterical g.
    instability g.
    intermittent double-step g.
    internal rotational g.
    intoeing g.
    jerky g.
    kinematic g.
    g. laboratory
    g. line
    listing g.
    g. lock splint (GLS)
    lurching g.
    marche à petits pas g.
    midstance period of g.
    g. and mobility
    myopathic g.
    narrow-base g.
    Oppenheim g.
    opposite foot-strike phase of g.
    opposite toe-off phase of g.
    out-toeing g.
    painful g.
    paraparetic g.
    parkinsonian g.
    g. pathomechanics
    g. pattern
    penguin g.
    petit pas g.
    Petren g.
    pigeon-toeing g.
    g. plate
    2-point g.
    3-point g.
    4-point g.
    propulsion g.
    push-off phase of g.
    reeling g.
    retropulsion of g.
    reversal of fore-aft shear phase
      of g.
    rigid g.
    scissor-leg g.
    scissors g.
    scraping toe g.
    short leg g.

    shuffling g.
    skater's g.
    slap foot g.
    slapping g.
    spastic g.
    spastic equinus g.
    stable g.
    staggering g.
    stamping g.
    stance phase of g.
    star g.
    station and g.
    g. and station
    steppage g.
    stiff g.
    stiff-knee g.
    stiff-legged g.
    stride length of g.
    strike phase of g.
    stuttering of g.
    swaying g.
    swing phase of g.
    swing-through g.
    swing-to g.
    tabetic g.
    tandem g.
    tiptoe g.
    Todd g.
    toe g.
    toe-heel g.
    toeing-in g.
    toeing-out g.
    toe-off phase of g.
    toe-toe g.
    toe-walking g.
    tottering g.
    g. training
    Trendelenburg g.
    tripoding g.
    uncoordinated g.
    unsteady g.
    waddling g.
    wide-based g.
gaiter cast
GaitKeeper cast shoe
GaitMaster low-profile frame
GAITRite mat
Galant
    G. sign
    G. test
Galante hip prosthesis
galaxy
    G. 900HS adjusting table
    G. McManis hylo table
Galeazzi
    G. fracture
    G. fracture-dislocation
    G. hip dislocation sign
    G. patellar operation

G. realignment
G. test
Galen scoliosis
Gallagher rasp
gallamine triethiodide
Gallannaugh plate
gall duct forceps
Gallie
G. ankle arthrodesis
G. approach
G. atlantoaxial arthrodesis
G. atlantoaxial fusion
G. atlantoaxial fusion technique
G. cervical fusion
G. fusion-using cable
G. needle
G. procedure
G. subtalar ankle fusion
G. subtalar fixation
G. wire fixation technique
G. wire fusion
G. wiring technique
gallium-67 scan
gallium citrate scan
Gallo traction
Gallows splint
GALOP
gait disorder, autoantibody, late-age
onset, polyneuropathy
GALOP syndrome
GALS
Gait, Arms, Legs, and Spine
GALS screening
Galt hand drill
galvanic
g. bath
g. electrode stimulator
high-voltage pulsed g.
g. skin response
g. stimulation
galvanism
high-voltage g.
low-voltage g. (LVG)
medical g.
surgical g.
Galveston
G. fixation with TSRH crosslink
G. metacarpal brace
G. Orientation and Amnesia Test
(GOAT)
G. pelvic fixation
G. plate

G. splint
G. technique
game
Boloxie OT Prehension G.
Cone checkers g.
g. knee
g. leg
gamekeeper's
g. injury
g. thumb
g. thumb dislocation
gamma
g. camera
g. camera imaging
G. locking nail
G. trochanteric locking nail
gamma-aminobutyric acid agonist
ganglion, pl. **ganglia**
Acrel g.
g. block
g. cyst
dorsal root g. (DRG)
intraosseous g.
metatarsophalangeal joint g.
periosteal g.
radiocapitellar joint g.
ganglionectomy
dorsal root g.
ganglioneuroma
ganglionic block
ganglionostomy
gangrene
dry g.
gas g.
ischemic g.
Meleney synergistic g.
peripheral g.
postnatal g.
Pott g.
Raynaud g.
synergistic g.
vascular g.
wet g.
gangrenosum
pyoderma g.
gangrenous necrosis
Ganley
G. modification of Keller
arthroplasty
G. splint
G. technique
G. tendon transfer

G

NOTES

Gant
- G. hip arthrodesis
- G. operation
- G. osteotomy

Ganz
- G. antishock pelvic fixator
- G. cup
- G. fixation
- G. periacetabular osteotomy

gap
- g. arthroplasty
- G. cup
- extension g.
- flexion g.
- flexion-extension g.
- fracture g.
- g. healing
- g. nonunion
- scapholunate g.

Garamycin Topical

Garceau
- G. cheilectomy
- G. tendon technique

Garceau-Brahms arthrodesis

Garcia wrist laxity criteria

garden
- G. alignment index
- G. angle
- G. femoral neck fracture
- G. femoral neck fracture classification
- G. screw
- g. spade deformity

Gardner
- G. bone forceps
- G. chair
- G. elevator
- G. operation
- G. syndrome

Gardner-Diamond syndrome

Gardner-Wells
- G.-W. fixation frame
- G.-W. tongs
- G.-W. tong traction

garment
- antishock g.
- compression g.
- console compression g.
- Elvarex compression g.
- Elvarex support g.
- g. hook
- pneumatic g.
- pneumatic antishock g. (PASG)
- support g.

Garré
- chronic sclerosing osteomyelitis of G.
- G. disease

- G. osteitis
- G. sclerosing osteomyelitis

Garrick test

Garrod
- G. disease
- G. fibromatosis

GARS
Gait Abnormality Rating Scale

GARS-M
Gait Abnormality Rating Scale Modified Version

garter strapping

Garth view

Gartland
- G. humeral supracondylar fracture classification
- G. procedure
- G. supracondylar fracture classification
- G. Universal radial fracture classification

GAS
General Adaption Syndrome

gas
- g. atomized dispersion strengthened (GADS)
- g. gangrene
- ionized g.
- g. sterilization

gasless
- balloon-assisted, endoscopic, retroperitoneal, g. (BERG)

gas-producing streptococcal infection

gastrocnemius
- g. angle
- g. bursitis
- g. equinus
- g. flap
- lateral head of g.
- g. lengthening
- g. muscle
- g. recession
- g. resistive exercise
- g. rupture
- g. soleus
- g. tendon
- g. tendon transfer

gastrocnemius-soleus
- g.-s. complex
- g.-s. contracture
- g.-s. fascial strip
- g.-s. gait
- g.-s. junction
- g.-s. muscle
- g.-s. muscle group
- g.-s. recession
- g.-s. stretching
- g.-s. tendon

gastrointestinal
    g. anastomosis (GIA)
    g. tract
gastrosoleal equinus
Gatch bed
gate control theory of pain
Gatellier-Chastang
    G.-C. ankle approach
    G.-C. incision
Gates-Glidden drill
gator plastic orthosis
Gaucher disease
gauge
    acetabular g.
    aneroid g.
    B&L pinch g.
    bone screw depth g.
    bone screw ruler g.
    Charnley femoral condyle radius g.
    Charnley socket g.
    clip g.
    Cloward depth g.
    Cobb g.
    CTS g.
    depth g.
    Durkan CTS g.
    finger g.
    force g.
    isometric strain g.
    Jamar hydraulic pinch g.
    measuring g.
    5.07 monofilament g.
    orthopaedic depth g.
    pain threshold g.
    Philips toe force g.
    pinch g.
    Preston pinch g.
    Rocabado posture g.
    Rosette strain g.
    screw depth g.
    socket g.
    spanner g.
    strain g.
    tourniquet g.
    uniaxial strain g.
    Vernier caliber g.
gauntlet
    AFG ankle/foot g.
    g. anesthesia
    g. atrophy
    g. bandage
    g. cast
    Jobst g.

    leather lacer g.
    wrist g.
gauze
    Adaptic g.
    Cover-Roll g.
    g. dressing
    iodoform g.
    Kerlix g.
    g. packing
    petrolatum g.
    plain g.
    pledget of g.
    Safe-Wrap g.
    g. sponge
    Surgitube tubular g.
    Telfa g.
    g. wrap
Gaynor-Hart
    G.-H. position
    G.-H. x-ray position of carpal
      tunnel
GCT
    giant cell tumor
GDLH posterior spinal system
GD Regainer System
gear
    shoe g.
gearshift probe
gear-stick sign
GEIN
    gradual elongation intramedullary nailing
Geissling rating scale
gel
    Adcon adhesive control g.
    Adcon-L anti-adhesion barrier g.
    Aquasonic Transmission G.
    atelocollagen g.
    Carrington Dermal wound g.
    g. cast
    Ceres' Secret aloe vera g.
    Crystal polymer g.
    g. cushion
    Flexall g.
    Gel Care self-adhesive g.
    Grafton DBM demineralized bone
      graft g.
    Lam IPM Wound G.
    Naftin g.
    osteoinductive enhanced-graft g.
    Oxiplex/SP g.
    g. pack
    silicone g.
    Silipos g.

G

NOTES

gel *(continued)*
    Silosheath g.
    sodium hyaluronate wound g.
    g. stump sock
    g. suspension sleeve
    g. tubing
    g. warmer
    wound g.
    g. wrap
gelatin
    g. compression boot
    g. foam
gelatinous
gelatin-resorcin-formalin glue
GelBand arm band
Gel-Bank patellar strap
Gelfoam
    G. cookie
    G. pack
    G. pledget
    G. stamp
    thrombin-soaked G.
Gel-Foam Ultra-Wedge cushion
Geliperm dressing
gelling phenomenon
Gelman
    G. foot operation
    G. foot procedure
Gelocast
    G. cast
    G. Unna boot compression dressing
    G. Unna boot compression wrap
Gelpi retractor
GelPort hand access laparoscopy
GELS
    gravity extension locking system
Gel-Sole shoe insert
gemellus, pl. **gemelli**
Gemini
    G. chiropractic table
    G. cup
    G. hip system prosthesis
    G. MKII mobile-bearing knee
      implant
Gem total knee system
GEN
    gradual elongation nailing
Genahist Oral
Gendron bariatric wheelchair
general
    g. ability
    G. Adaption Syndrome (GAS)
    g. adjustment
    g. capsular stretch
    g. endotracheal anesthesia
    g. thrust manipulation
generalized fibromatosis
generation
    G. II (GII)

    G. II 3DX brace
    G. II KAFO
    G. II knee brace
    G. II Unloader ADJ knee brace
    G. II Unloader Select knee brace
    Zest Anchor Advanced G. (ZAAG)
generator
    electrosurgical g.
Genesis
    G. arthroplasty hardware
    G. II foot/ankle system
    G. II foot system
    G. II mobile-bearing knee implant
    G. II total knee system
    G. knee prosthesis
    G. unicompartmental knee
genetic scoliosis
genicula (*pl. of* geniculum)
genicular
    g. artery
    g. neuralgia
geniculate
    g. artery
    medial g.
    g. neuralgia
geniculum, pl. **genicula**
genital system
genitofemoral nerve
Gennari band
genotypic chondrodysplasia
gentle
    G. Threads interference screw
    g. traction
GentleStep shoe
genu
    g. recurvatum
    g. valgum
    g. valgum deformity
    g. valgus
    g. varum
    g. varum deformity
    g. varus
Genucentric knee hinge
Genucom
    G. ACL laxity analysis system
    G. arthrometer
    G. knee flexion analysis system
Genutrain
    G. knee brace
    G. PE patellar realignment
    G. P3 knee support
Genzyme Tissue Repair
GeoFlex
    G. knee
    G. knee prosthesis
geographic destruction
Geo-Matt contour cushion
Geo-Mattress bariatric mattress

Geomedic
G. system
G. total knee prosthesis
geometric
g. device
g. supracondylar extension osteotomy
g. total knee prosthesis
Geo Rectangles spinal implant
George
G. line
G. test
Georgiade
G. fixation device
G. visor cervical collar
G. visor cervical traction
G. visor halo fixation
G. visor halo fixation apparatus
Gerard
G. prosthesis
G. resurfacing procedure
Gerber test
Gerbert osteotomy
Gerdy
G. ligament
G. tubercle
geriatric
g. chair trunk support
Löwenstein Occupational Therapy Cognitive Assessment - G. (LOTCA-G)
g. physical therapy
g. trauma
germicidal lamp
germinal matrix
germinative matrix
Gerota capsule
Gerson diet
Gerster
G. bone clamp
G. traction bar
Ger technique
Gertie ball
Gertzbein
G. classification of seat-belt injury
G. seat-belt injury classification
Gerzog bone mallet
Get-A-Grip grip
Ghajar guide
GHL
glenohumeral ligament
Ghon-Sachs complex
Ghon tubercle

GIA
gastrointestinal anastomosis
GIA staple
GIA stapler
Giannestras
G. modification of Lapidus technique
G. oblique metatarsal osteotomy
G. step-down modified osteotomy
giant
g. cell reaction
g. cell reparative granuloma
g. cell sarcoma
g. cell tumor (GCT)
g. cell tumor of tendon sheath
g. motor unit action potential
g. osteoid osteoma
g. popliteal synovial cyst
Gianturco
G. macrocoil
G. prosthesis
gibbosity
gibbous
gibbus
g. deformity
g. deformity of spine
Gibney
G. boot
G. fixation bandage
G. perispondylitis
G. taping
Gibson
G. approach
G. bandage
G. splint
Gibson-Piggott osteotomy
Giebel blade-plate
Giertz rib shears
Giertz-Shoemaker rib shears
Giertz-Stille scissors
Gifford mastoid retractor
gigantism
hyperpituitary g.
pituitary g.
gigas
pes g.
Gigli
G. saw
G. saw blade
G. saw guide
G. saw osteotomy
GII
Generation II

G

NOTES

GII (*continued*)
- GII EasyAnchor
- GII KAFO
- GII Snap-Pak anchor
- GII Unloader ADJ knee brace
- GII Unloader OA brace

Gilbert
- G. harvesting
- G. procedure
- G. scapular flap

Gilchrist
- G. splint
- G. test

Gilfillan humeral prosthesis
Giliberty
- G. acetabular prosthesis
- G. apparatus
- G. bipolar femoral head
- G. device
- G. femoral neck prosthesis
- G. hip prosthesis

gill
- G. arthrodesis
- G. massive sliding graft
- G. posterior bone block
- G. shelf procedure
- G. sliding graft technique

Gillet marching test
Gillette
- G. brace
- G. double-flexure ankle joint
- G. double-flexure ankle joint system
- G. joint orthosis
- G. joint prosthesis
- G. modification
- G. modification of ankle-foot orthosis

Gilliat-Summer nerve-damaged hand
Gillies
- G. bone graft
- G. bone hook
- G. pollicization
- G. prosthesis

Gillies-Dingman hook
Gillis suture
Gill-Manning-White spondylolisthesis
Gillquist
- G. procedure
- G. suction curette
- G. suction tube

Gill-Stein arthrodesis
Gilmer splint
Gilmore groin
Gimbel glove
gimpy
- g. knee
- g. leg

ginglymoarthrodial

ginglymoid joint
ginglymus
ginkgo biloba
Girard keratoprosthesis prosthesis
girdle
- Cadenza g.
- limb g.
- pectoral g.
- pelvic g.
- shoulder g.

Girdlestone
- G. hip procedure
- G. operation
- G. pseudarthrosis
- G. resection
- G. resection arthroplasty
- G. tendon transfer

Girdlestone-Taylor procedure
Gissane
- G. angle
- G. ankle fusion
- G. arthrodesis
- crucial angle of G.
- G. spike

give-way
- g.-w. phenomenon
- g.-w. weakness

giving
- g. way
- g. way of ankle
- g. way of knee

glabella
glabellar rasp
glacier
- G. ceramic 4-in-1 cutting guide
- G. ceramic knee cutting guide
- G. Pack

GLAD
- glenolabral articular disruption
- GLAD lesion

gladiatorum
- herpes g.
- tinea g.

gland
- eccrine sweat g.
- haversian g.
- parathyroid g.
- thyroid g.

Glasgow
- G. Coma Scale
- G. screw

Glasscock ear dressing
Glassman-Engh-Bobyn trochanteric slide
glatiramer acetate
Gleich
- G. osteotomy
- G. osteotomy for pes valgo planus

G-lengthening of semitendinosus tendon

glenohumeral
- g. adhesive capsulitis
- g. arthrodesis
- g. dislocation repair
- g. glide
- g. instability
- g. joint
- g. joint cohesion
- g. joint disease
- g. joint dislocation
- g. joint stability
- g. joint subluxation
- g. ligament (GHL)
- g. pain
- g. shift

glenoid
- g. alignment peg
- g. cartilage
- g. cavitary
- g. cavity
- g. component
- g. concavity
- g. drill
- g. drill guide
- g. fixation screw
- g. fossa
- g. fossa of scapula
- g. implant base impactor
- g. labrum
- lip of g.
- g. metal tray
- g. neck
- g. osteotomy
- g. point
- g. rim
- g. rim fracture
- g. slot

glenoid-reaming forceps
glenolabral
- g. articular disruption (GLAD)
- g. articular disruption lesion
- g. ovoid mass (GLOM)
- g. ovoid mass lesion
- g. ovoid mass sign

glenoplasty
- posterior g.
- Scott posterior g.

Gliadel implant
glide
- anterior g.
- anterior-inferior g.
- anterior-posterior g.
- cervical dorsal g.

- craniocaudal g.
- dorsal g.
- dynamic canal g.
- glenohumeral g.
- g. hole
- g. hole for screw placement
- g. hook
- inferior g.
- mushroom walker g.
- natural apophysial g.'s (NAGS)
- patellar g.
- posterior g.
- posterior-anterior g.
- self-sustained natural apophysial g.'s
- superior g.
- sustained natural apophysial g.'s (SNAGS)
- volar g.

glider
- g. cane
- g. cane board
- EasyStand 6000 g.
- G. II patient transfer system

gliding
- g. hinge joint
- g. hole
- g. layer
- g. mechanism
- g. principle

gliding-hole-first technique
glioma
gliosis
Glisson sling
global
- g. cavus
- g. equinus
- G. Fx shoulder fracture system
- g. metatarsus equinus
- G. total shoulder arthroplasty
- G. total shoulder arthroplasty system
- G. total shoulder implant

globose
GLOM
- glenolabral ovoid mass
- GLOM lesion
- GLOM sign

glomangiosarcoma
glomus tumor
glossopharyngeal neuralgia
glove
- g. anesthesia

G

NOTES

glove *(continued)*
    antivibration g.
    Biobrane g.
    Bio-Form g.
    carpal tunnel g.
    compression g.
    electrode g.
    finger flexion g.
    F&L attenuating g.
    flexion g.
    Gimbel g.
    Handeze fingerless g.
    impact g.
    Isotoner g.
    Jobst g.
    Kevlar g.
    Life Liner stick and cut-resistant g.
    Maxxus orthopaedic latex surgical g.
    Medak g.
    Medarmor puncture-resistant g.
    Necelon surgical g.
    peripheral nerve g.
    pressure g.
    Push-Ease wheelchair g.
    radial nerve g.
    SoftFlex computer g.
    Sorbothane antivibration g.
    surgical g.
    TheraKnit electrode g.
    Tubigrip g.
    vibration g.
    weighted g.
glove-and-stocking anesthesia
GLS
    gait lock splint
    GLS brace
    GLS suture anchor
glubionate
Gluck rib shears
glucocerebroside
glucocorticoid
gluconate
glucosteroid
glue
    cyanoacrylate g.
    gelatin-resorcin-formalin g.
    Histoacryl g.
    skin g.
    Tisseel fibrin g.
glued-to-the-floor phenomenon
glue-footed gait
glutamic-oxaloacetic transaminase
glutamic-pyruvic transaminase
glutaraldehyde
gluteal
    g. artery

    g. bonnet
    g. cleft
    g. fascia
    g. gait
    g. lurch
    g. nerve
    g. reflex
    g. region
    g. sulcus
gluteal/hamstring raise back exercise technique
gluteus
    g. maximus flap
    g. maximus gait
    g. maximus muscle
    g. maximus tensing test
    g. medius gait
    g. medius muscle
    g. medius paralysis
    g. minimus muscle
glycation
    nonenzymatic connective tissue g.
glycocalyx
glycogen sparing
glycosaminoglycan
GMFM
    Gross Motor Function Measure
G-myticin Topical
gnome's calf
goal
    rehabilitation g.
GOAT
    Galveston Orientation and Amnesia Test
goblet incision
Goethe bone
Gohil-Cavolo method
Golaski graft
gold
    g. probe
    g. salt
    g. sodium thiomalate
    g. therapy
    g. weight and wire spring implant material
Goldberg technique
golden
    G. closing wedge osteotomy
    G. Comfort orthotic
    G. Fitness orthotic
    G. mean testing system
Goldenberg footplate shoe
GoldenEye arthroscope
Goldenhar syndrome
gold-handled chuck
Goldman-Fristoe
    G.-F. test
    G.-F. test of articulation
Goldmar opponensplasty

Goldner
G. reconstruction
G. spinal arthrodesis
Goldner-Clippinger technique
gold-paneled chisel
GoldPoint
G. ACL functional knee brace
G. hinged knee brace
G. PCL functional knee brace
Goldstein
G. spinal fusion
G. spinal fusion technique
Goldthwait
G. brace
G. frame
G. sign
golfer
G. elbow
G. elbow test
Thera-Band Exercise System
for G.'s
G. wrist
Golf Exercise System
golf-stick dissector
Golgi
G. apparatus
G. device
G. tendon
G. tendon organ (GTO)
gonadotropin
human chorionic g.
gonalgia
gonarthritis
gonarthromeningitis
gonarthrosis
gonarthrotomy
gonatagra
gonatocele
gonial angle
goniometer
2-arm g.
electronic g.
EOC g.
finger g.
full-circle g.
O'Brien g.
orthopaedic g.
Polk finger g.
Sammons biplane g.
Scerratti g.
Sedan g.
universal full-circle manual g.
Zimmer g.

goniometric
goniometry
gonococcal
g. arthropathy
g. septic arthritis
gonococcic tenosynovitis
gonorrheal
g. heel
g. tenosynovitis
Gonstead
G. pelvic marking system
G. technique
gonycampsis
good
G. Grips utensil
G. 'N Bed wedge
G. rasp
Goode wrap
Goodman orthopaedic bed
Goodwin bone clamp
Goody's Headache Powders
goose-egg edema
gooseneck gouge
Go-Ped motorized scooter
Gordon
G. approach
G. joint injection technique
G. knee phenomenon
G. reflex
G. reflex sign
G. splint
G. squeeze test
Gordon-Broström single-contrast arthrogram
Gordon-Taylor hindquarter amputation
Gore
G. bit
G. smoother
G. smoother crucial tool
Gore-Tex
G.-T. anterior cruciate ligament
G.-T. interpositional arthroplasty
G.-T. knee prosthesis
G.-T. nonabsorbable suture
G.-T. waterproof cast liner
Gorham disease
Gosselin fracture
Gotfried percutaneous compression plating
Gottron
G. papule
G. sign
Gouffon pin fixation

G

NOTES

gouge
    Abbott g.
    Acufex g.
    Alexander g.
    Andrews g.
    Army bone g.
    arthroplasty g.
    Aufranc g.
    Bishop g.
    bone g.
    Buck-Gramcko g.
    Campbell g.
    Capener g.
    Capner g.
    Cobb spinal g.
    curved g.
    gooseneck g.
    Guy g.
    Hibbs g.
    Hoen g.
    Jewett g.
    Killian g.
    Lexer g.
    Lucas g.
    Metzenbaum g.
    Meyerding g.
    Moe g.
    Murphy g.
    orthopaedic g.
    oscillating g.
    Partsch g.
    Read g.
    Rubin g.
    Sheehan g.
    Smith-Petersen curved g.
    Smith-Petersen gooseneck g.
    Smith-Petersen straight g.
    Stagnara g.
    Stille bone g.
    straight g.
    swan-neck g.
    tendon g.
    U.S. Army g.
    Watson-Jones bone g.
    West bone g.
    Zielke g.
    Zimmer g.
Gould procedure
gout
    acute g.
    articular g.
    calcium g.
    chronic tophaceous g.
    latent stage of g.
    tophaceous g.
gouty
    g. arthritis
    g. diet

    g. node
    g. pain
    g. tophaceous deposit
    g. tophus
    g. tophus formation
Gowers
    G. maneuver
    G. muscular dystrophy
    G. phenomenon
    G. sign
    G. syndrome
GPS
    gravitational platelet separation
    GPS system
grab
    g. bar
    g. sign
grabber
    arthroscopic g.
    disc g.
    Tab G.
    tendon g.
grace
    G. method
    G. method of ratio of metatarsal length
    G. plate 4-hole adapter
gracilis
    g. flap
    g. muscle
    g. muscle graft
    g. procedure
    g. syndrome
    g. tendon
    g. test
graciloplasty
    stimulated g.
grade
    g. A, B, C1, C2, D mantle
    g. I, II oscillation
    Kellgren osteoarthritis g.
    Kendall muscle g.
    Meyerding g. I-III
    g.'s 1–5 of mobilization
    Risser g.
    Wagner g.
    Zachary sensory g.
graded
    g. Gore-Tex tape
    g. spinal anesthesia
gradient-recalled acquisition in steady state (GRASS)
grading
    activity g.
    g. of manipulation
    Meyerding g.
    osteoarthritis radiographic g.
    turf toe g.

gradual
    g. elongation intramedullary nailing (GEIN)
    g. elongation nailing (GEN)
graduated
    g. spinal block (GSB)
    g. tenotomy
graduated-height block
Graf
    G. classification
    G. stabilization system
Graflex material
graft
    AAA bone g.
    acetabular augmentation g.
    ACL g.
    advancement flap g.
    Albee bone g.
    allogenic bone g.
    allograft bone g.
    alloplastic g.
    antebrachial fascial g.
    anterior sliding tibial g.
    anterosuperior iliac spine g.
    autochthonous g.
    autogenous cancellous bone g.
    autogenous fibular g.
    autogenous patellar ligament g.
    autogenous quadrupled hamstring tendon g.
    autogenous semitendinosus-gracilis g.
    autologous cancellous bone g.
    autologous reverse g.
    autoplastic g.
    Banks bone g.
    barber-pole vein g.
    bicondylar g.
    bicortical iliac bone g.
    bicortical ilial strip g.
    bifid g.
    biopolymeric g.
    Blair-Brown skin g.
    bone autogenous g.
    bone block g.
    bone chip g.
    bone marrow g.
    bone peg g.
    bone replacement g.
    bone-tendon g.
    bone-tendon-bone g.
    bone-to-bone g.
    Bonfiglio bone g.

    bovine collagen g.
    Boyd dual-onlay bone g.
    BPB autologous g.
    BPTB g.
    Braun skin g.
    bridge g.
    bulk g.
    cable nerve g.
    cadaver bone g.
    calcaneal bone g.
    Calcitite g.
    calcium carbonate bone replacement g.
    calvarial free bone g.
    Campbell onlay bone g.
    cancellous chip bone g.
    cancellous insert g.
    cancellous morselized bone g.
    carbon fiber g.
    cartilage g.
    chemosterilized g.
    chip g.
    Chuinard autogenous bone g.
    Clancy patellar tendon g.
    clothespin spinal fusion g.
    composite rib g.
    composite skin g.
    consolidated g.
    g. containment system
    cortical bone g.
    cortical strut g.
    corticocancellous bone g.
    corticocancellous chip g.
    cutaneous g.
    cylindrical autologous dowel g.
    Dacron g.
    Daniel iliac bone g.
    Davis muscle-pedicle g.
    delayed g.
    demineralized bone g.
    devitalized bone g.
    diamond inlay bone g.
    double-looped gracilis g.
    Douglas skin g.
    g. dowel
    dowel bone g.
    Dragstedt skin g.
    g. driver
    dual onlay cortical bone g.
    dura mater g.
    Esser skin g.
    g. expulsion
    extraarticular g.

NOTES

graft *(continued)*
    fascial g.
    fascia lata freeze-thawed g.
    fascio-fat g.
    fat g.
    fatigue bone g.
    femoral-femoral bypass g.
    femorocrural g.
    femur g.
    fetal substantia nigra g.
    fibular onlay-inlay g.
    fibular strut g.
    filleted g.
    fillet local flap g.
    Fisk-Fernandez volar wedge bone g.
    g. fixation
    Flanagan-Burem apposing hemicylindric g.
    flap g.
    flat bone g.
    flexor tendon g.
    Forbes onlay bone g.
    g. fracture
    g. fragmentation
    free fat g.
    free skin g.
    freeze-dried g.
    freeze-thawed g.
    fresh-frozen g.
    full-thickness skin g. (FTSG)
    fusion g.
    Gillies bone g.
    Gill massive sliding g.
    Golaski g.
    gracilis muscle g.
    Grafton DBM crunch demineralized bone g.
    Grafton DBM flex demineralized bone g.
    Grafton DBM Matrix PLE demineralized bone g.
    Haldeman bone g.
    hamstring g.
    Harris superior acetabular g.
    g. harvest
    Hemashield enhanced g.
    hemicondylar g.
    hemicylindrical bone g.
    Henderson onlay bone g.
    Henry bone g.
    heterodermic g.
    heterogenous g.
    H-graft bone g.
    Hoaglund bone g.
    homogenous g.
    homologous g.
    homoplastic g.
    H-shaped g.
    Huntington bone g.
    iliac bone g. (IBG)
    iliac crest bone g. (ICBG)
    iliac crest bone free g.
    iliac crest-inlay g.
    iliac slot g.
    iliac strut bone g.
    iliotibial band g.
    g. impingement
    Inclan bone g.
    InFuse bone g.
    inlay bone g.
    insert g.
    interbody g.
    intercalary g.
    interpositional tricortical g.
    interposition bone g.
    intramedullary bone g.
    ipsilateral slide g.
    irradiation sterilized g.
    island g.
    isologous g.
    Isotec patellar tendon g.
    Judet g.
    jump g.
    keystone g.
    Krause-Wolfe skin g.
    Kutler V-Y flap g.
    LAD composite g.
    Langenskiöld bone g.
    lateral patellar autologous g.
    Lee anterosuperior iliac spine g.
    Lee bone g.
    ligamentous anterior dislocation composite g.
    load-bearing g.
    lyophilized bone g.
    Massie sliding g.
    massive sliding g.
    matchstick g.
    g. material
    g. material alternative
    Matti-Russe bone g.
    McFarland bone g.
    McMaster bone g.
    medullary bone g.
    meniscus g.
    mesh g.
    Meyers quadratus muscle-pedicle bone g.
    Millesi nerve g.
    Moberg dowel g.
    morcellized bone g.
    morcellized cancellous g.
    Mueller patellar tendon g.
    multiple cancellous chip g.
    muscle pedicle bone g.
    nail bed g.
    nerve g.

neurovascular island g.
Nicoll cancellous bone g.
Nicoll cancellous insert g.
nonisometric g.
nontubed closed distant flap g.
nontubed open distant flap g.
OATS g.
Ollier thick split free g.
Ollier-Thiersch skin g.
onlay bone g.
onlay cancellous iliac g.
OP-1 implant/bone g.
Opteform 100HT bone g.
osteoarticular g.
osteocartilaginous g.
osteochondral g.
osteogenic protein-1 bone g.
osteoperiosteal bone g.
Overton dowel g.
Papineau g.
particulate cancellous bone g.
patellar tendon g.
pedicle bone g.
pedicle fat g.
peg bone g.
percutaneous autogenous dowel
 bone g.
pericardium g.
peroneus brevis g.
Phemister onlay bone g.
pie-crusting skin g.
plantaris tendon g.
porous polyethylene g.
posterior bone g.
posterior cruciate ligament g.
posterolateral bone g.
powdered bone g.
g. preparation
prophylactic bone g.
prosthetic femorodistal g.
PTFE g.
rectus femoris g.
revascularization of g.
Reverdin epidermal free g.
rib g.
Russe bone g.
Ryerson bone g.
sandwiched iliac bone g.
scapular g.
segmental tendon g.
semitendinosus-gracilis g.
semitendinous g.
single-condylar g.

single-onlay cortical bone g.
single-stage tendon g.
skin g.
sliding bone g.
soft tissue g.
Soto-Hall bone g.
split calvarial bone g.
split-thickness skin g. (STSG)
Stark g.
g. strength
structural bone g.
g. structure
strut bone g.
subclavius tendon g.
Tait g.
temporal fascia g.
tendon g. (TG)
g. tension
tension-free Millesi nerve g.
textured allograft bone g.
Thiersch medium split free g.
Thiersch thin split free g.
Thomas extrapolated bar g.
tibial bone g.
tricortical iliac crest bone g.
tricortical ilial strip g.
tube flap g.
tubularization of g.
tumbler g.
vascularized bone g.
vascularized fibular g.
vascularized osteoseptocutaneous
 fibular autogenous g.
vascularized rib strut g.
VertiGraft textured allograft
 bone g.
wedge g.
Weiland iliac crest bone g.
Whitecloud-LaRocca fibular strut g.
Wilson bone g.
Wolfe hand surgery g.
Wolf full-thickness free g.
wraparound flap bone g.
Z-plasty local flap g.
graft-bony tunnel wall abrasion
Graftech
 G. structural allograft anterior ramp
 G. structural allograft cervical
 dowel
 G. structural allograft cervical
 spacer
 G. structural allograft posterior
 ramp

NOTES

grafted
> g. bone
> g. material

grafting vein

GraftJacket regenerative tissue repair matrix

Graftmaster device

Grafton
> G. bone matrix/marrow combination
> G. DBM crunch demineralized bone graft
> G. DBM demineralized bone graft gel
> G. DBM flex demineralized bone graft
> G. DBM Matrix demineralized bone graft plug
> G. DBM Matrix PLE demineralized bone graft
> G. DBM putty
> G. demineralized bone matrix putty material
> G. Plus DBM demineralized bone graft paste

Graham
> G. ankle arthrodesis
> G. muscle hook
> G. nerve hook
> G. traction

Grahamizer I exerciser

Gram-negative

Gram-positive

Gram stain

Granberg cervical traction system

Granberry
> G. frame
> G. traction

Grand Stand support stand

Grantham femur fracture classification

Grant, Surrall, and Lehman procedure

Granuflex dressing

granular
> g. cell myoblastoma
> g. histiocytosis

granulation
> extradural g.
> healing by g.
> g. phase
> g. tissue

granule
> ProOsteon Implant 500 g.

granuloma
> eosinophilic g.
> foreign body g.
> giant cell reparative g.
> Mignon eosinophilic g.
> pyogenic g.
> g. pyogenicum
> reparative g.

rheumatic g.
subperiosteal giant cell reparative g.
subungual g.
swimming pool g.
tubercular g.

granulomatosis
> Langerhans cell g.
> Wegener g.

granulomatous
> g. fungal infection
> g. mass
> g. myositis
> g. tenosynovitis

graph
> Moseley bone age g.
> Moseley straight line g.

Graphic Rating Scale (GRS)

graphospasm

Grashey view

grasp
> hook g.
> pinch g.
> prehension g.
> g. reflex
> thumb-pinch g.

grasper
> Acufex g.
> loose body g.
> pituitary g.

grasper-cutter
> Questus leading edge g.-c.

grasping
> g. forceps
> g. power
> g. suture

GRASS
> gradient-recalled acquisition in steady state

grasshopper
> g. patella
> G. positioner

Grass neurostimulator

grater reamer

Graves scapula

gravis
> myasthenia g.
> Tensilon test for myasthenia g.

gravitational
> g. insecurity
> g. line
> g. platelet separation (GPS)
> g. platelet separation system
> g. proprioception

gravity
> center of g. (CG, COG)
> g. drawer test
> g. equinus cast

g. extension locking system (GELS)
flex against g.
g. ground reaction force
g. inflow irrigation
line of g.
g. method
g. method of Stimson
g. plumb line
g. stress test

gravity-driven angle finder

gray

G. bone drill
g. matter
periaqueductal g. (PAG)
G. ramus communicans
G. reamer
G. revision instrument system

Grayson

G. ligament
G. ligament in hand

grease gun injury

great

g. sciatic nerve
g. toe
g. toe amputation
g. toe arthroplasty implant technique (GAIT)
g. toe bone
g. toe implant
g. toe implant prosthesis
g. toe push-off
g. toe reflex
g. vessel

greater

g. multangular
g. multangular bone
g. multangular ridge
g. pelvis
g. rhomboid muscle
g. trochanter
g. trochanteric apophysial arrest
g. trochanteric femoral fracture
g. tuberosity
g. tuberosity osteotomy

Greek foot

green

G. arthroplasty
G. muscle hook
G. and OʹBrien wrist function score
G. procedure
G. transfer

Green-Anderson growth table
Green-Banks technique
Greenberg clamp
Greene forceps
Greenfield

G. osteotomy
G. spinocerebellar ataxia classification

Green-Grice procedure
Green-Laird

G.-L. modification
G.-L. modification of Reverdin osteotomy

Green-O'Brien evaluation system
Green-Reverdin osteotomy
Green-Seligson-Henry (GSH)

G.-S.-H. nail

greenstick

g. dorsal proximal metatarsal osteotomy
g. fixation
g. fracture

Green-Watermann osteotomy
Greifer prosthesis
Greissinger

G. foot prosthesis
G. Multiaxis joint

Grelot

image en G.

grenade

g. thrower's arm
g. thrower's fracture

Greulich-Pyle

G.-P. bone age
G.-P. skeletal maturation stage
G.-P. technique

Grice

G. extraarticular subtalar arthrodesis
G. incision
G. procedure

Grice-Green

G.-G. extraarticular subtalar arthrodesis
G.-G. operation
G.-G. technique

grid

electrode g.
g. maze board
g. maze set
radiographic g.
Shar-Tek foot positioning g.

Grierson meniscal shaver

G

NOTES

griffe
  main en g.
Griffith incision
grimace test
grinder
  DePuy calcar g.
grinding test
grip
  dowel g.
  Get-A-Grip g.
  key g.
  g. lock
  pencil g.
  Posey g.
  Skil-Care cushion g.
  g. strength
  g. strength test
  syringe g.
  g. tester
  ulnar side g.
Grip-Ease device
Gripp
  G. squeeze ball
  G. squeeze ball hand exerciser
Gripper acetabular cup prosthesis
gripping exercises
GripTrack Commander strength tester
Grisactin Ultra
Grisel
  G. disease
  G. syndrome
Gristina-Webb total shoulder arthroplasty
Griswold distraction machine
grit-blasted prosthesis
Gritti
  G. amputation
  G. operation
Gritti-Stokes
  G.-S. amputation
  G.-S. distal thigh procedure
  G.-S. knee prosthesis
groin
  g. flap
  footballer's g.
  Gilmore g.
  g. pain
groin-to-ankle cast
grommet
  g. bone liner
  circumferential g.
  press-fit circumferential g.
  titanium circumferential g.
groove
  anular g.
  bicipital g.
  deltopectoral g.
  g. distal tibia
  femoral g.

fibular g.
flexor g.
intercollicular g.
intercondylar g.
intertubercular g.
nail g.
parasagittal g.
patellar g.
patellofemoral g.
peroneal g.
g. of Ranvier
spiral humeral g.
trochlear g.
grooved
  g. director
  g. dissector
  G. Pegboard Test
  g. protector
grooving
  g. osteotome
  g. reamer
gross
  g. fracture
  g. manipulation
  G. Motor Function Measure (GMFM)
Grosse-Kempf
  G.-K. interlocking medullary nail
  G.-K. interlocking medullary nailing
  G.-K. locking nail
  G.-K. tibial technique
ground
  g. electrode
  g. lamella
  purchase and press the g.
  g. reaction
  g. reaction force
group
  activity g.
  adductor muscle g.
  ancillary muscle g.
  AO g.
  g. fascicular repair
  gastrocnemius-soleus muscle g.
  levator ani g.
  muscle g. (MG)
  PROOF g.
  quadriceps muscle g.
grouped discharge
Grover
  G. meniscotome
  G. meniscus knife
Groves opponensplasty
growing pain
growth
  anchorage-dependent g.
  appositional g.
  g. arrest
  g. arrest line

asymmetrical g.
bone g.
g. center
g. center of bone
chondroosseous g.
ectopic bone g.
g. hormone
g. hormone hypersecretion
g. hormone resistance
latitudinal g.
physial g.
g. plate
g. plate abscess
g. plate fracture
g. plate injury
g. prediction
g. retardation
g. zone
GRS
Graphic Rating Scale
Gruca lower leg procedure
Gruca-Weiss spring
Gruen
G. mode
G. zone
gryphotic toenail
GSB
graduated spinal block
GSB elbow prosthesis
GSB expanded version for knee
prosthesis
GSH
Green-Seligson-Henry
GSH nail
G suit
GTO
Golgi tendon organ
GTS 2-piece implant system
guard
ankle g.
Cloward cervical drill g.
drill g.
fingertip g.
Freedom Palm G.
McDavid ankle g.
McDavid hinged knee g.
Omed vented instrument g.
PAL-Guard postamputation limb g.
palm g.
pin g.
Pro-Designed wrist g.
Progressive palm g.
Ullrich drill g.

guarded osteotome
guardian
G. limb salvage system
G. Red Dot walker
guarding
muscle g.
Guardsman femoral interference screw
Gubler tumor
Gudas
G. scarf Z-plasty
G. scarf Z-plasty osteotomy
Guepar hinged knee prosthesis
Guérin fracture
Guhl
G. distraction
G. technique
guide
Accu-Cut osteotomy g.
Accu-Line g.
acetabular cup peg drill g.
Achillon instrument g.
ACL drill g.
Acufex alignment g.
Acufex tibial g.
Adapteur multifunctional drill g.
adjustable angle g.
Adson drill g.
Adson saw g.
aiming g.
alignment g.
angel wing g.
apical axis g.
Arthrex femoral g.
Arthrex tibial g.
axis g.
Bailey-Gigli saw g.
Bailey saw g.
ball-tipped Küntscher g.
g. barrel
barrel g.
Blair saw g.
bone wire g.
Bow & Arrow cannulated drill g.
Bullseye femoral g.
g. bushing
calibrated pin g.
Cloward drill g.
contoured anterior spinal plate
drill g.
Cushing-Gigli saw g.
Cushing saw g.
cutter g.
Davis saw g.

G

NOTES

guide *(continued)*
    Delta Recon proximal drill g.
    DePuy femoral acetabular
      overlay g.
    distal femoral cutting g.
    drill g.
    eccentric drill g.
    Evolis femoral cutting g.
    extramedullary alignment g.
    femoral intramedullary g.
    femoral notch g.
    Ferkel C g.
    FIN pin g.
    Fisher g.
    fixed-offset g.
    front-entry g.
    Ghajar g.
    Gigli saw g.
    Glacier ceramic 4-in-1 cutting g.
    Glacier ceramic knee cutting g.
    glenoid drill g.
    handheld drill g.
    Hewson cruciate g.
    Hewson ligament drill g.
    Hoffmann pin g.
    g. hole
    Howell tibial g.
    humeral cutting g.
    intercondylar drill g.
    intramedullary g.
    Lebsche saw g.
    Levin drill g.
    ligature g.
    Lipscomb-Anderson drill g.
    long axial alignment g.
    long nail-mounted drill g.
    Modny g.
    nail-driving g.
    nail rotational g.
    neutral drill g.
    notch cutting g.
    nut alignment g.
    patellar drill g.
    patellar reamer g.
    patellar resection g.
    PCA cutting g.
    PCA medullary g.
    picket fence g.
    pin g.
    g. pin
    Poppen Gigli saw g.
    ProTrac alignment g.
    Puddu drill g.
    Raney saw g.
    reamer g.
    rear-entry ACL drill g.
    Reece osteotomy g.
    Richards angle g.
    Richards drill g.

    g. rod
    saw g.
    scaphoid screw g.
    Scott-RCE osteotomy g.
    screw angle g.
    Stader pin g.
    stationary angle g.
    Synthes wire g.
    targeting drill g.
    T-Bar g.
    telescopic view g.
    tibial cutting g.
    tibial drill g.
    tissue anchor g. (TAG)
    Todd-Wells g.
    tube g.
    tunnel drill g.
    tunnel locator g.
    Tworek screw g.
    Uslenghi drill g.
    g. wire
    wire and drill g.
    wound measuring g.
    Yasargil ligature g.
guideline
    AHCPR g.'s
    Böhler g.
    Hartel g.
    Letournel g.
guidepin, guide pin
    AO g.
    ball g.
    ball-point g.
    ball-tip g.
    beaded reamer g.
    calibrated g.
    femoral g.
    lateral g.
    nonbeaded g.
    precurved ball-tipped g.
    Rica wire g.
    Synthes g.
    threaded g.
    tibial g.
    Watson-Jones g.
guidewire, guide wire
    beaded g.
    drill-tipped g.
    Suretac g.
Guilford cervical brace
Guilford-Wright prosthesis
Guillain-Barré syndrome
Guilland sign
guillotine
    g. amputation
    Charnley femoral inlay g.
Guldmann Overhead Trac System
Guleke bone rongeur
Gulick II tape

Guller resection
gull-wing deformity
Gumboro disease
Gumley seat beat injury classification
gummatous
g. abscess
g. necrosis
gum rubber Martin bandage
gun
Arthrex meniscal dart g.
g. barrel sign
Biofix arrow g.
cement injection g.
CMW cement g.
Harris cement g.
heat g.
Reflex G.
rivet g.
staple g.
Sterivap cement g.
Gunderson
G. bone forceps
G. muscle forceps
Gunning splint
Gunn jaw winking
gunshot
g. fracture
g. wound
GunSlinger shoulder orthosis
gunstock deformity
Gunston
G. arthroplasty
G. polycentric knee prosthesis
Gunston-Hult knee prosthesis
Gurd
G. procedure
G. resection
Gustilo
G. classification of puncture wound
G. hip prosthesis
G. knee prosthesis
G. puncture wound classification
G. tibial fracture
G. tibial fracture classification
G. unconstrained prosthesis
Gustilo-Anderson
G.-A. open clavicular fracture

G.-A. open fracture classification
G.-A. tibial plafond fracture
classification
Gustilo-Kyle
G.-K. cementless total hip
arthroplasty
G.-K. femoral component
gutter
g. cast
g. splint
Guttmann
G. subtalar arthrodesis
G. technique
guy
G. gouge
g. suture
Guyon
G. amputation
G. canal
G. operation
G. tunnel release
G. tunnel syndrome
G/W Heel Lift, Inc. orthosis
gym
g. ball
Elite Power Station g.
hand g.
limb g.
Total G.
Zuni g.
gymball
Dyna-Disc g.
Exertools g.
Gymmy exercise unit
gymnastics
pommel horse g.
Swedish g.
Gymnastik ball
gymnast's wrist
Gymnic Plus exercise ball
Gynogen L.A. Injection
Gypsona
G. cast
G. cast material
Gyro-Flex upper extremity exerciser
Gyroscan superconducting MRI

NOTES

G

H

H buttress support patellofemoral brace
H reflex
H region
H wave
H1209 healing shoe
H1215 healing shoe
H2 blocker
HA
hallux abductus
hyaluronan
hydroxyapatite
HA 65101 implant metal
HA 65101 implant metal prosthesis
Haas
H. disease
H. operation
H. osteotomy
H. paralysis
habit scoliosis
habitual
h. control
h. dislocation
h. patella luxation
habituation
habitus
varus h.
Hackethal
H. intramedullary bouquet fixation
H. nail
H. stacked nailing technique
hacking
hacksaw
HA-coated hip implant
Haddad metatarsal osteotomy
Hadfield hand board
Hadley S-curve
Haemophilus
H. influenzae
H. parainfluenzae
Hafnia alvei
Hagie
H. hip pin
H. pin nail
H. sliding nail plate
HAGL
humeral avulsion of glenohumeral ligament
HAGL lesion
Haglund
H. bump
H. disease
H. exostosis

H. foot deformity
H. syndrome
Haglund-Stille plaster spreader
Hahn
H. bone nail
H. cleft
H. screw
Hahn-Steinthal
H.-S. capitellum fracture classification
H.-S. fracture
H.-S. fracture of capitellum
Haid
H. cervical plate
H. UBP system
H. Universal bone plate
hairline
h. crack
h. fracture
hairpin
h. knot
h. splint
Hajdu-Cheney syndrome
Hajdu staging system
Hajek
H. chisel
H. mallet
Hajek-Ballenger dissector
Hajek-Koffler bone punch forceps
Haldeman bone graft
Halder locking nail
half
h. ring
h. ring leg splint
half-and-half nail
half-circle plate
half-hitch arthroscopic knot
half-moon sign
half-pin
h.-p. external fixator
h.-p. fixation
half-shell splint
half-shoe
half-stitch arthroscopic knot
Halifax
H. clamp posterior cervical fixation
H. interlaminar clamp
H. interlaminar clamp kit
halisteresis phenomenon
Hall
H. air drill
H. air-driven oscillating saw
H. bur
H. double-hole spinal stapler
H. driver

H

Hall *(continued)*
    H. facet fusion
    H. Kalamchi shelf procedure
    H. mandibular implant system
    H. Micro-Aire drill
    H. Micro E power instrument
    H. modular acetabular reamer
      system
    H. Neurairtome
    H. power drill
    H. sagittal saw
    H. screwdriver
    H. series 4 large bone instrument
    H. spinal screw
    H. stepdown drill
    H. technique
    H. Versipower drill
    H. Versipower oscillating saw
    H. Versipower reamer
    H. Versipower reciprocating saw
Hall-Dundar drill
Halle bone curette
Hall-effect strain transducer
Hallpike maneuver
hallucal sesamoid
halluces (*pl. of* hallux)
hallucination
    stump h.
hallucis
    accessory abductor h.
    h. brevis tenodesis
    extensor h.
    hyperdynamic abductor h.
    h. longus laceration
hallux, pl. **halluces**
    h. abductovalgus (HAV)
    h. abductus (HA)
    clawed h.
    h. dolorosus
    dropped h.
    h. elevatus
    h. extensus
    hammer h.
    h. interphalangeal joint arthrodesis
    intrinsic minus h.
    h. IP joint
    h. limitus
    h. limitus deformity
    h. malleus
    h. metatarsophalangeal
      interphalangeal scale (HMIS)
    h. migration
    h. nail
    rectus h.
    h. rigidus
    h. rigidus arthrodesis
    h. sesamoid
    h. valgus (HV)
    h. valgus angle (HVA)

    h. valgus deformity
    h. valgus interphalangeus angle
    h. valgus-metatarsus primus varus
      complex
    h. valgus night splint
    h. valgus orthosis
    h. valgus procedure
    h. varus
    h. varus correction
    h. varus deformity
Hall-Zimmer power instrument
halo
    h. body jacket
    h. brace
    BRW head ring h.
    h. cast
    h. cervical orthosis
    h. cervical traction
    h. cervical traction system
    h. extension orthosis
    h. immobilization
    Lerman noninvasive h.
    h. nevus
    h. pedestal
    pericellular h.
    Perry-Nickel cranial h.
    h. pin
    h. ring
    h. sign
    h. traction jacket
    h. traction orthosis
    Twin Cities Lo-Profile h.
    h. vest
    h. vest apparatus
    h. vest device
halo-cast distraction
halo-dependent traction
halo-femoral
    h.-f. distraction
    h.-f. traction
halogen lamp
halo-gravity traction device
halo-Ilizarov distraction instrumentation
halo-pelvic
    h.-p. distraction
    h.-p. traction
halo-vest orthosis
halo-wheelchair traction
Halsey
    H. nail scissors
    H. needle holder
Halsted
    H. forceps
    H. maneuver
halter
    DePuy h.
    Diskard head h.
    head h.
    Repro head h.

h. traction
Upper 7 head h.
Zimfoam head h.
Zimmer head h.
hamartoma
cartilaginous h.
chondromatous h.
fibrous h.
leiomyomatous h.
lipofibromatous h.
neuromuscular h.
polymorphic h.
hamartomatous lesion
Hamas
H. technique
H. upper limb prosthesis
hamate
h. bone
hook of h.
h. hook
h. hook nonunion
h. ligament
h. tail fracture
hamate-lunate joint
hamatometacarpal ligament
Hamilton
H. apparatus
H. bandage
H. pelvic traction screw tractor
H. Rating Scale for Depression
H. ruler test
H. screw
H. traction
Hamilton-Russell traction
hammer
Babinski percussion h.
Berliner percussion h.
Buck neurological h.
Buck percussion h.
cervical/lumbar h.
Cloward h.
Davis percussion h.
Dejerine-Davis percussion h.
Dejerine percussion h.
h. digit syndrome
Epstein neurological h.
H. external fixation
h. finger
h. hallux
Küntscher h.
orthopaedic h.
OrthoVise with slap h.
percussion h.

reflex h.
slap h.
sliding h.
Taylor percussion h.
Troemner percussion h.
hammertoe (HT)
h. correction
h. correction with interphalangeal fusion
h. deformity
dynamic h.
fixed h.
flexible h.
h. repair
h. syndrome (HTS)
Hammon
H. foot operation
H. foot procedure
Hammond splint
hamstring
h. fixation technique
h. force
h. graft
h. lengthening
h. ligament augmentation
medial h.
h. muscle
h. reflex
h. release
h. stretcher
h. syndrome
h. tendon
h. tightness
hamstring-setting exercise
hamstrung knee
Hancock amputation
hand
accoucheur h.
all-median nerve h.
all-ulnar nerve h.
American Society for Surgery of the H. (ASSH)
h. amputation
h. anomaly
ape h.
apelike h.
artificial h.
baseball fracture of h.
bear's paw h.
h. block
h. board
h. brace
h. chuck

NOTES

H

319

hand *(continued)*
    claw h.
    cleft h.
    h. cock-up splint
    h. cone
    h. cuff
    Disabilities of Arm, Shoulder,
      and H. (DASH)
    h. dissector
    h. dominance
    dorsal venous arch of h.
    dorsum of h.
    h. drill
    h. elevator
    enchondroma of h.
    h. evaluation set
    h. exercise ball
    h. exerciser
    fell on outstretched h. (FOOSH)
    flat h.
    flexor retinaculum of h.
    flipper h.
    frostbite of h.
    h. function
    H. Functional Index (HFI)
    Gilliat-Summer nerve-damaged h.
    h. grasp strength
    Grayson ligament in h.
    h. grip dynamometer
    h. grip strength
    h. gym
    H. Helper
    H. Helper hand exerciser
    hemiplegic h.
    hypoplastic h.
    intrinsic minus h.
    intrinsic plus h.
    Krukenberg h.
    lobster-claw h.
    mirror h.
    mitten h.
    monkey fist h.
    Myobock artificial h.
    myopathy h.
    no man's land of h.
    oath h.
    obstetrician's h.
    opera-glass h.
    h. orthosis (HO)
    Otto Bock system electric h.
    outstretched h.
    pancake h.
    h. paralysis
    h. placement
    pretendinous band of h.
    h. prosthesis
    h. reconstruction
    h. rest
    h. saw

    skeleton h.
    spade h.
    spastic h.
    split h.
    spread h.
    tangential h.
    trident h.
    vaginal ligament of h.
    Volkmann claw h.
    h. volumeter
    web area of h.
    web border of h.
    writing h.
hand-arm vibration syndrome
handbag muscle
handball
    team h.
handbreadth
HandClens ultra antiseptic spray
handcuff disease
1-handed kitchen tool
handedness
Handeze fingerless glove
hand-foot syndrome
hand-foot-uterus syndrome
hand-glove prosthesis
handgrip
    h. ergometer
    h. exercise
handheld
    h. drill guide
    h. dynamometer (HHD)
    h. retractor
    h. weight (HHW)
hand-honed reverse cutting needle
handicap
    International Classification of
      Impairments, Disabilities, H.'s
      (ICIDH)
    Visual Analog Scale of H.
handle
    Bard-Parker h.
    Barton traction h.
    Beaver blade h.
    Charnley brace h.
    cup holder h.
    Dynagrip blade h.
    multisided blade h.
    Ortho-Grip silicone rubber h.
    stone basket screw mounted h.
    surgical knife h.
    Thera-Band h.
    Therap-Loop door h.
    T-pin h.
    traction h.
    Transfer Handle support h.
handlebar palsy
handle-type reamer
hand-operated drill

handpiece
> Coopervision irrigation/aspiration h.
> Max 3 electric h.
> reciprocating power h.

Hand-Schüller-Christian
> H.-S.-C. disease
> H.-S.-C. syndrome

hands-free crutch

handshake cast

handwriting
> Evaluation Tool of Children's H.

Handy-Buck traction

Hanger ComfortFlex knee prosthesis

hanging
> h. arm cast
> h. cast sling
> h. heel sign
> h. hip
> h. hip operation
> h. of limb
> h. toe operation

hangman's fracture

Hang Ups gravity boot

Hankin reduction

Hanna night splint

Hannover
> H. classification
> H. scoring system

Hansen
> H. disease
> H. fracture classification
> H. pin

Hansen-Street
> H.-S. driver-extractor
> H.-S. nail

Hanslik patellar prosthesis

Hansson
> Lars Ingvar H. (LIH)

Hapad
> H. felt insert
> H. heel pad
> H. heel wedge
> H. longitudinal metatarsal arch pad
> H. medial arch pad
> H. metatarsal arch
> H. metatarsal insole
> H. prefabricated wool felt pad
> H. scaphoid arch
> H. shoe insert

Happy podiatric bur

Hapset hydroxyapatite bone graft plaster

HAQ
> Headache Assessment Questionnaire
> HAQ Index

Hara infiltration block

hard
> h. callus stage
> h. collar
> h. corn
> h. disc
> h. socket

Hardcastle
> H. classification
> H. classification of tarsometatarsal joint injury

hardening
> work h.

Hardinge
> H. expansion bolt
> H. femoral approach
> H. lateral approach
> H. technique
> H. vastus lateralis procedure

hardware
> Genesis arthroplasty h.
> orthopaedic h.
> h. photopenia

hardy
> H. aluminum crutch
> H. hypophysial curette

Hardy-Clapham classification of sesamoid bones of foot

hare
> H. apparatus
> H. compact traction splint
> H. pin
> H. splint device
> H. traction

hark
> H. foot operation
> H. pes planus procedure

Harken prosthesis

Harloff cart

Harlow plate

Harmon
> H. cervical approach
> H. chisel
> H. hip reconstruction
> H. modified posterolateral approach
> H. procedure
> H. shoulder approach
> H. transfer
> H. transfer technique

harmonic imaging

NOTES

H

Harmony PLIF instrument set
Harms
    H. cage
    H. posterior cervical plate
Harms-Moss anterior thoracic
  instrumentation
harness
    figure-of-8 h.
    Forte h.
    Kicker Pavlik h.
    Pavlik h.
    weight-relieving Forte h.
    Wheaton Pavlik h.
    Zuni h.
Harold Crowe drill
Harpenden
    H. caliper
    H. dynamometer
Harpoon suture anchor
Harriluque technique
Harrington
    H. clamp forceps
    H. compression rod
    H. distraction instrumentation
    H. distraction outrigger
    H. distraction rod
    H. fixation device
    H. flat wrench
    H. hook clamp
    H. hook driver
    H. nail
    H. outrigger splint
    H. pedicle (bifid) hook
    H. rod clamp
    H. rod fixation
    H. rod and hook system
    H. rod instrumentation
    H. rod instrumentation compression
    H. rod instrumentation distraction
      outrigger device
    H. rod instrumentation failure
    H. rod instrumentation force
      application
    H. spinal elevator
    H. spreader
    H. total hip arthroplasty
Harrington-Kostuik
    H.-K. distraction device
    H.-K. instrumentation
Harrington-Luque technique
Harris
    H. anterolateral approach
    H. bolt
    H. brace-type reamer
    H. broach
    H. cemented hip prosthesis
    H. cement gun
    H. center-cutting acetabular reamer

    H. condylocephalic nail
    H. condylocephalic nailing
    H. condylocephalic rod
    H. criteria
    H. criteria for implant loosening
    H. Design femoral prosthesis
    H. Design-2 implant
    H. femoral component removal
    H. footprint mat
    H. growth arrest line
    H. Hemi Arm Sling
    H. hip line
    H. hip nail
    H. hip scale
    H. hip score (HHS)
    H. hip status system
    H. Infant Neuromotor Test (HINT)
    H. knotter
    H. lateral approach
    H. medullary nail
    H. Micromini prosthesis
    H. plate
    H. scope
    H. splint
    H. splint sling
    H. superior acetabular graft
    H. view
    H. wire tier
    H. 4-wire trochanter reattachment
Harris-Aufranc device
Harris-Beath
    H.-B. arthrodesis
    H.-B. axial calcaneus view
    H.-B. axial hindfoot x-ray
    H.-B. footprint
    H.-B. footprinting mat sign
    H.-B. footprint mat
    H.-B. operation
    H.-B. projection
Harris-Galante
    H.-G. acetabular cup
    H.-G. hip replacement acetabular
      component
    H.-G. I porous-coated acetabular
      component
    H.-G. porous hip prosthesis
    H.-G. stem
Harris-Mayo hip score
Harrison bone-holding forceps
Harrison-Nicolle polypropylene peg
Harris-Smith anterior interbody drill
Hartel guideline
Hart extension finger splint
Hartigan foramen
Hartmann
    H. bone rongeur
    H. mosquito forceps
Hartshill rectangle

harvest
>   graft h.
>   h. site

harvester
>   QuickDraw bone h.
>   tendon h.

harvesting
>   bone h.
>   Gilbert h.
>   Tamae h.
>   Weiland h.

Harvey wire-cutting scissors

Hass
>   H. osteotomy
>   H. procedure

Hastings
>   H. bipolar hemiarthroplasty
>   H. frame
>   H. hip prosthesis
>   H. open reduction

Hatcher pin

hatchet-head
>   h.-h. deformity
>   h.-h. shoulder

Hatfield bone curette

Hauser
>   H. Achilles lengthening procedure
>   H. ambulation index
>   H. bunionectomy
>   H. heel cord procedure
>   H. patellar operation
>   H. patellar realignment technique
>   H. patellar tendon procedure
>   H. realignment

Hausmann
>   H. weight rack
>   H. Work-Well work hardening
>   system

Hausted orthopaedic bed

Hautant test

HAV
>   hallux abductovalgus

haversian
>   h. bone remodeling
>   h. canal
>   h. gland
>   h. lamella
>   h. space
>   h. system
>   h. vessel

Hawaii Early Learning Profile (HELP)

Hawkeye
>   H. suture needle
>   H. suture needle for arthroscopy

Hawkins
>   H. impingement sign
>   H. line
>   H. procedure
>   H. talar fracture classification
>   H. talus fracture (type 1)
>   H. test

**Hawkins-Warren athlete's shoulder
  score**

Haygarth node

Hay lateral approach

Haynes pin

Haynes-Stellite (HS)
>   H.-S. 21 implant metal
>   H.-S. implant metal prosthesis

Hays hand retractor

hazard
>   job-related h.

H-block
>   Frost H-b.
>   H-b. nail surgery

HBO
>   hyperbaric oxygen
>   HBO therapy

HBS
>   headless bone screw
>   HBS bone screw system

HCA
>   heel cord advancement

HCl
>   hydrochloride

HCMI
>   Health Care Manufacturing Inc.
>   HCMI Chiropractic System

HCTU
>   home cervical traction unit

HD
>   Harris design
>   heloma durum

HD-2
>   HD-2 cemented hip prosthesis
>   HD-2 total hip prosthesis

head
>   abductor hallucis oblique h.
>   abductor hallucis transverse h.
>   Aequalis h.
>   avascular necrosis of femoral h.
>   (AVNFH)
>   BioPro ceramic TARA h.
>   h. brace

NOTES

H

head *(continued)*
    cartilaginous cap of phalangeal h.
    h. check
    cobalt-chromium h.
    collared femoral h.
    Continuum bipolar acetabular h.
    Copeland humeral resurfacing h.
    core decompression of femoral h.
    countersink screw h.
    DePuy Global Advantage shoulder eccentric humeral h.
    DePuy hip prosthesis with Scuderi h.
    femoral h.
    fibular h.
    first metatarsal h. (FMH)
    flat metatarsal h.
    h. fracture
    Giliberty bipolar femoral h.
    h. halter
    h. holder
    humeral h.
    infrared h.
    ischemic necrosis of femoral h. (INFH)
    J-FX bipolar h.
    long h.
    Matroc femoral h.
    metatarsal flat h.
    h. of patella
    phalangeal h.
    Phillips screw h.
    pseudometatarsal h.
    radial h.
    screw h.
    Scuderi h.
    talar h.
    terminal h.
    ulnar h.
    V40 forged femoral h.
    Vitox femoral h.
    Ziramic femoral h.
    zirconia orthopaedic prosthetic h.
    Zyranox femoral h.
headache
    H. Assessment Questionnaire (HAQ)
    cervicogenic h.
    exercise-related h.
head-at-risk sign
headed Bio-Corkscrew
head-first slide
head-halter traction
headholder
    Aesculap h.
headless
    h. bone screw (HBS)
    h. bone screw system

headlight
    Cogent LightWear h.
Headmaster collar
head-mounted display (HMD)
head-neck component
headrest
    doughnut h.
    h. extension
    Mayfield neurosurgical h.
    McConnell orthopaedic h.
    pin h.
    3-prong h.
head-shaft angle
head-splitting humeral fracture
head-stem offset
healed fracture
Healey revision acetabular component
healing
    bone h.
    cartilage h.
    contact h.
    h. by first intention
    fracture h.
    gap h.
    h. by granulation
    organizational phase of tendon h.
    per primam h.
    plasmatic phase of skin h.
    h. retardation
    h. by second intention
    h. shoe
    soft tissue h.
    spiritual h.
    tendon h.
    therapeutic ultrasound for tendon h.
Healos
    H. bone graft substitute
    H. synthetic bone grafting material
health
    H. Care Manufacturing Inc. (HCMI)
    H. O Meter Scale
Healthflex orthotic
Healthier seating cushion
Heal Well night splint
heart
    athlete's h.
    h. failure
    h. rate (HR)
heart-and-hand syndrome
heart-shaped buttocks
heat
    h. allodynia
    h. application
    h. cramp
    h. cramping
    damp h.
    h. fracture
    h. gain

h. gun
h. injury prevention
h. injury risk
h. loss
moist h.
H. Plus Massage lower body wrap
h. stress
h. stroke
h. syncope
h. therapy
heat-cured acrylic femoral head prosthesis
Heath mallet
heat-molded petroplastic ankle-foot orthosis
heavy
h. cross-slot screwdriver
h. side plate
heavy-duty
h.-d. femur plate
h.-d. 2-tooth retractor
Heberden
H. arthropathy
H. disease
H. node
H. nodosity
H. rheumatism
hebosteotomy
hebotomy
Hebra blade
Heck screw
Hector tendon
Hedrocel
H. cup
H. proximal tibia augmentation implant
H. tantalum metal structure
H. titanium screw
heel
anterior h.
black-dot h.
CarbonX active h.
h. compression syndrome
h. cord
h. cord advancement (HCA)
h. cord lengthening
h. cord stretch
h. cord stretching exercise
h. counter
cucumber h.
h. cup
cushion h.
h. cushion

h. equinus
h. eversion
h. fat pad
H. Free splint
gonorrheal h.
h. height
high-prow h.
H. Hugger therapeutic heel stabilizer
h. jar
jogger's h.
h. lift
h. lock
H. Minder foot elevator
h. pad pathology
h. pad thickening
painful h.
h. pain syndrome
policeman's h.
h. posting
h. prominence
prominent h.
h. raise exercise
reverse Thomas h.
h. rock exercise
rubber walking h.
SACH orthopaedic h.
h. sleeve
h. and sole insert
solid ankle, cushioned h. (SACH)
h. spike
h. spur
h. spur/plantar fasciitis syndrome
H. Spur Special
h. spur surgery
h. spur syndrome
h. stand
h. strike
h. tap test
tennis h.
h. tension
Thomas h.
h. valgus
h. varus
h. varus sign
h. walk
walking h.
h. wedge
wedge adjustable cushioned h. (WACH)
heel-and-toe
h.-a.-t. gait

NOTES

H

heel-and-toe *(continued)*
  h.-a.-t. walk
  h.-a.-t. walking
Heelbo decubitus heel/elbow protector
heel-contact
  h.-c. phase
  h.-c. phase of gait
Heelift
  H. suspension boot
  H. traction boot
heel-off
  h.-o. phase
  h.-o. phase of gait
heel-palm test
heel-rise test
heel-strike
  h.-s. phase
  h.-s. phase of gait
heel-tap reflex
heel-tip test
heel-toe
  h.-t. gait
  h.-t. pattern
  h.-t. runner
heel-to-knee test
heel-to-shin test
heel-to-toe medial shoe wedge
Heel-Up Boot suspension boot
HeelWedge healing shoe
Heerfort syndrome
Heermann alligator forceps
Hefty-bite pin cutter
Hegge pin
Heifetz procedure
height
  heel h.
  intervertebral disc h.
Hein rongeur
Heiple arthrodesis
Heiss soft tissue retractor
Helal
  H. flap arthroplasty
  H. modification
  H. osteotomy
Helbing sign
Helenca
  H. bandage
  H. binder
Helfet test
helical computed tomography
helicopod gait
helicopodia
Heliodorus bandage
**Helistat absorbable collagen hemostatic
  sponge**
helmet
  cranial h.
heloma
  h. durum (HD)

  h. molle (HM)
  h. vasculare
helotomy
HELP
  Hawaii Early Learning Profile
Helparm
  Swedish H.
helper
  Hand H.
hemangiectasia
  Klippel-Trenaunay
    osteohypertrophic h.
hemangioendothelioma
hemangioendotheliosarcoma
hemangioepithelioma
  epithelioid h.
hemangioma
  capillary h.
  cavernous h.
hemangiomatosis
hemangiopericytoma
hemangiosarcoma
hemarthrosis
  acute traumatic h.
  posttraumatic h.
  traumatic h.
Hemashield enhanced graft
hematogenous
  h. infection
  h. osteomyelitis
hematoma
  iliopsoas muscle h.
  intramedullary h.
  postoperative drainage-related h.
  pulsating h.
  sciatic nerve palsy h.
  subgluteal h.
  subungual h.
hematomyelia
hematorrhachis
hematosteon
hemianopsia
  homonymous h.
hemiarthroplasty
  Austin Moore h.
  Bateman h.
  Hastings bipolar h.
  I-beam hip h.
  large humeral head h.
  Miller-Galante I h.
  Neer h.
  prosthetic h.
  Smith-Petersen h.
hemiballism
hemicallotasis
hemic calculus
hemicondylar
  h. fracture
  h. graft

hemicord
hemicylindrical bone graft
hemidystonia
hemiepiphysiodesis
hemigigantism
hemihypertrophy
hemi-implant
    Dow Corning titanium h.-i.
hemi-interpositional implant
hemijoint arthroplasty
hemiknee
    Savastano h.
hemilaminectomy knife
hemimelia
    complete paraxial h.
    fibular h.
    paraxial h.
    partial h.
    radial h.
    tibial h.
hemimelic progressive osseous
  heteroplasia
hemiparetic gait
hemipelvectomy
    formal h.
    internal h.
hemipelvis
hemiphalangectomy
    Johnson h.
hemiplegia
    bilateral h.
    double h.
    spastic h.
    traumatic h.
hemiplegic
    h. amyotrophy
    h. foot
    h. gait
    h. hand
hemiprosthesis
    single-stemmed silicone h.
hemipulp flap
hemiresection interposition arthroplasty
hemisection
    triple h.
hemisemilaminotomy
hemi-silastic implant
hemispatial neglect
hemispherical
    h. pusher
    h. reamer
hemivertebra, pl. **hemivertebrae**
    balanced h.

    congenital h.
    thoracic hemivertebrae
    unbalanced h.
hemivertebral excision
hemochromatosis
hemodialysis-related arthropathy
hemogenesis
hemolymphangioma
hemolysis
    foot-strike h.
    intravascular h.
hemophilic
    h. arthritis
    h. arthropathy
    h. joint
hemorrhage
    intramedullary h.
    retroperitoneal h.
    subacute subperiosteal h.
hemorrhagic
    h. bulla
    h. osteomyelitis
    h. villous synovitis
hemosiderin deposition
hemostasis
hemostat
    blunt nose h.
    h. clamp
    Crile h.
    Kelly h.
    mosquito h.
    Nu-Knit absorbable h.
    orthopaedic h.
    Surgicel fibrillar h.
    Surgicel Nu-Knit absorbable h.
hemostatic
    h. forceps
    h. thoracic clamp
    Thrombostat topical h.
hemothorax
Hemovac
    H. Hydrocoat drain
    H. suction tube
Hendel guided osteotome
Henderson
    H. arthrodesis
    H. clamp approximator
    H. classification
    H. fracture
    H. lag screw
    H. onlay bone graft
    H. posterolateral approach

NOTES

H

Henderson *(continued)*
    H. posteromedial approach
    H. skin incision
Henderson-Jones
    H.-J. chondromatosis
    H.-J. disease
Hendler unitunnel technique
Hendren self-retaining retractor
Henle
    H. ligament
    trapezoid bone of H.
Hennessy knee brace
Henning
    H. cast spreader
    H. inside-to-outside technique
    H. instrument set
    H. mallet
    H. meniscal retractor
    H. plaster spreader
Henoch-Schönlein purpura
Henry
    H. acromioclavicular technique
    H. anterior strap approach
    H. anterolateral approach
    H. bone graft
    H. extensile approach
    H. incision
    H. knot
    knot of H.
    leash of H.
    ligament of H.
    master knot of H.
    H. muscle transfer
    H. paralysis
    H. posterior interosseous nerve
    approach
    H. posterior interosseous nerve
    exposure
    posterolateral approach of H.
    H. radial approach
    H. resection
Hensen plane
heparinized
    h. Ringer lactate solution
    h. saline flush
hepatotoxicity
herbal therapy
Herbert
    H. bone screw
    H. bone screw fixation
    H. bone screw system
    H. jig
    H. knee prosthesis
    H. saw
    H. scaphoid bone fracture
    H. scaphoid bone fracture
    classification
    H. scaphoid screw
    H. screw fixator

Herbert-Whipple bone screw
Hercules
    H. plaster shears
    H. TM drop-adjusting table
Herczel rib elevator
hereditaria
    myotonia h.
hereditary
    h. deforming chondrodysplasia
    h. essential myoclonus
    h. motor sensory neuropathy
    (HMSN)
    h. multiple exostosis
    h. neuropathic disease
    h. onychoosteodysplasia
    h. osteoonychodysplasia (HOOD)
    h. progressive arthroophthalmopathy
    h. sensory motor neuropathy (type
    I–III) (HSMN I–III)
    h. spinocerebellar ataxia
heredopathia atactica polyneuritiformis
Herendeen phenomenon
Heritage hip system
Hermes
    H. Evolution tricompartmental knee
    system
    H. total knee system
Hermodsson
    H. fracture
    H. internal rotation
    H. internal rotation technique
    H. tangential view
Hernandez-Ros bone staple
Herndon hip classification
hernia
    footballer's h.
    muscle h.
    sportsman's h.
    synovial h.
herniated
    h. disc
    h. intervertebral disc (HID)
    h. nucleus pulposus (HNP)
herniation
    central h.
    cervical midline disc h.
    contained disc h.
    disc h.
    intervertebral disc h.
    intraspongy nuclear disc h.
    midline disc h.
    noncontained disc h.
    phalangeal h.
    posterolateral h.
    synovial h.
    traumatic cervical disc h.
herpes
    h. gladiatorum
    h. simplex

herpetic whitlow
Herring lateral pillar classification
Herzenberg bolt
Herzmark frame
Hessco 300, 500 series hydrotherapy table
Hessing brace
heterodermic graft
heterogenesis
heterogenous graft
heterograft
heteroplasia
    hemimelic progressive osseous h.
    progressive osseous h.
heterotopic
    h. bone
    h. calcification
    h. ossification
    h. ossification prevention
Heuter-Volkmann law
Hewson
    H. breakaway pin
    H. cruciate guide
    H. drill
    H. ligament button
    H. ligament drill guide
    H. suture passer
    H. suture retriever
hex
    h. handle curette
    h. screw
    h. wrench
Hexadrol Phosphate
hexagonal slot-cap screw
Hexalite plastic
Hexcel
    H. knee prosthesis
    H. total condylar knee system
    H. total condylar prosthesis
Hexcelite
    H. cast
    H. sheet splint
Hex-Fix
    H.-F. Add-A-Clamp
    H.-F. external fixation
    H.-F. monolateral external fixator
    H.-F. Universal swivel clamp
hexhead
    h. bolt
    h. pin
    h. screwdriver
Hey
    H. amputation

    H. Groves clamp
    H. Groves fascia lata technique
    H. Groves-Kirk technique
    H. Groves ligament reconstruction technique
    H. Groves procedure
    H. internal derangement
    H. operation
Heyer-Schulte
    H.-S. antisiphon device
    H.-S. bur hole valve
    H.-S. wound drain
Heyman
    H. hip classification
    H. operation
    H. procedure
    H. technique
Heyman-Herndon
    H.-H. clubfoot operation
    H.-H. epiphysiodesis
    H.-H. procedure
    H.-H. release
Heyman-Herndon-Strong capsular release
HFI
    Hand Functional Index
HG
    HG multilock hip prosthesis
    HG multilock hip stem
hGH
    human growth hormone
HGO
    hip guidance orthosis
H-graft
    H-g. bone graft
    H-g. fusion
HHD
    handheld dynamometer
HHS
    Harris hip score
HHW
    handheld weight
Hi
    Darco Body Armor H.
    H. Speed Pulse lavage
HIAD
    high-impact aerobic dance
hiatal sign
hiatus
    adductor h.
    popliteal h.
Hibbs
    H. arthrodesis
    H. blade

NOTES

Hibbs *(continued)*
    H. bone-cutting forceps
    H. chisel
    H. chisel elevator
    H. curette
    H. curved osteotome
    H. extensor tendon transfer cavus deformity
    H. frame
    H. gouge
    H. mallet
    H. metatarsocalcaneal angle
    H. operation
    H. procedure
    H. retractor
    H. spinal fusion
    H. straight osteotome
    H. tendosuspension
hibernoma
Hibiclens
    H. scrub
    H. solution
    H. Topical
Hibistat Topical
Hick effect
hickory-stick fracture
Hicks lugged plate
HID
    herniated intervertebral disc
hidroacanthoma simplex
hierarchial
    h. ADL scales
    h. scales of ADLs
high
    h. heel shoe
    h. median-high radial palsy
    h. median-high ulnar palsy
    h. molecular weight polyethylene (HMWPE)
    h. muscular resistance bed
    h. performance silicone elastomer
    h. tibial osteotomy (HTO)
    h. toe box
    h. ulnar-high radial palsy
    h. velocity, low amplitude
high-air-loss bed
high-altitude
    h.-a. activity
    h.-a. adaptation
    h.-a. maladaption
high-assimilation pelvis
high-definition video display
high-density foam
high-energy
    h.-e. fracture
    h.-e. trauma
highest turbinated bone
high-frequency discharge

high-grade
    h.-g. spondylolisthesis
    h.-g. surface osteogenic sarcoma
    h.-g. ulcer
high-impact
    h.-i. activity
    h.-i. aerobic dance (HIAD)
high-level disinfectant
high-performance liquid chromatography (HPLC)
high-power athlete
high-pressure liquid chromatography (HPLC)
high-prow heel
high-resolution analysis
high-riding patella
high-risk factor
high-speed
    h.-s. bur
    h.-s. twist drill
high-steppage gait
high-tide walking brace
high-torque bur
high-velocity, low-amplitude thrust technique
high-voltage
    h.-v. galvanism
    h.-v. pulsed galvanic
    h.-v. pulsed galvanic stimulation (HVPGS)
    h.-v. pulsed stimulation (HVPS)
    h.-v. therapy (HVT)
hila (*pl. of* hilum)
hilar
Hilgenreiner
    H. angle
    H. brace
    H. horizontal Y line
Hilgenreiner-Perkins (H-P)
    H-P line
Hill Air-Drop HA90C table
Hillock arch
Hill-Rom orthopaedic bed
Hill-Sachs
    H.-S. deformity
    H.-S. fracture
    H.-S. lesion
    H.-S. shoulder dislocation
    H.-S. sign
    H.-S. view
hi-lo table
hilum, pl. **hila**
hilus
    neurovascular h.
    h. of tendon
Hinderer
    H. cartilage forceps
    H. malar prosthesis

hindfoot
- h. amputation
- h. anatomic variation
- h. arthrodesis
- h. cavus
- h. deformity
- h. excursion
- h. FPA
- h. instability
- h. joint complex
- h. kinematic
- lateral h.
- h. motion
- h. orthosis
- h. pronation
- h. reconstruction
- spastic varus h.
- h. supination
- h. valgus
- varus h.

hindfoot-midfoot collapse
hindquarter amputation
hinge
- h. abduction
- Adjusta-Wrist h.
- AHSC-Volz h.
- Arizona Health Sciences Center-
  Volz h.
- h. articulation
- h. axis concept
- Bahler h.
- Camber axis h. (CAH)
- Compass h.
- Dee elbow h.
- elbow h.
- flail-elbow h.
- Genucentric knee h.
- implant h.
- Kinematic rotation h.
- Kudo h.
- Lacey h.
- medial/plantar h.
- Noiles h.
- offset h.
- Quengel h.
- Rancho swivel h.
- h. rod
- rotating h.
- soft tissue h.
- stabilizing h.

hinged
- h. articulated fixator
- h. constrained knee prosthesis

- h. cylinder cast
- h. cylinder splint
- h. fragment
- h. great toe replacement prosthesis
- h. implant
- h. implant prosthesis
- h. joint
- h. knee brace
- h. Thomas splint
- h. total knee prosthesis

hinged-distraction apparatus
hinging
- hip h.

HINT
- Harris Infant Neuromotor Test

HIO
- hole-in-one
- HIO technique

hip
- h. abduction
- h. abduction stress test
- h. abductor strengthening exercise
- anthropometric total h. (ATH)
- h. arthroplasty
- h. avulsion fracture
- h. axis length
- biologically designed h. (BDH)
- h. bump
- h. bursitis
- h. capsule joint
- h. click
- h. compression screw
- congenital dislocation of h. (CDH)
- congenital dysplasia of h. (CDH)
- h. cup
- cup-on-cup arthroplasty of h.
- DePuy AML h.
- developmental dislocation of h.
  (DDH)
- developmental dysplasia of h.
  (DDH)
- h. disarticulation prosthesis
- h. disarticulation suspension
- h. dislocation
- h. dislocation classification
- dysplasia of h.
- h. dysplasia
- h. epiphysial injury
- h. extension
- h. extension exercise
- h. extension range of motion
- h. extensor gait
- h. flexion

NOTES

H

hip *(continued)*
>   h. flexion-extension
>   h. flexor contracture
>   h. fraction compaction drill
>   h. fracture compaction drill bit
> fused h.
>   h. guidance orthosis (HGO)
> hanging h.
>   h. hemipelvectomy suspension
>   h. hinge back exercise technique
>   h. hinging
> hockey player's h.
> irritable h.
> ischemic disease of growing h.
>   (IDGH)
>   h. joint angle (HJA)
>   h. joint aspiration under
>   fluoroscopic control
>   h. joint syndrome
> Kinamed anthropometric total h.
> Link anatomical h.
> Metasul metal-on-metal h.
>   h. mobility
> observation h.
>   h. orthosis (HO)
> pillow orthosis for h.
>   h. pin
>   h. pinning
>   h. pocket neuropathy
>   h. pointer
>   h. pointer contusion
> Precision total h.
>   h. reduction
>   h. replacement
>   h. replacement prosthesis
>   h. revision
> revision of total h.
>   h. roll
>   h. rotation
> Senegas approach to h.
>   h. skid
> snapping h.
>   h. spica
>   h. spica cast
>   h. subluxation
> tuberculosis of h.
> windblown h.
> windswept h.

HIPciser abduction splint
hipGRIP body positioning device
hip-knee-ankle (HKA)
>   h.-k.-a. angle

hip-knee-ankle-foot orthosis (HKAFO)
Hipokrat bimodular shoulder system
Hippocrates
>   H. bandage
>   H. manipulation

hippocratic
>   h. finger
>   h. maneuver

hipRAP postsurgical wound wrap
HipSaver protective underwear
hip-to-ankle
>   h.-t.-a. view
>   h.-t.-a. x-ray

Hirayma osteotomy
Hiroshim transfer
Hirsch
>   H. hypophysial punch
>   H. hypophysis punch forceps

Hirschberg
>   H. reflex
>   H. sign

Hirschhorn
>   H. compression approach
>   H. compression technique

Hirschtick utility shoulder splint
hirudin
His-Haas
>   H.-H. muscle transfer
>   H.-H. procedure

histiocytic tumor
histiocytoma
> angiomatoid malignant fibrous h.
>   (AMFH)
> fibrous h.
> malignant fibrous h.
> nevoid h.
> pleomorphic fibrous h.

histiocytosis
> granular h.
> Langerhans cell h.
> sinus h.

Histoacryl
>   H. glue
>   H. glue adhesive

histochemistry
Histofreezer
>   H. cryosurgical system
>   H. cryosurgical wart treatment kit

histogenesis
> distraction h.

histologic
histomorphometry
histopathology
> synovial h.

Histoplasma capsulatum
histoplasmosis
hitch
> ankle h.
> spinal h.

Hitchcock
>   H. arm procedure
>   H. stereotactic immobilization frame
>   H. tendon technique

hitch-hikers̐ thumb

Hi-Top
> H.-T. foot/ankle brace
> H.-T. foot/ankle walker
> H.-T. II adjustable walker
> H.-T. shoe

Hittenberger
> H. halo extension
> H. prosthesis

HJA
> hip joint angle

HJD
> Hospital for Joint Disease
> HJD total hip system

HKA
> hip-knee-ankle
> HKA angle

HKAFO
> hip-knee-ankle-foot orthosis

HLA
> human leukocyte antigen
> human lymphocyte antigen
> HLA B27-related
> spondyloarthropathy intersection
> syndrome

HLT-405 instrument adjusting table

HM
> heloma molle

HMD
> head-mounted display

HMIS
> hallux metatarsophalangeal
> interphalangeal scale

HMP
> hot moist pack

HMS
> hypermobility syndrome

HMSN
> hereditary motor sensory neuropathy

HMWPE
> high molecular weight polyethylene

HNA
> hypothalamoneurohypophysial axis

HNP
> herniated nucleus pulposus

HO
> hand orthosis
> hip orthosis

HOA
> hypertrophic osteoarthroscopy

Hoaglund bone graft

hobbling gait

Hobb view

hockey
> ice h.
> h. player's hip

hockey-stick
> h.-s. dissector
> h.-s. fracture
> h.-s. incision

Hodgen
> H. hip splint
> H. leg splint

Hodge plane

Hodgkinson acetabular component loosening criteria

Hodgson technique

Hodor-Dobbs procedure

Hoen
> H. clamp
> H. forceps
> H. gouge
> H. periosteal elevator
> H. retractor
> H. rongeur
> H. skull plate

Hoffa
> H. disease
> H. fat pad
> H. fracture
> H. massage
> H. operation
> H. sign
> H. syndrome
> H. tendon shortening
> H. tendon-shortening method
> H. test

Hoffa-Kastert disease

Hoffa-Lorenz operation

Hoffer
> H. ankle procedure
> H. split transfer

Hoffmann
> H. apex fixation pin
> H. approach
> H. C-series external fixator
> H. dynamic external fixator
> H. external fixation
> H. external fixation system
> H. frame
> H. II compact external fixation
> component
> H. ligament clamp
> H. metatarsal operation
> H. metatarsal procedure
> H. mini-lengthening fixation device

NOTES

H

Hoffmann *(continued)*
   H. muscular atrophy
   H. panmetatarsal head resection
   H. pin guide
   H. reflex
   H. sign
   H. syndrome
   H. transfixion pin
Hoffmann-Vidal
   H.-V. double frame
   H.-V. external fixation apparatus
   H.-V. external fixation device
   H.-V. external fixator
Hogg chair
**Hohl-Luck tibial plateau fracture
classification**
Hohl-Moore technique
**Hohl tibial condylar fracture
classification**
Hohmann
   H. bone retractor
   H. bunionectomy
   H. operation
   H. osteotomy
   H. procedure
**Hohmann-Thomasen metatarsal
osteotomy**
Hoke
   H. Achilles tendon lengthening
   H. Achilles tendon lengthening
    operation
   H. lumbar brace
   H. lumbar brace/corset
   H. lumbar corset
   H. osteotome
   H. procedure for tibial palsy
   H. tibial palsy procedure
   H. triple arthrodesis
   H. triple-section method
Hoke-Kite technique
Hoke-Martin traction
Hoke-Miller procedure
holder
   acetabular cup h.
   Alvarado knee h.
   arm h.
   arthroscopic leg h.
   Assistant Free orthopaedic
    needle h.
   Barraquer needle h.
   Böhler-Steinmann pin h.
   bone h.
   Castroviejo needle h.
   Charnley trochanter h.
   clamp h.
   Crile-Wood needle h.
   cup h.
   DeMartel-Wolfson clamp h.
   Donaghy angled suture needle h.

Drummond hook h.
Ferguson bone h.
Halsey needle h.
head h.
hook h.
hookbar h.
Jacobson needle h.
knee h.
leg h.
limb h.
Malis needle h.
Mayo-Hegar needle h.
microneedle h.
needle h.
neonatal tracheostomy tube h.
octopus h.
operative leg h.
OSI arthroscopic leg h.
pin h.
Rhoton needle h.
rod h.
Ryder needle h.
Sarot needle h.
Schmidt rod h.
shoulder h.
staple h.
thigh h.
tibial track h.
trochanter h.
TSRH hook h.
Wangensteen needle h.
washer h.
Watanabe pin h.
Webster needle h.
well-leg h.
Yasargil needle h.
holder/scissors
   Assistant Free orthopaedic
    needle h./s.
holding mitt
hold-relax
   h.-r. method
   h.-r. technique
Holdsworth spinal fracture classification
hole
   acetabular seating h.
   anchor h.
   anchoring h.
   blind anchorage h.
   bone hook with cable/wire h.
   bur h.
   cable/wire h.
   centering h.
   drill h.
   glide h.
   gliding h.
   guide h.
   lag screw thread h.
   offset drill h.

9-h. peg test
2-h. plate
5-h. plate
6-h. plate
7-h. plate
h. preparation method
3-hole
3-h. plate
3-h. suture tendon fixation
4-hole
4-h. Alta straight plate
4-h. side plate
10-hole blade-plate
hole-in-one (HIO)
h.-i.-o. technique
11-hole plate
holism
Hollander clog
Hollingshead Index
Hollister Hot/Ice knee blanket
hollow
h. back
h. bone
h. bone trephine
h. chisel
h. foot
h. foot clawfoot deformity
h. mill Asnis cannulated screw
h. mill drill
h. mill instrumentation
h. mill reamer
Hollywood
H. bed
H. bed extension hook set
H. roll technique
Holmes
H. operation
H. phenomenon
rebound phenomenon of H.
Holmes-Rahe Life Change Index
Holmes-Stewart phenomenon
holmium YAG laser
holorachischisis
Holscher
H. knee retractor
H. root retractor
Holstein fracture of humerus
Holstein-Lewis fracture
Holt
H. bolt
H. nail
H. nail plate
Holter traction

Holt-Oram dysplasia
Holzheimer retractor
Homans
H. sign
H. test
HOME
Home Observation and Measurement of the Environment
home
h. assessment
h. cervical traction unit (HCTU)
h. exercise program
h. medical equipment
H. Observation and Measurement of the Environment (HOME)
H. Ranger shoulder pulley
h. rehabilitation
h. spinal stabilization program
homeopathy
homeostasis
fluid h.
osseous h.
HomeStretch lumbar traction
HomeTrac
Saunders cervical H.
hominis
Dermatobia h.
homogenous graft
homograft
h. implant material
h. prosthesis
homolog
meniscus h.
homologous graft
homonymous hemianopsia
homoplastic graft
homuncular organization
homunculus
honeycomb pattern
HOOD
hereditary osteoonychodysplasia
hood
dorsal h.
extensor h.
retinacular h.
hoof bottom
hook
Acufex nerve h.
anatomic h.
h. approximator
APRL prosthetic h.
Austin Moore h.
Barr h.

NOTES

H

hook *(continued)*
    bifid h.
    h. blade
    h. blocker
    blunt h.
    Bobechko sliding barrel h.
    bone h.
    Boyes-Goodfellow h.
    button h.
    buttressed h.
    canted finger h.
    Carroll skin h.
    C-D h.
    h. clamp
    clawed pedicle h.
    closed Cotrel-Dubousset h.
    closed transverse process TSRH h.
    compression h.
    Culler h.
    Cushing dural h.
    h. dislodgment
    distraction h.
    h. distractor
    Dorrance h.
    double-open h.
    double-pronged skin h.
    down-angle h.
    downsized circular laminar h.
    drop-entry (closed body) h.
    Drummond h.
    dura h.
    Edwards h.
    Edwards-Levine h.
    Effler-Groves h.
    finger h.
    garment h.
    Gillies bone h.
    Gillies-Dingman h.
    glide h.
    Graham muscle h.
    Graham nerve h.
    h. grasp
    Green muscle h.
    h. of hamate
    hamate h.
    h. of hamate bone
    Harrington pedicle (bifid) h.
    H. hemi-harness shoulder
      immobilizer
    h. holder
    Hosmer Dorrance h.
    h. impactor
    Isola spinal implant system h.
    Jameson muscle h.
    Jannetta h.
    jig h.
    Joseph h.
    Keene compression h.
    Kennerdell-Maroon h.

Kilner h.
Kirby muscle h.
Knodt rod and h.
Küntscher nail-extracting h.
Lahey Clinic dural h.
Lambotte bone h.
laminar C-D h.
Leatherman h.
lyre-shaped finger h.
meniscus h.
Micro-One h.
Moe alar h.
Moss h.
multispan fracture h.
nail-extracting h.
nerve h.
neutral h.
O'Brien rib h.
Oesch h.
open C-D h.
Osher irrigating implant h.
PCL-oriented placement marking h.
pediatric C-D h.
pediatric TSRH h.
pedicle C-D h.
h. pin
h. plate
h. probe system
prosthetic h.
h. pusher
ribbed h.
right-angle h.
Rogozinski h.
h. rotary scissors
Selby I, II h.
sharp worm h.
side-opening laminar h.
h. site
skin h.
sliding barrel h.
split-finger h.
square-ended h.
T-handled h.
top-entry (open body) h.
traction h.
Trautman Locktite prosthetic h.
h. trial set screw
TSRH buttressed laminar h.
TSRH circular laminar h.
TSRH pedicle h.
TSRH trial h.
twist h.
Tyrell h.
up-angle h.
vessel h.
Vilex Ouchless H.
Volkmann bone h.
Yasargil spring h.

Zielke bifid h.
Zuelzer h.
hookbar holder
hooked
h. acromion
h. bone
h. foot
h. forefoot
h. intramedullary nail
h. knife
h. medullary nail
hook-end intramedullary pin
hookian region
hook-lying pectoral stretch exercise
hook-nail deformity
hook-pin fixation
hook-plate fixation
hook-rod
Cotrel-Dubousset h.-r.
Isola h.-r.
TSRH h.-r.
hook-to-screw L4-S1 compression construct
hoop stress fracture
Hoover
H. sign
H. test
hop
h. index
h. test
hope
Planning Alternative Tomorrows with H. (PATH)
Hopkins plaster knife
Hoppenfeld lateral approach
Hori technique
horizontal
h. cleavage
h. external rotation
h. fracture
h. gantry cut
h. mattress suture
h. meniscal tear
h. osteotomy
h. pedicle diameter
h. plane
h. platform support (HPS)
h. position
h. shoulder abduction exercise
h. Y line
hormone
adrenocorticotropic h. (ACTH)
growth h.

human growth h. (hGH)
thyrotropin-releasing h.
horn
anterior h.
bone graft shoe h.
central h.
cutaneous h.
enlarged frontal h.
posterior h.
shoulder h.
horse
charley h.
h. foot callus
horseback rider's knee
horse-hoof fracture nonunion
horseshoe
h. abscess
h. appearance
h. heel pad
h. patellofemoral brace
h. therapy table
horseshoe-shaped
h.-s. felt pad
h.-s. flap
horse-tail Achilles tendon tear
Horsley
H. bone cutter
H. bone-cutting forceps
H. bone rongeur
H. bone saw
H. bone wax
H. separator
Horsley-Stille
H.-S. bone-cutting forceps
H.-S. rib shears forceps
Horwitz
H. ankle fusion
H. ankle fusion approach
H. transmalleolar arthrodesis
Horwitz-Adams
H.-A. ankle fusion
H.-A. arthrodesis
HOS
human osteogenic sarcoma
hose
TED h.
Venosan support h.
Hosmer
H. above-knee rotator
H. Dorrance hook
H. Dorrance voluntary control 4-bar knee mechanism
H. Endurance knee

NOTES

337

Hosmer (*continued*)
    H. single-axis friction knee
    H. single-axis locking knee
    H. VC 4-bar knee orthosis
    H. WALK prosthesis
    H. weight-activated locking knee
hospital
    Imperial College, London H.
    H. for Joint Disease (HJD)
    H. for Special Surgery (HSS)
    H. for Special Surgery knee score
    H. for Special Surgery scale
    Texas Scottish Rite H. (TSRH)
    H. Trauma Index
host
    h. bone
    h. immune reaction
host-allograft junction
hot
    h. and cold contrast bath
    h. dog technique
    h. fomentation therapy
    h. joint
    h. knife
    h. moist pack (HMP)
    h. pack (HP)
    h. plate
    h. water bath
    h. weld
hot-cross-bun
    h.-c.-b. skull
    h.-c.-b. skull sign
hot/ice
    h./i. cold therapy cooler therapy device
    H./i. System III
Hotsy Cautery
hourglass
    h. capsulotomy
    h. constriction
    h. deformity
    h. vertebra
    h. vertebral body spacer
House-Dieter malleus nipper
household ambulatory
housemaid's knee
House reconstruction
Houston
    H. halo cervical support
    H. halo cervical traction
    H. halo traction cervical collar
    H. operation
Howard
    H. bone block
    H. technique
Howell tibial guide
Howmedica
    H. bone anchor
    H. cement

    H. cerclage
    H. cerclage cable
    H. Duracon implant
    H. ICS screw
    H. Kinematic II knee prosthesis
    H. knee instrumentation
    H. knee system
    H. Microfixation System drill bit
    H. Microfixation System forceps
    H. Microfixation System pliers
    H. monospherical implant
    H. monotube
    H. monotube external rotator
    H. PCA prosthesis
    H. total ankle system
    H. Universal compression screw
    H. Vitallium staple
    H. VSF fixation system
Howmedica-Osteonics instrument
Howorth
    H. approach
    H. procedure
    H. prosthesis
Howse
    H. prosthesis
    H. total hip replacement
Howship lacuna
Hoyer
    H. lift
    H. traction
HP
    hot pack
H-P
    Hilgenreiner-Perkins
    H-P line
HP-100
    HP-100 prosthetic finger
    HP-100 prosthetic finger joint
HPA
    hypothalamic-pituitary-adrenal
H.P. Acthar Gel
HPLC
    high-performance liquid chromatography
    high-pressure liquid chromatography
HPS
    horizontal platform support
    HPS II total hip prosthesis
HR
    heart rate
H-reflex
HS
    Haynes-Stellite
H-shaped
    H-s. capsular incision
    H-s. graft
    H-s. plate
HSMN I–III
    hereditary sensory motor neuropathy (type I–III)

HSS
    Hospital for Special Surgery
      HSS knee score
      HSS total condylar knee prosthesis

HT
    hammertoe
    Hubbard tank

HTO
    high tibial osteotomy
      HTO fixator
      HTO wedge human donor tissue
      allograft

HTS
    hammertoe syndrome

Hubbard
    H. bolt
    H. physical therapy tank
    H. side plate
    H. tank (HT)

hubbed needle

Huber
    H. abductor digiti quinti transfer
    H. adductor digiti quinti
    opponensplasty
    H. transfer of abductor digiti
    quinti

Hubscher maneuver

Huckstep nail

Hudson
    H. bone bur
    H. bone drill
    H. brace drill
    H. brace with bur
    H. bur
    H. chuck adapter
    H. forceps
    H. Hydrofloat Cushion
    H. TLSO brace

Hudson-Jones knee-cage brace

Hueter
    H. bandage
    H. line
    H. sign

Hughes fixation

Hughston
    H. Clinic injury classification
    H. external rotation recurvatum test
    H. knee evaluation
    H. knee jerk test
    H. knee score
    H. lateral compartment
    reconstruction
    H. plica test

    H. posterolateral drawer test
    H. posteromedial drawer test
    H. procedure
    H. realignment
    H. view

Hughston-Losee jerk test

human
    h. botfly
    h. cancellous bone
    h. chorionic gonadotropin
    h. cortical bone
    h. growth hormone (hGH)
    h. leukocyte antigen (HLA)
    h. lymphocyte antigen (HLA)
    h. osteogenic sarcoma (HOS)
    h. skin equivalent

humanism

Humby knife

humeral
    h. avulsion
    h. avulsion of glenohumeral
    ligament (HAGL)
    h. bone
    h. brace
    h. canal
    h. chondroblastoma
    h. circumflex vessel
    h. component
    h. condyle
    h. cutting guide
    h. device
    h. diaphysis
    h. epicondyle
    h. epicondylitis
    h. epiphysis
    h. fracture abduction splint
    h. fracture malunion
    h. head
    h. head retractor
    h. head-splitting fracture
    h. impactor
    h. mechanism
    h. neck
    h. physial fracture
    h. reamer
    h. saw
    h. shaft fracture
    h. supracondylar fracture

humeri (*pl. of* humerus)

humeroperoneal muscular dystrophy

humeroradial articulation

humerothoracic abduction

NOTES

H

humeroulnar
- h. angle
- h. articulation
- h. joint

humerus, pl. **humeri**
- articulatio humeri
- distal h.
- Holstein fracture of h.
- periarthrosis humeri
- proximal h.
- h. sulcus

humoral immunity

hump
- buffalo h.
- dowager's h.

humpback deformity

humpbacked spinal curvature

Humphry ligament

hunchback

Hungarian grip plate

Hungerford-Krackow-Kenna knee arthroplasty

Hungerford technique

hungry bone syndrome

hung-up knee jerk

hunter
- H. canal
- H. open cord tendon implant
- H. silastic prosthesis
- H. silastic rod
- H. tendon prosthesis

hunting
- h. reaction
- h. response

Huntington
- H. bone graft
- H. sign
- H. tibial technique

Hunt paradoxical phenomenon

Hunt-Thompson pantalar arthrodesis

Hurd bone-cutting forceps

Hurler
- H. disease
- H. polydystrophy
- H. syndrome

Hurler-Scheie
- H.-S. compound
- H.-S. syndrome

Husk bone rongeur

Hutchinson
- H. fracture
- melanotic whitlow of H.
- H. teeth

HV
- hallux valgus
- HV NightSplint splint
- HV SoftSplint splint

HVA
- hallux valgus angle

HVPGS
- high-voltage pulsed galvanic stimulation

HVPS
- high-voltage pulsed stimulation

HVT
- high-voltage therapy

hyaline
- h. cartilage
- h. cartilage detritus
- h. cartilage implant
- h. necrosis

hyalinization

hyalinum

hyaluronate

hyaluronidase

hybrid
- h. external fixator
- h. fixation
- h. fixation of hip replacement component
- h. total hip replacement

HybridFit
- H. total hip system
- H. total knee system

hydatid resonance

Hydra-Cadence
- H.-C. gait-control unit
- H.-C. knee prosthesis

Hydragrip clamp insert

hydrarthrodial

hydrarthrosis
- intermittent h.

hydrate

hydration status

hydraulic
- h. knee unit
- h. knee unit prosthesis
- h. test system

hydrisalic gel

Hydrisinol
- H. creme
- H. lotion

hydrobromide

hydrocele
- Dupuytren h.

hydrocephalus

hydrochloride (HCl)
- propoxyphene h.

hydrocodone
- h. and acetaminophen
- h. and aspirin
- h. bitartrate and ibuprofen
- h. and ibuprofen

hydrocollator
- H. heating unit
- H. pad
- H. steam pack

hydrocolloid occlusive dressing

Hydrocol wound dressing

HydroFlex arthroscopy irrigating system
hydrofloat cushion
hydrogen
    h. peroxide
    h. washout method
hydromassage table
hydromelia
Hydron Burn Bandage
hydrophilic dressing
hydrops canal
HydroSoothe recliner
hydrostatic pressure
HydroStat IR
hydrosyringomyelia
    communicating h.
hydrotherapy
    AquaMED dry h.
    dry h.
Hydro-Tone Bell
HydroTrack underwater treadmill
  system
hydroxyapatite (HA)
    h. adhesive
    h. bone
    h. bone replacement material
    calcium h. (CHA)
    h. cement
    coralline h.
    h. deposition disease
    h. implant material
    LLPS h.
    h. tetra-tri-calcium phosphate
hydroxyapatite-coated
    h.-c. ankle arthroplasty
    h.-c. porous alumni cement
    h.-c. stem
hydroxylapatite
    PureFix h.
25-hydroxyvitamin D
hygroma
    cystic h.
Hylamer
    H. enhanced ultra-high molecular
    weight polyethylene acetabular
    liner
    H. orthopaedic bearing polymer
Hyland's Leg Cramps with Quinine
hyoid bone
hypalgesia
hyperabduction
    h. maneuver
    h. syndrome test

hyperactive
    h. reflex
    h. response
hyperactivity
    physiological h.
hyperalgesia
hyperalimentation
hyperbaric
    h. oxygen (HBO)
    h. oxygen therapy
hypercalcemia
hypercortisolism
hyperdorsiflexion
hyperdynamic abductor hallucis
hyperemia
hyperemic
hyperesthesia
hyperesthetic
hyperextend
hyperextended knee gait
hyperextensibility
    joint h.
    h. of joint
hyperextension
    h. brace
    h. cast
    cruciform anterior spinal h.
    (CASH)
    h. deformity
    h. injury
    intraoperative neck h.
    h. orthosis
    rebound h.
    recurrent h.
    segmental h.
    h. stress
    h. teardrop fracture
    h. test
    h. trauma
hyperextension-hyperflexion injury
Hyperex thoracic orthosis
hyperflexed toe compartment syndrome
hyperflexion
    h. injury
    h. teardrop fracture
    h. trauma
hyperhidrosis, hyperidrosis
hyperintense
    h. signal
    h. zone
hyperkeratosis, pl. hyperkeratoses
    Kyrle h.
hyperkeratotic lesion

NOTES

H

hyperkyphoscoliosis
    neuropathic h.
hyperkyphosis
hyperlordosis
hypermobile
    h. flatfoot
    h. foot
    h. joint
    h. joint syndrome
    h. pes planovalgus
hypermobility
    compensatory h.
    joint h.
    h. syndrome (HMS)
hypernephroma
hyperosmotic
hyperosteoidosis
hyperostosis
    ankylosing spinal h.
    Caffey h.
    h. corticalis deformans
    diffuse idiopathic skeletal h.
    (DISH)
    flowing h.
    infantile cortical h.
    Morgagni h.
    sesamoid h.
    h. syndrome
hyperostotic
    h. bony fusion
    h. spondylosis
hyperparathyroidism
    brown tumor of h.
    h. tumor
hyperpathia
hyperphalangism
hyperphosphatasemic skeletal dysplasia
hyperpigmented lesion
hyperpituitary gigantism
hyperplantarflexion injury
hyperplasia
    epiphysial h.
    fibrous h.
hyperplastic
    h. bone
    h. chondrodysplasia
    h. osteoarthritis
hyperplastica
    synovitis h.
hyperpolarization
hyperpronation
hyperpyrexia
    malignant h.
hyperreflexia
    detrusor h.
hypersecretion
    growth hormone h.
hypersensitivity syndrome

hyperspectral near-infrared Raman imaging microscopy
hypertension
    calf h.
hyperthermia
    malignant h.
hyperthermic exercise-associated collapse
hypertonia
hypertonicity
hypertonus
hypertrophic
    h. arthritis
    h. cardiomyopathy
    h. chondrocyte
    h. exostosis
    h. flexor retinaculum
    h. granulation tissue
    h. interstitial neuropathy
    h. ligament
    h. osteoarthritis
    h. osteoarthroscopy (HOA)
    h. pulmonary osteoarthropathy
    h. scar
    h. skin
    h. spondylitis
    h. strength training
    h. synovitis
    h. vital nonunion
    h. zone
hypertrophica
    tenosynovitis h.
hypertrophied ligamentum flavum
hypertrophy
    bone h.
    cartilage h.
    cartilaginous h.
    endemic h.
    endosteal h.
    ligamentous-muscular h.
    smooth muscle h.
    uncinate h.
hypervascular
    h. fragment
    h. nonunion
hypesthesia, hypoesthesia
hypnoanalgesia
hypnoanesthesia
hypnopedia
hypnotic
    h. dissociation
    h. reinterpretation
    h. replacement
    h. therapy
hypoactive deep tendon reflex
hypoaldosteronism
    hyporeninemic h.
hypobaric
    H. microvalve

H. transfemoral system
H. transtibial system
hypochondriac region
hypochondriasis
hypochondroplasia
hypocycloidal ankle tomography
hypoechogenicity
hypoechoic intermetatarsal web space mass
hypoesthesia (*var. of* hypesthesia)
hypofibrinolysis
hypoflexibility of foot
hypogastric
   h. artery
   h. flap
hypoglossal nerve
hypointense signal
hypokinetic aberration
hypokyphosis
   right thoracic curve with h.
   thoracic h.
hypolordosis
   cervical h.
hypomelia
hypomobile
hyponychium
hypoosmotic
hypophalangism
   pedal h.
hypophosphatemic bone disease
hypophysial, hypophyseal
   h. c. curette
hypoplasia
   cartilage-hair h. (CHH)
   odontoid h.
   phalangeal h.
   skeletal h.
hypoplastic
   h. disc space
   h. finger

h. first rib
h. hand
h. thumb
hyporeninemic hypoaldosteronism
hypostatic abscess
hypotension
   exertional h.
   postexercise h.
hypotensive
   h. anesthesia
   h. surgery
hypothalamic-pituitary-adrenal (HPA)
   h.-p.-a. axis
hypothalamoneurohypophysial axis (HNA)
hypothenar
   h. eminence
   h. fascia
   h. hammertoe syndrome
   h. muscle
   h. reflex
hypothermia
hypothermic
hypothesis
   axoplasmic aberration h.
   instability h.
   neuroimmune h.
   somatoautonomic reflex h.
hypotonia
   congenital h.
hypotonic fluid
hypotonus
hypotrophic arthritis
HyProCure
   H. sinus tarsi implant
   H. sinus tarsi implant block
hysterical
   h. gait
   h. joint
   h. scoliosis

NOTES

IADL
    instrumental activities of daily living
Iamin hydrating gel
iatrogenic
    i. complication
    i. dural tear
    i. elevatus
    i. injury
    i. loss
    i. lumbar kyphosis
    i. osteomyelitis
I-beam
    I-b. cement punch
    I-b. hemiarthroplasty hip prosthesis
    I-b. hip hemiarthroplasty
    I-b. hip operation
    Jergesen I-b.
IBF
    Insall-Burstein-Freeman
    IBF knee instrument
IBG
    iliac bone graft
IBM
    inclusion body myositis
IBT
    inflatable bone tamp
    KyphX Elevate IBT
    KyphX Exact IBT
IC
    intermittent claudication
ICBG
    iliac crest bone graft
ICE
    ice, compression, elevation
ice
    i. application
    i., compression, elevation (ICE)
    i. hockey
    i. immersion
    Liquid I.
    i. massage
    N'ice Stretch night splint
    suspension system with Sealed I.
    i. pack
    i. skater's fracture
    I. Wedge hot/cold therapy wrap
I.C.E. Down cold pack
Iceflex Endurance suction suspension
  sleeve
Iceross Comfort Plus silicone gel liner
Icex socket
ichnogram
ICIDH
    International Classification of
    Impairments, Disabilities, Handicaps

icing
    cutaneous i.
ICLH
    ICLH ankle prosthesis
    ICLH double cup arthroplasty
    ICLH knee prosthesis
ICN
    inferior calcaneonavicular ligament
Icon pylon
ICRS
    Index Chemicus Registry System
    ICRS arthroscopic staging system
ICS
    inferior capsular shift
    intercostal space
ICT
    intermittent cervical traction
I&D
    incision and drainage
    irrigation and débridement
IDCN
    intermediate dorsal cutaneous nerve
Ideal spinal implant
Ideberg glenoid fracture classification
Identifit hip prosthesis
IDET
    intradiscal electrothermal treatment
    intradiscal electrothermal therapy
    IDET procedure
IDGH
    ischemic disease of growing hip
idiomuscular
idiopathic
    i. anterior knee pain
    i. arm pain
    i. avascular necrosis
    i. bone cavity
    i. erythromelalgia
    i. fracture
    i. genu valgum (IGV)
    i. hallux valgus
    i. hypertrophic osteoarthropathy
    (IHO)
    i. juvenile osteoporosis
    i. osteonecrosis
    i. polymyositis myopathy
    i. scoliosis
    i. skeletal
    i. skeletal hyperostosis syndrome
    i. toe-walker (ITW)
    i. toe walking
    i. transient osteoporosis
I disc
IDK
    internal derangement of knee

IDN
  interdigital neuroma
IEMG
  integrated rectified EMG
IFC
  interferential stimulation
I-Flow nerve block infusion kit
IGF
  insulin-like growth factor
IGF-binding protein
IGHL
  inferior glenohumeral ligament
    IGHL insertion
IGV
  idiopathic genu valgum
IHO
  idiopathic hypertrophic osteoarthropathy
IHW
  inner heel wedge
IKDC
  International Knee Documentation
  Committee
    IKDC form
    IKDC score
Ikuta
    I. clamp approximator
    I. fixation
    I. fixation device
    I. pectoralis major transfer
ILD
  ischemic limb disease
Ilfeld
    I. brace
    I. splint
    I. splint orthosis
Ilfeld-Gustafson splint
Ilfeld-Holder deformity
iliac
    i. apophysis
    i. apophysis sign
    i. apophysitis
    i. artery
    i. bone
    i. bone graft (IBG)
    i. buttressing procedure
    i. canal
    i. clamp
    i. compression test
    i. crest
    i. crest bone block
    i. crest bone free graft
    i. crest bone graft (ICBG)
    i. crest bone graft stabilization
    i. crest bridge
    i. crest dowel
    i. crest-inlay graft
    i. crest ossification
    i. epiphysis
    i. fixation

    i. oblique view
    i. osteocutaneous flap
    i. osteotomy
    i. post
    i. region
    i. screw
    i. slot graft
    i. spine
    i. strut bone graft
    i. tuberosity
    i. vein
    i. wing
    i. wing resection
iliacus
    i. dysfunction
    i. muscle
    i. syndrome
    i. test
ilial
iliococcygeus muscle
iliocostalis lumborum syndrome
iliocostal muscle
iliofemoral
    i. approach
    i. flap artery
    i. ligament
    i. pedicle flap
    i. thrombosis
    i. triangle
iliofemoroplasty
iliohypogastric nerve
ilioinguinal
    i. acetabular approach
    i. nerve
    i. syndrome
iliolumbar
    i. artery
    i. ligament
    i. vein
iliometer
iliopatellar
    i. band
    i. ligament
iliopectineal
    Bigelow i.
    i. bursitis
    i. line
iliopelvic
iliopsoas
    i. bursitis
    i. muscle
    i. muscle hematoma
    i. recession
    i. tendon
    i. test
    i. transfer
iliopubic
iliosacral
    i. articulation

i. and iliac fixation construct
i. implant
i. screw

iliospinal
iliotibial (IT)
i. band (ITB)
i. band fasciitis
i. band friction syndrome (ITBFS)
i. band graft
i. band graft augmentation
i. band tenodesis
i. band transfer
i. tract

iliotrochanteric ligament
ilioxiphopagus
ilium
AS i.
ASEx i.
ASIn i.
i. drainage
external i. (EI)
In/Ex I.
PIEx i.
PIIn i.
piriform sclerosis of i.
wing of i.

Ilizarov
I. ankle arthrodesis
I. ankle fusion technique
I. apparatus
I. circular external fixator
I. corticotomy
I. device
I. distractor
I. external fixation
I. external ring fixator
I. frame
I. hybrid fixator
I. limb lengthening
I. limb-lengthening system
I. limb-lengthening technique
I. method
I. procedure
I. ring
I. screw
I. tension-stress effect
I. wire

ILL
inequality in leg length
ill-fitting shoe
illness
National Foundation for
Depressive I. Inc.

illuminator
Cogent XL i.
IM
intermetatarsal
intramedullary
intramuscular
IM angle
IM joint
IMA
intermetatarsal angle
image
cockade i.
i. en Grelot
i. intensification
i. intensifier
postinjection i.
Image-I analysis software
imaging
bone-forming sarcoma bone i.
cine-magnetic resonance i. (cine-MRI)
color duplex i.
contrast medium-enhanced magnetic resonance i. (CME-MRI)
delayed bone i.
diagnostic i.
dipyridamole thallium i.
dynamic magnetic resonance i.
fixation i.
functional magnetic resonance i. (fMRI)
gadopentetate-dimeglumine-enhanced magnetic resonance i.
gamma camera i.
harmonic i.
indirect magnetic resonance arthrography nuclear bone i.
magnetic resonance i. (MRI)
magnetic source i. (MSI)
magnetization transfer magnetic resonance i. (mtMRI)
multiplanar virtual fluoroscopic i.
multiple line-scan i. (MLSI)
orthopantogram i.
orthoroentgenogram i.
radionucleotide i.
Raman spectroscopic i.
sagittal plane i.
trapezoidal i.
imbalance
fixed sagittal i.
isokinetic torque i.

NOTES

imbalance *(continued)*
  muscle i.
  rotator cuff i.
imbrication
  capsular i.
  MacNab line for facet i.
  medial capsular i.
imipenem and cilastatin
IML
  intermetacarpal ligament
immature
  i. bone
  skeletally i.
immediate
  i. amputation
  i. postoperative prosthesis (IPOP)
  i. postoperative stability (IPS)
  i. postsurgical fitting (IPSF)
immersion
  i. foot
  ice i.
immobilization
  cast i.
  i. degeneration
  external i.
  halo i.
  i. jacket
  joint i.
  i. method
  postoperative i.
  Rowe-Zarins shoulder i.
  sling i.
  sternal-occipital-mandibular i.
   (SOMI)
  Velcro i.
  Webril i.
immobilizer
  acromioclavicular i.
  ankle i.
  cast i.
  Comfort wrist i.
  DonJoy Ultrasling shoulder i.
  external i.
  Ezy Wrap shoulder i.
  Hook hemi-harness shoulder i.
  joint i.
  knee i.
  Kuz-Medics disposable knee i.
  long leg i.
  OEC knee i.
  Pedi-Wrap i.
  Plastazote-Kydex cervical i.
  postoperative i.
  QuickCast wrist i.
  Raymond shoulder i.
  sateen knee i.
  shoulder abduction i.
  single-panel knee i.
  sling i.

  Slingshot shoulder i.
  sternal-occipital-mandibular i.
  sternal-occipital-manubrial i.
  Tab-Strap knee i.
  thumb-wrist i.
  Trimline knee i.
  tri-panel knee i.
  Universal sling and swathe
   shoulder i.
  universal tri-panel knee i.
  Velcro i.
  Velpeau shoulder i.
  Watco knee i.
  Westfield acromioclavicular i.
  wrist i.
  Y-strap knee i.
  Zimmer knee i.
  Zinco thumb-wrist i.
immobilizing bandage
immovable
  i. articulation
  i. bandage
  i. joint
immune
  i. globulin
  i. system
immunity
  cell-mediated i.
  cellular i.
  humoral i.
immunoassay
  Alkphase-B i.
immunocompetence
immunogenicity
Immunomount
immunosuppression
  tolerogenic i.
immunosuppressive therapy
IMN
  intramedullary nailing
IMP
  innovative Medical Products
  Innovative Medical Products
  IMP bone screw targeter
  IMP knee positioning triangle
  IMP Steri-Clamp
  IMP surgical leg pedestal
  IMP turnstile casting stand
  IMP Universal knee positioner
  IMP Universal lateral positioner
impact
  i. biomechanics
  direct vertex i.
  i. glove
  i. mitt
  I. modular porous prosthesis
  I. modular total hip system
  I. total hip prosthesis
  I. total hip system

impacted
>   i. articular fracture
>   i. valgus fracture

impaction
>   atlantoaxial i.
>   i. cancellous autografting
>   digital i.
>   i. fracture

impactor
>   Austin Moore i.
>   bone i.
>   Cloward bone graft i.
>   Cohort spinal i.
>   Dawson-Yuhl i.
>   femoral i.
>   glenoid implant base i.
>   hook i.
>   humeral i.
>   Küntscher i.
>   Moe bone i.
>   mushroom i.
>   orthopaedic i.
>   i. rod
>   shell i.
>   Smith-Petersen i.
>   vertebral body i.

impactor-extractor
>   Fox i.-e.

impact-reducing pylon
impact-release binding on ski
impaired competitor policy
impairment
>   i. assessment
>   BFM i.
>   chronotropic i.
>   neurovascular i.
>   physical i.
>   sensory i.
>   visual-spatial ability i.

IMP-Capello arm support
impedance
>   bioelectrical i.
>   i. plethysmography

imperfecta
>   dentinogenesis i.
>   luxatio i.
>   osteogenesis i. (OI)

Imperial College, London Hospital
impingement
>   ankle i.
>   anterior ankle i.
>   anterior cord i.
>   anterior joint i.

anterior soft tissue i.
facet synovial i.
graft i.
lateral i.
i. lesion
i. pain
peroneal tendon i.
posterior i.
i. rod
roof i.
i. sign
i. spur
i. syndrome
i. test
tibiotalar i.
ulnocarpal i.

Impingement-Free Tibial Guide System
impinging exostosis
implant
>   Advanced mobile-bearing knee i.
>   i. alloy aluminum
>   AO-ASIF orthopaedic i.
>   i. arthroplasty
>   articulated chin i.
>   artificial joint i.
>   Ascension MCP finger joint i.
>   Ascension MCP total joint i.
>   BAK/Proximity interbody fusion i.
>   Bankart Tack i.
>   bicompartmental i.
>   BioAction great toe i.
>   bioactive i.
>   i. biocompatibility
>   BioCuff bioresorbable screw and
>   spiked washer i.
>   BioCuff C bioresorbable cannulated
>   screw and spike washer i.
>   BioCuff C bioresorbable spike
>   washer i.
>   biodegradable i.
>   Biodel i.
>   Biofix biodegradable i.
>   biomechanical failure of i.
>   Biomet custom i.
>   bioresorbable i.
>   BioSphere suture anchor i.
>   i. blank
>   bone i.
>   bovine collagen i.
>   Calnan-Nicolle finger i.
>   carbon i.
>   cartilage i.
>   Cartwright i.

NOTES

implant *(continued)*
    ceramic i.
    Charnley i.
    chromium i.
    chromium-cobalt-alloy i.
    CKS i.
    coated i.
    cobalt i.
    cobalt-chrome alloy and
      polyethylene i.
    cobalt-chromium i.
    i. collar
    condylar i.
    Continuum knee system i.
    Coonrad-Morrey i.
    Corail HA-coated stem hip i.
    COR/T i.
    CT-based CAD/CAM revision
      femoral i.
    curvilinear chin i.
    Custodis i.
    custom i.
    Cutter i.
    DePuy orthopaedic i.
    digital i.
    dorsal columella i.
    dorsal column stimulator i.
    double-stem silicone i.
    DTT i.
    Duracon knee i.
    Durallium i.
    Durapatite i.
    DynaGraft i.
    electrical i.
    Ewald-Walker knee i.
    i. failure
    i. fatigue
    fibrous tissue i.
    fin of the i.
    finger joint i.
    fixed anatomic patellar i.
    fixed bearing knee i.
    flail i.
    Flatt i.
    flexible digital i.
    flexible hinge i.
    i. forceps
    i. fracture
    Futura conical subtalar i.
    Futura flexible digital i.
    Futura metal hemi-toe i.
    Future i.
    Gemini MKII mobile-bearing
      knee i.
    Genesis II mobile-bearing knee i.
    gentamicin i.
    Geo Rectangles spinal i.
    Gliadel i.
    Global total shoulder i.

    great toe i.
    HA-coated hip i.
    Harris Design-2 i.
    Hedrocel proximal tibia
      augmentation i.
    hemi-interpositional i.
    hemi-silastic i.
    i. hinge
    hinged i.
    Howmedica Duracon i.
    Howmedica monospherical i.
    Hunter open cord tendon i.
    hyaline cartilage i.
    HyProCure sinus tarsi i.
    Ideal spinal i.
    iliosacral i.
    Insall-Burstein intracondylar knee i.
    Insall-Burstein total knee i.
    Interax Integrated Secure
      Asymmetric mobile-bearing
      knee i.
    Interpore i.
    joint i.
    Kalix flatfoot i.
    Kinetik great toe i. (KGTI)
    Kinetikos joint i.
    knee i.
    Koenig total great toe i.
    KPS bipolar vitallium-
      polyethylene i.
    LaPorta great toe i.
    Lawrence first metatarsophalangeal
      joint i.
    LCS total knee system i.
    i. loosening
    lumbar anterior-root stimulator i.
      (LARSI)
    i. material
    Maxwell-Brancheau arthroereisis i.
    McCutchen hip i.
    metacarpophalangeal i.
    i. metal
    metal-backed acetabular component
      hip i.
    metal-backed patellar i.
    metal hemi-toe i.
    metallic i.
    metal orthopaedic i.
    Metasul hip i.
    methyl methacrylate bead i.
    Microloc knee i.
    mobile-bearing knee i.
    modular i.
    Natural-Knee i.
    Neer II total shoulder system i.
    NeuFlex metacarpophalangeal
      joint i.
    NexGen knee i.
    Nexus i.

Niebauer i.
Niebauer-Cutter i.
OP-1 putty spinal fusion i.
OP-1 TM bone i.
orthobiologic i.
orthotic attachment i.
OsteoGen resorbable osteogenic
  bone-filling i.
Osteonics HA femoral i.
oxidized zirconium alloy on i.
Partnership i.
patellar resurfacing i.
pectoralis muscle i.
pedicle i.
percutaneous dorsal column
  stimulator i.
permanent i.
phalangeal i.
pin i.
plastic ball i.
PLLA i.
PMMA i.
polyglycolide i.
polylactide i.
polymethyl methacrylate i.
Polypin biodegradable pin i.
porous-coated i.
primus i.
processed carbon i.
Pro-Disc-C cervical artificial disc i.
Profix mobile-bearing knee i.
ProOsteon I. 500
pyrocarbon i.
i. reaction
i. removal
Restore cuff tear i.
Restore orthobiologic soft-tissue i.
rHead Recon i.
Rotaglide knee i.
rotating patellar i.
Schwaber otologic i.
Seeburger i.
self-aligning mobile-bearing knee i.
self-centering i.
self-sealing i.
Septacin i.
Sgarlato hammertoe i. (SHIP)
Sgarlato toe i.
Shaw-SHIP rod hammertoe i.
SHIP i.
silastic finger i.
silastic toe i.
silicone breast i.

silicone elastomer rubber ball i.
silicone MP i.
simple button patellar i.
single-stemmed toe i.
Sinterlock i.
Smart Screw bioabsorbable i.
spike washer i.
spinal i.
i. stage
STA-peg i.
StayFuse i.
i. stem
subtalar MBA i.
supraspinatus i.
Surgibone i.
Surgicel i.
i. survival rate
Sutter i.
Swanson carpal lunate i.
Swanson carpal scaphoid i.
Swanson finger joint i.
Swanson great toe i.
Swanson metacarpophalangeal i.
Swanson radial head i.
Swanson radiocarpal i.
Swanson small joint i.
Swanson trapezium i.
Swanson ulnar head i.
Swanson wrist joint i.
Swiss MP joint i.
Syed-Neblett i.
Syed template i.
synthetic bone i.
Techmedica i.
I. Technology LSF prosthesis
Teflon i.
TheraSeed i.
The Wedge bioresorbable
  interference-fit i.
TissueTak corkscrew i.
titanium i.
titanium-alloy i.
tobramycin-impregnated PMMA i.
toe i.
total knee i.
total ossicular reconstruction i.
Trac II knee i.
trial i.
tricompartmental i.
TSRH i.
UltraFix RC i.
UltraFix rotator cuff repair i.
unicompartmental knee i.

NOTES

implant *(continued)*
    Unilab Surgibone surgical i.
    Viladot i.
    vitallium i.
    Weber hip i.
    Weil i.
    Weil-modified Swanson i.
    Weil-type Swanson-design
      hammertoe i.
    white band on degenerated i.
    Wright monoblock titanium i.
    Zang metatarsal cap i.
    Zeichner i.
    Zymderm collagen i.
implantable
    i. bone anchor
    i. bone anchor device
    i. internal system
implantation
    autologous chondrocyte i. (ACI)
    collared press-fit femoral stem i.
    excision and i.
    1-level i.
    2-level i.
    3-level i.
    noncollared press-fit femoral
      stem i.
    periosteal i.
    screw i.
    vascular bundle i.
implant-cement interface
implanted bone growth stimulator
Implast
    I. adhesive
    I. bone cement
impression
    basilar i.
    i. defect
    i. fracture
imprinter
    foot i.
improvement
    maximal medical i. (MMI)
impulse
    afferent nerve i.
    efferent nerve i.
    i. inertial exercise trainer
    mobilization with i.
impulse-based nerve transmission
IMSC
    intramedullary supracondylar
      IMSC multihole nail
in
    in toto
    in vivo study
4-in-1
    4-i.-o. arthroplasty
    4-i.-o. cutting block
    4-i.-o. positioning block system

5-in-1
    5-i.-1 knee ligament repair
    5-i.-1 knee reconstruction
inactivity
    i. atrophy
    electrical i.
    physical i.
In-Bed AFO boot
InCare brace
incarial bone
incarnatus
    unguis i.
Incavo wire passer
incidence
    myelopathy i.
    nonunion i.
incise drape
incised wound
incision
    anteromedial i.
    Banks-Laufman i.
    Bardenheuer i.
    battledore i.
    bifrontal i.
    Brockman i.
    Brunner modified i.
    Brunner palmar i.
    Bruser skin i.
    Burns-Haney i.
    Burwell-Scott modification of
      Watson-Jones i.
    capsular i.
    Chang-Miltner i.
    Charnley i.
    chevron i.
    Cincinnati i.
    circumscribing i.
    Colonna-Ralston i.
    Couvelaire i.
    Crawford i.
    cruciate i.
    Cubbins i.
    Curtin i.
    curved i.
    curvilinear i.
    deltoid-splitting i.
    i. dilator
    dorsal linear i.
    dorsal longitudinal i.
    dorsal transverse i.
    dorsomedial i.
    double i.
    i. and drainage (I&D)
    DuVries i.
    Dwyer i.
    elliptical i.
    exploratory i.
    fascia-splitting i.
    fiber-splitting i.

fishmouth i.
Fowler-Philip i.
Gaenslen split-heel i.
Gatellier-Chastang i.
goblet i.
Grice i.
Griffith i.
Henderson skin i.
Henry i.
hockey-stick i.
H-shaped capsular i.
inverted-L lateral periosteal i.
inverted-Y i.
Jergesen i.
J-shaped skin i.
Kocher collar i.
Koenig-Schaefer i.
Langenbeck i.
lateral utility i.
lazy-C i.
lazy-L i.
lazy-S skin i.
L-curved i.
Loeffler-Ballard i.
longitudinal i.
L-shaped capsular i.
Ludloff i.
Mayfield i.
McLaughlin-Ryder i.
medial parapatellar i.
midaxillary line i.
muscle-splitting i.
Nicola i.
Ober i.
oblique i.
Ollier i.
palmar i.
parapatellar i.
parathenar i.
Picot i.
plantar longitudinal i.
posterior i.
posterolateral costotransversectomy i.
Pridie i.
4-i. procedure
5-i. procedure
racquet-shaped i.
relaxing i.
relieving i.
right-sided submandibular
  transverse i.
S i.
saber-cut i.

Seattle modification of Kocher i.
serpentine i.
S-flap i.
skin i.
skived i.
split i.
split heel i.
S-shaped i.
stab i.
straight i.
subfascial i.
Sutherland-Rowe i.
tangential i.
Texas T i.
thoracoabdominal i.
transverse i.
triradiate i.
T-shaped i.
Turco oblique posteromedial i.
universal i.
upright-Y i.
U-shaped i.
volar midline oblique i.
volar zigzag finger i.
V-shaped i.
Wagner skin i.
Watson-Jones i.
webspace i.
Westin-Hall i.
Y i.
Y-shaped i.
Y-V plasty i.
zigzag finger i.
Z-plasty i.

incisional
  i. biopsy
  i. neuroma
  i. skin-slough
incisive bone
Incisor arthroscopic blade
incisural notch
Inclan
  I. bone graft
  I. modification
  I. modification of Campbell ankle
  operation
  I. modification of Campbell ankle
  procedure
  I. posterior bone block
Inclan-Ober
  I.-O. arthroplasty
  I.-O. procedure

NOTES

inclination
    i. angle
    angle of thoracic i.
    thoracic i.
inclinometer
    Baseline Bubble i.
    Dualer Plus i.
    1-i. method
    2-i. method
inclinometry
    digital i.
inclusion
    i. body myositis (IBM)
    i. cyst
InCompass thoracolumbar spine fixation screw
incomplete
    i. amputation
    i. coalition
    i. dislocation
    i. fracture
    i. fracture of bone
    i. luxation
    i. paraplegia
    i. reduction
    i. syndactyly
    i. tear
incongruency
    subtalar joint i.
incongruent articulation
incongruity
    angle of i.
incontinence
    oral i.
    urinary i.
incoordination
incorporation
    bone graft i.
increased
    i. carrying angle
    i. depolymerization
    i. lateral joint space
increment after exercise
incremental response
incubation period
incudomalleolar
    i. articulation
    i. joint
incurvated
incurvatum reflex
independent
    i. exercise program
    i. transfer
index, pl. **indices**
    acetabular i.
    acetabular head i. (AHI)
    acromial spur i. (ASI)
    ADL i.
    indices of ADLs

alignment i.
alpha i.
ambulation i.
arch i.
arch-height i.
Arthritis Helplessness I. (AHI)
axial acetabular i. (AAI)
Barthel ADL i.
Benink tarsal i.
beta i.
body mass i. (BMI)
Caregiver Strain I. (CSI)
I. Chemicus Registry System (ICRS)
Chippaux-Smirak arch i.
Convery polyarticular disability i.
cortical i.
cyst i.
dynamic stability i.
Eyre-Brook epiphysial i.
femoral cortical i.
i. finger
i. finger abduction
Flower i.
Foot Function I. (FFI)
footprint i.
Functional Status I. (FSI)
Garden alignment i.
Hand Functional I. (HFI)
HAQ I.
Hauser ambulation i.
Hollingshead I.
Holmes-Rahe Life Change I.
hop i.
Hospital Trauma I.
Insall-Salvati patellar height i.
Ishihara cervical spine curve i.
Jette Functional Status i.
Katz ADL i.
Keitel i.
Kenny ADL i.
I. Knobber II massage tool
laxity i.
Lequesne Severity of Osteoarthritis I.
Life Satisfaction I. (LSI)
Lucas and Drucker Motor I.
malleolar i.
McDowell Impairment I. (MII)
McMurtry kinematic i.
i. metacarpophalangeal joint reconstruction
Motricity I.
Northwick Park I.
notch width i. (NWI)
Nottingham Extended ADL i.
Oswestry i.
PICA i.
Predictive Salvage I.

pressure excursion i.
I. prosthesis
Quetelet i.
i. ray amputation
Reimers hip position migration i.
Reimers instability i.
Reintegration to Normal Living i.
right and left ankle i.
Ritchie rheumatoid arthritis i.
Rivermead ADL i.
Rivermead Mobility I. (RMI)
Roland low back pain i.
sciatic function i. (SFI)
Singh osteoporosis i.
Spinal Cord Motor Index and
   Sensory Indices
Spotorno i.
Stahl i.
Takakura i.
talocalcaneal i.
toe i.
Waddell Chronic Back Pain
   Disability i.
Western Ontario Instability I.
   (WOSI)
Western Ontario and McMaster
   University osteoarthritis i.
Western Ontario Rotator Cuff I.
Wheelchair User's Shoulder Pain I.
   (WUSPI)

Indiana
   I. conservative prosthesis
   I. reamer
   I. tome carpal tunnel syndrome
      release system
   I. tome clip
   I. tome knife
indifferent electrode
indirect
   i. fracture
   i. magnetic resonance arthrography
      nuclear bone imaging
   i. manipulation
   i. reduction
   i. triangulation
Indochron E-R
indoleacetic acid
Indong Oh hip prosthesis
induction
   pain i.
inductive coupling device
indurated plantar keratoma (IPK)

induration
industry, pl. **industries**
   Duro-Med Industries (DMI)
inelastic
inequality
   anatomic leg length i.
   functional leg length i.
   leg length i. (LLI)
   i. in leg length (ILL)
Inerpan flexible burn dressing
inertia
   moment of i.
In/Ex Ilium
inextensibility
infant
   i. abduction splint
   i. clown cast shoe
   I.'s Feverall
   floppy i.
   Movement Assessment of I.'s
      (MAI)
   I.'s Silapap
infantile
   i. cortical hyperostosis
   i. dermal fibromatosis
   i. idiopathic scoliosis
   i. progressive spinal muscular
      atrophy
   i. tibia vara (ITV)
   i. trigger digit
infarct
   bone i.
infarction
   bone i.
   capsuloputaminal i.
   capsuloputaminocaudate i.
In-Fast bone screw system
infected
   i. bone
   i. nondraining nonunion
infection
   aerobic i.
   anaerobic i.
   aspergillosis i.
   blood-borne i.
   bone i.
   clostridial i.
   cryptococcal i.
   deep delayed i.
   deep wound i.
   epidural space i.
   fascial space i.
   felon i.

NOTES

infection *(continued)*
    fungal i.
    gas-producing streptococcal i.
    granulomatous fungal i.
    hematogenous i.
    Meleney i.
    musculoskeletal i.
    mycobacterial i.
    nontuberculous mycobacterial i.
    percutaneous bone marrow i.
    pin tract i.
    postoperative i.
    i. prevention
    pyogenic spinal i.
    spinal i.
    superficial i.
    suppurative joint i.
    tarsal joint i.
    webspace i.
infectious
    i. arthritis
    i. bulbar necrosis
    i. tenosynovitis
inferential therapy
inferior
    i. angle
    atraumatic, multidirectional, bilateral
      rehabilitation i. (AMBRI)
    i. band cruciform ligament
    i. calcaneal nerve
    i. calcaneonavicular ligament (ICN)
    i. capsular shift (ICS)
    i. capsular split technique
    i. costal sulcus
    i. extensor of foot
    i. extensor retinaculum
    i. facet
    i. gemelli muscle
    i. glenohumeral ligament (IGHL)
    i. glenohumeral ligament insertion
    i. glide
    i. ilioischial ligament
    i. laryngeal nerve
    i. leaf
    i. movement
    i. outline
    i. peroneal retinaculum
    i. process
    i. radioulnar joint
    i. ramus
    i. spur
    i. spurring
    i. thyroid artery
    i. tibiofibular joint
    i. tibiofibular repair
    i. vena cava
**inferoposterior acetabular capsule
  retractor**

infestation
    pressure ulcer-related maggot i.
INFH
    ischemic necrosis of femoral head
infiltrate
    fibrofatty i.
infiltration
    root i.
infinity
    I. femoral component
    I. hip system
    I. modular hip prosthesis
InFix interbody fusion system
inflamed synovial pouch
inflammation
    bursal i.
    i. management
    polyarticular symmetric tophaceous
     joint i.
    prepatellar bursa i.
    tendon i.
inflammatory
    i. arthropathy
    i. bowel disease associated arthritis
    i. fracture
    i. myositis
    i. phase
    i. scoliosis
    i. spondyloarthropathy
    i. synovitis
    i. tenovaginitis
inflatable
    i. bone tamp (IBT)
    i. elbow splint
inflexion point
inflow
    i. cannula
    vascular i.
infracalcaneal bursitis
infraclavicular
    i. region
    i. triangle
infraction fracture
infracture
infraganglionic injury
infraglenoid tuberosity
infragluteal
    i. creaking
    i. crease
infraisthmal
infrapatellar
    i. bursa
    i. bursitis
    i. contracture syndrome (IPCS)
    i. fat pad
    i. ligament
    i. plica
    i. strap
    i. tendinitis

i. tendon
i. tendon rupture
i. view
infrapatella tendinitis
infrared
i. applicator
i. head
i. light (IR)
i. light-emitting diode
i. therapy
i. thermography
infrascapular region
infraspinatus
i. muscle
i. tendinitis
i. tendon
infraspinous
i. fascia
i. region
infrasternal
infratrochlear
Infumorph Injection
InFuse
I. bone graft
I. bone graft/LT-Cage lumbar tapered fusion device
Infusible pressure infusion bag
infusion-aspiration drainage
infusion pump
Inge
I. retractor
I. spreader
Ingebrightsen traction
Inglis-Cooper release
Inglis-Pellicci elbow arthroplasty rating system
Inglis triaxial total elbow arthroplasty
Ingram
I. bony bridge resection
I. osteotomy
I. procedure
ingrowing toenail
ingrown
i. nail
i. toenail
ingrowth
bone i.
i. fixation
inguinal
i. approach
i. ligament
i. ligament syndrome
i. TEPP repair

inhalant anesthesia
inhalation anesthesia
inherent motion
inhibition test
inhibitive
i. cast
i. traction
inhibitor
aldose reductase i.
alpha-a_2-plasmin i.
anion transport i.
cholinesterase i.
monoamine oxidase-B i.
shoulder subluxation i. (SSI)
tissue i.
inhibitory postsynaptic potential
inhomogeneity
iniencephaly
inion bump
initial
i. manifestation
i. stance
initiation
i. feel
rhythmic i. (RI)
initiator drill
injection
alcohol i.
Black peroneal tendon sheath i.
cervical nerve root i.
chymopapain i.
epidural steroid i. (ESI)
extrafascial nerve i.
facet i.
Hyalgan i.
i. injury
intraarticular i.
intracranial pressure elevation joint i.
intramuscular i.
lumbar facet i.
lumbar nerve root i.
lumbar transforaminal epidural i.
nerve root i.
peroneal tendon sheath i.
procaine-phenol motor point i.
steroid i.
i. study
i. technique
tenosynovial i.
thecal i.
i. therapy
thoracic epidural i.

NOTES

injection *(continued)*
    trigger point i.
    zygapophysial joint i.
injurious energy input spearing
injury, pl. **injuries**
    acceleration/deceleration i.
    accessory nerve i.
    acquired brain i.
    acromioclavicular joint i.
    acute stretch i.
    i. algorithm
    ankle i.
    anular i.
    ASIA impairment scale for
      classification of spinal cord i.
    i. assessment
    athletic i.
    avulsion i.
    axial compression i.
    axial loading i.
    axillary nerve i.
    axonal i.
    ballistic i.
    barked i.
    bending toward the side of i.
    bicycle i.
    birth i.
    bladder i.
    brachial artery i.
    brachial plexus i.
    brachial plexus traction i. (BPTI)
    Brief Test of Head I. (BTHI)
    bunk bed i.
    burner i.
    burst i.
    calcaneocuboid joint nutcracker i.
    Callahan extension of cervical i.
    cervical nerve root i.
    cervical spinal i.
    cervical spine extension i.
    Chopart osseous joint i.
    chronic microtraumatic soft
      tissue i.
    closed kinetic chain i.
    closed soft tissue i.
    cocking i.
    cold i.
    2-column cervical spine i.
    3-column cervical spine i.
    compression-plus-torque cervical i.
    compressive flexion i.
    compressive hyperextension i.
    contrecoup i.
    crush i.
    i. culture paracetamol
    cuneiform i.
    Danis-Weber classification of
      ankle i.
    dashboard knee i.

    degloving i.
    diffuse axonal i. (DAI)
    discoligamentous i.
    distal tibial epiphysial i.
    distraction i.
    Drummond and Hastings cuboid
      extrusion i.
    dye punch i.
    elbow i.
    electrical i.
    epiphysial i.
    ergonomic i.
    Essex-Lopresti i.
    eversion i.
    explosion i.
    extensor tendon i.
    extravasation i.
    factitious i.
    femoral vein i.
    firearm i.
    flexion-distraction i.
    flexion-extension i.
    FOOSH i.
    forced flexion i.
    Foucher classification of
      epiphysial i.
    frostbite i.
    gamekeeper's i.
    Gertzbein classification of seat-
      belt i.
    grease gun i.
    growth plate i.
    Hardcastle classification of
      tarsometatarsal joint i.
    hip epiphysial i.
    hyperextension i.
    hyperextension-hyperflexion i.
    hyperflexion i.
    hyperplantarflexion i.
    iatrogenic i.
    infraganglionic i.
    injection i.
    interosseous nerve i.
    inversion ankle i.
    ipsilateral foot i.
    Klumpke i.
    knee ligamentous i.
    laryngeal nerve i.
    lateral compartment i.
    lateral compression i.
    lawn mower i.
    ligamentous i.
    Lisfranc i.
    long thoracic nerve i.
    low back i.
    lower plexus i.
    lumbar plexus i.
    lunate facet dye punch i.
    MacKinnon nerve i.

mangling i.
marching band i.
matrix i.
medial brachial cutaneous nerve i.
medial compartment i.
median nerve i.
meniscal i.
mesencephalic i.
metatarsophalangeal joint i.
midcarpal i.
middle column i.
missile i.
multiple injuries
muscle-tendon i.
musculocutaneous nerve i.
nail i.
nerve i.
neural i.
neurovascular i.
nutcracker i.
obturator nerve i.
Ontario Cohort of Running-
   Related I.
open-book pelvic i.
osteochondral i.
overuse i.
paint gun i.
paint thinner i.
i. pattern
pelvic i.
P-ER i.
perihamate i.
peripheral nerve i.
peripisiform i.
peritrapezial i.
peritrapezoidal i.
peroneal nerve i.
physial i.
pitching i.
plantarflexion i.
plantar plate i.
pleural i.
pneumatic tire i.
Poland classification of physial i.
posterior ligamentous i.
predictor of i.
pronation i.
pronation-abduction i.
pronation-eversion i.
pronation-eversion-external
   rotation i.
pseudogamekeeper's i.
pudendal nerve i.

Pugil stick i.
radial artery i.
radial nerve i.
radioulnar joint i.
recurrent laryngeal nerve i.
reperfusion i.
repetition strain i. (RSI)
repetitive stress i.
road burn i.
Rockwood classification of
   acromioclavicular i.
roller i.
Rosenthal classification of nail i.
rotator cuff i.
running-related i.
sacral plexus i.
sacroiliac joint i.
Sage-Salvatore classification of
   acromioclavicular joint i.
sailboarder i.
Salter-Harris classification of
   epiphysial plate i.
Salter-Harris tibial-fibular i.
sand toe i.
Scales of Cognitive Ability for
   Traumatic Brain I. (SCATBI)
scaphoid tuberosity i.
scapuloclavicular i.
sciatic nerve i.
seat-belt i.
sesamoid i.
I. Severity Score (ISS)
shearing i.
shotgun i.
sideswipe i.
skier's i.
snowboarding i.
softball sliding i.
soft tissue i.
spinal accessory nerve i.
spinal cord i. (SCI)
sports i.
stable cervical spine i.
steering wheel i.
sternoclavicular joint i.
stinger i.
straddle i.
strain-sprain i.
stress i.
stretch i.
subclavian artery i.
subclavian vein i.
subscapular artery i.

NOTES

injury *(continued)*
    subscapular nerve i.
    Sunderland classification of
      nerve i.
    Sunderland first-degree nerve i.
    supination i.
    supination-adduction i.
    supination-eversion i.
    supination-external rotation i.
    supination-inversion rotation i.
    supination-outward rotation i.
    supination-plantarflexion i.
    supraganglionic i.
    suprascapular nerve i.
    synovial i.
    talar neck class i. (I–III)
    tarsometatarsal joint i.
    thoracic duct i.
    thoracic nerve i.
    thoracoabdominal artery i.
    thoracodorsal nerve i.
    thoracolumbar spinal i.
    thoracolumbar spine flexion-
      distraction i.
    throwing i.
    tibial axial load i.
    tibial nerve i.
    tornado i.
    tracheal i.
    trampoline i.
    transcutaneous crush i.
    translation i.
    traumatic brain i. (TBI)
    traumatic burn i.
    turf toe i.
    ulnar artery i.
    ulnar collateral ligament i.
    ulnar nerve i.
    unstable cervical spine i.
    vascular i.
    vertebrobasilar i.
    Weber classification of physial i.
    weightbearing rotational i.
    whiplash i.
    wind-up i.
    wringer i.
**Inland Super Multi-Hite orthopaedic
bed**
inlay
    i. bone graft
    Sher diabetic shoe i.
inlet view
inner
    i. heel wedge (IHW)
    I. Lip Plate
    I. Lok ankle brace
    i. malleolus
    i. table

innervation
    muscle i.
    parasympathetic i.
    reciprocal i.
    somatic i.
    sympathetic i.
Innoboot splint
Innomed
    I. arthroplasty measuring system
    I. Assistant Free surgical
      instrument
    I. bone curette
innominate
    anterior i.
    i. bone
    i. bone resection
    left i.
    i. movement
    i. osteotomy
    posterior i.
    right posterior i.
    i. tilt
    i. vein
Innovasive
    I. bone anchor
    I. device
    I. fixation
innovation
    I. Sports bracing product
    I. Sports bracing support
innovative
    I. COR/T implant system
    I. Medical Products (IMP)
    I. Medical Products (IMP)
    I. Medical Products Steri-Clamp
inochondritis
inosculation phase
inotropism
**Inpatient Rehabilitation Facility–Patient
Assessment Instrument (IRFPAI)**
Inro surgical nail
Insall
    I. anterior approach
    I. anterior cruciate ligament
      reconstruction
    I. criteria
    I. ligament reconstruction technique
    I. patella alta method
    I. patellar injury classification
    I. procedure
    I. proximal realignment
    I. ratio
Insall-Burstein
    I.-B. II modular total knee system
    I.-B. intracondylar knee implant

I.-B. semiconstrained
tricompartmental knee prosthesis
I.-B. total knee implant
Insall-Burstein-Freeman (IBF)
I.-B.-F. knee arthroplasty
Insall-Hood reconstruction technique
Insall-Salvati
I.-S. measurement
I.-S. patellar height index
I.-S. ratio
insecurity
gravitational i.
insensate foot
insert
AliMed i.
angled bearing i.
articular i.
cancellous i.
clamp i.
cushioned shoe i.
custom-made i.
Durasul polyethylene, high wear
resistant acetabular i.
Energy Plus shoe i.
Gel-Sole shoe i.
i. graft
Hapad felt i.
Hapad shoe i.
heel and sole i.
Hydragrip clamp i.
Johnson & Johnson PFC cruciate-
substituting i.
New York University orthotic i.
NYU orthosis i.
Orthex Relievers shoe i.
orthotic shoe i.
Osteonics Scorpio i.
Poly-Dial i.
polyethylene tibial i.
polypropylene i.
POWERPoint orthotic shoe i.
Profix confirming tibial i.
retrieved i.
Roho solid seat i.
shoe i.
silicone gel socket i.
soft socket i.
sole i.
Spenco shoe i.
S-ROM Poly-Dial i.
thermomoldable i.
tibial i.
UCB shoe i.

viscoelastic heel i.
warm-and-form i.
inserter
Buck femoral cement restrictor i.
CDH cup i.
cement restrictor i.
cement spacer i.
cerclage wire i.
C-wire i.
deluxe FIN pin i.
Kirschner wire i.
Massie i.
prosthesis i.
Shaffner orthopaedic i.
spacer i.
staple i.
T-shaped i.
TSRH hook i.
inserter-extractor
compression i.-e.
insertion
anatomic i.
anomalous i.
Bosworth bone peg i.
C-D rod i.
deltoid i.
i. equipment
IGHL i.
inferior glenohumeral ligament i.
lag screw i.
ligamentous i.
oblique screw i.
pedicle screw i.
percutaneous pin i.
Pierrot-Murphy advancement i.
rerouting i.
screw i.
i. tendinopathy
insertional
i. Achilles tendinosis
i. activity
i. excursion
in-shoe transducer
inside-out
i.-o. Bankart shoulder instability
operation
i.-o. meniscal repair
i.-o. technique for establishing
ankle portal
i.-o. tissue repair technique
inside-to-outside technique
**Insight knee positioning and alignment
system**

NOTES

insole

Aliplast i.
Anti-Shox gel i.
Apex i.
Bestfoam i.
Comf-Orthotic 3/4-length i.
Comf-Orthotic sports replacement i.
Comf-Orthotic wool felt i.
Darco moldable i.
Diab-A-Foot rocker i.
Diab-A-Pad i.
Diab-A-Sole flat i.
Diab-A-Sole molded i.
Diabetic Diagnostic i.
D-Soles i.
EMED i.
Ever-Flex i.
Flat Foot i.
FlexiTherm diabetic diagnostic i.
Hapad metatarsal i.
Kinetic Wedge molded i.
molded postpartum i.
Orthex reliever i.
Plastazote i.
Plexidure i.
Poron 400 i.
PPT flat i.
PPT MXL soft molded i.
PPT Plastizote i.
PPT RX firm molded i.
ProThotics i.
PumpPals i.
Reflex Comfort i.
Sherform silicone i.
silicone i.
Sof Airr i.
SofSole Airr i.
Sorbothane i.
Spenco i.
S-Soles i.
TechnoGel i.
viscoelastic i.
Viscoped S i.

instability

ankle i.
i. of the ankle
anterior shoulder i.
anterolateral-anteromedial rotary i.
anterolateral rotary i. (ALRI)
anterolateral rotary knee i.
anteromedial-posteromedial rotary i.
anteromedial rotary i.
articular i.
atlantoaxial i.
atraumatic multidirectional i.
axial i.
capitate-lunate i.
carpal i.

Chrisman-Snook correction of
   ankle i.
chronic functional i.
chronic lateral ankle i.
collateral ligament i.
combined i.
congenital atlantoaxial i.
distal intercalated segment i. (DISI)
dorsal intercalated segment i.
   (DISI)
dorsiflexed intercalated segment i.
   (DISI)
DRUJ i.
extension i.
flexion i.
functional i.
i. gait
glenohumeral i.
hindfoot i.
i. hypothesis
intercalated segment i.
inversion i.
joint i.
knee i.
lateral rotatory ankle i.
lumbar spinal i.
lumbar spine i.
lunotriquetral i.
mechanical i.
medial column i.
membrane i.
midcarpal i. (MCI)
multidirectional i. (MDI)
open stabilization of traumatic
   anterior shoulder i.
osseous i.
patellar i.
pelvic i.
perilunar i.
1-plane i.
posterior shoulder i.
posterolateral rotary i.
posteromedial rotary i.
postural i.
progressive perilunar i.
push-pull i.
radiocarpal i.
rotary ankle i.
rotational i.
sagittal plane i.
scapholunate i.
shoulder i.
spinal i.
straight lateral i.
subtalar joint i.
thumb i.
tibiofibular joint i.
tibiotalar i.
traumatic anterior i.

traumatic anterior shoulder i.
triquetrolunate i.
valgus i.
varus-valgus i.
vertebral i.
volar flexed intercalated segment i.
  (VISI)
volar intercalary wrist i.
wrist i.
installation procedure
install method
Insta-Nerve device
instantaneous axis of rotation
instant cold pack
Instat collagen sponge
institute
  Podiatry I.
  Southern California Orthopaedic I.
  (SCOI)
**Instratek titanium cannulated small
  bone screw system**
Instron machine
instrument
  Accu-Line knee i.
  AccuSharp carpal tunnel release i.
  Achieve computer-assisted i.'s
  activating adjusting i. (AAI)
  Acufex arthroscopic i.
  Acufex MosaicPlasty i.
  American Academy of Orthopaedic
    Surgeons Pediatrics Outcomes I.
  Arthrex arthroscopy i.
  Arthroforce III hand i.
  arthroscopic laser i.
  Atlas orthogonal percussion i.
  AxyaWeld i.
  back range of motion i.
  battery-powered i.
  Collis TDR i.
  Command instrument system
    surgical i.
  Cotrel-Dubousset spinal i.
  Dreyfus prosthesis placement i.
  electrosurgical i.
  Femur Finder i.
  Friatec manual arthroscopy i.
  Hall Micro E power i.
  Hall series 4 large bone i.
  Hall-Zimmer power i.
  Howmedica-Osteonics i.
  IBF knee i.
  Innomed Assistant Free surgical i.

Inpatient Rehabilitation
  Facility–Patient Assessment I.
  (IRFPAI)
Kinetix i.
Kirschner surgical i.
laser i.
I. Makar biodegradable interference
  screw
microsurgical i.
Midas Rex pneumatic i.
i. migration
Mitek SuperAnchor i.
Monogram total knee i.
Nicolet Compass EMG i.
orthopaedic cutting i.
OrthoVise orthopaedic i.
oscilloscope i.
paraspinal skin temperature
  thermocouple i.
Partnership i.
passivation metal i.
PowerTrack II muscle testing i.
quadriceps-sparing, minimally
  invasive total knee i.
Rancho external fixation i.
reciprocal planing i.
RingLoc i.
ScoliTron i.
Shea prosthesis placement i.
single reference point i.
i., sponge, needle count
Steffee i.
Sulzer Orthopaedics i.
thermocouple i.
Ultra-Cut i.
Universal Minimally Invasive
  Assistant Free hip surgery i.'s
WeeFIM i.
Wiet graft-measuring i.
instrumental
  i. activities of daily living (IADL)
  i. ADLs
instrumentation
  Accu-Line knee i.
  Acufex arthroscopic i.
  anterior distraction i.
  anterior Zielke i.
  AO fixateur interne i.
  AO notched i.
  Apofix cervical i.
  Arthrotek Ellipticut hand i.
  biodegradable fixation i.
  bone-holding i.

NOTES

instrumentation *(continued)*
    cable-hook compression i.
    Caspar anterior i.
    C-D i.
    compression U-rod i.
    Cotrel-Dubousset pedicle screw i.
    distraction i.
    double Zielke i.
    Drummond spinal i.
    Dwyer spinal i.
    dynamic compression plate i.
    Edwards i.
    endoscopic carpal tunnel i.
    halo-Ilizarov distraction i.
    Harms-Moss anterior thoracic i.
    Harrington distraction i.
    Harrington-Kostuik i.
    Harrington rod i.
    hollow mill i.
    Howmedica knee i.
    Jacobs locking hook spinal rod i.
    Kaneda anterior spinal i.
    Kostuik-Harrington spinal i.
    locking hook i.
    Louis i.
    lumbar spine i.
    lumbosacral spine transpedicular i.
    Luque II segmental spinal i.
    Luque semirigid segmental spinal i.
    Mayfield i.
    McElroy i.
    modular i.
    Moreland total hip revision i.
    Moss i.
    multiple hook assembly C-D i.
    Passport i.
    posterior cervical spinal i.
    posterior distraction i.
    posterior hook-rod spinal i.
    Putti-Platt i.
    rod-sleeve i.
    sacral spine modular i.
    segmental spinal i. (SSI)
    Sielke i.
    skin-contact i.
    Smith-Richards i.
    spinal i.
    Steffee spinal i.
    Stryker power i.
    i. system
    total knee i.
    TSRH i.
    Universal sacral spine i.
    variable screw placement system i.
    VSP plate i.
    Wisconsin interspinous segmental
      spinal i.
    Zielke pedicular i.

insufficiency
    abductor i.
    active i.
    capsular length i.
    i. fracture
    ligamentous i.
    mechanical i.
    muscle i.
    passive i.
    peripheral vascular i.
    posterior tibial tendon i.
    PTT i.
    transverse plane motion i.
    vertebrobasilar i. (VBI)
insufflate
insulin-dependent diabetes mellitus
In-Tac bone-anchoring system
intact
    I. dressing
    neurologically i.
    neurovascularly i.
    i. neurovascular status
    i. peripheral pulses
    i. spinous lamina
    i. spinous process
intake
    dietary reference i. (DRI)
    energy i.
integral
    force-time i. (FTI)
    I. hip system
    I. Interlok femoral prosthesis
    pressure-time i. (PTI)
integrated
    I. Ankle orthotic ankle joint
    i. electromyography
    i. rectified EMG (IEMG)
    i. shape and imaging system
      (ISIS)
integration
    Beery-Buktenica Developmental Test
      of Visual-Motor I.
    body side i.
    DeGangi-Berk Test of Sensory I.
    Functional I. (FI)
    sensory i.
    visual-motor i. (VMI)
integrity
    I. acetabular cup
    I. acetabular cup prosthesis
    I. acetabular cup screw
    i. and alignment
    biochemical i.
    biomechanical i.
    bone plate i.
    maintenance of bone plate i.
    soft tissue i.
Intelect
    I. Combo stimulator/ultrasound

I. electric stimulator
I. laser system device
I. Legend stimulator
I. 600MP microcurrent stimulator
InteliJET fluid management system
Intelligent Prosthesis Plus prosthesis
IntelliTemp insulation material
intensification
    image i.
intensifier
    C-arm image i.
    image i.
intention
    first i.
    healing by first i.
    healing by second i.
    i. myoclonus
    primary i.
    second i.
    secondary i.
    i. tremor
intentional
    i. movement
    i. rotation
Intenzyme Forte
Inteq small joint suturing system
Inter
    I. Fix RP threaded spinal fusion
      cage device
    I. Fix threaded spinal fusion cage
      device
interaction
    surface shoe i.
    tibiofemoral i.
interarticular
    i. cartilage
    i. disc
    i. fracture
    i. joint
    i. ligament of head of rib
    i. sulcus
Interax
    I. Integrated Secure Asymmetric
      mobile-bearing knee implant
    I. total knee system
interbody
    i. arthrodesis
    i. fusion cage system
    i. graft
    i. rasp
    i. spinal fusion
intercalary
    i. allograft procedure

i. diaphysial allograft
i. graft
i. resection
i. segmental replacement
intercalated segment instability
intercarpal
    i. arthrodesis
    i. articulation
    i. joint
    i. ligament
    i. ligament capsulodesis
interchondral joint
interclavicular
    i. ligament
    i. notch
intercollicular groove
intercompartment fasciotome
intercondylar
    i. drill guide
    i. femoral fracture
    i. fossa
    i. groove
    i. humeral fracture
    i. notch
    i. process
    i. roof
    i. space
    i. tibial fracture
intercostal
    i. artery
    i. flap
    i. nerve
    i. nerve block
    i. neuralgia
    i. restriction
    i. space (ICS)
    i. vein
intercostobrachial nerve
intercritical time
intercuneiform joint
interdigital
    i. bone fusion
    i. corn
    i. ligament
    i. neoplasm
    i. nerve
    i. nerve bundle
    i. neuroma (IDN)
    i. webspace
interdischarge interval
interdisciplinary vocational evaluation
    program
interepicondylar axis

NOTES

interface
>acetabular prosthetic i.
>bone-cement i.
>bone-implant i.
>bone-peg i.
>bony i.
>cement i.
>cement-bone i.
>cup-cement i.
>fascial-muscle i.
>fat-blood i. (FBI)
>implant-cement i.
>long-term bone-instrumentation i.
>patient-table i.
>pin-bone i.
>prosthesis i.
>prosthesis-cement i.
>ShearBan low-friction i.
>shoe-foot i.
>soft tissue i.

interfacet
>i. wiring
>i. wiring and fusion

interfacetal dislocation
interfacial porosity
interfascicular
>i. epineurectomy
>i. epineurotomy
>i. neurolysis

interference
>i. fit
>i. fit fixation
>nerve i.
>i. pattern
>i. screw
>i. screw technique
>vertebrogenic i.

interferential
>i. current
>i. electrical stimulation
>i. stimulation (IFC)
>i. stimulator
>i. therapy

InterFix
>I. RP threaded spinal fusion cage
>I. titanium threaded spinal fusion cage

interfragmentary
>i. compression
>i. lag screw
>i. plate
>i. wire

intergluteal cleft
interilioabdominal amputation
interinnominate asymmetry
interinnominoabdominal
>i. amputation
>i. cleft

interlaminar clamp

interleukin-1 beta release
interline
>Lisfranc articular i.

interlocking
>i. acetabular cup
>distal i.
>i. medullary nail
>i. nailing
>proximal i.
>i. screw

intermaxillary bone
intermediary amputation
intermediate
>i. amputation
>i. bundle
>i. callus
>i. cast
>i. cuneiform fracture-dislocation
>i. disc
>i. disinfectant
>i. dorsal cutaneous nerve (IDCN)
>i. interference pattern
>i. lamella
>i. phalangectomy
>i. socket

Intermedics
>I. natural hip system
>I. Natural-Knee knee prosthesis

intermedius
>vastus i.

intermetacarpal
>i. articulation
>i. joint
>i. ligament (IML)

intermetatarsal (IM)
>i. angle (IMA)
>i. angle-reducing operation
>i. angle-reducing procedure
>i. artery
>i. bursa
>i. bursitis
>i. joint
>i. ligament
>i. nerve
>i. space
>i. vein

intermetatarsophalangeal
>i. bursa
>i. bursitis

intermittens
>dyskinesia i.
>myotonia congenita i.

intermittent
>i. arthralgia
>i. casting
>i. cervical traction (ICT)
>i. claudication (IC)
>i. double-step gait
>i. extremity pump

i. hydrarthrosis
i. impulse compression
i. paresthesia
i. pneumatic compression
i. torticollis

intermuscular
i. neuroma transposition
i. septum

internal
i. band
i. carotid artery
i. derangement
i. derangement of knee (IDK)
i. femoral rotation
i. fixation apparatus
i. fixation, closed reduction
i. fixation compression arthrodesis
i. fixation compression arthrodesis of ankle
i. fixation plate-screw system
i. fixation spring
i. fracture fixation
i. gel pad
i. hemipelvectomy
i. iliac artery
i. iliac vein
i. jugular vein
i. malleolus
i. movement
i. neurolysis
i. oblique muscle
posteroinferior i. (PIIn)
i. process
i. rotary component of force component
i. rotational gait
i. rotation deformity
i. rotation exercise
i. rotation in extension (IRE)
i. rotation in flexion (IRF)
i. rotator
i. snapping hip syndrome
i. spinal fixation
i. tibial torsion (ITT)
i. tibial torsion brace
i. tibiofibular torsion
i. topography
i. version

internal-external rotation
internally
i. fixed fracture
i. rotated

international
I. Classification of Impairments, Disabilities, Handicaps (ICIDH)
I. Classification for Surgery of the Hand in Tetraplegia
I. Knee Documentation Committee (IKDC)
I. Knee Documentation Committee form
I. Knee Documentation Committee knee scale
I. Knee Documentation Committee Subjective Knee Form
I. Knee Ligament
I. Knee Ligament Standard Evaluation questionnaire
I. Listing System
I. Society of Arthroscopy, Knee Surgery, and Orthopaedic Sports Medicine (ISAKOS)
I. 10-20 System

interne
AO-ASIF fixateur i.
AO fixateur i.
Dick AO fixateur i.

internervous plane
intern's
i. triangle
i. triangle in hip spica cast

internus
malleolus i.
metatarsus i.

interoceptor
postural i.

Inter-Op
I.-O. acetabular prosthesis
I.-O. acetabular shell
I.-O. hip prosthesis

interossei (*pl. of* interosseus)
interosseous
i. anastomosing channel
i. artery
i. branch
i. cartilage
i. compartment
i. cuneocuboid ligament
i. cuneometatarsal ligament
i. diastasis
i. intercuneiform ligament
i. ligament disruption
i. membrane (IOM)
i. metacarpal ligament
i. metatarsal ligament

NOTES

interosseous *(continued)*
    i. muscle
    i. nerve
    i. nerve injury
    i. nerve syndrome
    i. sacroiliac ligament
    i. talocalcaneal ligament (ITCL)
    i. tendon
    i. wire fixation
interosseum
interosseus, pl. **interossei**
interparietal bone
interpeak interval
interpedicular
    i. distance
    i. distance widening joint widening
interpediculate
interpeduncular
    i. notch
    i. space
interpelviabdominal amputation
interperiosteal fracture
interphalangeal (IP)
    i. abductus
    i. amputation
    i. arthrodesis
    i. arthroplasty
    i. articulation
    i. coalition
    distal i. (DIP)
    i. fusion
    i. joint (IPJ)
    i. joint dislocation
    i. joint space
    i. osteoarthritis
    proximal i. (PIP)
    proximal interphalangeal/distal i. (PIP/DIP)
    i. sesamoid management
    i. tenodesis
interphalangectomy
Interpore
    I. bone
    I. bone replacement material
    I. implant
interposed comminution
interposition
    i. bone graft
    ligament reconstruction with tendon i. (LRTI)
    i. membrane
    soft tissue i.
    tendon i.
interpositional
    i. arthroplasty
    i. tricortical graft
interpotential interval
interpubic disc
interquantile range

interregional displacement
interrupted
    i. LVG
    i. suture
intersacral canal
interscalene block
interscapular
    i. aching
    i. amputation
    i. reflex
interscapulothoracic forequarter amputation
Interseal
    I. acetabular cup
    I. Variant I–IV prosthesis
intersection syndrome
intersegmental
    i. fixation
    i. mobility
    i. motion
    i. movement
    i. range of motion palpation (IRMP)
    i. rotation
    i. traction chiropractic table
intersesamoidal
intersesamoid ligament
InterSpace
    I. hip spacer
    I. knee spacer
interspace (IS)
    atlantoodontoid i.
    wedging of vertebral i.
interspinal ligament
interspinous
    i. cable
    i. ligament
    i. process fusion
    i. pseudarthrosis
    i. segmental spinal instrumentation technique (ISSI)
    i. wiring
interstice
    bone i.
interstitial
    i. fluid
    i. lamella
    i. meniscal tear
    i. myofasciitis
interteardrop line
intertendinous vinculum
intertransverse
    i. fusion
    i. ligament
    i. process arthrodesis
intertrigo
intertrochanteric
    i. femoral fracture
    i. 4-part fracture

i. plate
i. varus osteotomy
Intertron therapy microprocessor
intertubercular
i. bursitis
i. groove
i. plane
i. sulcus
interval
acromiohumeral i. (AHI)
anterior atlantoodontoid i.
atlantoaxial i.
atlantodens i. (ADI)
atlas-dens i.
biceps i.
confidence i. (CI)
deltopectoral i.
interdischarge i.
interpeak i.
interpotential i.
Kocher i.
posterior atlantoodontoid i.
recruitment i.
response i.
scaphocapitate i.
Scheffé i.
i. training
trapeziodeltoid i.
intervening
i. connective tissue
i. muscle
intervention
late i.
prosthetic i.
rehabilitation i.
intervertebral
i. cartilage
i. disc
i. disc height
i. disc herniation
i. disc narrowing
i. disc nucleus signal
i. dysfunction
i. joint
i. motion
i. motor unit
i. notch
interview
School Setting I. (SSI)
Worker Role I. (WRI)
intervolar plate ligament
intoe
intoeing gait

intolerance
cold i.
exercise i.
fingertip cold i.
intorsion
intraacetabular
intraarticular
i. adhesion
i. arthrodesis
i. calcaneal fracture
i. cautery
i. cautery device
i. clavicle
i. disc
i. disc ligament
i. dislocation
i. fragment
i. hip fusion
i. injection
i. jamming
i. knee fusion
i. loose body
i. osteochondroma
i. osteoid osteoma
i. osteotomy
i. procedure
i. proximal tibial fracture
i. reconstruction
i. structure
intracapsular
i. ankylosis
i. excision
i. fracture
i. osteoid osteoma
i. osteotomy
i. rupture
Intracell
I. massage stick
I. mechanical muscle device
I. myofascial trigger-point device
I. Sprinter stick
I. trigger point massager
intrachondrial bone
intracompartmental
i. edema
i. ischemia
i. pressure
Intracone intramedullary reamer
intracortical
i. fibrous dysplasia
i. osteogenic sarcoma
i. radiolucent lesion

NOTES

intracranial pressure elevation joint injection
intractable plantar keratosis (IPK)
intracuticular stitch
intradermal suture
intradiscal, intradiskal
    i. electrothermal therapy (IDET)
    i. electrothermal therapy procedure
    i. electrothermal treatment (IDET)
    i. electrothermal treatment procedure
    i. pressure
intradural
    i. anastomosis
    i. dorsal spinal root rhizotomy
    i. tumor surgery
intraepiphysial osteotomy
Intrafix
    I. ACL tibial fastener
    I. fixation
    I. screw
intrafocal reduction technique
intraforaminal approach
intrafusal fiber
intralesional
    i. excision
    i. resection
    i. vascular resistance
intramedullary (IM)
    Ace i. (AIM)
    i. alignment jig
    i. alignment rod
    i. ANK nail
    i. bar
    i. bone graft
    i. bouquet fixation
    i. canal
    i. drill
    i. guide
    i. hematoma
    i. hemorrhage
    i. lesion
    i. nailing (IMN)
    i. pin
    i. reamer
    i. rod fixation
    i. saw
    i. skeletal kinetic distractor (ISKD)
    i. stem
    i. supracondylar (IMSC)
    i. supracondylar multihole nail
intramembranous
    i. formation
    i. ossification
intramuscular (IM)
    i. injection
    i. lengthening
    i. nerve transposition
    i. recording

intraneural
    i. fibrosis
    i. lipofibroma
intraoperative
    i. Cell Saver
    i. complication
    i. dural tear
    i. fluoroscopy
    i. fracture
    i. neck hyperextension
    i. roentgenography
    i. stress-relaxation
    i. view
    i. x-ray
intraorganically induced
intraosseous
    i. abscess
    i. circulation
    i. fixation
    i. ganglion
    i. lipoma
    i. lipomatosis
    i. membrane
    i. nerve transposition
    i. osteosarcoma
    i. pneumatocyst
    i. probe
    i. suture anchor
    i. therapy
    i. tibiofibular ligament
    i. tophaceous gouty invasion
    i. tumor
    i. vascular congestion
    i. venography
    i. wire
    i. wiring
90-90 intraosseous wire Nitinol flexible wire
intrapedicular fixation
intraperiosteal fracture
intraprosthetic
intrapyretic amputation
intrascaphoid angle
IntraSite dressing
intraspinous muscle
intraspongy nuclear disc herniation
intratendinous
intrathecal
    i. anesthesia
    i. neurolysis
intrathecally enhanced CT scan
intravascular hemolysis
intravenous
    i. block anesthesia
    i. pyelogram
    i. regional anesthesia (IVRA)
    i. therapy
intravertebral foramen (IVF)
Intrepid functional knee brace

intrinsic
- i. clubfoot
- i. contracture
- i. equilibrium
- finger i.
- i. function
- i. metatarsus primus elevatus
- i. minus deformity
- i. minus hallux
- i. minus hand
- i. minus position
- i. muscle
- i. muscle strength
- i. paralysis
- i. plus deformity
- i. plus hand
- i. restoration
- i. tightness test
- i. transverse connector
- i. transverse connector role

introducer
- Charnley i.
- Dumon-Gilliard prosthesis i.
- staple i.

intubation
- endotracheal i.

Invacare
- I. APM mattress
- I. Comfort-Mate extra cushion
- I. manual wheelchair
- I. padded shower chair
- I. vinyl transfer bench

invagination
- basilar i.
- endplate i.

invalid
- i. cushion
- i. ring

invasion
- intraosseous tophaceous gouty i.
- vascular i.

inventory
- Brief Pain I.
- Child Development I.
- Mayo-Portland Adaptability I.-3 (MPAI-3)
- Millon Behavioral Health I.
- Millon Clinical Multiaxial I.
- Multidimensional Pain i.
- Neurobehavioral Functioning I. (NFI)
- Pediatric Evaluation of Disability I. (PEDI)
- Vanderbilt Pain Management I.
- Westhaven Yale Multidimensional Pain I. (WHYMPI)

inversion
- ankle i.
- i. ankle injury
- i. ankle sprain
- i. ankle stress view
- fixed i.
- i. instability
- i. of muscle action
- restricted i.
- i. stress test

inversion-eversion
- ankle i.-e.
- i.-e. exercise
- i.-e. rotation

InvertaChair traction device

inverted
- i. champagne bottle leg
- i. Napoleon hat sign
- i. orthotics
- i. radial reflex
- i. scarf Z-osteotomy
- i. skin flap
- i. smile

inverted-L lateral periosteal incision

inverted-Y
- i.-Y Achilles tenotomy
- i.-Y fracture
- i.-Y incision

inverting knot technique

invertor force

Invertrac equipment

investing fascia

involucrum, pl. **involucra**

involuntary activity

involvement
- tumorous i.

inward rotation

Ioban Vi-Drape

iodine-labeled fibrinogen

iodoform gauze

iodoform-impregnated plastic sheet

iodophor solution

IOM
- interosseous membrane

Ionact antibacterial protection

ion-bombarded cobalt-chromium

IonGuard orthopaedic surface treatment

ionized
- i. gas
- i. gas field

NOTES

iontophoresis
>Dynaphor i.

ion transfer

iopamidol myelography

Iowa
>I. degenerative change
>I. hip score
>I. hip status rating system
>I. implant material
>I. internal prosthesis
>I. stem
>I. total hip prosthesis
>I. University periosteal elevator

IP
>interphalangeal
>IP joint

IPCS
>infrapatellar contracture syndrome

IPJ
>interphalangeal joint

IPK
>indurated plantar keratoma
>intractable plantar keratosis

I-plate

I-Plus
>I-P. system humeral fracture brace
>I-P. system ulnar fracture brace

Ipomax orthosis

IPOP
>immediate postoperative prosthesis

ipos
>i. arch support system
>i. forefoot relief orthosis
>i. heel relief orthosis
>i. heel relief shoe
>i. postoperative shoe

ipriflavone

IPS
>immediate postoperative stability
>IPS total hip system

IPSF
>immediate postsurgical fitting

ipsilateral
>i. approach
>i. femoral neck fracture
>i. femoral shaft fracture
>i. foot injury
>i. rotation
>i. side bending
>i. slide graft
>i. total elbow arthroplasty
>i. total shoulder arthroplasty

IR
>infrared light
>isotonic reversal

IRE
>internal rotation in extension

IRF
>internal rotation in flexion

IRFPAI
>Inpatient Rehabilitation Facility–Patient Assessment Instrument

iris scissors

IRMP
>intersegmental range of motion palpation

Irom
>I. bilateral splint
>I. Regal splint
>I. splint with shells

iron
>Jewett bending i.

iron-deficiency anemia

Ironman Triathlon Pro-Power massager

irradiation
>i. fibromatosis
>i. sterilized graft

irreducible
>i. fracture
>i. fracture dislocation

irregular
>i. articular surface
>i. bone
>i. potential

irregularity
>tendon i.

irregular-shaped lesion

irrigating solution

irrigation
>i. bulb
>i. burn
>closed i.
>closed suction i.
>i. and débridement (I&D)
>drip-suck i.
>gravity inflow i.
>Pulsavac i.
>i. solution
>i. suction
>Systec i.
>i. system
>i. tube
>WaterPik i.
>wound i.

irrigator
>Arthro-Flo i.
>Baumrucker clamp i.
>Fisch bone drill i.
>jet i.
>pulse i.

irritability
>nerve root i.
>soft tissue i.

irritable
>i. hip
>i. joint
>i. lesion
>i. symptom

irritation
  i. callus
  facet joint i.
  nerve root i.
  sciatic nerve i.
Irvine
  I. ankle
  I. ankle arthroplasty
  University of California, I. (UCI)
Irvine
Irwin osteotomy
IS
  interspace
Isaacs syndrome
ISAKOS
  International Society of Arthroscopy,
  Knee Surgery, and Orthopaedic Sports
  Medicine
Isch-Dish Plus cushion
ischemia
  capillary i.
  critical limb i. (CLI)
  exercise i.
  foot i.
  intracompartmental i.
  muscle i.
  myocardial i.
  myoneural i.
  postural i.
  tourniquet i.
  vasospastic i.
  Volkmann i.
  warm i.
ischemic
  i. compression
  i. contracture
  i. disease of growing hip (IDGH)
  i. foot
  i. forearm exercise test
  i. gangrene
  i. leg disease
  i. lesion
  i. limb
  i. limb disease (ILD)
  i. lumbago
  i. myositis
  i. necrosis
  i. necrosis of femoral head (INFH)
  i. tourniquet technique
  i. ulcer
ischia (*pl. of* ischium)
ischial
  i. bone

  i. bursitis
  i. containment socket
  i. spine
  i. tuberosity
  i. weightbearing leg brace
  i. weightbearing orthosis
  i. weightbearing prosthesis (IWP)
  i. weightbearing ring
ischial-bearing seat
ischialgia
ischial-gluteal weightbearing socket
ischiatic scoliosis
ischiectomy
ischioacetabular fracture
ischiodynia
ischiofemoral ligament
ischiogluteal
  i. bursa
  i. bursitis
ischiohebotomy
ischionitis
ischiopubic
  i. arch
  i. foramen
  i. ramus
ischiopubiotomy
ischiorectal
  i. abscess
  i. fossa
  i. region
ischium, pl. **ischia**
Iselin disease
Ishihara cervical spine curve index
Ishizuki unconstrained elbow prosthesis
ISIS
  integrated shape and imaging system
    ISIS screening
ISKD
  intramedullary skeletal kinetic distractor
    ISKD system
island
  i. adipofascial flap
  bone i.
  fibrin i.
  i. graft
  i. skin flap
Isobaric epidural/spinal anesthesia technique
Isocaine HCl
isodynamic
IsoDyn knee brace
isoelastic pelvic prosthesis

NOTES

isograft
 bone i.
isoinertial
isokinetic
 i. assessment
 concentric bilateral i.
 i. dynamometer
 i. dynamometry
 i. evaluation
 i. exercise
 i. joint apparatus
 i. knee extension
 i. movement
 i. performance
 i. resistance apparatus
 i. strength test maximal
 i. testing
 i. torque imbalance
 i. Unex III exerciser
Isola
 I. fixation system
 I. hook-rod
 I. spinal implant system accessory
 I. spinal implant system anchor
 I. spinal implant system application
 I. spinal implant system eye rod
 I. spinal implant system hook
 I. spinal implant system iliac post
 I. spinal implant system iliac
 screw
 I. spinal implant system plate-rod
 combination
 I. spinal instrumentation system
 I. vertebral screw
 I. wire
isolated
 i. avulsion
 i. dislocation
 i. modular tibial insert exchange
 i. paralysis
 i. zone
isolation drape
isolator
 Ankle I.
isologous graft
isometer
 I. bone graft placement site
 detector
 CA-5000 drill-guide i.
 PCL Protension i.
 tension i.
isometheptene mucate
isometric
 i. cervical extension strength
 i. contraction
 i. device
 i. exercise
 i. force
 i. motor testing

 i. point
 i. resistance
 i. strain gauge
 i. strength testing
 i. technique
 i. traction
 i. training
isometricity
isoniazid
isophendylate
Isoprene plastic splint
Iso-Quadron exerciser
Isostation B200
Isotechnologies B-200 low back machine
Isotec patellar tendon graft
IsoTis Orthobiologics Accell TMB
Isotoner glove
isotonic, pl. **isotonics**
 combination of isotonics (COI)
 i. contraction
 i. exercise
 i. machine
 i. motor testing
 i. resistance
 i. reversal (IR)
 i. traction
 i. training
isotope
 bone mineralization i.
 i. bone scan
isotropic disc
Isovue myelography
Israel
 I. rasp
 I. retractor
ISS
 Injury Severity Score
ISSI
 interspinous segmental spinal
 instrumentation technique
iStep FIT digital scanner
isthmic spondylolisthesis
isthmus, pl. **isthmi, isthmuses**
isuprel
IT
 iliotibial
ITB
 iliotibial band
 ITB fasciitis
ITBFS
 iliotibial band friction syndrome
ITCL
 interosseous talocalcaneal ligament
Itrel
 I. II, III spinal cord stimulation
 system
 I. programmed transmitter-receiver
ITT
 internal tibial torsion

ITV
    infantile tibia vara
ITW
    idiopathic toe-walker
Ivalon prosthesis
IVF
    intravertebral foramen
ivory
      i. bone

      i. osteoma
      i. phalanx sign
IVRA
    intravenous regional anesthesia
iWALKfree hands-free crutch
IWP
    ischial weightbearing prosthesis

NOTES

I

J

J board
J disc
J pad
J septum
J sign
jab and hook punch combination
Jaboulay amputation
Jaccoud
    J. arthritis
    J. arthropathy
    J. arthroplasty
    J. syndrome
Jace
    J. hand continuous passive motion
    unit
    J. shoulder exerciser
    J. W550 CPM device
jack
    J. Frost hot/cold pack
    J. test
    turnbuckle j.
    j. upper cut
jacket
    body j.
    Boston soft body j.
    cervicothoracic j.
    flexion body j.
    Frejka j.
    halo body j.
    halo traction j.
    immobilization j.
    Kydex body j.
    Lexan j.
    Low Profile plastic body j.
    LS^4 custom spinal j.
    Minerva cervical j.
    Orfizip body j.
    Orthoplast j.
    plastic body j.
    Prenyl j.
    Royalite body j.
    Sayre j.
    underarm body j.
    Vitrathene j.
    von Lackum transection shift j.
    Wilmington plastic j.
jackknife
    j. position
    j. test
The Jacknobber II
Jackson
    ankle scoring system of Baird
    and J.
    J. bone clamp

J. bone-extension clamp
J. bone-holding clamp
J. broad-blade staple forceps
J. compression test
J. dressing forceps
J. intervertebral disc rongeur
J. spinal surgery and imaging table
J. syndrome
J. tendon-seizing forceps
Jackson-Gorham syndrome
jacksonian epilepsy
Jackson-Pollock skinfold equation
Jackson-Pratt drain
Jacksonville sling
Jackson-Weiss syndrome
Jacobs
    J. chuck
    J. chuck adapter
    J. chuck drill
    J. chuck drive
    J. distraction rod
    J. locking hook spinal rod
    J. locking hook spinal rod
    instrumentation
    J. locking hook spinal rod
    instrumentation modification
    J. locking hook spinal rod
    technique
Jacob shift test
Jacobson
    J. bulldog clamp
    J. mosquito forceps
    J. needle holder
    J. resonator
    J. suture pusher
    J. system
Jacoby
    J. bunion splint
    J. heel splint
Jacquet fixator
Jadassohn-Lewandowsky syndrome
JAFAR
    Juvenile Arthritis Functional Assessment
    Report
Jaffe
    J. disease
    J. press-fit prosthesis
    J. procedure
Jaffe-Campanacci syndrome
jagged osteophyte
Jahss
    J. ankle dislocation classification
    J. classification of ankle dislocation
    J. maneuver

Jahss *(continued)*
J. metatarsophalangeal joint dislocation classification
J. 90-90 method
J. procedure
Jakob test
Jamaica Sandalthotics orthotic
Jamar
J. grip tester
J. hydraulic hand dynamometer
J. hydraulic pinch gauge
J. test
James
J. position
J. procedure
J. splint
J. wound forceps
Jameson
J. muscle clamp
J. muscle hook
jammed finger
jamming
intraarticular j.
Jamshidi needle
Janis tibialis posterior tendon dysfunction classification
Jannetta
J. duckbill elevator
J. hook
Jansen
J. bone curette
J. disease
J. metaphysial dysostosis
J. monopolar forceps
J. rasp
J. test
Jansey
J. procedure
J. technique
Jan van Breemen Function Questionnaire (JVBF)
Japanese Orthopaedic Association (JOA)
Japas
J. osteotomy
J. V-osteotomy
jar
heel j.
Jarcho-Levin syndrome
Jarell forceps
Jarit
J. anterior resection clamp
J. cartilage clamp
J. meniscal clamp
J. pin cutter
J. rotator
J. small bone-holding clamp
J. tendon-pulling forceps

JAS
Joint Activate Systems
JAS elbow motion device
javelin thrower's elbow
jaw
3-j. chuck
j. claudication
j. exerciser
j. opening reflex (JOR)
Jay
J. basic cushion
J. Combi cushion
J. J2 wheelchair
J. Rave cushion
J. Triad cushion
J. Xtreme cushion
JCE
job capacity evaluation
J-24 cervical orthosis
J-45 contraflexion orthosis
JCS
joint coordinate system
J2 cushion
Jeanie
J. Rub
J. Rub Massager
Jebsen
J. assessment
J. assessment of hand function
J. Hand Function Test
Jebsen-Taylor hand function test
Jefferson cervical burst fracture
Jeffery
J. radial fracture classification
J. technique
Jendrassik maneuver
Jergesen
J. I-beam
J. I-beam plate
J. incision
J. tapered plate
J. tube
jerk
Achilles j.
ankle j. (AJ)
biceps j. (BJ)
elbow j. (EJ)
j. finger
hung-up knee j.
knee j. (KJ)
patellar j. (PJ)
quadriceps j.
j. sign
supinator j.
tendon j.
j. test
triceps j. (TJ)
triceps surae j.
jerky gait

jersey finger
jet
- j. irrigator
- j. lavage
- Ortholav j.
- J. Vac cement dispenser

Jet-Air splint
Jeter lag/position screw
jet-pilot position
Jette Functional Status index
Jettmobile positioning and tumble form
jeweler's
- j. forceps
- j. thumb

Jewett
- J. bending iron
- J. contraflexion orthosis
- J. driver
- J. extractor
- J. gouge
- J. hyperextension orthosis
- J. nail
- J. nail overlay plate
- J. operation
- J. pick-up screw
- J. postfusion orthosis
- J. prosthesis
- J. thoracolumbosacral orthosis

Jewett-Benjamin
- J.-B. cervical brace
- J.-B. cervical orthosis

J-FX bipolar head
J-hook deformity
J-35 hyperextension orthosis
JIDC
- juvenile intervertebral disc calcification

jig
- chamfer cut j.
- Charnley tibial onlay j.
- cutting j.
- drilling j.
- external-alignment compression j.
- extramedullary tibial alignment j.
- femoral alignment j.
- fixation j.
- Herbert j.
- j. hook
- intramedullary alignment j.
- Miller-Galante j.
- Osteonics j.
- Plexiglas j.
- precompression j.

- spacer-tensor j.
- tibial j.

jing
- bifocal manipulative with distraction j.

J&J
- Johnson & Johnson
- J&J postoperative shoe
- J&J ulcer dressing

JMPT
- Journal of Manipulative and Physiological Therapeutics

JOA
- Japanese Orthopaedic Association
- JOA Scale

job
- j. capacity evaluation (JCE)
- j. redesign
- j. task analysis (JTA)

Jobert fossa
Jobe test
job-related hazard
Jobst
- J. air band
- J. appliance
- J. athrombotic pump
- J. boot
- J. brassiere
- J. gauntlet
- J. glove
- J. prosthesis
- J. stockings

jockey cap patella
Joerns orthopaedic bed
jogger's
- j. heel
- j. toe

jogging in place test
Johannesberg staple
Johannson lag screw
Johanson-Blizzard syndrome
Johansson fracture classification
John
- J. Barnes myofascial release
- J. C. Wilson arthrodesis

Johns
- J. Hopkins bulldog clamp
- J. Hopkins National Low Back Pain Study

Johnson
- J. chevron osteotomy
- J. hemiphalangectomy
- J. & Johnson (J&J)

NOTES

Johnson *(continued)*
    J. & Johnson PFC cruciate-substituting insert
    J. medial meniscal suturing
    J. pelvic fracture technique
    J. procedure
    J. pronator advancement
    J. resection arthroplasty
    J. screwdriver
    J. staple technique
    J. and Strom tibialis posterior tendon dysfunction classification

Johnson-Boseker scale
Johnson-Elloy accord unconstrained prosthesis
Johnson-Jahss classification of posterior tibial tendon tear
Johnson-Spiegl
    J.-S. procedure
    J.-S. tendon transfer
Johnston-Iowa hip prosthesis
joint
    AC j.
    acromioclavicular j.
    J. Activate Systems (JAS)
    adjustable dynamic j. (ADJ)
    amphidiarthrodial j.
    ankle j.
    anterior sternoclavicular j.
    apophysial j.
    j. arthrodesis
    j. arthrogram
    j. arthrography
    j. arthrometer
    j. arthropathy
    Ascension MCP total j.
    Ascension PIP total j.
    j. aspiration
    j. assessment
    atlantoaxial j.
    atlantooccipital j.
    atlantoodontoid j.
    bail-lock knee j.
    ball-and-socket j.
    basal j.
    beaking j.
    biaxial j.
    bilocular j.
    j. block
    Budin j.
    calcaneocuboid j.
    calcaneonavicular j.
    CAM Lock knee j.
    capitate-hamate j.
    capitate-lunate j.
    j. capsule
    j. capsule mechanoreceptor
    carpal-intercarpal j.
    carpometacarpal j.

carpophalangeal j.
cartilaginous j.
j. cavitation
j. cavity
CC j.
cervical j.
Charcot j.
j. chondroma
Chopart midtarsal j.
j. cinch
Clevisphere ankle j.
Clutton j.
CMC j.
coccygeal j.
3-j. complex
composite j.
compound j.
condyloid j.
j. congruence
congruent metatarsophalangeal j.
j. coordinate system (JCS)
coracoclavicular j.
costochondral j.
costotransverse j.
costovertebral j.
coxofemoral j.
cracking of j.
Cruveilhier j.
cubital j.
cubonavicular j.
cuneiform j.
cuneometatarsal j.
cuneonavicular j.
j. debris
j. deformity
j. degeneration
Delrin j.
j. depression fracture
diarthrodial j.
digital j.
DIP j.
j. disarticulation
j. disease
j. dislocation
j. disruption
distal interphalangeal j. (DIPJ)
distal radioulnar j. (DRUJ)
distal tibiofibular j.
j. distraction
j. distraction cuff
j. distractor
double-action ankle j.
double pearl-face hip j.
double-stem silicone lesser MP j.
dry j.
j. dysfunction
j. effusion
elastic knee cage with medial and lateral contoured knee j.'s

J

elbow j.
ellipsoid j.
enarthrodial j.
erythema of j.
extraarticular subtalar j.
facet j.
false j.
femoropatellar j.
femorotibial j. (FTJ)
fibrocartilaginous j.
fibrous j.
Fillauer dorsiflexion assist ankle j.
Fillauer PDC ankle j.
finger j.
flail j.
j. force
fourth metatarsophalangeal j.
freely movable j.
fringe j.
j. fulcrum
j. fusion
Gaffney j.
Gillette double-flexure ankle j.
ginglymoid j.
glenohumeral j.
gliding hinge j.
Greissinger Multiaxis j.
hallux IP j.
hamate-lunate j.
hemophilic j.
hinged j.
hip capsule j.
hot j.
HP-100 prosthetic finger j.
humeroulnar j.
hyperextensibility of j.
j. hyperextensibility
hypermobile j.
j. hypermobility
hysterical j.
IM j.
j. immobilization
j. immobilizer
immovable j.
j. implant
incudomalleolar j.
inferior radioulnar j.
inferior tibiofibular j.
j. instability
Integrated Ankle orthotic ankle j.
interarticular j.
intercarpal j.
interchondral j.

intercuneiform j.
intermetacarpal j.
intermetatarsal j.
j. internal derangement
interphalangeal j. (IPJ)
intervertebral j.
IP j.
irritable j.
j. kinematics
knee j.
lap j.
lateral atlantoaxial j.
j. lavage
j. laxity
lesser metatarsophalangeal j.
j. leveling
limited motion metal ankle j.
j. line
j. line pain
j. line tenderness
Lisfranc j.
locking of j.
LT j.
lumbosacral j.
lunocapitate j.
Luschka j.
j. manipulation
j. meniscoid
metacarpocapitate j.
metacarpocarpal j.
metacarpohamate j.
metacarpophalangeal j. (MPJ)
metacarpophysial j.
metacarpotrapezoid j.
Metasul j.
metatarsal j.
metatarsal-tarsal j.
metatarsocuboid j.
metatarsocuneiform j.
metatarsophalangeal j. (MTPJ)
metatarsosesamoid j.
j. mice
midcarpal j.
middle atlantoepistrophic j.
middle carpal j.
midfoot j.
midtarsal j.
j. mobility
j. mobilization
j. model
mortise and tenon j.
j. motion
movable j.

NOTES

joint *(continued)*
MTP j.
multiaxial j.
multiple-axis knee j.
naviculocuneiform j.
near-anatomic position of j.
neuropathic j.
neurotrophic j.
noncongruent metatarsophalangeal j.
nonsubluxated metatarsophalangeal j.
oblique metatarsocuneiform j.
occipital-atlantal j.
occipital-axis j.
occipitoatlantoaxial j.
Oklahoma ankle j.
j. osteoarthritis
Otto Bock 3R65 children's hydraulic knee j.
Otto Bock 3R45 modular knee j.
patellofemoral j.
pisotriquetral j.
pivot j.
plane j.
plastic limited-motion j.
j. play
polyaxial j.
j. popping
j. position sense (JPS)
proximal interphalangeal j. (PIPJ)
proximal tibiofibular j.
radiocapitellar j.
radiocarpal j.
radiohumeral j.
radiolunate j.
radioscaphoid j.
radioscapholunate j.
radioulnar j.
j. reconstruction
j. release
j. replacement surgery
j. rice
3R80 modular hydraulic knee j.
rotary j.
sacrococcygeal j.
sacroiliac j.
saddle-shaped j.
j. salvage procedure
scaphocapitate j.
scapholunate j.
scapuloclavicular j.
scapulothoracic j.
Scotty stainless ankle j.
Select j.
septic finger j.
sesamoidometatarsal j.
shoulder j.
SI j.
silastic finger j.
simple j.

single-axis ankle j.
single pearl-face hip j.
single smooth-face hip j.
S-K reconstruction of distal radioulnar j.
slip j.
solid ankle j.
j. space
j. spacer
spheroidal j.
spiral j.
j. sprain
stable hinge j.
sternoclavicular j. (SCJ)
sternocostal j.
j. stiffness
stifle j.
STT j.
subcrural j.
subluxated metatarsophalangeal j.
j. subluxation
subtalar j. (STJ)
superior radioulnar j.
superior tibiofibular j.
Sutter silicone metacarpophalangeal j.
suture pusher talofibular j.
Swanson finger j.
j. swelling
synarthrodial j.
synovial j.
talocalcaneal j.
talocalcaneonavicular j.
talocrural j.
talofibular j.
talonavicular j.
Tamarack flexure j.
tarsal j.
tarsometatarsal j.
temporomandibular j. (TMJ)
tibiofemoral j.
tibiofibular j.
tibiotalar j.
TN j.
total replacement j.
track-bound j.
transverse tarsal j.
trapeziometacarpal j.
trapeziotrapezoidal j.
triscaphe j.
trochoid j.
ulnocarpal j.
ulnohumeral j.
ulnomeniscotriquetral j.
Ultraflex dynamic j.
uncovertebral j.
uniaxial j.
unilocular j.
unstable j.

j. verrucous carcinoma
Virtual hip j.
von Gies j.
j. warmth
wedge-and-groove j.
weightbearing j.
j. wound
j. wrap
xiphisternal j.
zygapophysial j.
joint-destructive procedure
jointed
    double j.
Joint-Jack finger splint
joint-preservation surgery
joker
    j. dissector
    j. periosteal elevator
Jolly test
Jonas prosthesis
Jonell
    J. countertraction finger splint
    J. thumb splint
Jones
    J. abduction frame
    J. arm splint
    J. brace
    J. and Brackett anterior approach
    J. classification of congenital tibial deficiency
    J. cock-up toe operation
    J. compression cast
    J. compression pin
    J. compression plate
    J. congenital tibial deficiency classification
    J. diaphysial fracture classification
    J. dressing
    J. first toe repair
    J. fracture
    J. metacarpal splint
    J. position
    J. resection arthroplasty
    J. retinaculum reconstruction procedure
    J. scissors
    J. screw
    J. suspension traction
    J. tendosuspension
    J. thoracic clamp
    J. toe repair
    J. towel clamp
    J. traction splint
    J. transfer
    J. view
Jones-Ellison ACL reconstruction
Joplin
    J. bunionectomy
    J. operation
    J. toe prosthesis
JOR
    jaw opening reflex
Jordan frame
Joseph
    J. hook
    J. nasal rasp
    J. osteotome
    J. periosteal elevator
    J. periosteotome
    J. splint
Journal of Manipulative and Physiological Therapeutics (JMPT)
Jousto dropfoot splint, skid orthosis
JoyBags therapeutic heat pack
J-periosteal elevator
J-55 postfusion orthosis
JPS
    joint position sense
JRA
    juvenile rheumatoid arthritis
J.R. Moore procedure
J-shaped skin incision
JTA
    job task analysis
Judet
    J. epiphysial fracture classification
    J. graft
    J. hip status system
    J. pelvic x-ray view
    J. press-fit hip prosthesis
    J. quadricepsplasty
    J. radiograph
Juers-Lempert rongeur forceps
jugal
    j. bone
    j. suture
Julstro Self-Treatment system
jumbo
    j. acetabular cup
    j. uncemented cup acetabular component revision
jump
    j. graft
    j. sign
    squat j.

NOTES

jumper's
    j. knee
    j. knee position
jumping leg
junction
    allograft-host j.
    atlantooccipital j.
    beaked cervicomedullary j.
    cervicomedullary j.
    cervicothoracic j.
    femoral head-neck j.
    gastrocnemius-soleus j.
    host-allograft j.
    lumbosacral j.
    meniscocapsular j.
    meniscosynovial j.
    metaphysial-diaphysial j.
    musculotendinous j.
    myotendinous j.
    occipitocervical j.
    tarsometatarsal j.
    thoracolumbar j.
junctional
    j. fracture
    j. kyphosis
    j. nevus
junctura, pl. **juncturae**
Jüngling disease
Jung muscle
junior
    J. Strength Motrin
    J. Strength Panadol
Junod boot
Jurgan
    J. pin
    J. pin ball
    J. pin ball pin protector
    J. pin ball system
jury-rig
Juvara
    J. bunionectomy
    J. foot operation
    J. procedure
juvenile
    j. aponeurotic fibroma
    J. Arthritis Functional Assessment Report (JAFAR)

    j. bunion
    j. bunionectomy
    j. chronic arthritis
    j. discitis
    j. flatfoot pathomechanics
    j. hallux valgus
    j. hinge axis concept
    j. hyaline fibromatosis
    j. idiopathic scoliosis
    j. intervertebral disc calcification (JIDC)
    j. kyphosis
    j. muscular atrophy
    j. muscular dystrophy
    j. plantar dermatosis
    j. polyarthritis
    j. rheumatoid arthritis (JRA)
    j. thoracic kyphosis
    j. Tillaux fracture
    j. xanthogranuloma
juvenile-onset
    j.-o. ankylosing spondylitis
    j.-o. rheumatoid arthritis
juvenilis
    osteochondritis j.
    osteochondritis deformans j.
Jux-A-Cisor exerciser
juxtaarticular
    j. bone cyst
    j. fracture
    j. lesion
juxtaarticulation
juxtacortical
    j. chondroma
    j. chondrosarcoma
    j. fracture
juxtacubital reconstruction
juxtaepiphysial
juxtaspinal
Juzo
    J. brace
    J. Patellaligner brace
    J. support
J-Vac closed drainage system
JVBF
    Jan van Breemen Function Questionnaire

K

K blade
K needle

K2

K2 hemi toe implant system
K2 sensation prosthesis

K9 Scooter
Kadian Capsule
KAFO

knee-ankle-foot orthosis
Generation II KAFO
GII KAFO
PRAFO KAFO

Kager

K. fat pad
K. triangle

Kalamchi

K. classification
K. osteotomy

Kaleidoscope chair
Kalish

K. bunionectomy
K. bunionectomy modification
K. Duredge wire cutter
K. Duredge wire extractor
K. osteotomy

Kalix flatfoot implant
Kallassy

K. ankle support
K. brace
K. orthosis

Kaltenborn joint mobilization system
Kaltostat dressing
Kambin triangular working zone
Kampe corset
Kanavel

K. cock-up splint
K. sign
K. triangle

Kaneda

K. anterior spinal instrumentation
K. anterior spinal/scoliosis system
(KASS)
K. distraction device
K. plate
K. rod

Kantrowitz thoracic clamp
Kapandji

K. fracture
K. fracture of radius
K. pinning technique
K. thumb opposition score

Kapandji-Sauvé

K.-S. arthrodesis
K.-S. technique

Kapel

K. elbow dislocation technique
K. operation

Kaplan

K. modification
K. modification of Ruiz-Mora
procedure
K. oblique line
K. open reduction
K. osteotomy
K. sign
K. technique

Kaposi sarcoma
kappa receptor
Kaprelian easy-access tweezers (KEAT)
karate

Shotokan k.

karate-inspired aerobics
Karfoil splint
Karlsson

K. and Peterson scoring scale
K. procedure

Karsch-Neugebauer syndrome
Kasdan retractor
Kashin-Bek disease
Kashiwagi

K. resection
K. technique

KASS

Kaneda anterior spinal/scoliosis system

Kast syndrome
KAT

Kinesthetic Ability Trainer

Kates forefoot arthroplasty
Katz

K. ADL index
K. index of activities of daily
living

Kaufer tendon technique
Kaufmann technique
Kavanaugh-Brower-Mann fixation
Kawamura

K. dome osteotomy
K. pelvic osteotomy

Kay scissors
Kazanjian splint
KB

knee-bearing

Keane mobility bed
Kearns-Sayre syndrome
KEAT

Kaprelian easy-access tweezers

KED

Kendrick extrication device

K

keel
　All Poly Deltafit k.
　k. bone punch
　Deltafit K.
　k. of glenoid component
　k. and wing
keeled chest
Keene
　K. compression hook
　K. obturator
Keen sign
Kefurox Injection
Kehr
　K. procedure
　K. sign
Keitel index
Keithley clamp kit
Keith needle
Kelikian
　K. classification of nail deformity
　K. foot dressing
　K. modified Z bunionectomy
　K. modified Z osteotomy
　K. modified Z
　　osteotomy/bunionectomy
　K. nail deformity classification
　K. procedure
　K. push-up test
Keller
　K. arthroplasty
　K. bunionectomy
　K. bunionectomy with prosthesis
　K. foot operation
　K. hallux valgus operation
　K. procedure
　K. resection arthroplasty
Keller-Blake
　K.-B. half-ring splint
　K.-B. leg splint
Keller-Brandes
　K.-B. procedure
　K.-B. resection arthroplasty
Keller-Lelièvre arthroplasty
Keller-Mann resection arthroplasty
Keller-Mayo diabetic foot arthroplasty
Kellgren
　K. degenerative disc disease
　　criteria
　K. knee scale
　K. osteoarthritis grade
　K. sign
Kellgren-Lawrence grading system
Kellogg-Speed
　K.-S. lumbar spinal fusion
　K.-S. operation
Kelly
　K. clamp
　K. forceps
　K. hemostat

　K. peroneal tendon dislocation
　　procedure
　K. tendon lengthening osteotomy
Kelly-Keck osteotomy
Kelly-Kelly osteotomy
keloid scar
KELS
　Kohlman Evaluation of Living Skills
Kelsey unloading exercise therapy
Kelvin body
Kempf internal screw fixation
Kempson-Campanacci lesion
Kemp test
Ken
　K. driver
　K. driver-extractor
　K. screwdriver
　K. sliding nail
Kendall
　K. A-V impulse system
　K. muscle grade
Kendrick
　K. extrication device (KED)
　K. procedure
Kenna Knee Scale
Kennedy
　K. LAD
　K. ligament augmenting device
　K. ligament technique
　K. modification of Gallie ankle
　　fusion
　K. spillproof cup
Kennerdell-Maroon
　K.-M. elevator
　K.-M. hook
Kenny
　K. ADL index
　K. Self-Care Questionnaire
　K. treatment
Kenny-Caffey syndrome
Kenny-Howard
　K.-H. shoulder sling
　K.-H. splint
Keolar implant material
Keralyt Gel
Keramos ceramic/ceramic total hip system
Kerasal ointment
keratoderma blennorrhagica
keratolysis
keratolytic agent
keratoma
　indurated plantar k. (IPK)
keratome
　automated disposable k. (ADK)
　k. Beaver blade
keratoprosthesis
keratosis, pl. **keratoses**
　actinic k.

intractable plantar k. (IPK)
plantar k.
k. punctata
stucco k.

Kerboull acetabular reinforcement device

Kerlix
K. bandage
K. cast padding
K. dressing
K. gauze
K. wrap

Kern
K. bone-holding clamp
K. bone-holding forceps

Kernig
K. sign
K. test

Kern-Lane bone forceps
Kerpel bone curette
Kerr
K. abduction splint
K. electro-torque drill
K. hand drill
K. sign

Kerrison
K. chisel
K. curette
K. downbiting rongeur
K. punch

Kerr-Lagen abdominal support
Kessel-Bonney
K.-B. extension osteotomy
K.-B. procedure

Kessel plate
Kessler
K. external fixator
K. fixation device
K. grasping suture
K. metacarpal distractor
K. metacarpal lengthening
K. modified Achilles tendon repair
K. posterior tibial tendon transfer
K. posterior tibial tendon transfer operation
K. prosthesis
K. stitch
K. suture technique
K. traction
K. traction frame

Kessler-Tajima suture
Ketac cement
ketamine

Kevlar glove
Kevorkian curette
key
k. the cement
K. elevator
k. grip
K. intraarticular knee arthrodesis
K. periosteal elevator
k. pinch
K. rasp
k. release
K. wrist brace

keyboard
ErgoLogic k.
Kinesis k.
wave k.

keyboarder
MouseMitt k.

key-grip tenodesis
keyhole
k. approach
k. method
k. punch
k. tenodesis
k. tenodesis technique

Key-loc wrench
Key-Pred Injection
Key-Pred-SP Injection
keystone
k. of the calcar arch
k. graft
K. splint
k. structure

keyway
OEC lag screw component with k.

K-Fix Fixator system
KFS
Klippel-Feil syndrome

KGTI
Kinetik great toe implant

Khan-Lewis phonological analysis
kick bucket
kicker
K. Pavlik harness
K. Pavlik harness hip abduction brace

kick-point
Kid-Dee-Lite orthosis
Kidner
K. dissector
K. flatfoot
K. foot operation

K

NOTES

Kidner *(continued)*
  K. foot procedure
  K. lesion
kidney rest
Kiel bone
Kienböck
  K. atrophy
  K. disease
  K. dislocation
  K. phenomenon
Kikuchi-MacNap-Moreau approach
Kilfoyle humeral medial condylar
  fracture classification
Kilian line
Killian gouge
Kilner hook
Kiloh-Nevin
  K.-N. myopathy
  K.-N. ocular form of progressive
    muscular dystrophy
kilopond
kilovoltage potential
Kimerle anomaly
KinAir bed
Kinamed
  K. anthropometric total hip
  K. Exact-Fit ATH system
Kinast indirect reduction
Kin-Con
  K.-C. device
  K.-C. isokinetic exercise system
kinematic
  k. chain
  K. fully constrained
    tricompartmental knee prosthesis
  k. gait
  k. gait pattern
  k. gait pattern change
  hindfoot k.
  K. II condylar and stabilizer total
    knee system
  K. II rotating hinge knee system
  K. II rotating hinge total knee
    prosthesis
  k. index of McMurtry
  knee k.
  k. linkage
  K. rotation hinge
  k. study
kinematics
  joint k.
Kinemax
  K. modular condylar and stabilizer
    total knee system
  K. Plus knee prosthesis
  K. Plus total knee system
  K. removable fixation peg
  K. spacer
Kinemetric guide system

kineplastic amputation
kineplastics
kinesialgia
kinesiatrics
kinesiology
  applied k. (AK)
kinesiopathologic component
kinesiopathology
kinesipathist
Kinesis keyboard
kinesitherapy
kinesthesia
kinesthesiometer
kinesthetic
  K. Ability Trainer (KAT)
  k. awareness
  k. exercise
KineTec
  K. ECT system
  K. hip CPM machine
kinetic
  k. cervical spine
  k. chain
  k. energy
  k. energy theory
  k. foot pain
  k. gait analysis
  k. rehab device (KRD)
  k. splint
  K. Wedge molded insole
  K. Wedge orthotic
kinetics
Kinetik
  K. great toe implant (KGTI)
  K. great toe implant system
Kinetikos joint implant
Kinetix
  K. instrument
  K. instrument for carpal tunnel
    release
Kinetron muscle strengthening
  apparatus
king
  K. cervical brace
  K. cervical traction
  K. curve posterior correction (type
    IV)
  K. intraarticular hip fusion
  K. intraarticular hip fusion
    procedure
  K. maneuver
  K. open reduction
  K. scoliosis (type I–V)
  K. technique
  K. thoracic and lumbar curve
    (type I–IV)
  K. thoracic scoliosis classification
  k. wound forceps
King-Moe scoliosis

King-Richards dislocation technique
Kingsley Steplite foot
King-Steelquist hindquarter amputation
kinking
    catheter k.
    pedicular k.
Kinsbourne syndrome
Kirby muscle hook
Kirk
    K. distal thigh amputation
    K. distal thigh operation
    K. orthopaedic mallet
Kirkaldy-Willis
    K.-W. arthrodesis
    K.-W. operation
    K.-W. 3 phases of degeneration
Kirner deformity
Kirschenbaum
    K. foot positioner
    K. retractor
Kirschner
    K. apparatus
    K. bone drill
    K. device
    K. II-C shoulder system
    K. integrated shoulder system
    K. Medical Dimension hip
      replacement
    K. Medical Dimension prosthesis
    K. pin fixation
    K. skeletal traction
    K. stem
    K. surgical instrument
    K. tightener
    K. total shoulder prosthesis
    K. traction bow nut
    K. wire (K-wire)
    K. wire cutter
    K. wire drill
    K. wire driver
    K. wire fixation
    K. wire inserter
    K. wire pin
    K. wire placement
    K. wire tensioner
    K. wire traction bow
kissing
    k. lesions
    k. sequestra
    k. spines
Kistler force platform
kit
    Alpha suction attachment block k.

    Balcones Sensory Integration
      Screening K.
    BFO K.
    Bio-Dermal Hydrogel k.
    bone fixation k.
    Canadian Academy of Sports
      Medicine emergency k.
    carpal tunnel surgery relief k.
    Concept CTS Relief K.
    diabetic orthosis k.
    Digital Care k.
    Dr. Joseph's diabetic foot k.
    DynaPak electrode k.
    Elastafit tubing k.
    Elbow Injury Management K.
    Exerball k.
    Fillauer Scottish Rite orthosis k.
    Halifax interlaminar clamp k.
    Histofreezer cryosurgical wart
      treatment k.
    I-Flow nerve block infusion k.
    Keithley clamp k.
    Leukotape P combo pack taping k.
    MediCordz rehabilitation k.
    Merit final flexion k.
    nerve block infusion k.
    OsteoSet resorbable bead k.
    Oval-8 k.
    palmar swab k.
    parallel pin k.
    pelvic reconstruction k.
    portable diagnostic k.
    Posey bar k.
    resistive chair exercise k.
    sensory stimulation k.
    Shoulder Therapy K.
    Skin Care k.
    Tacticon peripheral neuropathy k.
    Unna-Flex Plus venous ulcer k.
    VersaFlex tubing k.
Kitaoka clinical rating scale
kite
    K. angle
    K. clubfoot cast
    K. and Lovell technique
    K. measurement
    K. metatarsal cast
    K. slipper
kitesurfing
KJ
    knee jerk

K

NOTES

Klebsiella
    K. *oxytoca*
    K. *pneumoniae*
Kleiger test
Klein
    K. drainage
    K. technique
Klein-Bell Activities of Daily Living Scale
Kleine-Levin syndrome
Kleinert
    K. modification
    K. postoperative traction brace
    K. repair
    K. splint
    K. technique of pulley reconstruction
Kleinert-Kutz
    K.-K. bone cutter
    K.-K. bone-cutting forceps
    K.-K. bone rongeur
    K.-K. clamp approximator
    K.-K. periosteal elevator
    K.-K. rasp
    K.-K. rongeur forceps
    K.-K. synovectomy rongeur
    K.-K. tendon forceps
    K.-K. tendon retriever
Kleinert-Ragnell retractor
Kleinman shear test
Klein-Vogelbach functional movement concept
Klemm nail
Klengall brace
Klenzak
    K. double-upright splint
    K. orthosis
    K. spring brace
Kline line
Kling
    K. adhesive dressing
    K. cervical brace
    K. elastic bandage
Klippel-Feil
    K.-F. malformation
    K.-F. segmentation defect
    K.-F. sign
    K.-F. syndrome (KFS)
Klippel-Trenaunay
    K.-T. osteohypertrophic hemangiectasia
    K.-T. syndrome
Klippel-Trenaunay-Weber syndrome
Kloehn craniofacial remodeling technique
Klumpke
    K. injury
    K. palsy
    K. plexopathy

Klüver-Bucy syndrome
KMFTR
    Kotz modular femur and tibia resection
KMO
    knee management orthosis
KMP
    K. femoral stem
    K. femoral stem prosthesis
knavel table
Knead-A-Ball exerciser
kneading massage
knee
    above k. (AK)
    acetabular k.
    ACL-deficient k.
    anatomic modular k. (AMK)
    anterior cruciate deficit k.
    k. arthrodesis
    k. arthroplasty
    k. arthroscopy
    Axiom total k.
    bicompartmental replacement of k.
    Biomet Ascent total k.
    k. bolster
    k. brace splint
    breaststroker's k.
    Brodie k.
    cadaveric k.
    k. cage brace
    carpenter's k.
    carpet layer's k.
    k. complex
    constant-friction k.
    constrained condylar k.
    Continuum P/S total k.
    k. contracture
    corner of k.
    deficient k.
    DePuy LCS mobile-bearing k.
    k. disarticulation amputation
    k. disarticulation suspension
    dislocated k.
    k. dislocation
    k. extension assist
    k. extension exercise
    k. extension orthosis
    k. extensor
    k. extensor system
    flail k.
    k. flexion
    k. flexion during stance phase motion gait determinant
    k. flexion-extension
    k. flexion reflex
    k. flexion stress test
    floating k.
    k. force
    k. fracture
    k. fusion

game k.
Genesis unicompartmental k.
GeoFlex k.
gimpy k.
giving way of k.
hamstrung k.
k. holder
horseback rider's k.
Hosmer Endurance k.
Hosmer single-axis friction k.
Hosmer single-axis locking k.
Hosmer weight-activated locking k.
housemaid's k.
k. immobilizer
k. immobilizer splint
k. implant
k. instability
k. instability test
internal derangement of k. (IDK)
k. jerk (KJ)
k. jerk reflex
k. jerk reflex test
k. joint
k. joint effusion
jumper's k.
k. kinematic
k. knob
k. laxity arthrometer
k. laxity test
k. ligament arthrometer
k. ligamentous injury
k. lock
locked k.
k. management orthosis (KMO)
Mauch Swing and Stance
  hydraulic k.
k. MD brace
Miller-Galante k.
mobile-bearing k.
Most Options system rotating hinge
  revision k.
motorcyclist's k.
moviegoer's k.
neuropathic k.
Noiles posterior stabilized k.
Noiles rotating hinge k.
k. orthosis (KO)
k. osteoarthritis
Otto Bock 3R60 EBS k.
Otto Bock 3R80 modular rotary
  hydraulic k.
Otto Bock Safety constant-
  friction k.

Oxford unicompartmental k.
PC Performer k.
K. Pillo
pneumatic 4-bar linkage k.
PolymerFriction total k.
porous-coated anatomic total k.
k. positioner
k. positioning triangle
posterior cruciate ligament of k.
press-fit condylar total k.
ProAdvantage k.
k. prosthesis
k. pump
k. pump exercise
k. retractor
k. rotation
runner's k.
k. saver
Seattle safety k.
self-aligning k. (SAL)
septic k.
k. signature system
single-axis friction k. (SAFK)
single-axis locking k. (SALK)
k. sleeve
K. Sleeve knee support
k. sling
snowstorm k.
K. Society Score
K. Society total knee arthroplasty
  roentgenography evaluation and
  scoring
k. stability
k. strike
tension band of k.
total condylar k.
Total Knee 2100 prosthetic k.
total rotating k. (TRK)
Translating and Congruent Mobile-
  Bearing K.
transverse ligament of k.
trick k.
USMC stance locking safety k.
valgus k.
varus k.
k. varus-valgus
voluntary control 4-bar k.
weight-activated locking k.
  (WALK)
windblown k.
wrenched k.
knee-ankle-foot orthosis (KAFO)
knee-bearing (KB)

NOTES

K

kneecap stabilizer
knee-chest
  k.-c. push
  k.-c. rocking
  k.-c. table
knee-control orthosis pad
Kneed-It kneeguard
knee-drop test
kneeGRIP
kneeguard
  Kneed-It k.
kneeling
  k. bench test
  k. position
  90-90 k. position
  k. reciprocal back exercise
    technique
KneeRanger hinged knee brace
kneeRAP wrap
Kniest syndrome
knife
  acetabular k.
  ACL graft k.
  amputation k.
  arthroscopic k.
  backward-cutting k.
  Ballenger swivel k.
  banana k.
  Bard-Parker k.
  bayonet k.
  Beaver cataract k.
  Beaver-DeBakey k.
  Bircher meniscus k.
  k. blade
  Blair k.
  Blount k.
  Bovie k.
  C k.
  cartilage k.
  cast k.
  Castroviejo bladebreaker k.
  Catlin amputating k.
  chondroplasty k.
  Collin amputating k.
  Crile k.
  cutting current k.
  discission k.
  Down epiphysial k.
  Downing cartilage k.
  Esmarch plaster k.
  forward-cutting k.
  Freiberg cartilage k.
  Freiberg meniscectomy k.
  full-radius resector k.
  Grover meniscus k.
  hemilaminectomy k.
  hooked k.
  Hopkins plaster k.
  hot k.

  Humby k.
  Indiana tome k.
  Langenbeck flap k.
  Langenbeck resection k.
  Lindvall-Stille k.
  Liston amputating k.
  Liston phalangeal k.
  Lowe-Breck cartilage k.
  Lowe-Breck meniscectomy k.
  Maltz cartilage k.
  McKeever cartilage k.
  meniscectomy k.
  meniscus k.
  Midas Rex k.
  Neff meniscus k.
  Oretorp retractable k.
  orthopaedic k.
  Reiner plaster k.
  retrograde-cutting hook-shaped k.
  Ridlon plaster k.
  rocker k.
  Salenius meniscus k.
  sculp k.
  semilunar cartilage k.
  serrated fine-cutting k.
  sheathed k.
  skiving k.
  Smillie-Beaver k.
  Smillie cartilage k.
  Smillie meniscal k.
  Smith cartilage k.
  Stryker cartilage k.
  tenotomy k.
  upward-cutting triangular k.
  Weck k.
  Yamanda myelotomy k.
knight
  K. back brace
  K. bone-cutting forceps
Knight-Taylor
  K.-T. thoracic brace
  K.-T. thoracolumbosacral orthosis
Knit-Rite suspension sleeve
knob
  knee k.
Knobber
  Original Index K. II
Knobble massager
knocked-down shoulder
knock-knee
  k.-k. brace
  k.-k. deformity
Knodt
  K. distraction rod
  K. rod and hook
knot
  arthroscopic k.
  hairpin k.
  half-hitch arthroscopic k.

half-stitch arthroscopic k.
k. of Henry
Henry k.
lockable arthroscopic k.
PDS k.
k. pusher
Revo k.
sliding k.
surfer's k.
wire k.
knotter
Harris k.
knotting forceps
Knott rod distraction device
Knowles
K. hip pin
K. pin nail
K. pinning
Knox
K. Cube Test
K. Preschool Play Scale
knuckle
k. bone
boxer's k.
k. pad
k. shaped
knuckle-bender splint
KO
knee orthosis
KobyGard system
Koby Isogard surgical treatment system
Kocher
K. clamp
K. classification
K. collar incision
K. curved-L approach
K. dissector
K. elevator
K. forceps
K. fracture
K. interval
K. lateral J approach
K. reduction
K. reduction of shoulder
dislocation
K. retractor
Kocher-Debré-Semelaigne syndrome
Kocher-Gibson posterolateral approach
Kocher-Langenbeck
K.-L. approach
K.-L. exposure

K.-L. ilioinguinal approach to
fracture repair
K.-L. ilioinguinal repair
Kocher-Lorenz
K.-L. capitellum fracture
classification
K.-L. fracture
K.-L. fracture of capitellum
Koch-Mason dressing
Kodel knee sling
Kodex drill
Koehler disease
Koenen periungual fibroma
Koenig
K. metatarsal broach
K. metatarsophalangeal joint
arthroplasty
K. MPJ prosthesis
K. nail-splitting scissors
K. rasp
K. total great toe implant
Koenig-Schaefer incision
Kofoed
K. Ankle Score
K. scoring system
Köhler
K. disease
K. fracture
K. hip protrusion grading scale
K. line
Köhler-Pellegrini-Stieda disease
**Kohlman Evaluation of Living Skills
(KELS)**
Kohs block
koilonychia
koilosternia
Kold Wrap
Kollagen dressing
Kolmogorov-Smirnov test
Kondoleon operation
König disease
Kool Kit cold therapy pack
Korean hand acupuncture
Korex cork sheet
Kortzeborn
K. hand operation
K. procedure
**Kostuik-Errico spinal stability
classification**
Kostuik-Harrington
K.-H. distraction system
K.-H. spinal instrumentation
Kostuik screw

K

NOTES

Kotz modular femur and tibia resection (KMFTR)
Koutsogiannis
    K. calcaneal displacement osteotomy
    K. procedure
KPS bipolar vitallium-polyethylene implant
Krackow
    K. Achilles tendon repair
    K. HTO blade staple
    K. locking loop technique
    K. locking suture technique
    K. maneuver
    K. point
    K. suture
Krackow-Thomas-Jones technique
Kramer
    K. modification
    K. modification of Hohmann osteotomy
Kraske position
Krause
    K. bone
    suture of K.
    ulnar collateral nerve of K.
Krause-Wolfe skin graft
KRD
    kinetic rehab device
    KRD L2000 rehab device
Kretschmer syndrome
Kreuscher
    K. bunionectomy
    K. operation
Kristiansen-Kofoed external fixation
Kronfeld pin
Kronner
    K. external fixation
    K. external fixation apparatus
    K. external fixation device
    K. ring fixation
Krukenberg
    K. amputation
    K. hand
    K. hand operation
    K. hand reconstruction
    K. procedure
Kruskal-Wallis test
KS 5 ACL brace
KSO brace
KT-1000
    KT-1000 foot stabilizer
    KT-1000 joint arthrometer
    KT-1000 knee ligament arthrometer
KT-1000/Jr arthrometer
KT-1000/s surgical arthrometer
KT-2000 knee ligament arthrometer

Kudo
    K. hinge
    K. unconstrained elbow prosthesis
Kugelberg reconstruction
Kugelberg-Welander
    K.-W. disease
    K.-W. juvenile spinal muscle atrophy
Kuhlman
    K. cervical traction device
    K. traction
Kumar
    K. application
    K. spica cast technique
Kümmell
    K. disease
    K. spondylitis
Küntscher
    K. awl
    K. drill
    K. extractor
    K. finisher
    K. hammer
    K. humeral prosthesis
    K. impactor
    K. medullary nailing
    K. modified knee arthrodesis
    K. nail
    K. nail driver
    K. nail-extracting hook
    K. ossimeter
    K. pin
    K. reamer
    K. rod
    K. technique
    K. traction apparatus
    K. traction device
Küntscher-Hudson brace
Kurosaka interference-fit screw
Kurtzke
    K. Expanded Disability scale
    K. functional system
    K. score
Kuschkin Ace wheelchair
Kuskokwim syndrome
Kutler
    K. double lateral advancement flap
    K. lateral V-Y flap
    K. V-Y flap
    K. V-Y flap graft
Kuwada Achilles tendon injury classification
Kuz-Medics disposable knee immobilizer
K-wire
    Kirschner wire
    K-wire driver
    K-wire fixation
    percutaneous K-wire
    K-wire placement

Kydex
- K. body jacket
- K. brace
- K. chairback orthosis

Kyle
- K. fracture classification
- K. fracture classification system
- K. internal fixation

kyllosis

kyphectomy
- Sharrard-type k.

kyphometer
- Debrunner k.

kyphoplasty

kyphorachitic pelvis

kyphoscoliorachitic pelvis

kyphoscoliosis
- neurofibromatosis k.
- k. secondary to neurofibromatosis
- severe k.
- thoracolumbar k.

kyphoscoliotic pelvis

kyphosing scoliosis

kyphosis
- acute angular k.
- adolescent k.
- anterior k.
- apprentice k.
- k. brace
- congenital k. (type I, II)
- k. correction
- k. correction surgery
- k. creation
- iatrogenic lumbar k.

junctional k.
juvenile k.
juvenile thoracic k.
long-radius k.
lumbar k.
lumbosacral k.
Luque rod fixation for k.
myelodysplastic k.
paralytic k.
postlaminectomy k.
postradiation k.
posttraumatic k.
rotational k.
sagittal k.
Scheuermann k.
Scheuermann juvenile k. (SJK)
short-radius k.
thoracic k.
thoracolumbar k.

kyphos resection

kyphotic
- k. angle
- k. angulation
- k. curve
- k. deformity
- k. deformity pathomechanics
- k. pelvis

kyphotone

KyphX
- K. Elevate IBT
- K. Exact IBT
- K. HV-R bone cement

Kyrle hyperkeratosis

kyrtorrhachic

K

NOTES

L
L plate
L rod
lab
laboratory
Orthopaedic Casting Lab (OCL)
laboratory (lab)
Army Prosthetics Research L. (APRL)
gait l.
University of California, Berkeley L. (UCBL)
labral
l. avulsion
l. lesion
l. tear
labrum, pl. **labra**
acetabular l.
anterior glenoid l.
articular l.
cartilaginous glenoid l.
glenoid l.
posterior glenoid l.
LAC
long arm cast
lace
l. closure
no-tie stretch l.
laced blucher of shoe
lace-lock ankle splint
lace-on brace
laceration
boot-top l.
burst-type l.
chevron l.
flexor tendon l.
hallucis longus l.
stellate nail bed l.
lacertus fibrosus
lace-up RocketSoc ankle brace
Lacey
L. fully constrained tricompartmental knee prosthesis
L. hinge
L. hinged knee prosthesis
L. rotating hinge arthroplasty
Lachman
L. maneuver
L. sign
L. test
Lac-Hydrin lotion
lacing ankle brace
laciniate ligament

lacrimal
l. bone
l. duct dilator
Lacroix
fibroosseous ring of L.
osseous ring of L.
L. osseous ring
lacrosse
lactate
blood l.
Ringer l.
l. threshold (LT)
lactic
l. acid
l. acidosis
l. acidosis threshold
Lactinol-E creme
Lactinol lotion
LactoSorb
L. orthopaedic wound material
L. resorbable copolymer
L. screw
lacuna, pl. **lacunae**
bone l.
cartilage l.
Howship l.
osseous l.
LAD
ligament augmentation device
ligamentous anterior dislocation
LAD composite graft
Kennedy LAD
ladder
finger l.
shoulder l.
l. splint
LAF
Leisure Activities Finder
Lafayette skinfold caliper
lag
l. screw
l. screw fixation
l. screw insertion
l. screw thread hole
Lahey
L. clamp
L. Clinic dural hook
Laing
L. concentric hip cup
L. H-beam nail
L. hip cup prosthesis
Lalonde
L. hook forceps
L. oblique fracture large bone clamp

L

Lalonde *(continued)*
  L. oblique fracture medium bone clamp
  L. oblique metacarpal fracture bone clamp
  L. small bone clamp
  L. tendon approximator
LAM
  limb accurate measurement
Lam
  L. inversion test
  L. IPM Wound Gel
lamb
  L. muscle transfer
  l. wool
  l. wool pad
Lambert cosine law
Lambert-Eaton myasthenic syndrome (LEMS)
Lambert-Lowman
  L.-L. bone clamp
  L.-L. chisel
Lambeth disability screening questionnaire
lamboid suture
Lambotte
  L. bone-holding clamp
  L. bone-holding forceps
  L. bone hook
  L. elevator
  L. osteotome
  L. principle
Lambrinudi
  L. dropfoot operation
  L. osteotomy
  L. splint
  L. technique
  L. triple arthrodesis
lamella, pl. **lamellae**
  articular bone l.
  basic l.
  circumferential l.
  concentric l.
  endosteal l.
  ground l.
  haversian l.
  intermediate l.
  interstitial l.
  osseous l.
  periosteal l.
lamellar
  l. bone
  l. pattern
  l. separation
  l. thickening
lamellated bone
lamellation
lamina, pl. **laminae**

  l. elevator
  intact spinous l.
laminagram
laminaplasty
  expansive l.
  Tsuji l.
  l. with extended foraminoplasty
laminar
  l. bone
  l. C-D hook
  l. cortex posterior aspect
  l. fracture
  l. spreader
laminectomized spine
laminectomy
  cervical spine l.
  l. chisel
  decompressive l.
  en bloc l.
  l. frame
  multilevel l.
  osteoplastic l.
  radial l.
laminoforaminotomy
laminoplasty
  distraction l.
laminotomy and discectomy
Lamis patellar clamp
lamp
  l. cord sign
  Derma-Wand germicidal l.
  germicidal l.
  halogen l.
Lance
  L. acetabuloplasty
  L. disease
  L. shelf procedure
Lanceford prosthesis
lancinating pain
lancing
Landeez all-terrain wheelchair
Landers-Foulks prosthesis
landmark
  anatomic l.
  bony l.
  pedicle l.
Landolt spreading forceps
Landouzy-Dejerine dystrophy
Landsmeer ligament
lane
  L. bone-holding clamp
  L. bone-holding forceps
  L. bone lever
  L. bone screw
  L. periosteal elevator
  L. plate
  L. procedure
  L. screwdriver
  L. screw-holding forceps

L. self-retaining bone-holding
forceps
Lanex screen
Lange
L. Achilles tendon reconstruction
L. bone retractor
L. hip reduction
L. operation
L. procedure
L. skinfold caliper
L. tendon lengthening
L. tendon-lengthening method
L. tendon lengthening and repair
Lange-Hohmann bone retractor
Langenbeck
L. amputation
L. anteromedial approach
L. bone-holding forceps
L. bone saw
L. flap knife
L. incision
L. metacarpal saw
L. operation
L. periosteal elevator
L. rasp
L. resection knife
L. retractor
L. triangle
Langenskiöld
L. bone graft
L. bony bridge resection
L. classification (stage I–VI)
L. fusion
L. grading system
L. osteotomy
L. procedure
Langer
L. axillary arch
L. axillary arch muscle
L. line
L. mesomelic dwarfism
Langerhans
L. cell granulomatosis
L. cell histiocytosis
Langoria sign
lap
l. joint
l. seatbelt fracture
laparoscopic surgeon's thumb
laparoscopy
GelPort hand access l.

laparotomy
l. sheet
l. sponge
Lapidus
L. alternating air-pressure mattress
L. arthrodesis
L. bed
L. bunionectomy
L. hammertoe technique
L. modified arthrodesis
L. operation
L. procedure
Lapidus-type correction
LaPorta
L. great toe implant
L. total toe prosthesis
lappet formation
L'Aprina topical spray
laptop cushion
large
l. callus Podi-Burr
l. Cobra retractor
l. composite allograft
l. egress cannula
l. humeral head hemiarthroplasty
l. nail Podi-Burr
large-bore inflow cannula
large-head humeral component
large-nail spicule bur
Lark scooter
Larmon
L. forefoot
L. forefoot arthroplasty
L. forefoot procedure
Laron dwarfism
Larrey
L. amputation
L. operation
Larsen
L. disease
L. hip score
L. lateral ankle stabilization
procedure
L. syndrome
L. tendon-holding forceps
Larsen-Johansson disease
LARSI
lumbar anterior-root stimulator implant
Lars Ingvar Hansson (LIH)
Larson
L. hip status system
L. ligament reconstruction
L. technique

NOTES

laryngeal
    l. nerve
    l. nerve injury
LAS
    local adaptation syndrome
LASA
    Lisfranc articular set angle
Laschal suture scissors
LASE
    laser-assisted spinal endoscopy
    LASE probe
Lasègue
    L. rebound test
    L. sign
laser
    l. acupuncture
    ArthroProbe arthroscopic l.
    l. arthroscopy
    Candela SPTL l.
    carbon dioxide l.
    cold l.
    diode l.
    l. Doppler flowmetry
    l. Doppler probe
    holmium YAG l.
    l. image custom arthroplasty
      (LICA)
    l. instrument
    low-energy l. (LEL)
    low-power l.
    l. nucleotomy
    l. partial matricectomy
    red light neon l.
    SilkTouch CO_2 l.
    Surgilase CO_2 l.
    Trimedyne Omnipulse holmium l.
    VersaPulse holmium l.
laser-assisted
    l.-a. capsular shift
    l.-a. capsulorrhaphy
    same-day microsurgical arthroscopic
      lateral-approach l.-a. (SMALL)
    l.-a. spinal endoscopy (LASE)
Laserflo BPM
LaserPen laser therapy
lashing suture
last normal vertebra (LNV)
lata, pl. **latae**
    fascia l.
    tensor fascia l. (TFL)
Latarjet procedure
late
    l. intervention
    l. response
    l. stage
    l. stance
latency
    l. of activation
    distal l.

    F l.
    motor l.
    onset l.
    peak l.
    proximal l.
    residual l.
    sensory peak l.
    terminal l.
latent
    l. diastasis
    l. period
    l. stage of gout
lateral
    l. acetabular shelf operation
    l. acromial border
    l. ankle sprain
    l. antebrachial cutaneous nerve
    l. anterior thoracic nerve
    l. arm flap
    l. aspiration
    l. atlantoaxial joint
    l. atlantooccipital ligament
    l. band
    l. band mobilization
    l. bending
    l. bending view
    l. bicipital sulcus
    l. block test
    l. bowing
    l. buttress support J patellofemoral
      brace
    l. calcaneal artery
    l. canal entrapment
    l. capsular release
    l. capsular sign
    l. cervical spine film
    l. closing wedge osteotomy
    l. collateral ligament (LCL)
    l. collateral sprain
    l. column calcaneal fracture
    l. column lengthening
    l. column lengthening surgery
    l. column syndrome
    l. common digital nerve
    l. compartment
    l. compartment disruption
    l. compartment injury
    l. compartment reconstruction
    l. compression (LC)
    l. compression force
    l. compression injury
    l. condylar fracture classification
    l. cord
    l. cortex
    l. corticospinal tract
    l. costotransverse ligament
    l. curvature
    l. decompression
    l. decubitus position

l. deltoid-splitting approach
l. deviation
l. deviation angle
l. disc protrusion
l. displacement osteotomy
l. distal femoral angle
l. drainage
l. electrical surface stimulation (LESS)
l. end
l. epicondyle
l. exostectomy
l. extensor expansion
l. extensor release
l. femoral condyle
l. femoral cutaneous nerve
l. femoral notch sign
l. flexion
l. flexion dynamic visual analysis
l. flexion malposition
l. flexion restriction
l. forefoot overload
l. full-spine radiographic examination
l. fusion
l. gap sign
l. guidepin
l. gutter syndrome
l. head of gastrocnemius
l. hindfoot
l. hip arthroscopy
l. hip rotation
l. humeral condyle fracture
l. humeral epicondylitis
l. hyperpressure syndrome
l. impingement
l. interosseous ligament
l. J approach
l. joint line
l. joint space
l. Kocher approach
l. listhesis
l. lumbar shift
l. lumbosacral ligament
l. malleolus
l. malleolus fracture
l. malleolus muscle
l. mass fracture
l. to medial screw
l. meniscectomy
l. meniscus
l. monopodal stance view
l. motion racket sport

l. oblique view
l. Ollier approach
l. opening wedge osteotomy
l. pad
l. parapatellar approach
l. park-bench position
l. patella displacement
l. patellar autologous graft
l. patellar compression syndrome
l. patellar facet
l. patellofemoral angle
l. pivot shift
l. pivot shift test
l. plantar artery
l. plantarflexion talar angle
l. plantar metatarsal angle
l. plantar nerve
l. plica
l. premalleolar bursitis
l. process
l. projection (LC)
l. quadruple complex
l. recess
l. recess stenosis (LRS)
l. retinaculum release
l. rhachotomy
l. roentgenogram
l. root pressure
l. rotary displacement
l. rotatory ankle instability
l. sacrococcygeal ligament
l. sesamoid
l. sesamoidectomy
l. shear
l. shelf
l. sling procedure
l. slip
l. slip angle
l. spring ligament
l. spring ligament of foot
l. spring-loaded lock
l. squeeze pinch
l. squeeze test
l. stability
l. step-up
l. superior genicular nerve
l. sway
l. talar-first metatarsal angle
l. talar process fracture
l. talocalcaneal ligament (LTC)
l. tarsometatarsal angle
l. tear
l. thigh flap

NOTES

lateral *(continued)*
    l. thoracic flap
    l. tibial condyle
    l. tibial plateau fracture
    l. tibial tubercle
    l. tilt stress ankle view
    l. tilt stress ankle x-ray
    l. transfer
    l. transmalleolar portal
    l. trap suture
    l. trunk shift
    l. tuberosity
    l. utility incision
    l. wedge
    l. wedge fracture
    l. weightbearing radiograph
lateralis
    malleolus l.
    vastus l. (VL)
    vastus medialis obliquus:vastus l.
      (VMO:VL)
laterality
    atlas l.
lateralization
laterally displaced fracture
lateral-to-medial thrust
lateroduction
lateropulsion
latex
    l. anaphylaxis
    l. cushion
latissimus
    l. dorsi
    l. dorsi flap
    l. dorsi muscle
Latitude curette
latitudinal growth
latticework
Lauenstein procedure
Lauge-Hansen
    L.-H. ankle fracture classification
    L.-H. stage II supination-eversion
      fracture
Laugier
    L. fracture
    L. sign
Laurence-Biedl syndrome
Laurence-Moon-Biedl
    L.-M.-B. law
    L.-M.-B. syndrome
Laurence-Moon syndrome
Lauren view
Laurin
    L. lateral patella displacement
    L. lateral patellofemoral angle
lavage
    bone l.
    CarboJet l.
    Hi Speed Pulse l.

    jet l.
    joint l.
    pulsatile jet l.
    pulsatile pressure l.
    Pulsavac l.
    pulsed l.
    Simpulse pulsing l.
    Simpulse S/I l.
law
    all-or-none l.
    Davis l.
    L. of Facilitation
    Heuter-Volkmann l.
    Lambert cosine l.
    Laurence-Moon-Biedl l.
    Ollier l.
    Palmerian l.
    Sherrington l.
    sports medicine l.
    von Schwann l.
    Wolff l.
lawn mower injury
Lawrence
    L. device
    L. first metatarsophalangeal joint
      implant
    L. view
Lawrence-Seip syndrome
Lawson-Thornton plate
Lawton procedure
laxity
    ankle l.
    collateral ligament l.
    congenital l.
    cruciate ligament l.
    l. index
    joint l.
    ligamentous l.
    radioscaphocapitate ligament l.
    subtalar l.
    l. to varus stress
layer
    cambium l.
    capsular l.
    gliding l.
    Ollier l.
    parietal tendon sheath l.
    periosteal cambium l.
    tangential l.
LazerSporin-C solution
lazy-C incision
lazy-L incision
lazy-S skin incision
**lazy-V deepithelialized turn-over
  fasciocutaneous flap**
L-Bolt
    TSRH L-B.
LBP
    low back pain

LBS
  Leisure Boredom Scale
LBW
  lean body weight
LC
  lateral compression
  lateral projection
LCC
  long calcaneocuboid
    LCC ligament
LCL
  lateral collateral ligament
LCPD
  Legg-Calvé-Perthes disease
LCR
  ligamentous and capsular repair
    LCR system
LCS
  low-contact stress
    LCS meniscal bearing
      semiconstrained prosthesis
    LCS mobile bearing knee system
    LCS New Jersey knee prosthesis
    LCS rotating platform
      semiconstrained prosthesis
    LCS substituting semiconstrained
      prosthesis
    LCS total knee system
    LCS total knee system implant
    LCS universal APG semiconstrained
      prosthesis
LCT
  liquid crystal thermography
L-curved incision
LDF
  lumbodorsal fascia
LE
  lower extremity
  lupus erythematosus
Le
    Le Dentu suture
    Le Fort amputation
    Le Fort fibular fracture
    Le Fort II fracture
    Le Fort I–III osteotomy
    Le Fort mandible fracture
    Le Fort-Wagstaffe fracture
LEA
  lower extremity amputation
Leach-Schepsis-Paul augmentation
lead
    Axxess spinal cord stimulation l.
    l. line

  l. pipe fracture
  l. synovitis
Leadbetter
  L. hip manipulation
  L. maneuver
  L. technique
leader
  tendon l.
  l.'s and trailers
lead-filled mallet
lead-line scan
leaf, pl. **leaves**
  inferior l.
  l. splint
  superior l.
leaf-spring
  AFO posterior l.-s.
  l.-s. brace
  plastic l.-s. (PLS)
leakage
  bony slurry l.
  chylous l.
lean
  antalgic l.
  l. body weight (LBW)
Leander
  L. chiropractic table
  L. motorized flexion table
leaning hop test
LEAP
  Lewis expandable adjustable prosthesis
  Lower Extremity Amputation Prevention
  LEAP monofilament test
  LEAP program
learning
  spinal l.
leash of Henry
leather
  l. ankle corset
  l. cuff
  l. lacer gauntlet
  l. orthosis
Leatherman hook
leaves (pl. of leaf)
Lebsche
  L. rongeur
  L. saw guide
  L. wire saw
LeCocq brace
Ledderhose disease
Ledraplastic exercise ball
Lee
  L. anterosuperior iliac spine graft

NOTES

Lee *(continued)*
    L. bone graft
    L. procedure
    L. reconstruction
    L. technique
leech
    American l.
    artificial l.
    medicinal l.
Leeds-Keio Dacron mesh replacement
Leeds spinal procedure
Lefferts rib shears
LEFS
    Lower Extremity Functional Scale
left
    l. erector spinae musculature
    l. innominate
    l. lateral flexion
    l. lower extremity (LLE)
    l. lower limb (LLL)
    l. lumbar convexity
    l. rotation
    l. thoracolumbar major curve
      pattern
    l. upper extremity (LUE)
    l. upper limb (LUL)
left-hand
    l.-h. dominance
    l.-h. dominant
left-right leg displacement
left-sided
    l.-s. nail
    l.-s. thoracotomy
leg
    anatomic short l.
    l. axis
    badger l.
    baker's l.
    bayonet l.
    bowed l.
    l. brace
    champagne bottle l.
    C-Leg System artificial l.
    l. compartment release
    l. decompression
    l. drift
    l. edema
    L. Extension Power Rig
    flaccid l.
    functional short l.
    game l.
    gimpy l.
    l. holder
    inverted champagne bottle l.
    jumping l.
    l. length
    l. length determination
    l. length discrepancy (LLD)
    l. lengthening

    l. length inequality (LLI)
    lusty l.
    nonpreferred l.
    paretic l.
    l. positioner
    l. press
    l. protection factor (LPF)
    restless l.
    rider's l.
    scissor l.
    short l.
    l. shortening
    l. sling
    stork l.
    stovepipe l.
    table short l.
    tennis l.
    l. traction
    unilateral spastic l.
    l. walking cast
1-leg
    1-l. hop for distance test
    1-l. stance test
Legasus support CPM device
leg-curl
    ankle joint l.-c.
legend
    L. ACL functional knee brace
    L. Hy-Lo adjusting table
    L. PCL functional knee brace
    L. stationary adjusting table
leg-foot-toe syndrome
Legg-Calvé-Perthes
    L.-C.-P. disease (LCPD)
    L.-C.-P. syndrome
Legg-Calvé-Waldenström
    L.-C.-W. disease
    L.-C.-W. syndrome
Legg-Perthes
    L.-P. disease
    L.-P. disease orthosis
    L.-P. shoe extension
    L.-P. sling
Legg procedure
legGRIP body positioning device
legholder
    Alvarado l.
    Arthroplasty Products Consultants
      foot and l.
    arthroscopic l.
    Bickel l.
    Cherf l.
    LH1000 arthroscopic l.
    lithotomy l.
    Low Profile l.
    operative l.
    Prep-Assist l.
    Surbaugh l.

SurgAssist surgical l.
Zollinger l.

leg-holding
    l.-h. apparatus
    l.-h. device

leg-lengthening device

Lehman technique

Leibinger
    L. Micro System drill bit
    L. Micro System plate cutter
    L. Micro System plate-holding
      forceps
    L. Profyle hand system

Leibolt technique

Leica model 1600 water-cooled diamond saw

Leichtenstern sign

Leinbach
    L. device
    L. femoral prosthesis
    L. hip prosthesis
    L. olecranon screw
    L. osteotome

leiomyomatous hamartoma

leisure
    L. Activities Finder (LAF)
    L. Boredom Scale (LBS)

Leksell
    L. adapter
    L. adapter to Mayfield device
    L. laminectomy rongeur
    L. rongeur forceps
    L. stereotactic arc

Leksell-Stille thoracic rongeur

LEL
    low-energy laser

Lelièvre osteotomy

Lema strap

Lemmon rib contractor

Lempert
    L. bone curette
    L. bone rongeur
    L. periosteal elevator
    L. rongeur forceps

LEMS
    Lambert-Eaton myasthenic syndrome

Lengemann wire

length
    distal parabola toe l.
    echo train l. (ETL)
    femur l. (FL)
    Grace method of ratio of
      metatarsal l.

hip axis l.
inequality in leg l. (ILL)
leg l.
limb l.
metatarsal l.
needle cord l.
pedicle screw cord l.
pedicle screw path l.
resting l.
l. of stay (LOS)
step l.
stride l.

lengthening
    Achilles tendon l.
    Anderson tibial l.
    aponeurotic l.
    Armistead ulnar l.
    calcaneal neck l.
    Codivilla tendon l.
    Compere l.
    l. contraction
    DeBastiani femoral l.
    distraction l.
    Evans calcaneal l.
    extensor tendon l.
    femoral l.
    fractional l.
    Frost posterior tibialis tendon l.
    gastrocnemius l.
    hamstring l.
    heel cord l.
    Hoke Achilles tendon l.
    Ilizarov limb l.
    intramuscular l.
    Kessler metacarpal l.
    Lange tendon l.
    lateral column l.
    leg l.
    limb l.
    limb-girdle l.
    metacarpal l.
    l. over nails procedure
    percutaneous heel cord l.
    percutaneous tendo Achillis l.
    posterior tibialis tendon l.
    l. reflex
    reverse undercutting l.
    Silfverskiöld Achilles tendon l.
    Spencer tendon l.
    step-cut l.
    Strayer l.
    subscapularis-capsular l.
    Tachdjian fractional l.

L

NOTES

lengthening *(continued)*
    Tachdjian hamstring l.
    tendo Achillis l. (TAL)
    tendo calcaneous l.
    tendon l.
    tibial l.
    transiliac l.
    ulnar l.
    Vulpius l.
    Wagner femoral l.
    Wagner tibial l.
    Warren-White Achilles tendon l.
    White tendo calcaneus l.
    Z-slide l.
length-tension curve
Lenke
    L. classification
    L. classification of adolescent
      idiopathic scoliosis
Lenox
    L. bucket
    L. Hill derotational knee brace
    L. Hill knee orthosis
    L. Hill Spectralite knee brace
lens
    Nikon SMZ 2T magnifying l.
lenticular bone
lenticularis
    dystonia l.
lentigo, pl. **lentigines**
    lentigines, electrocardiographic
      abnormalities, ocular hypertelorism,
      pulmonary stenosis, abnormalities
      of genitalia, retardation of
      growth, deafness (sensorineural)
      (LEOPARD)
    l. maligna
    l. maligna melanoma
Leo Bathlifter
Leone expansion screw
LEOPARD
    lentigines, electrocardiographic
      abnormalities, ocular hypertelorism,
      pulmonary stenosis, abnormalities of
      genitalia, retardation of growth,
      deafness (sensorineural)
    LEOPARD syndrome
Lepird procedure
L'Episcopo hip reconstruction
leptopodia
Lequesne Severity of Osteoarthritis
  Index
Lere bone mill
Leri
    L. disease
    L. pleonosteosis
    L. sign
    L. syndrome
Leriche syndrome

Leri-Weill
    L.-W. disease
    L.-W. syndrome
Lerman
    L. hinge brace
    L. multiligamentous knee control
      orthosis
    L. noninvasive halo
Lerman-Minerva collar
LeRoy clip-applying forceps
lesion
    acute traumatic l.
    ALPSA l.
    articular cartilage l.
    atlantoaxial l.
    Bankart shoulder l.
    Bennett l.
    BHAGL l.
    biceps interval l. (BIL)
    bone surface l.
    bony l.
    Brown-Séquard l.
    bubbly bone l.
    callosal l.
    cartilaginous l.
    chiropractic l.
    cleavage l.
    cyclops l.
    cystic bone l.
    desmoid l.
    destructive articular l.
    disc l.
    DREZ l.
    Essex-Lopresti l.
    expansile l.
    fibrous l.
    GLAD l.
    glenolabral articular disruption l.
    glenolabral ovoid mass l.
    GLOM l.
    HAGL l.
    hamartomatous l.
    Hill-Sachs l.
    hyperkeratotic l.
    hyperpigmented l.
    impingement l.
    intracortical radiolucent l.
    intramedullary l.
    irregular-shaped l.
    irritable l.
    ischemic l.
    juxtaarticular l.
    Kempson-Campanacci l.
    Kidner l.
    kissing l.'s
    labral l.
    l. lesion
    lytic l.
    lytic bone l.

meniscoid l.
metastatic bone l.
Monteggia equivalent l.
Morel-Lavelle l.
morphea-like l.
muscular l.
nail bed l.
neoplastic l.
nerve root l.
neuromechanical l.
nonlinear l.
Nora l.
occult talar l.
Osgood-Schlatter l.
osseous l.
osteoblastic l.
osteocartilaginous l.
osteochondral l.
osteopathic l.
paraosseous l.
parosteal l.
pedal hyperpigmented l.
Perthes l.
Perthes-Bankart l.
POLPSA l.
polyostotic bone l.
posterior labrocapsular periosteal
    sleeve avulsion l.
posterior-superior humeral head l.
postfracture l.
pseudoneoplastic l.
radiolucent l.
retroacetabular l.
reverse Bankart l.
reverse Hill-Sachs l.
rotator cuff l.
shoulder l.
Sinding-Larsen-Johansson l.
SLAP l.
soft tissue l.
Stener l.
striatal l.
subchondral l.
superior labrum anterior and
    posterior l.
transfer l.
transient l.
traumatic, unidirectional instability
    and Bankart l.
tuberculous l.
uncommitted metaphysial l.
upper motor neuron l.
vertebral l.

Wolin meniscoid l.
Woofry-Chandler classification of
    Osgood-Schlatter l.
Wrisberg l.
Leslie-Ryan anterior axillary approach
LESS
    lateral electrical surface stimulation
lesser
    l. metatarsal
    L. Metatarsophalangeal-
        Interphalangeal Scale (LMIS)
    l. metatarsophalangeal joint
    l. multangular
    l. multangular bone
    l. pelvis
    l. rhomboid muscle
    l. tarsal arthrodesis
    l. tarsus cavus
    l. toe
    l. trochanter
    l. trochanter fracture
    l. tuberosity
Lester muscle forceps
Letournel
    L. guideline
    L. plate
Letournel-Judet
    L.-J. acetabular fracture
        classification
    L.-J. approach
Letterer-Siwe disease
leukocyte scan
LeukoScan
Leukotape
    L. P combo pack taping kit
    L. P sportstape
    L. P stretch bandage
Leung thumb loss classification
levator
    l. ani group
    l. scapulae muscle
    l. scapulae syndrome
level
    l. of activity
    Allen Cognitive L. (ACL)
    comfort l.
    fat-fluid l.
    fluid-fluid l.
    l. foundation
    1-l. implantation
    2-l. implantation
    3-l. implantation
    long and short l.

L

NOTES

level *(continued)*
    myoinositol l.
    parathormone l.
    4-l. radiculopathy
    segmental l.
    sorbitol l.
    spinal l.
    transcutaneous oxygen l. (TCO_2)
    vertebral l.
leveling
    joint l.
level-specific chiropractic adjustment
lever
    l. arm
    Lane bone l.
levering
Levin drill guide
Levine
    L. Drennan angle
    L. Orthopaedic Outcomes
    Questionnaire
    L. patellar tendon strap
Levis arm splint
levoscoliosis scoliosis
Levy & Rappel foot orthosis
Lewin
    L. bone-holding clamp
    L. bone-holding forceps
    L. bunion dissector
    L. collar
    L. finger splint
    L. forceps
    L. punch test
    L. reverse Lasègue test
    L. snuff test
    L. spinal perforating forceps
    L. standing test
    L. supine test
Lewin-Gaenslen test
Lewin-Stern
    L.-S. finger splint
    L.-S. thumb splint
Lewis
    L. expandable adjustable prosthesis
    (LEAP)
    L. intercalary resection
    L. nail
    L. periosteal elevator
    L. periosteal rasp
    L. Trapezio prosthesis
Lewis-Prusik test
Lewit stretch technique
Lexan jacket
Lexer
    L. chisel
    L. gouge
    L. osteotome
Leyden-Möbius muscular dystrophy

Leyla
    L. arm
    L. bar
LFAC
    low-frequency alternating current
LFIT
    low-friction ion treatment
L-frame fixator
LH1000 arthroscopic legholder
Lhermitte
    L. sign
    L. syndrome
liability
    ergonomic assessment of risk
    and l. (EARLY)
LIAD
    low-impact aerobic dance
libectomy
    acetabular l.
liberator elevator
liberty
    L. CMC thumb brace
    L. One splint
    L. spinal system
LICA
    laser image custom arthroplasty
lichen
    l. nitidus
    l. planus
Lichtblau
    L. osteotomy
    L. tenotomy
Lichtman
    L. aseptic necrosis classification
    L. disease
    L. radiographic classification
    L. radiographic classification of
    Kienböck disease (stages I, II,
    IIIa, IIIb, IV)
    L. staging
    L. technique
    L. test
Lido
    L. Active Multijoint System
    L. isokinetic dynamometer
    L. lift
    L. lift and work set
    L. Passive Multijoint System
    L. WorkSET work simulator
Lidoback isokinetic dynamometry system
Lido-Gel topical anesthetic Hydrogel
Liebolt radioulnar technique
life
    Diabetic Quality of L.
    L. Liner stick and cut-resistant
    glove
    quality of l.
    L. Satisfaction Index (LSI)

LIFEC
>lumbar intersomatic fusion expandable cage

LifeGait partial weightbearing therapy device

Lifeline Wall Gym 2000 fitness system

Lifestride treadmill

lifestyle
>l. education (LSE)
>sedentary l.

lift
>BTE dynamic l.
>Calypso l.
>dead l.
>heel l.
>Hoyer l.
>Lido l.
>M/L l.
>shoe l.
>squat l.
>VuRyser monitor l.

lift-off
>foot l.-o.
>l.-o. of heel in walk
>l.-o. test
>tibial l.-o.
>varus-valgus l.-o.

Ligaclip applier

ligament
>accessory atlantoaxial l.
>accessory lateral collateral l.
>acromioclavicular l.
>acromiocoracoid l.
>adipose l.
>alar l.
>allograft reconstruction of fibular collateral l.
>l. anchor
>ankle inferior transverse l.
>anterior collateral l.
>anterior cruciate l. (ACL)
>anterior fibular l.
>anterior-inferior tibiofibular l.
>anterior longitudinal l. (ALL)
>anterior medial ankle l.
>anterior meniscofemoral l.
>anterior oblique l. (AOL)
>anterior sacrococcygeal l.
>anterior sacroiliac l.
>anterior talofibular l. (ATFL)
>anterior talotibial l.
>anterior tibiofibular l.
>anterior tibiotalar l.

anteroinferior glenohumeral l.
anteromedial glenohumeral l.
anterosuperior glenohumeral l.
anular l.
apical dental l.
arcuate popliteal l.
artificial l.
atlantal transverse l.
atlantoaxial l.
atlantooccipital l.
l. augmentation device (LAD)
avulsed l.
l. avulsion
Barkow l.
beak l.
Bertin l.
Bichat l.
bifurcate l.
Bigelow l.
bony humeral avulsion of glenohumeral l. (BHAGL)
Bourgery l.
Brodie l.
Burns l.
l. button
calcaneoastragaloid l.
calcaneoclavicular l.
calcaneocuboid l.
calcaneofibular l. (CFL)
calcaneonavicular l.
calcaneotibial l.
Caldani l.
Campbell l.
capital l.
capsular l.
carpal l.
carpometacarpal l.
CC l.
cervical mover l.
CH l.
checkrein l.
Chrisman-Snook reconstruction of ankle l.
Civinini l.
l. clamp
Cleland l.
collateral fibular l.
collateral radial l.
collateral tibial l.
collateral ulnar l.
Colles l.
congenital laxity of l.
conoid l.

NOTES

L

409

ligament *(continued)*
    coracoacromial l.
    coracoclavicular l.
    coracohumeral l.
    coronary l.
    corporotransverse inferior l.
    corporotransverse superior l.
    costoclavicular l.
    costotransverse l.
    cruciate l.
    Cruveilhier l.
    cuboideonavicular l.
    cuneonavicular l.
    DATT l.
    DCC l.
    deltoid l.
    deltotrapezius fascial l.
    dentate l.
    dorsoradial l. (DRL)
    DPTT l.
    dural l.
    l. elongation
    extraarticular knee l.
    extracapsular l.
    extrinsic l.
    fabellofibular l.
    falciform l.
    false l.
    fibular collateral l. (FCL)
    fibular sesamoidal l.
    fibulocalcaneal l.
    fibulotalar l.
    fibulotalocalcaneal l.
    first intermetacarpal l.
    flaval l.
    floating l.
    fracture-dislocation with anterior l.
    FTC l.
    Gerdy l.
    glenohumeral l. (GHL)
    Gore-Tex anterior cruciate l.
    Grayson l.
    hamate l.
    hamatometacarpal l.
    Henle l.
    l. of Henry
    humeral avulsion of
      glenohumeral l. (HAGL)
    Humphry l.
    hypertrophic l.
    iliofemoral l.
    iliolumbar l.
    iliopatellar l.
    iliotrochanteric l.
    inferior band cruciform l.
    inferior calcaneonavicular l. (ICN)
    inferior glenohumeral l. (IGHL)
    inferior ilioischial l.
    infrapatellar l.

inguinal l.
intercarpal l.
interclavicular l.
interdigital l.
intermetacarpal l. (IML)
intermetatarsal l.
International Knee L.
interosseous cuneocuboid l.
interosseous cuneometatarsal l.
interosseous intercuneiform l.
interosseous talocalcaneal l. (ITCL)
intersesamoid l.
interspinal l.
interspinous l.
intertransverse l.
intervolar plate l.
intraarticular disc l.
intraosseous tibiofibular l.
ischiofemoral l.
laciniate l.
Landsmeer l.
lateral atlantooccipital l.
lateral collateral l. (LCL)
lateral spring l.
lateral talocalcaneal l. (LTC)
LCC l.
limited proteoglycan matrix of l.
Lisfranc l.
long calcaneocuboid l.
longitudinal l.
long plantar l. (LPL)
LRL l.
LT l.
lumbocostal l.
lunotriquetral l.
medial collateral l. (MCL)
medial patellofemoral l. (MPFL)
medial sesamoid l.
medial ulnar collateral l. (MUCL)
meniscofemoral l.
meniscotibial l.
metacarpal l.
metacarpoglenoidal l.
metacarpophalangeal l.
metatarsal l.
metatarsosesamoid l.
middle glenohumeral l. (MGHL)
midline l.
natatory l.
navicular cuneiform l.
naviculocuneiform l.
nuchal l.
oblique popliteal l.
oblique retinacular l.
olecranon l.
orbicular l.
ossification of posterior
   longitudinal l. (OPLL)
patellar l.

patellofemoral l.
patellomeniscal l.
patellotibial l.
petroclinoid l.
pisiform metacarpal l.
pisohamate l.
pisometacarpal l.
plantar l.
popliteal l.
popliteofibular l.
posterior cruciate l. (PCL)
posterior inferior tibiofibular l.
posterior longitudinal l. (PLL)
posterior oblique l. (POL)
posterior talofibular l. (PTFL)
pubocapsular l.
pubofemoral l.
quadrate l.
radial collateral l. (RCL)
radiocapitate l.
radiocarpal l.
radiolunotriquetral l.
radioscaphocapitate l.
radioscaphoid l.
radioscapholunate l.
radiotriquetral l.
rearfoot l.
l. reconstruction
l. reconstruction with tendon
  interposition (LRTI)
l. replacement
retinacular l.
rhomboid l.
Robert l.
round l.
Rouviere l.
l. rupture sprain
sacrococcygeal l.
sacroiliac l.
sacrospinal l.
sacrospinous l.
sacrotuberal l.
sacrotuberous l.
scapholunate interosseous l.
scaphotrapezoid interosseous l.
scapular l.
scapulohumeral l.
SCC l.
sesamoid l.
sesamophalangeal l.
short calcaneocuboid l.
short plantar l. (SPL)
spinal posterior l.

spinal transverse l.
spinoglenoid l.
spiral oblique retinacular l.
spring l.
SRL l.
sternoclavicular l.
sternocostal l.
l. of Struthers
STT l.
subtalar interosseous l.
superior costotransverse l.
superomedial calcaneonavicular l.
supraspinous l.
syndesmotic l.
talocalcaneal l.
talofibular l.
talonavicular l.
tarsometatarsal l.
l. of tarsus
tectoral l.
tendinotrochanteric l.
tibial collateral l. (TCL)
tibial sesamoid l.
tibiocalcaneal l.
tibiofibular l.
tibionavicular l.
tibiospring l.
torn l.
trapezoid l.
traumatized l.
triangular l.
ulnar carpal collateral l.
ulnar collateral l. (UCL)
ulnocarpal l.
ulnolunate l.
ulnotriquetral l.
vaginal hand l.
vertebropelvic l.
Weitbrecht l.
l. of Wrisberg
yellow l.

ligamenta carpometacarpaliad dorsalia
ligament-bone
bone-patellar l.-b. (BPB)
l.-b. complex
ligamentoplasty
ligamentotaxis
multiplanar l.
ligamentous
l. ankylosis
l. anterior dislocation (LAD)
l. anterior dislocation composite
  graft

L

NOTES

ligamentous *(continued)*
  l. attachment
  l. attrition
  l. bouncing
  l. box
  l. and capsular repair (LCR)
  l. complex
  l. control brace
  l. disruption
  l. injury
  l. insertion
  l. instability test
  l. insufficiency
  l. laxity
  l. luxation
  l. release
  l. stability
  l. structure
  l. support tissue
  l. thickening
  l. weave procedure
ligamentous-muscular hypertrophy
ligament-scar matrix
ligamentum
  l. bifurcatum
  l. calcaneocuboideum
ligand adhesive
ligature
  l. carrier
  l. guide
  l. passer
  stick tie l.
light
  l. cast
  Cogent l.
  l. conductor
  l. cross-slot screwdriver
  infrared l. (IR)
  l. intensity training
  l. microscopy
  l. source
  therapeutic l.
  l. touch sensation
  l. touch test
  ultraviolet l.
  L. V sign
Lightplast athletic tape
LIH
  Lars Ingvar Hansson
  LIH hook pin
Likert and Borg scale
Lilienthal rib spreader
Lima external fixator
limb
  l. absence
  l. accurate measurement (LAM)
  artificial l.
  l. ataxia
  l. brace

  l. bud
  congenitally short l.
  l. girdle
  l. gym
  hanging of l.
  l. holder
  ischemic l.
  left lower l. (LLL)
  left upper l. (LUL)
  l. length
  l. length angulation
  l. length discrepancy
  l. length disparity
  l. lengthening
  phantom l.
  plantigrade l.
  posture of l.
  l. replantation
  residual l.
  right lower l. (RLL)
  right upper l. (RUL)
  l. salvage
  seal l.
  l. synergy
  Trow Bridge TerraRound sports l.
  Utah artificial l.
  4-l. Z-plasty
Limberg flap
limb-girdle
  l.-g. lengthening
  l.-g. muscular dystrophy
limb-girdle-trunk paresis
limb-salvage
  l.-s. procedure
  l.-s. surgery
limb-sparing operation
limbus
  l. annulare
  l. annularis
limied proteoglycan matrix
limit
  elastic l.
  endurance l.
  metal endurance l.
  motion l.
  L.'s of Stability (LOS)
  within functional l.'s (WFL)
limitation
  motion l.
  l. of motion (LOM)
  l. of movement
  protective l.
limited
  l. compression-dynamic compression
    plate
  l. fasciectomy
  l. intertarsal arthrodesis
  l. joint mobility (LJM)
  l. motion metal ankle joint

l. performance measure
l. proteoglycan matrix of ligament
limited-contact dynamic compression plate
limiter
Becker 655 motion control l.
motion control l.
limiting condition
limitus
bony hallux l.
cartilaginous hallux l.
hallux l.
McKeever arthrodesis for hallux l.
Regnauld free phalangeal base autograft for hallux l.
Z-slide lengthening in hallux l.
limp
antalgic l.
new-onset l.
Trendelenburg l.
LINAC
linear accelerator
Boston LINAC
University of Florida LINAC
Linberg syndrome
Lincoln-Oseretsky Motor Development Scale
Lindell classification
Lindemann bur
Lindeman procedure
Linder sign
Lindgren oblique osteotomy
Lindholm
L. Achilles lengthening procedure
L. open surgical tendon repair
L. technique
L. tendo calcaneus repair
Lindseth osteotomy
Lindsjö method
Lindvall-Stille knife
line
acetabular l.
AC-PC l.
action l.
Andren-von Rosen l.
anterior axillary l. (AAL)
anterior humeral l.
anterior spinal l.
antitension l.
AxyaWeld product l.
Beau l.
bisector l.
Blumensaat l.

Bryant l.
cement l.
cervical stress l.
Chamberlain l.
Chopart joint l.
cleavage l.
coronoid l.
cyma l.
l. of demarcation
divisionary l.
Duhot l.
epiphysial l.
Feiss l.
femoral head l. (FHL)
fracture l.
Fränkel white l.
gait l.
George l.
gravitational l.
l. of gravity
gravity plumb l.
growth arrest l.
Harris growth arrest l.
Harris hip l.
Hawkins l.
Hilgenreiner horizontal Y l.
Hilgenreiner-Perkins l.
horizontal Y l.
H-P l.
Hueter l.
iliopectineal l.
interteardrop l.
joint l.
Kaplan oblique l.
Kilian l.
Kline l.
Köhler l.
Langer l.
lateral joint l.
lead l.
Looser l.
lumbar gravitational l.
MacNab l.
Maquet l.
McGregor l.
McRae l.
Meary l.
medial joint l.
Meyer l.
Meyerding spondylolisthesis classification l.
midaxillary l. (MAL)
midheel l.

L

NOTES

413

line *(continued)*
    midmalleolar l.
    midsternal l. (MSL)
    Moloney l.
    Moyer l.
    Nélaton l.
    oblique metacarpal l.
    obturator/brim l.
    odontoid perpendicular l.
    Ogston l.
    parajugular l.
    parallel pitch l.'s
    Perkins-Ombredanne l.
    Perkins vertical l.
    physial l.
    plumb l.
    posterior axillary l. (PAL)
    posterior cervical l.
    radiocapitellar l.
    radiolucent l.
    relaxed skin tension l.
    Roser l.
    Roser-Nélaton l.
    sacral arcuate l.
    sacral horizontal plane l. (SHPL)
    sacroiliac l.
    sacroiliac symphysis l.
    Schoemaker l.
    sclerotic l.
    scurvy l.
    Shenton l.
    Shenton-Menard l.
    Skinner l.
    skin tension l.
    spinolaminar l.
    Sydney l.
    teardrop l.
    tibiofibular l.
    trapezoid l.
    trough l.
    Trümmerfeld l.
    Ullmann l.
    Wagner l.
    Wegner l.
    Whitesides l.
    Y l.
    Z l.
    l. of Zahn
linea
    l. aspera femoris
    l. semilunaris
Lineage acetabular cup
linear
    l. accelerator (LINAC)
    l. amputation
    l. analog pain scale
    l. capsulotomy
    l. fraction
    l. fracture

    L. hip stem
    l. osteotomy
    l. potentiometer
    l. scar
    L. total hip system
linear-variable-differential transducer
linebacker's arm
linen suture
liner
    acetabular l.
    acetabular prosthetic l.
    Alpha cushion l.
    Alps CustomPro custom l.
    bone l.
    cast l.
    cushion shoe l.
    DePuy acetabular l.
    Duraloc acetabular l.
    elevated rim acetabular l.
    Enduron acetabular l.
    Fillauer prosthesis l.
    Fillauer silicone suction l.
    Fillauer silicone suspension l.
    Gore-Tex waterproof cast l.
    grommet bone l.
    Hylamer enhanced ultra-high
      molecular weight polyethylene
      acetabular l.
    Iceross Comfort Plus silicone
      gel l.
    Medium-Plus alpha l.
    metal acetabular l.
    l. micromotion
    OrthoGel l.
    Plastazote shoe l.
    polyethylene l.
    Polysorb l.
    polyurethane l.
    Reflection l.
    RingLoc hip l.
    SiloLiner gel l.
    Spenco l.
    splint l.
    TEC l.
    USMC luxury l.
line-to-line reaming technique
Ling
    L. cemented hip prosthesis
    L. method
lingism
lingual
    l. artery
    l. vein
lining
    DePuy acetabular l.
    shoe l.
    Thermold heat moldable shoe l.
link
    L. acetabular cage

L. anatomical hip
4-bar l.
L. custom partial pelvis
replacement system
L. Endo-Model rotational knee
prosthesis
L. Endo-Model rotational knee
system
L. Lubinus SP II hip replacement
system
malleable l.
L. MP hip noncemented
reconstruction prosthesis
L. MP microporous hip stem
musculotendinous-osseous l.
offset l.
L. Orthopaedics device
L. Saddle Prosthesis Endo-Model
hip replacement system
L. Stack Split Splint
L. toe splint

linkage
kinematic l.
rod l.
linked potential
lint-free drape
Linton procedure
Linvatec
L. absorbable screw
L. arthroscopic infusion pump
L. arthroscopy product
L. bone anchor
L. driver
L. product
lion forceps
lion-jaw forceps
Lioresal Intrathecal
lip
l. of acetabulum
bone l.
l. of glenoid
l. of navicular
osteophytic bone l.
posterior l.
l. of tibia
lipid
l. inclusion cyst
l. tumor
lipoarthritis
lipoblastomatosis
lipocalcinogranulomatosis
lipochondrodystrophy

lipofibroma
intraneural l.
lipofibromatosis
lipofibromatous hamartoma
lipohemarthrosis
lipoma
endovaginal l.
intraosseous l.
pleomorphic l.
spindle cell l.
lipomatosis
intraosseous l.
lipomeningocele
liposarcoma
myxoid l.
myxoid-type l.
pleomorphic l.
round cell l.
round cell-type l.
well-differentiated myxoid l.
lipping
Lippman
L. hip prosthesis
L. screw
L. test
Lippman-Cobb technique
Lipscomb
L. metatarsophalangeal arthrodesis
L. modified McKeever arthrodesis
L. procedure
L. technique
Lipscomb-Anderson drill guide
liquid
l. cable
l. crystal thermography (LCT)
L. Ice
l. nitrogen cryotherapy
Lisch nodule
Lisfranc
L. amputation
L. arthrodesis
L. articular interline
L. articular set angle (LASA)
L. below-knee prosthesis
L. disarticulation
L. dislocation
L. fracture
L. fracture-dislocation
L. injury
L. joint
L. joint articulation
L. joint complex
L. ligament

L

NOTES

Lisfranc *(continued)*
  L. operation
  L. tubercle
Lissauer zone
list
  postural l.
Lister
  L. corn
  L. technique
  L. technique of pulley
    reconstruction
  L. tubercle
listhesis
  anterior-posterior l.
  lateral l.
listing
  dynamic l.
  l. gait
  static l.
Liston
  L. amputating knife
  L. bone-cutting forceps
  L. bone rongeur
  L. operation
  L. phalangeal knife
  L. shears
  L. splint
Liston-Key bone-cutting forceps
Liston-Key-Horsley rib shears
Liston-Littauer
  L.-L. bone-cutting forceps
  L.-L. rongeur
Liston-Stille bone-cutting forceps
LiteGait partial weightbearing gait
  therapy device
LiteNest portable seating system
lithotomy
  l. legholder
  l. position
Litt
  cloth tape occlusion method of L.
Littauer-Liston bone-cutting forceps
litter
  Neal-Robertson l.
Littig strut
little
  L. cargo vest
  l. finger
  L. Leaguer's elbow
  L. Leaguer's shoulder
  L. release
  L. syndrome
  L. technique
Littler
  L. operation
  L. opponensplasty
  L. pollicization
  L. technique
  wing excision of L.

Littler-Cooley
  L.-C. abductor digiti quinti transfer
  L.-C. muscle transfer
  L.-C. technique
livedo reticularis
Liverpool
  L. elbow prosthesis
  L. knee prosthesis
live splint
living
  activity of daily l. (ADL)
  Center for Independent L. (CIL)
  electronic aid for daily l. (EADL)
  extended activities of daily l.
    (EADL)
  instrumental activities of daily l.
    (IADL)
  Katz index of activities of daily l.
  Occupational Therapy Activities of
    Daily L. (OTADL)
Livingstone therapy
Livingston intramedullary bar
Liviscope scope
Livotrit Plus
LJM
  limited joint mobility
LLC
  long leg cast
LLD
  leg length discrepancy
LLE
  left lower extremity
LLI
  leg length inequality
LLL
  left lower limb
  lower fossa active, lateral knee pain, long
    leg on the side ipsilateral to the weak
    fossa
LLO
  lower limb orthosis
Llorente dissecting forceps
Lloyd
  L. adapter
  L. adapter for Smith-Petersen nail
  L. chiropractic table
  L. nail driver
Lloyd-Roberts
  L.-R. fracture
  L.-R. fracture technique
LLP
  lower limb prosthesis
LLPS
  low-load prolonged stretch
  low-pressure plasma spray
  LLPS hydroxyapatite
  LLPS hydroxyapatite adhesive
LLS
  long leg splint

LLWBC
long leg weightbearing cast
LLWC
long leg walking cast
LMB
LMB finger splint
LMB wire-foam economical resting
splint
LMIS
Lesser Metatarsophalangeal-
Interphalangeal Scale
LMJA
longitudinal midtarsal joint axis
L'Nard
L. boot
L. Multi Podus orthosis
L. thoracolumbosacral orthosis
LNS
localized nodular synovitis
LNV
last normal vertebra
Lo
L. Bak spinal support
L. Bak spinal support prosthesis
Darco Body Armor L.
L. Rider prosthetic foot
load
applied l.
axial compression l.
l. beam
bending l.
compression l.
critical l.
Euler l.
ramp l.
rotatory l.
l. and shift test
l. shift test
spinal axial l.
torque l.
torsional l.
l. transfer
load-and-shift maneuver
load-bearing graft
load-deflection curve
load-deformation curve
load-displacement
l.-d. curve
l.-d. plot
loading
anatomic l.
arch l.
axial l.

compression l.
concentric l.
cyclic l.
dynamic l.
eccentric l.
Edwards modular system
dynamic l.
fat l.
fracture callus l.
functional and anatomic l. (FAL)
l. mode
musculoskeletal l.
progressive l.
status l.
sustained l.
tension l.
l. time
vertical l.
load-sharing classification
load-to-grip displacement
Loban adhesive drape
Lobstein
L. disease
L. syndrome
lobster-claw
l.-c. deformity
l.-c. foot
l.-c. hand
lobster-type clamp
local
l. adaptation syndrome (LAS)
l. cavus
l. compression fracture
l. decompression fracture
l. epineurotomy
l. flap
l. radical resection
l. standby anesthesia
l. standby anesthesia technique
Localio procedure
localization
pedicle l.
localized
l. bone destruction
l. nodular synovitis (LNS)
l. nodular tenosynovitis
l. thermoregulation
localizer cast
locating pin
location
cervical sympathetic chain l.
pedicle l.

NOTES

locator
  Berman-Moorhead metal l.
  metal l.
locator/stimulator
  Pointer-Plus l./s.
lock
  Ball knee l.
  l. finger
  grip l.
  heel l.
  knee l.
  lateral spring-loaded l.
  Morse taper l.
  physiologic l.
  Ratchet Lock variable flexion
    knee l.
  spring-loaded knee l.
  VariLock socket l.
lockable arthroscopic knot
Locke
  L. bone clamp
  L. elevator
locked
  l. facet
  l. intramedullary osteosynthesis
  l. intramedullary osteosynthesis pin
  l. knee
  l. nailing
  l. scapula
Lockhart toe splint
locking
  anatomic medullary l. (AML)
  l. clamp
  l. disc
  distal l.
  l. hook instrumentation
  l. horizontal mattress suture
  l. of joint
  l. loop
  medullary l.
  l. nail
  l. nut
  l. peg
  l. pliers
  l. prosthesis
  proximal l.
  sacroiliac joint l.
  l. screw
locking-hook spinal rod
locking-position test
locking-suture technique
lockjaw
locknut wrench
lockout suture
locomotion
locomotor
  l. ataxia
  l. mechanism

  l. pattern
  l. system
LoCon-T
  L.-T distal radial plate
  L.-T distal radial plating system
Lodine XL
Loeffler-Ballard incision
Lofstrand crutch
log
  exercise l.
  Fin & Flipper exercise l.
  motor activity l.
Logan traction
logrolling maneuver
Lok-it screwdriver
LOM
  limitation of motion
  loss of motion
London unconstrained elbow prosthesis
Lone Star retractor system
long
  l. alignment rod
  l. arm brace
  l. arm cast (LAC)
  l. arm finger cast
  l. arm splint
  l. axial alignment guide
  l. axis
  l. axis of bone
  l. axis ray
  l. axis traction chiropractic table
  L. Beach pedicle screw
  l. bent-knee leg cast
  l. bone deficiency
  l. bone fracture
  l. bone osteomyelitis
  l. calcaneocuboid (LCC)
  l. calcaneocuboid ligament
  l. coarse bur
  l. curette
  l. deltopectoral approach
  l. extensor
  l. external rotator
  l. fibular muscle
  l. finger
  l. head
  l. head of biceps
  l. head biceps tendon
  l. leg arthropathy
  l. leg brace
  l. leg cast (LLC)
  l. leg hinged brace
  l. leg immobilizer
  l. leg orthosis
  l. leg splint (LLS)
  l. leg stockings
  l. leg walking cast (LLWC)
  l. leg weightbearing cast (LLWBC)

l. lever, low-amplitude type manipulation
l. nail-mounted drill guide
l. oblique fracture
l. opponens orthosis
l. plantar ligament (LPL)
l. posterior flap
l. radiolunate (LRL)
l. segment spinal fusion
l. and short level
l. stem (LS)
l. thoracic nerve injury
l. thoracic nerve palsy
l. toe flexor
l. tract sign
long-bone fixation
long-edge medullary nail
Longevity V-Lign hip prosthesis
longissimus colli muscle
longitudinal
l. arch stress
l. axis
l. blood supply
l. deficiency
l. displaced complete tear
l. distraction
l. epiphysial bracket
l. fracture
l. incision
l. incomplete intrameniscal tear
l. ligament
l. ligament rupture
l. member to anchor connector
l. member to longitudinal member connector
l. meniscal tear
l. midtarsal joint axis (LMJA)
l. plantar arch
l. ridge
l. spinal bar
l. split tear
l. tendon split
l. traction
long-jaw basket forceps
long-latency somatosensory evoked potential
long-radius kyphosis
long-stemmed powered bur
long-term bone-instrumentation interface
longus
abductor pollicis l. (APL)
adductor hallucis l.
l. capitis muscle

l. cervicis colli muscle
l. colli muscle
extensor carpi radialis l. (ECRL)
extensor digitorum l. (EDL)
extensor hallucis l. (EHL)
extensor pollicis l. (EPL)
flexor digitorum l. (FDL)
flexor hallucis l. (FHL)
flexor pollicis l. (FPL)
palmaris l. (PL)
peroneus l.
loop
Bunnell finger l.
l. circumferential wire
Duncan l.
figure-of-8 wire l.
finger l.
l. fixation
l. and hook strapping
locking l.
perineal l.
Ransford l.
l. scissors
thumb l.
toe l.
wire l.
loop-lock cock-up splint
loop-over wrap
loose
l. body grasper
l. cartilage
l. debris
l. fracture
l. fragment
l. joint body
L. knee procedure
L. procedure
l. shoulder
loosening
acetabular component l.
aseptic l.
Harris criteria for implant l.
implant l.
prosthetic l.
screw l.
sterile l.
Looser
L. line
L. zone
L. zone in insufficiency fracture
Looser-Milkman syndrome
Lo-Por vascular graft prosthesis

NOTES

LOPS
　loss of protective sensation
Lord
　L. cup
　L. press-fit hip prosthesis
　L. total hip arthrodesis
　L. total hip prosthesis
Lordex lumbar spine system
lordoscoliosis
lordosis
　cervical l.
　compensatory l.
　l. creation
　dorsal l.
　lumbar spine l.
　occipitocervical l.
　l. preservation
　reversal of cervical l.
　thoracic spine l.
lordotic
　l. curve
　l. pelvis
lordoticiser
　Posture Pump l.
Lorenz
　L. brace
　L. cast
　L. hip reduction
　L. operation
　L. osteosynthesis system
　L. osteotomy
　L. procedure
　L. sign
Lorenzo screw
Lore suction tube and tip-holding
　forceps
lorgnette
　main en l.
lorry driver's fracture
LOS
　length of stay
　Limits of Stability
Los Angeles
　University of California, L. A.
　(UCLA)
Losee
　L. knee instability test
　L. modification of MacIntosh
　technique
　L. sling and reef technique
loss
　blood l.
　bone l.
　l. of correction
　estimated blood l. (EBL)
　functional l.
　heat l.
　iatrogenic l.
　lumbar lordosis iatrogenic l.

　l. of motion (LOM)
　motor l.
　periprosthetic bone l.
　postmenopausal bone l.
　l. of protective sensation (LOPS)
　segmental bone l.
　sensory l.
LOTCA
　Löwenstein Occupational Therapy
　Cognitive Assessment
LOTCA-G
　Löwenstein Occupational Therapy
　Cognitive Assessment - Geriatric
Loth-Kirschner drill
lotion
　AmLactin l.
　Biotone Polar l.
　Criticaid l.
　Senuva l.
Lottes
　L. nailing
　L. pin
　L. triflanged medullary nail
lotus
　l. position
　l. unicompartment prosthesis
Loughheed and White procedure
Louis
　L. instrumentation
　L. plate
Louisiana
　L. ankle wrap technique
　L. State University (LSU)
　L. State University Medical Center
　(LSUMC)
loupe
　binocular l.
　l. magnification
　magnifying l.
　surgical l.
love
　L. nerve root retractor
　L. splint
Love-Adson periosteal elevator
Love-Gruenwald alligator forceps
Love-Kerrison rongeur forceps
Lovell clubfoot cast
Lovenox Injection
Lovett
　L. clinical scale of strength
　L. test
Lovibond angle
loving
　L. Comfort maternity support
　L. Comfort postpartum support
low
　l. back injury
　l. back neurosis
　l. back pain (LBP)

L. Back Pain Symptom Checklist
l. bone mass
l. cervical approach
l. impedance thermocouple
l. lumbar spine fracture
l. median-low ulnar palsy
L. Profile legholder
L. Profile plastic body jacket
l. quarter Blucher shoe
l. single thoracic curve
l. T humerus fracture
low-air-loss bed
low-arch foot
low-assimilation pelvis
low-contact
l.-c. dynamic compression plate
l.-c. stress (LCS)
l.-c. stress semiconstrained
prosthesis
Low-Dye
L. strapping
L. taping
L. taping technique
Lowe-Breck
L.-B. cartilage knife
L.-B. meniscectomy knife
Lowell
L. reduction
L. view
low-energy
l.-e. fracture
l.-e. laser (LEL)
Löwenstein
L. Occupational Therapy Cognitive
Assessment (LOTCA)
L. Occupational Therapy Cognitive
Assessment - Geriatric (LOTCA-
G)
L. view
lower
l. cervical spine
l. cervical spine fusion
l. cervical spine posterior
stabilization
l. cervical spine procedure
l. extremity (LE)
l. extremity amputation (LEA)
L. Extremity Amputation Prevention
(LEAP)
l. extremity bypass surgery
L. Extremity Functional Scale
(LEFS)
l. extremity noninvasive

l. extremity prosthesis
l. fossa active, lateral knee pain,
long leg on the side ipsilateral
to the weak fossa (LLL)
l. hand retractor
l. hook trial
l. limb dysmetria
l. limb orthosis (LLO)
l. limb prosthesis (LLP)
l. lumbar spine
l. nerve root compression
l. plexus injury
l. posterior lumbar spine and
sacrum surgery
l. sacral nerve root compression
(LSNRC)
l. thoracic pedicle
l. thoracic spine
**low-frequency alternating current
(LFAC)**
low-friction ion treatment (LFIT)
low-grade
l.-g. central osteogenic sarcoma
l.-g. ulcer
low-heeled shoe
low-impact aerobic dance (LIAD)
low-load prolonged stretch (LLPS)
Lowman
L. balance board
L. bone-holding clamp
L. bone-holding forceps
L. chisel
L. hand retractor
L. shelf procedure
Lowman-Gerster bone clamp
Lowman-Hoglund
L.-H. chisel
L.-H. clamp
low-neck femoral prosthesis
low-power laser
low-pressure
l.-p. plasma spray (LLPS)
l.-p. plasma-sprayed (LPPS)
low-profile
l.-p. cup
l.-p. dorsal plate
l.-p. femoral prosthesis
l.-p. halo traction
low-riding patella
low-set thumb
low-stress aerobic exercise
low-surface reactive
low-temperature plastic

NOTES

L

low-tide walking brace
low-turnover osteoporosis
low-viscosity bone cement
low-voltage galvanism (LVG)
loxoscelism
loxotomy
LP
  lumbar puncture
LPF
  leg protection factor
LPL
  long plantar ligament
L-plate
    Synthes mini L-p.
LPPS
  low-pressure plasma-sprayed
    LPPS hydroxyapatite fixation
LRL
  long radiolunate
    LRL ligament
L-rod
    Luque L-r.
LRS
  lateral recess stenosis
LRTI
  ligament reconstruction with tendon
    interposition
LS
  long stem
  lumbosacral
LS⁴ custom spinal jacket
LSE
  lifestyle education
L-shaped
    L-s. capsular incision
    L-s. capsulotomy
    L-s. osteotomy
    L-s. pad
    L-s. plate
    L-s. rod
    L-s. rotator cuff tear
LSI
  Life Satisfaction Index
    LSI Easy Stims self-adhesive
    electrode
    LSI silver self-adhesive disposable
    electrode
LSNRC
  lower sacral nerve root compression
LSO
  lumbosacral orthosis
L-spine
  lumbar spine
LSU
  Louisiana State University
    LSU reciprocation-gait orthosis
    LSU reciprocation-gait orthosis
    brace
    LSU reciprocator

LSUMC
  Louisiana State University Medical
  Center
    LSUMC classification
    LSUMC classification of motor
    and sensory function
LT
  lactate threshold
  lunotriquetral
    LT joint
    LT ligament
LTC
  lateral talocalcaneal ligament
LT-Cage lumbar tapered fusion device
Lubinus
    L. acetabular component
    L. AP hip system
    L. knee prosthesis
    L. SP II anatomically adapted hip
    system
Lucae bone mallet
Lucas
    L. chisel
    L. and Drucker Motor Index
    L. gouge
lucency
    cortical l.
    subchondral l.
    syndesmosis screw l.
lucent
luck
    L. bone drill
    L. hand procedure
    L. hip cup
    L. nail
    L. operation
Luck-Bishop bone saw
Ludington
    L. sign
    L. test
Ludloff
    L. bunionectomy
    L. incision
    L. medial approach
    L. operation
    L. osteotomy
    L. sign
    L. technique
Ludwig
    L. angle
    L. plane
LUE
  left upper extremity
Luer
    L. bone rongeur
    L. rongeur forceps
Luer-Lok needle
Luer-Whiting rongeur forceps

Luhr
    L. fixation system
    L. Microfixation cranial plate
    L. Microfixation System drill bit
    L. Microfixation System plate
      cutter
    L. Microfixation System plate-
      holding forceps
    L. Microfixation System pliers
    L. microplate
    L. miniplate
    L. pan plate
    L. screw

LUL
    left upper limb

lumbago
    ischemic l.

lumbago-mechanical instability syndrome

lumbar
    l. abscess
    l. accessory movement technique
    l. agenesis
    l. anesthesia
    l. anterior-root stimulator implant
      (LARSI)
    l. brace
    l. canal
    l. disc
    l. discectomy
    l. discography
    l. distraction manipulation
    l. epidural endoscopy
    l. extension
    l. extension test
    l. facet injection
    l. fascia
    l. flat back syndrome
    l. gravitational line
    l. intersomatic fusion expandable
      cage (LIFEC)
    l. kyphosis
    l. lateral flexion
    l. lateral flexion test
    l. lordosis iatrogenic loss
    l. lordosis preservation
    l. lordotic curve
    l. microtrauma
    l. nerve root injection
    l. olisthesis
    l. pedicle
    l. pedicle fixation
    l. pedicle marker
    l. pedicle screw

    l. plexus injury
    l. protective mechanism test
    l. puncture (LP)
    l. range of motion
    l. reflex
    l. region
    l. roll
    l. rotation
    l. rotation test
    l. sagittal mobility
    l. scoliosis
    l. spinal instability
    l. spine (L-spine)
    l. spine biopsy
    l. spine burst fracture
    l. spine decompression
    l. spine fusion
    l. spine instability
    l. spine instrumentation
    l. spine kyphotic deformity
    l. spine lordosis
    l. spine model
    l. spine pedicle diameter
    l. spine rotational stability
    l. spine segmental fixation
    l. spine transpedicular fixation
    l. spine trauma
    l. spine vertebral osteosynthesis
    l. spondylosis
    l. support cushion
    l. sympathectomy
    l. sympathetic block
    l. tapered-cage lumbar tapered
      fusion device
    l. thecoperitoneal shunt syndrome
    l. traction
    l. transforaminal epidural injection
    l. tumor
    l. vein
    l. vertebra
    l. vertebral interbody fusion

lumbarization
lumbocostal ligament
lumbodorsal
    l. fascia (LDF)
    l. support corset

Lumbo 90 home care traction system
lumbopelvic
    l. complex
    l. radiograph

lumbosacral (LS)
    l. brace
    l. cartilaginous system

NOTES

lumbosacral *(continued)*
    l. corset
    l. dislocation
    l. flexion
    l. fusion
    l. fusion elevator
    l. joint
    l. joint angle
    l. junction
    l. junction bone density
    l. junction fracture
    l. kyphosis
    l. mechanical syndrome
    l. orthosis (LSO)
    l. plexus
    l. radiculopathy
    l. series
    l. spine
    l. spine transpedicular
      instrumentation
    l. spondylolisthesis
    l. traction
    l. vertebra
Lumbotrain lumbosacral support
lumbrical
    l. bar
    l. intrinsic contracture
    l. muscle
    l. syndrome finger
    l. tendon
lumbricalis muscle
lumbrical-plus
    l.-p. finger
    l.-p. phenomenon
Lumex
    L. lightweight wheelchair
    L. Tub-Guard safety rail
    L. walker
Lunar
    L. DPX densitometer
    L. Expert densitometer
lunate
    l. acrylic cement wrist prosthesis
    l. bone
    l. dislocation
    l. facet dye punch injury
    l. fracture
    l. sinus
lunatomalacia
lunatotriquetral coalition
Lunceford-Pilliar-Engh hip prosthesis
Lund
    L. operation
    L. prototype unicompartment
      prosthesis
Lundholm
    L. plate
    L. screw

lunocapitate
    l. bone
    l. joint
lunotriquetral (LT)
    l. arthrodesis
    l. ballottement test
    l. dissociation
    l. fusion
    l. instability
    l. ligament
    l. shear test
lunula, pl. **lunulae**
Luongo hand retractor
lupus
    l. anticoagulant
    l. erythematosus (LE)
    l. erythematosus preparation
Luque
    L. cerclage wire
    L. fixation device
    L. II fixation system
    L. II plate
    L. II screw
    L. II segmental spinal
      instrumentation
    L. instrumentation concave
      technique
    L. instrumentation convex technique
    L. loop fixation
    L. L-rod
    L. pedicle screw
    L. rectangle
    L. ring
    L. rod
    L. rod bender
    L. rod fixation
    L. rod fixation for kyphosis
    L. rod migration
    L. segmental fixation
    L. semirigid segmental spinal
      instrumentation
    L. sublaminar wiring technique
    L. wiring
Luque-Galveston
    L.-G. fixation
    L.-G. post
    L.-G. rod
lurch
    abductor l.
    gluteal l.
    Trendelenburg l.
lurching gait
Luschka
    L. bursa
    L. joint
    L. muscle
Lusskin bone drill
Lust phenomenon
lusty leg

luxated bone
luxatio
>l. coxae congenita
>l. erecta
>l. erecta shoulder dislocation
>l. imperfecta

luxation
>atlantoaxial l.
>habitual patella l.
>incomplete l.
>ligamentous l.
>Malgaigne l.
>palmar l.
>patella l.

LVG
>low-voltage galvanism
>continuous LVG
>interrupted LVG

Lyden technique
Lyman-Smith traction
Lyme
>L. disease
>L. disease arthritis

lymphadenopathy
lymphangiography
lymphangioma
>cavernous l.

lymphangiosarcoma
lymphapress traction
lymphatic
lymphedema
>cancer treatment-related l.
>l. complex
>congenital l.
>descending l.
>factitious l.
>familial l.
>l. sling

lymphocyte count

lymphoma
>angiotropic l.
>primary l.

lymph vessel
Lynco
>L. biomechanical orthotic system
>L. foot orthosis

Lynn
>L. Achilles lengthening procedure
>L. Achilles tendon repair technique
>L. tendo calcaneus repair

Lynx wrist, hand, finger orthosis arm positioner splint
LYOfoam
>L. C dressing
>L. wound dressing

lyophilization of bone
lyophilized bone graft
lyre-shaped finger hook
Lyser
>trapezoid bone of L.

Lysholm
>L. knee function scoring scale
>L. knee joint instability scope
>L. knee scoring questionnaire
>L. knee test
>L. score

Lysholm-Gillquist
>L.-G. knee subjective function scale
>L.-G. knee subjective function score

lysis
lysosomal absorption
Lyte Fit orthotic
lytic
>l. bone lesion
>l. lesion

Lytle metacarpal splint

NOTES

L

M

    M band

    M wave

3M

    3M fiberglass cast

    3M Maxi Driver blade

    3M preparation

    3M skin drape

    3M staple

M/3

    middle third

M3-X extremity fixation system

mA

    milliampere

MAC

    Miami Acute Care

    monitored anesthesia control

    MAC cervical collar

MacAusland

    M. lumbar brace

    M. operation

    M. procedure

MacCarthy procedure

maceration

    cutaneous m.

Macewen

    M. classification

    M. drill

    M. osteotomy

Mache electromyogram setting

machine

    Accu-SPINA cervical
      decompression m.

    Accu-Tron microcurrent m.

    ankle exercise m.

    BackStrong lumbar extension m.

    Biodex isokinetic testing m.

    Bionx servohydraulic testing m.

    borazone blade cutting m.

    CamStar exercise m.

    continuous passive motion m.

    cooling m.

    CPM exerciser m.

    Cybex m.

    elliptical m.

    Griswold distraction m.

    Instron m.

    Isotechnologies B-200 low back m.

    isotonic m.

    KineTec hip CPM m.

    MB-900 AC m.

    Med-Fit Senior Circuit exercise m.

    MedX functional testing m.

    MedX Mark II lumbar
      extension m.

    MedX stretch m.

    Orthion traction m.

    Paramount total body plate-
      loaded m.

    passive motion m.

    Pec-Dec m.

    PodoFlex m.

    SAM spinal analysis m.

    Schwinn elliptical full body
      exercise m.

    m. screw

    spinal analysis m. (SAM)

    SurgiLav m.

    VersaClimber RX exercise m.

    Vivatek ultimate healing m.

    Wikco ankle m.

machine-gun-like pain

MacIntosh

    M. extraarticular tenodesis

    M. iliotibial band tenodesis

    M. lateral pivot shift test

    M. over-the-top ACL reconstruction

    M. over-the-top repair

    M. technique

    M. tibial plateau prosthesis

Mackenzie amputation

MacKinnon

    M. modification

    M. modification of Dellon ulnar
      nerve transposition

    M. nerve injury

Mackinnon-Dellon staging system

Maclaren mobile buggy

MacLean-Maxwell disease

MacLeod capsular rheumatism

MacNab

    M. line

    M. line for facet imbrication

    M. operation

    M. shoulder repair

MacNab-English shoulder prosthesis

MacNichol-Voutsinas classification

macroadhesion

macrobrachia

macrocheiria

macrocnemia

macrocoil

    Gianturco m.

macrodactalia

    m. reduction

    m. reduction procedure

macrodactylia, macrodactyly

    m. fibrolipomatosis

macrodactylia (continued)
    pedal m.
    progressive m.
macroelectromyography (macro-EMG)
macro-EMG
    macroelectromyography
    macro-EMG needle electrode
macronychia
MacroPore OS spinal system
macroradiograph
macrotrauma rehabilitation program
macularis eruptive perstans
Madajet XL jet-injection anesthesia system
Maddacare child bath seat
Maddacrawler prone support walker
Maddapult Asissto-Seat
Maddox rod test
Madelung
    M. deformity
    M. subluxation
madreporic
    m. coral
    m. hip prosthesis
Madura foot
maduromycosis
mafenide
    m. acetate
    m. acetate for burn
Maffucci
    M. disease
    M. syndrome
MAFO
    molded ankle-foot orthosis
    MAFO cane
Magerl
    M. hook-plate system
    M. plate-screw system
    M. posterior cervical screw fixation
    M. screw placement technique
    M. transarticular screw fixation
    M. translaminar facet screw fixation technique
magic
    m. angle effect
    m. angle phenomenon
    M. Wand vibrator
Magilligan measuring technique
Magna-FX cannulated screw system
MagnaPod pain relief magnet
MagnaScanner Picker Magnet
Magnassager
    M. massager
    M. massage tool
Magnatherm
    M. SSP electromagnetic therapy unit
    M. SSP pulse shortwave diathermy
Magnathotic orthotic

MagneCore magnetic therapy pad
magnesium
    m. deficiency
    m. salicylate
    m. sulfate
magnet
    ankle m.
    BIOflex medical m.
    Dyonics Golden Retriever m.
    elbow m.
    foot m.
    MagnaPod pain relief m.
    MagnaScanner Picker M.
    m. splint
    Tectonic m.
magnetic
    m. motion transducer
    m. resonance arteriography
    m. resonance arthrography
    m. resonance imaging (MRI)
    m. resonance neurography (MRN)
    m. resonance spectroscopy
    m. resonance venography
    m. retriever
    m. sensor
    m. source imaging (MSI)
    m. stimulation
    M. Support brace
    m. therapy
magnetization
    m. transfer
    m. transfer magnetic resonance imaging (mtMRI)
magnification
    loupe m.
    m. view
magnifying loupe
magnum
    M. 800 bed
    M. chisel
    M. curette
    foramen m.
    M. 101 Plus stimulator
    M. 101 Plus table
    M. 100 stimulator
    M. Tiger blade
magnus
    adductor m.
    nucleus raphe m. (NRM)
Magnuson
    M. abduction humeral splint
    M. débridement
    M. operation
    M. technique
    M. twist drill
    M. wire
Magnuson-Stack
    M.-S. arthroplasty
    M.-S. operation

M.-S. procedure
M.-S. shoulder arthrotomy
Ma-Griffith
M.-G. percutaneous Achilles tendon repair
M.-G. ruptured Achilles tendon repair
M.-G. technique
Mahan procedure
MAI
Movement Assessment of Infants
Maigne test
main
m. d'accoucheur
m. en crochet
m. en griffe
m. en lorgnette
m. fourchée
maintained contraction
maintenance of bone plate integrity
Maisel suppression theory
Maisonneuve
M. amputation
M. fibular fracture
M. sign
Maitland
M. manipulation
M. slump test
M. technique
Majestro-Ruda-Frost tendon technique
major
m. amputation
anterosuperior ilium m.
m. curve
m. fracture fragment
m. injury vector (MIV)
posteroinferior ilium m.
making
M. Action Plans (MAPs)
return-to-play sidelines decision m.
MAL
midaxillary line
malabsorption
maladaptation
soft tissue m.
maladaption
high-altitude m.
maladjustment
malakopathy
malalignment
dorsal m.
malicious m.
radial m.

rotational m.
varus m.
malangulation
malar
m. bone
m. fracture
Malawer
M. excision technique
M. resection
malaxation
Malcolm-Lynn
M.-L. C-RXF cervical retractor frame
M.-L. radiolucent spinal retraction system
Malcolm-Rand radiolucent headrest and retraction system
maldevelopment
male
m. reamer
m. washer
malformation
Arnold-Chiari m.
arteriovenous m.
Chiari m.
Klippel-Feil m.
medullary venous m. (MVM)
retromedullary arteriovenous m.
Malgaigne
M. amputation
M. luxation
M. pelvic fracture
Malibu
M. cervical orthosis
M. Sandalthotics orthotic
malicious malalignment
maligna
lentigo m.
malignancy
spinal m.
malignant
m. acetabular osteolysis
m. fasciculation
m. fibrous histiocytoma
m. fibrous xanthoma
m. hyperpyrexia
m. hyperthermia
m. melanoma
m. myeloid sarcoma
m. osteopetrosis
m. schwannoma
m. soft tissue tumor

M

NOTES

Malis
>M. CMC-II bipolar coagulator
>M. curette
>M. elevator
>M. hinge clamp
>M. jeweler bipolar forceps
>M. ligature passer
>M. needle holder

Malis-Jensen microbipolar forceps

malleable
>m. link
>m. metal finger splint
>structural aluminum m. (SAM)
>m. template

mallei (*pl. of* malleus)

malleolar
>m. chip fracture
>m. facet
>m. gel sleeve
>m. index
>m. osteotomy
>m. screw
>m. sulcus

Malleoloc
>M. anatomic ankle arthrosis
>M. ankle orthosis
>M. ankle support

malleolus, pl. **malleoli**
>bellybutton to medial m. (BB to MM)
>external m.
>m. externus
>fibular m.
>inner m.
>internal m.
>m. internus
>lateral m.
>m. lateralis
>medial m. (MM)
>m. medialis
>m. medialis tibiae
>outer m.
>posterior m.
>radial m.
>m. radialis
>tibial m.
>tip of medial m.
>ulnar m.
>m. ulnaris

Malleo-Med soft ankle support

malleotomy

Malleotrain ankle support

mallet
>Acufex m.
>Bergman m.
>bone m.
>boxwood m.
>cervical m.
>copper m.

Cottle m.
Crane m.
Doyen bone m.
m. finger
m. finger deformity
m. finger orthotic
m. fracture
Gerzog bone m.
Hajek m.
Heath m.
Henning m.
Hibbs m.
Kirk orthopaedic m.
lead-filled m.
Lucae bone m.
Mead m.
Meyerding m.
Miltex m.
Ombredanne m.
orthopaedic m.
polyethylene-faced m.
Richards m.
Rush m.
slotted m.
Steinbach m.
Swanson m.
m. thumb
m. toe
m. toe deformity
Williger bone m.

malleus, pl. **mallei**
>chirurgicum mallei
>hallux m.

malleus-incus prosthesis

Mallory
>M. prosthesis
>M. technique

Mallory-Head
>M.-H. femoral stem
>M.-H. I, II prosthesis
>M.-H. modular calcar system
>M.-H. porous primary femoral prosthesis
>M.-H. rasp
>M.-H. revision operation
>M.-H. total hip prosthesis
>M.-H. total hip revision

Malmö hip splint

malnutrition
>protein m.

malodorous foot

mal perforans ulcer

malposed vertebra

malposition
>extension m.
>flexion m.
>lateral flexion m.
>rotational m.

malreduction
    fracture m.
malrotation
Malteno tube implant material
maltracking patella
Maltz
    M. cartilage knife
    M. rasp
malum
    m. coxae senilis
    m. deformans
malunion
    angulatory m.
    calcaneal m.
    femoral shaft m.
    humeral fracture m.
    talar m.
    varus m.
malunited
    m. acetabulum
    m. calcaneus fracture
    m. forearm fracture
    m. radial fracture
mamillary process
management
    biologic fracture m.
    chiropractic m.
    conservative m.
    failure of conservative m.
    foot orthotic m.
    fracture m.
    inflammation m.
    interphalangeal sesamoid m.
    neuromechanical spinal
      chiropractic m.
    nonoperative orthopaedic m.
    nonsurgical m.
    preoperative m.
    pressure ulcer m.
    reflex tracheostomy m.
Mancini plate
mandible ossification
mandibular
    m. angle
    m. fracture
    m. nerve
    m. osteotomy
    m. spine
maneuver
    Adson m.
    Allen m.
    Allis m.
    Apley m.

    Bárány-Nylen m.
    Barlow m.
    Bigelow m.
    Bouvier m.
    Christiani m.
    circumduction m.
    closed manipulative m.
    costoclavicular m.
    Credé m.
    cross-leg Patrick m.
    Dandy m.
    Dix-Hallpike m.
    extension m.
    Finkelstein m.
    flexion-extension m.
    flexion-rotation-compression m.
    Foster-Kennedy m.
    Fowler m.
    Gowers m.
    Hallpike m.
    Halsted m.
    hippocratic m.
    Hubscher m.
    hyperabduction m.
    Jahss m.
    Jendrassik m.
    King m.
    Krackow m.
    Lachman m.
    Leadbetter m.
    load-and-shift m.
    logrolling m.
    manipulative m.
    McElvenny m.
    McKenzie extension m.
    McMurray circumduction m.
    McMurray twist m.
    Mendelsohn m.
    Meyn-Quigley m.
    military m.
    military brace m.
    milking m.
    Ortolani m.
    osteoclasis m.
    Parvin m.
    Patrick cross-leg m.
    Phalen m.
    postural fixation back m.
    Queckenstedt m.
    relative response attributable to
      the m. (RRAM)
    reverse Bigelow m.
    rotation-compression m.

M

NOTES

maneuver (*continued*)
    scalene m.
    Schreiber m.
    shear m.
    Slocum m.
    Smith m.
    Soto-Hall m.
    Spurling m.
    Steel m.
    Stimson m.
    twist m.
    Valsalva m.
    Walton m.
    Watson m.
    Whitman m.
    Wright m.
Mangled Extremity Severity Score (MESS)
mangling injury
manifestation
    initial m.
manipulable subluxation
manipulation
    m. of articulation
    back m.
    m. board
    chiropractic joint m.
    chiropractic manual m.
    closing wedge m.
    contact m.
    diversified m.
    fine m.
    general thrust m.
    grading of m.
    gross m.
    Hippocrates m.
    indirect m.
    joint m.
    Leadbetter hip m.
    long lever, low-amplitude type m.
    lumbar distraction m.
    Maitland m.
    medical m.
    myofascial m.
    noncontact m.
    opening wedge m.
    osteopathic m.
    passive joint m.
    rotational m.
    soft tissue m.
    specific thrust m.
    spinal m.
    target of m.
    thrust m.
    m. with distraction
manipulative
    m. maneuver
    m. procedure

    m. technique
    m. therapy
Mankin
    M. resection
    M. technique
Manktelow
    M. pectoralis major transfer
    M. transfer procedure
Mann
    M. bunionectomy
    M. modified McKeever arthrodesis
    M. procedure
    M. protocol
    M. resection arthroplasty
    M. technique
Mann-Coughlin-DuVries cheilectomy
Manske-McCarroll-Swanson centralization
Manske technique
Mantis retrograde forceps
mantle
    cement m.
    grade A, B, C1, C2, D m.
manual
    m. adjustment
    m. cavitation
    m. contact
    m. fracture reduction
    m. gun system
    m. locking knee prosthesis
    m. medicine
    m. muscle test
    m. muscle testing (MMT)
    m. pressure
    m. push-pull technique
    m. reflex neurotherapy
    m. resistance
    m. talar tilt
    m. therapy
    m. traction
    m. treatment
    m. wheelchair
    m. work
manubriosternal angle
manubrium, pl. **manubria**
manufacturing
    computer-aided design/computer-aided m. (CAD/CAM)
Manuflex external fixator
manus
    m. cava
    m. plana
    m. valga
    m. vara
ManuTrain active wrist support
MAP
    Miller Assessment for Preschoolers
    Multiaxial Assessment of Pain
Maple Leaf hip orthosis

mapping
  behavioral m.
  m. the defect
  dermatome m.
  MSI m.
  paraspinal m.
MAPs
  Making Action Plans
Maquet
  M. advancement
  M. dome osteotomy
  M. elevation
  M. elevation of tibial crest
  M. line
  M. procedure
  M. table extension
Maquet elevation
Maramed
  M. Miami fracture brace system
  M. ThermoFlex
marathoner's toe
marathon running
marble
  m. bone
  m. bone pin
Marcaine with epinephrine
march
  m. foot
  m. fracture
marche à petits pas gait
marching band injury
Marfan syndrome
margin
  anterior tibial m.
  fibular m.
marginal
  m. excision
  m. exostosis
  m. fracture
  m. osteophyte
  m. resection
margo, pl. **margines**
Marie-Bamberger disease
Marie-Charcot-Tooth disease
Marie-Foix sign
Marie-Strümpell
  M.-S. arthritis
  M.-S. disease
  M.-S. spondylitis
Marion screw
mark
  M. II Chandler total knee retractor
  M. II concave total knee retractor

M. II distal femur distractor
M. II femoral component extractor
M. III halo system
M. II Kodros radiolucent awl
M. II lateral collateral ligament
  retractor
M. II modular weight retractor
M. II Sorrells hip arthroplasty
M. II Sorrells hip arthroplasty
  retractor system
M. II S total knee retractor
M. II Stubbs short prong collateral
  ligament retractor
M. II Stulberg hip positioner
M. II Stulberg leg positioner
M. II tibial component extractor
M. II wide PCL knee retractor
M. II Wixson hip positioner
M. II Z knee retractor
Markell
  M. brace boot
  M. Mobility Health Clogs
  M. Mobility Shoes
  M. open-toe boot
  M. open-toe shoe
  M. tarso medius straight shoe
  M. tarso pronator outflare shoe
marker
  BB m.
  biochemical m.
  lumbar pedicle m.
  pedicle m.
  retroreflective m.
  skin m.
  tantalum-ball m.
  thoracic pedicle m.
  X-Act podiatric m.
Markham-Meyerding retractor
Markley retention pin
Marks-Bayne
  M.-B. technique
  M.-B. technique for thumb
    duplication
Markwalder
  M. bone rongeur
  M. rib forceps
Markwort ankle support
Marlex
  M. mesh
  M. methyl methacrylate prosthesis
Marlin
  M. cervical collar
  M. cervical orthosis

NOTES

M

Marmor
- M. modular knee prosthesis
- M. replacement

Marmor-Lynn fracture

maroon spoon

Maroteaux
- spondyloepiphysial dysplasia of M.

Maroteaux-Lamy
- M.-L. disease
- M.-L. syndrome

Marquardt
- M. angulation osteotomy
- M. bone rongeur

Marquet fracture table

marrow
- bone m.
- m. canal
- m. cavity
- m. disease
- m. edema
- m. nailing
- red m.
- m. stimulation
- yellow m.

MARS
- Modular Acetabular Revision System
- MARS revision acetabular component

Marshall
- M. Hall theory
- M. Hall theory of reflex action
- M. knee score
- M. ligament repair
- M. ligament repair technique
- M. patelloquadriceps tendon substitution

Marshall-McIntosh technique

Martel sign

martensitic stainless steel

Martin
- M. cartilage chisel
- M. cartilage clamp
- M. cartilage forceps
- M. cartilage scissors
- M. diamond wire cutter
- M. disease
- M. loop circumferential wire
- M. meniscal clamp
- M. muscular clamp
- M. osteotomy
- M. patellar wiring technique
- M. screw
- M. sheet rubber bandage

Martin-Gruber
- M.-G. anastomosis
- M.-G. connection

Martini bone curette

Marx osteoradionecrosis protocol

Mary
- angle of M.

Maryland
- M. Foot Score
- M. Foot Score Profile

MAS
- modified Ashworth scale

mason
- M. fracture
- M. fracture classification system
- M. radial head fracture classification
- M. splint

Mason-Allen
- M.-A. suture
- M.-A. Universal hand splint

mass
- bone m.
- bony m.
- cellular periosteal osteocartilaginous m.
- center of m.
- fat and fat-free m. (FFM)
- glenolabral ovoid m. (GLOM)
- granulomatous m.
- hypoechoic intermetatarsal web space m.
- low bone m.
- osteocartilaginous m.
- peak bone m.
- plantar-hindfoot-midfoot bony m.
- pre-Achilles m.
- radiodense m.
- soft tissue m.
- tumorous m.

massage
- aqua PT water m.
- m. ball
- callus m.
- connective tissue m. (CTM)
- m. cream
- cross-friction m.
- deep friction m.
- deep stroking and kneading m.
- effleurage m.
- friction m.
- Hoffa m.
- ice m.
- kneading m.
- m. oil
- pneumatic m.
- Shiatsu therapeutic m.
- Silhouette therapeutic m.
- soft tissue m.
- stimulating m.
- Swedish m.
- Teledyne Water Pik misting m.
- m. therapy
- M. Time Pro hydromassage table

transverse friction m.
vibratory m.

massager
AcuVibe m.
Body Sticks m.
Cryocup ice m.
Equalizer Pro m.
G5 Fleximatic
  massager/percussor m.
Intracell trigger point m.
Ironman Triathlon Pro-Power m.
Jeanie Rub M.
Knobble m.
Magnassager m.
Medisana M.
Morfam Quality Jeanie Rub m.
Omni Roller m.
Original Backnobber muscle m.
Original Index Knobber II m.
Power Pillow cervical m.
Reach Easy m.
Saso Variable Speed M.
Scrip Muscle Master m.
T-Bar trigger point m.
Thera Cane m.

massager/percussor
G5 Vibracare m./p.

masses sign
masseur
masseuse
Massie
M. driver
M. extractor
M. II nail
M. inserter
M. nail assembly
M. plate
M. screwdriver
M. sliding graft
M. sliding nail

massive
m. fibrolipoma
m. herniated disc
m. osteolysis
m. osteoplysis
m. sliding graft

Masson fasciotome
massotherapy
MAST
military antishock trousers

master
Balance M.
Body M.

m. cement
Cobra M.
m. knot of Henry
NeuroCom Balance M.
Pro Balance M.
M. screwdriver
Smart Balance M.
M. step foot prosthesis

Masterson
M. curved clamp
M. pelvic clamp
M. straight clamp

Master-Stim interferential stimulator
Mastin muscular clamp
Mastisol liquid adhesive
mastocytosis
mastoid
m. curette
m. process
m. rongeur

mat
Airex m.
air flow m.
AliMed sensor floor m.
AquaBodyCiser aquatic m.
aquatic m.
children's m.
Easyslide sliding m.
EMED-SF sensor m.
floor m.
footprint m.
GAITRite m.
Harris-Beath footprint m.
Harris footprint m.
Minislide sliding m.
Scoot-Gard m.
sliding m.
sting m.
m. table

matchstick
m. graft
m. test

mater
dura m.

material
acrylic implant m.
Alisoft splinting m.
allogenic lyophilized bone graft
  implant m.
AlloGro bone graft m.
alloplastic m.
alpha-BSM bone repair m.
alpha-BSM bone substitute m.

M

NOTES

material *(continued)*

aluminum oxide arthroplasty m.
American Society for Testing and M.'s (ASTM)
amorphous eosinophilic m.
Aquaplast splinting m.
Aquarelle hydrogel nucleus viscoelastic m.
bioabsorbable m.
bioceramic implant m.
bone implant m.
Bone Plast bone replacement m.
bone-tendon graft m.
Bonfiglio bone replacement m.
Calcitite graft m.
calcium carbonate graft m.
Carboplast II sheet orthotic m.
cellular response to implant m.
celluloid implant m.
CHAG bone graft substitute m.
composite m.
copolymer orthotic m.
corundum ceramic implant m.
Dacron synthetic ligament m.
DermAssist wound-filling m.
Dermatell hydrocolloid dressing m.
Durapatite bone replacement m.
Duraval Hook & Loop strap m.
DYNAfabric m.
Embarc bone repair m.
Ethrone implant m.
Evazote cushioning m.
m. failure break point
fibrillar absorbable hemostat m.
Fletching femoral hernia implant m.
gold weight and wire spring implant m.
Graflex m.
graft m.
grafted m.
Grafton demineralized bone matrix putty m.
Gypsona cast m.
Healos synthetic bone grafting m.
homograft implant m.
hydroxyapatite bone replacement m.
hydroxyapatite implant m.
implant m.
IntelliTemp insulation m.
Interpore bone replacement m.
Iowa implant m.
Keolar implant m.
LactoSorb orthopaedic wound m.
Malteno tube implant m.
methyl methacrylate implant m.
National Center to Improve Practice through Technology, Media, and M.'s

Nicoll bone replacement m.
NovaBone Bioglass bone grafting m.
Omega splinting m.
Ommaya reservoir implant m.
Opteform bone graft m.
OrthoDyn bone substitute m.
Ortho-Glass synthetic m.
Ortho-Jel impression m.
OsSatura synthetic bone graft substitution m.
Osteogenics BoneSource synthetic bone replacement m.
paraffin implant m.
Pe Lite thermoplastic crepe m.
Pelite thermoplastic crepe m.
PerioGlas bone graft m.
Plasti-Pore prosthetic m.
polyether implant m.
polyethylene implant m.
polyurethane implant m.
polyvinyl alcohol splinting m.
polyvinyl implant m.
Porocoat prosthetic m.
porous prosthetic m.
ProOsteon bone graft m.
Proplast I, II porous implant m.
Proplast prosthetic m.
purulent m.
Pyrost bone graft m.
Schepens hollow silicone hemisphere implant m.
Scutan temporary splint m.
Shearing posterior chamber implant m.
shell implant m.
silicone m.
Silon silicone thermoplastic splinting m.
solid buckling implant m.
solid silicone exoplant implant m.
Spitz-Holter valve implant m.
splinting m.
Stimoceiver implant m.
Synergy flexible splinting m.
synthetic m.
thermomoldable m.
ThermoSKY orthotic m.
tissue mandrel implant m.
titanium implant m.
Trilon multilayered m.
Unigraft bone graft m.
Unilab Surgibone bone replacement m.
Virtullene brace m.
viscoelastic m.
vitallium implant m.
Vitox alumina ceramic m.

zirconium oxide arthroplasty m.
Zorbacel shock-absorbing m.
Matev sign
Mathews
M. drill point
M. hand drill
M. load drill
M. olecranon fracture classification
Mathew scale
Mathieu rasp
Mathys prosthesis
matricectomy, matrixectomy
chemical m.
Frost partial m.
laser partial m.
partial m.
phenol m.
phenol-alcohol m.
Steindler m.
total m.
Winograd partial m.
Zadik total m.
matrix, pl. **matrices**
Accell Connexus bone m.
Accell DBM 100 bone m.
Accell TBM bone m.
Accell total bone m.
bone m.
Collagraft bone graft m.
demineralized bone m. (DBM)
germinal m.
germinative m.
GraftJacket regenerative tissue
repair m.
m. Grafton putty
m. injury
ligament-scar m.
limied proteoglycan m.
nail m.
proteoglycan m.
scaffold m.
m. seating system
sterile m.
total bone m. (TBM)
matrix-bone marrow slurry
matrixectomy (*var. of* matricectomy)
Matroc femoral head
Matrol femoral head prosthesis
Matson
M. Evaluation of Social Skills in
Individuals with Severe
Retardation (MESSIER)
M. periosteal elevator

M. procedure
M. rib elevator
Matson-Alexander rib elevator
Matta-Saucedo fixation
matter
gray m.
white m.
Matthew cross-leg clamp
Matthews-Green pin
matting
Dycem roll m.
Matti-Russe
M.-R. bone graft
M.-R. technique
mattress
Akros extended care m.
Akros pressure m.
AkroTech m.
antidecubitus m.
chiropractic m.
Clinisert m.
DeCube m.
m. double anchor footprint rotator
cuff tear repair
eggcrate m.
Geo-Mattress bariatric m.
Invacare APM m.
Lapidus alternating air-pressure m.
Nirvana m.
OptiMax Supreme pressure
reduction m.
overlay m.
PressureGuard m.
Q Star Voyager pressure
reduction m.
Rik fluid m.
Sofflex m.
Sof Matt pressure relieving m.
m. suture
Tempur-Pedic m.
Tempur-Pedic pressure relieving
Swedish m.
T-Foam m.
Tri-Float pressure reduction m.
Mattrix spinal cord stimulation system
maturation
accelerated bone m.
bone m.
delayed bone m.
m. phase
skeletal m.
m. zone

M

NOTES

maturity
    bone m.
    Oxford method for scoring
      skeletal m.
    skeletal m.
Mau
    M. bunionectomy
    M. and Ludloff procedure
    M. osteotomy
Mauch Swing and Stance hydraulic knee
Mauck
    M. knee procedure
    M. operation
Mauclaire disease
Maudsley test
max
    M. 3 electric handpiece
    Thera-Band M.
Maxi-Driver driver
MaxiFloat wheelchair cushion
maxillary
    m. fracture
    m. process
    m. spine
maxillectomy
    Cocke m.
    subtotal m.
maxillofacial bone screw
maxillotomy
    extended m.
Maxima II transcutaneous electrical nerve stimulator
maximal
    isokinetic strength test m.
    m. medical improvement (MMI)
    m. oxygen uptake
    m. stimulus
    m. voluntary contraction (MVC)
Maxim Modular Knee System
maximum
    m. conduction velocity
    m. control (MC)
    m. eversion velocity
    m. inversion velocity
    m. oxygen uptake
    m. pressure picture (MPP)
    m. radial bow
    repetition m. (RM)
    1-repetition m. (1-RM)
    M. Strength Desenex Antifungal
      Cream
    M. Strength Nytol
    m. voluntary effort (MVE)
    M. Voluntary Efforts Test
Maxon suture
Maxwell body

Maxwell-Brancheau
    M.-B. arthroereisis (MBA)
    M.-B. arthroereisis implant
Maxxus orthopaedic latex surgical glove
May anatomical bone plate
Mayday
    M. distal first metatarsal osteotomy
    M. distal first metatarsal osteotomy
      for hallux valgus
Mayer
    M. orthotic
    M. reflex
    M. splint
    M. transfer operation
Mayfield
    M. adapter
    M. device
    M. fixation frame
    M. forceps
    M. head rest
    M. incision
    M. instrumentation
    M. miniature clip applier
    M. neurosurgical headrest
    M. temporary aneurysm clip
      applier
Mayo
    M. ankle arthroplasty
    M. approach
    M. block anesthesia
    M. bunionectomy
    M. carpal instability classification
    M. clamp
    M. Clinic congruent elbow plate
    M. Clinic forefoot score
    M. Clinic hip scoring system
    M. elbow distraction device
    M. elbow fracture classification
    M. elbow performance score
    M. hallux valgus modified
      operation
    M. metatarsal head resection
    M. nerve block
    M. resection arthroplasty
    M. rigid cervical collar
    M. scissors
    M. semiconstrained elbow
      prosthesis
    M. total ankle prosthesis
    M. total elbow arthroplasty
Mayo-Collins retractor
Mayo-Hegar needle holder
Mayo-Portland Adaptability Inventory-3 (MPAI-3)
Mayo-Stone-Valenti hallux limitus/rigidus arthroplasty
Mayo-Thomas collar
Mazabraud syndrome

Mazas totally constrained elbow prosthesis
Mazet
  M. knee disarticulation
  M. technique
Mazur
  M. ankle elevation classification
  M. ankle evaluation
  M. ankle rating
  M. operation
MB-900 AC machine
MBA
  Maxwell-Brancheau arthroereisis
M-Brace knee brace
MBS
  Multi Balance System
    MBS snap-on orthotic
MC
  maximum control
  metacarpal
    MC walker brace
MCA
  motorcycle accident
McArdle
  M. disease
  M. syndrome
McAtee compression screw device
McBride
  M. bunionectomy
  M. bunion hallux valgus
  M. bunion hallux valgus operation
  M. femoral prosthesis
  M. hallux abductovalgus reduction
  M. hallux valgus reduction
  M. pin
  M. plate
  M. procedure
  M. tripod
  M. tripod pin traction
McCain
  M. TMJ arthroscopic system
  M. TMJ cannula
  M. TMJ curette
McCarthy
  M. hip distractor
  M. Scale of Children's Abilities
  M. test
McCarty hip procedure
McCash
  M. hand procedure
  M. hand surgery
McCauley foot procedure
McClintoch brace

McCollough internal tibial torsion brace
McConnell
  M. extensile approach
  M. median and ulnar nerve approach
  M. orthopaedic headrest
  M. patellofemoral treatment plan
  M. shoulder positioner
  M. taping technique method
  M. technique
McCullough retractor
McCune-Albright syndrome
McCutchen hip implant
McDavid
  M. ankle guard
  M. hinged knee guard
  M. knee brace
McDermott radiological classification
McDonald dissector
McDowell Impairment Index (MII)
McElroy
  M. curette
  M. instrumentation
McElvenny
  M. foot procedure
  M. maneuver
  M. technique
McFarland bone graft
McFarland-Osborne technique
McGee
  M. prosthesis needle
  M. splint
  M. wire-crimping forceps
McGee-Priest wire forceps
McGill
  M. pain checklist
  M. Pain Questionnaire
  M. pain scale
McGlamry
  M. elevator
  M. and Feldman modification
  M. procedure
McGlamry-Downey procedure
McGregor line
McGuire
  M. pelvic positioner
  M. rating
  M. score
MCI
  midcarpal instability
McIndoe
  M. bone rongeur

M

NOTES

McIndoe *(continued)*
    M. rongeur forceps
    M. scissors
McIntire splint
McIvor ENT retractor
McKay
    M. hip procedure
    M. osteotomy
McKay-Simons CSR
McKee
    M. brace
    M. femoral prosthesis
    M. totally constrained elbow
      prosthesis
    M. tri-fin nail
McKee-Farrar
    M.-F. acetabular cup
    M.-F. total hip arthroplasty
    M.-F. total hip prosthesis
McKeever
    M. arthrodesis for hallux limitus
    M. bunionectomy
    M. cartilage knife
    M. medullary clavicle fixation
    M. metatarsophalangeal arthrodesis
    M. metatarsophalangeal fusion
    M. open reduction
    M. operation
    M. patellar cap prosthesis
    M. patellar resurfacing device
    M. procedure
    M. vitallium knee prosthesis
McKeever-Buck fragment excision
McKenzie
    M. bone drill
    M. cervical roll
    M. enlarging bur
    M. extension exercise
    M. extension maneuver
    M. lumbar roll
    M. method
    M. night roll
    M. perforating twist drill
    M. Repex table
McKittrick transmetatarsal amputation
**McKusick-type metaphysial
  chondrodysplasia**
MCL
  medial collateral ligament
    MCL brace
McLaughlin
    M. acromioplasty
    M. approach
    M. arthroplasty
    M. carpal scaphoid screw
    M. modification of Bunnell pull-
      out suture
    M. nail
    M. operation

    M. osteosynthesis apparatus
    M. osteosynthesis device
    M. plate
    M. procedure
    M. subscapularis transfer
McLaughlin-Ryder incision
McLeod padded clavicular splint
McMaster bone graft
**McMaster-Toronto Arthritis Patient
  Preference Disability Questionnaire**
McMurray
    M. circumduction maneuver
    M. osteotomy
    M. sign
    M. test
    M. twist maneuver
McMurtry
  kinematic index of M.
    M. kinematic index
MCP
  metacarpophalangeal
    MCP finger joint prosthesis
MCR
  midcarpal radial
    MCR portal
McRae line
McReynolds
    M. driver
    M. driver-extractor
    M. method
    M. open fracture reduction
      technique
    M. open reduction
McShane-Leinberry-Fenlin acromioplasty
MCU
  midcarpal ulnar
    MCU portal
McWhorter posterior shoulder approach
MD
  muscular dystrophy
    MD brace
MDCN
  medial dorsal cutaneous nerve
MDI
  multidirectional instability
MDS MicroDebrider
M-DVPA
  Modified Dynamic Visual Processing
  Assessment
Mead
    M. bone rongeur
    M. mallet
    M. periosteal elevator
meal
  bone m.
MEAMS
  Middlesex Elderly Assessment of Mental
  state

mean
    m. flow velocity
    m. value
Mears sacroiliac plate
Meary
    M. line
    M. metatarsotalar angle
measure
    Canadian Occupational
      Performance M. (COPM)
    Child and Adolescent Social
      Perception M. (CASP)
    emergency closed manipulative m.
    functional assessment m. (FAM)
    functional independence m. (FIM)
    Gross Motor Function M. (GMFM)
    limited performance m.
    outcome m.
    parallel goniometric m.
    reconstructive m.
    standard goniometric m.
measured stress
measurement
    AccuSway balance m.
    Agliette m.
    alignment m.
    anthropometric m.
    appendicular bone mass m.
    arthrometer m.
    arthrometric knee laxity m.
    Blackburn-Peel m.
    bone density m.
    calcaneal compartment pressure m.
    clear space m.
    curve m.
    EMED-F foot-force m.
    foot central compartment
      pressure m.
    functional capacity m.
    Insall-Salvati m.
    Kite m.
    limb accurate m. (LAM)
    Mehta rib angle m.
    motion m.
    pain m.
    pedodynographic m.
    range of motion m.
    roof arc m.
    Schober m.
    skinfold m.
    spasticity m.
    tibiofibular overlap m.

    tissue pressure m.
    Zwipp subtalar joint instability m.
measurer
    Bunnell digital exertion m.
measuring
    m. gauge
    precise lesion m. (PLM)
mechanical
    m. agent
    m. axis
    combined m. (CM)
    m. dermatome
    m. dysfunction
    m. fixation
    m. instability
    m. instrument adjusting
    m. insufficiency
    m. low back pain syndrome
    m. modality
    m. pain threshold (MPTh)
    m. plate design
mechanics
    altered intervertebral m.
    altered regional m.
    body m.
    walking m.
mechanism
    abductor m.
    adhesion/cohesion m.
    Adjustable Leg and Ankle
      Repositioning M. (ALARM)
    4-bar linkage prosthetic knee m.
    capsuloligamentous m.
    central extensor m. (CEM)
    clamping m.
    Cook-Gordon m.
    m. of correction
    cranial-sacral respiratory m.
      (CRSM)
    digital extensor m.
    extensor hood m.
    fail-safe m.
    flexor m.
    gliding m.
    m. of growth arrest
    Hosmer Dorrance voluntary control
      4-bar knee m.
    humeral m.
    locomotor m.
    MicroStable liner locking m.
    neurotraumatic m.
    Noiles rotating hinge knee m.
    physiological venous pump m.

M

NOTES

mechanism *(continued)*
   post-and-cam m.
   primary cranial sacral
     respiratory m.
   quadriceps m.
   m. of reflex immunologic
     competence
   screw-home m.
   slider crank m.
   tendo Achillis m.
   terminal extensor m. (TEM)
   UHR locking ring m.
   Windlass m.
mechanoreceptor
   m. activity
   m. Golgi tendon organ
   joint capsule m.
   pacinian m.
   Ruffini m.
Meckel cavity
Mecring acetabluar prosthesis
Medak glove
Medarmor puncture-resistant glove
Mederma topical gel
Med-Fit
   M.-F. cranial-sacral table
   M.-F. Senior Circuit exercise
     machine
medial
   m. antebrachial cutaneous nerve
   m. articular nerve
   m. aspect
   m. aspiration
   m. bicipital sulcus
   m. bicortical screw
   m. border
   m. brachial cutaneous nerve injury
   m. brachial nerve
   m. calcaneal tubercle
   m. capsular imbrication
   m. capsular ligament
   m. capsulorrhaphy
   m. clear space
   m. closing wedge phalangeal
     osteotomy
   m. collateral ligament (MCL)
   m. collateral sprain
   m. column calcaneal fracture
   m. column instability
   m. compartment
   m. compartment disruption
   m. compartment injury
   m. cortical overlap technique
   m. crossover toe
   m. deviation
   m. deviation of second toe
   m. disc protrusion
   m. displacement
   m. displacement osteotomy

m. dorsal cutaneous nerve (MDCN)
m. drainage
m. eminence
m. eminence resection
m. end
m. epicondylar apophysis
m. epicondyle
m. epicondylectomy
m. epicondyle humeral fracture
m. epicondylitis
m. exostectomy
m. extensor expansion
m. femoral condyle
m. gastrocnemius bursitis
m. geniculate
m. geniculate artery
m. geniculate fascia
m. hamstring
m. head of gastrocnemius rupture
m. head-stem offset
m. heel-and-sole wedge
m. heel skive technique
m. heel wedge (MHW)
m. heel wedge orthosis
m. hip rotation
m. humeral condyle
m. joint line
m. longitudinal arch
m. malleolar fracture
m. malleolar/small bone fragment
   clamp
m. malleolus (MM)
m. malleolus cast
m. malleolus fixation
m. malleolus resection
m. malleolus of tibia
m. meniscectomy
m. meniscus
m. metacarpal bone
m. movement
m. nerve protector
m. neurovascular bundle
m. oblique (MO)
m. opening wedge osteotomy
m. outline
m. parapatellar arthrotomy
m. parapatellar capsular approach
m. parapatellar incision
m. patellar plica
m. patellofemoral ligament (MPFL)
m. plantar artery
m. plantar fasciocutaneous flap
m. plantar nerve
m. portal
m. proximal tibial angle
m. quadruple complex
m. ray adduction deformity
m. release
m. repair

m. rollover
m. rotation procedure
m. sesamoid
m. sesamoid ligament
m. shelf
m. shelf/medial plica
m. sole wedge
m. sole wedge orthosis
m. sole wedge shoe modification
m. stem pivot
m. sural cutaneous nerve
m. swivel dislocation
m. talocalcaneal bar
m. talocalcaneal ligament
m. talonavicular capsule
m. tennis elbow tendinosis
m. tibial epiphysiodesis
m. tibial flare
m. tibial stress syndrome (MTSS)
m. tibial syndrome (MTS)
m. torsion
m. T-strap
m. ulnar collateral ligament (MUCL)
m. unicortical screw
m. V-Y capsulotomy
m. wall

medialis
malleolus m.
m. pedis flap
vastus m.

medialization ratio

medial/lateral
m./l. femoral condyle
m./l. meniscus

medial/plantar hinge

median
m. nerve
m. nerve block
m. nerve compression
m. nerve entrapment
m. nerve injury
m. nerve palsy
m. neuropathy
m. raphe
m. sagittal plane

Medi-Band bandage

medical
m. adhesive
M. Design brace
m. elastomer X7-2320
M. Examination and Diagnostic Coding System (MEDICS)

m. galvanism
m. manipulation
M. Research Council (MRC)
m. subcutaneous reflection

medication
antiinflammatory m.
nonsteroidal antiinflammatory m.

medicinal leech

medicine
allopathic m.
alternative m.
American College of Sports M. (ACSM)
American Medical Society for Sports M. (AMSSM)
American Orthopaedic Society for Sports M. (AOSSM)
m. ball
Chinese m.
complimentary and alternative m. (CAM)
dance m.
doctor of podiatric m. (DPM)
electrodiagnostic m.
International Society of Arthroscopy, Knee Surgery, and Orthopaedic Sports M. (ISAKOS)
manual m.
Native American m.
occupational and environmental m. (OEM)
osteopathic m.
physical m. (PM)
podiatric m.
sports m.
vertebral m.

MediCordz rehabilitation kit

MEDICS
Medical Examination and Diagnostic Coding System

Medicus bed

Mediflow
M. waterbase pillow
M. Waterpillow

Mediloy
M. implant metal
M. implant metal prosthesis

mediolateral (M/L)
m. position
m. radiocarpal angle
m. stress
m. tilt

mediotarsal amputation

NOTES

M

Medipedic Multicentric knee brace
Mediplast
Medi Plus compression stockings
Medipore H surgical tape
Medi-Quick Topical Ointment
Medi-Rip dressing
MediRule II measuring device
Medisana Massager
Medi-Stim stimulator
meditation and mindfulness
medium
    Amipaque contrast m.
    m. callus Podi-Burr
    m. carbide cone bur
    dermatophyte test m. (DTM)
    m. fine bur
    Microfil contrast m.
    m. nail Podi-Burr
    m. profile femoral prosthesis
Medium-Plus alpha liner
medium-viscosity cement
medius
    digitus m.
MEDLS
  Milwaukee Evaluation of Daily Living
  Skills
Medmetric
    M. knee ligament arthrometer
    M. KT-1000 knee laxity
    arthrometer
Medoff
    M. axial compression screw
    M. sliding plate
Medralone Injection
Medrol
    M. Dosepak
    M. Oral
Medtronic spinal cord stimulation
  system
medulla, pl. **medullae**
medullary
    m. bone graft
    m. callus
    m. canal
    m. canal reamer
    m. cavity
    m. locking
    m. nail
    m. nail fixation
    m. nailing
    m. paraganglioma
    m. pin
    m. prosthesis
    m. saw
    m. venous malformation (MVM)
    m. vent tubing
medullectomy
medullization
medulloarthritis

medullostomy
    tarsal m.
MedX
    M. functional testing machine
    M. Mark II lumbar extension
    machine
    M. stretch machine
Meek
    M. clavicular strap
    M. pelvic traction belt
mefenamic acid
Mega-Air bed
megalodactyly
megaprosthesis
Mega Tilt and Turn bed
Mehta rib angle measurement
Meige syndrome
melagra
melalgia
melamine resin
melanoma
    acral lentiginous m.
    Breslow classification of m.
    Clark classification of m.
    lentigo maligna m.
    malignant m.
    metastatic m.
    nodular m.
    plantar malignant m.
melanosis circumscripta preblastomatosis
  of Dubreuilh
melanotic
    m. panaris
    m. whitlow of Hutchinson
Melaware flatware
Meleney
    M. infection
    M. synergistic gangrene
melioidosis
    musculoskeletal m.
melioidotic
Melone distal radius fracture
  classification
melon-seed body
melorheostosis
melosalgia
Melzack Pain Questionnaire
membrane
    anterior atlantooccipital m.
    atlantooccipital anterior m.
    basement m.
    cricothyroid m.
    m. instability
    interosseous m. (IOM)
    interposition m.
    intraosseous m.
    mucous m.
    periprosthetic m.
    Preclude spinal m.

spinal m.
suprasyndesmotic m.
synovial m.
m. tack
thickened synovial m.
trauma-induced m.

membranous
m. bone
m. ossification
m. osteogenesis

memory
m. board
cine m.
m. compression staple
m. splint

Mendel-Bekhterev
M.-B. reflex
M.-B. sign

Mendelsohn
M. maneuver
M. modification of matricectomy
suture technique

Menelaus triceps transfer
meningeal
m. nerve
m. syndrome

meningioma
meningism
meningismus
meningitis
meningocele
meningococcal purpura
meningoencephalomyelitis
meningomyelitis
meningomyelocele
meniscal
m. aponeurosis
m. arrow
m. autograft transplantation
m. clamp
m. curette
m. cutter
m. cyst
m. excision
m. flounce
m. injury
m. lateral tear
m. mirror
m. radial tear
m. repair
m. repair needle
m. scissors
m. spoon

m. staple
m. transverse tear

meniscectomy
arthroscopic m.
m. knife
lateral m.
medial m.
partial m.
Patel medial m.
m. scissors
subtotal lateral m.
total m.

menisci (*pl. of* meniscus)
meniscitis
meniscocapsular
m. junction
m. tear

meniscofemoral
m. capsule
m. ligament

meniscoid
m. entrapment
joint m.
m. lesion

meniscopexy
meniscoplasty
meniscorrhaphy
meniscosynovial junction
meniscotibial
m. capsule
m. ligament

meniscotome
Bircher m.
curved m.
Grover m.
Storz m.

meniscotomy chisel
meniscus, pl. **menisci**
M. Arrow fixation
bridge of m.
clefting of m.
degenerative m.
discoid lateral m.
m. forceps
frayed m.
fraying of m.
m. graft
m. homolog
m. hook
m. knife
lateral m.
medial m.
medial/lateral m.

M

NOTES

meniscus *(continued)*
    M. Mender II system
    peripheral m.
    resection of m.
    m. retractor
    m. scissors
    m. suturing
    torn m.
    trapped m.
Mennell
    M. sign
    M. test
MENS
    microamperage electrical nerve
      stimulation
    MENS unit
Mensor-Scheck
    M.-S. hanging-hip operation
    M.-S. technique
mental torticollis
mentor
    M. Self-Cath soft catheter
    M. tissue expander
mepacrine
Mephisto
    M. Mobils professional shoe
    M. speed lacing system
Mephisto speed lacing system
MEPP
    miniature end-plate potential
MERAC
    musculoskeletal evaluation, rehabilitation
    and conditioning
meralgia
merchant
    M. congruence angle
    M. and Dietz ankle score
    M. radiograph
    M. view
mercury
    millimeters of m. (mmHg)
meridian
    M. Intersegmental table
    M. ST femoral implant component
    m. therapy
Merit final flexion kit
Merkel cell
**Merland perimedullary arteriovenous
fistula classification**
Merle
    M. d'Aubigné hip score
    M. d'Aubigné and Postel hip
      rating scale
Merlin arthroscopy blade
Merocel pack
merry
    M. Walker
    M. Walker ambulation device

Mersilene
    M. Kessler stitch
    M. sling
    M. suture
    M. tape
Meryon sign
mesencephalic injury
mesenchymal
    m. cell
    m. chondrosarcoma
    m. tumor
mesenchyme
mesenchymoma
    pluripotential m.
mesenteric vasculitis
mesh
    chromium-cobalt m.
    m. graft
    Marlex m.
    metal m.
    sintered titanium m.
    stainless steel m.
    tantalum m.
mesher
    Zimmer skin graft m.
mesiodistal plane
mesocuneiform bone
mesotendineum
mesotendon
mesothenar muscle
MESS
    Mangled Extremity Severity Score
MESSIER
    Matson Evaluation of Social Skills in
      Individuals with Severe Retardation
MET
    metabolic equivalent of task
metabolic
    m. bone disease
    m. equivalent of task (MET)
    m. syndrome (MS)
    m. variable
metabolism
    energy m.
metacarpal (MC)
    m. amputation
    m. base
    m. beak
    m. block
    m. bone
    duplicated m.
    fifth m.
    first m.
    fourth m.
    m. lengthening
    m. ligament
    m. neck
    m. neck fracture
    m. osteotomy

second m.
third m.
thumb m.
metacarpectomy
metacarpocapitate joint
metacarpocarpal joint
metacarpoglenoidal ligament
metacarpohamate joint
metacarpophalangeal (MCP, MP)
    m. arthroscopy
    m. articulation
    m. dislocation
    m. implant
    m. joint (MPJ)
    m. joint arthroplasty
    m. ligament
metacarpophysial
    m. joint
    m. joint extension contracture
metacarpotrapezoid joint
metacarpus
metachromatic mucoid substance
metaepiphysis
metal
    m. acetabular liner
    Alivium implant m.
    Biophase implant m.
    Biotex implant m.
    m. clamp
    Coballoy implant m.
    Co-Cr-Mo alloy implant m.
    Co-Cr-W-Ni alloy implant m.
    m. endurance limit
    m. failure
    m. fatigue
    m. femoral head prosthesis
    m. foot plate
    HA 65101 implant m.
    Haynes-Stellite 21 implant m.
    m. hemi-toe implant
    m. hybrid orthosis
    implant m.
    m. implant corrosion
    m. locator
    m. measuring triangle
    Mediloy implant m.
    m. mesh
    Orthochrome implant m.
    m. orthopaedic implant
    m. pin
    porous m.
    Protasul implant m.
    m. pusher

m. pylon
Sinterlock implant m.
m. splint
tivanium implant m.
Vinertia implant m.
vitallium implant m.
Zimaloy implant m.
metal-backed
    m.-b. acetabular component
    m.-b. acetabular component hip implant
    m.-b. acetabular cup
    m.-b. acetabular shell
    m.-b. patellar implant
    m.-b. plastic-on-metal prosthesis
    m.-b. socket
metallic
    m. bead
    m. debris
    m. implant
metalloproteinase
    tissue inhibitor of m. (TIMP)
metallosis
metal-on-metal
    m.-o.-m. articulating intervertebral disc prosthesis
    m.-o.-m. design
metaphyses (*pl. of* metaphysis)
metaphysial
    m. abscess
    m. aclasis
    m. artery
    m. bone
    m. chondrodysplasia
    m. to diaphysial width ratio
    m. dysostosis
    m. fibrous cortical defect
    m. head resection
    m. head resection with prosthesis
    m. osteotomy
    m. shortening
    m. spike
    m. stapler
    m. tibial fracture
    m. tuberculosis
    m. wedge
metaphysial-articular nonunion
metaphysial-diaphysial
    m.-d. angle
    m.-d. junction
metaphysial-epiphysial angle
metaphysis, pl. **metaphyses**
    distal m.

NOTES

metaphysis (*continued*)
    femoral m.
    fibular m.
    funnelization of m.
    tibial m.
metaphysitis
metaplasia
    cartilaginous m.
    fibrous m.
    osteocartilaginous m.
metaplastic ossification
metastasis, pl. **metastases**
    bone m.
    bony m.
    osteoblastic m.
    Picker Magnascanner for bone m.
    spinal m.
metastatic
    m. bone lesion
    m. bone survey
    m. disease
    m. melanoma
    m. spinal tumor
Metasul
    M. hip joint component
    M. joint
    M. metal-on-metal hip
    M. metal-on-metal hip prosthesis
    system
metatarsal (MT)
    m. arch
    m. artery
    m. axis
    m. bar shoe modification
    m. base angle
    m. block
    m. bone
    m. callosity
    m. cookie
    m. cuneiform exostosis
    dorsiflexed m.
    m. flatfoot bar
    m. flat head
    m. fracture
    m. head extractor
    m. head osteotomy
    m. head resection
    m. joint
    m. length
    lesser m.
    m. ligament
    m. neck
    m. neck osteotomy
    m. oblique osteotomy
    m. ossification
    osteochondrosis of m.
    m. osteology
    m. overload syndrome
    m. pad

    m. parabola
    m. phalangeal angle
    m. proximal dome osteotomy
    m. ray
    m. Reverdin osteotomy
    m. shaft
    m. traction
    m. V-shaped osteotomy
metatarsalgia
    Morton m.
    secondary m.
    transfer m.
metatarsal-sesamoid arthrosis
metatarsal-tarsal joint
metatarsectomy
metatarsi (*pl. of* metatarsus)
metatarsocalcaneal angle
metatarsocuboid joint
metatarsocuneiform (MTC)
    m. angle
    m. arthrodesis
    m. articulation
    m. joint
    m. joint exostosis
    m. joint fusion
metatarsophalangeal (MT, MTP)
    m. arthroplasty
    m. capsulotomy
    m. creaking
    m. crease
    m. joint (MTPJ)
    m. joint arthrodesis
    m. joint capsule
    m. joint disarticulation
    m. joint dislocation
    m. joint fusion
    m. joint ganglion
    m. joint injury
    m. joint synovitis
    m. subluxation
metatarsophalangeal-interphalangeal scale
metatarsophalangealium
metatarsosesamoid
    m. joint
    m. ligament
metatarsotalar angle
metatarsus, pl. **metatarsi**
    m. abductus
    m. adductocavus
    m. adductovarus
    m. adductus (MTA)
    m. adductus angle
    m. adductus deformity
    m. cavus
    m. internus
    m. primus adductus (MPA)
    m. primus atavicus
    m. primus declination angle
    m. primus elevatus

m. primus equinus
m. primus osteotomy
m. primus varus (MPV)
m. primus varus deformity
m. rectus
m. valgus
m. varus (MTV)
m. varus deformity
metatropic dwarfism
metazonal region
Met Bar shoe modification
Metcalf spring drop brace
meter
Fischer pressure threshold m.
pinch m.
pressure threshold m.
methacrylate
antibiotic-impregnated
polymethyl m.
centrifuged methyl m.
methyl m.
polymethyl m. (PMMA)
m. resin
methemoglobin
methicillin-resistant Staphylococcus aureus (MRSA)
methocarbamol and aspirin
method
Abbott m.
antegrade m.
anthropometric m.
ARM m.
biofeedback-assisted m.
Bleck m.
Borggreve m.
Buck m.
Budin-Chandler m.
bundle-nailing m.
Burkhalter-Reyes m.
cable cerclage m.
Callahan m.
Carrel m.
Caton m.
Chamberlain m.
Chaput m.
Cobb m.
contoured adduction trochanteric-controlled alignment m. (CAT-CAM)
cup and cone m.
Delore m.
depth caliper-meter stick m.
disc diffusion m.

dynamic traction m.
Edinburgh m.
Elmslie-Trillat patellar realignment m.
Essex-Lopresti m.
extension block splinting m.
Fallat-Buckholz m.
Feldenkrais m.
Ferguson scoliosis measuring m.
Fick m.
Gohil-Cavolo m.
Grace m.
gravity m.
Hoffa tendon-shortening m.
Hoke triple-section m.
hold-relax m.
hole preparation m.
hydrogen washout m.
Ilizarov m.
immobilization m.
1-inclinometer m.
2-inclinometer m.
Insall patella alta m.
install m.
Jahss 90-90 m.
keyhole m.
Lange tendon-lengthening m.
Lindsjö m.
Ling m.
McConnell taping technique m.
McKenzie m.
McReynolds m.
Mose m.
Mosley anterior shoulder repair m.
nail length gauge m.
Neufeld dynamic m.
Oil-Red-O m.
OnTrack treatment m.
Oxford m.
Palmer m.
pedicle m.
m. of perpendiculars
Pilates exercise m.
pin-and-plaster m.
Ponseti clubfoot treatment m.
Ranawat-Dorr-Inglis m.
receptor-tonus m.
retrograde m.
Risser m.
Russe-Gerhardt m.
Schede m.
Schober m.
splinting m.

NOTES

method *(continued)*
    Stamm m.
    Stimson gravity m.
    Stulberg m.
    Tajima m.
    total mesenteric apron m.
    Trager m.
    Wagner limb lengthening m.
    Zwipp m.
methotrexate toxicity
methyl
    m. methacrylate
    m. methacrylate adhesive
    m. methacrylate bead
    m. methacrylate bead implant
    m. methacrylate cement
    m. methacrylate implant material
    m. salicylate
methylcellulose
methylene
    m. bisphenyl diisocyanate
    m. blue
    m. blue dye
    m. diphosphonate (MPD)
methylmalonic acid
methylprednisolone
    m. acetate
    m. sodium succinate
methylxanthine
Metrecom
    M. digitizer
    M. spinal analyzer
MetroGel Topical
Mettler
    M. electrotherapy
    M. Trio neuromuscular electrical
    stimulator
Metzenbaum
    M. chisel
    M. gouge
    M. scissors
Meuli arthroplasty
Meurig Williams plate
Meyer
    M. cervical orthosis
    M. dysplasia
    M. line
Meyer-Betz
    M.-B. disease
    M.-B. syndrome
Meyerding
    M. bone skid
    M. chisel
    M. curved osteotome
    M. gouge
    M. grade I-III
    M. grading
    M. grading of spondylolisthesis
    M. mallet

    M. retractor
    M. spondylolisthesis classification
    line
    M. straight osteotome
**Meyers-McKeever tibial fracture
classification**
**Meyers quadratus muscle-pedicle bone
graft**
Meyhoeffer bone curette
Meyn
    M. elbow reduction
    M. reduction of elbow dislocation
Meynet node
Meyn-Quigley maneuver
mezlocillin
MFA
    Musculoskeletal Function Assessment
    MFA questionnaire
M-F heel protector
MG
    muscle group
    MG II knee prosthesis
    MG II total knee system
MGHL
    middle glenohumeral ligament
    MGHL cord
MGH osteotome
MHOCE
    multiple hereditary osteochondral
    exostosis
MHW
    medial heel wedge
Miacalcin
    M. Injection
    M. nasal spray
Miami
    M. Acute Care (MAC)
    M. Acute cervical collar
    M. Acute collar cervical traction
    M. fracture brace
    M. J cervical collar
    M. J collar cervical traction
    M. TLSO scoliosis brace
Mibelli
    porokeratosis of M.
Micatin Topical
Mica 3x sleeve
mice (*pl. of* mouse)
Michaelis rhomboid
Michael Reese articulated prosthesis
Michel clip
Michele
    M. long-stem prosthesis
    M. test
    M. vertebral biopsy
    M. vertebral trephine
Michelson-Sequoia air drill
Michigan
    M. Bone Health Study

M. Hand Outcomes
M. Hand Outcomes Questionnaire
MiCOR
M. machine bone allograft
M. precision bone allograft
micro
M. QuickAnchor
M. Series wire driver
Micro-Aire
M.-A. débridement of bone surface
M.-A. drill
M.-A. oscillating saw
M.-A. osteotome
M.-A. reamer
microamperage
m. electrical nerve stimulation (MENS)
m. neural stimulation (MNS)
microanastomosis
microavulsion
MicroBite forceps
Microblator ArthroWand
microcirculation
microcoil
microcomputer upper limb exerciser (MULE)
microcrystalline collagen
microcurrent
m. electrode
m. therapy
MicroDebrider
MDS M.
Topaz M.
microdiscectomy
arthroscopic m. (AMD)
uniportal arthroscopic m.
MicroFET2
M. muscle tester
M. muscle testing device
Microfil contrast medium
Microfoam dressing
microfracture
microgeodic syndrome
micrographia
microinterlock
microirrigating cannula
microirrigator
MicroLite suture anchor
Microloc
M. knee implant
M. knee prosthesis
M. knee system

microlumbar
m. discectomy (MLD)
m. disc excision
m. discography
micromelic dwarfism
micrometric screw
Micro-Mill knee instrument system
MicroMite anchor suture
micromotion
liner m.
microneedle holder
microneurosurgical technique
Micro-One
M.-O. dissecting forceps
M.-O. hook
microoscillating saw
microparticulated protein product
MicroPhor iontophoretic drug delivery system
micropin
Pischel m.
Microplasty minimally invasive hip program
microplate
Luhr m.
micropodia
microprocessor
Intertron therapy m.
microsagittal saw
microsaw
Zimmer m.
microscissors
microscope
double binocular operating m.
operating m.
microscopy
confocal m.
hyperspectral near-infrared Raman imaging m.
light m.
transmission electron m.
Microsect
M. curette
M. shaver
MicroStable liner locking mechanism
microstaple
Barouk m.
microsurgical
m. discectomy (MSD)
m. instrument
m. thoracoscopic vertebrectomy
microtiter protein kinase assay

M

NOTES

microtrauma
  cervical m.
  lumbar m.
  repetitive m.
  thoracic m.
Micro-Two forceps
microvalve
  Hypobaric m.
microvascular
  m. clamp
  m. free muscle flap
  m. osseous transfer
  m. surgical anastomosis
microvasculature
Microvel prosthesis
microwave diathermy (MWD)
micro waveform
Micro-Z neuromuscular stimulator
Midas
  M. Rex acorn
  M. Rex bone cutter
  M. Rex bur
  M. Rex drill
  M. Rex instrumentation system
  M. Rex knife
  M. Rex pneumatic instrument
midaxillary
  m. line (MAL)
  m. line incision
midbody of vertebra
midcalf
midcarpal
  m. arthrodesis
  m. arthroscopy
  m. injury
  m. instability (MCI)
  m. joint
  m. portal
  m. radial (MCR)
  m. ulnar (MCU)
Middeldorpf
  M. splint
  M. triangle
middiaphysial axis
middle
  m. atlantoepistrophic joint
  m. carpal joint
  m. column injury
  m. ear barotrauma
  m. finger
  m. finger amputation
  m. finger test
  m. glenohumeral ligament (MGHL)
  m. raphe
  m. sacral artery
  m. sacral vein
  m. third (M/3)
  m. third of shaft

  m. thyroid vein
  m. tibial shaft fracture
Middlesex Elderly Assessment of
  Mental state (MEAMS)
midfacial fracture
midfemur
midfoot
  m. abductus
  m. adductus
  m. arthritis
  m. arthrodesis
  m. arthropathy
  m. cavus
  m. deformity
  m. fracture
  m. joint
  m. scale
midheel line
Midland
  M. multifunctional mat platform
  M. tilt table
midlatency SEP
midlateral
  m. approach
  m. capsule
  m. portal
midline
  m. disc herniation
  M. Hi-Lo Mat Platform
  m. ligament
  m. medial approach
  m. raphe
midmalleolar line
midmedial capsule
midnight fracture
midpalmar
  m. abscess
  m. space
midpatellar
  m. portal
  m. tendon
midsagittal plane
midshaft
  m. fracture
  m. metatarsal osteotomy
midstance period of gait
midsternal line (MSL)
midsubstance tear
midtarsal
  m. dome osteotomy
  m. joint
  m. osteoarthritis
  m. V osteotomy
midtarsus
midthigh amputation
Midwest Regional Spinal Cord Injury
  Center
Mignon eosinophilic granuloma

migration
m. of acetabular cup
brace m.
hallux m.
instrument m.
Luque rod m.
m. of prosthesis
rod m.
staple m.
trochanteric m.
migratory
m. arthralgia
m. arthritis
MII
McDowell Impairment Index
Mikasa subacromial bursography
Mikhail bone block
Mikulicz
M. angle
M. operation
M. pad
M. procedure
M. sponge
Mikulicz-Vladimiroff amputation
Milano Shoethotic footwear
Milch
M. condylar fracture classification
M. cuff resection
M. cuff resection of ulna
  technique
M. elbow fracture classification
M. elbow operation
M. elbow technique
M. fracture classification syndrome
M. plate
M. radioulnar joint repair
Miles
M. bone chisel
M. Nervine caplets
milestone
motor m.
Milford mallet finger technique
MiLIF
minimally invasive lumbar interbody
  fusion
military
m. antishock trousers (MAST)
m. brace maneuver
m. brace position
m. maneuver
m. posture test
m. tuck position
milk-alkali disease

milking
m. maneuver
m. sign
m. of vessel
milkmaid's
m. elbow
m. elbow dislocation
milkman's
m. pseudofracture
m. syndrome
milk test
mill
bone m.
Lere bone m.
OrthoBlend powered bone m.
mille
m. pattes screw
m. pattes technique
Millender arthroplasty
Millender-Nalebuff wrist arthrodesis
Miller
M. Assessment for Preschoolers
  (MAP)
M. flatfoot operation
M. foot procedure
M. rasp
Miller-Galante
M.-G. I condylar total knee system
M.-G. hip prosthesis
M.-G. I hemiarthroplasty
M.-G. II knee prosthesis
M.-G. jig
M.-G. knee
M.-G. knee arthroplasty
M.-G. revision knee system
Millesi
M. modified technique
M. nerve graft
milliampere (mA)
millimeter (mm)
m.'s of mercury (mmHg)
millimetric rule
milliner's needle
milling cutter
Millon
M. Behavioral Health Inventory
M. Clinical Multiaxial Inventory
Mills
M. dressing
M. test
Miltex
M. bone saw
M. mallet

NOTES

M

453

Miltex *(continued)*
    M. nail nipper
    M. wire twister
Milwaukee
    M. cervicothoracolumbosacral
    orthosis
    M. Evaluation of Daily Living
    Skills (MEDLS)
    M. scoliosis brace
    M. scoliosis orthosis
    M. shoulder syndrome
mimicry
    somatic visceral disease m.
Mimix bone replacement system
mimocausalgia
Minaar
    M. classification of coalition
    M. classification system
mind-body therapy
mineralization
Miner osteotome
miner's elbow
Minerva
    M. cast
    M. cervical brace
    M. cervical jacket
    M. fixation
    M. orthosis
    M. vest
mini
    m. AO screw
    m. applier
    M. Bio-Phase suture anchor
    M. Fragment Set
    M. GLS anchor
    m. lag screw system (MLS)
    M. Mental State Examination
    (MMSE)
**Mini-Acutrak small bone fixation
system**
miniature
    m. end-plate potential (MEPP)
    m. multipurpose clamp
mini-C-arm
    XiScan m.-C-a.
mini-core disease
minifixator
    articulate m.
minifragment
    m. plate fixation
    m. screw
mini-Hoffmann external fixator
mini-Hohmann podiatric retractor
mini-Kessler external fixator
mini-Lambotte osteotome
mini-Lexer osteotome
minimal incision plantar fasciotomy
minimally
    m. displaced fracture

    m. invasive lumbar interbody
    fusion (MiLIF)
minima patella
MiniMedBall hand exerciser
mini-meniscus blade
minimi
    abductor digiti m. (ADM)
    extensor digiti m. (EDM)
    opponens digiti m. (ODM)
minimum incision surgery (MIS)
minimus
    digitus m.
mini-open rotator cuff repair
mini-Orthofix fixator
mini-pilon fracture
miniplate
    Luhr m.
Mini-Revo Screws suture anchor
Mini-ROC anchor
Minislide sliding mat
ministaple
    Bio-R-Sorb resorbable poly-L-lactic
    acid m.
ministem shaft
mini-Stryker power drill
mini-Ullrich bone clamp
Minneapolis hip prosthesis
Minnesota
    Cognitive Assessment of M.
    (CAM)
    M. Manual Dexterity Test
    M. Rate of Manipulation test
    (MRMT)
    M. Spatial Relations Test
minor
    m. amputation
    m. curve
    M. sign
Minos air drill
6-minute walk test
Mira
    M. cautery
    M. drill
    M. reamer
Mirage Spinal System
mirror
    Apfelbaum m.
    dental m.
    m. hand
    meniscal m.
MIS
    minimum incision surgery
misalignment
miserable misalignment syndrome
missed fracture
misshapen
missile injury
Mital
    M. elbow release

M. elbow release operation
M. elbow release technique

Mitchell

M. bunionectomy
M. distal osteotomy
M. hallux valgus procedure
M. operation
M. osteotome
M. osteotomy/bunionectomy
M. posterior displacement osteotomy
M. step-down osteotomy

Mitek

M. absorbable anchor
M. anchor system
M. bone anchor
M. Fastin threaded anchor
M. GII easy anchor
M. GII Snap-Pak
M. GII suture anchor system
M. GL anchor
M. knotless anchor
M. ligament anchor
M. micro anchor
M. Micro QuickAnchor
M. Mini GLS anchor
M. Mini QuickAnchor
M. Panalok RC anchor
M. rotator cuff anchor
M. SuperAnchor instrument
M. Tacit threaded anchor
M. VAPR tissue removal system

mitella
miter technique
mitochondrial myopathy
mitochondrion, pl. **mitochondria**
mitt

holding m.
impact m.
motion control m.
paraffin m.
wash m.

mitten hand
Mittlemeier

M. ceramic hip prosthesis
M. noncemented femoral prosthesis

Mitutoyo digital caliper
MIV

major injury vector

mixed

m. amputation
m. connective tissue disease

m. connective tissue disorder
m. cord syndrome

mixer

MixEvac bone cement m.

MixEvac bone cement mixer
Mixter

M. forceps
M. ligature-carrier clamp
M. right-angle clamp

Miya hook ligature carrier
Miyakawa knee procedure
Mize-Bucholz-Grogan approach
Mizuno technique
MKG knee support
MKS II knee brace
M/L

mediolateral
M/L lift

MLD

microlumbar discectomy

MLS

mini lag screw system

MLSI

multiple line-scan imaging

MM

medial malleolus

mm

millimeter

mmHg

millimeters of mercury

MMI

maximal medical improvement

MMSE

Mini Mental State Examination

MMT

manual muscle testing

MNCV

motor nerve conduction velocity

MNS

microamperage neural stimulation

MO

medial oblique

Moberg

M. advancement flap
M. arthrodesis
M. deltoid muscle transfer
M. deltoid-to-triceps transfer
M. dowel graft
M. key-grip tenodesis
M. key-pinch procedure
M. osteotome
M. Picking Up Test

NOTES

M

Moberg *(continued)*
- M. screw
- M. splint

Mobic

mobile-bearing
- m.-b. knee
- m.-b. knee arthroplasty
- m.-b. knee implant

mobile wad

Mobilimb CPM device

mobility
- active m.
- m. aid
- coordinated m.
- fractured bone m.
- gait and m.
- hip m.
- intersegmental m.
- joint m.
- limited joint m. (LJM)
- lumbar sagittal m.
- muscle tissue m.
- passive m.
- rotation m.
- sacral m.
- sacroiliac joint m.
- sagittal m.
- segmental m.
- side-bending m.
- symphysial m.
- m. testing
- translation m.
- unisegmental m.
- vertical symphysial m.
- m. WHO Handicap Scale

mobilization
- ASTM augmented soft tissue m.
- augmented soft tissue m. (ASTM)
- Duran passive m.
- grades 1–5 of m.
- joint m.
- lateral band m.
- nonthrust m.
- soft tissue m.
- spinal joint m.
- m. with impulse

Mobils Professionals pedorthic footwear

modality
- deep heat m.
- electrical m.
- Fluidotherapy sterile dry heat m.
- mechanical m.
- nonthermal m.
- passive treatment m.
- superficial heat m.
- thermal m.

mode
- Gruen m.
- loading m.

model
- M. 810 axial closed-loop hydraulic mechanical testing
- Bennett pain m.
- corpectomy m.
- Currey m.
- Denis Browne 3-column m.
- family management m.
- foot m.
- joint m.
- lumbar spine m.
- M.'s of Media Representation of Disability
- Sandoz 4-phase m.
- Tanner developmental m.

modeling
- Ainsworth m.
- Anderson m.
- cortical bone m.

moderate-grade ulcer

modification
- Aufranc m.
- Bloom-Raney m.
- Bonfiglio m.
- Bunnell m.
- Burwell-Scott m.
- C-D screw m.
- chevron m.
- Chrisman-Snook technique m.
- dietary m.
- Downey m.
- Fairbanks technique with Sever m.
- Frank and Johnson m.
- Gillette m.
- Green-Laird m.
- Helal m.
- Inclan m.
- Jacobs locking hook spinal rod instrumentation m.
- Kalish bunionectomy m.
- Kaplan m.
- Kleinert m.
- Kramer m.
- MacKinnon m.
- McGlamry and Feldman m.
- medial sole wedge shoe m.
- metatarsal bar shoe m.
- Met Bar shoe m.
- Neer m.
- plasty m.
- Seattle m.
- Seddon m.
- Sequeira-Khanuja m.
- Sever m.
- shoe m.
- Stauffer m.
- Strickland m.
- Thompson m.

modified

M. American Shoulder and Elbow Surgeons Shoulder Patient Self-Evaluation Form patient questionnaire

m. Ashworth scale (MAS)

m. Boyd amputation

m. Boyd amputation of ankle and distal tibial physis

m. Boyd ankle arthrodesis

m. Boytchev procedure

m. Broström-Evans procedure

m. Broström procedure

m. Chrisman-Snook ankle reconstruction

m. Cocklin toe operation

m. Cotrel cast

m. Crawford Campbell inlaid bone-grafting technique

m. Darrach-type elevator

M. Dynamic Visual Processing Assessment (M-DVPA)

m. Fränkel classification

m. Fukuda-type retractor

m. Gait Abnormality Rating Scale

m. Grace plate

m. Harris hip score

m. Hoffmann quadrilateral external fixator

m. Hohmann bunionectomy

m. Hohmann osteotomy

m. Hoke-Miller flatfoot procedure

m. Kalish osteotomy

m. Keller resection arthroplasty

m. Kessler suture

m. Kessler-Tajima suture

m. Kienböck disease

m. Lapidus arthrodesis

m. Lapidus procedure

m. Mau bunionectomy

m. Mau osteotomy

m. McBride bunionectomy

m. mold and surface replacement arthroplasty

m. Moore hip locking prosthesis

m. Oppenheimer splint

m. 2-portal endoscopic carpal tunnel release

m. posterolateral approach

M. Rankin scale

m. Robert Jones dressing

m. Rowe shoulder score

m. Sillence classification

m. Stahl classification of Kienböck disease (stage I-V)

m. Stahl classification (stage I-V)

m. tonsillar prong

m. Wagner classification system

m. Watson-Jones ankle tenodesis

m. Wilson osteotomy

m. Z bunionectomy

m. Z osteotomy

Modny guide

modular

M. Acetabular Revision System (MARS)

m. Austin Moore hip prosthesis

m. hip implant component

m. implant

m. instrumentation

m. Iowa Precoat total hip prosthesis

m. large-head component

3R80 m. hydraulic knee joint

m. socket

m. S-ROM total hip system

m. unicompartmental knee prosthesis

modulation

central m.

peripheral m.

module

Allen Diagnostic M. (ADM)

Peak gait m.

Skills Assessment M. (SAM)

Modulock posterior spinal fixation

modulus

m. of elasticity

Young m.

Moe

M. alar hook

M. bone curette

M. bone impactor

M. gouge

M. intertrochanteric plate

M. modified Cotrel cast

M. modified Harrington rod

M. osteotome

M. scoliosis operation

M. scoliosis technique

M. square-end rod

M. system

Moe-Kettleson distribution

Moeller-Barlow disease

Moeltgen flexometer

Mogensen procedure

NOTES

M

Mohrenheim fossa
Mohr finger splint
Mohs technique
Moire topographic scoliosis assessment
moist
    m. heat
    m. heat therapy
    Restore Clean 'N M.
Molander-Olerud shoulder score
mold
    m. acetabular arthroplasty
    Aufranc concentric hip m.
    Biothotic orthotic m.
    caudad anterior m.
    cephalad anterior m.
molded
    AFO m.
    m. ankle-foot orthosis (MAFO)
    m. lumbosacral orthosis
    m. posterior plaster splint
    m. postpartum insole
    m. Thomas collar
molding
    compression m.
    elastomer skin m.
    polyethylene compression m.
    m. sock
Mold-In-Place back support
moleskin
    m. padding
    m. strip dressing
    m. traction tape
Molestick padding
Molesworth osteotomy
molle
    fibroma m.
    heloma m. (HM)
Moloney line
Molt periosteal elevator
molybdenum
    stainless steel and m. (SMO)
moment
    anterior bending m.
    m. arm
    m. of force
    m. of inertia
    3-point bending m.
    posterior bending m.
momentum
    angular m.
Momma-Too Maternity Support
MOM tractograph
Monarch knee brace
Monark
    M. bicycle
    M. Rehab Trainer
monarthric
monarthritis
    viral m.

monarticular synovitis
Mönckeberg sclerosis
Mondini dysplasia
Monistat-Derm Topical
monitor
    AccuGuide injection m.
    blood pressure m. (BPM)
    Brevio nerve conduction m.
    M. Master monitor support
    MyoTrac EMG biofeedback m.
    NervePace nerve conduction m.
    Polar wrist m.
    Tabs Elite mobility m.
    transcutaneous oxygen m. (TCOM)
    Vantage Performance m. (VPM)
monitored anesthesia control (MAC)
monitoring
    blood pressure m.
    fluorescein perfusion m.
    screw position perioperative m.
    somatosensory evoked potential m.
    spinal cord function
        intraoperative m.
MonitorMate monitor arm
monkey fist hand
monkey-paw
Monk hip prosthesis
monoamine oxidase-B inhibitor
monoarthritis
monoarticular septic arthritis
monoblock
    m. femoral component
    m. femoral stem prosthesis
monocane
monoclonal gammopathy
monodactyly
Monodos orthosis
monofilament
    calibrated m.
    5.07 m. gauge
    nylon m.
    m. pressure test
    Semmes-Weinstein m.
    Softip m.
    m. suture
    m. wire
    m. wire fixation
Monofixateur external fixator
Monogram total knee instrument
monolithic
    m. A1203 cup
    m. A1203 cup prosthesis
monomalleolar ankle fracture
mononeuritis multiplex
mononeuropathy
    diabetic femoral m.
    m. electrodiagnosis
    embolic m.
    m. multiplex

monophasic
- m. action potential
- m. endplate activity
- m. waveform

monoplace hyperbaric chamber

monoplegia
- monostotic m.

monopolar
- m. cautery
- m. needle recording electrode

monosodium urate crystal

monospherical total shoulder arthroplasty

monostotic
- m. fibrous dysplasia
- m. monoplegia

monosynaptic reflex arc

monotube
- M. external fixator system
- Howmedica m.

Monro bursa

Monteggia
- M. dislocation
- M. equivalent lesion
- M. forearm fracture
- M. fracture-dislocation
- M. fracture-dislocation of ulna

Montercaux fracture

Monticelli-Spinelli
- M.-S. circular external fixation system
- M.-S. distraction
- M.-S. distraction technique
- M.-S. distractor
- M.-S. fixator
- M.-S. frame
- M.-S. leg fixation

Montreal hip positioner

moon
- M. boot
- M. Boot brace
- M. Boot shoe
- M. Walker

Mooney
- M. brace
- M. cast

Moore
- M. bone drill
- M. bone elevator
- M. bone reamer
- M. driver
- M. femoral neck prosthesis
- M. fixation pin

- M. fracture
- M. hip endoprosthesis system
- M. hip prosthesis
- M. nail
- M. osteotomy
- M. osteotomy-osteoclasis
- M. posterior approach
- M. prosthesis extractor
- M. prosthesis-mortising chisel
- M. sliding nail plate
- M. stem
- M. technique
- M. template
- M. tibial plateau fracture classification

Moore-Southern approach

mooring

mop-end
- m.-e. Achilles tendon tear
- m.-e. appearance
- m.-e. mid-substance tear

Morand foot

morcellate

morcellation
- Robinson m.

morcellize

morcellized
- m. bone
- m. bone graft
- m. cancellous graft

Moreira plate

Moreland
- M. femoral component extractor
- M. osteotome
- M. total hip revision instrumentation

Moreland-Marder-Anspach femoral stem removal

Morel-Lavelle lesion

Morel syndrome

Moretz prosthesis

Morfam Quality Jeanie Rub massager

Morgagni hyperostosis

Morgan-Casscells meniscus suturing

morphea-like lesion

morphine
- m. pump
- m. sulfate

Morpho Exerciser

morphogenesis

morphogenetic protein

morphologically

M

NOTES

morphometry
  pedicle m.
Morquio
  M. disease
  M. sign
  M. syndrome
Morquio-Brailsford syndrome
Morquio-Ullrich
  M.-U. disease
  M.-U. syndrome
**Morrey elbow arthroplasty rating
  system**
Morris
  M. biphase screw
  M. retractor
Morrison
  M. neurovascular free flap
  M. technique
Morrissy
  M. percutaneous fixation of slipped
    epiphysis
  M. percutaneous slipped epiphysis
    fixation
Morscher cervical plate
Morse
  M. taper
  M. tapered prosthetic post
  M. taper lock
  M. taper lock of modular hip
    implant component
mortise
  ankle m.
  bone m.
  cuneiform m.
  m. and tenon joint
  tibial m.
  m. view
mortising chisel
Morton
  M. disease
  M. foot
  M. interdigital neuroma
  M. metatarsalgia
  M. neuralgia
  M. neurectomy
  M. neuroma
  M. neuroma neurolysis
  M. sign
  M. syndrome
  M. test
  M. toe
  M. toe support
mosaic
  m. arthroplasty
  m. plantar verruca
  m. wart
mosaicplasty
  arthroscopic m.

M. system
m. technique
Moseley
  M. bone age graph
  M. fasciotome
  M. glenoid rim prosthesis
  M. straight line graph
Mose method
Mosley
  M. anterior shoulder repair
  M. anterior shoulder repair method
mosquito
  m. clamp
  m. forceps
  m. hemostat
mosquito-tip grasping forceps
moss
  M. cage
  M. fixation system
  M. hook
  M. instrumentation
  M. rod
  M. screw
  M. technique
Mosso ergograph
mossy foot
**Most Options system rotating hinge
  revision knee**
moth-eaten destruction
Mother-Child Interaction checklist
Mother Jones dressing
Mother-To-Be
  M.-T.-B. abdominal support
  M.-T.-B. Support Maternity Support
motion
  accessory m.
  active ankle joint complex range
    of m.
  active-assisted range of m.
    (AAROM)
  active integral range of m.
    (AIROM)
  active and passive range of m.
  active range of m. (AROM)
  m. activity
  alternating range of m. (ARM)
  angular m.
  angulation m.
  ankle dorsiflexion range of m.
    (ADROM)
  ankle inversion-eversion range
    of m.
  AP translatory m.
  arc of m.
  axis of rib m.
  back range of m. (BROM)
  m. barrier
  bucket-handle rib m.
  cervical range of m. (CROM)

constant massive m.
continuous passive m. (CPM)
m. control
controlled ankle m. (CAM)
controlled range of m. (CRM)
m. control limiter
m. control mitt
m. control procedure
coupled m.
degrees-of-freedom joint m.
m. demand
distractive m.
double-flexion knee m.
end range of m.
Euler angle of wrist m.
frontal m.
full range of m. (FROM)
hindfoot m.
hip extension range of m.
inherent m.
intersegmental m.
intervertebral m.
joint m.
m. limit
m. limitation
limitation of m. (LOM)
loss of m. (LOM)
lumbar range of m.
m. measurement
osteokinematic m.
m. palpation
m. palpation screen
passive intervertebral m. (PIVM)
passive range of m. (PROM)
pattern of m.
m. performance
physiologic range of joint m.
pistoning m.
plantarflexory m.
protective limitation of range
 of m.
pump-handle rib m.
m. quality
range of m. (ROM)
rectilinear m.
m. response
restricted range of m.
restriction of m.
rib m.
rotary m.
sacroiliac joint m.
sagittal m.
scapulothoracic m.

m. segment
shoulder range of m.
m. slack
sling suspension range of m.
stable to m.
subtalar m.
synergistic finger m.
synergistic wrist m.
m. testing
m. therapy
toe range of m.
total active m. (TAM)
total eversion range of m.
total passive m. (TPM)
total range of m. (TROM)
translation m.
translatory m.
trial range of m.
triaxial m.
triplane m.
uninhibited ankle m.
valgus knee m.
m. velocity
winging m.
wrist m.
motion-preserving procedure
Motivator FTR2000 exerciser
motor
m. activity
m. activity log
m. branch
m. conduction velocity
m. deficit
m. development
m. dysfunction
m. examination
m. fascicle
m. function
m. function assessment
m. function deficit
m. latency
m. loss
m. milestone
m. neglect testing
m. nerve conduction velocity
 (MNCV)
m. neurectomy
m. neurolysis
m. neuronal pool
m. neuron disease
m. neuropathy
m. point
m. point block

M

NOTES

motor *(continued)*
    m. recovery
    m. reflex
    m. response
    m. restlessness
    m. and sensory neuropathy (type I–II)
    m. speech disorder
    m. strength
    m. unit
    m. unit action potential (MUAP)
    m. unit fraction
    m. unit potential (MUP)
    m. vehicle accident (MVA)
    m. weakness
motorcycle accident (MCA)
motorcyclist's knee
motorized
    m. bur
    m. meniscal cutter
    m. meniscal shaver
    m. reamer
    m. shaving system
    m. suction shaver
    m. trimmer
Moto-tool
    Dremel M.-t.
Motricity Index
mottled
mottling
Mouchet
    M. disease
    M. fracture
Mould arthroplasty
Moule screw pin
Mouradian
    M. humeral fixation system
    M. screw
mouse, pl. **mice**
    joint mice
    M. Nest mouse rest
mouse-ear appearance
MouseMitt keyboarder's
movable joint
move
    push-pull m.
movement
    active hip m.
    adventitious m.
    anterior-inferior m.
    anterior-posterior m.
    anterosuperior external ilium m. (ASEx)
    anterosuperior internal ilium m. (ASIn)
    arcuate m.
    m. artifact
    M. Assessment Battery for Children

    M. Assessment of Infants (MAI)
    assistive m.
    atlas-axis m.
    caliper rib m.
    compensatory m.
    m. disorder
    dissociation m.
    dynamic m.
    external ilium m.
    freedom of m.
    Frenkel m.
    inferior m.
    innominate m.
    intentional m.
    internal m.
    intersegmental m.
    isokinetic m.
    limitation of m.
    medial m.
    passive m.
    posteroinferior external m.
    posteroinferior internal m.
    primary or intentional m.
    primary rotation m.
    quasi-independent Y-axis m.
    resistive m.
    sagittal m.
    m. science
    Swedish m.
    total body m.
    trick m.
    unilateral posterior-anterior m.
    universal coronal m.
mover
    prime m.
moviegoer's knee
movie sign
moxa heat therapy
moxibustion heat therapy
Moyer line
Moynihan towel clamp
MP
    metacarpophalangeal
MPA
    metatarsus primus adductus
M-Pact
    M-P. cast cutter
    M-P. cast spreader
    M-P. cast vacuum
    M-P. flexible orthotic
MPAI-3
    Mayo-Portland Adaptability Inventory-3
MPD
    methylene diphosphonate
MPF
    myofascial pain syndrome
MPFL
    medial patellofemoral ligament

MPGR
    multiplanar gradient recalled
MPJ
    metacarpophalangeal joint
MPM
        MPM antimicrobial wound cleanser
        MPM bandage
MPP
    maximum pressure picture
M-Prednisol Injection
MPTh
    mechanical pain threshold
MPV
    metatarsus primus varus
MRC
    Medical Research Council
        MRC muscle function classification
MRI
    magnetic resonance imaging
        dynamic MRI
        flexion-extension MRI
        FONAR Stand-Up MRI
        Gyroscan superconducting MRI
        MRI testing
MRI-compatible plate and screw system
MRI-directed surgery
MRMT
    Minnesota Rate of Manipulation test
MRN
    magnetic resonance neurography
MRSA
    methicillin-resistant Staphylococcus
        aureus
MS
    metabolic syndrome
    multiple sclerosis
        MS Contin Oral
MS322 muscle stimulator
MSC cold pack
MSD
    microsurgical discectomy
MSI
    magnetic source imaging
        MSI mapping
MSIR Oral
MSL
    midsternal line
MT
    metatarsal
    metatarsophalangeal
    muscle testing
        MT bar

MTA
    metatarsus adductus
        MTA brace
MTC
    metatarsocuneiform
MTF
    Musculoskeletal Transplant Foundation
mtMRI
    magnetization transfer magnetic
        resonance imaging
MTP
    metatarsophalangeal
        MTP joint
MTPJ
    metatarsophalangeal joint
MTS
    medial tibial syndrome
MTSS
    medial tibial stress syndrome
MTV
    metatarsus varus
MUAP
    motor unit action potential
Muay Thai boxing
mucate
MUCL
    medial ulnar collateral ligament
mucoid degeneration
mucopolysaccharide
        sulfated m.
mucopolysaccharidosis,
    pl. **mucopolysaccharidoses**
mucous
        m. cyst
        m. membrane
mucus
Mudder sign
mud pack bath
Mueli wrist prosthesis
Mueller
        M. anterolateral femorotibial
            ligament tenodesis
        M. arthrodesis
        M. ATF ankle brace
        M. compression apparatus
        M. compression blade-plate
        M. cup
        M. distractor
        M. dual-lock hip prosthesis
        M. femoral supracondylar fracture
            classification
        M. fixation device
        M. hinged knee brace

M

NOTES

Mueller *(continued)*
    M. hip arthroplasty
    M. humerus fracture classification
    M. intertochanteric varus osteotomy
    M. knee operation
    M. knee procedure
    M. lateral compartment
    M. Lite ankle brace
    M. orthopaedic shoulder brace
    M. patellar tendon graft
    M. retractor
    M. template
    M. tibial fracture classification
    M. total hip replacement prosthesis
    M. transposition osteotomy
    M. Ultralite brace
    M. Weiss syndrome
    M. wrap-around knee brace
    M. wrench
Mueller-Charnley hip prosthesis
Mulder
    M. click
    M. sign
MULE
    microcomputer upper limb exerciser
    MULE upper limb exerciser
Mulholland and Gunn criteria
Müller
    M. intraarticular shoulder fusion
    M. osteotomy
    M. plate
    M. prosthesis
    M. saw
Mulligan silastic prosthesis
multangular
    m. bone
    greater m.
    lesser m.
    m. ridge fracture
multi
    M. Balance System (MBS)
    M. Podus boot
    M. Podus boot system
    M. Podus foot system
multiaction pin cutter
multiarticular
multiaxial
    M. Assessment of Pain (MAP)
    m. joint
    m. screw
multiaxis
    m. foot
    m. prosthesis
multiaxis ankle
MultiBoot orthosis
multicentric
    m. osteogenic sarcoma
    m. reticulohistiocytosis

Multidex chronic wound treatment system
Multidimensional Pain inventory
multidirectional instability (MDI)
multidisciplinary
multielectrode
multifidus
    m. muscle
    m. syndrome
Multiflex foot prosthesis
multifocal osteomyelitis
multifrequency
    m. probe
    m. transducer
multilead electrode
Multileaf Collimator
multilevel
    m. fracture
    m. fusion
    m. laminectomy
Multi-Lig knee brace
Multi-Lock
    M.-L. hand operating table
    M.-L. hip prosthesis
    M.-L. knee brace
multiloculated fluid collection
multipack
    Ortho-ice m.
multipartite
    m. fracture
    m. patella
multipennate muscle
multiplace hyperbaric chamber
multiplanar
    m. computed tomography scan
    m. CT scan
    m. deformity
    m. gradient recalled (MPGR)
    m. ligamentotaxis
    m. virtual fluoroscopic imaging
multiplane echo probe
multiple
    m. action cutter
    m. cancellous chip graft
    m. digits
    m. discharge
    m. enchondroma
    m. enchondromatosis
    m. epiphysial dysplasia
    m. finger
    m. flexible medullary nail
    m. fracture
    m. hereditary osteochondral exostosis (MHOCE)
    m. hook assembly
    m. hook assembly C-D instrumentation
    m. injuries
    m. line-scan imaging (MLSI)

m. myeloma
m. neurofibroma
m. osteochondromatosis
m. pinhole occluder
m. pterygium syndrome
m. ray
m. ray amputation
m. sclerosis (MS)
m. synostoses syndrome
m. tarsal coalitions
m. trauma
multiple-axis knee joint
multiple-point sacral fixation
multiplex
mononeuritis m.
mononeuropathy m.
myoclonus m.
paramyoclonus m.
multipolar bipolar cup
Multipulse 1000 compression pump
multipurpose
m. angled clamp
m. curved clamp
multiradius unconstrained prosthesis
multiray fracture
multisegmental
m. spinal distortion
m. spinal stenosis
multisided blade handle
multisized reamer
multispan fracture hook
multistaged carrier flap
Multitak
M. SS system
M. suture snap system
Mumford
M. procedure
M. resection
Mumford-Gurd arthroplasty
mummification necrosis
Munchmeyer disease
Munster cast
MUP
motor unit potential
Murphy
M. Achilles tendon advancement
M. brace
M. gouge
M. heel cord advancement
M. lateral approach
M. nail
M. osteotome
M. punch test

M. skid
M. sling
M. splint
Murphy-Lane bone skid
Murray
M. fixation
M. knee prosthesis
Murray-Jones arm splint
Murray-Thomas arm splint
muscle
abdominal m.
abductor digiti minimi m.
abductor digiti quinti m.
abductor hallucis m.
abductor pollicis brevis m.
abductor pollicis longus m.
accessory soleus m.
adductor hallucis m.
adductor pollicis m.
Aeby m.
agonist m.
agonistic m.
Albinus m.
m. analysis
anconeus m.
antagonistic m.
appendicular skeletal m. (ASM)
BBC m.'s
m. belly
biceps brachii m.
biceps femoris m.
bicipital m.
m. biopsy clamp
Bowman m.
brachialis m.
brachioradialis m.
buccinator m.
casserian m.
Casser perforated m.
Chassaignac axillary m.
m. contractility
m. contracture
m. contusion
coracobrachial m.
corrugator m.
m. cramp
cricopharyngeal sphincter m.
cucullaris m.
deepithelialized rectus abdominis m.
(DRAM)
deltoid m.
digastric m.
m. disorder

NOTES

M

465

muscle *(continued)*

dorsal interosseous m.
Dupré m.
ECRB m.
ECRL m.
ECU m.
EDB m.
EIP m.
elevator m.
emergency m.
m. energy
m. energy technique
epimeric m.
epitrochleoanconeus m.
extensor carpi radialis brevis m.
extensor carpi radialis longus m.
extensor carpi ulnaris m.
extensor communis m.
extensor digiti minimi m.
extensor digiti quinti m.
extensor digitorum brevis m.
extensor digitorum communis m.
extensor digitorum longus m.
extensor hallucis brevis m.
extensor hallucis longus m.
extensor indicis proprius m.
extensor pollicis brevis m.
extensor pollicis longus m.
extensor wad of 3 m.'s
external intercostal m.
external oblique m.
extrinsic m.
fascia of quadratus lumborum m.
m. fascicle
fast m.
femoral m.
m. fiber action potential
m. fiber conduction velocity
fibular m.
finger flexor m.
fixator m.
m. flap
flexor carpi radialis m.
flexor carpi ulnaris m.
flexor digiti quinti m.
flexor digitorum longus m.
flexor digitorum profundus m.
flexor digitorum sublimis m.
flexor digitorum superficialis m.
flexor hallucis brevis m.
flexor hallucis longus m.
flexor pollicis brevis m.
flexor pollicis longus m.
flexor wad of 5 m.'s
Folius m.
gastrocnemius m.
gastrocnemius-soleus m.
gluteus maximus m.
gluteus medius m.

gluteus minimus m.
gracilis m.
greater rhomboid m.
m. group (MG)
m. guarding
hamstring m.
handbag m.
m. hernia
hypothenar m.
iliacus m.
iliococcygeus m.
iliocostal m.
iliopsoas m.
m. imbalance
inferior gemelli m.
infraspinatus m.
m. innervation
m. insufficiency
internal oblique m.
interosseous m.
intervening m.
intraspinous m.
intrinsic m.
m. ischemia
Jung m.
Langer axillary arch m.
lateral malleolus m.
latissimus dorsi m.
lesser rhomboid m.
levator scapulae m.
long fibular m.
longissimus colli m.
longus capitis m.
longus cervicis colli m.
longus colli m.
lumbrical m.
lumbricalis m.
Luschka m.
mesothenar m.
multifidus m.
multipennate m.
m. and neurological stimulation
  electrotherapy device
nonstriated m.
oblique m.
obturator externus m.
obturator internus m.
omohyoid m.
opponens digiti quinti m.
opponens pollicis m.
palmar interosseous m.
palmaris digitorum superficialis m.
palmaris longus m.
paraspinal m.
paravertebral m.
m. patterning sequence
pectineus m.
pectoralis major m.
pectoralis minor m.

m. pedicle bone graft
peroneal m.
peroneus brevis m.
peroneus longus m.
peroneus quartus m.
peroneus tertius m.
Phillips m.
piriform m.
plantaris m.
platysma m.
m. play
pollicis longus m.
popliteal m.
postaxial m.
posterior deltoid m.
postural m.
preaxial m.
profundus m.
pronator quadratus m.
pronator teres m.
m. protein synthesis
psoas m.
quadrate m.
quadratus femoris m.
quadratus lumborum m.
quadratus plantae m.
quadriceps femoris m.
rectus abdominis m.
rectus femoris m.
red m.
m. relaxant
released ulnar intrinsic m.
m. repositioning
rhomboid m.
rider's m.
Riolan m.
rotator m.
M. Rub
sacrococcygeal m.
sacrospinal m.
sartorius m.
scalene m.
scapulohumeral m.
scapulothoracic m.
semimembranosus m.
semispinal m.
semitendinosus m.
serratus anterior m.
m. sheath
short fibular m.
shunt m.
Sibson m.
skeletal m.

m. slide
m. sliding operation
slow m.
smooth m.
soleus m.
somatic m.
m. spasm
m. spasticity
sphincter m.
m. spindle
spurt m.
sternocleidomastoid m.
sternohyoid m.
sternomastoid m.
sternothyroid m.
m. strain
strap m.
m. stretch reflex
striated m.
striped m.
subclavius m.
subcostal m.
suboccipital m.
subscapularis m.
subvertebral m.
supinator m.
supraspinatus m.
supraspinous m.
synergistic m.
teres major m.
teres minor m.
m. testing (MT)
thenar m.
third fibular m.
tibial m.
tibialis anterior m.
tibialis posterior m.
m. tissue mobility
toe extensor m.
toe flexor m.
m. tone
tonic m.
trachelomastoid m.
m. transfer
transversus abdominis m.
trapezius m.
triangular m.
triceps surae m.
tricipital m.
twitch m.
unipennate m.
unstriated m.
vastus intermedius m.

M

NOTES

muscle *(continued)*
    vastus lateralis m.
    vastus medialis m.
    vestigial m.
    voluntary m.
    white m.
    Wilson m.
    yoked m.
muscle-balancing procedure
muscle-plasty
    Speed V-Y m.-p.
muscle-setting exercise
muscle-splitting incision
muscle-strengthening exercise
muscle-tendon
    m.-t. attachment
    m.-t. injury
    m.-t. transplantation
muscle-to-bone suture
muscular
    m. atrophy
    m. attachment
    m. clamp
    m. contraction
    m. coordination
    m. cramp
    m. dystrophy (MD)
    m. lesion
    m. neurofibromatosis
    m. reeducation
    m. reflex
    m. rehabilitation
    m. tissue
    m. torticollis
    m. trophoneurosis
muscularity
musculature
    axial m.
    left erector spinae m.
    paraspinal m.
    paravertebral m.
    peroneal m.
    right erector spinae m.
musculoaponeurotic
musculocutaneous
    m. amputation
    m. free flap
    m. nerve
    m. nerve block
    m. nerve injury
    m. nerve paralysis
musculoelastic
musculofascial
musculointestinal
musculoligamentous
musculomembranous
musculophrenic
musculorum
    dystonia m.

musculoskeletal
    m. analysis
    m. evaluation, rehabilitation and
        conditioning (MERAC)
    M. Function Assessment (MFA)
    m. infection
    m. loading
    m. melioidosis
    M. Transplant Foundation (MTF)
    m. trauma
    M. Tumor Society
musculospiral paralysis
musculotendinous
    m. cuff
    m. flap
    m. junction
    m. system
    m. unit
musculotendinous-osseous link
Musgrave
    M. footprint pedobarograph
    M. Footprint System
mushroom
    m. impactor
    m. walker glide
mushy edema
musician's plight
muslin sling
Mustard iliopsoas transfer
mute toe sign
mutilans
    arthritis m.
    m. rheumatoid arthritis
mutilation
MV1, MV2 receptor
MVA
    motor vehicle accident
MVC
    maximal voluntary contraction
MVE
    maximum voluntary effort
MVM
    medullary venous malformation
MVP
    Biodex Multi-Joint System 3 MVP
MWD
    microwave diathermy
myalgia
myasthenia
    m. angiosclerotica
    m. gravis
myatonia
myatrophy
mycetoma
    Carter m.
    recurrent m.
Mycifradin Sulfate Topical
Mycitracin Topical

mycobacterial
    m. arthritis
    m. infection
Mycobacterium
    M. avium
    M. avium-intracellulare
    M. bovis
    M. chelonei
    M. fortuitum
    M. gordonae
    M. intracellulare
    M. kansasii
    M. marinum
    M. terrae
    M. tuberculosis
Mycocide
    M. NS
    M. NS antimicrobial solution
mycotic club nail
myectomy
myectopy
myelalgia
myelapoplexy
myelasthenia
myelatelia
myelatrophy
myelauxe
myelencephalitis
myelinated
myelinopathy
myelinosis
myelitis
    acute transverse m.
myeloblastoma
myelocele
myelocystocele
myelocystomeningocele
myelodiastasis
myelodysplasia
myelodysplastic kyphosis
myeloencephalitis
myelofibrosis
myelogenous callus
myelogram
myelographic
myelography
    air m.
    computer-assisted m. (CAM)
    iopamidol m.
    Isovue m.
    opaque m.
    oxygen m.
myelolipoma

myeloma
    multiple m.
    solitary m.
myelomalacia
myelomeningitis
myelomeningocele
myelomere
myeloneuritis
myeloparalysis
myelopathy
    cervical spondylotic m.
    m. incidence
    noncompressive m.
    progressive subacute m.
    radiation-related m.
    spinal stenotic m.
    transverse m.
    vacuolar m.
myelophthisis
myeloplegia
myeloproliferative disorder
myeloradiculitis
myeloradiculopathy
myelorrhagia
myelorrhaphy
    commissural m.
myelosclerosis
myelosyphilis
myelotomy
    Bischof m.
Myers knee retractor
mylohyoid
myoasthenia
myoblast
myoblastoma
    granular cell m.
Myobock
    M. artificial hand
    M. system
myobradia
myocardial
    m. bridging
    m. ischemia
myocele
myocelialgia
myocelitis
myocellulitis
myocerosis
myocervical collar
myoclasis
myoclonia
myoclonic epilepsy

M

NOTES

myoclonus
    action m.
    epileptic m.
    hereditary essential m.
    intention m.
    m. multiplex
    nocturnal m.
    palatal m.
    spinal m.
myocoele
myocrismus
myocutaneous
    m. flap
    transverse rectus abdominis m. (TRAM)
myocytoma
myodegeneration
myodemia
myodesis
myodiastasis
myodynamic
myodynamics
myodynia
myodysneuria
myodystonia
myodystrophia fetalis
myodystrophy
myoedema
myoelastic
myoelectrical
myoelectrically silent
myoelectric control prosthesis
myoencephalopathy
myofascia
myofascial
    m. closure
    m. manipulation
    m. pain
    m. pain syndrome (MPF)
    m. release
    m. tenderness
    m. trigger point
    m. unit
    m. unwinding
myofasciitis
    interstitial m.
myofibril
myofibroblast
myofibroma
myofibrosis
myofibrositis
myogelosis
myogenic
    m. paralysis
    m. tonus
    m. torticollis
myoglobinuria
    familial m.

myography
    acoustic m.
myohypertrophia
myoinositol level
myoischemia
myokerosis
myokinesis
myokymia
    exercise-induced m.
myokymic discharge
myolipoma
myologia
myology
myolysis
myoma
myomalacia
myomatosis
myomectomy, myomatectomy
myomelanosis
myonecrosis
    clostridial m.
myoneuralgia
myoneural ischemia
myoneurasthenia
myoneurectomy
myoneuroma
myoneurosis
myonosus
myopachynsis
myopalmus
myoparalysis
myoparesis
myopathic
    m. arthrogryposis
    m. atrophy
    m. gait
    m. motor unit potential
    m. paralysis
    m. recruitment
    m. scoliosis
myopathophysiology
myopathy
    acquired m.
    benign congenital m.
    carcinomatous m.
    centronuclear m.
    congenital m.
    exercise m.
    m. hand
    idiopathic polymyositis m.
    Kiloh-Nevin m.
    mitochondrial m.
    myotubular m.
    nemaline rod-body m.
    polymyositis m.
    postinfectious m.
    rheumatoid arthritis m.
    sarcotubular m.
    steroid m.

structural congenital m.
Welander distal m.
zebra body m.
zidovudine-induced m.
myophagism
myoplastic muscle stabilization
myoplasty
myopsychopathy
myorrhaphy
myorrhexis
myosarcoma
Myoscan sensor
myoschwannoma
myosclerosis
myositis
acute progressive m.
cervical tension m. (CTM)
clostridial m.
m. fibrosa
focal nodular m.
granulomatous m.
inclusion body m. (IBM)
inflammatory m.
ischemic m.
nodular m.
m. ossificans
m. ossificans progressiva
proliferative m.
rheumatoid m.
m. serosa
streptococcal m.
suppurative m.
tension m.
viral m.
myospasm
Myossage lotion
myostasis
myosteoma
myosthenic
myosthenometer
myosuture
myosynizesis
myotasis
myotatic
m. reflex
m. unit
myotendinous junction

myotenontoplasty
myotenositis
myotenotomy
myotomal pain
myotome
myotomy
myotonia
m. acquisita
m. atrophica
chondroplastic m.
m. congenita
m. congenita intermittens
congenital m.
drug-induced m.
m. dystrophica
m. hereditaria
Schwartz-Jampel m.
myotonic
m. discharge
m. muscular dystrophy
m. potential
myotonoid
myotonometer
myotonus
MyoTrac
M. device
M. EMG biofeedback monitor
M. single-channel
myotrophic
myotrophy
myotube
myotubular myopathy
myovascular
Mysono 201 portable ultrasound
Mysotrol hand sanitizer
mytenositis
myxedema
myxofibroma
myxoid
m. chondrosarcoma
m. cyst
m. liposarcoma
myxoid-type liposarcoma
myxoma
enchondromatous m.
soft tissue m.
myxosarcoma

M

NOTES

NA
neuropathic arthropathy
NAAP
National Arthritis Action Plan
Nada-Chair Back-Up portable back sling
NADD
National Association for Dually Diagnosed
NADPH
nicotinamide-adenine dinucleotide phosphate
Nafcil Injection
Naffziger
N. sign
N. syndrome
N. test
Nägele pelvis
NAGS
natural apophysial glides
reverse NAGS
nail
adjustable n.
Ainsworth modification of Massie n.
Albizzia intramedullary n.
Alta tibial n.
antegrade femoral n.
antegrade/retrograde compression n.
anteroposterior n.
AO slotted medullary n.
AP n.
n. assembly
Augustine boat n.
n. avulsion
Bailey-Dubow n.
Barr bolt n.
beak n.
n. bed
n. bed graft
n. bed hematoma evacuation
n. bed lesion
bent n.
Bickel intramedullary n.
Biomet ankle arthrodesis n.
blind medullary n.
boat n.
Böhler n.
brittle n.
Brooker double-locking unreamed tibial n.
Brooker femoral n.
Brooker-Wills n.
n. bur
Calandruccio n.

cannulated n.
centromedullary n.
Chandler unreamed interlocking tibial n.
Chick n.
Christensen interlocking n.
closed Küntscher n.
closed unlocked n.
cloverleaf Küntscher n.
clubbed n.
condylocephalic n.
crutch and belt femoral closed n.
Curry hip n.
n. deformity
Delitala T-nail n.
delta femoral n.
Delta Recon n.
delta tibial n.
Derby n.
Diamond n.
diamond-shaped medullary n.
digital n.
double-ended n.
double-hollow n.
n. drill
n. driver
n. dust
dynamic locking n.
dystrophic n.
Ender flexible medullary n.
n. extender
n. extension
extension n.
femoral neck n.
fissured n.
Fixion intramedullary humeral n.
4-flanged n.
flexible intramedullary n. (FIN)
flexible medullary n.
fluted Sampson n.
fluted titanium n.
n. fold
n. fold removal
Gamma locking n.
Gamma trochanteric locking n.
Green-Seligson-Henry n.
n. groove
n. groove callus
Grosse-Kempf interlocking medullary n.
Grosse-Kempf locking n.
GSH n.
Hackethal n.
Hagie pin n.
Hahn bone n.

N

nail *(continued)*
Halder locking n.
half-and-half n.
hallux n.
Hansen-Street n.
Harrington n.
Harris condylocephalic n.
Harris hip n.
Harris medullary n.
Holt n.
hooked intramedullary n.
hooked medullary n.
Huckstep n.
IMSC multihole n.
ingrown n.
n. injury
Inro surgical n.
interlocking medullary n.
intramedullary ANK n.
intramedullary supracondylar
  multihole n.
Jewett n.
Ken sliding n.
Klemm n.
Knowles pin n.
Küntscher n.
Laing H-beam n.
left-sided n.
n. length gauge method
Lewis n.
Lloyd adapter for Smith-Petersen n.
locking n.
long-edge medullary n.
Lottes triflanged medullary n.
Luck n.
Massie II n.
Massie sliding n.
n. matrix
n. matrix phenolization (NMP)
McKee tri-fin n.
McLaughlin n.
medullary n.
Moore n.
multiple flexible medullary n.
Murphy n.
mycotic club n.
nested n.
Neufeld n.
noncannulated n.
nonreamed n.
Nylok self-locking n.
onychocryptosis n.
open n.
open-section n.
Orthofix intramedullary n.
OrthoSorb pin n.
Palmer bone n.
PGP n.
Pidcock n.

pincer n.
Pitcock n.
n. plate
n. plate apparatus
n. plate device
n. plate fixation
n. plate removal
prebent n.
Pugh sliding n.
reamed n.
Recon n.
retrograde intramedullary n.
ReVision n.
Richards reconstruction n.
right-sided n.
n. root
n. rotational guide
Rush flexible medullary n.
Rush pin n.
Russell-Taylor delta tibial n.
Russell-Taylor interlocking
  medullary n.
Rydell n.
Sage forearm n.
Sage radial n.
Sage triangular n.
Sampson medullary n.
Sarmiento n.
Schneider medullary n.
Seidel humeral locking n.
self-broaching n.
self-locking n.
n. set
sliding n.
Slocum n.
slotted n.
Smillie n.
Smith-Petersen femoral neck n.
Smith-Petersen transarticular n.
specialized n.
spring-loaded n.
standard medullary n.
n. starter
static locking n.
Steinmann extension n.
Street forearm n.
striated n.
supracondylar medullary n.
n. suture
Sven-Johansson femoral neck n.
telescoping n.
Temple University n.
Terry n.
Thatcher n.
Thompson n.
Thornton n.
Tiemann n.
titanium n.
triangular medullary n.

triflanged Lottes n.
triflanged medullary n.
True/Flex intramedullary n.
turtle neck n.
Uniflex humeral n.
Uniflex intramedullary n.
Universal n.
Vector intertrochanteric n.
Venable-Stuck n.
Vesely-Street split n.
vitallium Küntscher n.
V-medullary n.
watch crystal n.
Watson-Jones n.
Webb bolt n.
Williams n.
Winograd technique for ingrown n.
Z fixation n.
Zickel subcondylar n.
Zickel subtrochanteric n.
Zickel supracondylar medullary n.
Zimmer telescoping n.
nail-bending device
nail-driving guide
nail-extracting hook
nailing
    antegrade n.
    blind medullary n.
    bundle nailing
    centromedullary n.
    closed Küntscher n.
    closed medullary n.
    condylocephalic n.
    crutch and belt femoral closed n.
    elastic stable intramedullary n.
      (ESIN)
    Ender n.
    exchange n.
    femoral n.
    fixator-augmented n.
    gradual elongation n. (GEN)
    gradual elongation intramedullary n.
      (GEIN)
    Grosse-Kempf interlocking
      medullary n.
    Harris condylocephalic n.
    interlocking n.
    intramedullary n. (IMN)
    Küntscher medullary n.
    locked n.
    Lottes n.
    marrow n.
    medullary n.

    open medullary n.
    retrograde n.
    static lock n.
    tibiocalcaneal medullary n.
    Vertstreken closed medullary n.
    Zickel n.
nail-mounted
    n.-m. compression device
    n.-m. targeting
nail-patella syndrome
nail-pulling forceps
nail-screw sideplate assembly
Nakamura
    N. brace
    N. disease
naked trabeculae
Nalebuff arthrodesis
Nalebuff-Millender lateral band
    mobilization technique
Nallpen Injection
naloxone hydrochloride
Namaqualand hip dysplasia
nana
    pelvis n.
nanocolloid
NAP
    nerve action potential
napkin
    n. ring calcar allograft
    n. ring compression
Napoleon hat sign
naprapathy
naproxen sodium
Nara arthroplasty
Naraghi-DeCoster reduction clamp
narrow
    n. AO dynamic compression plate
    n. Assistant Free retractor blade
    n. Cobra retractor
    n. double-prong acetabular retractor
    n. inferior acetabular retractor
    n. proximal femoral elevator
    n. toebox shoe
narrow-base gait
narrow-blade retractor
narrowed joint space
narrowing
    arthritic ankle joint n.
    n. of forefoot
    intervertebral disc n.
    n. of spinal canal
narrow-neck mini-Hohmann retractor

N

NOTES

nasal
> n. elevator
> n. spine

nascent motor unit potential

natatory
> n. cord
> n. ligament

national
> N. Academy on Aging Society
> N. Accessible Apartment Clearinghouse
> N. Aging Information Center
> N. Alliance for Blind Students
> N. Arthritis Action Plan (NAAP)
> N. Arthritis Data Workgroup
> N. Association for Dually Diagnosed (NADD)
> N. Association of Medical Equipment Suppliers
> N. Association for Rights, Protection, and Advocacy
> N. Center for Dissemination of Disability Research
> N. Center to Improve Practice through Technology, Media, and Materials
> N. Collegiate Athletic Association drug testing policy
> N. Collegiate Athletic Association prohibited drug
> N. Collegiate Athletic Association spine injury prevention rule
> N. Consumer Supporter Technical Assistance Center
> N. Council on Disability
> N. Depressive and Manic-Depressive Association
> N. Down Syndrome Society
> N. Empowerment Center
> N. Football Head and Neck Injury Registry
> N. Foundation of American Academy of Ophthalmology Public Service Programs
> N. Foundation for Depressive Illness Inc.
> N. Headache Foundation
> N. Hospice Organization
> N. Information Center for Children and Youth with Disabilities
> N. Institute of Arthritis and Musculoskeletal and Skin Diseases (NIAMS)
> N. Institute for Child Health and Human Development
> N. Lymphedema Network
> N. Maternal and Child Health Clearinghouse
> N. Mental Health Consumers' Self-Help Clearinghouse
> N. Operating Committee on Standards for Athletic Equipment (NOCSAE)
> N. Organization for Rare Disorders
> N. Osteoporosis Foundation
> N. Registry of Rehabilitation Technology supplier
> N. Rehabilitation Information Center
> N. Spinal Cord Injury Association
> N. Stroke Association

Nation Alliance for Research on Schizophrenia and Depression

Native American medicine

natural apophysial glides (NAGS)

Natural-Hip
> N.-H. prosthesis
> N.-H. system
> N.-H. titanium hip stem

naturalism

Natural-Knee
> N.-K. II system
> N.-K. implant
> N.-K. unconstrained prosthesis

Natural-Lok acetabular cup prosthesis

naturopathy

Naughton-Dunn triple arthrodesis

Nauth
> N. traction apparatus
> N. traction device

navicular
> accessory n.
> n. arthritis
> bifurcate n.
> n. body
> n. bone
> cartilaginous n.
> n. cookie in shoe
> cornuate n.
> n. cuneiform ligament
> divided n.
> n. dorsal lip fracture
> n. drop test
> n. to first metatarsal angle
> lip of n.
> n. osteonecrosis
> n. prominence
> protrusion of n.
> n. screw
> n. shoe cookie
> n. shoe pad
> tarsal n.
> n. tuberosity
> n. tuberosity fracture
> n. wedging

naviculectomy

naviculocapitate
  n. fracture
  n. fracture syndrome
naviculocuneiform
  n. breach
  n. coalition
  n. fusion
  n. joint
  n. joint arthrodesis
  n. ligament
Navigator power wheelchair
Navitrack computer-assisted surgery system
NC
  neurogenic claudication
NCAST feeding and teaching scales
NCS
  nerve conduction study
NCT
  nerve compression test
NCV
  nerve conduction velocity
Neal-Robertson litter
near-anatomic position of joint
near-constant frequency trains
near-far fashion
near-field potential
nearthrosis
NEB
  New England Baptist
  NEB acetabular cup
  NEB arthroplasty
  NEB total hip prosthesis
Necelon surgical glove
necessity
  fracture of n.
neck
  basal n.
  n. brace
  n. component
  congenital wry n.
  crick in the n.
  n. diameter
  femoral head and n.
  fibular n.
  n. fracture
  glenoid n.
  humeral n.
  metacarpal n.
  metatarsal n.
  n. pain syndrome
  phalangeal n.
  n. pillow

  radial n.
  n. reflex
  n. roll
  n. shaft
  skeletal wry n.
  supple n.
  surgical n.
  talar n.
  n. wrap
  wry n.
Neckcare pillow
Neck-Hugger cervical support pillow
neck-righting reflex
Neck-Roll aromatherapy hot/cold pack
neck-shaft angle (NSA)
Necktrac
  N. traction
  N. traction device
necrosis
  aseptic n.
  atraumatic n.
  avascular n. (AVN)
  bone n.
  bony n.
  bulbar n.
  central n.
  coagulation n.
  coagulative n.
  corticosteroid-induced avascular n.
  dry n.
  epiphysial aseptic n.
  epiphysial ischemic n.
  gangrenous n.
  gummatous n.
  hyaline n.
  idiopathic avascular n.
  infectious bulbar n.
  ischemic n.
  mummification n.
  Paget quiet n.
  pressure n.
  radiographic avascular n.
  septic n.
  skin n.
  steroid-induced avascular n.
  superficial n.
  total n.
  n. ustilaginea
  Zenker n.
necrotic
  n. bone
  n. skin
  n. tissue

NOTES

N

necroticans
    osteochondritis n.
necrotizing fasciitis
necrotomy
    osteoplastic n.
needle
    acupuncture n.
    atraumatic n.
    Beath n.
    Bergstrom n.
    Bier lumbar puncture n.
    n. biopsy
    bone biopsy n.
    bore n.
    bougie n.
    Bunnell tendon n.
    conventional cutting n.
    n. cord length
    cutting n.
    Deschamps n.
    diamond point n.
    discogram n.
    n. electrode
    Framer tendon-passing n.
    Gallie n.
    hand-honed reverse cutting n.
    Hawkeye suture n.
    n. holder
    hubbed n.
    Jamshidi n.
    K n.
    Keith n.
    Luer-Lok n.
    McGee prosthesis n.
    meniscal repair n.
    milliner's n.
    osteodysplasty of Melnick and N.'s
    n. placement
    Plum-Blossom acupuncture n.
    Quincke n.
    retrobulbar prosthesis n.
    reverse cutting n.
    ribbed n.
    Seirin acupuncture n.
    Sklar ligature n.
    spinal n.
    Stimuplex block n.
    swaged n.
    taper cut n.
    tapered n.
    tendon n.
    The Painless One acupuncture n.
    Thomas n.
    Tuohy lumbar puncture n.
    Verbrugge n.
    Veress n.
    Wangensteen n.
    Webster n.

needle-nose
    n.-n. rongeur
    n.-n. vise-grip pliers
needlescope
Neer
    N. acromioplasty
    N. acromioplasty for rotator cuff
    tear
    N. capsular shift procedure
    N. femur fracture classification
    N. hemiarthroplasty
    N. humeral replacement prosthesis
    N. humerus fracture classification
    N. II humeral component
    N. II shoulder system
    N. II total knee system
    N. II total shoulder system implant
    N. impingement sign
    N. impingement test
    N. lateral view
    N. modification
    N. open reduction
    N. posterior shoulder reconstruction
    N. ring
    N. shoulder fracture classification
    N. shoulder prosthesis (I, II)
    N. transscapular view
    N. umbrella prosthesis
    N. unconstrained shoulder
    arthroplasty
Neer-Horowitz
    N.-H. classification of humeral
    fracture
    N.-H. humerus fracture
    classification
Neff
    N. femorotibial nail system
    N. meniscus knife
negative
    n. afterpotential
    n. casting
    n. congruence angle
    n. impression cast
    n. ulnar variance (NUV)
    n. work
neglect
    hemispatial n.
    traumatic brain injury-related n.
    visual n.
neglected rupture
Neiguan point acupressure
Neisseria
    N. gonorrhoeae
    N. sicca
Neivert osteotome
Nélaton
    N. ankle dislocation
    N. line

N. operation
N. rubber tube drain
Nelson
N. finger exerciser
N. rib retractor
N. rib spreader
N. scissors
N. sign
nemaline rod-body myopathy
neoadjuvant chemotherapy
neocortex
NeoDecadron Topical
neoformation
nodular n.
neolimbus
Neomixin Topical
neomycin, polymyxin B, and hydrocortisone
neonatal
n. flatfoot
n. sandbag
n. septic arthritis
n. tracheostomy tube holder
neoplasm
bone n.
extensive n.
interdigital n.
neoplastic
n. fracture
n. lesion
n. osteoblast
Neoplush foam
neoprene
n. ankle support
n. back support
n. dressing
n. elbow sleeve
n. fabric
n. knee sleeve
n. shoe
n. wrist brace
n. wrist orthosis
n. wrist strap
Neoral Oral
Neosar Injection
Neosporin
N. Cream
N. Topical Ointment
Ne-Osteo bone morphogenic protein
neotendon
neovascularization
nerve
abductor digiti minimi n.

accessory n.
n. action potential (NAP)
antebrachial cutaneous n.
anterior thoracic n.
anterior tibial n.
Arnold n.
articular n.
axillary n.
n. block
n. block infusion kit
Bock n.
calcaneal n.
n. cap
cluneal n.
common digital n.
common peroneal n.
n. compression test (NCT)
n. conduction study (NCS)
n. conduction velocity (NCV)
n. conduction velocity test
n. crossing
cubital n.
cutaneous n.
deep peroneal n.
digital branch of plantar n.
dorsal cutaneous n.
dorsal scapular n.
dorsomedial cutaneous n.
n. ending
n. entrapment site
n. entrapment syndrome
n. entubulation
femoral cutaneous n.
n. fiber action potential
n. function test
genitofemoral n.
gluteal n.
n. graft
great sciatic n.
n. growth factor
n. hook
hypoglossal n.
iliohypogastric n.
ilioinguinal n.
inferior laryngeal n.
n. injury
intercostal n.
intercostobrachial n.
interdigital n.
n. interference
intermediate dorsal cutaneous n. (IDCN)
intermetatarsal n.

NOTES

nerve *(continued)*
   interosseous n.
   n. involvement testing
   laryngeal n.
   mandibular n.
   medial brachial n.
   medial dorsal cutaneous n. (MDCN)
   medial sural cutaneous n.
   median n.
   meningeal n.
   musculocutaneous n.
   obturator n.
   n. palsy
   pectoral n.
   peripheral n.
   peroneal n.
   phrenic n.
   plantar n.
   popliteal n.
   posterior tibial n. (PTN)
   radial digital n.
   radial sensory n.
   recurrent laryngeal n.
   recurrent meningeal n.
   regeneration of n.
   n. root
   n. root block
   n. root compression
   n. root decompression
   n. root entrapment
   n. root injection
   n. root irritability
   n. root irritation
   n. root lesion
   n. rootlet ablation
   n. root sheath
   sacral n.
   saphenous n.
   scapular n.
   sciatic n.
   sensorimotor n.
   sensory n.
   n. separator
   n. sheath tumor
   sinuvertebral n.
   somatic n.
   spinal accessory n.
   n. stretching
   superficial peroneal n.
   superficial radial n. (SRN)
   superior laryngeal n.
   suprascapular n.
   sural n.
   sympathetic n.
   thoracic n.
   thoracodorsal n.
   tibial n.
   n. tracing

   n. transmission
   n. transposition
   n. transposition surgery
   n. trunk action potential
   ulnar n. (UN)
   vagus n.
   vertebral n.
   n. wrapping
NervePace nerve conduction monitor
nervi erigentes
Nervoscope device
nested
   n. nail
   n. step stool
netting
   splint pan n.
network
   National Lymphedema N.
Neufeld
   N. apparatus
   N. cast
   N. device
   N. dynamic method
   N. nail
   N. pin
   N. plate
   N. roller traction
   N. screw
NeuFlex metacarpophalangeal joint implant
Neuhauser variant
Neumann syndrome
Neurain drill
Neurairtome
   N. drill
   Hall N.
neural
   n. arch resection technique
   n. crest
   n. element
   n. foramen
   n. foraminal stenosis (NFS)
   n. foraminotomy
   n. injury
   n. nevus
   n. strength training
   n. tension
   n. tissue
   n. tube defect
   n. tube defect-related anomaly of vertebra
   n. tumor
neuralgia
   adhesive n.
   brachial n.
   genicular n.
   geniculate n.
   glossopharyngeal n.
   intercostal n.

Morton n.
occipital n.
prepatellar n.
sciatic n.
stump n.
tension n.
traumatic prepatellar n.
trigeminal n.
vagoglossopharyngeal n.
vidian n.
neuralgic amyotrophy
neurapraxia
cervical cord n. (CCN)
Seddon n.
traction n.
transient n.
neurasthenia
neuraxial compression
neurectomy
adductor tenotomy and obturator n. (ATON)
Eggers n.
Morton n.
motor n.
obturator n.
Phelps n.
ulnar motor n.
neurilemoma
neuritic amyotrophy
neuritis
axial n.
brachial n.
obturator nerve n.
peripheral n.
pudendal n.
radicular n.
sciatic n.
suprascapular n.
sural n.
wallet n.
neuroablation
cryogenic n.
neuroablative
Neuro-Aide testing device
neuroanastomosis
neuroarthropathic foot
neuroarthropathy
atrophic n.
Charcot n.
neuroarticular
n. dysfunction

n. subluxation
n. syndrome
Neurobehavioral Functioning Inventory (NFI)
neurobiology
neuroblastoma
neurocentral synchondrosis
neurocirculation
NeuroCom Balance Master
neurocompressive disorder
neurocutaneous hand flap
neurodermatitis
neurodevelopmental
n. approach
n. training
n. treatment
NeuroDrape surgical drape
neurodystrophic
neuroectodermal tumor
neuroendocrine-immune connection
neurofibroma
multiple n.
nonplexiform cutaneous n.
plexiform n.
neurofibromatosis
formes frustes n.
n. kyphoscoliosis
kyphoscoliosis secondary to n.
muscular n.
type 1, 2 n.
neurofibrosarcoma
neurofibrositis
neurofunctional subluxation
neurogenic
n. arthrogryposis
n. atrophy
n. bladder
n. bowel
n. claudication (NC)
n. disease
n. disorder
n. fracture
n. motor evoked potential (NMEP)
n. scoliosis
n. shock
n. syndrome
n. torticollis
neurography
magnetic resonance n. (MRN)
neuroimmune hypothesis
neuroleptanalgesia
neuroleptic

N

NOTES

neurologic
- n. assessment
- n. complication
- n. deficit
- n. disorder
- n. examination
- n. function
- n. pain

neurological
- n. nerve conduction velocity examination
- n. physical therapy
- n. testing

neurologically intact

neurolysis
- alcohol n.
- chemical n.
- distal n.
- epidural n.
- external n.
- interfascicular n.
- internal n.
- intrathecal n.
- Morton neuroma n.
- motor n.
- phenol n.

neurolytic block

neuroma, pl. **neuromata**
- amputation stump n.
- bulb n.
- n. in continuity
- cutaneous n.
- dorsal n.
- false n.
- incisional n.
- interdigital n. (IDN)
- Morton n.
- Morton interdigital n.
- posttraumatic n.
- refractory n.
- n. sign
- spindle n.
- stump n.
- sural n.
- traumatic n.

neuromatosis

neuromatous

neuromechanical
- n. correction
- n. lesion
- n. spinal chiropractic management

neuromeningeal pathway

neuromuscular
- n. block
- n. component
- n. disease
- n. electrical stimulation (NMES)
- n. electrical stimulation therapy
- n. facilitation

- n. gait pattern
- n. gait pattern change
- n. hamartoma
- n. III stimulator
- n. junction disorder
- n. proprioceptive process
- n. reflex treatment
- n. scoliosis
- n. scoliosis orthotic treatment
- n. transfer

neuromusculoskeletal

neuromyotonia

neuromyotonic discharge

neuron
- fusimotor n.
- serotonergic n.

neuronitis
- Parsonage-Turner n.

neuropathic
- n. ankle
- n. arthritis
- n. arthropathy (NA)
- n. collapse
- n. foot
- n. foot deformity
- n. forefoot ulceration
- n. fracture
- n. hyperkyphoscoliosis
- n. joint
- n. joint disease
- n. joint dislocation
- n. knee
- n. motor unit potential
- n. osteoarthropathy
- n. recruitment
- n. spinal arthropathy
- n. ulcer

neuropathogenic

neuropathophysiology
- normalization of n.

neuropathy
- alcoholic n.
- amyloid n.
- brachial plexus n.
- chemotherapy-related n.
- compressive n.
- diabetic n.
- entrapment n.
- epineurial n.
- epineurial-perineurial n.
- fascicular n.
- hereditary motor sensory n. (HMSN)
- hereditary sensory motor n. (type I–III) (HSMN I–III)
- hip pocket n.
- hypertrophic interstitial n.
- median n.
- motor n.

motor and sensory n. (type I–II)
periepineurial n.
peripheral n.
peroneal n.
porphyritic n.
radiation-related n.
spontaneous median n.
sural n.
ulnar n.
neurophysiologic effect
neurophysiology
neuroplasty
neuroprosthesis
neuropsychological screening
neuroreflexive
neurorrhaphy
epineurial n.
perineurial n.
neurosis, pl. **neuroses**
low back n.
torsion n.
neuroskeletal
neurostimulator
Biotens n.
Grass n.
responsive n. (RNS)
Staodyne EMS+2 n.
neurosuture
neurosyphilis
neurotendinous
neurotherapy
manual reflex n.
neurothlipsis
neuroticism
neurotization
neurotmesis
Seddon n.
neurotomy
neurotraumatic mechanism
neurotripsy
neurotrophic
n. atrophy
n. factor
n. food ulcer
n. fracture
n. joint
n. ulceration
Neurotube bioabsorbable nerve conduit
neurovascular (NV)
n. anatomy
n. bundle
n. complication
n. corn

n. dystrophy
n. free flap
n. hilus
n. impairment
n. injury
n. island graft
n. status
n. structure
neurovascularly intact
neutral
n. angle
n. anteversion
n. drill guide
n. hip position
n. hook
n. position splint
n. rotation
n. triangle
n. wrist curl
n. zone (NZ)
neutralization
anterior n.
n. parameter
n. plate
n. plate fixation
neutron radiography
nevi (*pl. of* nevus)
Neviaser
N. acromioclavicular technique
N. arthroplasty
N. classification of frozen shoulder
N. frozen shoulder classification
N. operation
N. portal
N. test
N. theory
Nevin ankle brace
nevoid histiocytoma
nevus, pl. **nevi**
new
n. bone
n. bone formation
N. England Baptist (NEB)
N. England Baptist acetabular cup
N. England Baptist hip arthroplasty
N. England scoliosis brace
n. happy bur
N. Jersey ankle
N. Jersey hemiarthroplasty
prosthesis
N. Jersey LCS shoulder prosthesis
N. Jersey LCS total knee
prosthesis

N

NOTES

new (continued)
    N. Mind Set toe splint
    N. Schwinn 900 bicycle
    N. Schwinn elliptical bicycle
    N. Versaback gym ball
    N. York diagnostic criteria
    N. York diagnostic criteria
    classification
    N. York diagnostic criteria for
    rheumatoid arthritis
    N. York Orthopaedic front-opening
    orthosis
    N. York University (NYU)
    N. York University orthotic insert
newer-generation device
Newington
    N. brace
    N. orthosis
newly woven bone
Newman
    N. plate
    N. radial fracture
    N. radial neck and head fracture
    classification
Newman-Keuls procedure
new-onset limp
Newport
    N. hip system
    N. MC hip orthosis
    N. MC hip orthosis brace
Newton
    N. ankle prosthesis
    N. force
newtonian body
newton-meter
    concentric plantar flexion peak
    torque n.-m.
89-newton test
Nexerciser Plus
NexGen
    N. complete knee replacement
    system
    N. complete knee system
    N. component
    N. knee implant
    N. offset stem extension
Nex-Link spinal fixation system
Nextep knee brace
Nexus
    N. hip prosthesis
    N. implant
    N. wheelchair seating system
NFI
    Neurobehavioral Functioning Inventory
NFS
    neural foraminal stenosis
NIAMS
    National Institute of Arthritis and
    Musculoskeletal and Skin Diseases

N'ice
    N. Stretch night splint
    N. Stretch night splint suspension
    system with Sealed Ice
Nicholas
    N. ligament technique
    N. manual muscle tester
    N. 5-in-1 reconstruction
    N. 5-in-1 reconstruction technique
Nickelplast blank
nickel-titanium (NiTi)
Nicola
    N. arthroplasty
    N. forceps
    N. incision
    N. scissors
    N. shoulder operation
    N. shoulder procedure
Nicoladoni suture
Nicolet Compass EMG instrument
Nicoll
    N. bone
    N. bone replacement material
    N. cancellous bone graft
    N. cancellous insert graft
    N. classification
    N. extractor
    N. fracture operation
    N. fracture repair procedure
    N. plate
    N. rasp
    N. tendon prosthesis
nicotinamide-adenine dinucleotide
  phosphate (NADPH)
NIDJD
    noninflammatory degenerative joint
    disease
nidus
    radiolucent n.
Niebauer
    N. finger-joint replacement
    prosthesis
    N. implant
    N. metacarpophalangeal joint
    silastic prosthesis
    N. trapeziometacarpal arthroplasty
    N. trapezium replacement prosthesis
Niebauer-Cutter
    N.-C. implant
    N.-C. prosthesis
Niebauer-King technique
Niemann-Pick disease
Nievergelt-Pearlman syndrome
night
    n. brace
    n. splint
    n. splinting
    N. Splint support
Nightimer carpal tunnel support

nightstick fracture
night-walker fracture
nigricans
    acanthosis n.
Nikon SMZ 2T magnifying lens
Nilsson lateral ankle stabilization
  procedure
Nimmo receptor-tonus technique
nipper
    English anvil nail n.
    House-Dieter malleus n.
    Miltex nail n.
    n.'s nail drill
Niro
    N. bone-cutting forceps
    N. wire-twisting forceps
Nirschl
    N. operation
    N. technique
Nirvana mattress
Nitalloy
NiTi
    nickel-titanium
    NiTi alloy
nitidus
    lichen n.
nitinol
nitrofurazone
nitrogen
    n. balance
    urinary n.
nitroglycerin
nitroprusside
Nitro wheelchair
NMEP
    neurogenic motor evoked potential
NMES
    neuromuscular electrical stimulation
    NMES therapy
NMP
    nail matrix phenolization
NMR
    nuclear magnetic resonance
no
    no man's land of hand
    no touch rule
Nobel test
nociception
nociceptive
    n. receptor
    n. transmission
nociceptor
    n. agent

    angry backfiring C n.
    bombardment by n.
NOCSAE
    National Operating Committee on
    Standards for Athletic Equipment
nocturnal myoclonus
node
    Bouchard n.
    gouty n.
    Haygarth n.
    Heberden n.
    Meynet n.
    Osler n.
    Parrot n.
    Schmorl n.
nodosa
    arthritis n.
    panarteritis n.
    polyarteritis n.
nodose rheumatism
nodosity
    Heberden n.
nodular
    n. fasciitis
    n. melanoma
    n. myositis
    n. neoformation
    n. tenosynovitis
nodularity
    tendon n.
nodulation
nodule
    Bouchard n.
    Lisch n.
    rheumatoid n.
    Schmorl n.
    synovial n.
    tendon n.
NOF
    nonossifying fibroma
NoHands Mouse-Foot-Operated
  Computer Mouse System
Noiles
    N. fully constrained
    tricompartmental knee prosthesis
    N. hinge
    N. posterior stabilized knee
    N. rotating hinge knee
    N. rotating hinge knee mechanism
noise
    endplate n.
Nolan system collimator mounted
  contact shield

N

NOTES

nomenclature
    dynamic listing n.
    static listing n.
nomogram
nonabsorbable suture
nonadherent gauze dressing
nonambulation
no-name, no-fame bursa
nonarticular
    n. arthritis
    n. distal radial fracture
nonaugmented repair
nonbeaded guidepin
nonbeveled
nonbipedal
noncannulated nail
noncemented total hip arthroplasty
noncollared press-fit femoral stem
  implantation
noncompliance
noncompressive myelopathy
noncongruent metatarsophalangeal joint
noncontact manipulation
noncontained
    n. disc
    n. disc herniation
noncontiguous fracture
noncontractile
nondermatomal pattern
nondisplaced fracture
nondissociative
    carpal instability, n. (CIND)
nonenzymatic connective tissue glycation
nonfenestrated stem
nonfluency
nonfused arthrodesis
nonglabrous skin
nonhinged
    n. knee prosthesis
    n. linked prosthesis
nonimpulsed base nerve transmission
noninflammatory degenerative joint
  disease (NIDJD)
non-insulin-dependent diabetes mellitus
noninvasive
    lower extremity n.
    n. technique
nonisometric graft
nonlamellar bone
nonlamellated bone
nonlinear lesion
nonloadbearing
    n. bone fracture
    n. fractured bone
nonloop fixation
nonmanipulable subluxation
nonnarcotic analgesic

nonoperative
    n. orthopaedic management
    n. treatment
nonorganic physical sign
nonosseous
    n. tarsal coalition
    n. tissue trauma
nonossified tarsal navicular cartilage
nonossifying fibroma (NOF)
nonosteoconductive bone-void filler
nonosteogenic fibroma
nonphysial fracture
nonpitting edema
nonplexiform cutaneous neurofibroma
nonporous-coated endoprosthesis
nonporous sheet
nonpreferred leg
nonradicular pattern
nonreactive nonunion
nonreamed nail
nonreconstructable
nonreplantable amputation
nonrotational burst fracture
non-self-tapping screw
nonspasmodic torticollis
nonspecific
    n. arthralgia
    n. cardiomyopathy
nonstanding lateral oblique view
nonsteroidal
    n. antiinflammatory drug (NSAID)
    n. antiinflammatory medication
nonstriated muscle
nonstructural curve
nonsubluxated metatarsophalangeal joint
nonsubperiosteal cortical defect
nonsuppurative
    n. osteitis
    n. osteomyelitis
nonsurgical management
nonthermal modality
nonthreaded
    n. pin
    n. wire
nonthrust mobilization
nontotal-contact disorder
nontraumatic
    n. idiopathic osteonecrosis
    n. synovitis
nontubed
    n. closed distant flap graft
    n. open distant flap graft
nontuberculous mycobacterial infection
nonunion
    atrophic n.
    avascular n.
    bayonet n.
    bioelectrical repair of delayed
      union or n.

defect n.
draining infected n.
dry infected n.
elephant-foot fracture n.
fracture fragment n.
n. of fracture site
n. fracture trauma
gap n.
hamate hook n.
n. horse-hoof fracture
horse-hoof fracture n.
hypertrophic vital n.
hypervascular n.
n. incidence
infected nondraining n.
n. long-bone fracture
metaphysial-articular n.
nonreactive n.
oligotrophic fracture n.
n. osteomyelitis
n. rate
reactive n.
scaphoid n.
supracondylar n.
symptomatic n.
synovial n.
talar body n.
n. torsion wedge fracture
torsion wedge fracture n.
vascular n.
wedge n.
nonunited fracture
nonwalking cast
nonweightbearing (NWB)
n. brace
n. crutch walk
n. crutch walking
n. view
n. x-ray
Nora lesion
NordiCare
N. Back Therapy System
N. Enabler exerciser
N. Strider exerciser
NordicTrack
N. Motion Analyzer
N. ski exerciser
no-reflow phenomenon
Norgaard view
Norgesic Forte
Norian SRS cement
Noritate Cream

Norland
N. bone densitometer
N. bone densitometry
normal
n. anatomic position
n. last shoe
n. lordotic curve
upper limits of n.
normalization of neuropathophysiology
Normalize press-fit hip prosthesis
Norman
N. tibial bolt
N. tibial pin
normoxia
Norm testing and rehabilitation system
north
N. American blastomycosis
N. American Malignant
Hyperthermia protocol
N. American Riding for
Handicapped Association
Northville brace
Northwick
N. Park Index
N. Park Index of Independence in
ADL
Norton
N. ball reamer
N. scale
Norwich press-fit prosthesis
Norwood iliotibial band tenodesis
nose
anteater n.
no-stretch RocketSoc brace
notariorum
paralysis n.
notch
acetabular n.
A-frame n.
clavicular n.
coracoid n.
costal n.
cotyloid n.
cuboid n.
n. cut
n. cutting guide
incisural n.
interclavicular n.
intercondylar n.
interpeduncular n.
intervertebral n.
radial sigmoid n.
scapular n.

N

NOTES

notch *(continued)*
    sciatic n.
    semilunar n.
    sigmoid n.
    spinoglenoid n.
    suprasternal n.
    trochlear n.
    ulnar n.
    vertebral n.
    n. view
    n. width index (NWI)
notcher device
notchplasty
    n. blade
    n. procedure
Nothnagel acroparesthesia
no-tie stretch lace
notochord
    persistent n.
no-touch technique
Nottingham Extended ADL index
nourished
    well developed, well n. (WDWN, WD WN)
NovaBone Bioglass bone grafting material
Novagel gel sheet
Novocain Injection
Novus
    N. LC threaded interbody fusion cage
    N. LT titanium threaded interbody fusion cage
Noyes flexion rotation drawer test
nozzle
    suction n.
NRM
    nucleus raphe magnus
NRS
    numeric rating scale
NSA
    neck-shaft angle
NSAID
    nonsteroidal antiinflammatory drug
N-telopeptide (NTx)
N-Terface dressing
NTx
    N-telopeptide
Nu
    N. Gauze bandage
    N. Gauze dressing
    N. Gauze packing
nubbin
nuchal
    n. ligament
    n. region
    n. rigidity
nuclear
    n. arthrogram

    n. magnetic resonance (NMR)
    n. magnetic resonance scan
nuclei (*pl. of* nucleus)
Nucleotome
    N. probe
    N. system
nucleotomy
    laser n.
    percutaneous n.
nucleus, pl. **nuclei**
    force n.
    periaqueductal gray n.
    prosthetic disc n. (PDN)
    n. pulposus
    pulpy n.
    n. raphe magnus (NRM)
nudge
    n. control
    n. control on prosthesis
Nu-Knit absorbable hemostat
numeric rating scale (NRS)
NuPulse device
Nurick
    N. classification of spondylosis
    N. spondylosis classification
Nurolon suture
nursemaid's elbow
Nussbaum bracelet
NuStep
    N. exerciser
    N. total body recumbent stepper
nut
    n. alignment guide
    Close Encounter n.
    Kirschner traction bow n.
    locking n.
    nylon n.
    traction bow n.
    VDS hex n.
nutation
    counter n.
nutcracker
    n. fracture
    n. injury
    n. sign
NutraFill hydrophilic dressing
NutraStat wound dressing
nutrient
    n. artery
    n. flap
nutrition
    parenteral n.
    tissue n.
    total parenteral n. (TPN)
nutritional osteomalacia
NUV
    negative ulnar variance
Nuwave transcutaneous electrical nerve stimulator

NV
 neurovascular
NWB
 nonweightbearing
NWI
 notch width index
Nylatex
 N. strap
 N. wrap
Nylok self-locking nail
nylon
 n. monofilament

 n. nut
 n. suture
 n. teaspoon
NYU
 New York University
 NYU orthosis insert
NYU-Hosmer
 NYU-H. electric elbow
 NYU-H. prehension actuator
NZ
 neutral zone

NOTES

N

OBrien bone clamp
OA
    osteoarthritis
        OA knee brace
OAdjuster knee brace
OAE
    otoacoustic emission
OAP
    osteoarthropathy
OAR
    Ottawa Ankle Rule
oarsman's wrist
OAS
    Oral Analogue Scale
OASIS
    osteotomy analysis simulation software
    Outcome and Assessment Information
    Set
Oasis wound dressing
OAsys knee brace
oath hand
OATS
    osteochondral autograft transfer system
        OATS graft
        OATS procedure
        OATS technique
OAV
    oculoauriculovertebral
OAWO
    opening abductory wedge osteotomy
Ober
    O. anterior transfer
    O. incision
    O. operation
    O. posterior drainage
    O. release
    O. tendon technique
    O. test
obese
    o. bed
    o. knee osteoarthritis
    o. support
    o. walker
objective sign
OBLA
    onset of blood lactate accumulation
obligate translation
oblique
    o. amputation
    o. bandage
    o. closing wedge osteotomy
    (OCWO)
    o. displacement
    o. facet wiring
    o. fracture

    o. incision
    medial o. (MO)
    o. meniscal tear
    o. metacarpal line
    o. metatarsocuneiform joint
    o. midtarsal joint axis (OMJA)
    o. muscle
    o. osteotomy for tibial deformity
    o. osteotomy with derotation
    o. popliteal ligament
    o. proximal phalangeal osteotomy
    o. retinacular ligament
    o. retinacular ligament tightness
    test
    o. screw insertion
    o. slide osteotomy
    o. view
    o. wire
    o. wiring facet
obliquity
    o. fracture
    pelvic o.
    reverse o.
obliquus
    vastus medialis obliquus (VMO)
obliterans
    arteriosclerosis o.
    endarteritis o.
oblong polyethylene acetabular cup
O₂Boot
O'Brien
    O. capsular shift procedure
    O. goniometer
    O. pelvic halo operation
    O. radial fracture classification
    O. rib hook
    O. staple
observation hip
obstetrician's hand
obturator
    o. artery
    o. avulsion fracture
    blunt o.
    conical o.
    core biopsy o.
    o. externus muscle
    o. internus muscle
    o. internus tendon
    Keene o.
    o. nerve
    o. nerve injury
    o. nerve neuritis
    o. neurectomy
    o. oblique view
    o. sign

O

obturator *(continued)*
    o. sleeve
    o. sulcus
obturator/brim line
Obus back support
Obwegeser
    O. sagittal mandibular osteotomy
    O. sagittal mandibular osteotomy technique
Obwegeser-Dalpont internal screw fixation
OCAIRS
    Occupational Circumstances Assessment-Interview Rating Scale
occipital
    o. bone
    o. condyle
    o. condyle fracture
    o. neuralgia
    o. region
occipital-atlantal joint
occipital-atlantoaxial complex
occipital-axis joint
occipital-fiber analysis
occipitoatlantal dislocation
occipitoatlantoaxial
    o. fusion
    o. joint
    o. joint complex
occipitocervical
    o. angle
    o. arthrodesis
    o. articulation
    o. fixation
    o. fusion
    o. junction
    o. lordosis
    o. plate
    o. stabilization
occluder
    multiple pinhole o.
Occlusal-HP wart medication
occlusal splint
occlusive dressing
occult
    o. fracture
    o. primary malignant tumor
    o. talar lesion
occulta
    spina bifida o. (SBO)
occupation
    sedentary o.
occupational
    o. behavior
    O. Circumstances Assessment-Interview Rating Scale (OCAIRS)
    o. and environmental medicine (OEM)

    O. Performance History Interview - Second Version (OPHI-II)
    O. Questionnaire (OQ)
    o. rating
    o. risk
    o. role
    o. science
    o. stress syndrome (OSS)
    o. therapy (OT)
    O. Therapy Activities of Daily Living (OTADL)
occupation-related disorder
OCD
    osteochondritis dissecans
ochronosis
ochronotic
    o. arthritis
    o. arthropathy
OCL
    Orthopaedic Casting Lab
    OCL volar splint
O'Connor
    O. finger dexterity test
    O. operating arthroscope
    O. tweezer dexterity test
OCT
    optimal cutting temperature
    OCT compound
OctaFix occipital fixation system
octagon roll
Octocaine Injection
octopus holder
OCTR
    open carpal tunnel release
ocular
    o. prosthesis
    o. scoliosis
    o. sign
oculoauriculovertebral (OAV)
    o. dysplasia
oculoplethysmography (OPG)
Ocutricin Topical Ointment
OCWO
    oblique closing wedge osteotomy
OD
    osteochondritis dissecans
Oden peroneal tendon subluxation classification
Odland ankle prosthesis
ODM
    opponens digiti minimi
O'Donoghue
    O. ACL reconstruction
    O. cotton cast
    O. dressing
    O. facetectomy
    O. knee splint
    O. procedure
    O. stirrup splint

O. test
triad of O.
unhappy triad of O.

odontoid
o. agenesis
o. condyle
o. condyle fracture
o. fracture internal fixation
o. fracture stabilization
o. hypoplasia
o. perpendicular line
o. process
o. process osteosynthesis
o. x-ray view

odontoid-axial area
odontoidectomy
ODQ
opponens digiti quinti

O'Driscoll posterolateral pivot test
OEC
OEC knee immobilizer
OEC lag screw component
OEC lag screw component with
keyway
OEC Mini 6600 imaging system
OEC popliteal pad
OEC splint
OEC wrist/forearm support

Oehler symptom
OEM
occupational and environmental medicine

Oesch hook
offloading knee brace
offset
o. cane
o. cap
o. drill hole
femoral o.
head-stem o.
o. hinge
o. link
medial head-stem o.
o. suspension feeder

offset-V
o.-V osteotomy
o.-V procedure

Ogata technique
Ogden
O. Anchor soft tissue device
O. bone anchor
O. epiphysial fracture classification
O. fracture classification system
O. knee dislocation classification

O. plate
O. plate system
O. tissue reattachment mini system

Ogee acetabular component
Ogston
O. line
O. operation

Oh
Oh cemented hip prosthesis
Oh press-fit hip prosthesis

Oh-Spectron prosthesis
OI
osteogenesis imperfecta

OIC
osteogenesis imperfecta congenita

OIF
Osteogenesis Imperfecta Foundation

oil
Decubitene oxygenated o.
massage o.

Oil-Red-O method
OIT
osteogenesis imperfecta tarda

OKCE
open kinetic chain exercise

Oklahoma
O. ankle joint
O. ankle joint orthosis
O. ankle prosthesis
O. cable system

OKQ
Osteoporosis Knowledge Questionnaire

old
o. fracture
o. man's back
o. smoothie bur
o. unreduced dislocation

olecranarthritis
olecranarthrocace
olecranarthropathy
olecranization
olecranoid
olecranon
o. bursa
o. bursitis
o. fossa
o. ligament
o. osteochondritis
o. process
o. region
o. tip fracture

oleic acid
oleoma

O

NOTES

Olerud
>> O. internal fixator
>> O. and Molander fracture classification
>> O. pedicle fixation system
>> O. PSF fixation system
>> O. PSF rod
>> O. PSF screw
>> O. transpedicular fixation

oligoarthritis
>> undifferentiated o.

oligoarticular
>> o. arthritis
>> o. disease

oligodendroglioma
oligotrophic fracture nonunion
olisthesis
>> anterior o.
>> degenerative o.
>> lumbar o.
>> progressive o.
>> rotatory o.

olisthetic vertebra
olisthy
Olivecrona
>> O. clip-applying and removing forceps
>> O. rasp

olive-shaped bur
olive wire
Ollier
>> O. approach
>> O. arthrodesis approach
>> O. disease
>> O. dyschondroplasia
>> O. incision
>> O. lateral approach
>> O. law
>> O. layer
>> O. operation
>> O. osteochondromatosis
>> O. rake retractor
>> O. syndrome
>> O. technique
>> O. thick split free graft

Ollier-Thiersch skin graft
O'Malley jaw fracture splint
Ombredanne mallet
Omed vented instrument guard
omega
>> O. compression hip screw system
>> O. Plus compression hip system
>> O. splinting material

Omega-3 dietary supplement
omental flap
Omer-Capen carpectomy
OMJA
>> oblique midtarsal joint axis

Ommaya
>> O. reservoir device
>> O. reservoir implant material

Omni
>> O. knee brace
>> O. Roller massager

Omniace RT3200N electromyographic amplifier
Omniderm dressing
Omnifit
>> O. dual geometry microstructured prosthesis
>> O. HA hip stem prosthesis
>> O. HA hip stent
>> O. knee prosthesis
>> O. Plus hip system
>> O. PSL microstructured prosthesis
>> O. total knee system

Omnifit-C stem
OmniFlex
>> O. hip prosthesis
>> O. knee orthosis

Omni-Flexor
>> O.-F. device
>> O.-F. wrist exerciser

Omnisense 7000S bone sonometer
Omnitron exercise testing
omoclavicular
omodynia
omohyoid muscle
omosternum
Omotrain active shoulder support
omovertebral bone
OMS Oral
OMT
>> osteomanipulative therapy
>> osteopathic manipulative therapy

Oncovin injection
one
>> o. and one-half spica cast
>> o. wound-one scar concept

one-half
>> o.-h. patellar tendon transplant
>> o.-h. spica cast

Ongoing Ambulating AFO boot
onlay
>> o. bone graft
>> o. bone graft cast
>> o. cancellous iliac graft

onset
>> o. of blood lactate accumulation (OBLA)
>> delayed o.
>> o. frequency
>> o. latency

Ontario Cohort of Running-Related Injury

OnTrack
    O. system
    O. treatment method
onychauxis
onychectomy
onychoclavus
onychocryptosis nail
onychodystrophy
onychogryphosis
onycholysis
onychomadesis
onychomycosis
    proximal subungual o. (PSO)
    subungual o.
    superficial white o. (SWO)
onychomycotic toenail
onychoosteodysplasia
    hereditary o.
onychophosis
onychotomy
Ony-Clear
    O.-C. Nail
    O.-C. Spray
onyxis
OP
    opponens pollicis
OP-1
    osteogenic protein-1
    OP-1 implant/bone graft
    OP-1 putty spinal fusion implant
    OP-1 TM bone implant
opaque
    o. arthrography
    o. myelography
    o. synovium
OPC Synergy
open
    o. amputation
    o. base wedge osteotomy
    o. base wedge
    osteotomy/bunionectomy
    o. biopsy
    o. bone graft epiphysiodesis
    o. carpal tunnel release (OCTR)
    o. C-D hook
    o. disc surgery
    o. dislocation
    o. double-decked hook cervical
    system
    o. drainage
    o. exit foramen
    o. fracture (type I, II, III, IIIA,
    IIIB, IIIC)

    o. fracture wound drain
    o. kinematic chain
    o. kinetic chain exercise (OKCE)
    o. medullary nailing
    o. nail
    o. palm technique
    o. pinning
    o. reduction
    o. reduction of fracture
    o. reduction and internal fixation
    (ORIF)
    o. stabilization
    o. stabilization of traumatic anterior
    shoulder instability
    o. tenotomy
    o. wedge (OW)
    o. wound
open-air splint
open-book
    o.-b. fracture
    o.-b. pelvic injury
open-bowl cement technique
open-break fracture
open-chain exercise
open-end wrench
opening
    o. abductory wedge osteotomy
    (OAWO)
    Sierra 2-load voluntary o.
    voluntary o. (VO)
    o. wedge manipulation
    o. wedge manipulation and
    reapplication of plaster
    o. wedge osteotomy
open-section nail
open-staple capsulorrhaphy
open-toe shoe
opera-glass hand
operating
    o. microscope
    o. room
    o. time
operation
    Abbe o.
    Abbott o.
    Abbott-Lucas shoulder o.
    Adams hip o.
    Adelmann o.
    Akin o.
    Albee o.
    Albee-Delbert o.
    Albert knee o.
    Alouette o.

NOTES

operation *(continued)*

Amstutz resurfacing o.
Anderson o.
Annandale o.
anterior ankle shift o.
Armistead ulnar lengthening o.
ASIF screw fixation o.
Aufranc-Turner o.
Auto-Implant o.
Avila o.
Axer o.
Badgley o.
Baker patellar advancement o.
Baker translocation o.
Bankart o.
Bankart-Putti-Platt o.
Barker o.
Barr tendon transfer o.
Barsky o.
Barwell o.
Bateman shoulder o.
Bennett quadriceps plastic o.
Bent o.
Berger o.
Bier o.
Blundell-Jones o.
Bora o.
Bosworth shelf o.
Boyd o.
Brahms foot o.
bridle posterior tibial tendon
    transfer o.
Bristow o.
Brittain o.
Brockman foot o.
Brooks cervical fusion o.
Broström-Gould ankle instability o.
Brown knee approach o.
Buck o.
Bunnell posterior tibial tendon
    transfer o.
Butler fifth toe o.
Campbell ankle o.
Carnesale hip approach o.
Cave o.
centralization of radius o.
Chopart o.
Cloward o.
Cocklin toe o.
Codivilla o.
Cole o.
Colonna shelf o.
Compere o.
Conn o.
Contour DF-80 total hip o.
Cotrel-Dubousset derotation o.
Credo o.
Crutchfield o.
Cubbins o.

Davies-Colley o.
Diamond-Gould syndactyly o.
Dickson o.
Dickson-Diveley foot o.
Dieffenbach o.
Dunn hip o.
Dupuytren o.
Durham flatfoot o.
DuVries modified McBride hallux
    valgus o.
Dwyer clawfoot o.
Eden-Hybbinette o.
Eggers o.
Ellis Jones peroneal tendon o.
Elmslie-Cholmeley foot o.
Elmslie peroneal tendon o.
Elmslie-Trillat patellar o.
Evans ankle joint instability o.
Farmer o.
flap o.
French supracondylar fracture o.
Frost foot o.
Galeazzi patellar o.
Gant o.
Gardner o.
Gelman foot o.
Girdlestone o.
Grice-Green o.
Gritti o.
Guyon o.
Haas o.
Hammon foot o.
hanging hip o.
hanging toe o.
Hark foot o.
Harris-Beath o.
Hauser patellar o.
Hey o.
Heyman o.
Heyman-Herndon clubfoot o.
Hibbs o.
Hoffa o.
Hoffa-Lorenz o.
Hoffmann metatarsal o.
Hohmann o.
Hoke Achilles tendon
    lengthening o.
Holmes o.
Houston o.
I-beam hip o.
Inclan modification of Campbell
    ankle o.
inside-out Bankart shoulder
    instability o.
intermetatarsal angle-reducing o.
Jewett o.
Jones cock-up toe o.
Joplin o.
Juvara foot o.

Kapel o.
Keller foot o.
Keller hallux valgus o.
Kellogg-Speed o.
Kessler posterior tibial tendon
transfer o.
Kidner foot o.
Kirkaldy-Willis o.
Kirk distal thigh o.
Kondoleon o.
Kortzeborn hand o.
Kreuscher o.
Krukenberg hand o.
Lambrinudi dropfoot o.
Lange o.
Langenbeck o.
Lapidus o.
Larrey o.
lateral acetabular shelf o.
limb-sparing o.
Lisfranc o.
Liston o.
Littler o.
Lorenz o.
Luck o.
Ludloff o.
Lund o.
MacAusland o.
MacNab o.
Magnuson o.
Magnuson-Stack o.
Mallory-Head revision o.
Mauck o.
Mayer transfer o.
Mayo hallux valgus modified o.
Mazur o.
McBride bunion hallux valgus o.
McKeever o.
McLaughlin o.
Mensor-Scheck hanging-hip o.
Mikulicz o.
Milch elbow o.
Miller flatfoot o.
Mital elbow release o.
Mitchell o.
modified Cocklin toe o.
Moe scoliosis o.
Mueller knee o.
muscle sliding o.
Nélaton o.
Neviaser o.
Nicola shoulder o.
Nicoll fracture o.

Nirschl o.
Ober o.
O'Brien pelvic halo o.
Ogston o.
Ollier o.
Osgood o.
Overholt o.
over-the-top knee o.
Paci o.
Pauwels o.
Pheasant elbow o.
Phelps o.
Phemister o.
Putti-Platt o.
resurfacing o.
reverse Mauck knee o.
revision total hip o.
Ridlon o.
Rose foot o.
Roux-Goldthwait o.
Sargent knee o.
Sayre o.
Schanz o.
screw fixation o.
Selig hip o.
Smith-Robinson o.
Sofield femoral deficiency o.
Souter hip o.
Stener-Gunterberg hip o.
Stewart arm o.
subcutaneous o.
Suppan foot o.
Sutherland hip o.
Syme o.
Tharies hip replacement o.
T-plasty modification of Bankart
shoulder o.
Vulpius equinus deformity o.
Weaver-Dunn acromioclavicular o.
West and Soto-Hall patella o.
Zadik foot o.
Zickel subtrochanteric fracture o.

operative
o. ankylosis
o. arthroscopy
o. arthrotomy
o. leg holder
o. legholder
o. roentgenogram
o. site

OPG
oculoplethysmography
O'Phelan technique

NOTES

OPHI-II
Occupational Performance History
Interview - Second Version
opiate receptor antagonist
Opiela brace
opioid
o. antagonist
o. receptor
opisthenar
opisthotonic position
OPLL
ossification of posterior longitudinal
ligament
Opmi microscopic drape
Oppenheim
O. amyotonia
O. brace
O. disease
O. gait
O. reflex
O. sign
O. syndrome
Oppenheimer
O. sign
O. spring wire
O. spring wire splint
O. with reverse knuckle-bender
splint
Oppociser
O. exercise device
O. hand exerciser
opponens
o. bar
o. digiti minimi (ODM)
o. digiti quinti (ODQ)
o. digiti quinti muscle
o. orthosis
o. pollicis (OP)
o. pollicis muscle
o. splint
o. transfer
opponensplasty
abductor digiti minimi o.
abductor digiti quinti o.
Bunnell o.
Camitz o.
Goldmar o.
Groves o.
Huber adductor digiti quinti o.
Littler o.
Phalen-Miller o.
ring sublimis o.
Riordan finger o.
opposite
o. foot-strike phase
o. foot-strike phase of gait
o. toe-off phase
o. toe-off phase of gait

opposition
o. contracture
finger o.
o. test
thumb o.
Opraflex
O. drape
O. dressing
OpSite wound dressing
opsonic activity
Opteform
O. bone graft material
O. 100HT bone graft
Optetrak
O. comprehensive knee system
O. total knee replacement system
optical
o. stereophotogrammetry
o. trapping
Opti-Curve therapeutic pillow
Opti-Fix
O.-F. femoral prosthesis
O.-F. hip stem
O.-F. II acetabular cup
O.-F. I, II prosthesis
O.-F. total hip system
optimal
o. alignment
o. cutting temperature (OCT)
**OptiMax Supreme pressure reduction
mattress**
optimizing motion palpation
option
O. hip system
O. Orthotic Series
optoelectric
o. measuring apparatus
o. measuring system
o. signal detection apparatus
Optotrak motion measurement system
OPTP
Orthopaedic Physical Therapy Products
OPTP Slant
OQ
Occupational Questionnaire
O'Rahilly limb deficiency classification
oral
O. Analogue Scale (OAS)
o. incontinence
o. nutritional supplement
Oramorph SR Oral
Oratec chisel
Orateck device
orbicular
o. ligament
o. zone
orbit
angular process of o.
Orbital shoulder stabilizer brace

Orbiter treadmill
orbitosphenoidal bone
order of activation
ordinal classification
Oregon Poly II ankle prosthesis
Oretorp retractable knife
Orfit splint
Orfizip
    O. body jacket
    O. knee cast
    O. wrist cast
organ
    Golgi tendon o. (GTO)
    mechanoreceptor Golgi tendon o.
organic dysfunction
organization
    homuncular o.
    National Hospice O.
organizational
    o. phase
    o. phase of tendon healing
orientation
    phalangeal articular o.
    visual o.
    o. WHO Handicap Scale
ORIF
    open reduction and internal fixation
origin
    adductor o.
    deltoid o.
    fever of undetermined o. (FUO)
    flexor-pronator o.
    tripartite muscle o.
original
    O. Backnobber massage tool
    O. Backnobber muscle massager
    O. Index Knobber II
    O. Index Knobber II massager
    O. Index Knobber II massage tool
    O. Jacknobber II muscle-massage
    device
Orion anterior cervical plate
Oris pin
Orlando hip-knee-ankle-foot orthosis
ORLAU
    Orthotic Research and Locomotor
    Assessment Unit
    ORLAU swivel walker
    ORLAU swivel walker orthosis
Orlon with Lycra stump sock
Ormandy screw
Ormco pin

ORN
    osteoradionecrosis
oropharyngeal approach
Orozco plate
orphenadrine, aspirin, and caffeine
Orthairtome
    O. II drill
    O. wire driver
Orthawear antiembolism stockings
orthesis
orthetics
Orth-evac
    O.-e. autotransfusion system
    O.-e. postoperative transfusion
    system
Orthex
    O. cannulated bone screw
    O. reliever insole
    O. Relievers shoe insert
Orthion traction machine
Ortho
    O. DX electromedical stimulator
    O. DX stimulator for knee
    rehabilitation
Ortho-Arch II orthotic
orthobiologic implant
Ortho-Biotic recliner
OrthoBlast
    O. osteoinductive bioimplant
    O. paste
OrthoBlend powered bone mill
OrthoBone pillow
Ortho-Cel pad
Orthochrome
    O. implant metal
    O. implant metal prosthesis
Orthocomp cement
orthodigita
Orthodoc presurgical planning system
orthodox procedure
orthodromic velocity
OrthoDyn bone substitute material
Orthodyne Enhancer unit
Orthofit 9000, 9001 orthotic
Orthofix
    O. apparatus
    O. Cervical-Stim bone growth
    stimulator
    O. external fixation device
    O. intramedullary nail
    O. ISKD device
    O. M-100 distractor

O

NOTES

Orthofix *(continued)*
    O. monolateral femoral external fixator
    O. Ogden anchor
    O. pin
    O. prosthesis
    O. screw
Orthoflex
    O. dressing
    O. elastic plaster bandage
Ortho-Foam
    O.-F. elbow/heel pad
    O.-F. protector
Orthofuse implantable growth stimulator
OrthoGel liner
OrthoGen bone growth stimulator
Orthogenesis LPS limb preservation prosthesis system
Ortho-Glass
    O.-G. splint
    O.-G. synthetic material
Ortho-Grip silicone rubber handle
Ortho-ice multipack
Ortho-Jel impression material
orthokinetic exercise
orthokinetics
    orthopaedic o.
Orthokinetics travel chair
Ortho-last splint
Ortholav
    O. irrigation and suction device
    O. jet
Ortholen sheet
Ortholign spinal orthosis
Ortholoc
    O. Advantim revision knee system
    O. Advantim total knee system
    O. II unconstrained prosthesis
    O. implant metal prosthesis
OrthoLogic
    O. 1000 bone growth stimulation
    O. 1000 bone growth stimulator
orthomechanical
orthomechanotherapy
Orthomedics
    O. brace
    O. Stretch and Heel splint
    O. Ultra-Guard hip orthosis
orthomelic
Orthomerica
    O. TC AFO system
    O. UFO
Orthomet
    O. Axiom total knee system
    O. Perfecta total hip system
Orthomite II adhesive
Ortho-Mold
    O.-M. lumbar body

    O.-M. spinal brace
    O.-M. splint
orthomolecular medicine/megavitamin therapy
orthonormal diameter
orthopaedic, orthopedic
    Advanta O.'s
    o. bed
    o. bone file
    o. broach
    o. bur
    O. Casting Lab (OCL)
    o. cement
    o. chisel
    o. curette
    o. cutting instrument
    damage-control o.'s
    o. depth gauge
    o. dynamometer
    Encore O.'s
    o. evaluation
    evidence-based o.'s
    o. felt
    o. forceps
    o. goniometer
    o. gouge
    o. hammer
    o. hardware
    o. hemostat
    o. impactor
    o. knife
    o. mallet
    o. orthokinetics
    o. osteotome
    o. oxford shoe
    pediatric o.'s
    O. Physical Therapy Products (OPTP)
    O. Positioning Seat
    o. propeller
    o. prosthesis
    o. rasp
    o. reamer
    o. rehabilitation
    o. retractor
    o. rongeur
    o. scissors
    o. shoulder elevator
    o. stockinette
    o. strap clavicular splint
    Sulzer O.'s
    o. surgery
    o. surgical file
    o. surgical pliers
    o. surgical stripper
    O. Systems Inc. (OSI)
    o. table
    O. Trauma Association classification

orthopaedist, orthopedist
OrthoPak
    O. bone growth stimulator system
    O. II bone growth stimulator
Ortho-Pal body support
orthopantogram imaging
OrthoPAT system
orthopedic (*var. of* orthopaedic)
orthopedist (*var. of* orthopaedist)
orthopercussion
ortho physical therapy
Orthoplast
    O. dressing
    O. fracture brace
    O. isoprene splint
    O. jacket
    O. plastic
    O. slipper cast
orthoPLUG soft bone plug
orthopod
orthopraxis
orthopraxy spurious spinous process
orthoRaps postsurgical wound wrap
orthoroentgenogram imaging
orthoroentgenography
Orthoset radiopaque bone cement
orthosis, pl. **orthoses**
    abduction hip o.
    accommodative o.
    Adjustable Advanced Reciprocating
      Gait O. (ARGO)
    A-frame o.
    airplane splint o.
    AliCork Foot O.
    AliMed o.
    Aliplast custom-molded foot o.
    ambulation training o.
    Amfit custom o.
    ankle o. (AO)
    ankle contracture o.
    ankle-foot o. (AFO)
    ankle-foot plastic o.
    ankle stabilizing o. (ASO)
    anteroposterior control o.
    Anti-Shox o.
    Atlanta brace o.
    Atlanta-Scottish Rite abduction o.
    bail-lock knee joint o.
    balanced forearm o. (BFO)
    balance padding o.
    bar-and-shoe o.
    Bauerfeind Malleolic Ankle O.
    Beaufort seating o.

    Bebax o.
    Bennett o.
    BFO O.
    BioCast wrist/hand o.
    Biothotic foot o.
    Boston brace thoracolumbosacral o.
    Boston postoperative hip o.
    cable-twister o.
    calcaneal spur cookie o.
    Caligamed ankle o.
    caliper o.
    Canadian Knee O.
    CASH thoracolumbosacral o.
    C-bar o.
    cervical o. (CO)
    cervical thoracic o.
    cervicothoracic o. (CTO)
    cervicothoracolumbosacral o.
      (CTLSO)
    chairback lumbosacral o.
    clavicle o.
    cock-up splint o.
    Comfy Elbow O.
    Comfy Knee O.
    Controller shoulder o.
    copolymer ankle-foot o.
    corrective o.
    Craig-Scott o.
    cruciform anterior spinal
      hyperextension o.
    CTLSO o.
    Daytona cervical o.
    DDH o.
    Denis Browne bar foot o.
    developmental dislocated hip o.
    Diabetic D-Sole foot o.
    dial-lock o.
    dorsiflexion assist ankle joint
      ankle-foot o.
    o. drop-lock ring
    dual-photon electrospinal o.
    DuraBoot o.
    Dynamic elbow o.
    Dynamic knee o.
    Dynamic wrist o.
    elastic knee cage o.
    elastic twister o.
    elbow o. (EO)
    elbow-wrist-hand o. (EWHO)
    Engen extension o.
    Engen palmar finger o.
    externally powered tenodesis o.
    E-Z arm abduction o.

O

NOTES

orthosis *(continued)*

figure-of-8 thoracic o.
Fillauer bar foot o.
FirmFlex custom o.
Flex Foam o.
flexible o.
flexion-extension control cervical o.
flexor hinge o.
floor-reaction ankle-foot o.
foot o. (FO)
Foot Levelers o.
Frejka pillow o.
front-opening o.
gator plastic o.
Gillette joint o.
Gillette modification of ankle-foot o.
GunSlinger shoulder o.
G/W Heel Lift, Inc. o.
hallux valgus o.
halo cervical o.
halo extension o.
halo traction o.
halo-vest o.
hand o. (HO)
heat-molded petroplastic ankle-foot o.
hindfoot o.
hip o. (HO)
hip guidance o. (HGO)
hip-knee-ankle-foot o. (HKAFO)
Hosmer VC 4-bar knee o.
hyperextension o.
Hyperex thoracic o.
Ilfeld splint o.
Ipomax o.
ipos forefoot relief o.
ipos heel relief o.
ischial weightbearing o.
J-24 cervical o.
J-45 contraflexion o.
Jewett-Benjamin cervical o.
Jewett contraflexion o.
Jewett hyperextension o.
Jewett postfusion o.
Jewett thoracolumbosacral o.
J-35 hyperextension o.
Jousto dropfoot splint, skid o.
J-55 postfusion o.
Kallassy o.
Kid-Dee-Lite o.
Klenzak o.
knee o. (KO)
knee-ankle-foot o. (KAFO)
knee extension o.
knee management o. (KMO)
Knight-Taylor thoracolumbosacral o.
Kydex chairback o.
L.A. cervical o.

leather o.
Legg-Perthes disease o.
Lenox Hill knee o.
Lerman multiligamentous knee control o.
Levy & Rappel foot o.
L'Nard Multi Podus o.
L'Nard thoracolumbosacral o.
long leg o.
long opponens o.
lower limb o. (LLO)
LSU reciprocation-gait o.
lumbosacral o. (LSO)
Lynco foot o.
Malibu cervical o.
Malleoloc ankle o.
Maple Leaf hip o.
Marlin cervical o.
medial heel wedge o.
medial sole wedge o.
metal hybrid o.
Meyer cervical o.
Milwaukee cervicothoracolumbosacral o.
Milwaukee scoliosis o.
Minerva o.
molded ankle-foot o. (MAFO)
molded lumbosacral o.
Monodos o.
MultiBoot o.
neoprene wrist o.
Newington o.
Newport MC hip o.
New York Orthopaedic front-opening o.
Oklahoma ankle joint o.
OmniFlex knee o.
opponens o.
Orlando hip-knee-ankle-foot o.
ORLAU swivel walker o.
Ortholign spinal o.
Orthomedics Ultra-Guard hip o.
o. overlapped uprights
overlapped uprights in o.
parapodium o.
passive prehension o. (PPO)
patellar tendon-bearing o. (PTBO)
patellar tendon weightbearing brace o.
patellar tracking o.
patellofemoral o.
pediatric pressure relief ankle foot o.
Phelps o.
pillow o.
plantar arch support o.
plantar fasciitis o. (PFO)
Plastazote cervical collar o.
plastic ankle-foot o.

plastic floor reaction ankle-foot o.
pneumatic o.
polypropylene ankle-foot o.
polypropylene glycol-ankle-foot o.
  (PPG-AFO)
polypropylene glycol-
  thoracolumbosacral o. (PPG-TLSO)
poster o.
2-poster cervical o.
4-poster cervical o.
posterior leaf-spring ankle-foot o.
postoperative lumbosacral o.
prehension o.
pressure-relieving o.
Profile Sitting O.
Pro-glide o.
Progressive ankle o.
prosthesis and o. (P&O)
PTB ankle-foot o.
PTB plastic o.
Pucci pediatrics hand o.
Pucci rehab knee o.
reciprocal finger prehension o.
reciprocation gait o. (RGO)
resting o.
rib belt o.
rigid o.
Rochester hip-knee-ankle-foot o.
SACH o.
sacroiliac o. (SIO)
safety pin o.
Sawa shoulder o.
Scottish Rite hip o.
Seattle o.
Select joint o.
semirigid polypropylene ankle-
  foot o.
serial stretch orthoses
Shaeffer rigid o.
short leg o.
short opponens o.
shoulder o. (SO)
shoulder-elbow-wrist-hand o.
  (SEWHO)
single-photon electrospinal o.
skull-occiput-mandibular
  immobilization o.
Slim Option shoe o.
soft collar cervical o.
SOLEutions custom o.
SOMI o.
spinal o. (SO)
Sport-Stirrup o.

spring-loaded lock o.
spring-wire ankle-foot o.
standard shell ankle-foot o.
standing frame o.
static o.
steel sole plate o.
sternal-occipital-mandibular
  immobilizer o.
sternooccipital mandibular
  immobilizer o.
supramalleolar o. (SMO)
Swede-O-Universal o.
Swedish knee cage o.
Tachdjian o.
Taylor thoracolumbosacral o.
tenodesis o.
themoplastic ankle-foot o.
therapeutic o.
Thera-Pos elbow o.
Therapy Carrot Finger O. (TCFO)
Thomas collar cervical o.
Thomas heel o.
thoracic o. (TO)
thoracic spine o.
thoracolumbar o.
thoracolumbosacral o. (TLSO)
Tib-Transformer o.
TIRR foot-ankle o.
ToeOFF o.
tone-reducing ankle-foot o.
  (TRAFO)
Toronto parapodium o.
total contact o. (TCO)
total contact bivalve ankle-foot o.
total hip stabilization o.
TPE ankle-foot o.
TPE biomechanical foot o.
TRAFO o.
Transpire wrist o.
trilateral knee-ankle-foot o.
trunk-hip-knee-ankle-foot o.
  (THKAFO)
turnbuckle wrist o.
UCB foot o.
UCBL o.
UCOlite o.
Ultrabrace knee o.
underarm o.
University of California Berkeley
  Laboratory o.
upper limb o. (ULO)
VAPC dorsiflexion assist o.
Vari-Duct hip and knee o.

NOTES

orthosis *(continued)*
    Viscoheel K, N o.
    Viscolas o.
    von Rosen splint hip o.
    weight-relieving o.
    Williams o.
    wrist-driven flexor hinge o.
    wrist-driven lateral prehension o.
    wrist-driven wrist-hand o.
    wrist-hand o. (WHO)
    XPE foot o.
    Zinco ankle o.

Orthosleep Pillow
OrthoSorb
    O. absorbable pin
    O. pin fixation
    O. pin nail
    O. rod

orthostatic
Orthotech Controller knee brace
orthotic
    Aerodyn o.
    Alden CDI o.
    Alznner o.
    Amfit o.
    Anti-Shox sports o.
    o. attachment implant
    BIOflex o.
    Biofoot o.
    BioSole-GEL o.
    Biothotic o.
    Blake inverted o.'s
    Blanke inverted tibialis posterior
      tendon o.
    Blue Line o.
    o. coiled spring twister
    custom-molded o.'s
    DesignLine o.
    o. device
    Diab-A-Thotics o.
    DressFlex o.
    DSIS o.
    D-Soles o.
    Dual AFO Boot o.
    Duraleve custom molded foot o.
    Extreme foot o.
    FirmFlex custom o.
    FlexiSport o.
    Foot Levelers custom o.
    Footmaster o.
    functional o.
    Golden Comfort o.
    Golden Fitness o.
    Healthflex o.
    inverted o.'s
    Jamaica Sandalthotics o.
    Kinetic Wedge o.
    Lyte Fit o.
    Magnathotic o.

    Malibu Sandalthotics o.
    mallet finger o.
    Mayer o.
    MBS snap-on o.
    M-Pact flexible o.
    Ortho-Arch II o.
    Orthofit 9000, 9001 o.
    ParFlex o.
    o. plate
    Powerstep o.'s
    PRAFO adjustable o.
    PreCustom O.
    pressure-relief ankle-foot o.
      (PRAFO)
    ProLite Plus runner's o.
    prosthetic and o. (P&O)
    Pro Support Systems o.
    Pucci Air o.
    QuikFormables o.
    Rediform o.
    O. Research and Locomotor
      Assessment Unit (ORLAU)
    Rohadur o.
    SACH o.
    SAFE o.
    Sandalthotics postural support o.
    shoe o.
    o. shoe insert
    Slimthetics o.
    Sof Sole motion control o.
    Soft Super Sport o.
    Soft Support Preforms o.
    SOLEutions soft plus o.
    SOLEutions sport shell o.
    solid ankle, cushioned heel o.
    Sporthotics o.
    Sport Preforms o.
    Sport-Rite o.'s
    stationary attachment flexible
      endoskeletal o.
    Stratos o.
    Superfeet Custom Pre-Fabricated O.
    Superform Contours o.
    Super Jock n' Jill store
      Superfeet o.
    Supralen cradle o.
    Supralen Schaefer o.
    Swiss Balance o.
    Thermo HK/Rohadur o.
    Thermo HK/Tepefom o.
    Thinline uncovered o.
    total contact shell ankle-foot o.
    UCOheal o.
    UltraStep o.
    Universal plantar fasciitis o. (UFO)
    Wire-Foam O.
    XO-soft-sole o.
orthotist
orthotome resector

Ortho-Trac
    O.-T. adhesive skin traction
    bandage
    O.-T. pneumatic vest
orthotripsy
    OssaTron o.
Orthotron exerciser
OrthoTurn standing transfer aid
Ortho-Vent
    O.-V. bandage
    O.-V. traction
OrthoVise
    O. orthopaedic instrument
    O. with slap hammer
OrthoWedge healing shoe
Ortho-Yomy facebow
Ortolani
    O. click
    O. maneuver
    O. sign
Orudis KT
os
    os acromiale
    os calcis pin fixation
    os peroneum
    os styloideum
    os trigonum fracture
OS-5/Plus 2 knee brace
Osada
    O. portable electric handpiece
    system
    O. portable handpiece system
    O. saw
Osborne
    O. fascia
    O. plate
    O. posterior approach
    O. punch
Osborne-Cotterill
    O.-C. elbow dislocation
    O.-C. elbow technique
Oscar ultrasonic bone cement removal
    system
oscillating
    o. gouge
    o. saw
oscillation
    grade I, II o.
oscillator
oscilloscope instrument
Osebold-Remondini syndrome
Osgood
    O. modified technique

    O. operation
    O. rotational osteotomy
Osgood-Schlatter
    O.-S. disease
    O.-S. knee brace
    O.-S. lesion
    O.-S. syndrome
Osher irrigating implant hook
OSI
    Orthopaedic Systems Inc.
    OSI arthroscopic leg holder
    OSI extremity elevator
    OSI laxity tester
    OSI modular table system
    OSI Well Leg Support
OSI-Schlein shoulder positioner
Osler node
OsmoCyte island wound-care dressing
Osmond-Clarke technique
osphyomyelitis
osphyotomy
OSS
    occupational stress syndrome
ossa tarsi
OssaTron
    O. noninvasive extracorporeal shock
    wave therapy device
    O. orthotripsy
    O. Orthotripter device
    O. shock wave
    O. shock wave therapy system
OsSatura synthetic bone graft
    substitution material
osseoaponeurotic
osseocartilaginous thoracic cage
Osseodent surgical drill
osseofibrous
osseointegrated prosthesis
osseointegration
osseomucoid
osseous
    o. adjustment
    o. attachment
    o. bridge
    o. bridge prevention
    o. coalition
    o. defect
    o. drift
    o. dystrophy
    o. equinus
    o. foraminal encroachment
    o. homeostasis
    o. instability

NOTES

O

osseous *(continued)*
  o. lacuna
  o. lamella
  o. lesion
  o. patella outgrowth
  o. pin
  o. prominence
  o. ring
  o. ring of Lacroix
  o. structure
  o. tissue
  o. trabecula
  o. tunnel
ossicle
  accessory o.
  talonavicular o.
ossicular chain replacement prosthesis
ossiferous
ossific
ossificans
  myositis o.
  osteitis o.
  pelvospondylitis o.
  periostitis o.
ossification
  bilateral heterotopic o.
  bipartite o.
  Brooker classification of
    heterotopic o. (I–IV)
  cartilaginous o.
  ectopic o.
  enchondral o.
  endochondral o.
  endplate o.
  heterotopic o.
  iliac crest o.
  intramembranous o.
  mandible o.
  membranous o.
  metaplastic o.
  metatarsal o.
  periarticular heterotopic o.
  perichondral o.
  periosteal o.
  pisiform o.
  o. of posterior longitudinal
    ligament (OPLL)
  o. primary center
  o. secondary center
  trapezium o.
  trapezoid o.
  triquetrum o.
ossification-associated fracture
ossifluent abscess
ossiform
ossify
ossifying fibroma
ossimeter
  Küntscher o.

Ostase
  Access O.
ostealgia
ostealgic
osteal resonance
ostectomy
  fibular o.
  partial o.
osteitis
  alveolar o.
  condensing o.
  o. deformans
  o. distal phalanx
  Garré o.
  o. necroticans pubis
  nonsuppurative o.
  o. ossificans
  pagetoid o.
  o. pubis
  rarefying o.
  sclerosing nonsuppurative o.
  suppurative o.
ostemia
ostempyesis
osteoanagenesis
OsteoAnalyzer device
osteoanesthesia
osteoaneurysm
Osteoarc-Guide II
OsteoArthritic knee brace
osteoarthritic knee pain
osteoarthritis (OA)
  ankle o.
  o. deformans
  o. deformans endemica
  degenerative o.
  endemic o.
  erosive o.
  o. grading classification
  hyperplastic o.
  hypertrophic o.
  interphalangeal o.
  joint o.
  knee o.
  midtarsal o.
  obese knee o.
  o. padded night sleeve brace
  posttraumatic o.
  primary degenerative o.
  o. radiographic grading
  tarsometatarsal o.
  traumatic o.
osteoarthropathy (OAP)
  hypertrophic pulmonary o.
  idiopathic hypertrophic o. (IHO)
  neuropathic o.
  pneumogenic o.
  pulmonary o.

pustulotic o.
tabetic o.
osteoarthroscopy
hypertrophic o. (HOA)
osteoarthrosis
posttraumatic o.
osteoarthrotomy
osteoarticular
o. allograft
o. allograft transplantation
o. defect
o. graft
o. pathology
o. tuberculosis
Osteo Bi-Flex
osteoblast
neoplastic o.
o. proliferation fluorometric assay
osteoblastic
o. bone regeneration
o. lesion
o. metastasis
o. osteogenic sarcoma
osteoblastoma
spinal o.
Osteobond copolymer bone cement
Osteo-B Plus
osteobunionectomy
osteocachexia
osteocalcin injection
osteocampsia
OsteoCap hip prosthesis
osteocartilaginous
o. exostosis
o. graft
o. lesion
o. loose body
o. mass
o. metaplasia
osteochondral
o. allograft
o. autograft transfer system
(OATS)
o. contusion
o. defect
o. fracture arthrography
o. fracture of dome of talus
o. fragment
o. graft
o. injury
o. lesion
o. non-load-bearing bone fracture

o. prominence
o. ridge
osteochondritis
capitellar o.
crushing o.
o. deformans juvenilis
o. deformans juvenilis dorsi
o. dissecans (OCD, OD)
epiphysial o.
o. juvenilis
o. necroticans
olecranon o.
puncture wound o.
syphilitic o.
osteochondroarthropathy
osteochondrodesmodysplasia
osteochondrodysplasia
osteochondrodystrophia deformans
osteochondrodystrophy
osteochondrofibroma
osteochondrolysis
osteochondroma
congenital o.
epiphysial o.
excision of o.
intraarticular o.
pedunculated o.
sessile-type o.
osteochondromatosis
multiple o.
Ollier o.
synovial o.
osteochondromatous dysplasia
osteochondromyxoma
osteochondropathy
osteochondrophyte
osteochondrosarcoma
osteochondrosis
o. deformans tibiae
o. of metatarsal
osteochondrotic loose body
osteochrondral slice fracture
Osteo-clage cable system
osteoclasis
Blount technique for o.
o. maneuver
osteoclast
Collin o.
Rizzoli o.
o. tension staple
osteoclastic
o. erosion

O

NOTES

osteoclastic *(continued)*
    o. giant cell
    o. resorption
osteoclast-mediated
    o.-m. bone
    o.-m. osteoporosis
osteoclastoma
osteoconduction
osteocutaneous free flap
osteocystoma
osteocyte
osteodesmosis
osteodiastasis
osteodistractor
    Ace/Normed o.
osteodynia
osteodysplasty of Melnick and Needles
osteodystrophy
    Albright hereditary o.
    azotemic o.
    parathyroid o.
    pulmonary o.
    renal o.
osteoectasia
    familial o.
osteoectomy
osteoenchondroma
osteoepiphysis
osteofascial compartment
osteofibrochondrosarcoma
osteofibroma
osteofibromatosis
osteofibrosis
osteofibrous dysplasia
Osteofil allograft paste
OsteoGen
    O. bone growth stimulation
    O. implantable bone growth
      stimulator
    O. resorbable osteogenic bone-
      filling implant
osteogenesis
    distraction o.
    endochondral o.
    o. imperfecta (OI)
    o. imperfecta congenita (OIC)
    O. Imperfecta Foundation (OIF)
    o. imperfecta tarda (OIT)
    membranous o.
    periosteal o.
osteogenic
    o. cell
    o. fibroma
    o. osteomalacia
    o. protein-1 (OP-1)
    o. protein-1 bone graft
    o. sarcoma
    o. scoliosis

Osteogenics BoneSource synthetic bone
   replacement material
OsteoGram
    O. bone density test
    O. 2000 densitometer
osteohalisteresis
osteohydatidosis
osteoid
    calcified o.
    o. osteoma
    o. seam
    unmineralized o.
osteoinduction
osteoinductive enhanced-graft gel
osteokinematic motion
osteokinematics
osteolipochondroma
osteolipoma
Osteolock
    O. acetabular component
    O. HA femoral component
    O. hip prosthesis
    Precision O.
osteology
    metatarsal o.
osteolysis
    acetabular o.
    atraumatic o.
    debris-incited o.
    debris-induced o.
    familial expansile o.
    femoral o.
    malignant acetabular o.
    massive o.
    posttraumatic o.
    pubic o.
osteolytic sarcoma
osteoma
    cavalryman's o.
    compact o.
    o. durum
    o. eburneum
    giant osteoid o.
    intraarticular osteoid o.
    intracapsular osteoid o.
    ivory o.
    osteoid o.
    parosteal o.
    solitary o.
    o. spongiosum
    subperiosteal-paraarticular–type
      osteoid o.
osteomalacia
    nutritional o.
    osteogenic o.
    renal tubular o.
    senile o.
osteomalacic pelvis
osteomanipulative therapy (OMT)

Osteomark bone-loss urine test
osteomatoid
osteomatosis
Osteomed screw
osteomesopyknosis
osteometry
osteomusculocutaneous flap
osteomyelitic
    o. cloaca formation
    o. sinus
osteomyelitis
    Ackerman criteria for o.
    acute hematogenous o. (AHO)
    anaerobic o.
    ankle o.
    blastomycotic o.
    chloramphenicol o.
    cystic o.
    femoral o.
    Gaenslen o.
    Garré sclerosing o.
    hematogenous o.
    hemorrhagic o.
    iatrogenic o.
    long bone o.
    multifocal o.
    nonsuppurative o.
    nonunion o.
    pedal o.
    pin-tract o.
    postfracture o.
    posttraumatic chronic o.
    primary subacute o.
    probe test for o.
    pyogenic vertebral o.
    sclerosing nonsuppurative o.
    secondary hematogenous o.
    spinal o.
    subacute hematogenous o.
    suppurative o.
    synovitis-acne-pustulosis-
     hyperostosis o. (SAPHO)
    tuberculous spinal o.
    tuberculous vertebral o.
    typhoid o.
    vertebral o.
osteomyelodysplasia
osteon
osteonal
    o. bone union
    o. lamellar bone
Osteone air drill

osteonecrosis
    dysbaric o.
    femoral head o.
    Ficat classification of femoral
     head o.
    idiopathic o.
    navicular o.
    nontraumatic idiopathic o.
    posttraumatic o.
    steroid-induced o.
osteoneuralgia
Osteonics
    O. acetabular cup
    O. acetabular dome hole plug
    O. HA femoral implant
    O. hip prosthesis
    O. jig
    O. Omnifit-C stem
    O. Omnifit-HA component
    O. Omnifit-HA hip stem
    O. Scorpio insert
    O. Scorpio posterior cruciate
     retaining total knee system
    Stryker Howmedica O.
osteoonychodysplasia
    hereditary o. (HOOD)
Osteopatch
    O. bone density test
    O. transdermal patch
osteopathia striata
osteopathic
    o. lesion
    o. manipulation
    o. manipulative therapy (OMT)
    o. manipulative treatment
    o. medicine
    o. scoliosis
osteopathology
osteopathy
    alimentary o.
osteopenia
    transient o.
osteopenic
    o. bone
    o. bone stock
osteoperiosteal
    o. bone graft
    o. flap
osteoperiostitis
osteopetrorickets
osteopetrosis
    malignant o.
osteophlebitis

O

NOTES

osteophore
osteophyte
    apophysial joint o.
    bony o.
    bridging o.
    o. elevator
    o. formation
    fringe of o.
    jagged o.
    marginal o.
    posterior o.
osteophytic
    o. bone lip
    o. spur
osteophytosis
osteoplaque
osteoplastic
    o. amputation
    o. flap clamp
    o. laminectomy
    o. necrotomy
    o. reconstruction
osteoplasty
osteoplysis
    massive o.
osteopoikilosis
osteopoikilotic
osteoporosis
    disuse o.
    dual photon densitometry test
      for o.
    femoral o.
    idiopathic juvenile o.
    idiopathic transient o.
    O. Knowledge Questionnaire (OKQ)
    low-turnover o.
    osteoclast-mediated o.
    posttraumatic o.
    o. pseudoglioma syndrome
    regional migratory o.
    secondary o.
    senile o.
    Singh index of o.
    transient o.
osteoporotic
    o. ankle fracture
    o. bone
    o. fracture risk
    o. spine
Osteopower modular handpiece system
osteoprogenitor cell
osteoprotegerin
osteoradionecrosis (ORN)
osteorrhagia
osteorrhaphy
osteosarcoma
    conventional o.
    extraskeletal o.
    intraosseous o.

    parosteal o.
    periosteal o.
    recurrent parosteal o.
    secondary o.
    spinal o.
    telangiectatic o.
OsteoSet
    O. bone filler
    O. bone graft substitute
    O. resorbable bead kit
OsteoSet-T medicated bone graft
  substitute
osteosis
osteospongioma
OsteoStat
    O. disposable power tool
    O. single-use power surgical
      equipment
Osteo-Stim
    O.-S. implantable bone growth
      stimulation
    O.-S. implantable bone growth
      stimulator
osteosuture
osteosynovitis
osteosynthesis
    anterior column o.
    locked intramedullary o.
    lumbar spine vertebral o.
    odontoid process o.
    plate-screw o.
    posterior column o.
    thoracic spine vertebral o.
    thoracolumbar spine vertebral o.
    vertebral o.
    Wagner multiple K-wire o.
osteotabes
osteotelangiectasia
osteothrombophlebitis
osteothrombosis
OsteoTite bone screw
osteotome
    AcuDriver o.
    Acufex o.
    air compression o.
    Albee o.
    Alexander costal o.
    Anderson-Neivert o.
    Andrews o.
    Army o.
    arthroscopic o.
    Aufranc o.
    backcutting o.
    bayonet o.
    Blount o.
    Bowen o.
    box o.
    Campbell o.
    Cavin o.

Cebotome o.
Cherry o.
Cinelli o.
Clayton o.
Cloward spinal fusion o.
Cobb o.
Compere o.
Cottle o.
Crane o.
curved o.
Dautrey o.
Dingman o.
disposable 1-piece o.
Epker o.
fine o.
grooving o.
guarded o.
Hendel guided o.
Hibbs curved o.
Hibbs straight o.
Hoke o.
Joseph o.
Lambotte o.
Leinbach o.
Lexer o.
Meyerding curved o.
Meyerding straight o.
MGH o.
Micro-Aire o.
Miner o.
mini-Lambotte o.
mini-Lexer o.
Mitchell o.
Moberg o.
Moe o.
Moreland o.
Murphy o.
Neivert o.
orthopaedic o.
Padgett o.
Parkes o.
Peck o.
Rhoton o.
Rish o.
rotary o.
Sheehan o.
Silver o.
Simmons o.
Smith-Petersen curved o.
Smith-Petersen straight o.
Stille o.
straight o.
Swanson o.

Swiss pattern o.
thin o.
unguarded o.
U.S. Army o.
Weck o.
West o.
osteotomize
osteotomized bone
osteotomy
Abbott-Gill o.
abduction o.
abductory midfoot o.
abductory wedge o.
acetabular shelf o.
adduction o.
Agliette supracondylar o.
Akin proximal phalangeal o.
Akron midtarsal o.
Amspacher-Messenbaugh closing
  wedge o.
Amstutz-Wilson o.
o. analysis simulation software
  (OASIS)
angulation o.
anterior calcaneal o.
arcuate o.
Austin o.
Axer lateral opening wedge o.
Axer varus derotational o.
Bailey-Dubow o.
Baker-Hill o.
Balacescu closing wedge o.
ball-and-socket trochanteric o.
Barouk microscrew with
  shortening o.
barrel-stave o.
basal chevron o.
basal closing wedge o.
base of neck o.
base wedge o.
basilar closing wedge metatarsal o.
basilar crescentic o.
basilar plantarflexory metatarsal o.
Bellemore-Barrett closing wedge o.
Berens o.
Berman-Gartland metatarsal o.
Bernese periacetabular o.
bifurcation o.
biplane Dwyer o.
biplane trochanteric o.
biplaning of o.
block o.
Blount displacement o.

O

NOTES

osteotomy *(continued)*

Blundell-Jones hip o.
Blundell-Jones varus o.
Bonney-Kessel dorsiflexionary tilt-up o.
Booth wire o.
Brackett o.
Brett o.
o. bunionectomy
calcaneal L o.
calcaneal sliding corrective o.
Campbell tibial o.
Canale o.
canal innominate o.
capital crescentic shelf o.
Carstan reverse wedge o.
Cartam-Treander reverse wedge o.
Chambers o.
chevron o.
chevron-Akin double o.
chevron modification of Mitchell o.
Chiari innominate o.
closed base wedge o. (CBWO)
closed intramedullary o.
closing abductory-wedge o. (CAWO)
closing base-wedge o.
closing wedge greenstick dorsal proximal metatarsal o.
closing wedge high tibial o. (CWHTO)
Cole o.
compensatory basilar o.
compromise o.
controlled rotational o.
corrective lengthening o.
countersinking o.
Coventry distal femoral o.
Coventry proximal tibial o.
Coventry vagal o.
Crawford L-shaped o.
Crego femoral o.
crescentic base wedge o.
crescentic basilar first metatarsal o.
crescentic calcaneal o.
crescentic shelf o. (CSO)
crescent-shaped o.
cuboid-calcaneal o.
cuboid wedge o.
cuneiform o.
cup-and-ball o.
curved o.
cylindrical o.
decompressive o.
Dega pelvic o.
delayed femoral o.
derotational o.
dial pelvic o.
dial periacetabular o.

diaphysial o.
Dickson geometric o.
Dillwyn-Evans o.
Dimon o.
Dimon-Hughston intertrochanteric o.
displacement anterior cavus V o.
distal L o.
distal oblique sliding o.
dome proximal tibial o.
dome-shaped o.
dorsal V o.
dorsiflexion metatarsal o.
dorsiflexory wedge o.
double o.
Dunn o.
Dwyer o.
Dwyer calcaneal o.
elevating o.
Elizabethtown o.
Elmslie-Trillat o.
Emmon o.
epiphysial-metaphysial o.
Eppright dial o.
Estersohn o.
Evans anterior opening wedge calcaneal o.
eversion o.
extended slide trochanteric o.
extension o.
failed femoral o.
femoral derotation o.
Fernandez o.
fibular o.
Fish cuneiform o.
flexion o.
Fowler o.
free-floating o.
French lateral closing-wedge o.
Fulkerson oblique tibial tubercle o.
Gant o.
Ganz periacetabular o.
geometric supracondylar extension o.
Gerbert o.
Giannestras oblique metatarsal o.
Giannestras step-down modified o.
Gibson-Piggott o.
Gigli saw o.
Gleich o.
glenoid o.
Golden closing wedge o.
greater tuberosity o.
Greenfield o.
Green-Laird modification of Reverdin o.
Green-Reverdin o.
greenstick dorsal proximal metatarsal o.
Green-Watermann o.

Gudas scarf Z-plasty o.
Haas o.
Haddad metatarsal o.
Hass o.
Helal o.
high tibial o. (HTO)
Hirayma o.
Hohmann o.
Hohmann-Thomasen metatarsal o.
horizontal o.
iliac o.
Ingram o.
innominate o.
intertrochanteric varus o.
intraarticular o.
intracapsular o.
intraepiphysial o.
Irwin o.
Japas o.
Johnson chevron o.
Kalamchi o.
Kalish o.
Kaplan o.
Kawamura dome o.
Kawamura pelvic o.
Kelikian modified Z o.
Kelly-Keck o.
Kelly-Kelly o.
Kelly tendon lengthening o.
Kessel-Bonney extension o.
Koutsogiannis calcaneal
  displacement o.
Kramer modification of
  Hohmann o.
Lambrinudi o.
Langenskiöld o.
Le Fort I–III o.
Lelièvre o.
Lichtblau o.
Lindgren oblique o.
Lindseth o.
linear o.
Lorenz o.
L-shaped o.
Ludloff o.
Macewen o.
malleolar o.
mandibular o.
Maquet dome o.
Marquardt angulation o.
Martin o.
Mau o.
Mayday distal first metatarsal o.

McKay o.
McMurray o.
metacarpal o.
metaphysial o.
metatarsal head o.
metatarsal neck o.
metatarsal oblique o.
metatarsal proximal dome o.
metatarsal Reverdin o.
metatarsal V-shaped o.
metatarsus primus o.
midshaft metatarsal o.
midtarsal dome o.
midtarsal V o.
Mitchell distal o.
Mitchell posterior displacement o.
Mitchell step-down o.
modified Hohmann o.
modified Kalish o.
modified Mau o.
modified Wilson o.
modified Z o.
Molesworth o.
Moore o.
Mueller intertochanteric varus o.
Mueller transposition o.
Müller o.
oblique closing wedge o. (OCWO)
oblique proximal phalangeal o.
oblique slide o.
Obwegeser sagittal mandibular o.
offset-V o.
open base wedge o.
opening abductory wedge o.
  (OAWO)
opening wedge o.
Osgood rotational o.
Pauwels proximal o.
Pauwels valgus o.
Pauwels Y o.
pedicle subtraction o.
peg-in-hole o.
Peimer reduction o.
pelvic o.
Pemberton pericapsular o.
percutaneous o.
periacetabular o.
pericapsular o.
phalangeal o.
Phemister o.
o. pin
plantarflexor proximal metatarsal o.
plantarflexory o.

NOTES

O

osteotomy *(continued)*
    Platou o.
    posterior calcaneal displacement o.
    posterior iliac o.
    posterior spinal wedge o.
    Potts eversion o.
    Potts tibial o.
    radial recession o.
    radial wedge o.
    Rappaport o.
    rearfoot o.
    reduction o.
    Regnauld o.
    Reverdin o.
    Reverdin-Green o.
    Reverdin-Laird o.
    reverse Austin o.
    reverse closing base wedge o.
    reverse Dillwyn-Evans calcaneal o.
    rotational scarf o.
    Roux o.
    sagittal split o.
    sagittal Z o.
    Sakoff o.
    Salter innominate o.
    Salter pelvic o.
    Samilson crescentic calcaneal o.
    sandwich o.
    Sarmiento intertrochanteric o.
    Scanz o.
    scarf Z o.
    Schanz angulation o.
    Schanz femoral o.
    Schanz-type proximal femoral
      valgization o.
    Schede hip o.
    Schwartz dorsiflexory o.
    segmental alveolar o.
    shortening o.
    Siffert intraepiphysial o.
    Simmonds-Menelaus metatarsal o.
    Simmonds-Menelaus proximal
      phalangeal o.
    Simmons o.
    Smith-Petersen o.
    Sofield o.
    Southwick biplane trochanteric o.
    Speed o.
    spike o.
    spinal o.
    Sponsel oblique o.
    Stamm metatarsal o.
    Steel triple innominate o.
    Steel triradiate o.
    step o.
    step-cut o.
    step-down o.
    subcapital o.
    subcondylar o.

    subtraction o.
    subtrochanteric o.
    Sugioka transtrochanteric
      rotational o.
    supracondylar femoral
      derotational o.
    supracondylar varus o.
    supramalleolar derotational o.
    supramalleolar varus derotation o.
    supratubercular wedge o.
    Sutherland-Greenfield o.
    Swanson o.
    talar neck o.
    talocalcaneal o.
    tarsal wedge o.
    tendon lengthening o.
    Thompson telescoping V o.
    through-and-through V-shaped
      horizontal o.
    tibial tuberosity o.
    total maxillary o.
    translational o.
    transpedal multiplanar wedge o.
    transtrochanteric rotational o.
    transtrochanteric valgus o. (TVO)
    trapezoidal resection o.
    Trillat o.
    triplane o.
    triple innominate o.
    trochanteric o.
    tubercle o.
    U o.
    unplanned valgus o.
    V o.
    Vanore o.
    varus rotational o. (VRO)
    varus rotation shortening o.
    vertical sagittal split o. (VSO)
    visor o.
    visor/sandwich o.
    V-shaped o.
    Wagdy double-V o.
    Waterman o.
    Weber humeral o.
    Weber subcapital o.
    wedge o.
    Weil o.
    Whitman o.
    Wilson double oblique o.
    Wilson oblique displacement o.
    Wiltse ankle o.
    Wiltse varus supramalleolar o.
    Y o.
    Yancey o.
    Youngswick o.
    Yu o.

osteotomy/bunionectomy
    base wedge o./b.
    closed wedge o./b.

crescentic base wedge o./b.
Kelikian modified Z o./b.
Mitchell o./b.
open base wedge o./b.
rotational scarf o./b.
scarf Z o./b.
supertubercular wedge o./b.
osteotomy-osteoclasis
Moore o.-o.
osteotribe
osteotripsy
osteotrite
Osteotron stimulator for bone union
osteotylus
OsteoView
O. digital bone densitometer
O. 2000 imaging system
O. x-ray device
ostium, pl. **ostia**
ostraceous
ostracosis
Ostrum-Furst syndrome
Ostrup harvesting technique
Oswestry
O. Disability Score
O. index
O. Low Back Pain Disability
Oswestry-O'Brien spinal stapler
OT
occupational therapy
OTADL
Occupational Therapy Activities of Daily
Living
otoacoustic emission (OAE)
Ottawa Ankle Rule (OAR)
Otto
O. Bock 1A30 Greissinger Plus
foot
O. Bock 1D25 Dynamic Plus foot
O. Bock dynamic prosthesis
O. Bock MOBIS mobility system
O. Bock 3R65 children's hydraulic
knee joint
O. Bock 3R60 EBS knee
O. Bock 3R45 modular knee joint
O. Bock 3R80 modular rotary
hydraulic knee
O. Bock Safety constant-friction
knee
O. Bock system electric hand
O. disease
O. pelvis
O. pelvis dislocation

Oudard procedure
out
draped o.
step out, turn o. (SOTO)
toeing o.
outcome
O. and Assessment Information Set
(OASIS)
o. measure
Michigan Hand O.'s
Outerbridge
O. classification
O. degenerative arthritis staging
O. ridge
O. scale
Outerbridge-Kashiwagi procedure
outer malleolus
outflow cannula
outgrowth
osseous patella o.
outlet
cervical o.
supraspinatus o.
o. view
outline
inferior o.
medial o.
out-of-cast ankle brace
outpatient
o. physical therapy
o. rehabilitation
outpouching
synovial o.
output
cardiac o.
urinary o.
outrigger
o. arm
o. cast
dorsal wrist splint with o.
Harrington distraction o.
o. splint
O. wire
outside-in technique
outside-the-boot brace
outside-to-outside arthroscopy technique
outsole
outstretched hand
out-toeing gait
outward rotation
Ovadia-Beals tibial plafond fracture
classification

O

NOTES

Oval-8
O.-8 kit
O.-8 ring splint
O.-8 sizing set
oval
o. amputation
o. curved-cup curette
o. washer
over-bed table
Overcast cast cover
overcorrection
overdistraction
Overdyke hip prosthesis
overextension
overflexion
overgrowth
bony o.
terminal o.
overhead
o. exercise test
o. olecranon traction
o. pulley
Overholt
O. clip-applying forceps
O. operation
overhydration
fluid o.
overlap
tibiofibular o.
overlapped uprights in orthosis
overlapping fifth toe
overlay
Bodyline sleeper mattress o.
o. drafting
o. mattress
o. plate
Stimulite honeycomb mattress o.
x-ray o.
overload
compression o.
lateral forefoot o.
progressive o.
torsional o.
overmotivation
overpull
overreaching
overriding fifth toe
oversewn
oversize tennis shoe
over-straight toe
overstrain
overstretch weakness

over-the-door traction unit
over-the-top
o.-t.-t. knee operation
o.-t.-t. knee procedure
o.-t.-t. position
Overton dowel graft
overtraining syndrome
over-tying wire
overuse
o. injury
o. injury assessment
o. syndrome
OW
open wedge
Owen gauze dressing
Owens silk
Oxford
O. fixator
O. meniscal unicompartmental knee system
O. meniscal unicompartment prosthesis
O. method
O. method for scoring skeletal maturity
O. uncompartmental device
O. unicompartmental knee
oxidation
carbohydrate o.
fat o.
oxide
ethylene o.
oxidized
o. zirconium
o. zirconium alloy on implant
oximeter
pulse o.
Oxiplex/SP
O./SP bioresorbable product
O./SP gel
Oxycel oxidized cellulose
oxygen
dysbaric o.
epiphysial o.
hyperbaric o. (HBO)
o. myelography
o. seizure
o. tension
o. therapy
transcutaneous o.
oxymorphone hydrochloride
oyster-shell brace

P

passive

P/3

proximal third

PA

posteroanterior

Paas disease

PaBA anchor

Paced Auditory Serial Addition test (PASAT)

pachydactylia

pachydactylous

pachydactyly

pachyonychia congenita

pachyperiostitis

pachypodous

pacinian mechanoreceptor

Paci operation

pack

Adaptic p.
Arctic Blaze hot/cold p.
Avitene p.
Back-Ease aromatherapy hot/cold p.
Baxter personal Von-Loc ice p.
BodyIce cold p.
cold p.
Coldhot p.
Colpacs p.
cool p.
CP2 inflatable cold p.
DynaHeat hot p.
gel p.
Gelfoam p.
Glacier P.
6-p. hand exercise
hot p. (HP)
hot moist p. (HMP)
Hydrocollator steam p.
ice p.
I.C.E. Down cold p.
instant cold p.
Jack Frost hot/cold p.
JoyBags therapeutic heat p.
Kool Kit cold therapy p.
Merocel p.
MSC cold p.
Neck-Roll aromatherapy hot/cold p.
Polar P.
Softouch Cold/Hot P.
P. technique
TheraBeads microwaveable moist heat p.
Thera-Med cold p.
Thermal P.
ThermalSoft hot & cold p.'s
Thermophore hot p.
Ultimate Cold N' Hot P.
vaginal p.
Whitehall Glacier P.

Pack-Ehrlich deep iliac dissection

packing

Adaptic p.
gauze p.
Nu Gauze p.
wound p.

Pacs

Boo-Boo P.

PACU

postanesthesia care unit

pad

ABD p.
abdominal lap p.
Achilles heel p.
Airex balance p.
AirLITE support p.
Aliplast p.
alternating pressure p.
antidecubitus p.
aperture p.
Aquaflex gel p.
Aquatech cast p.
Aquatherm bed p.
Arthropor cup p.
artificial fat p.
balance p.
Bauerfeind silicone heel p.
buttocks p.
buttress p.
calcaneal fat p.
Charnley foam suture p.
cloverleaf met foot p.
cold p.
crest buttress p.
dancer's p.
digital p.
distal star p.
elbow p.
fat p.
fibrocartilaginous p.
finger p.
fingertip p.
foam p.
foveal fat p.
Hapad heel p.
Hapad longitudinal metatarsal arch p.
Hapad medial arch p.
Hapad prefabricated wool felt p.
heel fat p.
Hoffa fat p.

P

pad (*continued*)
    horseshoe heel p.
    horseshoe-shaped felt p.
    Hydrocollator p.
    infrapatellar fat p.
    internal gel p.
    J p.
    Kager fat p.
    knee-control orthosis p.
    knuckle p.
    lamb's wool p.
    lateral p.
    L-shaped p.
    MagneCore magnetic therapy p.
    metatarsal p.
    Mikulicz p.
    navicular shoe p.
    OEC popliteal p.
    Ortho-Cel p.
    Ortho-Foam elbow/heel p.
    painful heel p.
    patellar fat p.
    patellar orthosis p.
    Pedi-Cushions p.
    Pedifix crest p.
    Pedifix hammertoe p.
    Pen/Alps distal p.
    plantar fat p.
    pre-Achilles fat p.
    prefabricated wool felt p.
    premalleolar fat p.
    pubic p.
    Redigrip knee p.
    reticulated polyurethane p.
    retropatellar fat p.
    Roho heel p.
    scalene fat p.
    scaphoid shoe p.
    Scholl p.
    second skin p.
    sensor p.
    shock-absorbent heel p.
    shoe heel p.
    silicone p.
    Silipos digital p.
    Sof-Rol cast p.
    Sof Sole Sof Gel heel p.
    Sorbothane recoil p.
    S'port Max stabilization p.
    spur p.
    Staph-Chek p.
    supracondylar p.
    Sure Sport p.
    T-Foam bed p.
    Thermapad p.
    Thermophore moist heat p.
    thickness of heel p.
    Vac-Pac p.
    valgus knee control p.
    varus knee control p.
    Zimfoam p.

padded
    p. aluminum splint
    p. board splint
    p. bolster
    p. button
    p. clamp
    p. plywood splint
    p. tongue blade splint

padding
    biplane p.
    cast p.
    contoured felt p.
    cotton cast p.
    Delta-Rol cast p.
    felt p.
    Kerlix cast p.
    moleskin p.
    Molestick p.
    pressure relief p.
    Protouch synthetic orthopaedic p.
    QuickStick p.
    Reston p.
    Sifoam p.
    splint p.
    Therafoam p.
    Thero-Skin gel p.
    Webril cotton p.

Padgett
    P. electric dermatome
    P. osteotome
    P. prosthesis

pad/protector

PAG
    periaqueductal gray

Pagddu procedure

Paget
    P. disease
    P. juvenile syndrome
    P. osteitis deformans
    P. quiet necrosis
    P. test

Paget-associated osteogenic sarcoma

pagetoid
    p. bone
    p. osteitis

Paget-Schrötter syndrome

pain
    aches and p.'s
    Achilles tendon p.
    aching p.
    acute p.
    adolescent back p.
    AHCPR guidelines for treatment of acute low back p.
    amputation-related bone p.
    p., asymmetry, range, tone, special test (PARTS)

p. at rest
back p.
bandlike p.
Behavioral Assessment of P. (BAP)
boring p.
burning p.
causalgic p.
cervical myofascial p.
chronic low back p. (CLBP)
chronic subtalar joint p.
contralateral p.
p. control infusion pump
cross leg p.
deafferentation p.
dermatomal p.
discogenic neck p.
p. drawing
dull aching p.
p. dysfunction syndrome
endogenous p.
epicritic p.
exercise-induced breast p.
fibromyalgic p.
functional back p.
gate control theory of p.
glenohumeral p.
gouty p.
groin p.
growing p.
idiopathic anterior knee p.
idiopathic arm p.
impingement p.
p. induction
joint line p.
kinetic foot p.
lancinating p.
low back p. (LBP)
machine-gun-like p.
p. measurement
Multiaxial Assessment of P. (MAP)
myofascial p.
myotomal p.
neurologic p.
osteoarthritic knee p.
patellofemoral p. (PFP)
perimalleolar p.
periscapulitis shoulder p.
persistent p.
phantom limb p.
pillar p.
plantar p.
postherpetic p.
postoperative p.

posttraumatic p.
prickling p.
primary focus of p.
Pronex pneumatic device for
  cervical p.
p. provocation test
radicular p.
recalcitrant p.
referred neuritic p.
referred trigger point p.
rest p. (RP)
Roland index of low back p.
scapulothoracic p.
sclerotomal p.
searing p.
shooting p.
splintlike p.
static foot p.
sympathetically mediated p.
p. threshold gauge
ticlike p.
vise like p.
volley of p.
p. with weightbearing
pain-all-over syndrome
PainFree pump
painful
  p. arc
  p. arc sign
  p. arc syndrome
  p. femoral head prosthesis
  p. gait
  p. heel
  p. heel pad
  p. minor intervertebral dysfunction
    (PMID)
  p. spur
  p. stump
  p. toe
pain-related sleep disturbance
paint
  p. gun injury
  p. thinner injury
paired
  p. discharge
  p. response
  p. scintigraphy
  p. stimulus
Pak
  Apollo hot/cold P.
PAL
  posterior axillary line

NOTES

P

Palacos
P. cement adhesive
P. radiopaque bone cement
P. R bone cement
palatal myoclonus
palatine bone
Palex expansion screw
Paley classification
PAL-Guard postamputation limb guard
palindromic
p. arthropathy
p. rheumatism
palliation
palliative care
pallor
palm
p. guard
p. space
palmar
p. advancement flap
p. aponeurosis
p. approach
p. arch
p. carpal ligament
p. carpometacarpal ligament
p. clip
p. cock-up splint
p. creaking
p. crease
p. cross-finger flap
p. fascia
p. fasciotomy
p. fibromatosis
p. flexion
p. grasp reflex
p. incision
p. intercarpal deltoid ligament
p. interosseous muscle
p. luxation
p. metacarpal ligament
p. pinch
p. plate
p. radiocarpal ligament
p. swab kit
p. synovectomy
p. tilt
p. T-plate
p. ulnocarpal ligament
p. wrist
p. wrist splint
palmaris
p. digitorum superficialis muscle
p. longus (PL)
p. longus muscle
p. longus tendon
palmature
Palmer
P. bone nail
P. method

P. primary fracture
P. screw
P. technique
P. transscaphoid perilunar
dislocation
P. triangular fibrocartilage complex
lesion classification
Palmerian
P. law
P. philosophy
palm-to-axilla dressing
palm-up test
palpable band
palpation
p. of anterior superior iliac spine
digital p.
end-feel p.
flat p.
p. of iliac crest
intersegmental range of motion p.
(IRMP)
motion p.
optimizing motion p.
pincer p.
p. of posterior superior iliac spine
screening p.
static p.
p. testing
palpatory
p. diagnosis
p. examination
p. skill
p. technique
p. technique for joint assessment
PALS
Pediatric Advanced Life Support
palsy
ataxic cerebral p.
athetoid cerebral p.
backpack p.
Bell p.
brachial plexus p.
cerebral p. (CP)
combined nerve p.
crutch p.
drummer-boy p.
Duchenne-Erb p.
dyskinetic cerebral p.
Erb p.
Erb-Duchenne p.
flaccid cerebral p.
handlebar p.
high median-high radial p.
high median-high ulnar p.
high ulnar-high radial p.
Hoke procedure for tibial p.
Klumpke p.
long thoracic nerve p.
low median-low ulnar p.

median nerve p.
nerve p.
peripheral nerve p.
peroneal nerve p.
posterior interosseous nerve p.
postnatal cerebral p.
prisoner's p.
progressive supranuclear p.
pseudobulbar p.
radial nerve p.
Saturday night p.
sciatic p.
spastic cerebral p.
tardy ulnar p.
thenar p.
thoracic nerve p.
tourniquet p.
ulnar nerve p.

Paltrinieri-Trentani
P.-T. prosthesis
P.-T. resurfacing

Palumbo
P. ankle stabilizer
P. dynamic patellar brace
P. knee brace
P. knee support
P. patella tracker
P. stabilizing brace

pamidronate
Panacryl suture
Panafil ointment
Panafil-White ointment
Panalok absorbable suture anchor
panaris
melanotic p.
panarteritis nodosa
panarthritis
panastragaloid arthrodesis
pancake hand
panclavicular dislocation
pancreatic enzyme therapy
pandemic
Panje voice button prosthesis
panmetatarsal
p. head resection
p. tendon suspension
Panner disease
panniculus adiposus
pannus
p. deformity
p. of synovium
Panogauze Hydrogel wound dressing
panosteitis

Panoview
P. arthroscope
P. arthroscopic system
panplexopathy
pan splint
pant
prophylactic abduction p.
pantalar
p. ankle fusion
p. arthrodesis
pantalocrural
p. arthritic destruction
p. arthritis
pantaloon
p. brace
p. spica cast
p. walking cast
Pantopaque
pantrapezial arthritis
pants-over-vest
p.-o.-v. capsulorrhaphy
p.-o.-v. technique
panty
Cadenza p.
PAOD
peripheral arterial occlusive disease
papain-urea-chlorophyllin copper complex debriding and healing ointment
Papavasiliou olecranon fracture classification
papaverine
papillary adenoma
Papineau
P. graft
P. technique
papule
Gottron p.
piezogenic p.
papyrus
Edwin Smith p.
PAR
postanesthesia recovery
paraaminosalicylic acid
paraarticular
p. arthrodesis
p. calcification
Parabath paraffin heat treatment
parabola
metatarsal p.
Para-Care paraffin therapy bath
paracervical

NOTES

P

parachute
    Corkscrew P.
    p. jumper's dislocation
    p. reflex
    p. technique
    p. test
    p. therapy
parachutist ankle brace
paradoxical
    p. ankle reflex
    p. breathing
    p. extensor reflex
    p. flexor reflex
    p. lumbrical-plus finger
    p. patellar reflex
    p. triceps reflex
paraffin
    p. bath (PB)
    p. heat therapy
    p. implant material
    p. mitt
    p. treatment
    p. wax therapeutic application
Parafon
    P. Forte
    P. Forte DSC
paraganglioma
    medullary p.
paraglenoid sulcus
parajugular line
parallel
    p. goniometric measure
    p. pin kit
    p. pitch lines
    p. squat exercise
parallelism
parallelogram electrogoniometer
paralysis, pl. **paralyses**
    adductor pollicis p.
    p. agitans
    atrophic muscular p.
    backpack p.
    brachial plexus p.
    Chaves-Rapp p.
    common peroneal nerve p.
    compression p.
    cruciate p.
    crutch p.
    Cruveilhier p.
    Dewar-Harris p.
    Dickson p.
    familial periodic p.
    femoral nerve p.
    flaccid p.
    gluteus medius p.
    Haas p.
    hand p.
    Henry p.
    intrinsic p.

    isolated p.
    musculocutaneous nerve p.
    musculospiral p.
    myogenic p.
    myopathic p.
    p. notariorum
    peripheral p.
    peroneal p.
    Pott p.
    pressure p.
    Remak p.
    rucksack p.
    serratus anterior p.
    spastic p.
    spinomuscular p.
    tourniquet p.
    ulnar nerve p.
    Vastamäki p.
    Volkmann ischemic p.
    Whitman p.
    writer's p.
paralytic
    p. chest
    p. contracture
    p. foot
    p. kyphosis
    p. scoliosis
paramalleolar artery
ParaMax
    P. ACL guide system
    P. angled driver
paramedian
    p. approach
    p. sagittal plane
parameniscus
parameter
    angular p.
    clinical p.
    neutralization p.
    radiographic p.
    rotational p.
    translational p.
paramethasone acetate
paramount
    P. total body plate-loaded machine
    P. 3-way press bench
paramyoclonus multiplex
paramyotonia congenita
paraneoplastic neuromuscular syndrome
paraosseous lesion
paraparesis
paraparetic gait
parapatellar
    p. approach
    p. arthrotomy
    p. incision
    p. plica
    p. synovitis
paraphysiological space

paraphysiologic zone
paraplegia
    incomplete p.
    postoperative p.
    Pott p.
    spastic p.
    traumatic p.
parapodium orthosis
pararectus approach
parasacral block
parasagittal
    p. groove
    p. scar
parascapular flap
paraspinal
    p. abscess
    p. approach
    p. mapping
    p. muscle
    p. muscle spasm
    p. musculature
    p. point
    p. rod application
    p. skin temperature thermocouple
      instrument
paraspinous muscular spasm
parasympathetic
    p. innervation
    p. nervous system (PNS)
parasympatholytic
paratenon
paratenonitis
parathenar incision
parathormone level
parathyroid
    p. gland
    p. osteodystrophy
paratonia
paratrooper fracture
paravertebral
    p. abscess
    p. block
    p. muscle
    p. muscle spasm
    p. musculature
    p. sympathetic chain
paraxial hemimelia
Pare elbow dislocation reduction
parenteral nutrition
paresis
    limb-girdle-trunk p.
paresthesia, pl. **paresthesias**
    Berger p.

    intermittent p.
    saddle p.
paresthetica
    cheiralgia p.
paretic leg
ParFlex orthotic
Parham
    P. band
    P. support
Parham-Martin
    P.-M. band
    P.-M. bone-holding clamp
    P.-M. fracture apparatus
    P.-M. fracture device
parietal
    p. bone
    p. pleura
    p. tendon sheath layer
    p. tuberosity
Paris
    elastic plaster of P.
    P. manual therapy table
    plaster of P. (POP)
park
    P. aneurysm
    transverse line of P.
Parkes osteotome
Parkinson disease
parkinsonian gait
Parona space
paronychia bur
parosteal
    p. chondrosarcoma
    p. lesion
    p. osteogenic sarcoma
    p. osteoma
    p. osteosarcoma
parosteitis
parosteosis
paroxysmal burning
PAR-Q
    Physical Activity Readiness
    Questionnaire
parquetry set
Parrish-Mann hammertoe technique
Parrish procedure
parrot
    p. foot
    P. node
    P. pseudoparalysis
parrot-beak tear
parry fracture

NOTES

P

pars
  p. defect
  p. interarticularis fracture
Parsonage-Aldren-Turner syndrome
Parsonage-Turner
  P.-T. neuronitis
  P.-T. syndrome
2-part
  2-p. Apley test
  2-p. fracture
4-part
  4-p. fracture
  4-p. variant
1-part fracture
3-part fracture
partial
  p. adactyly
  p. ankylosis
  p. aphalangia
  p. cervical vertebrectomy
  p. discectomy
  p. dislocation
  p. fasciectomy
  p. fibulectomy
  p. hand amputation
  p. hemimelia
  p. matricectomy
  p. meniscectomy
  p. ossicular
    reconstruction/replacement
    prosthesis
  p. ossicular replacement prosthesis
    (PORP)
  p. ostectomy
  p. patellectomy
  p. sit-ups back exercise technique
  p. thromboplastin time (PTT)
  p. weightbearing (PWB)
partially
  p. necrotic osseous trabecula
  p. threaded pin
participation
  sports p.
particle of bone
particulate
  p. cancellous bone graft
  p. synovitis
  p. wear debris
partnership
  P. implant
  P. instrument
  P. system
partridge
  P. band
  P. strap
PARTS
  pain, asymmetry, range, tone, special test

Partsch
  P. chisel
  P. gouge
Parvin
  P. gravity technique
  P. maneuver
  P. reduction
PASA
  proximal articular set angle
PASAT
  Paced Auditory Serial Addition test
PASG
  pneumatic antishock garment
passage
  adiabatic fast p.
  wire p.
passer
  Batzdorf cervical wire p.
  Brand tendon p.
  Bunnell tendon p.
  Charnley wire p.
  Concept 2-pin p.
  curved p.
  DeMayo suture p.
  Framer tendon p.
  Hewson suture p.
  Incavo wire p.
  ligature p.
  Malis ligature p.
  Shuttle-Relay suture p.
  suture p.
  tendon p.
  Wedeen wire p.
  wire p.
passing suture
passivation metal instrument
passive (P)
  p. accessory motion test
  p. assistance exercise
  p. dorsiflexion
  p. gliding technique
  p. insufficiency
  p. intervertebral motion (PIVM)
  p. joint manipulation
  p. mobility
  p. mobility testing
  p. motion device
  p. motion machine
  p. movement
  p. night stretch splint
  p. patellar glide test
  p. patellar tilt test
  p. physiological test
  p. physiotherapy
  p. plantarflexion
  p. positioning device
  p. prehension orthosis (PPO)
  p. range of motion (PROM)
  p. range of motion exercise

p. resistive exercise
p. restraint
p. spacer
p. straight leg raising
p. stretch
p. stretch exercise
p. traction table
p. treatment modality
Passow chisel
Passport instrumentation
paste
    absorbable collagen p. (ACP)
    allograft p.
    bone p.
    Coe-pak p.
    electrode p.
    Grafton Plus DBM demineralized
      bone graft p.
    OrthoBlast p.
    Osteofil allograft p.
    Regenafil allograft p.
    Unna p.
Pasteurella multocida
PAT
    Physical Ability Test
Patau syndrome
patch
    Carrel p.
    p. dressing
    felt p.
patella, pl. **patellae**
    absent p.
    p. alta
    apex patellae
    apex of head of p.
    p. baja
    p. ballottement
    p. bipartita
    bipartite p.
    p. bone saw
    chondromalacia patellae
    p. cubiti
    p. cup
    débridement p.
    dislocated p.
    p. displacement
    floating p.
    grasshopper p.
    head of p.
    high-riding p.
    jockey cap p.
    low-riding p.
    p. luxation

maltracking p.
minima p.
multipartite p.
plastic p.
prosthetic p.
P. Pusher
skyline x-ray view of p.
slipping p.
squinting p.
subluxing p.
superior pole of p.
p. tracker
p. turndown approach
undersurface of p.
patellalgia
Patellaligner knee brace
patellapexy
patellaplasty
patellar
    p. advancement
    p. affection
    p. aligner
    p. alignment
    p. apprehension sign
    p. apprehension test
    p. band
    P. Band knee protector
    p. bar
    p. bone-tendon-bone autograft
    p. bursa
    p. bursitis
    p. button
    p. cement clamp
    p. chondromalacia
    p. clonus
    p. clunk syndrome
    p. contour
    p. dislocation cast
    p. drill guide
    p. edge
    p. fat pad
    p. fossa
    p. glide
    p. glide test
    p. groove
    p. hesitation sign
    p. inhibition test
    p. instability
    p. intraarticular dislocation
    p. jerk (PJ)
    p. ligament
    p. ligament-patellar ratio
    p. malalignment syndrome

NOTES

P

patellar *(continued)*
    p. orthosis pad
    p. pair syndrome
    p. plug
    p. portal
    p. realignment
    p. reamer guide
    p. reamer shaft
    p. reduction clamp
    p. reflex
    p. region
    p. resection guide
    p. resurfacing
    p. resurfacing implant
    p. retinacula release
    p. retinaculum
    p. retraction test
    p. rotation
    p. shelf
    p. skyline view
    p. sleeve fracture
    p. stabilizer
    p. stabilizing brace (PSB)
    p. subluxation
    p. taping
    p. tap test
    p. tendinitis
    p. tendon
    p. tendon-bearing (PTB)
    p. tendon-bearing below-knee
      prosthesis
    p. tendon-bearing brace
    p. tendon-bearing orthosis (PTBO)
    p. tendon-bearing-supracondylar
    p. tendon-bearing-supracondylar-
      suprapatellar (PTB-SC-SP)
    p. tendon-bearing suspension
      (PTBS)
    p. tendon bone block
    p. tendon graft
    p. tendon repair
    p. tendon socket (PTS)
    p. tendon stabilization (PTS)
    p. tendon substitution
    p. tendon transfer (PTT)
    p. tendon weightbearing brace
      orthosis
    p. tendon weightbearing cast
    p. tracking
    p. tracking orthosis
    p. transplant
    p. tuberosity
patellectomy
    partial p.
    total p.
    West-Soto-Hall p.
patelloadductor reflex
patellofemoral
    p. alignment

    p. angle
    p. arthritis
    p. articulation
    p. brace
    p. compartment
    p. congruence
    p. crepitation
    p. disorder
    p. dysarthrosis
    p. dysfunction (PFD)
    p. dysplasia
    p. groove
    p. groove cartilage
    p. joint
    p. joint radiography
    p. joint reaction force
    p. ligament
    p. orthosis
    p. pain (PFP)
    p. pain syndrome (PPS)
    p. realignment
    p. stress syndrome
patellomeniscal ligament
patelloplasty
patelloquadriceps
    p. tendon
    p. tendon substitution
patellotibial ligament
Patel medial meniscectomy
Paterson
    P. procedure
    P. technique
PATH
    Planning Alternative Tomorrows with
      Hope
PathFinder pedicle screw
Pathfinder prosthetic foot
pathogenesis
pathognomonic sign
pathokinesiologic
pathologic
    p. amputation
    p. barrier
    p. dislocation
    p. fracture
    p. reflex
    p. spondylolisthesis
pathological plica
pathology
    bone p.
    heel pad p.
    osteoarticular p.
pathomechanical state
pathomechanics
    gait p.
    juvenile flatfoot p.
    kyphotic deformity p.
    spinal fusion p.
pathomechanism

pathway
    neuromeningeal p.
patient
    p. positioning
    Test of Orientation for
        Rehabilitation P.'s (TORP)
patient-controlled
    p.-c. analgesia (PCA)
    p.-c. anesthesia (PCA)
patient-on-table friction
patient-resisted internal rotation
patient-table interface
Patrick
    P. cross-leg maneuver
    P. drill
    P. sign
    P. test
    P. trigger area
Patrick/FABERE test
Patten-Bottom-Perthes brace
pattern
    AO fracture p.
    calcaneal gait p.
    cloverleaf p.
    Collimator plugging p.
    compression p.
    corduroy cloth p.
    curve p. (type I, II)
    dermatomal p.
    DISI collapse p.
    double major curve p.
    facilitation p.
    firing p.
    fracture p.
    full interference p.
    gait p.
    heel-toe p.
    honeycomb p.
    injury p.
    interference p.
    intermediate interference p.
    kinematic gait p.
    lamellar p.
    left thoracolumbar major curve p.
    locomotor p.
    p. of motion
    neuromuscular gait p.
    nondermatomal p.
    nonradicular p.
    plantar pressure p.
    PNF p.
    2-point step-to gait p.
    polka-dot p.

    posterior depression p.
    primitive locomotor p.
    recruitment p.
    reduced interference p.
    right thoracic, left lumbar curve p.
    right thoracic, left thoracolumbar
        curve p.
    right thoracic minor curve p.
    single ray p.
    single-unit p.
    storiform p.
    stretch p.
    p. of thrust
    whorled p.
patterning
    Aston p.
PattStrap knee support
patty
    cement p.
    cottonoid p.
pauciarticular arthritis
Paufique blade
Paulos ligament technique
Paulson knee retractor
Paulus plate
Pauly point
Pauwels
    P. angle
    P. femoral neck fracture
        classification
    P. fracture
    P. operation
    P. proximal osteotomy
    P. technique
    P. valgus osteotomy
    P. Y osteotomy
Pauzat disease
Pavlik
    P. bandage
    P. harness
    P. harness splint
    P. sling
Pavlov ratio
Payr sign
PB
    paraffin bath
    peroneus brevis
PBS
    peroneus brevis split
PC
    PC Performer knee
    PC Performer knee prosthesis

NOTES

P

PCA
   patient-controlled analgesia
   patient-controlled anesthesia
   porous-coated anatomic
      PCA cutting guide
      PCA hip stem
      PCA medullary guide
      PCA Original prosthesis
      PCA primary total knee system
      PCA Standard prosthesis
      PCA total hip replacement
      PCA unconstrained tricompartmental prosthesis
      PCA unicompartmental knee prosthesis
      PCA Universal total knee instrument system
PCB
   proximal communicating branch
PCE
   physical capacity evaluation
PCL
   posterior cruciate ligament
      PCL Protension isometer
PCL-oriented
      PCL-o. placement (POP)
      PCL-o. placement marking hook
PDA
   plantar digital artery
pDEXA x-ray peripheral bone densitometer
PDGF
   platelet-derived growth factor
PDLS
   physical daily living skills
PDN
   prosthetic disc nucleus
      PDN device
PDS
   polydioxanone suture
      PDS band
      PDS knot
      PDS suture
pDXA
   peripheral dual-energy x-ray absorptiometry
Peabody
      P. and Munro procedure
      P. splint
peacock
      P. transposing index ray
      P. transposing technique
peak
      P. anterior compression plate system
      p. bone mass
      p. dorsiflexion torque
      P. Fixation System
      P. gait module

      p. height velocity (PHV)
      p. latency
      P. Motus Motion Measurement System
      p. pressure
      p. torque
      p. torque test
peak-pressure analysis
Pean clamp
pear bur
pear-shaped
      p.-s. body
      p.-s. vertebra
Pearson
      P. attachment to Thomas splint
      P. intramedullary saw
      P. splint attachment
Pease-Thomson traction
Pebax
      P. counter unit
      P. fastening strap
PEC
      PEC modular total knee system
      PEC total hip system
Pec-Dec machine
Peck osteotome
pectineus muscle
pectoral
      p. girdle
      p. nerve
      p. reflex
pectoralis
      p. major flap
      p. major muscle
      p. minor muscle
      p. muscle implant
pectus
      p. carinatum
      p. excavatum
      p. recurvatum
pedal
      p. disability benefit
      p. exerciser
      p. hyperpigmented lesion
      p. hypophalangism
      p. macrodactylia
      p. osteomyelitis
Pedar
      P. in-shoe measurement system
      P. pressure insole system
      P. pressure measurement system
PED block
pedestal, pedistal
      Body P.
      cast equipped with rubber p.
      halo p.
      IMP surgical leg p.
      rubber p.
      shelf p.

p. sign
surgical leg p.
pedestaled
pedestrian accident
PEDI
Pediatric Evaluation of Disability Inventory
Pediapred Oral
pediatric
P. Advanced Life Support (PALS)
p. blade-plate
p. C-D hook
p. Cotrel-Dubousset rod
P. Evaluation of Disability Inventory (PEDI)
p. flatfoot
p. nutritional formula
p. orthopaedics
p. physical therapy
p. PRAFO brace
p. pressure relief ankle foot orthosis
p. system
p. TSRH hook
P. Ultrasound Bone Analyzer
pedicle
adjoining p.
p. anatomy
p. axis angle
p. bone graft
p. C-D hook
p. clamp
p. connector
contralateral hypoplastic/agenetic p.
p. cortex disruption
p. diameter
p. entrance point
p. erosion
p. fat graft
p. finder
p. fracture
p. groin flap
p. implant
p. landmark
p. localization
p. location
lower thoracic p.
lumbar p.
p. marker
p. method
p. morphometry
p. plate
p. screw

p. screw breakage
p. screw construct
p. screw cord length
p. screw fixation
p. screw hardware prominence
p. screw insertion
p. screw linkage design
p. screw path length
p. screw plating
p. screw pull-out strength
p. screw system
p. sounder
p. sounding probe
p. subtraction osteotomy
thoracic p.
p. of vertebral arch
pedicled
p. fibular transfer
p. transplant
Pedic sponge
pedicular
p. fixation
p. kinking
pediculosis
pedicure
Pedi-Cushions pad
Pedi-Dri topical powder
Pedifix
P. crest pad
P. forefoot compression sleeve
P. hammertoe pad
Pedilen polyurethane foam
Pediplast
P. cushion
P. moldable footcare compound
Pedi-Pro Topical
pedis
calcar p.
pollex p.
porta p.
tinea p.
pedistal (*var. of* pedestal)
Pedi-Wrap immobilizer
pedobarogram
pedobarograph
Biokinetics p.
EMED-SF p.
Musgrave footprint p.
pedobarographic analysis
pedobarography
dynamic p. (DPB)
pedodynamometer
pedodynograph

NOTES

P

529

pedodynographic
    p. examination
    p. measurement
pedogram
pedograph
pedography
pedometer
Pedors orthopaedic shoe
pedorthics
pedorthist peritenon
pedorthotic
pedorthotist
pedoscope
Pedrialle template
pedunculated
    p. loose body
    p. osteochondroma
PEER
    pronation-eversion-external rotation
Peet Z-plasty
peg
    anchoring p.
    p. base plate
    Beath bone intramedullary p.
    bone p.
    p. bone graft
    p. device
    fiber-metal p.
    fibular p.
    fixation p.
    glenoid alignment p.
    Harrison-Nicolle polypropylene p.
    Kinemax removable fixation p.
    locking p.
    polyethylene p.
    stringing p.
    subtalar joint arthroereisis p. (STA-peg)
peg-and-socket technique
pegboard
    p. lateral positioning device
    Purdue p.
pegged tibial prosthesis
pegging
    bone p.
peg-in-hole
    p.-i.-h. arthroereisis
    p.-i.-h. osteotomy
Peimer reduction osteotomy
Pe Lite thermoplastic crepe material
Pelite thermoplastic crepe material
Pelken sign
Pellegrini disease
Pellegrini-Stieda disease
pellet
    calcium hydroxyapatite p.
pelves (*pl. of* pelvis)
pelvic
    p. abscess

p. angle
p. avulsion fracture
p. band
p. bench
p. block
p. brace
p. brim
p. C clamp
p. circumference
p. discontinuity
p. drainage
p. effluent
p. fixation
p. flexion contracture (PFC)
p. floor exercise
p. fracture frame
p. girdle
p. hyperextension traction
p. injury
p. instability
p. kinematic chain
p. lateral shift
p. lateral tilt
p. obliquity
p. osteotomy
p. pain and organic dysfunction
p. plane
p. reconstruction kit
p. region bursitis
p. region contusion
p. rim fracture
p. ring
p. ring dysfunction
p. ring fracture
p. rock (PR)
p. rock test
p. rotation
p. rotation motion gait determinant
p. shift motion gait determinant
p. side-shift
p. sling
p. splint
p. splinting
p. straddle fracture
p. tilt motion gait determinant
p. traction belt
p. unleveling
pelvic-femoral angle
pelvis, pl. **pelves**
    achondroplastic p.
    assimilation p.
    beaked p.
    bony p.
    caoutchouc p.
    cordate p.
    cordiform p.
    coxalgic p.
    dual drop p. (DDP)
    dwarf p.

false p.
frozen p.
greater p.
high-assimilation p.
kyphorachitic p.
kyphoscoliorachitic p.
kyphoscoliotic p.
kyphotic p.
lesser p.
lordotic p.
low-assimilation p.
Nägele p.
p. nana
osteomalacic p.
Otto p.
Prague p.
pseudoosteomalacic p.
rachitic p.
Rokitansky p.
rostrate p.
rubber p.
scoliotic p.
split p.
spondylolisthetic p.
sprung p.
p. spuria
stove-in p.
pelvofemoral muscular dystrophy
pelvospondylitis ossificans
Pemberton
P. acetabuloplasty
P. pericapsular osteotomy
P. spur-crushing clamp
PEMF
peripheral nerve cutaneous field
pulsating electromagnetic field
pulsed electromagnetic field
PEMF bone growth stimulation
pen
STA-Pen writer p.
weighted p.
Pen/Alps distal pad
pencil
p. and cup deformity
electrosurgical p.
p. grip
skin p.
sterile p.
penciling of ribs on x-ray
pencil-tip drill
Penco Walker Sleds
pendulum exercise

penetrating
p. drill
p. fracture
penetration
anterior cortex p.
penetrator
Arthrex P.
Penfield
P. 4 dissector
P. periosteal elevator
penguin gait
Penlac
P. Nail Lacquer
P. Nail Lacquer topical solution
Pennal classification
pennation angle
Penn finger drill
Pennig dynamic wrist fixator
Pennsylvania bimanual work sample
Penrose drain
Pentothal Sodium
pentoxifylline
peptic ulcer
peptide
atrial natriuretic p.
brain natriuretic p. (BNP)
chemotactic p.
peptido-leukotriene
P-ER
pronation-external rotation
P-ER injury
peracetic acid
perception
constant-touch p.
p. deficit
visual p.
PercScope percutaneous discectomy
percussion
p. hammer
p. sign
p. tenderness
Trömner p.
Percuss-O-Matic jackhammer device
percutaneous
p. Achilles tendon repair
p. autogenous dowel bone graft
p. bone marrow infection
p. core bone biopsy
p. corticotomy
p. dorsal column stimulator implant
p. epiphysiodesis
p. fixation
p. heel cord lengthening

NOTES

P

percutaneous *(continued)*
    p. K-wire
    p. lumbar discectomy
    p. needle placement
    p. nucleotomy
    p. osteotomy
    p. pin
    p. pin insertion
    p. pinning
    p. pinning of fracture
    p. plantar fasciotomy (PPF)
    p. reduction
    p. stapling
    p. tendo Achillis lengthening
    p. tenotomy
    p. transcaudal epidural endoscopy
    p. transmalleolar drilling
Percy
    P. amputating saw
    P. amputation retractor
    P. plate
Perez postoperative pain scale
Perfecta
    P. femoral stem
    P. hip prosthesis
    P. I, II prosthesis
    P. total hip system
PerFixation
    P. screw
    P. system
perforating
    p. artery
    p. bur
    p. forceps
    p. fracture
    p. twist drill
perforation
    attritional p.
    cortical p.
    femoral cortical p.
perforator
    Boyd p.
    Dodd p.
    p. drill
Performance
performance
    p. area
    P. Assessment of Self-Care Skills
    p. component
    p. context
    Fugl-Meyer Evaluation of
      Physical P.
    functional p.
    isokinetic p.
    P. knee prosthesis
    P. modular total knee system
    motion p.
    safety p.
    Test of Infant Motor P. (TIMP)

    P. unicompartmental knee system
    P. Wrap knee support
performance-enhancing steroid
performer ultralight knee brace
perfusion
    digital blood p.
    pulsatile hypothermic p.
periacetabular osteotomy
perianal
    p. sensation
    p. skin
periaqueductal
    p. gray (PAG)
    p. gray nucleus
periarthritis
periarthrosis humeri
periarticular
    p. abscess
    p. calcification
    p. fibrositis
    p. fracture
    p. heterotopic ossification
    p. tissue
pericapsular osteotomy
pericapsulitis
pericardium graft
pericellular halo
perichondral
    p. circulation
    p. ossification
    p. ring
perichondrium
pericyte
    Zimmerman p.
periepineurial neuropathy
perihamate injury
perilesional bone
Peri-Loc prosthesis
perilunar
    p. instability
    p. transscaphoid dislocation
perilunate
    p. carpal dislocation
    p. fracture-dislocation (PLFD)
perilymphatic fistula (PLF)
perimalleolar pain
perimeniscal cyst
perimysial
perimysiitis
perimysium
perinea (*pl. of* perineum)
perineal
    p. flexure
    p. loop
    p. post
    p. sensation
perineometer
    Peritron p.
perineum, pl. perinea

perineural
p. block
p. fibroma (PNR)
p. fibrosis
p. tissue
perineurial neurorrhaphy
perineurium, pl. **perineuria**
period
absolute refractory p.
functional refractory p.
incubation p.
latent p.
postinjury p.
refractory p.
relative refractory p.
silent p.
periodic arthralgia
periodization of training
PerioGlas bone graft material
perionychium
perioperative
p. antibiotic therapy
p. autotransfusion system
p. reduction
periostalgia
chronic p.
periostea (pl. of periosteum)
periosteal
p. arthritis
p. band
p. bone collar
p. button
p. cambium layer
p. chondroma
p. chondrosarcoma
p. desmoid
p. elevation
p. elevator
p. fibroma
p. ganglion
p. implantation
p. lamella
p. new bone
p. new bone formation
p. ossification
p. osteogenesis
p. osteosarcoma
p. reaction
round-tapped p.
p. sarcoma
p. sleeve
p. tissue
p. vessel

periosteopathy
periosteoplastic amputation
periosteotome
Alexander costal p.
Alexander-Farabeuf p.
Ballenger p.
Brown p.
costal p.
elevator p.
Fomon p.
Joseph p.
periosteotomy
periosteum, pl. **periostea**
periostitis
florid reactive p.
p. ossificans
suppurative p.
periostotome
periostotomy
peripatellar
p. retinacular support
p. tendinitis
peripheral
p. arterial occlusive disease (PAOD)
p. arteriography
p. artery
p. capsule
p. chemical sympathectomy
p. dual-energy x-ray absorptiometry (pDXA)
p. gangrene
p. meniscus
p. modulation
p. nerve
p. nerve block
p. nerve block anesthesia
p. nerve cutaneous field (PEMF)
p. nerve entrapment
p. nerve glove
p. nerve injury
p. nerve palsy
p. nerve tumor classification
p. nervous system (PNS)
p. neuritis
p. neurocompressive disorder
p. neuropathy
p. paralysis
p. polyneuritis
p. vascular disease (PVD)
p. vascular insufficiency
p. vascular obstructive disease

NOTES

P

peripheral *(continued)*
    p. vascular surgery (PVS)
    p. vascular system (PVS)
peripisiform injury
peripolar zone
periprosthetic
    p. bone loss
    p. bone resorption
    p. fracture
    p. membrane
    p. radiolucency
periscapulitis shoulder pain
perispondylitis
    Gibney p.
peritendinitis
    Achilles p.
    p. crepitans
    p. serosa
peritendinous scar
peritendon
peritenon
    pedorthist p.
peritoneum
peritrapezial
    p. arthritis
    p. injury
peritrapezoidal injury
peritrochanteric fracture
Peritron perineometer
periungual fibroma
PER-IV fracture
Perkins
    P. test
    P. traction
    P. vertical line
Perkins-Ombredanne line
Perlstein brace
Perma-Hand silk suture
Permalock
    Weber P.
Perman cartilage forceps
permanent
    p. callus
    p. disability
    p. implant
    p. partial disability (PPD)
    p. partial disability rating
    p. and total disability (PTD)
peroneal
    p. artery
    p. bupivacaine injection
    p. compartment syndrome
    p. dislocation
    p. groove
    p. island flap
    p. muscle
    p. muscle spasm
    p. muscular atrophy
    p. musculature

    p. nerve
    p. nerve entrapment
    p. nerve injury
    p. nerve palsy
    p. neuropathy
    p. paralysis
    p. retinaculum
    p. sign
    p. sinus
    p. spastic flatfoot
    p. strengthening exercise
    p. tendinitis
    p. tendon
    p. tendon displacement
    p. tendon impingement
    p. tendon procedure
    p. tendon sheath injection
    p. tendon subluxation
    p. tenolysis
    p. tenosynovitis
    p. tunnel
    p. tunnel compression test
    p. vein
peronealis
    trochlea p.
peroneum
    os p.
peroneus
    p. brevis (PB)
    p. brevis elongation
    p. brevis graft
    p. brevis to longus anastomosis
    p. brevis muscle
    p. brevis split (PBS)
    p. brevis tendon
    p. brevis transfer
    p. longus
    p. longus muscle
    p. longus tendinopathy (PLT)
    p. longus tendon
    p. quartus muscle
    p. tertius muscle
    p. tertius tendon
peroxide
    p. flush
    hydrogen p.
perpendicular
    method of p.'s
    p. strumming
per primam healing
Perrin-Ferraton disease
Perry
    P. extensile anterior approach
    P. sensor
    P. technique
Perry-Nickel cranial halo
Persian slipper foot
persistent
    p. clonus

p. notochord
p. occiput/atlas disrelationship
p. pain
p. sciatic artery
perstans
macularis eruptive p.
Perthes
P. disease
P. epiphysis
P. lesion
P. procedure
P. reamer
P. tourniquet test
Perthes-Bankart lesion
pertrochanteric fracture
perturbation
perverted function
pes
p. adductus
p. anserinus
p. anserinus syndrome
p. anserinus transplant
p. arcuatus
p. arcuatus clawfoot deformity
p. calcaneus
p. cavovalgus
p. cavovarus
p. cavus
p. cavus clawfoot deformity
p. equinovalgus
p. equinovarus
p. equinovarus adductus
p. equinus
p. febricitans
p. gigas
p. planovalgus
p. plano valgus
p. planovalgus abductus
p. planovalgus deformity
p. plantigrade planus
p. planus deformity
p. pronatus
p. valgo planus
p. valgo planus deformity
p. valgus planus
p. varus
PET
positron emission tomography
PET electrotherapy
petaling the cast
petechia, pl. **petechiae**

Peterson
P. syndrome
P. traction
PET/Eurotech Generation 2000 table
petit
p. pas gait
P. triangle
Petren gait
Petrie spica cast
pétrissage
petroclinoid ligament
petrolatum gauze
petroleum gauze dressing
petrosal bone
petrous temporal bone
Pettibon chiropractic procedure
PFA
proximal reference axis
PFC
pelvic flexion contracture
PFC curved unconstrained
prosthesis
PFC femoral prosthesis
PFC hip stem
PFC modular total knee system
PFC offset tibial tray
PFC Sigma knee system
PFC TC3 modular knee system
PFC total hip replacement system
PFD
patellofemoral dysfunction
polyurethane foam dressing
Pfeiffer syndrome
PFFD
proximal focal femoral deficiency
Pfitzner theory of coalition formation
PF Night Splint II splint
PFO
plantar fasciitis orthosis
PFO night splint
PFP
patellofemoral pain
PFT
postoperative flexor tendon
PFT traction brace
PGA-PLA
polyglycolic acid-polylactic acid
PGA-PLA biomaterial
PGP
PGP flexible nail system
PGP nail
PGS-3000 pulsed galvanic stimulator
phagocytosis

NOTES

P

phalangeal
  p. articular orientation
  p. articulation
  p. bone
  p. clamp
  p. condylectomy
  p. degloving
  p. diaphysial fracture
  p. dislocation
  p. fracture fixation
  p. head
  p. herniation
  p. hypoplasia
  p. implant
  p. malunion correction
  p. microgeodic syndrome
  p. neck
  p. osteotomy
  p. polydactyly
  p. synostosis
phalangectomy
  intermediate p.
phalanges (*pl. of* phalanx)
phalangization
phalangophalangeal amputation
phalanx, pl. **phalanges**
  accessory p.
  delta p.
  distal p. (DP)
  osteitis distal p.
  proximal p. (PP)
  tufted p.
  waist of p.
Phalen
  P. maneuver
  P. position
  P. wrist flexion test
Phalen-Miller opponensplasty
phantom
  p. frame
  p. limb
  p. limb pain
  p. limb syndrome
  p. pain phenomenon
  p. sensation
phantosmia
pharmacodynamic
pharmacokinetic
pharyngeal tissue
phase
  blood pool p.
  3-p. bone scan
  double-leg stance p.
  p. 2 elbow program
  fibroblastic p.
  flexor p.
  foot-strike p.
  granulation p.
  heel-contact p.

  heel-off p.
  heel-strike p.
  inflammatory p.
  inosculation p.
  maturation p.
  opposite foot-strike p.
  opposite toe-off p.
  organizational p.
  plasmatic p.
  propulsive p.
  push-off p.
  remodeling p.
  reparative p.
  stance p.
  swing p.
  toe-off p.
pheasant
  P. discotome
  P. elbow operation
  P. elbow technique
Phelps
  P. brace
  P. neurectomy
  P. operation
  P. orthosis
  P. partial resection
  P. scapulectomy
  P. splint
Phemister
  P. acromioclavicular pin fixation
  P. biopsy trephine
  P. elevator
  P. medial approach
  P. medial approach to tibia
  P. onlay bone graft
  P. onlay bone graft technique
  P. operation
  P. osteotomy
  P. posteromedial approach
  P. rasp
Phemister-Bonfiglio technique
Phenaphen With Codeine
Phendry Oral
phenol
  p. cauterization
  p. chemosurgery
  P. EZ swab
  p. matricectomy
  p. neurolysis
phenol-alcohol matricectomy
phenolization
  nail matrix p. (NMP)
phenomenon, pl. **phenomena**
  bioelectric p.
  brake p.
  Burner p.
  combined flexion p.
  compression p.
  crankshaft p.

gelling p.
give-way p.
glued-to-the-floor p.
Gordon knee p.
Gowers p.
halisteresis p.
Herendeen p.
Holmes p.
Holmes-Stewart p.
Hunt paradoxical p.
Kienböck p.
lumbrical-plus p.
Lust p.
magic angle p.
no-reflow p.
phantom pain p.
pivot shift p.
pronation p.
Queckenstedt p.
radial p.
Raynaud p.
referred anatomic p.
referred trigger point p.
relaxation p.
release p.
Rust p.
spontaneous vacuum p.
staircase p.
temporary cavity p.
tibial p.
toe p.
vacuum p.
Valleix p.
vertebral steal p.
Westphal p.
wind-up p.
phenylephrine
phenyltoloxamine
Philadelphia
P. cervical collar
P. collar cervical support
P. collar cervical traction
P. Plastizote cervical brace
P. rigid collar
Philips
P. Angiodiagnostics 96 apparatus
P. linear accelerator
P. toe force gauge
Phillips
P. head screw
P. head screwdriver
P. muscle
P. recessed-head screw

P. screw head
P. splint
philosophy
Palmerian p.
phlebography
phlebolith
phlebothrombosis
phlogistic agent
phocomelia
complete p.
distal p.
proximal p.
phocomelic dwarfism
Phoenix
P. foot system
P. Outrigger splint
P. total hip prosthesis
phonological analysis
phonophoresis
hydrocortisone p.
p. plantarflexion
ultrasound p.
Phoresor
P. II iontophoretic drug delivery
system
P. PM900 iontophoresis system
phosphatase
alkaline p.
bone-specific alkaline p. (BSAP)
tartrate resistant acid p. (TRAP)
phosphate
calcium p.
hydroxyapatite tetra-tri-calcium p.
nicotinamide-adenine dinucleotide p.
(NADPH)
technetium-99m p.
tetracalcium p.
tricalcium p.
phosphatidylcholine
dipalmitoyl p. (DPPC)
phospholipid
photoactive naphthalimide compound
photogrammetry
x-ray p.
photon densitometry
photopenia
hardware p.
photoplethysmography (PPG)
digital p.
phrenic nerve
phthinoid chest
PHV
peak height velocity

NOTES

phycomycosis
physes (*pl. of* physis)
physial, physeal
    p. angle
    p. bar
    p. bridge
    p. cartilage
    p. closure
    p. damage
    p. disruption
    p. distraction
    p. growth
    p. injury
    p. line
    p. mamillary process
    p. plate fracture
    p. region
    p. scar
    p. stapling
physiatric
physiatrics
physiatrist
physiatry
physical
    P. Ability Test (PAT)
    p. activity
    P. Activity Readiness Questionnaire (PAR-Q)
    p. agent
    p. capacity evaluation (PCE)
    p. condition, upper limb function, lower limb function, sensory component, excretory function, support function (PULSES)
    p. daily living skills (PDLS)
    p. examination
    p. impairment
    p. inactivity
    p. independence WHO Handicap Scale
    p. medicine (PM)
    p. medicine and rehabilitation (PMR)
    p. realignment
    p. therapy (PT)
    p. therapy table
    p. training (PT)
    p. work
    p. work capacity (PWC)
physiognomy
PhysioGymnic exercise ball
physiologic
    p. barrier
    p. flatfoot
    p. lock
    p. lock of motion segment
    p. range of joint motion
    p. response

    p. saline
    p. valgus
physiological
    p. hyperactivity
    p. venous pump mechanism
PhysioLogics Alpha Lipoic Acid
physiology
    exercise p.
physiolysis
    central p.
Physio-Roll-R-Cise
Physio-Roll VisuaLiser exercise ball
Physio-Stim Lite bone growth stimulator
physiotherapist
physiotherapy
    active p.
    aqua PT dry p.
    passive p.
physique
    ectomesomorphic p.
    ectomorphic p.
physis, pl. physes
    distal tibial p.
    p. fracture
    modified Boyd amputation of ankle and distal tibial p.
phytoestrogen
phytonadione
phytonutrient
PI
    posteroinferior
piano key sign
piano-wire dorsiflexion brace
PICA
    posterior inferior cerebellar artery
    PICA index
pick
    P. chisel
    dental p.
Picker Magnascanner for bone metastasis
picket
    p. fence guide
    P. Fence leg positioner
pick-up
    p.-u. forceps
    p.-u. test
Picot incision
picture
    p. frame appearance
    maximum pressure p. (MPP)
Pidcock
    P. nail
    P. pin
piecemeal
pie-crusting skin graft
Piedmont fracture
Pierrot-Murphy advancement insertion

PIEx
    posteroinferior external
      PIEx ilium
      PIEx subluxation
piezoelectric
    p. accelerometer
    p. potential
Piezo electro-needleless stimulator
piezogenic papule
Piffard curette
pigeon
    p. breast
    p. chest
pigeon-toeing gait
pigmented
    p. nodular synovitis
    p. nodular synovitis of tendon
      sheath
    p. villonodular bursitis
    p. villonodular synovitis (PVNS,
      PVS)
pigtail tendon stripper
PIIn
    posteroinferior internal
      PIIn ilium
      PIIn subluxation
Pilates
    P. exercise method
    P. method exercise
pillar
    articular p.
    p. pain
    p. tenderness
Pillet hand prosthesis
Pilliar
    P. prosthesis
    P. total hip replacement
Pillo
    Knee P.
Pillo-Pedic cervical traction pillow
pillow
    abduction p.
    antibacterial p.
    Bio-Gel decubitus p.
    Bodynapper Comfort P.
    Capello slim-line abduction p.
    Carter elevation p.
    Carter foam p.
    cervical sleep p.
    cervical support p.
    cervical traction p.
    p. collar
    Comfort Club tub p.

    Comfort-U total body p.
    Crescent Complete Sleeper p.
    Crescent memory p.
    Crescent-Pillo p.
    D-Core support p.
    Dream P.
    elevation p.
    Flip-Flop p.
    foam p.
    foot p.
    p. fracture
    Frejka p.
    Mediflow waterbase p.
    neck p.
    Neckcare p.
    Neck-Hugger cervical support p.
    Opti-Curve therapeutic p.
    OrthoBone p.
    p. orthosis
    p. orthosis for hip
    Orthosleep P.
    Pillo-Pedic cervical traction p.
    Pillo-Wedge p.
    Pron p.
    shoulder abduction p.
    Silicore foot p.
    snooze p.
    Softeze water p.
    p. splint
    Tempur-Pedic pressure relieving
      Swedish p.
    T-Foam p.
    Theracloud p.
    Therapeutica Sleeping P.
    Therasleep Cervical P.
    Tri-Core cervical support p.
    Wal-Pil-O neck p.
Pillo-Wedge pillow
pill rolling tremor
pilomotor
    p. dysfunction
    p. response
pilon
    p. fracture
    p. fracture classification
pilonidal dimple
Pil-O-Splint wrist splint
pilot
    p. bur
    p. drill
    P. point screw
pin
    A p.

NOTES

P

pin *(continued)*

absorbable polymeric p.
absorbable polyparadioxanone p.
Ace p.
Acufex distractor p.
alignment p.
Allofix freeze-dried cortical
  bone p.
Apex p.
Arthrex zebra p.
arum fixation p.
ASIF screw p.
Asnis p.
Austin Moore p.
p. ball system
Barr p.
beaded hip p.
Beath p.
Belos compression p.
Bilos p.
Biofix system p.
bioresorbable p.
Böhler p.
Böhler-Knowles hip p.
Böhler-Steinmann p.
Bohlman p.
breakaway p.
Breck p.
buttress p.
calcaneal p.
calibrated p.
Canakis beaded hip p.
cancellous p.
Charnley p.
p. chuck
p. clamp
clavicle p.
cloverleaf p.
Co-Cr-Mo p.
collapsible p.
Compere threaded p.
Compton clavicle p.
Conley p.
cortical p.
Craig p.
p. crimper
Crowe pilot point on Steinmann p.
Crowe tip p.
Crutchfield p.
p. cutter
Davis p.
Day fixation p.
DCS p.
deluxe FIN p.
Denham p.
DePuy p.
derotational p.
Deyerle II p.
distraction p.

drill p.
Ender p.
p. external fixator
Fahey p.
femoral guide p.
Fischer transfixing p.
Fisher half p.
p. fixation
fixation p.
Freebody p.
freeze-dried bone p.
friction lock p.
p. guard
p. guide
Hagie hip p.
halo p.
Hansen p.
Hare p.
Hatcher p.
Haynes p.
p. headrest
Hegge p.
Hewson breakaway p.
hexhead p.
hip p.
Hoffmann apex fixation p.
Hoffmann transfixion p.
p. holder
hook p.
hook-end intramedullary p.
p. implant
intramedullary p.
Jones compression p.
Jurgan p.
Kirschner wire p.
Knowles hip p.
Kronfeld p.
Küntscher p.
LIH hook p.
locating p.
locked intramedullary
  osteosynthesis p.
Lottes p.
marble bone p.
Markley retention p.
Matthews-Green p.
McBride p.
medullary p.
metal p.
Moore fixation p.
Moule screw p.
Neufeld p.
nonthreaded p.
Norman tibial p.
Oris p.
Ormco p.
Orthofix p.
OrthoSorb absorbable p.
osseous p.

osteotomy p.
partially threaded p.
percutaneous p.
Pidcock p.
Pugh hip p.
rasp p.
resorbable polydioxanon p.
resorbable polymer p.
restorative p.
p. retractor
ReUnite orthopaedic p.
Rhinelander p.
Riordan p.
Risser p.
Rush p.
Rush intramedullary fixation p.
Safir p.
Sage p.
Scand p.
Schanz p.
Schneider p.
Schweitzer p.
self-broaching p.
self-tapering p.
Serrato forearm p.
Shriners p.
p. site
skeletal p.
p. sleeve
Smart P.
SmartPin/PLLA p.
Smillie p.
Smith-Petersen fracture p.
SMO Moore p.
smooth Steinmann p.
Snap fixation p.
SOC p.
socket p.
spring p.
Stader p.
Steinmann fixation p.
Street medullary p.
strut-type p.
p. suture
Tachdjian p.
tapered p.
threaded Steinmann p.
tibial p.
titanium half p.
p. track
p. tract infection
traction p.
transarticular p.

transcapitellar p.
transfixing p.
trochanteric p.
Turner p.
Tutofix cortical p.
union broach retention p.
Varney p.
p. vise
von Saal medullary p.
Walker hollow quill p.
Watanabe p.
Webb p.
p. wheel
wrench p.
Z p.
Zimfoam p.
Zimmer p.

pin-and-plaster
   p.-a.-p. fixation
   p.-a.-p. method
pin-bone interface
pincement
pincer
   p. nail
   p. nail formation
   p. palpation
   p. testing
pinch
   p. callus
   p. gauge
   P. Gauge and Jackson Strength
     Evaluation System
   p. grasp
   key p.
   lateral squeeze p.
   p. meter
   palmar p.
   p. power
   p. restoration
   p. strength
   tip p.
   tip-to-tip p.
   p. tree
pinchometer
   Prestop p.
ping-pong
   p.-p. bone
   p.-p. fracture
Pinkus
   fibroepithelioma of P.
Pinna-Cal ipriflavone
Pinnacle acetabular cup system
Pinn-ACL guide system

NOTES

P

Pinn anterior cruciate ligament guide system
pinning
    Asnis p.
    closed p.
    hip p.
    Knowles p.
    open p.
    percutaneous p.
    Sherk-Probst percutaneous p.
    Sofield p.
    Wagner closed p.
pinpoint ulceration
pinprick
    p. hyperalgesia test
    p. sensation
pin-seating forceps
pin-to-bar clamp
Pinto distractor
pin-tract osteomyelitis
pinwheel
    Cleanwheel disposable
    neurological p.
    Safe-T-Wheel p.
    P. System
    Wartenberg p.
Piotrowski sign
PIP
    proximal interphalangeal
    PIP articulation
    PIP flexion creaking
PIP/DIP
    proximal interphalangeal/distal
    interphalangeal
    PIP/DIP strap
piperacillin/tazobactam therapy
pipe tree
PIPJ
    proximal interphalangeal joint
Pipkin
    P. fracture classification system
    P. posterior hip dislocation
    classification
    P. subclassification of Epstein-
    Thomas classification
Pipkin-type femoral head fracture
pi-plate dorsal distal radius plate
Pirie
    P. bone
    talonavicular ossicle of P.
piriform
    p. muscle
    p. sclerosis
    p. sclerosis of ilium
piriformis
    p. sign
    p. syndrome
Pirogoff amputation
Pischel micropin

pisiform
    p. bone
    p. bursa
    p. metacarpal ligament
    p. ossification
pisohamate ligament
pisometacarpal ligament
pisotriquetral
    p. arthritis
    p. joint
pistol-grip hand drill
piston
    cannulated expulsion p.
    p. prosthesis
    p. sign
pistoning motion
pitch
    calcaneal p.
pitching injury
Pitcock nail
pitted cartilage
pitting edema
Pittsburgh pelvic frame
pituitary
    p. gigantism
    p. grasper
    p. rongeur
PIVM
    passive intervertebral motion
    PIVM testing
pivot
    Accu-Line dual p.
    calcar p.
    p. of calcar
    p. joint
    medial stem p.
    P. Plate rehabilitation plate
    P. Pole walking device
    p. shift phenomenon
    p. shift sign
    p. shift test
    p. sport activity
pivoting
    p. and cutting activity
    p. sports
PJ
    patellar jerk
PL
    palmaris longus
placement
    bone graft p.
    electrode p.
    glide hole for screw p.
    hand p.
    Kirschner wire p.
    K-wire p.
    needle p.
    PCL-oriented p. (POP)
    percutaneous needle p.

plate p.
portal p.
posterolateral bone graft p.
p. reflex
rod p.
sacral screw p.
screw p.
variable screw p. (VSP)
placing reflex
plafond
p. fracture
tibial p.
varus p.
plain
p. gauze
p. pattern plate
p. rotary scissors
p. screwdriver
p. tissue forceps
Plak-Vac oral suction brush
plan
Making Action P.'s (MAPs)
McConnell patellofemoral
treatment p.
National Arthritis Action P.
(NAAP)
preoperative p.
plana
coxa p.
manus p.
vertebra p.
plane
AC-PC p.
anatomic p.
axial p.
coronal p.
3-p. deformity
facet p.
fascial p.
flexion-extension p.
Frankfort horizontal p.
frontal p.
Hensen p.
Hodge p.
horizontal p.
internervous p.
intertubercular p.
p. joint
Ludwig p.
median sagittal p.
mesiodistal p.
midsagittal p.
paramedian sagittal p.

pelvic p.
primary movement p.
sagittal p.
scapulothoracic guiding p.
spinous p.
sternoxiphoid p.
subcostal p.
suprasternal p.
thigh-shank p.
thoracic p.
transverse p.
varus-valgus p.
vertical p.
1-plane
1-p. bilateral external fixator
1-p. bilateral frame
1-p. deformity
1-p. instability
1-p. unilateral external fixator
1-p. unilateral frame
2-plane
2-p. bilateral external fixator
2-p. bilateral frame
2-p. deformity
2-p. fluoroscopy
2-p. roentgenogram
2-p. unilateral external fixator
2-p. unilateral frame
planer
calcar p.
Rubin bone p.
Rubin cartilage p.
plane-type acromioclavicular articulation
planning
P. Alternative Tomorrows with
Hope (PATH)
preoperative p.
rehabilitation p.
Planostretch stockings
planovalgus
p. deformity
p. foot
hypermobile pes p.
pes p.
talipes p.
plantalgia
plantar
p. angulation
p. aponeurosis
p. approach
p. arch support orthosis
p. arterial arch
p. artery

NOTES

P

plantar *(continued)*
> p. artery flap
> p. axial view
> p. Babinski response
> p. bone
> p. bony prominence
> p. bromidrosis
> p. buckling
> p. calcaneal spur
> p. calcaneocuboid ligament
> p. calcaneonavicular ligament
> p. calcaneonavicular ligament-tibialis posterior tendon advancement
> p. callosity
> p. capsular release
> p. capsule
> p. capsuloligamentous complex
> p. compartment
> p. condylectomy
> p. corn
> p. cuboideonavicular ligament
> p. cuneocuboid ligament
> p. cuneonavicular ligament
> p. dermatosis
> p. digital artery (PDA)
> p. ecchymosis sign
> p. fascia
> p. fascial release
> p. fasciitis
> p. fasciitis night splint
> p. fasciitis orthosis (PFO)
> p. fasciitis syndrome
> p. fasciitis taping
> p. fasciotomy
> p. fat pad
> p. fibromatosis
> p. foot
> p. grasp reflex
> p. intercuneiform ligament
> p. keratosis
> p. lateral base
> p. ligament
> p. longitudinal incision
> p. malignant melanoma
> p. metatarsal angle
> p. metatarsal artery
> p. metatarsal ligament
> p. nerve
> p. pain
> p. plate
> p. plate injury
> p. plate release
> p. pressure
> p. pressure pattern
> p. reflex
> p. shift
> p. spring ligament
> p. stress ankle x-ray

> p. sweating
> p. tarsometatarsal ligament
> p. tendopathy
> p. toe pulp
> p. transposition
> p. ulcer
> p. vault
> p. V infiltration block
> p. V-Y advancement flap
> p. wart (PW)

plantar-dorsiflexion
plantarflex
plantarflexed stress radiograph
plantarflexing
plantarflexion
> p. injury
> phonophoresis p.
> p. stress view
> p. torque

plantarflexion-inversion deformity
plantarflexion-inversion test
plantarflexor
> p. proximal metatarsal osteotomy
> p. reflex

plantarflexory
> p. motion
> p. osteotomy

plantar-hindfoot-midfoot bony mass
plantaris
> p. muscle
> p. tendon
> p. tendon graft

plantar-lateral release
plantar-medial release
plantarward
plantigrade
> p. foot
> p. limb
> p. platform

planus
> collapsing pes valgo p.
> flexible pes p.
> Gleich osteotomy for pes valgo p.
> lichen p.
> pes plantigrade p.
> pes valgo p.
> pes valgus p.
> rigid pes p.
> talipes p.

plasma
> p. beta-endorphin
> p. cell dyscrasia
> coagulated p.
> p. volume shift

plasmacytoma
> aggressive solitary p.
> extramedullary p.

Plasmanate

plasma-sprayed
    low-pressure p.-s. (LPPS)
    p.-s. titanium
plasmatic
    p. phase
    p. phase of skin healing
plasmin
Plasmodium falciparum
plast
    Putti bone p.
Plastalume
    P. bulb-ended splint
    P. straight splint
Plastazote
    P. arch support
    P. blank
    P. cervical collar
    P. cervical collar orthosis
    P. foam
    P. foot bed
    P. insole
    P. orthotic device
    P. shoe liner
Plastazote-Kydex cervical immobilizer
plaster
    Batchelor p.
    p. cast application burn
    closing wedge manipulation and
      reapplication of p.
    Hapset hydroxyapatite bone graft p.
    opening wedge manipulation and
      reapplication of p.
    p. of Paris (POP)
    p. of Paris bandage
    p. of Paris cast
    p. of Paris splint
    p. saw
    p. slab splint
    p. sole
    p. sore
    p. toe cap
    Velpeau p.
    x-ray in p. (XIP)
    x-ray out of p. (XOP)
    Zoroc p.
plastic
    p. achillotenotomy
    p. ankle-foot orthosis
    p. ball implant
    p. body jacket
    p. bowing fracture
    p. cast
    p. collar

    p. deformation
    p. end cap
    p. femoral plug
    p. floor reaction ankle-foot orthosis
    p. heel cup
    Hexalite p.
    p. leaf-spring (PLS)
    p. limited-motion joint
    low-temperature p.
    p. marrow canal restrictor
    Orthoplast p.
    p. patella
    p. repair
    p. strain
    thermolabile p.
    unitary p.
PlastiCast adjustable joint cast system
plasticity
    connective tissue p.
    cortical p.
Plasticor prosthesis
Plasti-Pore
    P.-P. ossicular replacement
      prosthesis
    P.-P. prosthetic material
Plastiport
    P. TORP
    P. TORP prosthesis
Plast-O-Fit thermoplastic bandage
plasty
    Bosworth-type reverse p.
    Coleman p.
    Durham p.
    flap p.
    p. modification
    rotation p.
    side-swing p.
    skin p.
    trans-bone p.
    V-Y p.
    Y-V p.
plate
    4-hole Alta straight p.
    4-hole side p.
    acetabular reconstruction p.
    AcroMed VSP p.
    Acumed congruent clavicle p.
    alar p.
    Alta condylar buttress p.
    Alta distal fracture p.
    anchor p.
    angled compression p.
    Ant-Cer dynamic cervical p.

NOTES

P

plate (*continued*)

anterior cervical p. (ACP)
anterior sacroiliac joint p.
antiglide p.
AO-ASIF compression p.
AO contoured T p.
AO dynamic compression p.
AO hook p.
AO-Morscher p.
AO reconstruction p.
AO semitubular p.
AO small fragment p.
AO spoon p.
Armstrong p.
ASIF broad dynamic compression bone p.
ASIF T-p.
athletic shoe carbon fiber p.
autocompression p.
avulsion of nail p.
axial p.
Badgley p.
Bagby angled compression p.
barrel p.
Batchelor p.
Becton Colles fracture p.
p. bender
biodegradable p.
Blount blade p.
bone flap fixation p.
Bosworth spine p.
Boyd side p.
bridge p.
broad AO dynamic compression p.
Burns p.
butterfly-shaped monoblock vertebral p.
buttress pie p.
buttress-type p.
Calandruccio side p.
Calcanea fracture p.
calcaneal Y p.
cap-and-anchor p.
carbon fiber-reinforced p.
cartilaginous growth p.
Caspar cervical p.
cervical p.
cloverleaf p.
coaptation p.
cobra-head p.
Collison p.
compression p.
Concise side p.
condylar p.
connecting p.
Continuum total knee base p.
contoured anterior spinal p. (CASP)
contoured T-plate p.

cortical p.
craniocervical p.
crosslink p.
cruciform tibial base p.
C-shaped p.
p. cutter
3D p.
deck p.
DePuy p.
Deyerle p.
dorsal p.
double Cobra p.
double-H p.
Driessen hinged p.
p. driver
dual p.
Dwyer-Hall p.
dynamic compression p. (DCP)
eccentric dynamic compression p. (EDCP)
Eggers bone p.
Elliott femoral condyle blade p.
end p.
epiphysial growth p.
femoral p.
ferromagnetic metal p.
fibrocartilaginous p.
p. fixation
flat p.
flexor p.
foot p., footplate
force p.
frontal p.
fusion p.
gait p.
Gallannaugh p.
Galveston p.
growth p.
Hagie sliding nail p.
Haid cervical p.
Haid Universal bone p.
half-circle p.
Harlow p.
Harms posterior cervical p.
Harris p.
heavy-duty femur p.
heavy side p.
Hicks lugged p.
Hoen skull p.
2-hole p.
3-hole p.
5-hole p.
6-hole p.
7-hole p.
11-hole p.
17-hole p.
Holt nail p.
hook p.
hot p.

H-shaped p.
Hubbard side p.
Hungarian grip p.
Inner Lip P.
interfragmentary p.
intertrochanteric p.
Jergesen I-beam p.
Jergesen tapered p.
Jewett nail overlay p.
Jones compression p.
Kaneda p.
Kessel p.
L p.
Lane p.
Lawson-Thornton p.
Letournel p.
limited compression-dynamic
  compression p.
limited-contact dynamic
  compression p.
LoCon-T distal radial p.
Louis p.
low-contact dynamic compression p.
low-profile dorsal p.
L-shaped p.
Luhr Microfixation cranial p.
Luhr pan p.
Lundholm p.
Luque II p.
Mancini p.
Massie p.
May anatomical bone p.
Mayo Clinic congruent elbow p.
McBride p.
McLaughlin p.
Mears sacroiliac p.
Medoff sliding p.
metal foot p.
Meurig Williams p.
Milch p.
modified Grace p.
Moe intertrochanteric p.
Moore sliding nail p.
Moreira p.
Morscher cervical p.
Müller p.
nail p.
narrow AO dynamic
  compression p.
Neufeld p.
neutralization p.
Newman p.
Nicoll p.

occipitocervical p.
Ogden p.
Orion anterior cervical p.
Orozco p.
orthotic p.
Osborne p.
overlay p.
palmar p.
Paulus p.
pedicle p.
peg base p.
Percy p.
pi-plate dorsal distal radius p.
Pivot Plate rehabilitation p.
p. placement
plain pattern p.
plantar p.
Polytechnic foot-pressure
  measuring p.
precurved p.
pressure p.
protection p.
pterygoid p.
Pugh p.
pylon attachment p.
quadrangular positioning p.
reconstruction p.
resorbable p.
Richards-Hirschhorn p.
Rohadur gait p.
roof p.
round-hole compression p.
Roy-Camille p.
SC-AcuFix ThinLine p.
Schweitzer spring p.
semitubular compression p.
Senn p.
serpentine p.
Sherman bone p.
side p.
Simmons p.
slide p.
slotted femur p.
Smith-Petersen intertrochanteric p.
SMO p.
p. spacer washer
spinous process p.
spoon p.
spring p.
stabilization p.
stainless steel p.
static compression p.
Steffee pedicle p.

NOTES

plate *(continued)*
    Steffee screw p.
    stem base p.
    subchondral p.
    supracondylar p.
    symmetrical thoracic vertebral p.
    symmetric sacral p.
    Synthes dorsal distal radius p.
    Synthes pie p.
    Syracuse anterior I p.
    Tacoma sacral p.
    tarsal p.
    T buttress p.
    tectal p.
    Temple University p.
    tendon p.
    tension band p.
    thoracolumbosacral p.
    Thornton nail p.
    tibial base p.
    titanium hollow screw
      osseointegrating reconstruction p.
      (THORP)
    titanium mandibular p.
    toe p.
    Townley tibial plateau p.
    Townsend-Gilfillan p.
    trial base p.
    T-shaped AO p.
    TSRH p.
    tubular bone p.
    Tupman p.
    twisted p.
    UCBL foot p.
    universal bone p. (UBP)
    Uslenghi p.
    variable screw p. (VSP)
    V blade p.
    Venable p.
    vertebral end p.
    vitallium Luhr p.
    V nail p.
    volar T p.
    VSP p.
    Wainwright p.
    Weber antiglide p.
    Wenger p.
    Whitman p.
    Wilson p.
    wing p.
    Wright p.
    Wurzburg p.
    X p.
    X-10 Crosslink p.
    X-shaped p.
    Y bone p.
    Y-shaped p.
    Zimmer side p.
    Zimmer Y p.
    Z-shaped p.
    Zuelzer hook p.

plateau
    bicondylar tibial p.
    p. fracture
    proximal tibial p.
    tibial p.

plateaued
plate-holding forceps
platelet
    p. concentrate
    p. count
platelet-derived growth factor (PDGF)
platelike atelectasis
plate-screw
    p.-s. fixation
    p.-s. osteosynthesis
    p.-s. system
platform
    p. crutch
    Kistler force p.
    Midland multifunctional mat p.
    Midline Hi-Lo Mat P.
    plantigrade p.
    Velcro-Lock mat p.
plating
    compression p.
    diaphysial p.
    Gotfried percutaneous
      compression p.
    pedicle screw p.
    posterior spinal p.
    variable spinal p. (VSP)
Platinum stationary table
Platou osteotomy
platybasia
platysma muscle
platyspondylia, platyspondylisis
play
    end p.
    excessive joint p.
    joint p.
    muscle p.
    return to p. (RTP)
playfulness
    Child Behaviors Inventory of P.
      (CBI)
    Test of P. (ToP)
Playmaker
    P. functional knee brace
    P. support
PlayTuf knee brace
PLB
    primary lymphoma of bone
pledget
    Betadine-soaked p.
    p. dressing
    p. of gauze
    Gelfoam p.

pleomorphic
p. fibrous histiocytoma
p. lipoma
p. liposarcoma
p. rhabdomyosarcoma

pleonosteosis
Leri p.

plethysmography
digital p.
impedance p.

pleura, pl. **pleurae**
parietal p.

pleural injury

Plexidure insole

plexiform
p. fibrohistiocytic tumor
p. neurofibroma

Plexiglas
P. jig
P. spacer

PlexiPulse
P. DVT prophylaxis system
P. intermittent pneumatic
compression device

plexitis

plexopathy
brachial p.
congenital p.
Klumpke p.

plexus, pl. **plexuses**
p. block
brachial p.
cervical p.
fascial p.
lumbosacral p.
sacral p.
subdermal p.

PLF
perilymphatic fistula

PLFD
perilunate fracture-dislocation

plica, pl. **plicae**
bucket-handle p.
infrapatellar p.
lateral p.
medial patellar p.
medial shelf/medial p.
parapatellar p.
pathological p.
suprapatellar p.
symptomatic synovial p.
p. syndrome
synovial p.

tendon p.
p. test

plication
capsular p.
disc p.
soft tissue p.

plicectomy

pliers
Compaction p.
extraction p.
Howmedica Microfixation
System p.
locking p.
Luhr Microfixation System p.
needle-nose vise-grip p.
orthopaedic surgical p.
Power-Grip p.
slip-joint p.
Sontec p.
square-end p.
Storz Microsystems p.
Synthes Microsystems p.
wire bending p.

PLIF
posterior lumbar interbody fusion
posterolateral interbody fusion

plight
musician's p.

plinth

PLL
posterior longitudinal ligament

PLLA
poly-L-lactic acid

PLM
precise lesion measuring
PLM device

plombage
bone p.

plot
load-displacement p.

plotter
X-Y p.

PLS
plastic leaf-spring

PLT
peroneus longus tendinopathy

plug
bone femoral p.
bone-graft p.
Buck p.
calcaneal bone p.
cement p.
p. cutter

NOTES

P

plug (*continued*)
    Exeter intramedullary bone p.
    femoral p.
    Grafton DBM Matrix demineralized bone graft p.
    orthoPLUG soft bone p.
    Osteonics acetabular dome hole p.
    patellar p.
    plastic femoral p.
    polyethylene femoral Buck p.
plumb
    p. line
    p. line analysis
plumbism
Plum-Blossom acupuncture needle
Plummer-Vinson syndrome
plunger
    dome p.
plunger-type femoral pressurizer
pluripotential
    p. mesenchymal tumor
    p. mesenchymoma
plus
    Nexerciser P.
    Steri-Cuff P.
Plyoback Rebounder
plyometric
    p. exercise
    p. resistance
plyometrics
Plyo-Sled exerciser
Plystan prosthesis
PM
    physical medicine
PMA
    progressive muscular atrophy
PMD
    progressive muscular dystrophy
PMID
    painful minor intervertebral dysfunction
PMMA
    polymethyl methacrylate
    PMMA bone cement
    PMMA centralizer
    PMMA implant
PMR
    physical medicine and rehabilitation
    polymyalgia rheumatica
    posteromedial release
PMT
    PMT halo system
    PMT halo system brace
PneuGel
    P. ankle brace
    P. ankle wrap
    P. shoulder wrap
Pneu Knee brace
pneumarthrosis

pneumatic
    p. ankle tourniquet
    p. antishock garment (PASG)
    p. 4-bar linkage knee
    p. compression boot
    p. compression sleeve
    p. compression stockings
    p. compression therapy
    p. drill accessory
    p. external compression device
    p. garment
    p. massage
    p. orthosis
    p. pedal compression
    p. peripheral circulation improvement device (PPCID)
    p. resistance exercise
    p. splint
    p. tire injury
    p. tourniquet
    p. tourniquet cuff
pneumatocyst
    intraosseous p.
pneumoarthrogram
pneumoarthrography
pneumogenic osteoarthropathy
pneumonitis
pneumothermomassage
pneumothorax
Pneu-trac
    P.-t. cervical collar
    P.-t. neck brace
PNF
    proprioceptive neuromuscular facilitation
    proprioceptive neuromuscular fasciculation
    PNF exercise
    PNF pattern
    PNF technique
PNR
    perineural fibroma
PNS
    parasympathetic nervous system
    peripheral nervous system
P&O
    prosthesis and orthosis
    prosthetic and orthotic
podalgia
podarthritis
podedema
podiatric
    p. bur
    p. medicine
podiatrist
podiatry
    P. Institute
    P. Institute procedure

P. Institute procedures for ankle arthrodesis

P. Institute rasp

PodiAxis orthopaedic sole

Podi-Burr

large callus P.-B.

large nail P.-B.

medium callus P.-B.

medium nail P.-B.

P.-B. nail bur

podismus

poditis

pododynamometer

pododynia

PodoFlex

P. machine

P. reflexology device

podogeriatrics

podogram

podograph

podologist

podology

podomechanotherapy

podometer

podopediatrics

podospasm

Podospray

Darco P.

P. nail drill system

P. podiatry drill

Pogon chair

Pogrund lateral approach

point

acupuncture p.

anchoring p.

associated myofascial trigger p.

back shu paraspinal p.

bleeding p.

break p.

cannulated drill p.

carbon steel drill p.

contact p.

cookbook stimulation of acupuncture p.'s

Crowe pilot p.

Crutchfield drill p.

dorsal p.

drill p.

electrodesiccated bleeding p.

end p.

entry p.

Erb p.

glenoid p.

inflexion p.

isometric p.

6-p. knee brace

Krackow p.

material failure break p.

Mathews drill p.

motor p.

myofascial trigger p.

paraspinal p.

Pauly p.

pedicle entrance p.

pressure p.

p. and pressure systems

primary myofascial trigger p.

referred p.

satellite myofascial trigger p.

secondary myofascial trigger p.

single reference p.

Steinmann pin with Crowe pilot p.

tender p. (TeP)

p. tenderness

trigger p.

Trousseau p.

twist drill p.

Universal drill p.

vector p.

2-point

2-p. discrimination

2-p. discrimination test

2-p. gait

2-p. nerve block

2-p. step-to gait pattern

3-point

3-p. bending moment

3-p. gait

3-p. pressure cast

3-p. pressure system

3-p. pressure technique

3-p. skeletal traction

4-point

4-p. fixation

4-p. gait

4-p. IROM brace

4-p. IROM splint

4-p. SuperSport functional knee brace

4-p. walker

pointed

p. awl

p. toe shoe

pointer

hip p.

shoulder p.

NOTES

P

Pointer-Plus locator/stimulator
pointillage
point-of-reduction clamp
Poirier
    space of P.
Poisson ratio
poker
    p. back
    p. spine
POL
    posterior oblique ligament
Poland
    P. anomaly
    P. classification of physial injury
    P. epiphysial fracture classification
    P. syndrome
polar
    P. Care 500 cryotherapy device
    P. Pack
    P. Wrap cold therapy
    P. wrist monitor
    p. zone
Polaris knee rehab brace
polarization
Polar-Mate coagulator
Polarus
    P. humeral rod
    P. Plus humeral fixation system
    P. positional humeral fixation
       system
pole
    Exerstrider walking p.
    walking p.
policeman's heel
policy
    impaired competitor p.
    National Collegiate Athletic
       Association drug testing p.
    P. and Review Committee for
       Human Research
polio
poliomyelitis treatment
polka-dot pattern
Polk finger goniometer
pollex
    p. abductus
    p. pedis
pollicis
    adductor p.
    p. longus muscle
    opponens p. (OP)
pollicization
    Buck-Gramcko p.
    Gillies p.
    Littler p.
    Riordan p.
pollicized ray
Pollock sign

POLPSA
    posterior labrocapsular periosteal sleeve
      avulsion
    POLPSA lesion
polyacetal resin
polyarteritis nodosa
polyarthric
polyarthritis
    juvenile p.
    vertebral p.
polyarthropathy
polyarticular
    p. juvenile rheumatoid arthritis
    p. symmetric tophaceous joint
      inflammation
polyaxial
    p. cervical screw
    p. joint
    p. system
polybutester suture
polybutilate-coated polyester
Polycel bone composite prosthesis
polycentric
    P. Hinged Ulnar Deviation Splint
    p. knee prosthesis
    p. rotation
    p. unconstrained prosthesis
    P. and Wide-Track knee system
polydactylous cleft foot
polydactyly
    central p.
    phalangeal p.
    postaxial p.
    preaxial p.
    short rib p.
    thumb p.
    Wassel classification of thumb p.
Polydek suture
Polyderm hydrophilic polyurethane foam
  dressing
Poly-Dial
    P.-D. insert
    P.-D. prosthesis
    P.-D. socket
polydioxanone suture (PDS)
polydystrophy
    Hurler p.
polyester
    Dacron p.
    polybutilate-coated p.
    p. suture
polyether implant material
polyethylene
    ArCom processed p.
    p. button
    carbon fiber-reinforced p.
    p. compression molding
    p. debris
    p. drain

Durasul p.
extruded bar p.
p. femoral Buck plug
p. femoral Buck plug procedure
p. foam
high molecular weight p.
  (HMWPE)
p. implant material
p. liner
p. liner implant component
p. patellar implant prosthesis
p. peg
porous p.
p. proximal brim in quadrilateral
  contour
p. sleeve
p. socket
p. suture
p. talar prosthesis
p. tibial insert
ultrahigh molecular weight p.
  (UHMWPE)
polyethylene-faced
p.-f. driver
p.-f. mallet
Polyform splint
polygalactic acid suture
polyglactin suture
polyglycolide implant
polyglyconate suture
polylactide
p. absorbable screw
p. implant
poly-L-lactic acid (PLLA)
Poly-Lock bonding
PolyMem wound care dressing
polymer
biodegradable synthetic p.
cold-curing p.
Hylamer orthopaedic bearing p.
self-curing p.
viscoelastic p.
PolymerFriction total knee
polymeric
p. debris
p. dressing
polymerization of bone cement
polymetatarsalia
polymethyl
p. methacrylate (PMMA)
p. methacrylate bone cement
p. methacrylate implant
polymethylmethacrylate biomaterial

polymorphic hamartoma
polymyalgia rheumatica (PMR)
polymyositis myopathy
polyneuritiformis
heredopathia atactica p.
polyneuritis
peripheral p.
polyneuropathy
gait disorder, autoantibody, late-age
  onset, p. (GALOP)
sensory p.
polyolefin elastomer
polyostotic
p. bone lesion
p. fibrous dysplasia
polyp
fibroepithelial p.
polyphasic action potential
Polypin biodegradable pin implant
polypropylene
p. ankle-foot orthosis
p. glycol-ankle-foot orthosis (PPG-
  AFO)
p. glycol-thoracolumbosacral orthosis
  (PPG-TLSO)
p. insert
p. prosthesis
p. suture
polyradiculoneuropathy
acute inflammatory demyelinating p.
  (AIDP)
polyradiculopathy
acute inflammatory p.
diabetic p.
polyserositis
Polyskin dressing
Polysonic ultrasound lotion
Polysorb
P. heel cup
P. liner
P. meniscal stapler XLS
P. suture
Polysporin Topical
Polystim electrode
Polytechnic foot-pressure measuring
  plate
polytetrafluoroethylene (PTFE)
expanded p. (EPTFE)
polytomography
polytrauma algorithm
polyurethane
p. bandage
p. cast

NOTES

P

553

polyurethane *(continued)*
    p. foam dressing (PFD)
    p. implant material
    p. liner
polyvinyl
    p. alcohol
    p. alcohol splint
    p. alcohol splinting material
    p. chloride (PVC)
    p. implant material
PolyWic dressing
pommel
    p. cushion
    p. horse gymnastics
Poncet
    P. disease
    P. rheumatism
poncho restraint
pond
    P. adjustable splint
    p. fracture
Ponseti
    P. clubfoot treatment method
    P. splint
    P. technique
Pontenza arthrodesis
pontine micturition center
Pontocaine With Dextrose Injection
pontoon spica cast
pool
    Aquaciser p.
    AquaMotion p.
    aquatic therapy p.
    Endless Pool physical therapy p.
    Ferno custom therapy p.
    motor neuronal p.
    SwimEx p.
    p. therapy
poor
    p. alignment
    p. bone stock
    p. cosmesis
POP
  PCL-oriented placement
  plaster of Paris
    POP cast
pop
    p. rivet
    P. Rivet fixation system
Popeye arm
popliteal
    p. angle
    p. artery
    p. block
    p. crease
    p. entrapment syndrome
    p. fascia
    p. flexion creaking
    p. fossa

    p. fossa entrapment
    p. fossa neural blockade
    p. hiatus
    p. ligament
    p. muscle
    p. nerve
    p. pressure sign
    p. pterygium syndrome
    p. recess
    p. region
    p. sciatic nerve block
    p. space
    p. tendon
    p. vein
    p. vessel
popliteofibular ligament
popliteomeniscal fascicle
popliteus
    p. bypass
    p. tendinitis
    p. tendon
popoff suture
Poppen
    P. forceps
    P. Gigli saw guide
    P. ridge sensitometer
popping
    joint p.
porcine prosthesis
PORD
  posterior reduction device
porencephalic cyst
Porocoat
    P. AML noncemented prosthesis
    P. porous coating
    P. prosthetic material
    Tri-Lock total hip prosthesis
    with P.
Poro-in-between sole
porokeratoma
porokeratosis, pl. **porokeratoses**
    p. of Mibelli
poroma
    eccrine p.
Porometal noncemented femoral
  prosthesis
Poron
    P. cellular urethane
    P. 400 insole
poroplastic splint
porosity
    interfacial p.
porotic bone
porous
    p. cementless component
    p. coating
    p. ingrowth fixation
    p. metal
    p. polyethylene

p. polyethylene graft
p. prosthetic material
p. sheet
p. surfaced prosthesis
porous-coated
p.-c. acetabular cup
p.-c. anatomic (PCA)
p.-c. anatomic prosthesis
p.-c. anatomic total hip
replacement
p.-c. anatomic total knee
p.-c. component
p.-c. femur prosthesis
p.-c. hip prosthesis
p.-c. implant
PORP
partial ossicular replacement prosthesis
Richards hydroxyapatite PORP
porphyria
porphyritic neuropathy
portable
p. C-arm image intensifier
fluoroscopy
p. diagnostic kit
P. Topical Hyperbaric Oxygen
Extremity Chamber
portal
1–2 p.
3–4 p.
4–5 p.
p. accessory
ankle p.
anterior p.
anterocentral arthroscopic p.
anteroinferior p.
anterolateral p.
anteromedial p.
arthroscopic entry p.
Caspari arthroscopic p.
central transpatellar tendon p.
desktop therapy p.
direct lateral p.
inside-out technique for establishing
ankle p.
lateral transmalleolar p.
MCR p.
MCU p.
medial p.
midcarpal p.
midlateral p.
midpatellar p.
Neviaser p.
patellar p.

p. placement
posterior p.
posteroinferior p.
posterolateral p.
posteromedial p.
P. Pro 2 treatment chair
proximal midpatellar medial and
lateral p.'s
radiocarpal p.
stab wound arthroscopic entry p.
straight posterior p.
subacromial p.
superior p.
superolateral outflow p.
superomedial p.
suprapatellar p.
Swedish p.
6-p. synovectomy
2-p. technique
3-p. technique
transmalleolar p.
transpatellar tendon p.
transtendocalcaneus p.
6U p.
Wilmington arthroscopic p.
porta pedis
Porter-Richardson-Vainio
P.-R.-V. synovectomy
P.-R.-V. technique
portion
accessory p.
cord p.
devitalized p.
proximal p.
Portmann drill
portmanteau procedure
Portola Valley Scale
port-wine stain
Porzett splint
Posada fracture
Posey
P. bar kit
P. bed cradle
P. belt
P. drop seat
P. grip
P. Palm Cone
P. sling
Positex knee wedge
position
anatomic p.
angular p.
antiembolic p.

NOTES

position *(continued)*
    arch and slouch p.
    barber chair p.
    bayonet fracture p.
    beach chair p.
    Bonner p.
    Brickner p.
    cottonloader p.
    decubitus p.
    de Kleyn p.
    dorsal lithotomy p.
    dorsal recumbent p.
    dorsiflexion-plantar flexion p.
    empty can p.
    equinus p.
    erect p.
    figure-of-4 p.
    fist p.
    flexed p.
    Fowler p.
    frog-leg p.
    full lateral p.
    p. of function
    Gaynor-Hart p.
    horizontal p.
    intrinsic minus p.
    jackknife p.
    James p.
    jet-pilot p.
    Jones p.
    jumper's knee p.
    kneeling p.
    90-90 kneeling p.
    Kraske p.
    lateral decubitus p.
    lateral park-bench p.
    lithotomy p.
    lotus p.
    mediolateral p.
    military brace p.
    military tuck p.
    neutral hip p.
    normal anatomic p.
    opisthotonic p.
    over-the-top p.
    Phalen p.
    prayer p.
    prone p.
    proximal bow p.
    quasistatic stressed p.
    rectus p.
    recumbent p.
    resting calcaneal stance p. (RCSP)
    reverse Trendelenburg p.
    scissor-leg p.
    semi-Fowler p.
    semisitting p.
    p. sense
    side-lying p.

    side-posture p.
    Sims p.
    sitting p.
    sniffer's p.
    p. in space
    spinal fusion p.
    subtalar joint neutral p. (STNP)
    supine p.
    three-quarters prone p.
    tibial sesamoid p. (TSP)
    translational p.
    Trendelenburg p.
    x-ray p.

positional
    p. dyskinesia
    p. release therapy

positioner
    acetabular cup p.
    Allen arthroscopic elbow p.
    Allen arthroscopic knee p.
    Allen arthroscopic wrist p.
    arm p.
    Assistant Free Stulberg leg p.
    Bareskin knee p.
    Biomet Second Assistant knee p.
    cup p.
    DeMay hip p.
    De Mayo hip p.
    Grasshopper p.
    IMP Universal knee p.
    IMP Universal lateral p.
    Kirschenbaum foot p.
    knee p.
    leg p.
    Mark II Stulberg hip p.
    Mark II Stulberg leg p.
    Mark II Wixson hip p.
    McConnell shoulder p.
    McGuire pelvic p.
    Montreal hip p.
    OSI-Schlein shoulder p.
    Picket Fence leg p.
    Prep-Assist p.
    Profex arthroscopic leg p.
    Schlein shoulder p.
    shoulder abduction p.
    Stulberg hip p.
    Stulberg Mark II leg p.
    SurgAssist leg p.
    Ther-A-Shapes p.
    Universal knee p.
    Universal lateral p.
    Vac-Pac p.
    Wixson hip p.

positioning
    patient p.
    proper neck p.

positive
    p. ability

p. afterpotential
p. impingement sign
p. rim sign
p. sharp wave
p. supporting reflex
p. ulnar variance (PUV)

positron

p. emission tomographic scan
p. emission tomography (PET)

post

extrinsic rearfoot p.
iliac p.
Isola spinal implant system iliac p.
Luque-Galveston p.
Morse tapered prosthetic p.
perineal p.
status p.
thumb p.
P. total shoulder arthroplasty

postactivation

p. depression
p. exhaustion
p. facilitation
p. potentiation

postacute sprain
Postalume finger splint
post-and-cam mechanism
postanesthesia

p. care unit (PACU)
p. recovery (PAR)

postaxial

p. muscle
p. polydactyly

postcalcaneal bursitis
postcast compression reflex
postcasting syndrome
postcompetition rehabilitation
postconcussive syndrome
Postel

P. coxarthropathy
P. hip status system

2-poster

2-p. brace
2-p. cervical orthosis

4-poster

4-p. cervical brace
4-p. cervical orthosis
4-p. frame

posterior

anterior and p. (AP)
p. to anterior screw
p. apprehension test
p. arch

p. arch fracture
p. atlantoaxial arthrodesis
p. atlantoodontoid interval
p. axillary line (PAL)
p. bending moment
p. bone block
p. bone graft
p. bow
p. calcaneal displacement osteotomy
p. capsule
p. capsulorrhaphy
p. capsulotomy
p. cervical fixation
p. cervical fusion
p. cervical line
p. cervical spinal instrumentation
p. colliculus
p. column fracture
p. column osteosynthesis
p. column sign
p. compartment
p. component
p. construct
p. cord syndrome
p. costotransversectomy approach
p. cruciate
p. cruciate condylar knee system
p. cruciate ligament (PCL)
p. cruciate ligament graft
p. cruciate ligament of knee
p. cruciate ligament tear
p. cruciate sprain
p. curvature
p. deltoid muscle
p. deltoid-to-triceps transfer
p. depression pattern
p. distraction instrumentation
p. drainage
p. drawer sign
p. drawer test
p. element
p. element fracture
p. endplate
p. facet
p. facet dislocation
p. facet displacement
p. femoral cutaneous nerve
p. fixation system biomechanics
p. flap
p. flap technique
p. fracture-dislocation
p. glenoid elevator
p. glenoid labrum

NOTES

P

posterior *(continued)*
    p. glenoplasty
    p. glide
    p. hiatal sign
    p. hip dislocation
    p. hook-rod spinal instrumentation
    p. horn
    p. horn meniscal tear
    p. iliac osteotomy
    p. iliofemoral technique
    p. impingement
    p. impingement syndrome
    p. incision
    p. inferior cerebellar artery (PICA)
    p. inferior tibiofibular ligament
    p. innominate
    p. innominate rotation
    p. interosseous branch
    p. interosseous nerve
    p. interosseous nerve approach
    p. interosseous nerve compression
      syndrome
    p. interosseous nerve entrapment
    p. interosseous nerve palsy
    p. interspinous wiring
    p. inverted-U approach
    p. joint syndrome
    p. knee pull syndrome
    p. labrocapsular periosteal sleeve
      avulsion (POLPSA)
    p. labrocapsular periosteal sleeve
      avulsion lesion
    p. leaf-spring ankle-foot orthosis
    p. ligamentous injury
    p. lip
    p. longitudinal fiber region
    p. longitudinal ligament (PLL)
    p. lower cervical spine stabilization
    p. lower cervical spine surgery
    p. lumbar interbody fusion (PLIF)
    p. lumbar interbody fusion surgery
    p. lumbar spine and sacrum
      surgery
    p. malleolus
    p. meniscofemoral ligament
    p. midline approach
    p. mold splint
    p. nerve decompression
    p. oblique fiber region
    p. oblique ligament (POL)
    p. oblique meniscal tear
    p. oblique sprain
    p. occipitocervical approach
    p. osteophyte
    p. pelvic tilt
    p. pharyngeal abscess
    p. portal
    p. process fracture

    p. radial collateral artery
    p. reduction device (PORD)
    p. release
    p. rhizotomy
    p. rod system
    p. rotation on left side
    p. rotation on right side
    p. sacroiliac ligament
    p. sacroiliac spine (PSIS)
    p. sag sign
    p. screw fixation
    p. segmental fixation
    p. shoulder approach
    p. shoulder dislocation
    p. shoulder instability
    p. spinal fusion
    p. spinal plating
    p. spinal wedge osteotomy
    p. spur
    p. stability
    p. stress test
    p. subluxation test
    p. superior humeral head defect
    p. superior iliac spine (PSIS)
    superior labrum anterior and p.
      (SLAP)
    p. talar process fracture
    p. talofibular ligament (PTFL)
    p. thigh bar
    p. tibial artery
    p. tibialis tendon lengthening
    p. tibial nerve (PTN)
    p. tibial nerve entrapment
    p. tibial pulse (PTP)
    p. tibial spine
    p. tibial tendinitis (PTT)
    p. tibial tendinopathy
    p. tibial tendon (PTT)
    p. tibial tendon dysfunction
      (PTTD)
    p. tibial tendon insufficiency
    p. tibial tendon transfer
    p. tibiofibular ligament
    p. tibiotalar ligament
    p. translation
    p. transolecranon approach
    p. triangle
    p. tuberosity
    p. upper cervical spine surgery
    p. wall fracture
posterior-anterior
    p.-a. glide
    p.-a. pressure
    p.-a. screw
posterior-inferior
    p.-i. capsular shift procedure
    p.-i. spine
posteriorly

posterior-superior
    p.-s. humeral head lesion
    p.-s. oblique projection
posteroanterior (PA)
posterodistal
posteroinferior (PI)
    p. external (PIEx)
    p. external movement
    p. ilium major
    p. internal (PIIn)
    p. internal movement
    p. portal
posterolateral
    p. approach
    p. approach of Henry
    p. arthrodesis
    p. aspect
    p. bone graft
    p. bone graft placement
    p. bundle
    p. capsule
    p. compartment
    p. costotransversectomy incision
    p. costotransversectomy technique
    p. decompression
    p. drainage
    p. drawer sign
    p. drawer test
    p. herniation
    p. interbody fusion (PLIF)
    p. lumbosacral fusion
    p. pivot test
    p. portal
    p. release
    p. rotary instability
    p. spine fusion
    p. structure
posteromedial
    p. approach
    p. bow
    p. bundle
    p. capsule
    p. compartment
    p. corner
    p. dislocation
    p. drainage
    p. drawer sign
    p. pivot-shift test
    p. portal
    p. region
    p. release (PMR)
    p. release of clubfoot
    p. rotary instability

posteroproximal
poster orthosis
postexercise hypotension
postfracture
    p. cyst
    p. lesion
    p. osteomyelitis
    p. swelling
    p. syndrome
postfusion brace
postganglionic technique
postherpetic pain
postinfectious
    p. arthritis
    p. myopathy
posting
    heel p.
    strip p.
    wedge p.
postinjection image
postinjury period
postirradiation
    p. fracture
    p. osteogenic sarcoma
postisometric
    p. relaxation
    p. relaxation traction technique
    p. stretch technique
postlaminectomy
    p. kyphosis
    p. 2-level spondylolisthesis
postmenopausal
    p. arthritis
    p. bone loss
postmortem fracture
postnatal
    p. cerebral palsy
    p. gangrene
postoperative
    p. antibiotic
    p. bracing
    p. casting
    p. complication
    p. corticosteroid
    p. drainage-related hematoma
    p. dressing
    p. extubation
    p. flexor tendon (PFT)
    p. fracture
    p. immobilization
    p. immobilizer
    p. infection
    p. lumbosacral orthosis

NOTES

P

postoperative *(continued)*
    p. pain
    p. paraplegia
    p. radiograph
    p. regimen
    p. shoe
    p. synovitis
    p. therapy
    p. wound care
postphlebitis syndrome
postpoliomyelitic contracture
postpolio syndrome
postpyelomyelitis syndrome
postradiation kyphosis
postreduction x-ray
poststatic dyskinesia (PSDK)
postsurgical heel condition
posttetanic
    p. exhaustion
    p. facilitation
    p. potentiation
posttraumatic
    p. algodystrophic syndrome
    p. angulation
    p. apoplexy
    p. arthritis
    p. arthrosis
    p. cavus
    p. chronic cord syndrome
    p. chronic osteomyelitis
    p. degenerative disease
    p. dystrophy
    p. edema
    p. epilepsy
    p. flatfoot
    p. hemarthrosis
    p. kyphosis
    p. neuroma
    p. osteoarthritis
    p. osteoarthrosis
    p. osteolysis
    p. osteonecrosis
    p. osteoporosis
    p. pain
    p. sacroiliac dysfunction
    p. spinal deformity
    p. syringomyelia
postulnar bone
postural
    p. analysis
    p. balance
    p. complex
    p. component
    p. control
    p. development
    p. exteroceptor
    p. fixation back maneuver
    p. instability
    p. interoceptor

    p. ischemia
    p. list
    p. muscle
    p. receptor
    p. reflex
    p. strain
    p. sway
    p. syndrome
    p. tremor
    p. variation
Postura wheelchair cushion
posture
    batrachian p.
    benediction p.
    cavus p.
    P. Curve lumbar cushion
    decerebrate p.
    decorticate p.
    p. education
    forward flexion p.
    forward head p.
    p. of limb
    P. Pump lordoticiser
    P. Pump Spine Trainer
    recumbent p.
    P. S'port
    p. Wedge seat cushion
Posture-Rite lap desk
posturing
    equinovarus p.
posturography
    computerized dynamic p. (CDP)
potassium-40 count
potential
    action p. (AP)
    auditory evoked p. (AEP)
    bioelectric p.
    biphasic action p.
    bizarre repetitive p.
    brainstem auditory evoked p.
     (BAEP)
    brief, small, abundant p. (BSAP)
    brief, small, abundant,
     polyphasic p. (BSAPP)
    complex motor unit action p.
    compound mixed nerve action p.
    compound motor nerve action p.
    compound muscle action p.
     (CMAP)
    compound muscle-motor action p.
     (CMAP)
    compound sensory nerve action p.
    denervation p.
    dermatosensory evoked p.
    electrical p.
    electrokinetic p.
    endplate p. (EPP)
    evoked compound muscle action p.
    excitatory postsynaptic p.

far-field p.
fasciculation p.
fibrillation p.
giant motor unit action p.
inhibitory postsynaptic p.
irregular p.
kilovoltage p.
linked p.
long-latency somatosensory evoked p.
miniature end-plate p. (MEPP)
monophasic action p.
motor unit p. (MUP)
motor unit action p. (MUAP)
muscle fiber action p.
myopathic motor unit p.
myotonic p.
nascent motor unit p.
near-field p.
nerve action p. (NAP)
nerve fiber action p.
nerve trunk action p.
neurogenic motor evoked p. (NMEP)
neuropathic motor unit p.
piezoelectric p.
polyphasic action p.
pseudopolyphasic action p.
regeneration motor unit p.
resting membrane p.
satellite p.
sensory evoked p.
sensory nerve action p. (SNAP)
serrated action p.
short-latency somatosensory evoked p.
somatosensory evoked p. (SEP, SSEP)
spinal evoked p.
streaming p.
tetraphasic action p.
triphasic action p.
visual evoked p.

potentiation
postactivation p.
posttetanic p.

potentiometer
linear p.

Pott
P. abscess
P. ankle fracture
P. disease
P. dwarfism

P. gangrene
P. paralysis
P. paraplegia
P. puffy tumor
P. spinal curvature

Potter arthrodesis
Potts
P. eversion osteotomy
P. splint
P. tibial osteotomy

Potts-Smith dressing forceps
pouce flottant thumb
pouch
antibiotic bead p.
bead p.
inflamed synovial p.
suprapatellar p.

pouch-type sling
Poulet disease
poundal
pounds of traction
Poupart inguinal ligament
Pouteau
P. fracture
P. syndrome

powder
p. board
thrombin p.

powdered bone graft
power
P. Anthro Shoe
p. bone saw
p. bur
p. drill
grasping p.
p. oscillating saw
P. Pillow cervical massager
pinch p.
P. Play knee brace
P. Pogo stationary exerciser
p. rasp
p. reamer
thumb pinch p.
P. Trainer cycle
P. Web hand exerciser
P. Web Jr. exerciser
p. wheelchair

Powerbelt exercise system
PowerCut drill blade
power-driven
p.-d. reamer
p.-d. saw
powered metaphysial stapler

NOTES

P

Powerflex
    P. CMP exerciser
    P. tape
Power-Grip pliers
Powermatic table
POWERPoint orthotic shoe insert
PowerStar bipolar scissors
Powerstep
    P. foot support
    P. orthotics
PowerTrack II muscle testing
  instrument
PP
    proximal phalanx
PPCID
    pneumatic peripheral circulation
      improvement device
      PPCID slippers
PPD
    permanent partial disability
      PPD rating
PPF
    percutaneous plantar fasciotomy
PPG
    photoplethysmography
PPG-AFO
    polypropylene glycol-ankle-foot orthosis
      PPG-AFO brace
PPG-TLSO
    polypropylene glycol-thoracolumbosacral
      orthosis
      PPG-TLSO brace
PPO
    passive prehension orthosis
PPS
    patellofemoral pain syndrome
    prospective payment system
PPT
    professional protective technology
      PPT flat insole
      PPT gel stirrup ankle support
      PPT insole system
      PPT MXL soft molded insole
      PPT orthotic device
      PPT Plastizote insole
      PPT RX firm molded insole
      PPT sheet
      PPT soft tissue orthotic system
PQ
    pronator quadratus
      PQ premium heel cup
PR
    pelvic rock
    progressive-resistive exercise
practitioner
    scientific p.
PRAFO
    pressure-relief ankle-foot orthotic
      PRAFO adjustable orthotic

      PRAFO KAFO
      PRAFO PKA KAFO attachment
Prague pelvis
Pratt
    P. open reduction
    P. symptom
    P. T-clamp
    P. technique
prayer
    p. position
    p. view
PRE
    progressive-resistive exercise
preacher curl
pre-Achilles
    p.-A. bursa
    p.-A. bursitis
    p.-A. fat pad
    p.-A. mass
preassembled metal-backed socket
preaxial
    p. muscle
    p. polydactyly
prebent nail
precaution
    cardiac p.'s
    universal p.'s
precise lesion measuring (PLM)
precision
    P. hip stem
    P. Osteolock
    P. Osteolock femoral component
      system
    P. Osteolock femoral prosthesis
    P. Osteolock fixation
    P. Osteolock hip prosthesis
    P. spinal cord stimulator
    P. Strata hip system
    P. total hip
Preclude spinal membrane
precoat
    P. hip prosthesis
    P. Plus femoral prosthesis
precompression jig
precontoured unit rod
precurved
    p. ball-tipped guidepin
    p. plate
PreCustom Orthotic
Predcor-TBA Injection
prediction
    Anderson-Green growth p.
    growth p.
Predictive Salvage Index
predictor of injury
predislocation syndrome
predisposition
    congenital p.
Prednisol TBA Injection

preemptive blockade technique
prefabricated wool felt pad
preganglionic
 p. sympathectomy
 p. technique
prehallux
 external p.
 p. osseous prominence
prehension
 p. force
 p. grasp
 p. orthosis
preinterparietal bone
Preiser disease
preload
Prelone Oral
premalleolar
 p. bursitis
 p. fat pad
premanipulative testing
premature
 p. closure
 p. consolidation
Premier press fit prosthesis
prenatal dislocation
Prenyl jacket
preoperative
 p. antibiotic
 p. drawing
 p. evaluation
 p. management
 p. plan
 p. planning
 p. roentgenography
 p. tomography
preparation
 bone-patellar tendon-bone p.
 facet joint p.
 graft p.
 lupus erythematosus p.
 3M p.
 rod contour p.
 skin p.
 Spälteholz p.
 wire contour p.
Prep-Assist
 P.-A. legholder
 P.-A. positioner
prepatellar
 p. bursa
 p. bursa inflammation
 p. bursitis
 p. neuralgia

Prep-IM
presacral block
Presbyterian Hospital T-clamp
preschooler
 Miller Assessment for P.'s (MAP)
prescription
 ACSM Guidelines for Exercise
  Testing and P.
 P. Strength Desenex
preservation
 lordosis p.
 lumbar lordosis p.
prespondylolisthesis
press
 CamStar power leg p.
 p. fit
 leg p.
 Shuttle MVP leg p.
 supine chest p.
 p. up
press-fit
 p.-f. acetabular implant insertion
  technique
 p.-f. circumferential grommet
 p.-f. condylar knee arthroplasty
 p.-f. condylar total knee
 p.-f. condylar total knee prosthesis
 p.-f. cup
 p.-f. femoral component
 p.-f. fixation
 p.-f. stem
 p.-f. total condylar knee system
pressure
 p. algometer
 ankle systolic p.
 blood p.
 bone marrow p. (BMP)
 central posterior-anterior p.
 compartmental p.
 p. cushion
 disc p.
 Doppler ankle systolic p.
 p. epiphysis
 p. excursion index
 forefoot peak p.
 p. fracture
 p. glove
 hydrostatic p.
 intracompartmental p.
 intradiscal p.
 lateral root p.
 manual p.
 p. necrosis

NOTES

P

pressure *(continued)*
    p. paralysis
    peak p.
    plantar p.
    p. plate
    p. point
    posterior-anterior p.
    p. relief padding
    p. relief shoe
    Rolfing p.
    P. Sentinel reamer
    sequential p.
    p. sore
    systolic blood p.
    p. therapy
    p. threshold
    p. threshold meter
    tissue p.
    toe p.
    p. tolerance
    tourniquet p.
    p. transducer
    p. transducer-monitor system
    p. ulcer assessment
    p. ulcer classification
    p. ulcer cleansing
    p. ulcer dressing
    p. ulcer (grade I-IV)
    p. ulcer management
    p. ulcer prevention
    p. ulcer-related maggot infestation
    ultraviolet light p.
PressureGuard mattress
pressure-relief
    p.-r. ankle-foot orthotic (PRAFO)
    p.-r. cushion
pressure-relieving orthosis
pressure-sensitive
    p.-s. area
    p.-s. tissue
Pressure-Specified Sensory Device
pressure-time integral (PTI)
pressure-tolerant tissue
pressurized cement
pressurizer
    acetabular p.
    plunger-type femoral p.
Preston
    P. ligamentum flavum forceps
    P. overhead pulley
    P. pinch gauge
    P. screw
    P. Traveler CPM exerciser
Prestop pinchometer
pretarget filtration system
pretendinous
    p. band
    p. band of hand
    p. cord

pretibial
    p. bearing (PTB)
    p. buttress (PTB)
    p. edema
Prevacare
    P. moisturizing cream
    P. spray
prevention
    heat injury p.
    heterotopic ossification p.
    infection p.
    Lower Extremity Amputation P.
    (LEAP)
    osseous bridge p.
    pressure ulcer p.
    rod rotation p.
Prevent Recurrence of Osteoporotic Fractures (PROOF)
prevertebral space
PRICE
    protection, restricted activity, ice, compression, elevation
Price muscular biopsy clamp
prickling pain
Pridie
    P. ankle arthrodesis
    P. incision
Primaderm dressing
Primapore wound dressing
primary
    p. amputation
    p. arthroplasty
    p. bone union
    p. center
    p. closure
    p. cranial sacral respiratory mechanism
    p. curve
    p. cystic arthrosis
    p. degenerative arthritis
    p. degenerative osteoarthritis
    p. focus of pain
    p. hip replacement
    p. intention
    p. or intentional movement
    p. lymphoma
    p. lymphoma of bone (PLB)
    p. movement plane
    p. myofascial trigger point
    p. peroneus longus tendinopathy
    p. progressive amyotrophy
    p. repair
    p. rotation movement
    p. sequestrum
    p. spongiosa
    p. stem (PS)
    p. subacute osteomyelitis
    p. subtalar arthrodesis

p. tumor
p. x-ray beam
prime mover
Primer modified Unna boot
primitive
p. bone
p. dislocation
p. locomotor pattern
p. reflex
primus
digitus p.
P. flexible great toe
p. implant
princeps pollicis artery
principal stress
principle
anatomic fracture reduction p.
axial compression p.
biomechanical p.
Enneking p.
gliding p.
Lambotte p.
SAID p.
spherical gliding p.
prism
Fresnel p.
prisoner's palsy
Pritchard
P. II elbow prosthesis
P. total elbow prosthesis
Pritchard-Walker
P.-W. semiconstrained elbow
prosthesis
P.-W. total elbow prosthesis
Pritsch talar osteochondroma
classification
prizm
p. Electro-Mesh Sock electrode
p. Electro-Mesh Z-Stim-II
stimulator
Pro
P. Balance Master
P. Osteon 500 bone graft
substitute
P. Support Systems orthotic
Pro-8 ankle brace
ProAdvantage knee
probability
bone cyst fracture p.
probe
Acufex p.
angled p.
arthroscopic p.

Bipolar Circumactive P. (BICAP)
blunt-tip p.
Bunnell dissecting p.
Bunnell forwarding p.
calibrated p.
dissecting p.
free-spinning p.
gearshift p.
gold p.
intraosseous p.
LASE p.
laser Doppler p.
multifrequency p.
multiplane echo p.
Nucleotome p.
pedicle sounding p.
reverse-cutting meniscal p.
skin temperature monitoring p.
spinning p.
p. test
p. test for osteomyelitis
triple-frequency p.
ultrasonic p.
Woodson p.
probe-to-bone test
problem area
procaine-phenol motor point injection
procallus formation
Procardia XL
Procase Ankle-Lock brace
procedure
Adams p.
Akin p.
Albee shelf p.
Albizzia leg-lengthening p.
AMBRI p.
anchovy p.
Anderson-Fowler p.
antenna p.
anterior stabilization p.
AO p.
arthroscopic transglenoid suture
stabilization p.
articulatory p.
Auto-Implant p.
Axer-Clark p.
Badgley combination p.
Baker Achilles tendon
lengthening p.
BAK laparoscopic p.
Bankart p.
Bankhart p.
Barsky p.

NOTES

procedure *(continued)*

Bartlett p.
Basic I, II cranial adjusting p.
Baxter-D'Astous p.
beefburger p.
Bell-Tawse p.
Bennett quadriceps plastic p.
Bentson p.
Berman-Gartland p.
B.H. Moore p.
Bilhaut-Cloquet p.
Blair p.
Blatt p.
bone block p.
bony p.
Bose p.
Bosworth shelf p.
Boyd-McLeod p.
Boytchev p.
Brahms p.
Braun p.
Bridle p.
Bristow p.
Bristow-Helfet p.
Bristow-Latarjet p.
Bristow-May p.
Brockman p.
Broström p.
Broström-Evans p.
Bryan p.
buttressing p.
Calandriello p.
callus distraction p.
Campbell ankle p.
capsular imbrication p.
capsular shift p.
Carticel implant p.
Castle p.
Chambers p.
Chandler p.
Charnley ankle fusion p.
checkrein p.
chevron p.
Chiari shelf p.
chiropractic adjustment p.
Chrisman-Snook weave p.
Clayton p.
Cobb tibialis posterior tendon
  dysfunction p.
Cole p.
Connolly p.
Copeland-Howard shoulder p.
core drilling p.
Cotting ingrown nail p.
Cotton p.
Cracchiolo p.
Cummins p.
curative soft tissue p.
Darrach p.

Das Gupta p.
debulking p.
degloving p.
denervation p.
DePalma staple p.
Dewar posterior cervical fixation p.
Dickson-Diveley p.
Dorrance p.
Downey-McGlamery p.
Downey-Rubin overlapping toe
  repair p.
DREZ p.
Durham p.
DuVries p.
Dwyer p.
Eden-Hybbinette p.
Eden-Lange p.
Edwards p.
eggshell p.
Elmslie-Cholmeley p.
Elmslie peroneal tendon p.
Elmslie-Trillat patellar p.
Elmslie weave p.
Engebretsen p.
Evans p.
Eve reconstructive p.
extraarticular Grice p.
failed p.
Fairbanks-Sever p.
femoral Buck plug p.
femorodistal bypass p.
Ficat p.
Fired-Hendel p.
forage p.
Fowler p.
Frank and Johnson modification of
  Heyman p.
Froimson p.
Froimson-Oh arm p.
Frost foot p.
Fulford p.
Gallie p.
Gartland p.
Gelman foot p.
Gerard resurfacing p.
Gilbert p.
Gillquist p.
Gill shelf p.
Girdlestone hip p.
Girdlestone-Taylor p.
Gould p.
gracilis p.
Grant, Surrall, and Lehman p.
Green p.
Green-Grice p.
Grice p.
Gritti-Stokes distal thigh p.
Gruca lower leg p.
Gurd p.

Hall Kalamchi shelf p.
hallux valgus p.
Hammon foot p.
Hardinge vastus lateralis p.
Hark pes planus p.
Harmon p.
Hass p.
Hauser Achilles lengthening p.
Hauser heel cord p.
Hauser patellar tendon p.
Hawkins p.
Heifetz p.
Hey Groves p.
Heyman p.
Heyman-Herndon p.
Hibbs p.
His-Haas p.
Hitchcock arm p.
Hodor-Dobbs p.
Hoffer ankle p.
Hoffmann metatarsal p.
Hohmann p.
Hoke-Miller p.
Hoke tibial palsy p.
Howorth p.
Hughston p.
IDET p.
iliac buttressing p.
Ilizarov p.
4-incision p.
5-incision p.
Inclan modification of Campbell
  ankle p.
Inclan-Ober p.
Ingram p.
Insall p.
installation p.
intercalary allograft p.
intermetatarsal angle-reducing p.
intraarticular p.
intradiscal electrothermal therapy p.
intradiscal electrothermal
  treatment p.
Jaffe p.
Jahss p.
James p.
Jansey p.
Johnson p.
Johnson-Spiegl p.
joint-destructive p.
joint salvage p.
Jones retinaculum reconstruction p.
J.R. Moore p.

Juvara p.
Kaplan modification of Ruiz-
  Mora p.
Karlsson p.
Kehr p.
Kelikian p.
Keller p.
Keller-Brandes p.
Kelly peroneal tendon
  dislocation p.
Kendrick p.
Kessel-Bonney p.
Kidner foot p.
King intraarticular hip fusion p.
Kortzeborn p.
Koutsogiannis p.
Krukenberg p.
Lance shelf p.
Lane p.
Lange p.
Langenskiöld p.
Lapidus p.
Larmon forefoot p.
Larsen lateral ankle stabilization p.
Latarjet p.
lateral sling p.
Lauenstein p.
Lawton p.
Lee p.
Leeds spinal p.
Legg p.
lengthening over nails p.
Lepird p.
ligamentous weave p.
limb-salvage p.
Lindeman p.
Lindholm Achilles lengthening p.
Linton p.
Lipscomb p.
Localio p.
Loose p.
Loose knee p.
Lorenz p.
Loughheed and White p.
lower cervical spine p.
Lowman shelf p.
Luck hand p.
Lynn Achilles lengthening p.
MacAusland p.
MacCarthy p.
macrodactalia reduction p.
Magnuson-Stack p.
Mahan p.

NOTES

P

procedure *(continued)*
    manipulative p.
    Manktelow transfer p.
    Mann p.
    Maquet p.
    Matson p.
    Mauck knee p.
    Mau and Ludloff p.
    McBride p.
    McCarty hip p.
    McCash hand p.
    McCauley foot p.
    McElvenny foot p.
    McGlamry p.
    McGlamry-Downey p.
    McKay hip p.
    McKeever p.
    McLaughlin p.
    medial rotation p.
    Mikulicz p.
    Miller foot p.
    Mitchell hallux valgus p.
    Miyakawa knee p.
    Moberg key-pinch p.
    modified Boytchev p.
    modified Broström p.
    modified Broström-Evans p.
    modified Hoke-Miller flatfoot p.
    modified Lapidus p.
    Mogensen p.
    motion control p.
    motion-preserving p.
    Mueller knee p.
    Mumford p.
    muscle-balancing p.
    Neer capsular shift p.
    Newman-Keuls p.
    Nicola shoulder p.
    Nicoll fracture repair p.
    Nilsson lateral ankle stabilization p.
    notchplasty p.
    OATS p.
    O'Brien capsular shift p.
    O'Donoghue p.
    offset-V p.
    orthodox p.
    Oudard p.
    Outerbridge-Kashiwagi p.
    over-the-top knee p.
    Pagddu p.
    Parrish p.
    Paterson p.
    Peabody and Munro p.
    peroneal tendon p.
    Perthes p.
    Pettibon chiropractic p.
    Podiatry Institute p.
    polyethylene femoral Buck plug p.
    portmanteau p.

    posterior-inferior capsular shift p.
    Proxiderm p.
    Putti-Platt shoulder p.
    realignment p.
    reefing p.
    Regnauld p.
    resurfacing p.
    Reverdin-Green foot p.
    Reverdin-Green-Laird p.
    reverse Jones p.
    reverse Mauck knee p.
    reverse Putti-Platt p.
    revision p.
    Ridlon p.
    Roaf, Kirkaldy-Willis, and
      Cattero p.
    Rockwood p.
    Root p.
    Rose foot p.
    Roux-Goldthwait p.
    Ruiz-Mora p.
    Ryerson p.
    sacroiliac buttressing p.
    Saha p.
    salvage p.
    Samilson p.
    sartorial slide p.
    Sauvé-Kapandji p.
    Schrock p.
    Scuderi p.
    Selakovich p.
    semitendinosus p.
    sequential p.
    Sgarlato hammertoe implant p.
    Sham p.
    shelf p.
    short lever specific contact p.
    Silfverskiöld p.
    Silver p.
    Skoog p.
    sling p.
    Slocum knee p.
    Somerville p.
    Souter hip p.
    Southwick slide p.
    spinal fusion p.
    spinal locking p.
    Spira p.
    Spittler p.
    SPLATT p.
    split anterior tibial tendon p.
    stabilization of chevron p.
    Stack shoulder p.
    staged p.
    staggered p.
    Staheli shelf p.
    Stamm p.
    STA-peg p.
    Steindler p.

Steytler-Van Der Walt p.
Stone p.
Strayer Achilles lengthening p.
Stromeyer Achilles tenotomy p.
Sutherland hip p.
Syme p.
Tachdjian p.
Taylor p.
tendon checkrein p.
terminal Syme p.
Thomas p.
Thomas-Thompson p.
Thompson-Terwilliger p.
Tikhoff-Linberg radical arm p.
p. time
Trillat p.
triple-wire p.
Tsai-Stillwell p.
TUBS p.
upper cervical spine p.
Valenti p.
Van Ness p.
Verebelyi-Ogston decancellation p.
VertiLok 2-stage closure p.
Vulpius p.
Vulpius-Stoffel p.
wafer p.
Wallenberg p.
Watson-Jones p.
Weaver-Dunn p.
Webb p.
Weber p.
Weston shelf p.
White slide p.
Whitman talectomy p.
Williams p.
Wilson p.
Woodward p.
Yoke transposition p.
Young p.
Youngswick p.
Youngswick-Austin metatarsal
    head p.
Yount p.
Zadik foot p.
Zancolli clawhand deformity p.
Zancolli lasso p.
Zancolli static lock p.
Zarins-Rowe p.
process
abnormal posterior talar p.
absent spinous p.
acromion p.

articular p.
bifid spinous p.
BioCleanse tissue sterilization p.
bone destructive p.
bony p.
capitular p.
casting p.
Civinini p.
cleft spinous p.
clinoid p.
condyloid p.
conoid p.
coracoacromial p.
coracoid p.
coronoid p.
cubital p.
deficient spinous p.
dislocation of articular p.
inferior p.
intact spinous p.
intercondylar p.
internal p.
lateral p.
mamillary p.
mastoid p.
maxillary p.
neuromuscular proprioceptive p.
odontoid p.
olecranon p.
orthopraxy spurious spinous p.
physial mamillary p.
proprioceptive p.
sacralized transverse p.
spinous p.
spurious articular p.
Steida bony p.
styloid p.
superior p.
supracondylar p.
talar p.
talus lateral posterior p.
transverse p.
Tutoplast p.
unciform p.
ungual p.
xiphoid p.
Zimmer PMMA precoat p.
processed carbon implant
procession
fast imaging with steady p. (FISP)
ProCol bovine bioprosthesis tendon
procurvatum deformity
ProCyte transparent dressing

NOTES

P

Proderm topical spray
Pro-Designed wrist guard
ProDisc
> P. I disc prosthesis
> P. lumbar total disc replacement
> P. spinal disc prosthesis

Pro-Disc-C cervical artificial disc implant
product
> Body Glove orthopaedic p.
> cyclooxygenase p.
> Fortitude Ti titanium spinal fixation p.
> Fortitude Vue titanium spinal fixation p.
> Innovation Sports bracing p.
> Innovative Medical P.'s (IMP)
> Linvatec p.
> Linvatec arthroscopy p.
> microparticulated protein p.
> Orthopaedic Physical Therapy P.'s (OPTP)
> Oxiplex/SP bioresorbable p.
> resistive exercise p.'s (REP)

production
> bone p.
> torque p.

professional protective technology (PPT)
Profex
> P. arthroscopic leg positioner
> P. arthroscopic tourniquet

proficiency
> Bruininks-Oseretsky Test of Motor P.

profile
> acromial p.
> Functional Limitation P. (FLP)
> Hawaii Early Learning P. (HELP)
> P. hip prosthesis
> P. hip stem
> Maryland Foot Score P.
> PULSES p.
> reduced p. (RP)
> risk factor p.
> P. Sitting Orthosis
> Staheli rotational p.
> surface p.
> P. total hip system
> wrist speed p.

Profix
> P. confirming tibial insert
> P. metaphysial tibial stem
> P. mobile-bearing knee implant
> P. nonporous tibial base
> P. porous femoral component
> P. total knee replacement system

ProFlex wrist support
ProFlo vascular compression therapy

Profore
> P. Four-Layer bandage system
> P. wound dressing

ProForma prosthesis
profunda
> p. brachii artery
> p. femoris

profundus
> p. advancement
> p. artery fracture
> flexor digitorum p. (FDP)
> p. muscle
> p. tendon

Pro-glide
> P.-g. orthosis
> P.-g. splint

program
> Abaqus modeling p.
> aquatic exercise p.
> aquatic stabilization p.
> Camp Diversity arthritis p.
> Carpal Care rehabilitative p.
> exercise p.
> flexibility conditioning p.
> home exercise p.
> home spinal stabilization p.
> independent exercise p.
> interdisciplinary vocational evaluation p.
> LEAP p.
> macrotrauma rehabilitation p.
> Microplasty minimally invasive hip p.
> National Foundation of American Academy of Ophthalmology Public Service P.'s
> phase 2 elbow p.
> rehabilitation therapeutic p.
> Rothman Institute total hip p.
> 4-star exercise p.
> stretching p.
> TotalGym Exercise P.
> trunk stabilization rehabilitation p.
> Ultimate Hand Helper strengthening p.
> walking p.
> weight-training p.
> Westcott Pyramid P.
> Williams exercise p.
> work hardening p.

programmable VariGrip II prosthetic control system
progression
> curve p.
> p. to full weightbearing
> p. of training
> p. walking component

progressiva
> dysbasia lordotica p.

fibrodysplasia ossificans p.
fibrositis ossificans p.
fibrous dysplasia ossificans p.
myositis ossificans p.

progressive
p. Ambulation Scale
p. ankle orthosis
p. diaphysial dysplasia
p. loading
p. lumbar extension rehabilitation
p. macrodactylia
p. muscle relaxation
p. muscular atrophy (PMA)
p. muscular dystrophy (PMD)
p. myositis fibrosa
p. neurologic disorder
p. nuclear amyotrophy
p. olisthesis
p. osseous heteroplasia
p. overload
p. palm guard
p. perilunar instability
p. resistance brace
p. resistance training
p. spinal amyotrophy
p. subacute myelopathy
p. supranuclear palsy
p. systemic sclerosis
p. weight
p. weightbearing
progressively larger reamer
progressive-resistance exercise
progressive-resistive exercise (PR, PRE)
Progress splint
proinflammatory state
projection
axial calcaneal p.
axial sesamoid p.
bursal p.
cephaloscapular p.
convergence p.
dorsoplantar p.
Harris-Beath p.
lateral p. (LC)
posterior-superior oblique p.
stress dorsiflexion p.
prolapse
disc p.
Prolene suture
proliferating zone
proliferation
angiofibroblastic p.

bizarre parosteal
osteochondromatous p. (BPOP)
fibroblastic p.
reactive periosteal p.
p. therapy
villous lipomatous p.
proliferative
p. arthritis
p. fasciitis
p. myositis
p. synovitis
Proline Stomatex shoulder brace
ProLite Plus runner's orthotic
prolonged insertional activity
prolotherapy
PROM
passive range of motion
prominence
heel p.
navicular p.
osseous p.
osteochondral p.
pedicle screw hardware p.
plantar bony p.
prehallux osseous p.
rotational p.
tibial tubercle p.
prominent
p. heel
p. spur
Promogran matrix wound dressing
promontory, promontorium
sacral p.
Promos modular shoulder system
pronate
pronated
p. foot
p. pes cavus
p. straight flatfoot
pronation
p. contracture
p. control
p. of foot
hindfoot p.
p. injury
p. phenomenon
p. sign
p. spring-control device
subtalar p.
p. and supination
pronation-abduction
p.-a. fracture
p.-a. injury

NOTES

P

pronation-eversion
> p.-e. fracture
> p.-e. injury

pronation-eversion-external
> p.-e.-e. rotation (PEER)
> p.-e.-e. rotation fracture
> p.-e.-e. rotation injury
> p.-e.-e. rotation injury of ankle

pronation-external rotation (P-ER)
pronation/spring control (PSC)
pronation-supination
pronator
> p. drift
> p. drill
> p. quadratus (PQ)
> p. quadratus muscle
> p. reflex
> p. teres (PT)
> p. teres muscle
> p. teres release
> p. teres syndrome
> p. teres tendon

pronatory gait
pronatus
> pes p.

prone
> p. blocking technique
> p. extension test
> p. external rotation test
> p. knee-bend test
> p. knee flexion test
> p. position
> p. rectus test
> p. reduction
> p. sacral push
> p. scapular retraction exercise

Pronex
> P. home traction
> P. patient controlled pneumatic traction device
> P. pneumatic cervical traction
> P. pneumatic device for cervical pain

prong
> 4-p. finger splint
> modified tonsillar p.
> 5-p. rake blade retractor

2-prong
> 2-p. rake retractor
> 2-p. stem finger prosthesis

3-prong
> 3-p. headrest
> 3-p. rake blade retractor

pronometer
Pron pillow
Pronto cement

PROOF
> Prevent Recurrence of Osteoporotic Fractures
> PROOF group

ProOsteon
> P. bone graft material
> P. Implant 500
> P. implant 500 coralline hydroxyapatite bone void filler
> P. Implant 500 granule

Propac
> Champ Insulated P. II

propagation velocity
Propel cannulated interference screw
propeller
> orthopaedic p.

proper
> p. digital nerve branch
> p. neck positioning

properitoneal space
properly seated
property
> elastic p.
> elongation p.

prophylactic
> p. abduction pants
> p. antibiotic
> p. antibiotic therapy
> p. anticoagulation
> p. bone graft
> p. fasciotomy
> p. operative stabilization
> p. resection
> p. skeletal fixation
> p. taping

prophylaxis, pl. **prophylaxes**
> deep venous thrombosis p.
> dextran p.
> DVT p.

Propionibacterium acnes
propionic acid
Proplast
> P. HA
> P. I, II porous implant material
> P. prosthesis
> P. prosthetic material

proportionate dwarfism
proprioception
> gravitational p.

proprioceptive
> p. deficit
> p. exercise
> p. neuromuscular facilitation (PNF)
> p. neuromuscular facilitation approach
> p. neuromuscular fasciculation (PNF)
> p. process

p. rehabilitation
p. training
proprioceptor
propriosensory training
proprius
extensor indicis p. (EIP)
p. tendon
Prop'R Toes hammertoe cushion
propulsion
p. biomechanics
p. gait
propulsive phase
prospective payment system (PPS)
prostaglandin
PROSTALAC
prosthetic antibiotic-loaded acrylic
cement
PROSTALAC temporary hip
prosthesis
PROSTALAC total hip prosthesis
PROSTALAC total joint prosthesis
prosternation
prosthesis, pl. **prostheses**
above-knee p.
Accolade hip p.
acetabular p.
acrylic bar p.
ACS Gemini p.
ACS Profile p.
ACS Star p.
AcuMatch M Series modular
femoral hip p.
advanced mobile-bearing p.
Advance PS total knee p.
Advantim total knee p.
Advantim unconstrained p.
Aequalis humeral p.
Aequalis reversed shoulder p.
Aesculap-PM noncemented
femoral p.
AGC femoral p.
AGC knee p.
AGC tibial p.
AHP digital p.
AHSC elbow p.
AHSC-Volz elbow p.
Airlite p.
Airprene hinged knee p.
AK p.
Alivium implant metal p.
Allen-Brown p.
Allurion foot p.
alumina cemented total hip p.

alumina-on-alumina total hip p.
AMC total wrist p.
American Heyer-Schulte chin p.
American Heyer-Schulte-Hinderer
malar p.
American Heyer-Schulte Radovan
tissue expander p.
AMK unconstrained p.
AML Plus p.
AML Tang femoral p.
AML total hip p.
Amstutz cemented hip p.
Anametric total knee p.
Anatomic Precoat hip p.
anatomic surface p.
Anderson acetabular p.
ankle p.
Apollo hip p.
APR acetabular p.
APR femoral p.
APR II p.
APRL hand p.
Arafiles elbow p.
Arthropor cup p.
Arthropor II acetabular p.
Atlas modular humeral p.
Attenborough total knee p.
Aufranc cobra hip p.
Aufranc-Turner cemented hip p.
Austin Moore femoral head p.
Autophor ceramic total hip p.
Autophor femoral p.
Avanta MCP joint implant
finger p.
Averett hip p.
Averill press fit p.
Balance hip p.
ball-and-socket ankle p.
Bankart shoulder p.
Bantam CDH p.
4-bar linkage on knee p.
4-bar polycentric knee p.
Bateman femoral neck p.
Bateman finger p.
Bateman UPF II bipolar p.
Bateman UPF II shoulder p.
BDH p.
Beachcomber waterproof p.
bead-blasted p.
Bechtol hip p.
Bechtol shoulder p.
Bechtol system p.
Becker hand p.

NOTES

P

prosthesis *(continued)*

Beck-Steffee total ankle p.
below-elbow p.
below-knee p.
Bi-Angular shoulder p.
Biaxial Weave composite p.
bicentric p.
bicompartmental knee implant p.
bicondylar ankle p.
bicondylar knee p.
Bi-Metric hip p.
Bi-Metric Interlok femoral p.
Bi-Metric porous primary
   femoral p.
Bio-Chromatic hand p.
Bioclad with pegs reinforced
   acetabular p.
BioFit Press-Fit acetabular p.
Bioglass p.
Bio-Groove acetabular p.
Bio-Groove Macrobond HA
   femoral p.
Biomet AGC knee p.
Biomet hip p.
Biometric p.
Biomet total toe p.
Bio-Modular shoulder p.
Biophase implant metal p.
Biotex implant metal p.
bipolar femoral head p.
bipolar hip replacement p.
Björk p.
BK p.
Blauth knee p.
Blazina p.
Bock knee p.
Bombelli-Mathys-Morscher hip p.
bone p.
bovine collagen material p.
Brigham p.
Bryan total knee implant p.
Buchholz p.
Buechel-Pappas total ankle p.
Byars mandibular p.
CAD/CAM p.
CAD femoral stem p.
Caffinière trapeziometacarpal p.
Calandruccio cemented hip p.
calcar replacement femoral p.
Callender technique hip p.
Calnan-Nicolle finger p.
Calnan-Nicolle
   metatarsophalangeal p.
Calnan-Nicolle synthetic joint p.
camouflage p.
Canadian hip disarticulation p.
Capello press-fit p.
capitellocondylar unconstrained
   elbow p.

Carbon Copy high performance
   foot p.
Carbon Copy HP foot p.
Carbon Copy II foot p.
Carbon Copy II Light p.
Cardona keratoprosthesis p.
carpal lunate implant p.
carpal scaphoid implant p.
Cathcart Orthocentric hip p.
CDH Precoat Plus hip p.
cemented hip p.
cementless p.
Centralign precoat hip p.
ceramic femoral head p.
ceramic ossicular p.
Ceramion p.
CFS hip p.
Charnley acetabular cup p.
Charnley cemented p.
Charnley-Hastings p.
Charnley low-friction hip p.
Charnley-Müller hip p.
Charnley total hip p.
Chatzidakis hinged Vitallium
   implant p.
CHD p.
Chopart partial foot p.
Choyce MK II keratoprosthesis p.
Christiansen hip p.
Cinch instant suction B.K. p.
Cintor knee p.
Cirrus foot p.
clamshell p.
Clayton p.
C-Leg lower limb p.
Cloutier unconstrained knee p.
coated p.
Coballoy implant metal p.
cobalt-chromium-alloy p.
Co-Cr-Mo alloy p.
Co-Cr-W-Ni alloy p.
Cofield shoulder p.
cold-mold p.
cold-weld femoral p.
collar-calcar support femoral p.
College Park TruStep foot p.
Compartmental II knee p.
p. component
p. component subsidence
compression-molded p.
computer-assisted design/computer-
   assisted manufacturing p.
Conaxial ankle p.
conoidal ankle p.
constrained hinged knee p.
constrained nonhinged knee p.
Continuum unconstrained p.
Contour internal p.
conventional single-axis knee p.

Coonrad hinged p.
Coonrad-II p.
Coonrad-Morrey elbow p.
Coonrad semiconstrained elbow p.
Corail press-fit p.
CPT p.
crimped Dacron p.
cruciate condylar unconstrained p.
cruciate-retaining p.
cruciate-sacrificing p.
p. cup
custom p.
custom-threaded p.
Dacron p.
DANA shoulder p.
d'Aubigné femoral p.
Deane unconstrained knee p.
DeBakey p.
debonded femoral stem p.
Dee totally constrained elbow p.
p. dehiscence
de La Caffinière
  trapeziometacarpal p.
DeLaura knee p.
DeLaura-Verner knee p.
DePalma hip p.
DePuy AML Porocoat stem p.
DePuy hip p.
Deune knee p.
digital p.
Dimension-C femoral stem p.
Dimension hip p.
direct-impact p.
distal radioulnar joint p.
doffing p.
donning p.
Dorrance hand p.
Dow Corning Wright finger
  joint p.
p. driver
DRUJ p.
dual-lock total hip p.
Duocentric p.
Duocondylar knee p.
Duo-Lock hip p.
duopatellar unconstrained p.
Dupaco knee p.
Duracon p.
Duraloc p.
Dycor Geriatric ADL single axis
  foot p.
Dynaplex knee p.

Eaton trapezium finger joint
  replacement p.
Edwards seamless p.
E-2 foot p.
Eftekhar-Charnley hip p.
Eftekhar long-stem p.
Eicher femoral p.
Eicher hip p.
Eilers-Armstrong unicompartmental
  knee p.
elbow p.
Endolite p.
Endo-Model hinged knee p.
Endo-Model rotating knee joint p.
Endo-Model sled p.
Endo rotating knee joint p.
energy storing foot p.
Engh porous metal hip p.
Englehardt femoral p.
English-McNab shoulder p.
Entegra p.
EPTFE graft p.
Eriksson knee p.
Evolution hip p.
Ewald unconstrained elbow p.
Exeter cemented hip p.
Exeter-Femora press fit p.
femoral neck p.
finger joint implant p.
Finney p.
Finney-Flexirod p.
Finn hinged knee p.
fixed femoral head p.
flanged revision p.
Flatt finger-joint p.
Flatt finger-thumb p.
Flex-Foot Modular III p.
Flex H/A total ossicular p.
Flex-Sprint p.
Flex-Walk p.
Flex-Walk II p.
fluid p.
foot p.
forearm lift-assist p.
forged cobalt-chromium alloy p.
Free-Flow system p.
Freeman-high neck press fit p.
Freeman modular total hip p.
Freeman-Samuelson knee p.
Freeman-Swanson knee p.
F.R. Thompson femoral p.
fully constrained tricompartmental
  knee p.

NOTES

P

575

prosthesis *(continued)*
Gaffney ankle p.
Galante hip p.
Gemini hip system p.
Genesis knee p.
GeoFlex knee p.
Geomedic total knee p.
geometric total knee p.
Gerard p.
Gianturco p.
Gilfillan humeral p.
Giliberty acetabular p.
Giliberty femoral neck p.
Giliberty hip p.
Gillette joint p.
Gillies p.
Girard keratoprosthesis p.
Gore-Tex knee p.
great toe implant p.
Greifer p.
Greissinger foot p.
Gripper acetabular cup p.
grit-blasted p.
Gritti-Stokes knee p.
GSB elbow p.
GSB expanded version for knee p.
Guepar hinged knee p.
Guilford-Wright p.
Gunston-Hult knee p.
Gunston polycentric knee p.
Gustilo hip p.
Gustilo knee p.
Gustilo unconstrained p.
HA 65101 implant metal p.
Hamas upper limb p.
hand p.
hand-glove p.
Hanger ComfortFlex knee p.
Hanslik patellar p.
Harken p.
Harris cemented hip p.
Harris Design femoral p.
Harris-Galante porous hip p.
Harris Micromini p.
Hastings hip p.
Haynes-Stellite implant metal p.
HD-2 cemented hip p.
HD-2 total hip p.
heat-cured acrylic femoral head p.
Herbert knee p.
Hexcel knee p.
Hexcel total condylar p.
HG multilock hip p.
Hinderer malar p.
hinged constrained knee p.
hinged great toe replacement p.
hinged implant p.
hinged total knee p.
hip disarticulation p.

hip replacement p.
Hittenberger p.
homograft p.
Hosmer WALK p.
Howmedica Kinematic II knee p.
Howmedica PCA p.
Howorth p.
Howse p.
HPS II total hip p.
HSS total condylar knee p.
Hunter silastic p.
Hunter tendon p.
Hydra-Cadence knee p.
hydraulic knee unit p.
I-beam hemiarthroplasty hip p.
ICLH ankle p.
ICLH knee p.
Identifit hip p.
immediate postoperative p. (IPOP)
Impact modular porous p.
Impact total hip p.
Implant Technology LSF p.
Index p.
Indiana conservative p.
Indong Oh hip p.
Infinity modular hip p.
Insall-Burstein semiconstrained
  tricompartmental knee p.
p. inserter
Integral Interlok femoral p.
Integrity acetabular cup p.
Intelligent Prosthesis Plus p.
p. interface
Intermedics Natural-Knee knee p.
Inter-Op acetabular p.
Inter-Op hip p.
Interseal Variant I–IV p.
Iowa internal p.
Iowa total hip p.
ischial weightbearing p. (IWP)
Ishizuki unconstrained elbow p.
isoelastic pelvic p.
Ivalon p.
Jaffe press-fit p.
Jewett p.
Jobst p.
Johnson-Elloy accord
  unconstrained p.
Johnston-Iowa hip p.
Jonas p.
Joplin toe p.
Judet press-fit hip p.
Keller bunionectomy with p.
Kessler p.
Kinematic fully constrained
  tricompartmental knee p.
Kinematic II rotating hinge total
  knee p.
Kinemax Plus knee p.

Kirschner Medical Dimension p.
Kirschner total shoulder p.
KMP femoral stem p.
knee p.
Koenig MPJ p.
K2 sensation p.
Kudo unconstrained elbow p.
Küntscher humeral p.
Lacey fully constrained
  tricompartmental knee p.
Lacey hinged knee p.
Laing hip cup p.
Lanceford p.
Landers-Foulks p.
LaPorta total toe p.
LCS meniscal bearing
  semiconstrained p.
LCS New Jersey knee p.
LCS rotating platform
  semiconstrained p.
LCS substituting semiconstrained p.
LCS universal APG
  semiconstrained p.
Leinbach femoral p.
Leinbach hip p.
Lewis expandable adjustable p.
  (LEAP)
Lewis Trapezio p.
Ling cemented hip p.
Link Endo-Model rotational
  knee p.
Link MP hip noncemented
  reconstruction p.
Lippman hip p.
Lisfranc below-knee p.
Liverpool elbow p.
Liverpool knee p.
Lo Bak spinal support p.
locking p.
London unconstrained elbow p.
Longevity V-Lign hip p.
Lo-Por vascular graft p.
Lord press-fit hip p.
Lord total hip p.
Lotus unicompartment p.
low-contact stress
  semiconstrained p.
lower extremity p.
lower limb p. (LLP)
low-neck femoral p.
low-profile femoral p.
Lubinus knee p.
lunate acrylic cement wrist p.

Lunceford-Pilliar-Engh hip p.
Lund prototype unicompartment p.
MacIntosh tibial plateau p.
MacNab-English shoulder p.
madreporic hip p.
malleus-incus p.
Mallory p.
Mallory-Head I, II p.
Mallory-Head porous primary
  femoral p.
Mallory-Head total hip p.
manual locking knee p.
Marlex methyl methacrylate p.
Marmor modular knee p.
Master step foot p.
Mathys p.
Matrol femoral head p.
Mayo semiconstrained elbow p.
Mayo total ankle p.
Mazas totally constrained elbow p.
McBride femoral p.
McKee-Farrar total hip p.
McKee femoral p.
McKee totally constrained elbow p.
McKeever patellar cap p.
McKeever vitallium knee p.
MCP finger joint p.
Mecring acetabluar p.
Mediloy implant metal p.
medium profile femoral p.
medullary p.
metal-backed plastic-on-metal p.
metal femoral head p.
metal-on-metal articulating
  intervertebral disc p.
metaphysial head resection with p.
MG II knee p.
Michael Reese articulated p.
Michele long-stem p.
Microloc knee p.
Microvel p.
migration of p.
Miller-Galante hip p.
Miller-Galante II knee p.
Minneapolis hip p.
Mittlemeier ceramic hip p.
Mittlemeier noncemented femoral p.
modified Moore hip locking p.
modular Austin Moore hip p.
modular Iowa Precoat total hip p.
modular unicompartmental knee p.
Monk hip p.
monoblock femoral stem p.

NOTES

P

prosthesis *(continued)*
monolithic A1203 cup p.
Moore femoral neck p.
Moore hip p.
Moretz p.
Moseley glenoid rim p.
Mueli wrist p.
Mueller-Charnley hip p.
Mueller dual-lock hip p.
Mueller total hip replacement p.
Müller p.
Mulligan silastic p.
multiaxis p.
Multiflex foot p.
Multi-Lock hip p.
multiradius unconstrained p.
Murray knee p.
myoelectric control p.
Natural-Hip p.
Natural-Knee unconstrained p.
Natural-Lok acetabular cup p.
NEB total hip p.
Neer humeral replacement p.
Neer shoulder p. (I, II)
Neer umbrella p.
New Jersey hemiarthroplasty p.
New Jersey LCS shoulder p.
New Jersey LCS total knee p.
Newton ankle p.
Nexus hip p.
Nicoll tendon p.
Niebauer-Cutter p.
Niebauer finger-joint replacement p.
Niebauer metacarpophalangeal joint
  silastic p.
Niebauer trapezium replacement p.
Noiles fully constrained
  tricompartmental knee p.
nonhinged knee p.
nonhinged linked p.
Normalize press-fit hip p.
Norwich press-fit p.
nudge control on p.
ocular p.
Odland ankle p.
Oh cemented hip p.
Oh press-fit hip p.
Oh-Spectron p.
Oklahoma ankle p.
Omnifit dual geometry
  microstructured p.
Omnifit HA hip stem p.
Omnifit knee p.
Omnifit PSL microstructured p.
OmniFlex hip p.
Opti-Fix femoral p.
Opti-Fix I, II p.
Oregon Poly II ankle p.
Orthochrome implant metal p.

Orthofix p.
Ortholoc implant metal p.
Ortholoc II unconstrained p.
orthopaedic p.
p. and orthosis (P&O)
osseointegrated p.
ossicular chain replacement p.
OsteoCap hip p.
Osteolock hip p.
Osteonics hip p.
Otto Bock dynamic p.
Overdyke hip p.
Oxford meniscal unicompartment p.
Padgett p.
painful femoral head p.
Paltrinieri-Trentani p.
Panje voice button p.
partial ossicular
  reconstruction/replacement p.
partial ossicular replacement p.
  (PORP)
patellar tendon-bearing below-
  knee p.
PCA Original p.
PCA Standard p.
PCA unconstrained
  tricompartmental p.
PCA unicompartmental knee p.
PC Performer knee p.
pegged tibial p.
Perfecta hip p.
Perfecta I, II p.
Performance knee p.
Peri-Loc p.
PFC curved unconstrained p.
PFC femoral p.
Phoenix total hip p.
Pillet hand p.
Pilliar p.
piston p.
Plasticor p.
Plasti-Pore ossicular replacement p.
Plastiport TORP p.
Plystan p.
Polycel bone composite p.
polycentric knee p.
polycentric unconstrained p.
Poly-Dial p.
polyethylene patellar implant p.
polyethylene talar p.
polypropylene p.
porcine p.
Porocoat AML noncemented p.
Porometal noncemented femoral p.
porous-coated anatomic p.
porous-coated femur p.
porous-coated hip p.
porous surfaced p.
Precision Osteolock femoral p.

Precision Osteolock hip p.
precoat hip p.
Precoat Plus femoral p.
Premier press fit p.
press-fit condylar total knee p.
Pritchard II elbow p.
Pritchard total elbow p.
Pritchard-Walker semiconstrained
  elbow p.
Pritchard-Walker total elbow p.
ProDisc I disc p.
ProDisc spinal disc p.
Profile hip p.
ProForma p.
2-prong stem finger p.
Proplast p.
PROSTALAC temporary hip p.
PROSTALAC total hip p.
PROSTALAC total joint p.
prosthetic antibiotic-loaded acrylic
  cement total joint p.
Protasul femoral p.
Protasul-10 noncemented femoral p.
Protasul-64 WF Zweymuller
  femoral p.
Protek p.
provisional p.
proximal humeral p.
proximal third femoral p.
PTB-SC-SP p.
PTB supracondylar p.
PTB suprapatellar p.
PTS soft wedge p.
pyrocarbon p.
Quantum Foot p.
radial head implant p.
Radovan tissue expander p.
Ranawat-Burstein hip p.
Randelli shoulder p.
Rastelli p.
Reflection I p.
Reflection Interfit p.
Reflection V p.
Re-Flex VSP p.
Repiphysis p.
retaining knee p.
Reverdin p.
reversed shoulder p.
Richards hip p.
Richards maximum contact cruciate-
  sparing p.
Richard Smith p.

Richards Spectron metal-backed
  acetabular p.
Richards Zirconia femoral head p.
Ring knee p.
Ring total hip p.
Ring UPM press-fit p.
RMC p.
RM isoelastic hip p.
Robert Brigham semiconstrained p.
Robert Brigham total knee p.
Roper-Day p.
Rosenfeld hip p.
rotating femoral head p.
rotating hinge knee p.
rotating knee joint p.
Rothman Institute femoral p.
Roy-Camille p.
SACH foot p.
sacrificing knee p.
saddle p.
SAF p.
SAFE II p.
Salzer p.
Sampson p.
Sarmiento STH-2 hip p.
Sauerbruch p.
Savastano Hemi-Knee p.
Savastano unconstrained p.
Savastano unicompartment p.
Sbarbaro hip p.
Sbarbaro tibial plateau p.
Scarborough p.
Schlein semiconstrained elbow p.
Schlein total elbow p.
Schlein trisurface ankle p.
Schuknecht Gelfoam wire p.
Schuknecht Teflon wire piston p.
seating of p.
Seattle foot p.
Secur-Fit HA PSL X'tra p.
Select ankle p.
Select modular shoulder p.
self-bearing ceramic hip p.
self-centering Universal hip p.
semiconstrained tricompartmental
  knee p.
Sense-of-Feel p.
SensorHand p.
Sharrard-Trentani p.
Shaw-Sgarlato hammertoe
  implant p.
Sheehan knee p.
Sherfee p.

NOTES

579

prosthesis *(continued)*
Shier knee p.
shoulder disarticulation p.
silastic ball spacer p.
silastic radial head p.
silastic thumb p.
Silflex intramedullary p.
silicone trapezium p.
single-axis ankle p.
sintered implant p.
Sinterlock implant metal p.
Sivash hip p.
SMA p.
Smith ankle p.
Smith-Petersen hip cup p.
SMO p.
solid ankle, cushioned heel p.
Solution p.
Souter-Strathclyde elbow p.
Souter unconstrained elbow p.
Spectron hip p.
Speed radius cap p.
spherocentric fully constrained
  tricompartmental knee p.
Spotorno hip p.
Springlite lower limb p.
S-ROM Arthropor I–III p.
S-ROM Arthropor oblong p.
S-ROM femoral stem p.
S-ROM hip p.
S-ROM super cup p.
S-ROM ZZT I, II p.
stainless steel implant metal p.
Stanmore shoulder p.
Stanmore totally constrained
  elbow p.
STAR ankle joint p.
stemmed tibial p.
Stenzel rod p.
Stevens-Street elbow p.
St. Georg-Buchholz ankle p.
St. Georg fully constrained p.
St. Georg sledge
  unicompartment p.
STH-2 hip p.
St. Jude p.
Street-Stevens humeral p.
substituting knee p.
suction suspension p.
Sulzer p.
SuperCup acetabular cup p.
Sure-Flex p.
surgical p.
Surgitek p.
Sutter double-stem silicone
  implant p.
Sutter MCP finger joint p.
Swanson finger joint p.
Swanson flexible hallux valgus p.

Swanson great toe p.
Swanson metacarpal p.
Swanson metatarsal p.
Swanson silastic elbow p.
Swanson T-shaped great toe
  silastic p.
Swanson wrist p.
Syme amputation p.
Syme foot p.
Synatomic total knee p.
synthetic p.
Taperloc femoral p.
TARA total hip p.
Target p.
Tavernetti-Tennant knee p.
TCCK unconstrained knee p.
Teflon tri-leaflet p.
p. template
tendon p.
Thackray hip p.
Tharies hip replacement p.
thermomechanical implant metal p.
T28 hip p.
Thompson femoral neck p.
Thompson hemiarthroplasty hip p.
threaded titanium acetabular p.
thrust plate p. (TPP)
Ti-Bac II hip p.
tibial plateau p.
Ti/CoCr hip p.
Ti-Con p.
Tilastin hip p.
Tillman p.
Titan cemented hip p.
titanium hip p.
titanium implant p.
Ti-Thread p.
Titian hip p.
tivanium hip p.
tivanium implant metal p.
TMA p.
toe p.
TORP p.
total articular replacement
  arthroplasty p.
Total Concept ankle/foot p.
total condylar p. III (TCP III)
total condylar III fully
  constrained p.
total condylar knee p.
total condylar semiconstrained
  tricompartmental p.
total hip replacement p.
total joint replacement p.
total knee replacement p.
total ossicular replacement p.
  (TORP)
Total Shock p.
Townley-horizontal platform p.

Townley TARA p.
Townley total knee p.
TPR ankle p.
Trac II knee p.
transfemoral modular p.
transtibial immediate
  postoperative p.
trapezial p.
trapeziometacarpal joint
  replacement p.
trapezium implant p.
Trapezoidal-28 hip p.
Trapezoidal-28 internal p.
TR-28 hip p.
Triad p.
trial p.
Tri-Axial p.
triaxial semiconstrained elbow p.
tricompartmental knee p.
Tricon-M cruciate-sparing p.
Tricon-M patellar p.
trileaflet p.
Tri-Lock press-fit p.
Trilogy p.
Tronzo p.
Trow Bridge Terra-Round all-
  terrain p.
trunnion-bearing hip p.
TruStep foot p.
TTAP p.
TTAP-ST acetabular p.
TT Pylon p.
Turner p.
UCI ankle p.
UCI unconstrained p.
UHMWPE p.
ulnar head implant p.
Ultimate knee p.
unconstrained tricompartmental
  knee p.
unicompartmental knee p.
unicondylar p.
Universal I, II p.
Universal femoral head p.
Universal hip p.
upper extremity myoelectric p.
upper limb p. (ULP)
Valls hip p.
Vanghetti limb p.
Varikopf hip p.
VerSys p.
Viladot p.
Vinertia implant metal p.

vitallium humeral replacement p.
Volz wrist p.
Wadsworth unconstrained elbow p.
Wagner p.
Walldius Vitallium mechanical
  knee p.
Warsaw hip p.
Waugh knee p.
Waugh total ankle replacement p.
Wayfarer modifiable foot p.
Weller total hip joint p.
well-seated p.
Whitesides Ortholoc II condylar
  femoral p.
Whitesides total knee p.
William Harris hip p.
Wilson-Burstein hip internal p.
Wright knee p.
Wright titanium p.
wrist joint implant p.
Xenophor femoral p.
Young hinged knee p.
Zimaloy femoral head p.
Zimaloy implant metal p.
Zimmer Centralign Precoat hip p.
Zimmer hip p.
Zimmer shoulder p.
Zimmer tibial p.
zirconia femoral head p.
zirconia orthopaedic p.
zirconium oxide ceramic p.
Z-stent p.
ZTT I, II acetabular cup p.
Zweymuller cementless hip p.
prosthesis-cement interface
prosthetic
  p. ambulation
  American Board of Certification of
    Orthotics and P.'s
  American Hand P.'s (AHP)
  p. antibiotic-loaded acrylic cement
    (PROSTALAC)
  p. antibiotic-loaded acrylic cement
    total joint prosthesis
  p. arthroplasty
  Cirrus foot p.
  p. cone
  p. design
  p. disc nucleus (PDN)
  p. disc nucleus device
  p. femorodistal graft
  p. finger
  p. fitting

NOTES

P

prosthetic *(continued)*
    p. foam
    p. foot
    p. gait training
    p. hemiarthroplasty
    p. hook
    p. intervention
    p. loosening
    p. and orthotic (P&O)
    p. patella
    P. Problem Inventory Scale
    P. Problem Inventory Scale
      classification
    p. replacement
    p. sock
    p. socket
    p. spacer
    p. speech aid
    p. stance phase shock
    p. stem lateral fin
    p. support
    p. training
Flex-Walk
    F.-W. II prosthesis
    F.-W. prosthesis
    F.-W. II prosthetic foot
prosthetist
prosthetist/orthotist
ProStretch exerciser
Protasul
    P. femoral prosthesis
    P. implant metal
Protasul-10 noncemented femoral prosthesis
Protasul-64 WF Zweymuller femoral prosthesis
Pro-Tec patellar tendon strap
protection
    digital artery p.
    Ionact antibacterial p.
    p. plate
    p., restricted activity, ice, compression, elevation (PRICE)
protective
    p. extension reaction
    p. limitation
    p. limitation of range of motion
    p. sensation
    p. shield
    p. weightbearing
protector
    Air-Limb amputation p.
    Alvarado collateral ligament p.
    ankle ligament p. (ALP)
    Bandage Gard cast p.
    Cast Gard cast p.
    grooved p.
    Heelbo decubitus heel/elbow p.
    Jurgan pin ball pin p.

    medial nerve p.
    P. meniscus suturing system
    M-F heel p.
    Ortho-Foam p.
    Patellar Band knee p.
    Roho heel p.
    Seal-Tight cast p.
    ShowerSafe waterproof cast and bandage p.
    The Heeler inflatable heel p.
    tissue p.
Protecto splint
Protege manual flexion distraction table
protein
    bone morphogenetic p. (BMP)
    cartilage oligomeric matrix p. (COMP)
    C-reactive p.
    dietary p.
    IGF-binding p.
    p. malnutrition
    morphogenetic p.
    Ne-Osteo bone morphogenic p.
    soluble *N*-eythyl-maleimide sensitive factor attachment p. (SNAP)
protein-1
    osteogenic p.-1 (OP-1)
protein-based bone graft substitute
Protek prosthesis
proteoglycan
    p. matrix
    p. synthesis
Proteus
    P. mirabilis
    P. syndrome
prothelen set
ProThotics insole
prothrombin time (PT)
prothrombotic state
protocol
    Bruce p.
    Evans-Burkhalter p.
    Mann p.
    Marx osteoradionecrosis p.
    North American Malignant Hyperthermia p.
    p. of Walsh
proton density
Protonic brace
Protoplast cement
prototype design
Protouch synthetic orthopaedic padding
ProTrac
    P. alignment guide
    P. cruciate reconstruction system
    P. measurement device
    P. system for knee surgery
protraction

protractor
    arthrodial p.
    triplanar p.
    Zimmer p.
protruding disc
protrusio
    p. acetabuli
    p. cage
    p. deformity
    p. ring
    p. shell
protrusion
    central disc p.
    disc p.
    p. distance
    lateral disc p.
    medial disc p.
    p. of navicular
protuberans
    dermatofibrosarcoma p.
    enchondroma p.
proud flesh
Providence Scoliosis System
provisional
    p. amputation
    p. calcification
    p. callus
    p. fixation
    P. Fixation TC-100 plating system
    p. prosthesis
    p. stabilization
Proxiderm
    P. procedure
    P. wound closure system
proximal
    p. anular pulley
    p. anular pulley of thumb
    p. articular facet angle
    p. articular set angle (PASA)
    p. bow position
    p. carpal row
    p. cement spacer
    p. chevron osteotomy
    p. communicating branch (PCB)
    p. compression test
    p. and distal realignment
    p. and distal screw
    p. dome osteotomy
    p. drill-guide assembly
    p. end tibia fracture
    p. femoral elevator
    p. femoral epiphysiolysis
    p. femoral focal deficiency

    p. femoral fracture
    p. femoral metaphysial shortening
    p. femoral osteotomy
    p. femoral resection
    p. femur
    p. fibula
    p. fibular facet
    p. first metatarsal osteotomy
    p. focal femoral deficiency (PFFD)
    p. humeral fracture
    p. humeral prosthesis
    p. humerus
    p. interlocking
    p. interphalangeal (PIP)
    p. interphalangeal/distal
      interphalangeal (PIP/DIP)
    p. interphalangeal joint (PIPJ)
    p. interphalangeal joint approach
    p. intrinsic release
    p. latency
    p. level amputation
    p. locking
    p. medial brim
    p. metatarsal approach
    p. metatarsal osteotomy
    p. midpatellar medial and lateral
      portals
    p. nerve release
    p. phalangeal epiphysiodesis
    p. phalangeal osteotomy
    p. phalanx (PP)
    p. phalanx osteotomy
    p. phocomelia
    p. portion
    p. radioulnar articulation
    p. radius
    p. reference axis (PFA)
    p. row carpectomy
    p. set angle deviation
    p. subungual onychomycosis (PSO)
    p. tendon rupture
    p. thigh band
    p. third (P/3)
    p. third femoral prosthesis
    p. third of shaft
    p. tibia
    p. tibial metaphysial fracture
    p. tibial osteotomy
    p. tibial plateau
    p. tibiofibular joint
    p. tibiofibular joint dislocation
    p. tibiofibular subluxation
    p. tibiofibular synostosis

NOTES

P

proximal (*continued*)
    p. ulna
    p. Wagner metaphysial shortening
proximal-to-distal
    p.-t.-d. dissection technique
    p.-t.-d. ring
proximoataxia
proximolateral
prune-belly syndrome
PS
    primary stem
PSB
    patellar stabilizing brace
PSC
    pronation/spring control
PSDK
    poststatic dyskinesia
pseudankylosis
pseudarthrosis, pseudoarthrosis
    ball-and-socket giant p.
    closed p.
    congenital tibial p.
    documented p.
    extraarticular p.
    failed back syndrome with
      documented p.
    fibular p.
    Girdlestone p.
    interspinous p.
    radial p.
    p. rate
    p. repair
    synovial p.
    tibial p.
pseudoacetabulum
pseudoachondroplasia
pseudoanemia
    athlete's p.
    dilutional p.
pseudoaneurysm
pseudoarthritis
    ball-and-socket giant p.
    congenital p.
pseudoarthrosis (*var. of* pseudarthrosis)
pseudoarticulation
pseudo-Babinski sign
pseudoboutonnière deformity
pseudobulbar palsy
pseudocapsule chondrosarcoma
pseudoclaudication
pseudoclawing
pseudocortex
pseudocoxalgia
pseudocyst
    calcaneal p.
pseudodislocation
pseudoephedrine and ibuprofen
pseudoepiphysis
pseudoexostosis

pseudofacilitation
pseudofracture
    milkman's p.
pseudogamekeeper's injury
pseudogout
pseudohead
pseudo-Hurler deformity
pseudohypertrophic dystrophy
pseudohypertrophy
pseudohypoparathyroidism
pseudo-Jones fracture
pseudometatarsal head
pseudomyotonic discharge
pseudoneoplastic lesion
pseudoneuroma
pseudoosteomalacic pelvis
pseudoosteomyelitis
pseudoparalysis
    congenital atonic p.
    Parrot p.
pseudoperiosteal reaction
pseudopodia
pseudopodium
pseudopolyphasic action potential
pseudo-Pott disease
pseudoradicular syndrome
pseudosarcomatous
    p. fasciitis
    p. fibromatosis
    p. reaction
pseudostability test
pseudosubluxation
pseudotendon
pseudothrombophlebitis (PTP)
pseudotumorous mucin deposition
pseudovarus
    cubitus p.
PSIS
    posterior sacroiliac spine
    posterior superior iliac spine
PSO
    proximal subungual onychomycosis
psoas
    p. abscess
    p. muscle
    p. tendon syndrome
Psoralen-UVA therapy
psoriasis
    arthritis-associated p.
psoriatic arthritis
psychogenic equinovarus
psychological adjustment
psychometrics
psychomotor
psychoneuroimmunology
psychosomatic
PT
    physical therapy
    physical training

pronator teres
prothrombin time
    PT pulse
    PT tilt table
PTB
    patellar tendon-bearing
    pretibial bearing
    pretibial buttress
        PTB ankle-foot orthosis
        PTB brace
        PTB cast
        PTB plastic orthosis
        PTB supracondylar prosthesis
        PTB suprapatellar prosthesis
PTBO
    patellar tendon-bearing orthosis
PTBS
    patellar tendon-bearing suspension
PTB-SC-SP
    patellar tendon-bearing-supracondylar-
      suprapatellar
        PTB-SC-SP prosthesis
PTD
    permanent and total disability
pterotic bone
pterygium colli
pterygoid
    p. bone
    p. chest
    p. plate
PTFE
    polytetrafluoroethylene
      PTFE graft
PTFL
    posterior talofibular ligament
PTI
    pressure-time integral
PTN
    posterior tibial nerve
PTP
    posterior tibial pulse
    pseudothrombophlebitis
PTS
    patellar tendon socket
    patellar tendon stabilization
        PTS knee brace
        PTS soft wedge prosthesis
PTT
    partial thromboplastin time
    patellar tendon transfer
    posterior tibial tendinitis
    posterior tibial tendon
        PTT insufficiency

PTTD
    posterior tibial tendon dysfunction
pubalgia
    athletic p.
pubic
    p. bone
    p. diastasis
    p. fascia
    p. osteolysis
    p. pad
    p. ramus
    p. symphysis
pubiotomy
pubis
    osteitis p.
    osteitis necroticans p.
    symphysis p.
puboanalis
pubocapsular ligament
pubococcygeus
pubofemoral ligament
puboischial area
puborectalis
Pucci
    P. Air orthotic
    P. pediatrics hand orthosis
    P. rehab knee orthosis
    P. splint
pucker sign
Puddu
    P. drill guide
    P. osteotomy system
    P. tendon technique
pudendal
    p. artery
    p. block
    p. nerve injury
    p. neuritis
Pudenz flushing chamber
puerperal synovitis
Pugh
    P. driver
    P. hip pin
    P. plate
    P. sliding nail
    P. traction
Pugil stick injury
Puka chisel
Pul-Ez
    P.-E. exerciser
    P.-E. shoulder pulley

NOTES

P

pull
>p. screw
>spinous p.

pulled elbow

puller
>Ultra-Drive plug p.

pulley
>anular p. (A1–A4)
>cruciate p. (C1–C3)
>p. exercise
>fibroosseous p.
>Flex Ranger stretch cable with p.
>Home Ranger shoulder p.
>overhead p.
>Preston overhead p.
>proximal anular p.
>Pul-Ez shoulder p.
>Range-Master p.
>p. reconstruction
>Saba p.
>shoulder p.
>weights and p.'s

pull-out
>p.-o. button
>p.-o. strength
>p.-o. suture

pulmonary
>p. atelectasis
>p. barotrauma
>p. complication
>p. embolism
>p. osteoarthropathy
>p. osteodystrophy

pulp
>p. amputation
>p. approach
>finger p.
>p. flap
>plantar toe p.
>p. traction

pulposus
>herniated nucleus p. (HNP)
>nucleus p.

pulpy nucleus

pulsatile
>p. hypothermic perfusion
>p. jet lavage
>p. pneumatic plantar-compression
> device
>p. pressure lavage

pulsating
>p. electromagnetic field (PEMF)
>p. hematoma

Pulsavac
>P. III wound débridement system
>P. irrigation
>P. lavage

pulse
>blood volume p. (BVP)

>dorsalis pedis p.
>dorsal pedal p.
>DP p.
>intact peripheral p.'s
>p. irrigator
>p. oximeter
>posterior tibial p. (PTP)
>PT p.
>p. status-pull test
>p. volume recorder (PVR)

pulsed
>p. diathermy
>p. electric magnetic field bone
> growth stimulation
>p. electromagnetic field (PEMF)
>p. galvanic stimulator
>p. lavage
>p. short-wave therapy
>p. ultrasound

pulselessness

PULSES
>physical condition, upper limb function,
>lower limb function, sensory
>component, excretory function, support
>function
>PULSES profile
>PULSES Profile for Comprehensive
> Rehabilitation

Pulvertaft
>P. end-to-end suture
>P. fish-mouth stitch
>P. interweave suture
>P. weave tendon repair technique

pulvinar
>p. fibrofatty debris
>p. region

pumice stone

pump
>Alzet continuous infusion
> osmotic p.
>ankle rehabilitation p.
>arthroscopic p.
>A-V Impulse foot p.
>p. bump
>p. bump area
>p. bump deformity
>p. bump exostosis
>cement p.
>compression p.
>continuous wave arthroscopy p.
>extremity p.
>EZ hand p.
>infusion p.
>intermittent extremity p.
>P. It Up pneumatic socket volume
> management system
>Jobst athrombotic p.
>knee p.
>Linvatec arthroscopic infusion p.

morphine p.
Multipulse 1000 compression p.
pain control infusion p.
PainFree p.
sequential extremity p.
Vacumix vacuum p.
vacuum p.
venous foot p.
pump-handle rib motion
PumpPals insole
punch
Acufex rotary p.
arthroscopic p.
p. biopsy
bone graft p.
bone hole p.
boxer's p.
Caspari suture p.
Casselberry suture p.
cervical laminectomy p.
Charnley femoral prosthesis neck p.
cruciate p.
Deyerle p.
p. drunk syndrome
p. forceps
Hirsch hypophysial p.
I-beam cement p.
keel bone p.
Kerrison p.
keyhole p.
Osborne p.
rotary p.
Rowe glenoid p.
Schlesinger p.
suction p.
suture p.
tibial p.
tubular p.
punctata
chondrodysplasia p.
keratosis p.
puncture
p. fracture
lumbar p. (LP)
spinal p.
p. wound
p. wound osteochondritis
Puno-Winter-Byrd (PWB)
P.-W.-B. system
purchase
bony p.

compression locking anchor with secondary p. (CLASP)
p. and press the ground
secondary p.
socket p.
toe-ground p.
Purdue pegboard
pure
p. limb apraxia limb asymmetry
p. syndactyly
PureFix hydroxylapatite
purine metabolism
Puros Accugraft
purposeful activity
purpura
p. fulminans
Henoch-Schönlein p.
meningococcal p.
purse-string
pursestring suture
purulent
p. material
p. synovitis
push
p. cuff
knee-chest p.
P. medical brace
prone sacral p.
spinous p.
Push-Ease
P.-E. Quad Cuff
P.-E. wheelchair glove
pusher
Charnley femoral prosthesis p.
femoral component p.
hemispherical p.
hook p.
Jacobson suture p.
knot p.
metal p.
Patella P.
Revo loop handle knot p.
suture p.
push-off
great toe p.-o.
p.-o. by great toe
p.-o. phase
p.-o. phase of gait
p.-o. velocity
push-pull
p.-p. activity
p.-p. ankle stress view
p.-p. hip view

NOTES

P

push-pull (continued)
    p.-p. instability
    p.-p. move
    p.-p. test
push-up
    p.-u. block
    p.-u. test
pustulotic osteoarthropathy
putative segmental instantaneous axis of rotation
Puth abduction splint
Putti
    P. bone plast
    P. bone rasp
    P. knee arthrodesis
    P. posterior approach
    P. posterior bone block
    scapular sign of P.
    P. sign
    P. splint
Putti-Platt
    P.-P. arthroplasty
    P.-P. instrumentation
    P.-P. operation
    P.-P. shoulder procedure
putty
    AliMed p.
    AlloMatrix bone graft p.
    AlloMatrix injectable p.
    BeOK hand exercise p.
    Blue Brand Therapy P.
    bone graft p.
    color-coded therapy p.
    exercise p.
    Flexi-Grip exercise p.
    Grafton DBM p.
    matrix Grafton p.
    Thera-Plast p.
    Therapy P.
PUV
    positive ulnar variance
PVC
    polyvinyl chloride
    PVC drain
    PVC tubing
PVD
    peripheral vascular disease
    PVD dressing
PVNS
    pigmented villonodular synovitis
PVR
    pulse volume recorder
PVS
    peripheral vascular surgery
    peripheral vascular system
    pigmented villonodular synovitis
PW
    plantar wart

PWB
    partial weightbearing
    Puno-Winter-Byrd
        PWB transpedicular spine fixation system
PWC
    physical work capacity
pyarthrosis
PyC
    pyrolytic carbon
pycnodysostosis
PYD
    pyridinium collagen crosslink
    pyridinoline collagen crosslink
pyelogram
    intravenous p.
pyknodysostosis
Pyle
    bone age according to Greulich and P.
    P. disease
pylon
    AirStance p.
    p. attachment plate
    Icon p.
    impact-reducing p.
    P. intramedullary nail system
    metal p.
    Stratus impact-reducing p.
    vertical shock p.
pyocyanin
pyoderma gangrenosum
pyogenic
    p. arthritis
    p. bursitis
    p. granuloma
    p. spinal infection
    p. vertebral osteomyelitis
pyogenicum
    granuloma p.
pyomyositis
    staphylococcal p.
Pyramesh cage
pyramid
    p. attachment
    suction p.
pyramidal
    p. fracture
    p. tract
Pyrenochaeta romeroi
pyridinium collagen crosslink (PYD)
pyridinoline collagen crosslink (PYD)
Pyrilinks-D urine assay
pyrocarbon
    p. implant
    p. prosthesis
pyrolytic
    p. carbon (PyC)
    p. carbon device

Pyrost bone graft material

NOTES

Q

Q angle
Q disc
Q Star Voyager pressure reduction
  mattress

Q angle
QCT
  quantitative computed tomography
QDR-1500 bone densitometer
QDR-2000 bone densitometer
QF
  quadratus femoris
QIF
  Quadriplegia Index of Function
qigong
Qingyangshen (QYS)
QLV
  quasilinear viscoelastic
    QLV theory
QNA
  quadriceps neutral angle
QNST
  Quick Neurological Screening Test
Q-Ray bracelet
**QRS Quantronic Resonance pulsating
  magnetic field**
QSAC
  quadrant sparing acetabular component
QSART
  quantitative sudomotor axon reflex test
QST
  quantitative sensory testing
quad
  q. bar
  q. board
  q. cane
quadrangular
  q. cartilage
  q. positioning plate
quadrant
  Q. advanced shoulder brace
  q. of death
  q. sparing acetabular component
    (QSAC)
  q. test
quadrate
  q. ligament
  q. ligament of Denuce
  q. muscle
quadratus
  q. femoris (QF)
  q. femoris fascia
  q. femoris muscle
  q. lumborum muscle
  q. lumborum syndrome

q. plantae muscle
pronator q. (PQ)
quadriceps
  q. active test
  q. angle
  q. aponeurosis
  q. apron
  q. atrophy
  q. contraction test
  q. contracture
  q. contusion
  q. De Lorme boot
  q. femoris muscle
  q. femoris muscle cast
  q. jerk
  q. mechanism
  q. muscle group
  q. neutral angle (QNA)
  q. reflex
  q. strengthening exercise
  q. tendon
  q. wasting
quadricepsplasty
  Coonse-Adams q.
  Judet q.
  Thompson q.
  V-Y q.
quadriceps-setting exercise
**quadriceps-sparing, minimally invasive
  total knee instrument**
Quadriflex
quadrilateral
  q. brim
  q. frame
  q. ischial weightbearing socket
  q. space syndrome
quadriparesis
quadripartite bone
quadriplegia
  Q. Index of Function (QIF)
  spastic q.
  transient q.
quadriplegic
quadruped back exercise technique
quadruple
  q. amputation
  q. complex
Quadtro
  Q. cushion
  Q. cushion with Isoflap valve
QualCare knee brace
QualCraft
  Q. ankle support
  Q. short elastic wrist support

QualCraft *(continued)*
    Q. splint
    Q. strap
quality
    Agency for Healthcare Research and Q. (AHRQ)
    q. of life
    motion q.
    Q. of Well-Being Scale
quantitative
    q. computed tomography (QCT)
    q. mechanical pain testing
    q. sensory testing (QST)
    q. sudomotor axon reflex test (QSART)
    q. ultrasound (QUS)
quantity
    scalar q.
    vector q.
Quantum
    Q. foot
    Q. Foot prosthesis
    Q. 400 traction
Quartzo device
quasi-independent Y-axis movement
quasilinear viscoelastic (QLV)
quasistatic stressed position
Quebec Back Pain Disability Scale
Queckenstedt
    Q. maneuver
    Q. phenomenon
    Q. sign
    Q. test
Queckenstedt-Stookey test
Quengel
    Q. apparatus
    Q. cast
    Q. device
    Q. hinge
Quénu-Küss tarsometatarsal injury classification
Quénu nail plate removal technique
Quervain disease
question
    Enneking q.
questionnaire
    American Academy of Orthopaedic Surgeons/Hip Society Q.
    Behavioral Assessment of Pain Q.
    Children's Comprehensive Pain Q. (CCPQ)
    Cincinnati knee scoring q.
    Clinical Analysis Q. (CAQ)
    Community Integration Q. (CIQ)
    Coping Strategies Q. (CSQ)
    DASH q.
    Disabilities of Arm, Shoulder, and Hand q.
    disability screening q.

    Foot Function Index q.
    Foot Health Status Q.
    Functional Status Q. (FSQ)
    Headache Assessment Q. (HAQ)
    International Knee Ligament Standard Evaluation q.
    Jan van Breemen Function Q. (JVBF)
    Kenny Self-Care Q.
    Lambeth disability screening q.
    Levine Orthopaedic Outcomes Q.
    Lysholm knee scoring q.
    McGill Pain Q.
    McMaster-Toronto Arthritis Patient Preference Disability Q.
    Melzack Pain Q.
    MFA q.
    Michigan Hand Outcomes Q.
    Modified American Shoulder and Elbow Surgeons Shoulder Patient Self-Evaluation Form patient q.
    Occupational Q. (OQ)
    Osteoporosis Knowledge Q. (OKQ)
    Physical Activity Readiness Q. (PAR-Q)
    Roland-Morris Q. (RMQ)
    Short Musculoskeletal Function Assessment q.
    Shoulder Pain and Disability Index patient q.
    Shoulder Severity Index patient q.
    Simple Shoulder Test patient q.
    Subjective Shoulder Rating Scale patient q.
    Varni-Thompson Pediatric Pain Q.
Questus leading edge grasper-cutter
Quetelet index
quick
    Q. Neurological Screening Test (QNST)
    q. stretch
QuickAnchor
    Micro Q.
    Mitek Micro Q.
    Mitek Mini Q.
Quickbox container
QuickCast
    Q. splint
    Q. wrist immobilizer
QuickDraw bone harvester
Quickie
    Q. Carbon wheelchair
    Q. EX wheelchair
    Q. GPS wheelchair
    Q. GP Swing-Away wheelchair
    Q. GPV wheelchair
    Q. Kidz wheelchair
    Q. Recliner wheelchair
    Q. Ti wheelchair

Quick-Sil silicone system
QuickStick padding
QuickTack periosteal fixation system
quiescence
quiet hip disease
Quigley traction
QuikFormables orthotic
Quik splint
Quinby pelvic fracture classification
Quincke needle
Quinsana Plus

quinti
  abductor digiti q. (ADQ)
  extensor digiti q. (EDQ)
  Huber transfer of abductor
    digiti q.
  opponens digiti q. (ODQ)
quotient
  acetabular head q.
QUS
  quantitative ultrasound
QUS-2 calcaneal ultrasonometer

NOTES

RA
> rheumatoid arthritis
>> RA factor
>> RA test

rabbeting

Rabideau Kitchen Evaluation - Revised (RKE-R)

race-pace exercise

rachicentesis, rachiocentesis

rachilysis

rachiochysis

rachiodynia

rachiokyphosis

rachiomyelitis

rachioparalysis

rachiopathy

rachioplegia

rachioscoliosis

rachiotome

rachiotomy, rachitomy

rachisagra

rachischisis

rachitic
> r. cat-back
> r. pelvis
> r. rosary sign
> r. scoliosis

rachitomy (*var. of* rachiotomy)

rack
> Hausmann weight r.

racket amputation

racquetball

racquet-shaped incision

RADAR
> Rapid Assessment of Disease Activity in Rheumatology

radial
> r. agenesis
> r. antebrachial region
> r. artery
> r. artery injury
> r. bearing
> r. bone
> r. bursa
> r. carpal collateral ligament
> r. clubhand
> r. collateral ligament (RCL)
> r. collateral ligament complex (RCLC)
> r. column
> r. deficiency
> r. deviation
> r. digital nerve
> r. drift

> r. epicondylalgia
> r. forearm flap
> r. fracture reduction
> r. head
> r. head anlage
> r. head-capitellum view
> r. head dislocation
> r. head fracture
> r. head implant prosthesis
> r. head subluxation
> r. hemimelia
> R. Hinged Ulnar Deviation Splint
> r. laminectomy
> r. malalignment
> r. malleolus
> r. meniscal tear
> r. metacarpal ligament
> midcarpal r. (MCR)
> r. neck
> r. neck fracture
> r. nerve glove
> r. nerve injury
> r. nerve palsy
> r. phenomenon
> r. pseudarthrosis
> r. ray defect
> r. recession osteotomy
> r. reflex
> r. sensory nerve
> r. sensory nerve entrapment syndrome
> r. shaft
> r. sigmoid notch
> r. slab splint
> r. styloid fracture
> r. sulcus
> r. trial
> r. tuberosity
> r. tunnel
> r. tunnel syndrome
> r. wedge osteotomy
> r. wrist extensor
> r. wrist extensor tendinitis

radial-based flap

radialis
> flexor carpi r. (FCR)
> malleolus r.
> r. sign

radialized

radians per second (rad/s)

radiate
> r. carpal ligament
> r. ligament of head of rib
> r. sternocostal ligament

radiation
  r. therapy
  thorny r.
radiation-related
  r.-r. myelopathy
  r.-r. neuropathy
radiatum
radical
  r. approach
  r. compartmental excision
  r. flexor release
  r. nail bed ablation
  r. palmar fasciectomy
  r. resection
radicotomy
radicular
  r. artery
  r. neuritis
  r. pain
radiculectomy
radiculitis
  acute brachial r.
  cervical r.
radiculomyelopathy
radiculoneuritis
radiculopathy
  cervical r.
  4-level r.
  lumbosacral r.
radicurogram
radii (*pl. of* radius)
radioactive
  r. iodine-labeled fibrinogen
  r. xenon clearance
radiocapitate ligament
radiocapitellar
  r. articulation
  r. joint
  r. joint ganglion
  r. line
  r. subluxation
radiocarpal
  r. angle
  r. arthritis
  r. arthrodesis
  r. arthroscopy
  r. articulation
  r. dislocation
  r. instability
  r. joint
  r. ligament
  r. portal
radiodense mass
radiodiagnostic study
radiogram
radiograph
  anterior drawer stress r.
  cross-table lateral r.
  dorsoplantar r.

frog-leg lateral r.
Judet r.
lateral weightbearing r.
lumbopelvic r.
Merchant r.
plantarflexed stress r.
postoperative r.
skyline r.
spot r.
stress r.
tangential standing r.
Velpeau axillary r.
weightbearing dorsoplantar r.
weightbearing tangential r.
West Point axillary lateral r.
radiographic
  r. avascular necrosis
  r. examination
  r. grid
  r. parameter
radiography
  biplanar r.
  Broden stress r.
  carpometacarpal joint r.
  elbow r.
  flat plate r.
  flexion-extension r.
  neutron r.
  patellofemoral joint r.
  scanogram r.
  serendipity view in shoulder r.
  shoulder r.
  stress r.
  upright skeletal r.
radiohumeral
  r. articulation
  r. bursa
  r. bursitis
  r. epicondylitis
  r. joint
radioisotope
  r. clearance assay
  r. gallium scan
  r. indium-labeled white blood cell
  scan
  r. technetium scan
  r. thallium
radiolucency
  periprosthetic r.
radiolucent
  r. awl
  r. lesion
  r. line
  r. nidus
  r. roll
  r. sound
  r. splint
  r. wrist fixation system

radiolunate
 r. fusion
 r. joint
 long r. (LRL)
 short r. (SRL)
radiolunotriquetral ligament
radionucleotide imaging
radionuclide bone scan
radiopaque bone cement
radioscaphocapitate (RSC)
 r. ligament
 r. ligament laxity
radioscaphoid
 r. articulation
 r. fusion
 r. joint
 r. ligament
radioscapholunate
 r. joint
 r. ligament
radiotherapy
 coxa vara deformity pelvic r.
radiotranslucent rod
radiotriquetral ligament
radioulnar
 r. articulation
 r. dislocation
 r. dissociation
 r. joint
 r. joint injury
 r. subluxation
 r. surface
 r. synostosis (type I, II)
radius, pl. **radii**
 absent r.
 r. of angulation
 anular ligament of r.
 r. of curvature
 distal r.
 Kapandji fracture of r.
 proximal r.
 thrombocytopenia-absent r. (TAR)
Radley-Liebig-Brown approach
Radovan tissue expander prosthesis
rad/s
 radians per second
ragged-red fiber
Ragnell retractor
rail
 Bed-Bar support r.
 Lumex Tub-Guard safety r.
Raimiste sign
Raimondi hemostatic forceps

Rainbow cast sandal
raise
 crossed straight leg r.
 resisted straight leg r.
 single-leg toe r.
raising
 contralateral straight leg r.
 crossed straight leg r. (CSLR)
 diurnal variation in straight leg r.
 passive straight leg r.
 straight leg r. (SLR)
 well-leg r.
rake-handle effect
rake retractor
rales and rhonchi
Ralks
 R. bone drill
 R. fingernail drill
Raman spectroscopic imaging
ramp
 Graftech structural allograft
  anterior r.
 Graftech structural allograft
  posterior r.
 r. load
ramus, pl. **rami**
 dorsal r.
 inferior r.
 ischiopubic r.
 pubic r.
Ranawat-Burstein
 R.-B. hip prosthesis
 R.-B. porous stem
Ranawat classification
Ranawat-Dorr-Inglis method
Rancho
 R. ankle foot control device
 R. anklet foot control apparatus
 R. Cube System
 R. external fixation instrument
 R. swivel hinge
Ranchos Los Amigos Scale
Rand
 R. Functional Limitations Battery
 R. Physical Capacities Battery
Randelli shoulder prosthesis
random pattern flap
Raney
 R. bone drill
 R. flexion jacket brace
 R. perforator drill
 R. saw guide

R

NOTES

Raney-Crutchfield
- R.-C. tongs
- R.-C. tong traction

range
- r. of excursion
- r. of extension
- interquantile r.
- r. of motion (ROM)
- r. of motion brace
- r. of motion exercise
- r. of motion measurement
- r. of motion rehabilitation
- r. of motion restriction
- r. of motion testing
- r. of motion therapeutic stretching
- r. of motion therapy

Range-Master pulley
Ranke complex
Ransford
- R. loop
- R. Pain Drawing

Ranvier
- groove of R.
- zone of R.

Rapamune
raphe
- anterolateral r.
- median r.
- middle r.
- midline r.

Rapid Assessment of Disease Activity in Rheumatology (RADAR)
RAP-n-roll
Rappaport osteotomy
rarefaction
rarefying osteitis
RAS
- rhythmic auditory stimulation

Rascal scooter
rasp, raspatory
- Acufex convex r.
- Alexander r.
- Alexander-Farabeuf r.
- angled r.
- Arthrofile orthopaedic r.
- Aufricht glabellar r.
- Austin Moore r.
- Bacon r.
- bell r.
- Black r.
- Bristow r.
- Brown r.
- carbon-tungsten r.
- Charnley r.
- convex r.
- Coryllos r.
- Cottle r.
- custom r.
- DePuy r.
- diamond r.
- Doyen costal r.
- Doyen rib r.
- Endotrac r.
- Epstein bone r.
- Farabeuf bone r.
- Farabeuf-Lambotte r.
- femoral r.
- first rib r.
- Fisher r.
- Fomon r.
- Gallagher r.
- glabellar r.
- Good r.
- interbody r.
- Israel r.
- Jansen r.
- Joseph nasal r.
- Key r.
- Kleinert-Kutz r.
- Koenig r.
- Langenbeck r.
- Lewis periosteal r.
- Mallory-Head r.
- Maltz r.
- Mathieu r.
- Miller r.
- Nicoll r.
- Olivecrona r.
- orthopaedic r.
- Phemister r.
- r. pin
- Podiatry Institute r.
- power r.
- Putti bone r.
- rib r.
- Rubin r.
- Thompson r.
- triangular r.
- ulnar r.
- Yasargil micro r.
- Zollner r.

raspatory
Rastelli prosthesis
ratchet
- r. clamp
- r. flexor tenodesis splint
- R. Lock variable flexion knee lock

ratcheting T-handle
ratchet-type brace
ratchety weakness
rate
- basal metabolic r. (BMR)
- erythrocyte sedimentation r. (ESR)
- firing r.
- fusion nonunion r.
- heart r. (HR)
- implant survival r.
- nonunion r.

R

pseudarthrosis r.
resting heart r. (RHR)
sedimentation r.
steady state heart r. (SSHR)
strontium-85 resorption r.
vertebral osteosynthesis fusion r.
volumetric wear r.
Westergren sedimentation r.

rated perceived exertion (RPE)
Rath treatment table
rating
American Shoulder and Elbow
  Surgeons r.
Fitzgerald r.
Mazur ankle r.
McGuire r.
occupational r.
r. of perceived exertion (RPE)
permanent partial disability r.
PPD r.

ratio
AB/AD r.
abductor/adductor r.
ankle-brachial pressure r.
arch-height r.
Blackburne r.
Blackburn-Peel r.
bone age r.
bone and limb growth velocity r.'s
Brattström condylar height r.
canal-to-calcar isthmus r.
carpal height r.
Dorr r.
ER/IR r.
external rotation/internal rotation r.
femoral head-neck r.
femur length to abdominal
  circumference r. (FL/AC)
FL/AC r.
Insall r.
Insall-Salvati r.
medialization r.
metaphysial to diaphysial width r.
patellar ligament-patellar r.
Pavlov r.
Poisson r.
respiratory exchange r.
r. scale in rehabilitation testing
VMO:VL EMG r.
waist-to-hip r.

Ratliff avascular necrosis classification
rat-tooth forceps

Rauchfuss
R. sling
R. triangle
rave
fracture en r.
raw bone
ray
r. amputation
r. axis
border r.
central r.
finger r.
long axis r.
metatarsal r.
multiple r.
Peacock transposing index r.
plantarflexed
pollicized r.
r. resection
R. screw
stiff r.
R. TFC threaded fusion cage
transposing index r.

Rayhack technique
Raymond shoulder immobilizer
Raynaud
R. disease
R. gangrene
R. phenomenon
R. syndrome
Rayport muscular biopsy clamp
Ray-Tec sponge
razor
RazorVac ArthroWand
RBANS
Repeatable Battery for the Assessment of
  Neuropsychological status
RBMT
Rivermead Behavioral Memory Test
RBMT-E
Rivermead Behavioral Memory Test-
  Extended Version
RC
rehabilitation counseling
Role checklist
rotator cuff
RCB
rotator cuff buttress
RCL
radial collateral ligament
RCLC
radial collateral ligament complex

NOTES

RCSP
  resting calcaneal stance position
reabsorption
  bony r.
Reach Easy massager
reacher
  Double Duty cane r.
  E-Z R.
reaction
  compensation r.
  epidermophytid r.
  equilibrium r.
  exaggeration r.
  r. force
  foreign body r.
  giant cell r.
  ground r.
  host immune r.
  hunting r.
  implant r.
  periosteal r.
  protective extension r.
  pseudoperiosteal r.
  pseudosarcomatous r.
  r. time
  vagal r.
reactive
  r. arthritis
  r. bone formation
  low-surface r.
  r. nonunion
  r. periosteal proliferation
  r. synovitis
Read gouge
Real-EaSE neck and shoulder relaxer
realignment
  distal r.
  Elmslie-Trillat r.
  Galeazzi r.
  Genutrain PE patellar r.
  Hauser r.
  Hughston r.
  Insall proximal r.
  patellar r.
  patellofemoral r.
  physical r.
  r. procedure
  proximal and distal r.
  Roux-Goldthwait r.
Reality Orientation Chart
reamed
  r. nail
  sequentially r.
reamer
  acetabular r.
  acorn r.
  Aequalis r.
  Anspach r.
  Arthrex coring r.

Aufranc r.
Austin Moore r.
ball r.
blunt tapered T-handled r.
bone r.
r. brace
brace-type r.
calcar r.
Campbell r.
chamfer r.
Charnley deepening r.
Charnley expanding r.
Charnley taper r.
Charnley trochanter r.
cheese-grater hemispherical r.
Christmas tree r.
r. clamp
concave-surface r.
congruous cup-shaped r.
conical r.
Con-Nex r.
corrugated r.
cup r.
debris-retaining r.
deepening r.
DePuy r.
end-cutting r.
expanding r.
female r.
femoral head bone removal r.
fenestrated r.
flexible medullary r.
fluted r.
grater r.
Gray r.
grooving r.
r. guide
Hall Versipower r.
handle-type r.
Harris brace-type r.
Harris center-cutting acetabular r.
hemispherical r.
hollow mill r.
humeral r.
Indiana r.
Intracone intramedullary r.
intramedullary r.
Küntscher r.
male r.
medullary canal r.
Micro-Aire r.
Mira r.
Moore bone r.
motorized r.
multisized r.
Norton ball r.
orthopaedic r.
Perthes r.
power r.

R

power-driven r.
Pressure Sentinel r.
progressively larger r.
Richards r.
rigid r.
Rush rod awl r.
Smith-Petersen r.
spherical r.
spiral cortical r.
spiral trochanteric r.
spot-face r.
step-cut r.
straight power r.
Swanson r.
tapered r.
tapered hand r.
T-handled r.
triangular bone r.
triple r.
trochanteric r.
Wagner acetabular r.
reaming awl
reamputation
reanastomosis of blood supply
rear-entry ACL drill guide
rearfoot
r. deformity
r. ligament
r. osteotomy
r. stability system (RSS)
r. valgus
r. varus
re-arthroscoped
reassessment
reattachment
Amstutz r.
Doll trochanteric r.
Harris 4-wire trochanter r.
4-wire trochanter r.
Rebel knee brace
rebound
r. hyperextension
r. phenomenon of Holmes
r. tenderness
rebounder
Plyoback R.
recalcitrant
r. neuropathic ulcer
r. pain
r. plantar fasciitis
recalled
multiplanar gradient r. (MPGR)
ReCap femoral resurfacing system

receiver operating characteristic
recent dislocation
receptor
delta r.
epicritic r.
epsilon r.
kappa r.
MV1, MV2 r.
nociceptive r.
opioid r.
postural r.
sensory nerve action potential r.
(SNARE)
sigma r.
SNAP r.
stretch r.
receptor-tonus method
recess
acetabular r.
anular periradial r.
Flatt r.
lateral r.
popliteal r.
ulnar synovial r.
recession
Bleck iliopsoas r.
endoscopic gastrocnemius r.
gastrocnemius r.
gastrocnemius-soleus r.
iliopsoas r.
Strayer gastrocnemius r.
Strayer gastrocnemius-soleus r.
tongue-in-groove r.
ulnar r.
recipient
r. site
r. team
reciprocal
r. arm raise back exercise
technique
r. finger prehension orthosis
r. innervation
r. isokinetic testing
r. planing instrument
r. relaxation
r. stimulation
reciprocating
r. motor saw
r. power handpiece
reciprocation gait orthosis (RGO)
reciprocator
LSU r.
Recklinghausen disease

NOTES

recliner
    HydroSoothe r.
    Ortho-Biotic r.
reclining frame wheelchair
recoil
    elastic r.
recombinant human erythropoietin
Recon
    R. nail
    R. proximal drill guide bolt
reconstituted depolymerized heparin
reconstruction
    ACL r.
    Allman modification of Evans
      ankle r.
    allograft r.
    Andrews iliotibial band r.
    ankle r.
    anterior capsulolabral r. (ACLR)
    arthroscopically assisted anterior
      cruciate ligament r.
    arthroscopic transhumeral r.
    augmented r.
    autogenous patellar tendon r.
    backfilling r.
    Bankart r.
    bifurcated vein graft for
      vascular r.
    bilobed flap r.
    Bristow shoulder r.
    Broström ligament r.
    Brown knee joint r.
    Bunnell technique of pulley r.
    capsular r.
    capsular-shift r.
    Cho anterior cruciate ligament r.
    Chrisman-Snook r.
    Clancy-Andrews r.
    Clancy cruciate ligament r.
    complex acetabular r.
    cruciate ligament r.
    d'Aubigné femoral r.
    d'Aubigné resection r.
    Eaton-Littler ligament r.
    Ellison lateral knee r.
    Elmslie r.
    endoscopic anterior cruciate
      ligament r.
    Eriksson cruciate ligament r.
    Evans calcaneal r.
    Evans lateral ankle r.
    exogenous r.
    extraarticular r.
    Goldner r.
    hand r.
    Harmon hip r.
    hindfoot r.
    House r.
    Hughston lateral compartment r.

    index metacarpophalangeal joint r.
    Insall anterior cruciate ligament r.
    intraarticular r.
    joint r.
    Jones-Ellison ACL r.
    juxtacubital r.
    Kleinert technique of pulley r.
    5-in-1 knee r.
    Krukenberg hand r.
    Kugelberg r.
    Lange Achilles tendon r.
    Larson ligament r.
    lateral compartment r.
    Lee r.
    L'Episcopo hip r.
    ligament r.
    Lister technique of pulley r.
    MacIntosh over-the-top ACL r.
    modified Chrisman-Snook ankle r.
    Neer posterior shoulder r.
    Nicholas 5-in-1 r.
    O'Donoghue ACL r.
    osteoplastic r.
    r. plate
    pulley r.
    Rosenberg endoscopic anterior
      cruciate ligament r.
    Sauve-Kapandji distal radioulnar
      joint r.
    Silfverskiöld Achilles tendon r.
    S-K r.
    2-stage tendon graft r.
    sternoclavicular joint r.
    sural island flap for foot and
      ankle r.
    surgical r.
    Swanson r.
    tenoplastic r.
    thumb r.
    Torg knee r.
    total ossicular r.
    Verdan osteoplastic thumb r.
    Vulpius Achilles tendon r.
    Watson-Jones r.
    Whitman femoral neck r.
    Zancolli r.
reconstructive measure
recorder
    pulse volume r. (PVR)
recording
    r. electrode
    intramuscular r.
recovery
    fluid attenuation inversion r.
      (FLAIR)
    functional r.
    motor r.
    r. phase rehabilitation
    postanesthesia r. (PAR)

r. room (RR)

short time inversion r. (STIR)

recreational therapy (RT)

recrudescence

recruitment

r. frequency

r. interval

myopathic r.

neuropathic r.

r. pattern

rectangle

Hartshill r.

Luque r.

rectangular

r. amputation

r. awl

r. frame

rectilinear

r. bone scan

r. motion

rectus

r. abdominis flap

r. abdominis muscle

r. adductor syndrome

r. femoris

r. femoris contracture

r. femoris flap

r. femoris graft

r. femoris muscle

r. femoris tendon

r. foot type

r. hallux

metatarsus r.

r. position

r. sheath

recumbency

recumbent

r. bicycle

r. cycle

r. position

r. posture

recurrent

r. disorder

r. hyperextension

r. laryngeal nerve

r. laryngeal nerve injury

r. median nerve block

r. meningeal nerve

r. mycetoma

r. parosteal osteosarcoma

r. patellar dislocation

r. synovitis

recurvatum

r. angulation deformity

cubitus r.

genu r.

pectus r.

r. test

red

R. Cross freeze-dried allograft

r. light neon laser

r. marrow

r. muscle

r. response

Reddihough scale

redesign

job r.

Redi-Around finger splint

Rediform orthotic

Redigrip

R. knee pad

R. pressure bandage

Redi-Trac

R.-T. traction apparatus

R.-T. traction device

Redi-Vac cast cutter

red-red meniscal zone

redressement forcé

redresser

dual pin r.

redressment

reduced

r. interference pattern

r. profile (RP)

reducible

reduction

Ace bandage r.

Agee force-couple splint r.

Allen r.

anatomic r.

Aston cartilage r.

Barsky macrodactyly r.

Becton open r.

Bell-Tawse open r.

calcaneal fracture r.

closed r. (CR)

concentric r.

congruent r.

Cooper r.

cotton elbow r.

Crego hip r.

Crosby r.

Cubbins open r.

r. deformity

delayed open r.

NOTES

reduction *(continued)*
>> Eaton closed r.
>> Essex-Lopresti open r.
>> external fixation r. (EX-FI-RE)
>> femoral neck fracture r.
>> Ferguson hip r.
>> r. fixation
>> Flynn femoral neck fracture r.
>> force-couple splint r.
>> r. forceps
>> Fowles open r.
>> fracture r.
>> r. of fracture
>> fracture-dislocation r.
>> frame of r.
>> Hankin r.
>> Hastings open r.
>> hip r.
>> incomplete r.
>> indirect r.
>> internal fixation, closed r.
>> Kaplan open r.
>> Kinast indirect r.
>> King open r.
>> Kocher r.
>> Lange hip r.
>> Lorenz hip r.
>> Lowell r.
>> macrodactalia r.
>> manual fracture r.
>> McBride hallux abductovalgus r.
>> McBride hallux valgus r.
>> McKeever open r.
>> McReynolds open r.
>> Meyn elbow r.
>> Neer open r.
>> open r.
>> r. osteotomy
>> Pare elbow dislocation r.
>> Parvin r.
>> percutaneous r.
>> perioperative r.
>> Pratt open r.
>> prone r.
>> radial fracture r.
>> Ridlon hip r.
>> r. ring
>> shoulder r.
>> side posture r.
>> spondylolisthesis r.
>> stable r.
>> sternoclavicular joint r.
>> Stimson r.
>> surgical r.
>> swan-neck deformity r.
>> r. syndactyly
>> r. technique
>> tibiofibular joint r.

>> trial r.
>> Wayne County r.

red-white meniscal zone
Reebok
>> R. shoe
>> R. Slide System
>> R. Step System

Reece
>> R. orthopaedic shoe
>> R. osteotomy guide

Reed cast belt
reeducation
>> muscular r.

reefing
>> capsular r.
>> r. procedure

reel foot
reeling gait
Reese
>> R. dermatome
>> R. osteotomy guide system

reevaluate
reexploration
reference
>> biomechanical frame of r.
>> r. electrode

referred
>> r. anatomic phenomenon
>> r. neuritic pain
>> r. point
>> r. trigger point pain
>> r. trigger point phenomenon

refill
>> capillary r.

reflection
>> Campbell triceps r.
>> r. ceramic acetabular system
>> r. Interfit prosthesis
>> r. Interfit shell
>> r. I prosthesis
>> r. I, V, FSO acetabular cup
>> r. liner
>> medical subcutaneous r.
>> vertebral neural r.
>> r. V prosthesis

Re-Flex
>> R.-F. VSP artificial foot
>> R.-F. VSP prosthesis

reflex
>> absent r.
>> accommodation r.
>> Achilles tendon r.
>> r. action
>> adductor r.
>> anal r.
>> ankle jerk r.
>> antagonistic r.
>> r. anterior cervical plate system
>> aponeurotic r.

r. arc
arthrokinetic r.
asymmetric incurvatum r.
asymmetric tonic neck r. (ATNR)
automatic neonatal walking r.
axon r.
Babinski r.
Bekhterev deep r.
Bekhterev-Mendel r.
biceps r.
blink r.
body righting r.
brachioradialis r.
Brain r.
Brudzinski r.
bulbocavernosus r.
Chaddock r.
r. Comfort insole
cremasteric r.
crossed adductor r.
crossed extensor r.
crossed flexor r.
cry r.
cutaneous axon r.
deep tendon r. (DTR)
delayed r.
deltoid r.
depressed r.
derotational r.
r. development
digital r.
dorsal r.
elbow r.
equilibrium r.
r. examination
r. exercise and rehabilitation
  equipment
extensor thrust r.
external hamstring r.
external oblique r.
femoral r.
finger-thumb r.
flexor withdrawal r.
r. function
gluteal r.
Gordon r.
grasp r.
great toe r.
r. Gun
H r.
r. hammer
hamstring r.
heel-tap r.

Hirschberg r.
Hoffmann r.
hyperactive r.
hypoactive deep tendon r.
hypothenar r.
r. immunologic competence
incurvatum r.
interscapular r.
inverted radial r.
jaw opening r. (JOR)
knee flexion r.
knee jerk r.
lengthening r.
lumbar r.
Mayer r.
Mendel-Bekhterev r.
motor r.
muscle stretch r.
muscular r.
r. muscular contraction
myotatic r.
neck r.
neck-righting r.
r. neurovascular dystrophy
Oppenheim r.
palmar grasp r.
parachute r.
patellar r.
patelloadductor r.
pathologic r.
pectoral r.
placement r.
placing r.
plantar r.
positive supporting r.
postcast compression r.
postural r.
primitive r.
pronator r.
quadriceps r.
radial r.
r. rebound component of whiplash
Remak r.
righting r.
Romberg r.
scapular r.
scapulohumeral r.
slow stretch r.
sole r.
sole-tap r.
somatoautonomic r. (SAR)
somatosomatic r.
Stookey r.

R

NOTES

reflex *(continued)*
    stretch r.
    sudomotor startle r.
    supinator jerk r.
    supinator longus r.
    suprapatellar r.
    r. sympathetic dystrophy (RSD)
    r. sympathetic dystrophy syndrome (RSDS)
    tarsophalangeal r.
    tendon r.
    r. therapy
    r. threshold
    tibioadductor r.
    tilting r.
    toe r.
    tonic neck r.
    r. tracheostomy management
    triceps surae r.
    ulnar r.
    vertebra prominens r.
    vertical suspension r.
    vestibulospinal r.
    viscerosomatic r.
    von Bekhterev r.
    wrist flexion r.
ReFlexion first MPJ implant system
reflexogenic
reflexology
refractory
    r. neuroma
    r. period
refracture
Refsum syndrome
refusion
Regal Acrylic/Stretch prosthetic sock
Regenafil allograft paste
regenerated fibroblast
regeneration
    r. motor unit potential
    r. of nerve
    osteoblastic bone r.
    tibial bone defect r.
    r. torus
Regen flexion exercise
regimen
    postoperative r.
region
    axillary r.
    basilar r.
    calcaneal r.
    cervical r.
    deltoid r.
    diaphysial r.
    elbow r.
    femoral r.
    gluteal r.
    H r.
    hookian r.

    hypochondriac r.
    iliac r.
    infraclavicular r.
    infrascapular r.
    infraspinous r.
    ischiorectal r.
    lumbar r.
    metazonal r.
    nuchal r.
    occipital r.
    olecranon r.
    patellar r.
    physial r.
    popliteal r.
    posterior longitudinal fiber r.
    posterior oblique fiber r.
    posteromedial r.
    pulvinar r.
    radial antebrachial r.
    sinus tarsi r.
    superomedial r.
    true acetabular r.
    ulnar antebrachial r.
    volar antebrachial r.
regional
    r. anesthesia
    r. block
    r. migratory osteoporosis
registration
    sensory r.
registry
    National Football Head and Neck Injury R.
Regnauld
    R. enclavement
    R. free phalangeal base autograft for hallux limitus
    R. free phalangeal bone autograft
    R. hallux rigidus classification
    R. modification of Keller arthroplasty
    R. osteotomy
    R. procedure
Regnauld-type great toe degeneration
0.01% Regranex Gel
regular
    r. stem
    R. Strength Bayer Enteric 500 Aspirin
rehabilitation
    acute phase r.
    aquatic r.
    r. assessment
    r. care
    community r.
    r. counseling (RC)
    cryotherapy r.
    day treatment r.
    electrical stimulation r.

R. Engineering and Assistive Technology Society of North America (RESNA)
r. flexibility exercise
free weight r.
functional phase r.
r. goal
home r.
R. Impairment Category (RIC)
r. intervention
r. muscle strengthening
muscular r.
Ortho DX stimulator for knee r.
orthopaedic r.
outpatient r.
physical medicine and r. (PMR)
r. planning
postcompetition r.
progressive lumbar extension r.
proprioceptive r.
PULSES Profile for Comprehensive R.
range of motion r.
recovery phase r.
remote locomotor r.
Safety Assessment of Function and the Environment for R. (SAFER)
Stage model of industrial r.
Synergy joint r.
r. therapeutic program
r. treatment
vocational r. (VR)

rehabilitator
Ankle Isolator ankle r.

Rehab TROM brace
Reichenheim technique
Reichert-Mundinger stereotactic device
Reimers
R. hip position migration index
R. instability index

reimplantation
Reiner
R. bone rongeur
R. plaster knife

Reinert acetabular extensile approach
reinforcement
acetabular r.
Bragard r.
r. ring

reinnervation
Reintegration to Normal Living index
reinterpretation
hypnotic r.

Reiter
R. disease
R. syndrome

ReJuveness scar treatment
rekindling test
relapsing ankle sprain
relation to subadjacent segment
relative
r. refractory period
r. response attributable to the maneuver (RRAM)
r. risk (RR)

Relax-A-Bac posture support
relaxant
muscle r.
skeletal muscle r.

relaxation
ferromagnetic r.
r. phenomenon
postisometric r.
progressive muscle r.
reciprocal r.
r. response
r. training

relaxed skin tension line
relaxer
Real-EaSE neck and shoulder r.

relaxing incision
Re-Lax-O chiropractic table
release
adductor tendon and lateral capsular r.
Agee carpal tunnel r.
anterior hip r.
anterior shoulder r.
anterolateral r.
Baxter nerve r.
Beaty lateral r.
bipolar r.
brevis r.
Brown 2-portal carpal tunnel r.
capsular r.
carpal tunnel r. (CTR)
Chow endoscopic carpal tunnel r.
circumferential r.
clubfoot r.
complete subtalar r. (CSR)
direct-vision carpal tunnel r.
distal intrinsic r.
distal soft tissue r. (DSTR)
Dupuytren contracture r.
Eberle contracture r.
endoscopic carpal tunnel r. (ECTR)

NOTES

R

release *(continued)*
 Endotrac endoscopic carpal
  tunnel r.
 extensor hood r.
 fascial r.
 Ferkel bipolar r.
 flexor hallucis longus tendon r.
 flexor plate r.
 flexor-pronator origin r.
 Guyon tunnel r.
 hamstring r.
 Heyman-Herndon r.
 Heyman-Herndon-Strong capsular r.
 Inglis-Cooper r.
 interleukin-1 beta r.
 John Barnes myofascial r.
 joint r.
 key r.
 Kinetix instrument for carpal
  tunnel r.
 lateral capsular r.
 lateral extensor r.
 lateral retinaculum r.
 leg compartment r.
 ligamentous r.
 Little r.
 medial r.
 Mital elbow r.
 modified 2-portal endoscopic carpal
  tunnel r.
 myofascial r.
 Ober r.
 open carpal tunnel r. (OCTR)
 patellar retinacula r.
 r. phenomenon
 plantar capsular r.
 plantar fascial r.
 plantar-lateral r.
 plantar-medial r.
 plantar plate r.
 posterior r.
 posterolateral r.
 posteromedial r. (PMR)
 pronator teres r.
 proximal intrinsic r.
 proximal nerve r.
 radical flexor r.
 retinacular r.
 retrogeniculate hamstring r.
 Sengupta quadriceps r.
 Siegel hip r.
 Snow-Littler r.
 soft tissue r.
 spinal fascial r.
 tarsal tunnel r. (TTR)
 tendon r.
 triceps surae r.
 trigger finger r.

 trigger thumb r.
 Turco clubfoot r.
 Turco posteromedial r.
 Ueba r.
 ulnar nerve r.
 unipolar r.
 Z-plasty r.
released ulnar intrinsic muscle
Reliance CM femoral implant
 component
relieving incision
relocation test
Relton-Hall frame
Remak
 R. paralysis
 R. reflex
remedial exercise
remediation
 biokinetic r.
Remifemin herbal product
Remimembranosus complex
remobilization
remodeling
 bone r.
 cortical bone r.
 haversian bone r.
 r. phase
 simultaneous r.
remote
 r. locomotor rehabilitation
 r. pedicle flap
removable cast
removal
 Cameron femoral component r.
 cast r.
 cement r.
 Collis-Dubrul femoral stem r.
 r. of excess cement
 femoral component r.
 femoral stem r.
 Harris femoral component r.
 implant r.
 Moreland-Marder-Anspach femoral
  stem r.
 nail fold r.
 nail plate r.
 stem r.
 Winograd nail plate r.
remover
 Biomet Ultra-Drive cement r.
 Craig pin r.
renal
 r. osteodystrophy
 r. tubular osteomalacia
Renaut body
Renee creak sign
Renolux convertible car seat
reoperation

REP
resistive exercise products
REP Bands exercise band
repair
Achilles tendon r. (ATR)
ACL r.
acromioclavicular joint r.
all-inside r.
arthroscopic Bankart r.
Atasoy-type flap for nail injury r.
augmented r.
Bankart shoulder r.
Becker tendon r.
bioabsorbable tack r.
bioelectrical r.
Black r.
bone graft r.
Bosworth tendo calcaneus r.
Boyd-Anderson biceps tendon r.
brachial plexus r.
Broström lateral ankle ligament r.
Bunnell tendon r.
capsule r.
capsulolabral r.
Caspari r.
Chonstruct chondral r.
delayed primary r.
dog-ear r.
dural r.
DuVries hammertoe r.
dynamic r.
end-to-end tendon r.
end-to-side r.
epineural r.
extensor tendon r.
fascicular r.
first toe Jones r.
fixed hammertoe deformity r.
flexor tendon r.
fracture r.
Froimson-Oh r.
Genzyme Tissue R.
glenohumeral dislocation r.
group fascicular r.
hammertoe r.
inferior tibiofibular r.
inguinal TEPP r.
inside-out meniscal r.
Jones first toe r.
Jones toe r.
Kessler modified Achilles tendon r.
Kleinert r.
5-in-1 knee ligament r.

Kocher-Langenbeck ilioinguinal r.
Kocher-Langenbeck ilioinguinal
approach to fracture r.
Krackow Achilles tendon r.
Lange tendon lengthening and r.
ligamentous and capsular r. (LCR)
Lindholm open surgical tendon r.
Lindholm tendo calcaneus r.
Lynn tendo calcaneus r.
MacIntosh over-the-top r.
MacNab shoulder r.
Ma-Griffith percutaneous Achilles
tendon r.
Ma-Griffith ruptured Achilles
tendon r.
Marshall ligament r.
mattress double anchor footprint
rotator cuff tear r.
medial r.
meniscal r.
Milch radioulnar joint r.
mini-open rotator cuff r.
Mosley anterior shoulder r.
nonaugmented r.
patellar tendon r.
percutaneous Achilles tendon r.
plastic r.
primary r.
pseudarthrosis r.
Revo rotator cuff r.
rod fracture r.
rotator cuff r.
Scuder r.
semitendinosus augmentation of
patellar tendon r.
Sever-L'Episcopo shoulder r.
shoulder r.
1-sided dog-ear r.
Speed sternoclavicular r.
Staples r.
Strickland tendon r.
suture anchor shoulder r.
sutureless avascular meniscal r.
tendon r.
Teuffer tendo calcaneus r.
tissue r.
total extraperitoneal r. (TEPP)
transacromial coracoacromial
ligament r.
transglenoid suture r.
triad knee r.
triple ligamentous r.
Tsuge tendon r.

R

NOTES

repair *(continued)*
    vertical loop suture technique for meniscus r.
    volar plate r.
    Watson-Jones fracture r.
    Zone Specific II meniscal r.
reparative
    r. granuloma
    r. phase
Repeatable Battery for the Assessment of Neuropsychological status (RBANS)
repeated
    r. quick stretch (RQS)
    r. quick stretch from elongation (RQS-E)
    r. quick stretch superimposed upon an existing contraction (RQS-SEC)
reperfusion injury
repetition
    r. maximum (RM)
    r. strain injury (RSI)
    r. time (TR)
1-repetition maximum (1-RM)
repetitive
    r. discharge
    r. exercise
    r. microtrauma
    r. nerve stimulation
    r. nerve stimulator (RNS)
    r. strain disorder
    r. stress disorder
    r. stress injury
    r. stress syndrome (RSS)
    r. trauma
    r. trauma disorder (RTD)
Repicci II knee replacement
Repiphysis prosthesis
replacement
    allograft ligament r.
    alumina bioceramic joint r.
    Amstutz total hip r.
    anatomic porous r. (APR)
    Ascension MCP total joint r.
    Ascension PIP total joint r.
    Averill total hip r.
    bicompartmental r.
    r. bone
    Buechel-Pappas total ankle r.
    calcar r.
    Capello total hip r.
    cementless total hip r.
    Charnley total hip r.
    dynamic double tendon r.
    elbow r.
    electrolyte r.
    Engh total hip r.
    Ewald total elbow r.
    facet r.

    failed joint r.
    hip r.
    Howse total hip r.
    hybrid total hip r.
    hypnotic r.
    intercalary segmental r.
    Kirschner Medical Dimension hip r.
    Leeds-Keio Dacron mesh r.
    ligament r.
    Marmor r.
    PCA total hip r.
    Pilliar total hip r.
    porous-coated anatomic total hip r.
    primary hip r.
    ProDisc lumbar total disc r.
    prosthetic r.
    Repicci II knee r.
    revision r.
    Ring UPM total hip r.
    Ring UPM total knee r.
    SAF hip r.
    Scandinavian total ankle r. (STAR)
    Scarborough total hip r.
    self-articulating femoral hip r.
    self-bearing ceramic total hip r.
    Stanmore knee r.
    Stanmore total hip r.
    surface r.
    Tharies hip r.
    tile plate facet r.
    r. tissue
    total ankle r. (TAR)
    total hip r. (THR)
    total joint r. (TJR)
    total knee r. (TKR)
    tricompartmental r.
    TR-28 total hip r.
    unicompartmental knee r.
    universal head r. (UHR)
    Vanguard Uni unicompartmental knew r.
replantable amputation
replantation
    r. of amputated digit
    autogenous meniscal cartilage r.
    r. bandage
    r. of finger
    limb r.
RepliCare wound dressing
Replica total hip replacement system
repolarization
report
    Juvenile Arthritis Functional Assessment R. (JAFAR)
repositioner
    Wilson-Cook prosthesis r.
repositioning
    muscle r.

reproducibility
reproducible
Repro head halter
requirement
    therapeutic r.
rerouted tendon
rerouting
    Blair-Omer r.
    r. insertion
    Zancolli biceps tendon r.
research
    Agency for Health Care Policy
      and R. (AHCPR)
    Alvarado Orthopaedic R.
    Foundation for Chiropractic
      Education and R. (FCER)
    National Center for Dissemination
      of Disability R.
    Policy and Review Committee for
      Human R.
    The Institute for Rehabilitation R.
      (TIRR)
resectable
resecting fracture
resection
    anterior tarsal r.
    r. arthrodesis
    r. arthroplasty
    Badgley iliac wing r.
    bar r.
    bone r.
    bony bridge r.
    calcaneal r.
    calcaneonavicular bar r.
    Carrell r.
    caudal lamina r.
    Clayton procedure with
      panmetatarsal head r.
    cuff r.
    Darrach r.
    r. dermodesis
    Dillwyn-Evans r.
    distal femoral r.
    DuVries r.
    en bloc r.
    epiphysial bar r.
    extraarticular r.
    femoral r.
    fibular head r.
    first rib r.
    Girdlestone r.
    Guller r.
    Gurd r.

R

    Henry r.
    Hoffmann panmetatarsal head r.
    iliac wing r.
    Ingram bony bridge r. ·
    innominate bone r.
    intercalary r.
    intralesional r.
    Kashiwagi r.
    Kotz modular femur and tibia r.
      (KMFTR)
    kyphos r.
    Langenskiöld bony bridge r.
    Lewis intercalary r.
    local radical r.
    Malawer r.
    Mankin r.
    marginal r.
    Mayo metatarsal head r.
    medial eminence r.
    medial malleolus r.
    r. of meniscus
    metaphysial head r.
    metatarsal head r.
    Milch cuff r.
    Mumford r.
    panmetatarsal head r.
    Phelps partial r.
    prophylactic r.
    proximal femoral r.
    radical r.
    ray r.
    Rockwood r.
    Thompson r.
    Tikhoff-Linberg shoulder girdle r.
    transoral odontoid r.
    tumor r.
    vertebral body stapling wedge r.
    wafer distal ulna r.
    Weaver-Dunn r.
    wedge r.
    wedge matrix r. (WMR)
resection-arthrodesis
    Enneking r.-a.
resection-realignment
resector
    Accu-Line femoral r.
    Accu-Line tibial r.
    r. blade
    femoral r.
    full-radius r.
    orthotome r.
    synovial r.
    tibial r.

NOTES

residence ridge
residual
r. cement
r. heel equinus
r. hindfoot equinus
r. latency
r. limb
r. tension
residuum, pl. **residua**
resilience
resin
melamine r.
methacrylate r.
polyacetal r.
Resist-A-Band exercise band
resistance
growth hormone r.
intralesional vascular r.
isometric r.
isotonic r.
manual r.
plyometric r.
strength against r.
R. Support Formula
Thera-Band System of
Progressive R.
r. training
resistant clubfoot
Resist-A-Tube exercise band
resisted
r. active flexion
r. dorsiflexion
r. external rotation
r. straight leg raise
r. straight leg raise test
resistive
r. chair exercise kit
r. exercise
r. exercise products (REP)
r. exerciser
r. exercise table
r. movement
r. weighed column
RESNA
Rehabilitation Engineering and Assistive
Technology Society of North America
resonance
field focused nuclear magnetic r.
(FONAR)
hydatid r.
nuclear magnetic r. (NMR)
osteal r.
resonator
Jacobson r.
resorbable
r. ceramic
r. graft containment system
r. plate
r. polydioxanon pin

r. polymer pin
r. polymer screw
r. scaffold
resorption
bone r.
osteoclastic r.
periprosthetic bone r.
tuftal r.
resource
Assessment of Living Skills
and R.'s (ALSAR)
respiratory exchange ratio
Respond II muscle stimulator
response
acute inflammatory r.
average evoked r.
axon r.
biochemical r.
blink r.
brainstem auditory evoked r.
(BAER)
cellular level r.
decremental r.
delayed r.
evoked r.
foreign body r.
F-wave r.
galvanic skin r.
hunting r.
hyperactive r.
incremental r.
r. interval
late r.
motion r.
motor r.
paired r.
physiologic r.
pilomotor r.
plantar Babinski r.
red r.
R. rehabilitation and fitness
equipment
relaxation r.
sensory r.
tissue-level r.
visual evoked r.
responsive neurostimulator (RNS)
rest
bed r.
Chiroflow back r.
Core Hibak R.
Core Lobak R.
Core Sitback R.
foot r.
hand r.
r., ice, compression, elevation
(RICE)
kidney r.
Mayfield head r.

Mouse Nest mouse r.
r. pain (RP)
pain at r.

Restcue bed

resting
r. calcaneal stance position (RCSP)
r. foot sling
r. forefoot supination angle
r. heart rate (RHR)
r. length
r. membrane potential
r. orthosis
r. pan splint
r. shear stiffness
r. tremor
r. zone

restless leg

restlessness
motor r.

Reston
R. dressing
R. padding

restoration
r. acetabular system
functional r.
r. GAP acetabular cup
intrinsic r.
pinch r.
r. Secur-Fit X'tra acetabular shell

Restoration-HA hip system

restorative pin

restore
R. ACL guide system
R. AF
R. AF antifungal lotion
R. AF antimicrobial skin cleanser
R. AF antimicrobial solution
r. CalciCare dressing
R. Clean 'N Moist
R. cuff tear implant
R. orthobiologic soft-tissue implant

restraint
active r.
passive r.
poncho r.
universal canvas body r.

restricted
r. inversion
r. range of motion

restriction
extension r.
flexion r.

intercostal r.
lateral flexion r.
r. of motion
range of motion r.
rotational r.
skin r.
soft tissue r.
talocrural r.

restrictive bandage

restrictor
BioStop G bone cement r.
cement r.
femoral canal r.
plastic marrow canal r.

result
false-negative r.

resurfacing
Achilles tendon r.
Amstutz r.
bone r.
r. operation
Paltrinieri-Trentani r.
patellar r.
r. procedure
Salzer r.

resurrection bone

retainer
Thermoskin heat r.

retaining knee prosthesis

retardation
deafness, onychoosteodystrophy,
mental r. (DOOR)
growth r.
healing r.
Matson Evaluation of Social Skills
in Individuals with Severe R.
(MESSIER)

retention
r. drill
r. suture

reticula (*pl. of* reticulum)

reticular
r. bone bruise
r. cell sarcoma

reticularis
livedo r.

reticulated polyurethane pad

reticulin stain

reticulocytosis
cerebroside r.

reticuloendothelial system

reticuloendotheliosis

R

NOTES

reticulohistiocytosis
    multicentric r.
reticulum, pl. **reticula**
    endoplasmic r.
    sarcoplasmic r.
retinacular
    r. artery
    r. hood
    r. ligament
    r. release
retinaculum, pl. **retinacula**
    caudal r.
    extensor r.
    flexor r.
    hypertrophic flexor r.
    inferior extensor r.
    inferior peroneal r.
    patellar r.
    peroneal r.
    superior extensor r.
    superior peroneal r. (SPR)
    Weitbrecht r.
retraction
    Schink metatarsal r.
retractor
    Adson cerebellar r.
    Adson hemilaminectomy r.
    Allport r.
    Alm wound r.
    amputation r.
    APC hip r.
    appendiceal r.
    Army-Navy r.
    Assistant Free long prong collateral
      ligament r.
    Assistant Free Shubbs short prong
      collateral ligament r.
    Assistant Free wide PCL r.
    Aufranc cobra r.
    Badgley laminectomy r.
    Balfour self-retaining r.
    Ballantine hemilaminectomy r.
    Bankart r.
    Beckman r.
    Bennett bone r.
    Bennett tibial r.
    Bertin hip r.
    blade-point r.
    blade-spike r.
    Blount anvil r.
    Blount knee r.
    Bodnar r.
    Boyle-Davis r.
    Busenkell posterior hip r.
    Campbell nerve root r.
    Carroll-Bennett r.
    Carroll hand r.
    Caspar r.
    cerebellar r.

Chandler knee r.
Charnley horizontal r.
Charnley initial incision r.
Charnley knee r.
Charnley pin r.
Charnley self-retaining r.
Cloward blade r.
cobra r.
Collis r.
Collis-Taylor r.
Cooley rib r.
crank frame r.
Crego r.
curved r.
Cushing r.
Darrach r.
Deaver r.
deep r.
D'Errico r.
digital self-retaining r.
Doane knee r.
double bent Hohmann acetabular r.
double-ended right-angle r.
Downey hemilaminectomy r.
Dozier radiolucent Bennett r.
dual nerve root suction r.
East-West r.
Elite Farley r.
extra-depth posterior acetabular r.
extra-large hip r.
Fahey r.
fat pad r.
Finochietto rib r.
flat r.
FlexPosure endoscopic r.
Fukuda humeral head r.
Gelpi r.
Gifford mastoid r.
handheld r.
Hays hand r.
heavy-duty 2-tooth r.
Heiss soft tissue r.
Hendren self-retaining r.
Henning meniscal r.
Hibbs r.
Hoen r.
Hohmann bone r.
Holscher knee r.
Holscher root r.
Holzheimer r.
humeral head r.
inferoposterior acetabular capsule r.
Inge r.
Israel r.
Kasdan r.
Kirschenbaum r.
Kleinert-Ragnell r.
knee r.
Kocher r.

Lange bone r.
Lange-Hohmann bone r.
Langenbeck r.
large Cobra r.
Love nerve root r.
lower hand r.
Lowman hand r.
Luongo hand r.
Markham-Meyerding r.
Mark II Chandler total knee r.
Mark II concave total knee r.
Mark II lateral collateral
  ligament r.
Mark II modular weight r.
Mark II S total knee r.
Mark II Stubbs short prong
  collateral ligament r.
Mark II wide PCL knee r.
Mark II Z knee r.
Mayo-Collins r.
McCullough r.
McIvor ENT r.
meniscus r.
Meyerding r.
mini-Hohmann podiatric r.
modified Fukuda-type r.
Morris r.
Mueller r.
Myers knee r.
narrow-blade r.
narrow Cobra r.
narrow double-prong acetabular r.
narrow inferior acetabular r.
narrow-neck mini-Hohmann r.
Nelson rib r.
Ollier rake r.
orthopaedic r.
Paulson knee r.
Percy amputation r.
pin r.
2-prong rake r.
3-prong rake blade r.
5-prong rake blade r.
Ragnell r.
rake r.
rib r.
ribbon r.
Richardson r.
ring r.
Rosenberg r.
Rowe humeral head r.
Sauerbruch r.
Scholten sternal r.

Scoville r.
Seeburger r.
self-retaining r.
Senn r.
sharp r.
Sherwin knee r.
Sims r.
single-prong broad acetabular r.
skid humeral head r.
Smillie knee r.
Sofield r.
soft tissue blade r.
Southwick two-tined r.
standard 2-inch blade r.
standard 4-inch blade r.
stiff ribbon r.
Tang r.
Taylor r.
thin glenoid r.
tibial r.
Tupper hand-holder and r.
upper hand r.
U-shaped r.
Verbrugge-Hohmann bone r.
Volkmann rake r.
Wagner r.
Watanabe r.
Weit-Arner r.
Weitlaner r.
3-2 Weitlaner self-retaining r.
Wichman r.
Williams self-retaining r.
Wilson gonad r.
Wink r.
Z r.
retractor-narrow
  bent Hohman r.-n.
retractor-wide
  bent Hohman r.-w.
retraining
  VMO r.
retrieved insert
retriever
  Carroll tendon r.
  Hewson suture r.
  Kleinert-Kutz tendon r.
  magnetic r.
retroacetabular lesion
retro-Achilles bursa
retrobulbar prosthesis needle
retrocalcaneal
  r. bursa
  r. bursitis

NOTES

retrocalcaneal *(continued)*
r. disorder
r. exostosis
r. spur
retrocalcaneobursitis
retrodisplaced fracture
retroflexion
tibial r.
retrogeniculate hamstring release
retrograde
r. AXT
r. Beaver blade
r. degeneration
r. drilling
r. intramedullary nail
r. meniscal blade
r. method
r. nailing
retrograde-cutting hook-shaped knife
retrolisthesed fragment
retrolisthesis positional dyskinesia
retromedullary arteriovenous malformation
retropatellar
r. fat pad
r. fat pad contracture
retroperitoneal
r. approach
r. decompression
r. fibrosis
r. hemorrhage
r. space
retropharyngeal
r. abscess
r. approach
r. fascial cleft
r. space
retropulsed
r. bone excision
r. bony fragment
retropulsion of gait
retroreflective marker
retrosacral fascia
retrospondylolisthesis
retrosternal
r. abscess
r. dislocation
retrotorsion
femoral r.
tibial r.
retrovascular cord
retroversion
r. of acetabular cup
angle of r.
femoral r.
tibial r.
Rett syndrome

return
r. to play (RTP)
r. of sensation
return-to-play
r.-t.-p. consideration
r.-t.-p. injury assessment
r.-t.-p. musculoskeletal assessment
r.-t.-p. sidelines decision making
reulceration
ReUnite
R. hand fixation
R. orthopaedic pin
R. orthopaedic screw
R. resorbable orthopaedic fixation system
revascularization
endosteal r.
r. of graft
revascularized tissue
Revelation hip system
Reverdin
R. bunionectomy
R. epidermal free graft
R. osteotomy
R. prosthesis
Reverdin-Green
R.-G. bunionectomy
R.-G. foot procedure
R.-G. osteotomy
Reverdin-Green-Laird procedure
Reverdin-Laird
R.-L. bunionectomy
R.-L. osteotomy
Reverdin-McBride bunionectomy
reversal
r. of antagonist (ROA)
r. of cervical lordosis
r. of fore-aft shear phase of gait
isotonic r. (IR)
stabilizing r. (SR)
reverse
r. Austin osteotomy
r. Bankart lesion
r. Barton fracture
r. Bigelow maneuver
r. buckling
r. closing base wedge osteotomy
r. Colles fracture
r. cross-finger flap
r. cutting needle
r. Dillwyn-Evans calcaneal osteotomy
r. forearm island flap
r. Hill-Sachs defect
r. Hill-Sachs lesion
r. Hill-Sachs sign
r. Jones procedure
r. knuckle-bender splint
r. Lachman test

r. Lasègue test
r. last shoe
r. lunge back exercise technique
r. Mauck knee operation
r. Mauck knee procedure
r. Monteggia fracture
r. NAGS
r. obliquity
r. obliquity fracture
r. pivot shift
r. pivot shift test
r. Putti-Platt procedure
r. tennis elbow
r. Thomas heel
r. Trendelenburg position
r. undercutting lengthening
r. wedge technique
r. windlass
r. wrist curl
reverse-cutting meniscal probe
reversed shoulder prosthesis
reverse-flow flap
reverse-threaded screw
**reversible ischemic neurologic disability
(RIND)**
revised
Rabideau Kitchen Evaluation - R.
(RKE-R)
Symptoms Checklist 90 R. (SCL-90R)
Vineland Adaptive Behavior
Scales, R. (VABS)
revision
r. arthroplasty
exploration and r.
hip r.
r. hip arthroplasty
r. hip replacement
R. hip stem
jumbo uncemented cup acetabular
component r.
Mallory-Head total hip r.
r. procedure
stump r.
total hip r.
r. of total hip
r. total hip operation
ReVision nail
Revo
R. knot
R. loop handle knot pusher
R. retrievable cancellous screw
R. rotator cuff repair

R. rotator cuff repair system
R. suture anchor
Rezaian
R. external fixation
R. external fixation apparatus
R. external fixation device
R. interbody device
R. spinal fixator
RGO
reciprocation gait orthosis
rhabdomyolysis
exertional r.
rhabdomyoma
rhabdomyosarcoma
alveolar r.
embryonal r.
pleomorphic r.
R-Hab lighter weight ankle
rhachotomy
Capener lateral r.
decompression r.
lateral r.
rHead
r. implant system
r. Recon implant
rheobase
rheostosis
rheumatic
r. fever
r. granuloma
r. scoliosis
rheumatica
polymyalgia r. (PMR)
rheumatism
Besnier r.
chronic r.
Heberden r.
MacLeod capsular r.
nodose r.
palindromic r.
Poncet r.
tuberculous r.
World Health
Organization/International League
Against R. (WHO/LAR)
rheumatismal edema
rheumatoid
r. arthritis (RA)
r. arthritis factor
r. arthritis myopathy
r. arthritis synovitis
r. cyst
r. deformity

NOTES

rheumatoid *(continued)*
>r. disease
>r. disorder
>r. foot
>r. myositis
>r. nodule
>r. spondylitis
>r. vasculitis

rheumatologic disorder
rheumatologist
rheumatology
>American College of R. (ACR)
>Rapid Assessment of Disease
>>Activity in R. (RADAR)

Rhinelander pin
Rhino Triangle polypropylene hip abduction brace
rhizomelic spondylosis
rhizomelic-type chondrodysplasia
rhizomesomelic bone dysplasia
rhizotomy
>intradural dorsal spinal root r.
>posterior r.
>selective posterior r. (SPR)

RHOCS
>right-handed orthogonal coordinate
>system

rhomboid
>r. flap
>r. ligament
>Michaelis r.
>r. muscle

rhonchus, pl. **rhonchi**
>rales and rhonchi

Rhoton
>R. elevator
>R. enucleator
>R. needle holder
>R. osteotome

RHR
>resting heart rate

Rhus toxicodendron
rhythm
>scapulohumeral r.

rhythmic
>r. auditory stimulation (RAS)
>r. handgrip work
>r. initiation (RI)
>r. initiation technique
>r. stabilization

RI
>rhythmic initiation

rib
>r. approximator
>bed of r.
>r. belt
>r. belt orthosis
>bicipital r.
>bucket-handle r.

>r. cage
>cervical r.
>r. contractor
>r. contusion
>costochondral junction of r.'s
>r. cutter
>r. drill
>r. elevator
>false r.
>r. fixation
>floating r.
>r. forceps
>r. fracture
>r. graft
>hypoplastic first r.
>interarticular ligament of head
>>of r.
>r. motion
>radiate ligament of head of r.
>r. rasp
>r. retractor
>rudimentary r.
>slipping r.
>spurious r.
>sternal r.
>Stiller r.
>true r.
>vertebral r.
>vertebrocostal r.
>vertebrosternal r.

ribbed
>r. hook
>r. needle

ribbed-sole shoe
Ribbing disease
Ribble bandage
ribbon
>r. retractor
>r. sign

ribonucleoprotein (RNP)
rib-vertebral angle
RIC
>Rehabilitation Impairment Category

Rica
>R. bone drill
>R. wire guidepin

Ricard amputation
RICE
>rest, ice, compression, elevation

rice
>r. body
>joint r.

"Rice Krispie" crepitation
Richards
>R. angle guide
>R. arthrodesis
>R. bone clamp
>R. classic compression hip screw
>R. Colles external fixator

R. drill guide
R. fixation staple
R. fixator system
R. hip endoprosthesis system
R. hip prosthesis
R. hydroxyapatite PORP
R. lag screw
R. lag screw device
R. locking rod
R. Lovejoy bone drill
R. mallet
R. maximum contact (RMC)
R. maximum contact cruciate-sparing prosthesis
R. modular hip system
R. modular stem
R. pistol-grip drill
R. reamer
R. reconstruction nail
R. sideplate
R. Solcotrans orthopaedic drainage-reinfusion system
R. Spectron metal-backed acetabular prosthesis
R. Zirconia femoral head prosthesis
Richards-Hirschhorn plate
Richard Smith prosthesis
Richardson
R. retractor
R. rod
R. subtalar arthrodesis
Riche-Cannieu
R.-C. anastomosis
R.-C. connection
Riches artery forceps
Richet
R. bandage
R. tibial-astragalocalcaneal canal
Richie brace
Richmond
R. bolt
R. subarachnoid screw
R. subarachnoid screw sensor
R. subarachnoid twist drill
Richter
R. bone drill
R. bone screwdriver
rickets
adult r.
florid r.
vitamin D-dependent r. (VDDR)
vitamin D-resistant r. (VDRR)
rickshaw rehabilitation exerciser

Rideau technique
rider's
r. bone
r. bursa
r. leg
r. muscle
r. sprain
r. tendon
ridge
dorsal r.
epicondylar r.
greater multangular r.
longitudinal r.
osteochondral r.
Outerbridge r.
residence r.
talar r.
trapezial r.
vastus lateralis r.
Ridlon
R. hip reduction
R. operation
R. plaster knife
R. procedure
Riecken PQ premium heel cup
rig
Leg Extension Power R.
right
r. ankle bur
r. erector spinae musculature
r. lateral flexion
r. and left ankle index
r. lower extremity (RLE)
r. lower limb (RLL)
r. posterior innominate
r. rotation
r. thoracic curve
r. thoracic curve with hypokyphosis
r. thoracic, left lumbar curve pattern
r. thoracic, left thoracolumbar curve pattern
r. thoracic minor curve pattern
r. upper extremity (RUE)
r. upper limb (RUL)
r. ventricular cardiomyopathy
right-angle
r.-a. dental drill
r.-a. hook
right-hand
r.-h. dominance
r.-h. dominant

NOTES

right-handed orthogonal coordinate system (RHOCS)
righting
> r. reflex
> trunk r.

right/left
> r./l. discrimination
> r./l. timing

right-sided
> r.-s. nail
> r.-s. submandibular transverse incision
> r.-s. thoracotomy

rigid
> r. bar
> r. below-knee cast
> r. body
> r. collar
> r. curve
> r. curve scoliosis
> r. dressing
> r. equinovarus deformity
> r. flatfoot
> r. flatfoot deformity
> r. foot
> r. foot cavus
> r. frame wheelchair
> r. gait
> r. internal fixation
> r. metal pelvic band
> r. orthosis
> r. pedicle screw
> r. pes planus
> r. postoperative brace
> r. reamer
> r. rockerbottom (RRB)
> r. round back
> r. sound

rigidity
> C-D instrumentation r.
> cogwheel r.
> Cotrel pedicle screw r.
> nuchal r.
> spinal fixation r.
> torsional r.

rigidus
> hallux r.

Rik
> R. fluid mattress
> R. FootHugger fluid heel boot

Riley-Day syndrome
rim
> acetabular r.
> alar r.
> glenoid r.
> sclerotic marginal r.
> r. sign
> tibial r.

Rincoe
> R. human action bionic
> R. human action bionic ankle

RIND
> reversible ischemic neurologic disability

ring
> Ace-Colles half r.
> arterial r.
> r. block anesthesia
> carbon fiber half r.
> cartilaginous r.
> Charnley centering r.
> congenital r.
> constriction r.
> cricoid r.
> r. curette
> r. cushion
> doughnut r.
> drop-lock r.
> epiphysial r.
> r. external fixator
> extracapsular arterial r.
> fibroosseous r.
> r. finger
> r. finger–small finger syndactyly
> Fischer r.
> foam r.
> r. forceps
> r. fracture
> half r.
> halo r.
> Ilizarov r.
> invalid r.
> ischial weightbearing r.
> R. knee prosthesis
> Lacroix osseous r.
> Luque r.
> r. man shoulder
> Neer r.
> orthosis drop-lock r.
> osseous r.
> pelvic r.
> perichondral r.
> protrusio r.
> proximal-to-distal r.
> reduction r.
> reinforcement r.
> r. retractor
> r. sign
> r. structure
> r. sublimis opponensplasty
> r. syndrome
> R. total hip prosthesis
> R. UPM press-fit prosthesis
> R. UPM total hip replacement
> R. UPM total knee replacement
> V1 halo r.

ringer
    R. arthroscopy
    R. lactate
RingLoc
    R. acetabular series
    R. hip liner
    R. instrument
Riolan
    R. bone
    R. muscle
Riordan
    R. club hand classification
    R. finger flexion
    R. finger opponensplasty
    R. pin
    R. pollicization
    R. sign
    R. tendon transfer technique
Ripped Fuel
rise
    single heel r.
    r. time
Riseborough-Radin
    R.-R. fracture classification system
    R.-R. intercondylar fracture
      classification
riser
    stress r.
Rish osteotome
risk
    ergonomic r.
    r. factor profile
    fracture r.
    heat injury r.
    occupational r.
    osteoporotic fracture r.
    relative r. (RR)
Risser
    R. category
    R. classification
    R. classification of scoliosis
    R. frame
    R. grade
    R. localizer scoliosis cast
    R. method
    R. pin
    R. sign (grade 1-4)
    R. stage
    R. technique
    R. turnbuckle cast
Risser-Ferguson technique

Ritchie
    R. brace
    R. rheumatoid arthritis index
Rivermead
    R. ADL index
    R. Behavioral Memory Test
      (RBMT)
    R. Behavioral Memory Test-
      Extended Version (RBMT-E)
    R. Mobility Index (RMI)
    R. Motor Assessment
rivet
    r. gun
    pop r.
Rizzoli osteoclast
RKE-R
    Rabideau Kitchen Evaluation - Revised
RLE
    right lower extremity
RLL
    right lower limb
RM
    repetition maximum
    RM isoelastic hip prosthesis
1-RM
    1-repetition maximum
RMC
    Richards maximum contact
    RMC knee replacement device
    RMC prosthesis
RMI
    Rivermead Mobility Index
RMQ
    Roland-Morris Questionnaire
RNS
    repetitive nerve stimulator
    responsive neurostimulator
R/O
    rule out
ROA
    reversal of antagonist
road burn injury
Roaf, Kirkaldy-Willis, and Cattero procedure
Robert
    R. Brigham semiconstrained
      prosthesis
    R. Brigham total knee prosthesis
    R. Jones bandage
    R. Jones dressing
    R. Jones splint
    R. ligament
    R. view

R

NOTES

Roberts
- R. approach
- R. technique

Robinson
- R. anterior cervical discectomy
- R. anterior cervical fusion
- R. arthrometer
- R. arthroplasty
- R. cervical spine fusion
- R. morcellation
- R. spinal arthrodesis

Robinson-Smith
- R.-S. anterior cervical approach
- R.-S. spinal arthrodesis

Robinson-Southwick
- R.-S. fusion
- R.-S. fusion technique

Robins-Riley spinal fusion
Robodoc robot
robot
- Robodoc r.

robotic
robust rheumatoid arthritis
Rocabado posture gauge
ROC anchor
Rochester
- R. bone trephine device
- R. compression system
- R. harvest bone cutter
- R. hip-knee-ankle-foot orthosis
- R. lamina elevator
- R. recipient bone cutter
- R. spinal elevator

Rochester-Carmalt forceps
Rochester-Ochsner forceps
Rochester-Pean forceps
rock
- R. ankle exercise board
- pelvic r. (PR)
- R. & Roller exercise board

rocker
- r. balance square
- r. bar
- r. board
- r. boot
- Carolina r.
- r. knife
- Uniplane r.

rockerbottom
- r. flatfoot
- r. flatfoot deformity
- r. foot
- rigid r. (RRB)
- r. shoe
- r. sole

RocketSoc ankle brace
rocking
- knee-chest r.

Rockwood
- R. anterior acromioplasty
- R. classification
- R. classification of acromioclavicular injury
- R. posterior capsulorrhaphy
- R. procedure
- R. resection
- R. shoulder screw

Rockwood-Green technique
rocky boat exerciser
rod
- alignment guide r.
- Alta advance tibial/humeral r.
- Alta CFX reconstruction r.
- Alta tibial-humeral r.
- aluminum master r.
- Amset R-F r.
- auto-reinforced polyglycolide r.
- Bailey-Dubow r.
- r. bender
- r. bending
- Bickel intramedullary r.
- centralizing r.
- r. clamp
- cold rolled r.
- compression r.
- concave r.
- r. contour preparation
- convex r.
- Cotrel-Dubousset r.
- Dacron-impregnated silicone r.
- degradable polyglycolide r.
- delta r.
- distraction r.
- r. distraction device
- double-L spinal r.
- Edwards D-L modular screw r.
- Edwards-Levine r.
- Edwards modular system Universal r.
- Ender r.
- Enneking r.
- Fixateur Interne r.
- flared spinal r.
- fluted medullary r.
- r. fracture repair
- guide r.
- Harrington compression r.
- Harrington distraction r.
- Harris condylocephalic r.
- hinge r.
- r. holder
- Hunter silastic r.
- impactor r.
- impingement r.
- intramedullary alignment r.
- Isola spinal implant system eye r.
- Jacobs distraction r.

Jacobs locking hook spinal r.
Kaneda r.
Knodt distraction r.
Küntscher r.
L r.
r. linkage
locking-hook spinal r.
long alignment r.
L-shaped r.
Luque r.
Luque-Galveston r.
r. migration
Moe modified Harrington r.
Moe square-end r.
Moss r.
Olerud PSF r.
OrthoSorb r.
pediatric Cotrel-Dubousset r.
PGA r.
r. placement
Polarus humeral r.
precontoured unit r.
radiotranslucent r.
Richards locking r.
Richardson r.
r. rotation prevention
round-ended distraction r.
Rush r.
Russell-Taylor delta r.
Sage r.
Sampson r.
Schneider r.
screw alignment r.
Selby I, II r.
Serrato forearm r.
Shaw-SHIP r.
Sheffield r.
silicone-dacron tendon r.
r. sleeve fixation
spinal fixation r.
square-ended distraction r.
stainless steel r. (SST)
Stenzel r.
straight threaded r.
surgical r.
R. TAG suture anchor system
telescoping medullary r.
r. template
tendon r.
threaded r.
U Luque vertebral r.
unit spinal r.

V-A alignment r.
VDS compression r.
VSF r.
Williams r.
Wiltse system aluminum master r.
Wiltse system spinal r.
Wissinger r.
Zickel r.
Zielke r.
rod-hook construct
rod-mounted
   r.-m. targeting apparatus
   r.-m. targeting device
rod-sleeve instrumentation
Roeder manipulative aptitude test device
roentgen
   r. stereophotogrammetric analysis (RSA)
   r. stereophotogrammetry
roentgenogram
   biplane r.
   lateral r.
   operative r.
   2-plane r.
   templating r.
roentgenography
   intraoperative r.
   preoperative r.
   stress r.
roentgenometrics
roentgen-stereophotogrammatic study
Roger
   R. Anderson compression device
   R. Anderson external fixation apparatus
   R. Anderson external fixation device
   R. Anderson external fixator
   R. Anderson fixation
   R. Anderson splint
   R. Anderson stabilization device
   R. Anderson system
   R. Anderson table
   R. Anderson traction
Rogers cervical fusion technique
Rogozinski
   R. hook
   R. screw system
   R. spinal fixation
   R. spinal fixation system
   R. spinal rod system

R

NOTES

Rohadur
    R. gait plate
    R. orthotic
Roho
    R. bed
    R. heel pad
    R. heel protector
    R. Pack-It cushion
    R. pediatric seating system
    R. solid seat insert
Rokitansky pelvis
Rolaids Calcium Rich
Roland
    R. index of low back pain
    R. low back pain index
Roland low back pain index
Roland-Morris Questionnaire (RMQ)
Rolando fracture
role
    R. checklist (RC)
    intrinsic transverse connector r.
    occupational r.
Rolfing
    R. therapy
    R. treatment
Rolimeter
    Aircast R.
roll
    cervical r.
    chest r.
    r. control bolster
    cotton r.
    Dutchman's r.
    Feldenkrais foam r.
    Fluftex gauze r.
    hip r.
    lumbar r.
    McKenzie cervical r.
    McKenzie lumbar r.
    McKenzie night r.
    neck r.
    octagon r.
    radiolucent r.
    Skillbuilder half r.
    r. stitch
    towel r.
    Tumble Forms r.
Roll-A-Bout 4-wheel walker
Rollator Nova walker
rollback
    femoral r.
rolled felt
roller
    r. bandage
    r. injury
    Sorbothane rice sheller r.
RollerBack self-massage device
rolling
    skin r.

Rollocane
rollover
    medial r.
Rolyan
    R. AquaForm wrist and thumb
     spica splint
    R. arm elevator
    R. foot support
    R. Gel Shell spica splint
    R. Reach N Range Pulley System
    R. TakeOff Sprint brace
    R. tibial fracture brace
Rolz device
ROM
    range of motion
    ROM knee brace
    ROM therapy
    ROM walker brace
Roman arch
Romano curved drilling system
Romberg
    R. reflex
    R. sign
    R. test
Rome criteria
rongeur
    Adson r.
    angled jaw r.
    angled pituitary r.
    angular bone r.
    Bacon bone r.
    Baer bone r.
    Bane bone r.
    Bane-Hartmann bone r.
    basket r.
    bayonet r.
    Beyer r.
    Blumenthal bone r.
    bone-nibbling r.
    bone punch r.
    Bruening-Citelli r.
    Campbell r.
    cervical r.
    Cicherelli bone r.
    Cintor bone r.
    Cleveland bone r.
    Cloward intervertebral disc r.
    Codman-Kerrison laminectomy r.
    Cohen r.
    Colclough laminectomy r.
    Corbett bone r.
    curved bone r.
    Cushing disc r.
    Dale first rib r.
    Dean bone r.
    Decker r.
    Defourmentel bone r.
    disc r.
    double-action r.

downbiting r.
duckbill r.
Echlin bone r.
Echlin duckbill r.
Echlin-Luer r.
Ferris-Smith r.
Ferris-Smith-Kerrison
  laminectomy r.
Ferris-Smith-Spurling disc r.
Fisch bone r.
flat-bottomed Kerrison r.
r. forceps
Friedman bone r.
Guleke bone r.
Hartmann bone r.
Hein r.
Hoen r.
Horsley bone r.
Husk bone r.
Jackson intervertebral disc r.
Kerrison downbiting r.
Kleinert-Kutz bone r.
Kleinert-Kutz synovectomy r.
Lebsche r.
Leksell laminectomy r.
Leksell-Stille thoracic r.
Lempert bone r.
Liston bone r.
Liston-Littauer r.
Luer bone r.
Markwalder bone r.
Marquardt bone r.
mastoid r.
McIndoe bone r.
Mead bone r.
needle-nose r.
orthopaedic r.
pituitary r.
Reiner bone r.
Ruskin r.
Ruskin-Liston bone r.
Ruskin-Rowland bone r.
Schell bone r.
Schlesinger cervical r.
Schlesinger intervertebral disc r.
Semb bone r.
Semb-Stille bone r.
Shearer r.
single-action r.
Smith-Petersen r.
Spurling r.
Spurling-Kerrison upbiting and
  downbiting r.

Stille r.
Stille-Horsley bone r.
Stille-Luer bone r.
Stille-Luer duckbill r.
Stille-Luer-Echlin r.
Stille-Ruskin bone r.
straight bone r.
straight pituitary r.
Super Cut laminectomy r.
synovial r.
upbiting r.
upcut r.
Watson-Williams intervertebral
  disc r.
Weil-Blakesley intervertebral disc r.
Wilde intervertebral disc r.
rongeured
Rood technique
roof
acetabular r.
r. arc measurement
r. impingement
intercondylar r.
r. plate
r. wedge
roofplasty
**roof-reinforcement ring hip arthroplasty
  component**
room
Allender vertical laminar flow r.
Charnley laminar flow r.
operating r.
recovery r. (RR)
surgical dressing r. (SDR)
training r.
Roos
R. approach
R. overhead exercise test
R. rib cutter
root
r. anomaly
r. canal broach
cervical r.
r. infiltration
nail r.
nerve r.
R. procedure
r. tension sign
rootlet
rope
r. stretching device
Roper-Day prosthesis
ropey

NOTES

ropiness
rose
    R. foot operation
    R. foot procedure
Rosen
    R. bur
    R. elevator
    R. splint
Rosenberg
    R. endoscopic anterior cruciate
     ligament reconstruction
    R. retractor
    R. view
Rosenfeld hip prosthesis
Rosenthal
    R. classification
    R. classification of nail injury
Roser line
Roser-Nélaton line
rosette
    r. Beaver blade
    R. strain gauge
rostrate pelvis
Rotablator rotating bur
Rotaflex exerciser
Rotaglide
    R. knee implant
    R. lubricating solution
    R. total knee system
rotary
    r. ankle instability
    r. basket
    r. basket forceps
    r. bur
    r. control
    r. deviation
    r. displacement
    r. drawer test
    r. instability test
    r. joint
    r. motion
    r. osteotome
    r. punch
    r. stability
rotated
    externally r.
    internally r.
rotating
    r. basket shaver
    r. bur
    r. drill
    r. femoral head prosthesis
    r. hinge
    r. hinge knee prosthesis
    r. knee joint prosthesis
    r. patellar implant
    r. turner
rotating drill

rotation
    abduction and external r. (ABER)
    abduction-external r. (AER)
    abnormal instantaneous axis of r.
    anatomical hip center of r.
    anterior innominate r.
    axial r.
    r. axis
    axis of r.
    Borggreve limb r.
    center of axial r.
    cervical general r.
    cervical specific r.
    r. device
    r. drawer test
    eccentric axis of ankle r.
    r. exercise
    external r.
    external rotation/internal r. (ER/IR)
    flexion, abduction, external r.
     (FABER)
    flexion, adduction, internal r.
     (FADIR)
    foot r.
    forced passive internal r.
    functional axial r.
    Hermodsson internal r.
    hip r.
    horizontal external r.
    instantaneous axis of r.
    intentional r.
    internal-external r.
    internal femoral r.
    intersegmental r.
    inversion-eversion r.
    inward r.
    ipsilateral r.
    knee r.
    lateral hip r.
    left r.
    lumbar r.
    medial hip r.
    r. mobility
    neutral r.
    outward r.
    patellar r.
    patient-resisted internal r.
    pelvic r.
    r. plasty
    polycentric r.
    posterior innominate r.
    pronation-eversion-external r.
     (PEER)
    pronation-external r. (P-ER)
    putative segmental instantaneous
     axis of r.
    r. recurvatum test
    resisted external r.
    right r.

sagittal r.
spine r.
supination-external r. (SER)
supination-external r. IV
synchronous scapuloclavicular r.
r. testing
thoracolumbosacral orthosis—flexion, extension, lateral bending, and transverse r. (TLSO-FELR)
tibiofibular r.
vertebral r.

rotational
r. alignment
r. burst fracture
r. contracture
r. correction
r. deformity
r. flap
r. instability
r. kyphosis
r. malalignment
r. malposition
r. manipulation
r. parameter
r. prominence
r. restriction
r. scarf osteotomy
r. scarf osteotomy/bunionectomy
r. scoliosis

rotation-compression maneuver
rotationplasty
tibial hindfoot osteomusculocutaneous r.
Van Ness r.
Winkelmann r.

rotator
r. cuff (RC)
r. cuff buttress (RCB)
r. cuff calcific tendinitis
r. cuff calcified deposit
r. cuff contusion
r. cuff degeneration
r. cuff function
r. cuff imbalance
r. cuff impingement syndrome
r. cuff injury
r. cuff lesion
r. cuff repair
r. cuff tear
r. cuff tear arthroplasty
r. cuff tendinopathy
r. cuff tendon
external r.

Hosmer above-knee r.
Howmedica monotube external r.
internal r.
Jarit r.
long external r.
r. muscle
short external r.
r. unit

rotatores syndrome
rotatory
r. atlantoaxial subluxation
r. load
r. olisthesis
r. torque

rotatory-variable-differential transducer
RotaWire guide wire
Rotes joint mobility scale
Rothman
R. Institute femoral prosthesis
R. Institute total hip program

Roto-Rest bed
RotorloC absorbable rotator cuff suture anchor
rotoscoliosis
rototome
Rotter-Erb syndrome
roughened cartilage
roughening
roughen the surface
rouleaux formation
round
r. bur
r. cell liposarcoma
r. cell-type liposarcoma
r. ligament
r. shoulder
r. shoulder deformity

roundback stem
round-ended distraction rod
round-hole compression plate
round-tapped
r.-t. elevator
r.-t. periosteal

Rousek
R. extender
R. extraction set
R. extractor

Rousso stitch
Roussy-Lévy
R.-L. disease
R.-L. syndrome

Rouviere ligament

NOTES

Roux
 R. osteotomy
 R. sign
Roux-duToit staple capsulorrhaphy
Roux-Goldthwait
 R.-G. operation
 R.-G. procedure
 R.-G. realignment
row
 carpal r.
 proximal carpal r.
Rowe
 R. blanket
 R. calcaneal fracture classification
 R. disimpaction forceps
 R. fusion
 R. glenoid punch
 R. glenoid-reaming forceps
 R. humeral head retractor
 R. modified-Harrison forceps
 R. posterior shoulder approach
Rowe-Harrison bone-holding forceps
Rowe-Zarins shoulder immobilization
rowing and sculling
Roxanol
 R. Rescudose
 R. SR Oral
Royalite body jacket
Roy-Camille
 R.-C. plate
 R.-C. posterior screw plate fixation
 R.-C. prosthesis
Roylan ergonomic hand exerciser
Royle-Thompson transfer technique
RP
 reduced profile
 rest pain
RPE
 rated perceived exertion
 rating of perceived exertion
RQS
 repeated quick stretch
RQS-E
 repeated quick stretch from elongation
RQS-SEC
 repeated quick stretch superimposed upon an existing contraction
RR
 recovery room
 relative risk
RRAM
 relative response attributable to the maneuver
RRB
 rigid rockerbottom
RSA
 roentgen stereophotogrammetric analysis
RSC
 radioscaphocapitate

RSD
 reflex sympathetic dystrophy
RSDS
 reflex sympathetic dystrophy syndrome
RSI
 repetition strain injury
RSS
 rearfoot stability system
 repetitive stress syndrome
RT
 recreational therapy
RTD
 repetitive trauma disorder
RTP
 return to play
rub
 friction r.
 Jeanie R.
rubber
 r. band traction
 r. bolster
 r. drain
 r. held cup
 r. pedestal
 r. pelvis
 r. shod
 r. shod clamp
 r. sling
 r. sole cast walker
 r. spacer
 r. walking heel
 r. wedge walker
Rubbermaid adjustable bath/shower seat
Rubin
 R. bone planer
 R. cartilage planer
 R. gouge
 R. rasp
Rubinstein-Taybi syndrome
rubor
rucksack paralysis
rudimentary
 r. bone
 r. rib
RUE
 right upper extremity
Ruedi-Allgower
 R.-A. classification
 R.-A. tibial plafond fracture
Ruedi fracture
Ruffini mechanoreceptor
rugby jersey finger
rugger
 r. jersey sign
 r. jersey spine
Ruiz-Mora
 R.-M. correction
 R.-M. procedure

RUL
> right upper limb

rule
>> millimetric r.
>> National Collegiate Athletic Association spine injury prevention r.
>> no touch r.
>> Ottawa Ankle R. (OAR)
>> r. out (R/O)

ruler
>> Berndt hip r.
>> ulnar r.

Rumel
>> R. aluminum bridge splint
>> R. myocardial clamp
>> R. rubber clamp
>> R. thoracic clamp

runner
>> r. bump
>> heel-toe r.
>> r. knee
>> Sprint R.
>> r. toe

running
>> marathon r.
>> r. suture
>> treadmill r.

running-related injury

rupture
>> Achilles tendon r. (ATR)
>> adductor longus muscle r.
>> anterior talofibular ligament r.
>> buttonhole r.
>> closed r.
>> collateral ligament r.
>> crescentic r.
>> cruciate ligament r.
>> distal biceps brachii tendon r.
>> extracapsular r.
>> flexor tendon r.
>> gastrocnemius r.
>> infrapatellar tendon r.
>> intracapsular r.
>> longitudinal ligament r.
>> medial head of gastrocnemius r.
>> neglected r.
>> proximal tendon r.
>> spontaneous r.
>> stress r.
>> subscapularis r.
>> syndesmosis r.
>> tendon r.

>> transverse ligament r.
>> ulnar collateral ligament r.

ruptured
>> r. disc
>> r. disc excision

rush
>> R. bender
>> R. bone clamp
>> R. driver
>> R. driver-bender-extractor
>> R. extender
>> R. flexible medullary nail
>> R. intramedullary fixation pin
>> R. mallet
>> R. pin
>> R. pin nail
>> R. pin reamer awl
>> R. rod
>> R. rod awl reamer

Ruskin
>> R. bone-cutting forceps
>> R. bone-splitting forceps
>> R. rongeur
>> R. rongeur forceps

Ruskin-Liston
>> R.-L. bone-cutting forceps
>> R.-L. bone rongeur

Ruskin-Rowland
>> R.-R. bone-cutting forceps
>> R.-R. bone rongeur

Russe
>> R. bone graft
>> R. classification
>> R. technique

Russe-Gerhardt method

Russell
>> R. fibular head autograft
>> R. skeletal traction
>> R. splint

Russell-Silver dwarfism

Russell-Taylor
>> R.-T. classification
>> R.-T. delta rod
>> R.-T. delta tibial nail
>> R.-T. femoral interlocking nail system
>> R.-T. interlocking medullary nail
>> R.-T. screw

Russian
>> R. forceps
>> R. waveform

rust
>> R. amputation saw

NOTES

rust *(continued)*
- R. disease
- R. phenomenon
- R. sign
- R. syndrome

Ruta graveolens
Rüter classification
R-Value exercise ball

Rx Comfort sock
Rydell nail
Ryder needle holder
Ryerson
- R. bone graft
- R. procedure
- R. technique
- R. triple arthrodesis

SA
   skeletal age
SAARD
   slow-acting antirheumatic drug
Saba pulley
Sabel cast walker
saber
   S. Bisector ArthroWand
   s. shin
   s. shin deformity
   s. tibia
saber-cut
   s.-c. approach
   s.-c. incision
Sabolich above-knee socket system
SAC
   short arm cast
   sideline assessment of concussion
   space available for cord
sac
   bursal s.
   common dural s.
   thecal s.
SACH
   solid ankle, cushioned heel
      SACH foot
      SACH foot adapter
      SACH foot prosthesis
      SACH orthopaedic heel
      SACH orthosis
      SACH orthotic
Sach nerve separator
saclike cavity
sacra (*pl. of* sacrum)
sacral
   s. agenesis
   s. ala
   s. alar screw
   s. approach
   s. arcuate line
   s. artery
   s. bar technique
   s. base angle
   s. base distortion
   s. block
   s. bone
   s. bone tip
   s. bursa
   s. canal
   s. cyst
   s. dermatome
   s. fracture
   s. fusion screw fixation
   s. horizontal plane line (SHPL)
   s. mobility

   s. nerve
   s. nerve root sparing
   s. pedicle screw
   s. pedicle screw fixation
   s. plexus
   s. plexus injury
   s. promontory
   s. screw placement
   s. segment
   s. slope
   s. spine
   s. spine decompression
   s. spine fixation
   s. spine fusion
   s. spine modular instrumentation
   s. spine stabilization
   s. support
   s. tilt
   s. triangle
   s. tuberosity
   s. vertebra
sacralgia
sacralization
sacralized transverse process
sacrectomy
sacrificing knee prosthesis
sacrococcygeal
   s. abscess
   s. articulation
   s. chordoma
   s. joint
   s. ligament
   s. muscle
sacrodynia
sacrofemoral angle
sacrohorizontal angle
sacroiliac (SI)
   s. approach
   s. articulation
   s. belt
   s. binder
   s. block
   s. buttressing procedure
   s. disarticulation
   s. dislocation
   s. dysfunction
   s. extension fixation
   s. flexion fixation
   s. fracture
   s. hypermobility syndrome
   s. joint
   s. joint arthropathy
   s. joint disease
   s. joint fusion

S

sacroiliac (continued)
s. joint inflammatory spondyloarthropathy
s. joint injury
s. joint locking
s. joint mobility
s. joint motion
s. joint syndrome
s. ligament
s. line
s. orthosis (SIO)
s. subluxation
s. symphysis line
sacroiliac-iliosacral dysfunction
sacroiliitis
sacrooccipital technique (SOT)
sacrospinal
s. ligament
s. muscle
sacrospinalum
sacrospinous ligament
sacrotomy
sacrotuberal ligament
sacrotuberous ligament
sacrovertebral angle
sacrum, pl. **sacra**
transverse process of s.
saddle
s. back
basal block cervical s.
s. block anesthesia
cervical s.
s. clamp
Cloward surgical s.
s. cushion
s. paresthesia
s. prosthesis
s. sore
saddlebag
Seidel s.
saddle-shaped joint
SAF
self-articulating femoral
SAF hip replacement
SAF prosthesis
SAFE
solid ankle flexible endoskeletal
stationary attachment flexible endoskeletal
SAFE foot
SAFE II prosthesis
SAFE orthotic
SAFER
Safety Assessment of Function and the Environment for Rehabilitation
Safe-T mate anti-rollback device
Safe-T-Wheel pinwheel

safety
S. Assessment of Function and the Environment for Rehabilitation (SAFER)
ergonomic s.
s. performance
s. pin orthosis
s. pin splint
safety-bolt suture
Safe-Wrap gauze
SAFHS
sonic accelerated fracture healing system
SAFHS ultrasound device
Safir pin
SAFK
single-axis friction knee
sag
sling seat s.
s. test
tibial s.
sage
S. cheilectomy
S. driver
S. driver-extractor
S. extractor
S. forearm nail
S. pin
S. radial nail
S. rod
S. triangular nail
Sage-Clark cheilectomy
Sager traction splint
Sage-Salvatore classification of acromioclavicular joint injury
sagittal
s. anatomic alignment
s. band
s. conventional spin-echo proton-density sequence
s. deformity
s. kyphosis
s. mobility
s. motion
s. movement
s. pedicle angle
s. pedicle diameter
s. plane
s. plane displacement
s. plane imaging
s. plane instability
s. roll spondylolisthesis
s. rotation
s. spinal canal diameter
s. split osteotomy
s. stress test
s. stress x-ray
s. surgical saw
s. Z osteotomy

Saha
   S. procedure
   S. shoulder muscle classification
   S. transfer technique
Sahara
   S. clinical bone sonometer
   S. portable bone densitometer
SAID
   specific adaptation to imposed demand
   SAID principle
sailboarder injury
Sakellarides calcaneal fracture classification
Sakoff osteotomy
SAL
   self-aligning knee
Salenius meniscus knife
salicylic
   s. acid
   s. acid and lactic acid
   s. acid and propylene glycol
salicylsalicylic acid
salient angle
saline
   s. acceptance test
   physiologic s.
   s. solution
saline-enhanced
   s.-e. arthrography
   s.-e. MR arthrogram
   s.-e. MR arthrography of shoulder
SALK
   single-axis locking knee
salmon calcitonin
Salmonella
   Salmonella arthritis
   Salmonella osteomyelitis
Salmonine Injection
salt
   gold s.
Salter
   S. criteria
   S. epiphysial fracture classification
   S. fracture
   S. innominate osteotomy
   S. pelvic osteotomy
   S. sling
   S. technique
Salter-Harris
   S.-H. classification of epiphysial plate injury
   S.-H. fracture (type I–VI)
   S.-H. tibial-fibular injury

   S.-H. tibial-fibular injury classification
Salter-Harris-Rang epiphysial fracture classification
Salter-Thompson classification
Saltiel brace
salvage
   s. ankle arthrodesis
   diabetic limb s.
   s. fusion
   limb s.
   s. procedure
Salzer
   S. prosthesis
   S. resurfacing
SAM
   Skills Assessment Module
   spinal analysis machine
   structural aluminum malleable
   SAM spinal analysis machine
   SAM splint
Sam
   S. Jr. posture analyzer
   S. splint
same-day microsurgical arthroscopic lateral-approach laser-assisted (SMALL)
Samilson
   S. crescentic calcaneal osteotomy
   S. procedure
   sliding plane osteotomy of S.
Sammons biplane goniometer
sample
   Pennsylvania bimanual work s.
   Valpar Component Work S.'s
Sampson
   S. medullary nail
   S. prosthesis
   S. rod
Samuels forceps
SANC
   short arm navicular cast
sand
   s. toe
   s. toe injury
sandal
   Benefoot & Birkenstock orthotic s.
   Exercise S.
   Rainbow cast s.
sandalthotics
   Foot Levelers s.
   S. postural support orthotic

NOTES

S

sandbag
    neonatal s.
sandbagging long bone fracture
Sanders
    S. CT Classification
    S. fracture
    S. intraarticular calcaneal fracture
    classification
    S. type
Sandimmune
    S. Injection
    S. Oral
Sandoz
    S. 4-phase model
    S. 4-phase model of spinal
    degeneration
sandwiched iliac bone graft
sandwich osteotomy
Sanfilippo syndrome
Sangeorzan
    S. internal fixation
    S. navicular fracture
sanguineous
Sani-Grinder
sanitizer
Sani Vac
Santa Casa distractor
SAOF
    Self-Assessment of Occupational
    Functioning
saphenous
    s. artery
    s. flap
    s. nerve
    s. vein
SAPHO
    synovitis-acne-pustulosis-hyperostosis
    osteomyelitis
    SAPHO syndrome
sapphire
    S. table
    S. View arthroscope
SAR
    somatoautonomic reflex
Saratoga cycle
Sarbo sign
sarcoid
    s. arthritis
    Boeck s.
sarcoidosis
sarcoma
    alveolar soft-part s.
    bicompartmental soft tissue s.
    botryoid s.
    chondroblastic s.
    clear cell s.
    deep intracompartmental soft
    tissue s.
    epithelioid s.

    Ewing s.
    extracompartmental soft tissue s.
    fascial s.
    femoral s.
    fibroblastic s.
    giant cell s.
    high-grade surface osteogenic s.
    human osteogenic s. (HOS)
    intracortical osteogenic s.
    Kaposi s.
    low-grade central osteogenic s.
    malignant myeloid s.
    multicentric osteogenic s.
    osteoblastic osteogenic s.
    osteogenic s.
    osteolytic s.
    Paget-associated osteogenic s.
    parosteal osteogenic s.
    periosteal s.
    postirradiation osteogenic s.
    reticular cell s.
    sclerosa osteoblastic osteogenic s.
    small cell osteogenic s.
    soft tissue s.
    subcutaneous intracompartmental
    soft tissue s.
    synovial cell s.
sarcomatous change
sarcopenia
sarcoplasmic reticulum
sarcotubular myopathy
Sargent knee operation
Sarmiento
    S. fracture brace
    S. intertrochanteric osteotomy
    S. nail
    S. short leg patellar tendon-bearing
    cast
    S. STH-2 hip prosthesis
    S. trochanteric fracture technique
Sarot needle holder
sartorial slide procedure
sartorius
    s. muscle
    s. tendon
SAS
    short arm splint
    shoulder arm system
    SAS II brace
    SAS shoe
Saso Variable Speed Massager
Sat-A-Lite contoured wedge seat
cushion
sateen knee immobilizer
satellite
    s. myofascial trigger point
    s. potential
Saticon tube camera
Satinsky clamp

Satterlee
    S. amputating saw
    S. bone saw
saturation
    arterial oxygen s.
    fat s.
Saturday night palsy
Saturn carpal tunnel splint
saucerization
    discoid meniscus s.
Saucony shoe
Sauerbruch
    S. prosthesis
    S. retractor
    S. rib elevator
    S. rib forceps
    S. rib shears
Saunders
    S. cervical HomeTrac
    S. mobilization wedge
    S. traction
sausage
    s. digit
    s. finger
    s. toe
Sauvé-Kapandji
    S.-K. arthroplasty
    S.-K. procedure
Sauve-Kapandji distal radioulnar joint reconstruction
Savastano
    S. hemiknee
    S. Hemi-Knee prosthesis
    S. unconstrained prosthesis
    S. unicompartment prosthesis
saver
    intraoperative Cell S.
    knee s.
saw
    Adams s.
    Adson wire s.
    Aesculap s.
    air-driven oscillating s.
    amputation s.
    Bailey wire s.
    bayonet s.
    Beaver s.
    Bier amputation s.
    Bishop s.
    bone s.
    Charriere amputation s.
    Charriere bone s.
    circular s.

Cottle s.
counter rotating s.
crescentic s.
crosscut s.
Delrin-handle bone s.
DeMartel wire s.
electric cast s.
end-cutting reciprocating s.
Engel plaster s.
fine-tooth electric s.
Gigli s.
s. guide
Hall air-driven oscillating s.
Hall sagittal s.
Hall Versipower oscillating s.
Hall Versipower reciprocating s.
hand s.
Herbert s.
Horsley bone s.
humeral s.
intramedullary s.
Langenbeck bone s.
Langenbeck metacarpal s.
Lebsche wire s.
Leica model 1600 water-cooled
    diamond s.
Luck-Bishop bone s.
medullary s.
Micro-Aire oscillating s.
microoscillating s.
microsagittal s.
Miltex bone s.
Müller s.
Osada s.
oscillating s.
patella bone s.
Pearson intramedullary s.
Percy amputating s.
plaster s.
power bone s.
power-driven s.
power oscillating s.
reciprocating motor s.
Rust amputation s.
sagittal surgical s.
Satterlee amputating s.
Satterlee bone s.
single-blade s.
single-sided bone s.
Skil s.
Sklar bone s.
Stryker s.
Tuke s.

S

NOTES

saw *(continued)*
    twin-blade oscillating s.
    Weiss amputation s.
    Zimmer oscillating s.
Sawa
    S. shoulder brace
    S. shoulder orthosis
sawblade
    Stablecut s.
sawcut
SAXT
    slow axoplasmic transport
Sayre
    S. bandage
    S. elevator
    S. jacket
    S. operation
    S. splint
    S. suspension apparatus
    S. suspension traction
Sbarbaro
    S. hip prosthesis
    S. spica cast
    S. tibial plateau prosthesis
SBO
    spina bifida occulta
SB+ testing and treatment
SB– testing and treatment
SC
    sternoclavicular
    supracondylar
    SC suspension
SC-AcuFix
    SC-A. anterior cervical plate
      system
    SC-A. ThinLine plate
scaffold
    bioabsorbable mesh s.
    collagen s.
    s. matrix
    resorbable s.
Scaglietti
    S. closed reduction technique
    S. procedure scale
scalar
    s. classification
    s. quantity
scale
    Abbreviated Injury S. (AIS)
    Abnormal Involuntary Movement S.
      (AIMS)
    Activity Index and Meaningfulness
      of Activity S.
    Adelaar-Williams-Gould 10-point s.
    Adolescent and Pediatric Pain
      Tool S.
    Adult Nowicki Strickland Internal
      External Control S. (ANSIE)
    Adult Playfulness S.

Alberta Infant Motor S.'s (AIMS)
Allen Semantic Differential S.
American Musculoskeletal Tumor
    Society rating s.
American Orthopaedic Foot and
    Ankle Society Ankle-Hindfoot S.
American Shoulder and Elbow
    Surgeons s.
American Spinal Injury Association
    impairment s.
Angus-Cowell s.
ankle-hindfoot s.
Arthritis Impact Measurement S.
    (AIMS)
Arthritis Quality of Life S.
Ashworth s.
ASIA impairment s.
balance beam s.
Behavior Assessment Rating S.
    (BASC)
Berg Balance S.
Borg Numerical Pain S.
Boyd modification of Tardieu
    spastic measurement s.
Braden risk assessment s.
Broberg-Morrey elbow function s.
Charnley-Merle d'Aubigné disability
    grading s.
Charnley pain and function
    grading s.
Children's Handwriting
    Evaluation S. (CHES)
Clyde Mood s.
S.'s of Cognitive Ability for
    Traumatic Brain Injury (SCATBI)
Crowe hip s.
DASH s.
Disabilities of Arm, Shoulder, and
    Hand s.
disability s.
economic self-sufficiency WHO
    Handicap S.
Edinburgh Rehabilitation Status S.
    (ERSS)
Exercise Self-Efficacy S.
Expanded Disability Status S.
    (EDSS)
foot and ankle severity s. (FASS)
French s.
Gait Abnormality Rating S.
    (GARS)
Geissling rating s.
Glasgow Coma S.
Graphic Rating S. (GRS)
hallux metatarsophalangeal
    interphalangeal s. (HMIS)
Harris hip s.
Health O Meter S.
hierarchial ADL s.'s

Hospital for Special Surgery s.
International Knee Documentation
  Committee knee s.
JOA S.
Johnson-Boseker s.
Karlsson and Peterson scoring s.
Kellgren knee s.
Kenna Knee S.
Kitaoka clinical rating s.
Klein-Bell Activities of Daily
  Living S.
Knox Preschool Play S.
Köhler hip protrusion grading s.
Kurtzke Expanded Disability s.
Leisure Boredom S. (LBS)
Lesser Metatarsophalangeal-
  Interphalangeal S. (LMIS)
Likert and Borg s.
Lincoln-Oseretsky Motor
  Development S.
linear analog pain s.
Lower Extremity Functional S.
  (LEFS)
Lysholm-Gillquist knee subjective
  function s.
Lysholm knee function scoring s.
Mathew s.
McGill pain s.
Merle d'Aubigné and Postel hip
  rating s.
metatarsophalangeal-
  interphalangeal s.
midfoot s.
mobility WHO Handicap S.
modified Ashworth s. (MAS)
modified Gait Abnormality
  Rating S.
Modified Rankin s.
NCAST feeding and teaching s.'s
Norton s.
numeric rating s. (NRS)
Occupational Circumstances
  Assessment-Interview Rating S.
  (OCAIRS)
Oral Analogue S. (OAS)
orientation WHO Handicap S.
Outerbridge s.
Perez postoperative pain s.
physical independence WHO
  Handicap S.
Portola Valley S.
Progressive Ambulation S.
Prosthetic Problem Inventory S.

Quality of Well-Being S.
Quebec Back Pain Disability S.
Ranchos Los Amigos S.
Reddihough s.
Rotes joint mobility s.
Scaglietti procedure s.
Severin hip dysplasia s.
Social Integration World Health
  Organization Handicap S.
Social Interaction S. (SIS)
Sports Activity S.
Stanford Hypnotic Clinical S.
Steinberg rating s.
Symptoms and Sports Participation
  Rating S.
Tardieu spasticity measurement s.
Tegner activity rating s.
The Experience of Leisure S.
  (TELS)
The Knee Society clinical-rating s.
UCLA Shoulder Rating s.
visual analog s.
Volpicelli functional ambulation s.
Wechsler Adult Intelligence s.
Wechsler Memory s.
Work Environment Impact S.
  (WEIS)

scalene
  s. block
  s. fat pad
  s. maneuver
  s. muscle
scalenotomy
scalenus anterior syndrome
scalloping
  endosteal s.
  s. of vertebra
  vertebral s.
scalpel
  Bard-Parker s.
scalprum
scan
  adenosine thallium s.
  bone s.
  CT s.
  DEXA s.
  DXA s.
  gallium-67 s.
  gallium citrate s.
  intrathecally enhanced CT s.
  isotope bone s.
  lead-line s.
  leukocyte s.

NOTES

S

scan *(continued)*
- multiplanar computed tomography s.
- multiplanar CT s.
- nuclear magnetic resonance s.
- 3-phase bone s.
- positron emission tomographic s.
- radioisotope gallium s.
- radioisotope indium-labeled white blood cell s.
- radioisotope technetium s.
- radionuclide bone s.
- rectilinear bone s.
- seratec s.
- technetium-99m diphosphonate s.
- technetium-99m methylene diphosphate bone s.
- technetium-99m pyrophosphate s.
- technetium-99m sulfur colloid s.
- thallium s.
- triple-phase isotope bone s.
- white blood cell s.

Scandinavian total ankle replacement (STAR)

Scand pin

scanner
- Acoma s.
- All-Tronics s.
- iStep FIT digital s.
- thermographic s.

scanning
- s. densitometry
- s. EMG

scanogram
- s. of lower extremity
- s. radiography

scanography

Scanz osteotomy

scaphocapitate
- s. fusion
- s. interval
- s. joint
- s. syndrome

scaphocapitolunate arthrodesis (SCL)

scaphoid
- s. arch
- bipartite s.
- s. bone
- carpal s.
- s. cookie in shoe
- s. fracture
- s. humpback deformity
- s. lift test
- s. nonunion
- s. scapula
- s. screw guide
- s. shift test
- s. shoe cookie
- s. shoe pad
- s. tuberosity injury
- waist of s.

scaphoiditis

scaphoid-lunate

scapholunate (SL)
- s. advanced collapse (SLAC)
- s. angle
- s. arthritis collapse (SLAC)
- s. dissociation
- s. gap
- s. instability
- s. interosseous ligament
- s. joint

scaphotrapeziotrapezoid arthrodesis

scaphotrapezoid interosseous ligament

scaphotrapezoid-trapezial (STT)

scapula, pl. **scapulae**
- alar s.
- s. alata
- body of s.
- s. elevata
- elevated s.
- glenoid fossa of s.
- Graves s.
- locked s.
- scaphoid s.
- snapping s.
- winging of s.

scapulalgia

scapular
- s. approximation test
- s. border
- s. dysfunction
- s. elevation
- s. elevation test
- s. flap
- s. fracture
- s. graft
- s. ligament
- s. nerve
- s. notch
- s. peroneal atrophy
- s. reflex
- s. sign of Putti
- s. winging

scapulectomy
- Das Gupta s.
- Phelps s.

scapuloclavicular
- s. articulation
- s. injury
- s. joint

scapulocostal syndrome

scapulodynia

scapulohumeral
- s. atrophy
- s. bursa
- s. ligament
- s. muscle

s. reflex
s. rhythm
scapulolateral view
scapuloperoneal syndrome
scapulopexy
scapulothoracic
s. arthrodesis
s. bursitis
s. dissociation
s. fusion
s. guiding plane
s. joint
s. motion
s. muscle
s. pain
scapulovertebral border
scar
area s.
s. band
s. formation
hypertrophic s.
keloid s.
linear s.
parasagittal s.
peritendinous s.
physial s.
s. tissue
Scarborough
S. prosthesis
S. total hip replacement
scarf
s. bandage
s. osteotomy bunionectomy
s. Z osteotomy
s. Z osteotomy/bunionectomy
s. Z-plasty
scarlatinal synovitis
Scarpa fascia
scarring
s. cosmesis
s. effect
epineural s.
s. and furrowing
SCATBI
Scales of Cognitive Ability for Traumatic
Brain Injury
SCATBI Assessment
SCC
short calcaneocuboid
SCC ligament
SCD
sequential compression device
SCD stockings

Scerratti goniometer
SCFE
slipped capital femoral epiphysis
Schaffer squeeze
Schanz
S. angulation osteotomy
S. collar
S. collar brace
S. disease
S. dressing
S. femoral osteotomy
S. operation
S. pin
S. screw
S. syndrome
Schanz-type proximal femoral
valgization osteotomy
Schatzker
S. fracture
S. fracture classification system
S. tibial plateau fracture
classification
Schauwecker
S. patellar tension band wire
S. patellar wiring
S. patellar wiring technique
Schede
S. bone curette
S. hip osteotomy
S. method
Scheffé
S. interval
S. test
Scheie syndrome
Schell bone rongeur
Schepens hollow silicone hemisphere
implant material
Scherisorb dressing
Scher nail biopsy
Scheuermann
S. disease
S. dystrophic spondylosis
S. juvenile kyphosis (SJK)
S. kyphosis
S. syndrome
Schiek Belt
Schink metatarsal retraction
Schlatter disease
Schlatter-Osgood disease
Schlein
S. clamp
S. elbow arthroplasty
S. semiconstrained elbow prosthesis

S

NOTES

Schlein (*continued*)
  S. shoulder positioner
  S. total elbow prosthesis
  S. trisurface ankle prosthesis
Schlesinger
  S. cervical punch forceps
  S. cervical rongeur
  S. intervertebral disc rongeur
  S. punch
  S. rongeur forceps
  S. sign
Schmeisser
  S. spica
  S. spica cast
Schmid
  S. disease
  S. metaphysial dysostosis
Schmidt rod holder
Schmitt fan
Schmorl
  S. disease
  S. node
  S. nodule
Schneider
  S. driver-extractor
  S. extractor
  S. extractor-driver
  S. fixation
  S. hip arthrodesis
  S. medullary nail
  S. nail driver
  S. pin
  S. rod
Schnute wedge resection technique
Schober
  S. measurement
  S. method
  S. technique
  S. test
  S. test of lumbar flexion
Schoemaker line
Scholl pad
Scholten sternal retractor
School Setting Interview (SSI)
Schreiber maneuver
Schrock
  S. arthroplasty
  S. procedure
Schrudde rotational flap
Schuind external fixation
Schuknecht
  S. Gelfoam wire prosthesis
  S. Teflon wire piston prosthesis
Schultze acroparesthesia
Schwaber otologic implant
Schwann
  S. cell
  S. tumor

schwannoma
  cellular s.
  collagenous s.
  malignant s.
Schwartz
  S. clip-applying forceps
  S. dorsiflexory osteotomy
  S. syndrome
  S. temporary clamp-applying
    forceps
Schwartze chisel
Schwartz-Jampel
  S.-J. myotonia
  S.-J. syndrome
Schwarz finger extension bow
Schweitzer
  S. pin
  S. spring plate
Schwinn
  S. Air-Dyne bicycle
  S. bi-directional Windjammer upper
    body cycle
  S. elliptical full body exercise
    machine
  S. Fitness Advisor
  S. Spinner bicycle
  S. 900 stationary bicycle
SCI
  spinal cord injury
sciatic
  s. foramen
  s. function index (SFI)
  s. leg block
  s. nerve
  s. nerve block
  s. nerve injury
  s. nerve irritation
  s. nerve palsy hematoma
  s. neuralgia
  s. neuritis
  s. notch
  s. palsy
  s. scoliosis
  s. tension sign
sciatica
science
  exercise s.
  movement s.
  occupational s.
scientific practitioner
scientist-practitioner
scintigraphy
  bone s.
  combined s.
  indium-111 s.
  paired s.
  triphase technetium s.

scissor-leg
  s.-l. gait
  s.-l. position
scissor leg
scissors
  Acufex s.
  adventitial s.
  arthroscopic s.
  Aslan endoscopic s.
  Assistant Free orthopaedic s.
  Babcock wire-cutting s.
  Bantam wire-cutting s.
  Beebe wire-cutting s.
  Bellucci alligator s.
  blunt-tip iris s.
  cartilage s.
  collar and crown s.
  Crafoord thoracic s.
  crown and collar s.
  curved Mayo s.
  Dean s.
  dissecting s.
  Fiskars s.
  s. gait
  Giertz-Stille s.
  Halsey nail s.
  Harvey wire-cutting s.
  hook rotary s.
  iris s.
  Jones s.
  Kay s.
  Koenig nail-splitting s.
  Laschal suture s.
  loop s.
  Martin cartilage s.
  Mayo s.
  McIndoe s.
  meniscal s.
  meniscectomy s.
  meniscus s.
  Metzenbaum s.
  s. nail drill
  Nelson s.
  Nicola s.
  orthopaedic s.
  plain rotary s.
  PowerStar bipolar s.
  serrated s.
  Sistron s.
  Sistrunk s.
  Slip-N-Snip s.
  Smillie meniscal s.
  Smith s.
  Stephen s.
  straight s.
  suture s.
  tissue s.
  Walton s.
  Webster meniscectomy s.
  Weck microsuture cutting s.
  Weller cartilage s.
  wire-cutting s.
SCIWORA
  spinal cord injury without radiographic
    abnormality
SCJ
  sternoclavicular joint
SCL
  scaphocapitolunate arthrodesis
scleroderma
  focal s.
sclerosa osteoblastic osteogenic sarcoma
sclerosing
  s. nonsuppurative osteitis
  s. nonsuppurative osteomyelitis
sclerosis, pl. scleroses
  amyotrophic lateral s. (ALS)
  anterolateral s. (ALS)
  Baló s.
  bone s.
  diaphysial s.
  endplate s.
  Mönckeberg s.
  multiple s. (MS)
  piriform s.
  progressive systemic s.
  subchondral s.
  systemic s.
  zonal s.
sclerotic
  s. bone
  s. line
  s. marginal rim
  s. segment
sclerotomal pain
sclerotome pain chart
SCL-90R
  Symptoms Checklist 90 Revised
SCOI
  Southern California Orthopaedic Institute
    SCOI arthroscopic tenodesis
    SCOI shoulder brace
scoliokyphosis
scoliometer
scoliosis
  adolescent s.

S

NOTES

scoliosis *(continued)*
 adolescent idiopathic s. (AIS)
 adult s.
 s. angle
 bregmatic bone Brissaud s.
 Brissaud s.
 s. cast
 cicatricial s.
 Cobb method for measuring s.
 compensatory s.
 congenital s.
 s. correction
 s. correction with Dwyer cable
 Cotrel s.
 coxitic s.
 curve progression in s.
 degenerative lumbar s.
 dextrorotary s.
 dextroscoliosis s.
 double major curve s.
 double thoracic curve s.
 Dwyer correction of s.
 electrical surface stimulation
  treatment for s.
 empyemic s.
 endoscopic correction of s.
 Fergusson method for measuring s.
 s. fixation
 fracture with s.
 functional s.
 Galen s.
 genetic s.
 habit s.
 hysterical s.
 idiopathic s.
 infantile idiopathic s.
 inflammatory s.
 ischiatic s.
 juvenile idiopathic s.
 King-Moe s.
 King s. (type I–V)
 kyphosing s.
 Lenke classification of adolescent
  idiopathic s.
 levoscoliosis s.
 lumbar s.
 myopathic s.
 neurogenic s.
 neuromuscular s.
 ocular s.
 s. operating frame
 osteogenic s.
 osteopathic s.
 s. overlap brace
 paralytic s.
 rachitic s.
 S. Research Society Hughston knee
  scope
 rheumatic s.

 rigid curve s.
 Risser classification of s.
 rotational s.
 sciatic s.
 s. spinal fusion
 static s.
 structural s.
 s. surgery
 thoracic curve s.
 thoracogenic s.
 thoracolumbar idiopathic s.
 thoracolumbar spine s.
 uncompensated rotary s.
 Winter-King-Moe s.

scoliotic
 s. curve
 s. curve fixation
 s. pelvis

scoliotone

ScoliTron instrument

scooter
 Go-Ped motorized s.
 K9 S.
 Lark s.
 Rascal s.

Scoot-Gard mat

scope
 Doppler s.
 Endoflex endoscopic lumbar
  discectomy s.
 Harris s.
 Liviscope s.
 Lysholm knee joint instability s.
 Scoliosis Research Society
  Hughston knee s.

SCORE
 Simple Calculated Osteoporosis Risk
  Estimation

score
 AAOS Knee Society Clinical
  Rating S.
 American Knee Society s.
 AOFAS s.
 ASES shoulder s.
 Ashworth muscle spasticity s.
 Bandi patellofemoral s.
 Carter-Rowe shoulder s.
 Catterall hip s.
 Champion Trauma S. (CTS)
 Charnley hip s.
 composite knee s.
 d'Aubigné-Postel postoperative
  function s.
 duPont Bunion Rating S.
 Fries rheumatoid arthritis s.
 Fulkerson functional knee s.
 Functional Rating S.
 Green and OʹBrien wrist
  function s.

Harris hip s. (HHS)
Harris-Mayo hip s.
Hawkins-Warren athlete's
shoulder s.
Hospital for Special Surgery
knee s.
HSS knee s.
Hughston knee s.
IKDC s.
Injury Severity S. (ISS)
Iowa hip s.
Kapandji thumb opposition s.
Knee Society S.
Kofoed Ankle S.
Kurtzke s.
Larsen hip s.
Lysholm s.
Lysholm-Gillquist knee subjective
function s.
Mangled Extremity Severity S.
(MESS)
Marshall knee s.
Maryland Foot S.
Mayo Clinic forefoot s.
Mayo elbow performance s.
McGuire s.
Merchant and Dietz ankle s.
Merle d'Aubigné hip s.
modified Harris hip s.
modified Rowe shoulder s.
Molander-Olerud shoulder s.
Oswestry Disability S.
Sherman s.
skeletal injury s.
T s.
Tegner knee reconstruction
activity s.
trauma s.
Z s.
scored cartilage
scoring
Knee Society total knee
arthroplasty roentgenography
evaluation and s.
Scorpio total knee system
Scotchcast
S. 2 cast tape
S. length splinting system
scotoma, pl. **scotomata**
absolute s.
Scott
S. ankle splint
S. arthroplasty

S. double-strap ankle support
S. elastic ankle strap
S. glenoplasty technique
S. hinged knee support
S. humeral splint
S. posterior glenoplasty
S. Uniform tennis elbow splint
S. wrist wrap
Scottish
S. Rite brace
S. Rite hip orthosis
S. Rite splint
Scott-RCE osteotomy guide
scotty
s. dog sign
s. stainless ankle joint
scout film
Scoville
S. curette
S. retractor
Scranton transmalleolar arthrodesis
scraper
Bradley femoral canal
preparation s.
scraping toe gait
scratch test
screen
ACL S.
Allen Cognitive Level S. (ACLS)
Fast Lanex rare earth s.
Lanex s.
motion palpation s.
split s.
screening
Gait, Arms, Legs, and Spine s.
GALS s.
ISIS s.
neuropsychological s.
s. palpation
screw
Absolute absorbable s.
Ace s.
AcroMed s.
alar s.
s. alignment bar
s. alignment rod
Alta cancellous s.
Alta cortical s.
Alta cross-locking s.
Alta lag s.
Alta supracondylar s.
Alta transverse s.
Ambi hip s.

NOTES

screw *(continued)*

Amset R-F s.
anchor s.
s. angle guide
s. angulation
AO-ASIF s.
AO cancellous s.
AO cortex s.
AO lag s.
AO spongiosa s.
Arthrex sheathed interference s.
arthrodesis s.
ASIF cancellous s.
ASIF cortical s.
ASIF malleolar s.
Asnis III cannulated s.
Aten olecranon s.
Autogenesis automator for
  Ilizarov s.
axial compression s.
s. backout
Barouk cannulated bone s.
Basile hip s.
Bechtol s.
bicortical s.
Bio-Absorbable interference s.
BioCuff C bioresorbable
  cannulated s.
Bio-Interference tibial s.
Biologically Quiet interference s.
Bionx absorbable cannulated s.
Bionx self-reinforced PLLA
  smart s.
BioRCI bioabsorbable s.
bioresorbable s.
BioScrew absorbable interference s.
BioSorbFX SR self-reinforced plate
  and s.
Bold compression s.
Bone Mulch s.
Bosworth coracoclavicular s.
s. breakage
buttress thread s.
Campbell cannulated s.
cancellous bone s.
cannulated bone s.
cannulated cancellous lag s.
cannulated hip s.
carpal scaphoid s.
Carrell-Girard s.
Caspar cervical s.
CD Horizon M8 multiaxial s.
chrome-cobalt s.
Clearfix s.
Cohort bone s.
Collison s.
compression hip s.
compression lag s.
s. compressor

Concise compression hip s.
coracoclavicular s.
cortex s.
cortical ASIF s.
cortical bone s.
cortical cancellous s.
Cotrel pedicle s.
Coventry s.
crossing s.'s
cross-locking s.
crown drill s.
cruciate head bone s.
cruciform head bone s.
Cubbins s.
s. depth calibrator
s. depth gauge
DePuy interference s.
s. design
Deyerle interlocking s.
distal locking s.
distraction s.
double-threaded Herbert s.
dual-threaded s.
Duo-Drive s.
Dwyer spinal s.
Dynamic condylar s. (DCS)
dynamic hip s. (DHS)
ECT bone s.
Edwards modular system
  spinal/sacral s.
Eggers s.
encased s.
EndoFix bioabsorbable
  interference s.
Endo-FixL s.
s. epiphysiodesis
expansion s.
Fabian s.
femoral head cork s.
Fixateur Interne s.
fixation s.
s. fixation
s. fixation operation
flute of cannulated s.
foreign body s.
FRS s.
s. fusion
Garden s.
Gentle Threads interference s.
Glasgow s.
glenoid fixation s.
Guardsman femoral interference s.
Hahn s.
Hall spinal s.
Hamilton s.
s. head
headless bone s. (HBS)
Heck s.
Hedrocel titanium s.

Henderson lag s.
Herbert bone s.
Herbert scaphoid s.
Herbert-Whipple bone s.
hex s.
hexagonal slot-cap s.
hip compression s.
hollow mill Asnis cannulated s.
hook trial set s.
Howmedica ICS s.
Howmedica Universal
  compression s.
iliac s.
iliosacral s.
Ilizarov s.
s. implantation
InCompass thoracolumbar spine
  fixation s.
s. insertion
s. insertion technique
Instrument Makar biodegradable
  interference s.
Integrity acetabular cup s.
interference s.
interfragmentary lag s.
interlocking s.
Intrafix s.
Isola spinal implant system iliac s.
Isola vertebral s.
Jeter lag/position s.
Jewett pick-up s.
Johannson lag s.
Jones s.
Kostuik s.
Kurosaka interference-fit s.
LactoSorb s.
lag s.
Lane bone s.
lateral to medial s.
Leinbach olecranon s.
Leone expansion s.
Linvatec absorbable s.
Lippman s.
locking s.
Long Beach pedicle s.
s. loosening
Lorenzo s.
Luhr s.
lumbar pedicle s.
Lundholm s.
Luque II s.
Luque pedicle s.
machine s.

malleolar s.
Marion s.
Martin s.
maxillofacial bone s.
McLaughlin carpal scaphoid s.
medial bicortical s.
medial unicortical s.
Medoff axial compression s.
micrometric s.
mille pattes s.
mini AO s.
minifragment s.
Moberg s.
Morris biphase s.
Moss s.
Mouradian s.
multiaxial s.
navicular s.
Neufeld s.
non-self-tapping s.
Olerud PSF s.
Ormandy s.
Orthex cannulated bone s.
Orthofix s.
Osteomed s.
OsteoTite bone s.
Palex expansion s.
Palmer s.
PathFinder pedicle s.
pedicle s.
PerFixation s.
PGA s.
Phillips head s.
Phillips recessed-head s.
Pilot point s.
s. placement
s. placement C-guide
polyaxial cervical s.
polylactide absorbable s.
s. position perioperative monitoring
posterior to anterior s.
posterior-anterior s.
Preston s.
Propel cannulated interference s.
proximal and distal s.
pull s.
Ray s.
resorbable polymer s.
ReUnite orthopaedic s.
reverse-threaded s.
Revo retrievable cancellous s.
Richards classic compression hip s.
Richards lag s.

S

NOTES

screw *(continued)*
    Richmond subarachnoid s.
    rigid pedicle s.
    Rockwood shoulder s.
    Russell-Taylor s.
    sacral alar s.
    sacral pedicle s.
    Schanz s.
    Scuderi s.
    Selby I, II s.
    self-tapping bone s.
    SemiFix s.
    set s.
    Shanz s.
    Sharpey s.
    sheathed interference s.
    Shelton bone s.
    Sherman bone s.
    Simmons double-hole spinal s.
    Simmons-Martin s.
    sliding compression hip s.
    small fragment s.
    small-headed s.
    spherical-headed s.
    spongiosa s.
    s. stabilization
    stainless steel s.
    Steffee plate and s.
    step s.
    Storz s.
    s. stripout
    Stryker lag s.
    subarticular s.
    superior thoracic pedicle s.
    supracondylar s.
    Swiss cancellous s.
    syndesmotic s.
    Synthes compression hip s.
    Talon compression hip s.
    s. tap
    4-tap s.
    Thatcher s.
    thoracolumbar pedicle s.
    Thornton s.
    threaded cancellous s.
    thumb s.
    tibial head s.
    tibia-pro-fibula s.
    s. tip
    titanium s.
    tivanium cancellous bone s.
    s. toggle
    s. torque
    Townley bone graft s.
    Townsend-Gilfillan s.
    traction tongs s.
    transarticular s.
    transfixion s.
    translaminar facet s.
    transpedicular s.
    transverse s.
    triangulated pedicle s.
    Trinion meniscus s.
    TSRH pedicle s.
    tulip pedicle s.
    Tunneloc bone mulch s.
    Twist-Off S.
    unicortical s.
    Universal fixation s.
    Uppsala s.
    Vari-Angle s.
    varus-valgus adjustment s.
    VDS s.
    Venable s.
    Vilex F-Series dual-thread s.
    Virgin hip s.
    vitallium s.
    VSF s.
    Wagner-Schanz s.
    Weise jack s.
    Wiltse pedicle s.
    wood s.
    Woodruff s.
    Wurzburg s.
    Yuan s.
    Zimmer compression hip s.
    Zuelzer s.
screw-and-keel fixation
screw-and-plate fixation
screw-and-wire fixation
screwdriver
    Allen head s.
    automatic s.
    Becker s.
    Bio-Interference s.
    Bosworth s.
    cannulated s.
    Children's Hospital s.
    Collison s.
    cross-slot s.
    cruciform s.
    Cubbins bone s.
    DePuy s.
    Dorsey screw-holding s.
    double-slot s.
    European-style s.
    Flatt self-retaining s.
    Hall s.
    heavy cross-slot s.
    hexhead s.
    Johnson s.
    Ken s.
    Lane s.
    light cross-slot s.
    Lok-it s.
    Massie s.
    Master s.
    Phillips head s.

plain s.
Richter bone s.
self-retaining s.
Sherman s.
single cross-slot s.
single-slot s.
skull plate s.
straight hex s.
Stryker s.
torque s.
Trinkle s.
Universal hex s.
VDS s.
White s.
Williams s.
Woodruff s.
Zimmer s.
screw-holding forceps
screw-home mechanism
screw-in ceramic acetabular cup
Screw-Lok tap
screw-plate
    s.-p. approach
    Calandruccio impaction s.-p.
    s.-p. fixation
    Zimmer impaction s.-p.
screw-rod
    Wiltse s.-r.
screw-to-screw compression construct
Scrip Muscle Master massager
scroll bone
scrub
    Hibiclens s.
SCS
    spinal canal stenosis
    spinal cord stimulator
SCSP, SC-SP
    supracondylar-suprapatellar
Scuderi
    S. head
    S. procedure
    S. screw
    S. technique
Scuder repair
sculling
    rowing and s.
Scully
    S. Hip S'port
    S. Hip S'port hip device
sculp
    Concise cementing s.
    s. knife

Scultetus
    S. bandage
    S. binder
scurvy line
Scutan temporary splint material
S-cutting block
Scytalidium
    S. dimidiatum
    S. hyalinum
SD
    shoulder disarticulation
    SD sorb staple
SDD
    sterile dry dressing
SDR
    surgical dressing room
Seaber forceps
seal-fin deformity
seal limb
Seal-Tight cast protector
seam
    osteoid s.
searching big toe
searing pain
seat
    antithrust s.
    Backjoy s.
    Carrie car s.
    Comfy toilet lift s.
    s. cushion
    Dream Ride car s.
    ischial-bearing s.
    Maddacare child bath s.
    Orthopaedic Positioning S.
    Posey drop s.
    Renolux convertible car s.
    Rubbermaid adjustable
      bath/shower s.
    Snug s.
    Special S.
    Spelcast car s.
    Tall-ette toilet s.
    Tubsider Kneeling S.
seat-belt injury
seated
    S. Cable Row exerciser
    s. flexion test
    s. hamstring curl
    properly s.
    s. root test
    s. scapular retraction exercise
seating
    s. aid

S

NOTES

seating *(continued)*
- s. chisel
- s. cushion
- s. of prosthesis
- trial s.
- s. wedge

Seattle
- S. foot prosthesis
- S. modification
- S. modification of Kocher incision
- S. orthosis
- S. safety knee
- S. splint

Sebileau periosteal elevator
Seconal Injection
second
- s. cervical vertebra
- cycle per s. (cps, c/sec)
- s. impact syndrome
- s. intention
- s. metacarpal
- s. metatarsal artery
- s. metatarsophalangeal joint arthrodesis
- radians per s. (rad/s)
- s. skin pad

secondary
- s. amputation
- s. bone union
- s. center
- s. closure
- s. disability
- s. erythromelalgia
- s. fracture
- s. hematogenous osteomyelitis
- s. hip-spine syndrome
- s. intention
- s. metatarsalgia
- s. myofascial trigger point
- s. osteoporosis
- s. osteosarcoma
- s. posttraumatic syringomyelia
- s. purchase
- s. stabilizer

second-generation cementing technique
second-look arthroscopy
section
- bar s.
- calcaneonavicular bar s.

sectioning
- sequential s.

Secure Yet Gentle surgical dressing system
Secur-Fit HA PSL X'tra prosthesis
Sedan goniometer
sedation therapy
Seddon
- S. classification
- S. coin test

- S. dorsal spine costotransversectomy
- S. modification
- S. neurapraxia
- S. neurotmesis
- S. technique

sedentary
- s. lifestyle
- s. occupation
- s. work

Sedillot periosteal elevator
sedimentation rate
Seeburger
- S. implant
- S. retractor

segment
- apical s.
- central s.
- motion s.
- physiologic lock of motion s.
- relation to subadjacent s.
- sacral s.
- sclerotic s.
- spinal s.
- subadjacent s.
- vertebral motion s.

segmental
- s. alveolar osteotomy
- s. bone defect
- s. bone loss
- s. compression construct
- s. deficiency
- s. dysfunction
- s. fixation
- s. fracture
- s. hyperextension
- s. level
- s. mobility
- s. mobility testing
- s. motion testing
- s. spinal correction system (SSCS)
- s. spinal instrumentation (SSI)
- s. tendon graft

segmentally demineralized bone technology
segmentation
- s. defect
- supernumerary lumbar s.

segmented orthopaedic system total hip and knee system
Segond tibial avulsion fracture
Séguin fracture
Seidel
- S. bone-holding clamp
- S. humeral locking nail
- S. intramedullary fixation
- S. nail
- S. saddlebag

Seinsheimer femoral fracture classification

Seirin acupuncture needle
seismotherapy
seizing forceps
seizure
  acute repetitive s. (ARS)
  oxygen s.
Selakovich procedure
Selby
  S. I, II fixation system
  S. I, II hook
  S. I, II rod
  S. I, II screw
select
  S. ankle prosthesis
  S. joint
  S. joint orthosis
  S. modular shoulder prosthesis
  S. shoulder system
selection
  bone plate s.
  Edwards modular system
    construct s.
selective
  s. posterior rhizotomy (SPR)
  Theraform S.'s
  s. thoracic spine fusion
Selectively Lockable knee brace
selenium sulfide
self-adhering varus/valgus wedge
self-aligning
  s.-a. knee (SAL)
  s.-a. mobile-bearing knee implant
self-articulating
  s.-a. femoral (SAF)
  s.-a. femoral hip replacement
Self-Assessment of Occupational
  Functioning (SAOF)
self-bearing
  s.-b. ceramic hip prosthesis
  s.-b. ceramic total hip replacement
self-broaching
  s.-b. nail
  s.-b. pin
self-care
self-centering
  s.-c. bone-holding forceps
  s.-c. implant
  s.-c. Universal hip prosthesis
self-curing polymer
self-efficacy
  exercise s.-e.
self-help ability
self-locking nail

self-mutilation
self-propelling wheelchair
self-reinforcing polylevolactic acid (SR-
  PLLA)
self-retaining
  s.-r. bone-holding forceps
  s.-r. clamp
  s.-r. retractor
  s.-r. screwdriver
self-sealing
  s.-s. cannula
  s.-s. implant
self-sustained natural apophysial glides
self-tapering pin
self-tapping bone screw
Selig hip operation
Sell-Frank-Johnson
  S.-F.-J. extensor shift
  S.-F.-J. extensor shift technique
Sellors rib contractor
Selverstone rongeur forceps
Semb
  S. bone forceps
  S. bone-holding clamp
  S. bone rongeur
  S. rib forceps
Semb-Stille bone rongeur
sEMG
  surface electromyography
semicanal of humerus sulcus
semicircular flap amputation
semiconstrained
  s. total elbow arthroplasty
  s. tricompartmental knee prosthesis
SemiFix screw
semiflexion
semi-Fowler position
semilunar
  s. bone
  s. cartilage
  s. cartilage knife
  s. notch
  s. sulcus
semilunaris
  linea s.
semiluxation
semimembranosus
  s. bursitis
  s. muscle
  s. tendinitis
  s. tendon
semiopen sliding tenotomy

S

NOTES

semirigid
- s. ankle brace
- s. fiberglass cast (SRF)
- s. polypropylene ankle-foot orthosis
- s. postoperative dressing
- s. shell

semisitting position
semispinal muscle
semisupinated oblique view
semi-suture-loop technique
semitendinosus
- s. augmentation of patellar tendon repair
- s. muscle
- s. procedure
- s. technique
- s. tendon
- s. tendon transfer
- s. tenodesis

semitendinosus-gracilis graft
semitendinous graft
semitubular
- s. blade-plate
- s. compression plate

Semmes-Weinstein
- S.-W. monofilament
- S.-W. monofilament pressure esthesiometry
- S.-W. monofilament pressure test

Senegas
- S. approach to hip
- S. hip approach

senescence
Sengupta quadriceps release
senile
- s. hallux valgus
- s. hip disease
- s. osteomalacia
- s. osteoporosis
- s. subcapital fracture

senilis
- coxa s.
- malum coxae s.

Senn
- S. plate
- S. retractor

senna
sensation
- altered s.
- catching s.
- diminished s.
- epicritic s.
- exteroceptive s.
- light touch s.
- loss of protective s. (LOPS)
- perianal s.
- perineal s.
- phantom s.
- pinprick s.

- protective s.
- return of s.
- sharp s.
- shocklike s.
- touch s.
- vibration s.

sense
- joint position s. (JPS)
- position s.
- vibration s.

Sense-of-Feel prosthesis
sensibility recovery sequence
sensitivity
- vibration s.

sensitometer
- Poppen ridge s.

sensor
- capacitive s.
- DermaTemp infrared thermographic s.
- magnetic s.
- Myoscan s.
- s. pad
- Perry s.
- Richmond subarachnoid screw s.
- Servo Pro force s.

SensorHand prosthesis
sensorimotor, sensory motor
- s. deficit
- s. nerve
- s. stimulation approach

sensorineural, sensory/neural
- s. abnormality

sensory
- s. awareness
- s. component
- s. deficit
- s. delay
- s. evoked potential
- s. examination
- s. fascicle
- s. function
- s. impairment
- s. integration
- S. Integration and Praxis test (SIPT)
- s. loss
- s. motor
- s. nerve
- s. nerve action potential (SNAP)
- s. nerve action potential receptor (SNARE)
- s. nerve conduction velocity
- S. Organization test (SOT)
- s. peak latency
- s. polyneuropathy
- s. registration
- s. response
- s. stimulation kit

sensory-motor training
sensory/neural (*var. of* sensorineural)
sentinel fracture
Senuva lotion
Seoffert triple arthrodesis
SEP
    somatosensory evoked potential
    microneurography
    midlatency SEP
separation
    AC joint s.
    acromioclavicular s.
    articular mass s.
    atlantoaxial s.
    degree of s.
    fracture fragment s.
    gravitational platelet s. (GPS)
    lamellar s.
    shoulder s.
    sternoclavicular joint s.
    transepiphysial s.
separator
    abduction knee s.
    finger s.
    Horsley s.
    nerve s.
    Sach nerve s.
    toe s.
sepsis
Septacin implant
septal forceps
septic
    s. arthritis
    s. bursitis
    s. finger joint
    s. knee
    s. necrosis
SeptiCare antimicrobial wound cleanser
Septisol solution
Septobal bead
septum, pl. septa
    Bigelow s.
    fascial s.
    intermuscular s.
    J s.
    Septa Topical Ointment
    vertical s.
Sequeira-Khanuja modification
sequela, pl. sequelae
sequence
    axial fat-suppressed turbo spin-echo
      T2-weighted s.
    Carr-Purcell s.

Carr-Purcell-Meiboom-Gill s.
coronal T1-weighted s.
fat-suppressed turbo spin-echo T2-
    weighted s.
muscle patterning s.
sagittal conventional spin-echo
    proton-density s.
sensibility recovery s.
standard imaging s.
T2-weighted dual-echo s.
sequencing bead patterns set
sequential
    s. compression
    s. compression device (SCD)
    s. extremity pump
    s. foot compression device (SFCD)
    s. pneumatic compression boot
    s. pneumatic pump traction
    s. pressure
    s. procedure
    s. sectioning
sequentially reamed
sequestered disc
sequestra (*pl. of* sequestrum)
sequestral
sequestrated disc
sequestration
sequestrectomy
sequestrotomy
sequestrum, pl. sequestra
    avascular s.
    bone s.
    bony s.
    button s.
    s. forceps
    kissing sequestra
    primary s.
    tuberculous s.
SER
    supination-external rotation
    SER IV fracture
sera (*pl. of* serum)
Seradge hand exercises
Serafin technique
seratec scan
serendipity
    s. view
    s. view in shoulder radiography
serial
    s. casting
    s. stretch orthoses
    s. wedge cast

S

NOTES

series
- Davis s.
- lumbosacral s.
- Option Orthotic S.
- RingLoc acetabular s.
- Valpar component work sample s.

Serola sacroiliac belt

seroma

seronegative
- s. arthropathy
- s. enthesopathy and arthropathy syndrome
- s. rheumatoid arthritis

seropositive rheumatoid arthritis

serosa
- myositis s.
- peritendinitis s.

serosanguineous

serotonergic neuron

serous
- s. abscess
- s. synovitis

serpentine
- s. foam collar
- s. foot
- s. incision
- s. plate

serrated
- s. action potential
- s. fine-cutting knife
- s. scissors

Serratia marcescens

serration

Serrato
- S. forearm pin
- S. forearm rod

serratus
- s. anterior flap
- s. anterior muscle
- s. anterior paralysis

serum, pl. **sera**
- s. calcium

service
- Carticel cartilage-cell culturing s.

Servo Pro force sensor

Servox device

sesamoid
- accessory s.
- bipartite tibial s.
- s. bone
- s. clamp
- s. disruption
- fibular s.
- s. fracture
- hallucal s.
- hallux s.
- s. hyperostosis
- s. injury
- lateral s.

- s. ligament
- medial s.
- tibial s.
- tibial hallux s.

sesamoidectomy
- s. dissector
- fibular s.
- lateral s.

sesamoiditis

sesamoidometatarsal joint

sesamophalangeal ligament

sessile

sessile-type osteochondroma

set
- acetabular trial s.
- ACL guide s.
- aluminum contouring template s.
- s. angle
- s. angle of toe
- AO minifragment s.
- Bankart shoulder repair s.
- bone drill s.
- Brown-Mueller T-fastener s.
- Catalyst anterior instrument s.
- Craig vertebral biopsy s.
- Entrex small joint arthroscopy instrument s.
- grid maze s.
- hand evaluation s.
- Harmony PLIF instrument s.
- Henning instrument s.
- Hollywood bed extension hook s.
- Lido lift and work s.
- Mini Fragment S.
- nail s.
- Outcome and Assessment Information S. (OASIS)
- Oval-8 sizing s.
- parquetry s.
- prothelen s.
- Rousek extraction s.
- s. screw
- sequencing bead patterns s.
- SmartPin instrument s.
- Stille bone drill s.
- Stille-pattern trephine and bone drill s.
- vari-balance board s.
- volumeter s.

set-hold adjustment

Seton hip brace

Setopress dressing

setter
- bone plug s.

setting
- bone s.
- Mache electromyogram s.

Seutin plaster shears

Sever
  S. disease
  S. modification
  S. modification of Fairbank
    technique
severance
  severe s.
severe
  s. kyphoscoliosis
  s. rigid thoracic curve
  s. severance
Severin
  S. classification
  S. hip criteria
  S. hip dysplasia scale
  S. radiographic classification system
Sever-L'Episcopo
  S.-L. repair of shoulder
  S.-L. shoulder repair
SEWHO
  shoulder-elbow-wrist-hand orthosis
sex-linked muscular dystrophy
SFA
  superficial femoral artery
SFCD
  sequential foot compression device
SFEMG
  single-fiber electromyography
SFI
  sciatic function index
S-flap incision
Sgarlato
  S. device
  S. hammertoe implant (SHIP)
  S. hammertoe implant procedure
  S. toe implant
shadow
  elliptical overlap s.
  s. shield
shadowing
  acoustical s.
**Shadow-Line ACF spine retractor
  system**
Shaeffer rigid orthosis
Shaffner orthopaedic inserter
shaft
  bone s.
  Cloward drill s.
  distal third of s.
  femoral s.
  s. fracture
  metatarsal s.
  middle third of s.

ministem s.
neck s.
patellar reamer s.
proximal third of s.
radial s.
Sham procedure
shank
  s. bone
  extended steel s.
  steel s.
  Zimmer-Hudson s.
Shanz screw
shape
  Erlenmeyer flask s.
  familial s.
Shapiro
  S. classification
  S. classification of mechanisms of
    growth arrest
sharing
  Edwards modular system load s.
Shark pediatric wheelchair
sharp
  acetabular angle of S.
  S. acetabular angle
  s. dissection
  s. retractor
  s. sensation
  s. trocar
  s. worm hook
sharp/dull discrimination
Sharpey
  S. fiber
  S. screw
sharp-pointed wire
Sharp-Purser Test
SharpShooter
  S. tissue repair system
  S. tissue repair technique
Sharrard
  S. posterior transfer
  S. transfer technique
Sharrard-Trentani prosthesis
Sharrard-type kyphectomy
Shar-Tek foot positioning grid
shaver
  arthroscopic s.
  automated s.
  Cuda s.
  cutting s.
  Dyonics s.
  Grierson meniscal s.
  Microsect s.

S

NOTES

shaver (*continued*)
    motorized meniscal s.
    motorized suction s.
    rotating basket s.
    sucker s.
    synovial s.
shaving
    arthroscopic s.
    femoral condylar s.
    s. system
Shaw-Sgarlato hammertoe implant prosthesis
Shaw-SHIP
    S.-SHIP rod
    S.-SHIP rod hammertoe implant
shea
    S. drill
    s. prosthesis placement instrument
shear
    airplane s.'s
    anterior s.
    Baer rib s.'s
    Bethune-Coryllos rib s.'s
    Bethune rib s.'s
    biarticular bone s.'s
    Brunner rib s.'s
    Brunn plaster s.'s
    Collins rib s.'s
    Cooley rib s.'s
    Esmarch plaster s.'s
    Felt s.'s
    s. fracture
    Giertz rib s.'s
    Giertz-Shoemaker rib s.'s
    Gluck rib s.'s
    Hercules plaster s.'s
    lateral s.
    Lefferts rib s.'s
    Liston s.'s
    Liston-Key-Horsley rib s.'s
    s. maneuver
    Sauerbruch rib s.'s
    Seutin plaster s.'s
    s. stiffness
    Stille plaster s.'s
    s. strain
    s. stress
    s. test
    s. testing
    vertical s. (VS)
ShearBan low-friction interface
Shearer rongeur
shearing
    s. callosity
    s. callus
    s. force
    s. injury
    S. posterior chamber implant material

shearling surface
shear-off device
sheath
    arthroscopic s.
    carotid s.
    digital flexor tendon s.
    Endius bipolar s.
    fascia s.
    femoral s.
    fibroosseous s.
    flexor tendon s.
    giant cell tumor of tendon s.
    muscle s.
    nerve root s.
    pigmented nodular synovitis of tendon s.
    rectus s.
    synovial s.
    tendinous s.
    tendon s.
    tenosynovial s.
    visceral tendon s.
sheathed
    s. interference screw
    s. knife
sheath/liner
    Silipos Distal Dip prosthetic s./l.
Sheehan
    S. chisel
    S. gouge
    S. knee prosthesis
    S. osteotome
sheepskin
sheet
    Alpha flat s.
    Antishear gel s.
    Barrier lower extremity s.
    s. cork
    iodoform-impregnated plastic s.
    Korex cork s.
    laparotomy s.
    nonporous s.
    Novagel gel s.
    Ortholen s.
    porous s.
    PPT s.
    sterile s.
sheeting
    Carboplast II s.
    silastic s.
    sterile s.
Sheffield
    S. hand elevator
    S. rod
    S. support
shelf
    s. acetabuloplasty
    Blumer s.
    s. flexion

lateral s.
medial s.
patellar s.
s. pedestal
s. procedure
shell
acetabular s.
AFO standard s.
s. allograft
calf s.
s. impactor
s. implant material
Inter-Op acetabular s.
Irom splint with s.'s
metal-backed acetabular s.
protrusio s.
Reflection Interfit s.
Restoration Secur-Fit X'tra
acetabular s.
semirigid s.
S-ROM contained s.
thigh s.
total hip articular replacement by
internal eccentric s.'s (THARIES)
Unna paste s.
shelling off of cartilage
Shelton
S. bone screw
S. femoral fracture classification
shelving
Shenton line
Shenton-Menard line
shepherd
s. crook deformity
S. fracture
S. internal screw fixation
Sher diabetic shoe inlay
Sherfee prosthesis
Sherform silicone insole
Sherk-Probst percutaneous pinning
Sherlock threaded suture anchor
Sherman
S. block test
S. bone plate
S. bone screw
S. remote podiatric vacuum system
S. score
S. screwdriver
Sherman-Stille drill
Sherrington law
Sherwin knee retractor
ShiatsuBACK back support
Shiatsu therapeutic massage

shield
AME pin site s.
arthroscopic s.
bunion s.
contact s.
Nolan system collimator mounted
contact s.
protective s.
shadow s.
Sof-Gel palm s.
Sportelli system collimator mounted
contact s.
shielding
stress s.
Shier knee prosthesis
Shifrin wire twister
shift
anterior talus s.
atraumatic, multidirectional, bilateral
rehabilitation inferior capsular s.
capsular s.
glenohumeral s.
inferior capsular s. (ICS)
laser-assisted capsular s.
lateral lumbar s.
lateral pivot s.
lateral trunk s.
pelvic lateral s.
plantar s.
plasma volume s.
reverse pivot s.
Sell-Frank-Johnson extensor s.
s. sign
talar s.
s. test
trochanteric s.
trunk s.
shifter
AliMed Conductive Patient S.
shifting
vessel s.
shin
s. bone
saber s.
s. splint
shingling
SHIP
Sgarlato hammertoe implant
SHIP implant
Shirley drain
shirt
EZ "T" orthopaedic s.
shish kebab technique

S

NOTES

shock

s. absorption
s. artifact
neurogenic s.
prosthetic stance phase s.
spinal s.
s. treatment
vasogenic s.

shock-absorbent

s.-a. heel pad
s.-a. sole

shock-absorbing shoe
shocklike sensation
Shockmaster heel cushion
shock-wave therapy (SWT)
shod

rubber s.

shoe

accommodative s.
AccuTread s.
Acor Quikform I, II s.
Ambulator H1200 healing s.
Ambulatory s.
Anywear s.
Apex Ambulator s.
Ariat s.
arthritic s.
Asics Gel-MC s.
balmoral laced s.
Bebax s.
Bevin s.
Birkenstock s.
Blucher laced s.
broad-toed s.
Brooks s.
calcaneal spur pad in s.
Canfield s.
cast s.
Comed postoperative s.
s. cookie
corrective s.
custom-made s.
custom-molded s.
cutout s.
Dansko s.
Darco Medical-Surgical s.
Darco OrthoWedge healing s.
Darco Softie s.
Darco surgical s.
Darco Wedge s.
depth inlay s.
Depth orthopaedic s.
s. dermatitis
diabetic pressure relief s.
Dynaslipper night s.
extended-counter s.
extended steel-shank s.
s. extension
extra-depth s.

s. filler
GaitKeeper cast s.
s. gear
GentleStep s.
Goldenberg footplate s.
healing s.
s. heel pad
HeelWedge healing s.
H1209 healing s.
H1215 healing s.
high heel s.
Hi-Top s.
ill-fitting s.
infant clown cast s.
s. insert
ipos heel relief s.
ipos postoperative s.
J&J postoperative s.
laced blucher of s.
s. lift
s. lining
low-heeled s.
low quarter Blucher s.
Markell Mobility S.'s
Markell open-toe s.
Markell tarso medius straight s.
Markell tarso pronator outflare s.
Mephisto Mobils professional s.
s. modification
Moon Boot s.
narrow toebox s.
navicular cookie in s.
neoprene s.
normal last s.
open-toe s.
orthopaedic oxford s.
s. orthotic
OrthoWedge healing s.
oversize tennis s.
Pedors orthopaedic s.
pointed toe s.
postoperative s.
Power Anthro S.
pressure relief s.
Reebok s.
Reece orthopaedic s.
reverse last s.
ribbed-sole s.
rockerbottom s.
SAS s.
Saucony s.
scaphoid cookie in s.
shock-absorbing s.
Softie s.
soft-vamp s.
s. sole
space s.
stiff-soled s.
straight last s.

s. stretcher
tarsal pronator s.
Terrmocork diabetic s.
Thera-Medic s.
therapeutic s.
torque heel s.
Tru-Fit custom-molded s.
Tru-Mold s.
Urban Walkers s.
vamp of s.
Vibram rockerbottom s.
Viking postoperative s.
Viva s.
WACH orthopaedic s.
s. wear
Weaver rockerbottom s.
s. wedge
wedge adjustable cushioned heel s.
wedged s.
wide toebox s.
wooden s.
wooden-soled s.
Xsensibles s.
Xtra Depth s.
Zimmer postoperative s.
Zohar s.

shoe-foot interface
Shoemaker lateral approach
shooting pain
short

s. arm brace
s. arm cast (SAC)
s. arm fiberglass cast
s. arm gauntlet cast
s. arm navicular cast (SANC)
s. arm splint (SAS)
s. arm sugar-tong splint
s. bone
s. calcaneocuboid (SCC)
s. calcaneocuboid ligament
s. coarse bur
s. curette
s. external rotator
s. fibula
s. fibular muscle
s. fine bur
s. head of biceps
s. leg
s. leg caliper brace
s. leg cast (SLC)
s. leg double-upright brace
s. leg gait

s. leg orthosis
s. leg plaster cast
s. leg splint
s. leg syndrome
s. leg walker
s. leg walking brace
s. leg walking cast (SLWC)
s. lever accessory movement
technique
s. lever specific contact procedure
S. Musculoskeletal Function
Assessment (SMFA)
S. Musculoskeletal Function
Assessment questionnaire
s. oblique fracture
s. opponens orthosis
s. plantar ligament (SPL)
s. radiolunate (SRL)
s. rib polydactyly
s. segment spinal fusion
s. stature
s. thumb
s. time inversion recovery (STIR)
s. walking cast
s. Z bunionectomy

short-acting block anesthesia
shortened foot
shortening

Achilles tendon s.
closed femoral diaphysial s.
s. collectomy
s. contraction
digital s.
distal Wagner femoral
metaphysial s.
femoral metaphysial s.
fibula s.
fibular s.
Hoffa tendon s.
leg s.
metaphysial s.
s. osteotomy
proximal femoral metaphysial s.
proximal Wagner metaphysial s.
skeleton s.
tibial diaphysial s.
Wagner femoral metaphysial s.

short-latency somatosensory evoked
potential
short-limb dwarfism
short-radius kyphosis
shortwave diathermy (SWD)

NOTES

S

shot
> fast low-angle s. (FLASH)
> s. wadding

shotgun injury

Shotokan karate

shoulder
> s. abduction immobilizer
> s. abduction pillow
> s. abduction positioner
> s. abduction test
> s. amputation
> s. ankylosis
> apprehension s.
> s. apprehension sign
> archer's s.
> s. arm system (SAS)
> s. arthrodesis
> s. arthroplasty
> baseball s.
> Bigliani/Flatow complete s.
> s. blade
> s. bone
> bull's eye s.
> s. clock
> s. complex
> s. contracture
> s. controller
> s. cuff
> s. deformity
> s. depression test
> s. disarticulation (SD)
> s. disarticulation prosthesis
> s. dislocation
> s. dome
> double contrast arthrotomography of s.
> drop s.
> s. dystopia
> s. Ease abduction support
> flail s.
> floating s.
> football player s.'s
> frozen s.
> s. girdle
> hatchet-head s.
> s. holder
> s. horn
> s. impingement sign
> s. instability
> s. joint
> s. joint effusion
> knocked-down s.
> s. ladder
> s. lesion
> Little Leaguer's s.
> loose s.
> Neviaser classification of frozen s.
> s. orthosis (SO)

> s. Pain and Disability Index patient questionnaire
> s. pointer
> s. pulley
> s. radiography
> s. range of motion
> s. reduction
> s. repair
> ring man s.
> s. ROM arc
> round s.
> s. saddle sling
> saline-enhanced MR arthrography of s.
> s. separation
> s. Severity Index patient questionnaire
> Sever-L'Episcopo repair of s.
> s. spica cast
> s. spica splint
> stubbed s.
> s. subluxation
> s. subluxation inhibitor (SSI)
> s. subluxation inhibitor brace
> swimmer's s.
> tennis s.
> terrible triad of s.
> s. Therapy Kit
> weightlifter's s.
> s. wheel

shoulder-elbow-wrist-hand orthosis (SEWHO)

shoulder-girdle syndrome

shoulder-hand-finger syndrome

shoulder-hand syndrome

shoulder-pad sign

shoulderRAP postsurgical wound wrap

shoulder-to-head check

ShowerSafe
> S. waterproof cast and bandage cover
> S. waterproof cast and bandage protector

SHPL
> sacral horizontal plane line

Shriners pin

shrinker
> stump s.

shucking

shuck test

shuffling gait

shunt
> s. muscle
> Sundt s.
> ventriculoperitoneal s.

Shur-Band self-closure elastic bandage

shuttle
> s. Balance trainer
> s. cardiomuscular conditioner

Caspari s.
s. MiniClinic resistance system
s. MVP leg press
Shuttle-Relay suture passer
Shutt Mantis retrograde forceps
Shwachman syndrome
Shy-Drager syndrome
SI
sacroiliac
SI belt
SI joint
sialoprotein
bone s.
sibilant
Sibson
S. fascia
S. muscle
sicca
caries s.
synovitis s.
sickle-cell anemia
sickle-shape Beaver blade
sick scapula syndrome
side
s. bending
crest sign s.
s. cutter
dollar sign s.
s. lunge back exercise technique
s. plate
posterior rotation on left s.
posterior rotation on right s.
s. posture reduction
side-bending
s.-b. barrier
s.-b. mobility
side-cut pin cutter
side-cutting
s.-c. basket forceps
s.-c. blade
s.-c. bur
s.-c. Swanson bar
1-sided dog-ear repair
side-glide test
side-jump test
Sidekick foot support
sideline
s. assessment
s. assessment of concussion (SAC)
s.'s triage
side-lying
s.-l. back exercise technique
s.-l. hip abductor

s.-l. iliac compression test
s.-l. position
side-opening laminar hook
sideplate
s. barrel
barreled s.
compression s.
Richards s.
sliding compression screw with s.
side-posture position
side-shift
pelvic s.-s.
side-specific chiropractic adjustment
side-swing plasty
sideswipe
s. elbow fracture
s. injury
Siegel hip release
Sielke instrumentation
Siemens
S. linear accelerator
S. Sonocur Basic extracorporeal
shockwave therapy system
Sierra 2-load voluntary opening
Siffert intraepiphysial osteotomy
Sifoam padding
sighting device
sigma receptor
sigmoid notch
sign
abduction s.
Achilles bulge s.
Adam s.
adduction s.
Adson s.
alien hand s.
Allen s.
Allis s.
Amoss s.
André Thomas s.
Anghelescu s.
antecedent s.
anterior drawer s.
anterior foot draw s.
anterior hiatal s.
anterior tibial s.
anvil s.
Apley s.
apprehension s.
arterial occlusion s.
Ashhurst s.
augmented Tinel s.
Babinski s.

S

NOTES

sign *(continued)*

Bancroft s.
Barlow s.
Bassett s.
Battle s.
bayonet s.
Beevor s.
benediction attitude s.
bite s.
Bloomberg s.
bone bruise s.
bottle s.
Bouchard s.
bowstring s.
bow-tie s.
Bragard s.
Brudzinski s.
Bryant s.
Burton s.
C s.
camelback s.
Carman meniscus s.
cement-wedge s.
Chaddock s.
Chinese red line s.
choppy sea s.
Clark s.
clawhand s.
Cleeman s.
click s.
Codman s.
cogwheel s.
Collier s.
comma s.
commemorative s.
Comolli s.
contralateral s.
Coopernail s.
crescent s.
crest s.
cupid's bow contour s.
Dawbarn s.
deep lateral femoral notch s.
Dejerine s.
Demianoff s.
Desault s.
Destot s.
dimple s.
divot s.
dollar s.
doll's eye s.
double-arc s.
double camelback s.
double PCL s.
drawer s.
drivethrough s.
drop-arm s.
Dupuytren s.
Earle s.

Egawa s.
Erichsen s.
eye s.
FABERE s.
FADIR s.
Fairbanks s.
Fajersztajn crossed sciatic s.
fallen-fragment s.
fallen-leaf s.
fan s.
fat-blood interface s.
fat pad s.
FBI s.
finger in balloon s.
Finkelstein s.
fishtail s.
flag s.
Fleck s.
flipped meniscus s.
fluid s.
Forestier bowstring s.
Fränkel s.
Froment paper s.
Gaenslen s.
Gage s.
Galant s.
Galeazzi hip dislocation s.
gear-stick s.
glenolabral ovoid mass s.
GLOM s.
Goldthwait s.
Gordon reflex s.
Gottron s.
Gowers s.
grab s.
Guilland s.
gun barrel s.
half-moon s.
halo s.
hanging heel s.
Harris-Beath footprinting mat s.
Hawkins impingement s.
head-at-risk s.
heel varus s.
Helbing s.
hiatal s.
Hill-Sachs s.
Hirschberg s.
Hoffa s.
Hoffmann s.
Homans s.
Hoover s.
hot-cross-bun skull s.
Hueter s.
Huntington s.
iliac apophysis s.
impingement s.
inverted Napoleon hat s.
ivory phalanx s.

J s.
jerk s.
jump s.
Kanavel s.
Kaplan s.
Keen s.
Kehr s.
Kellgren s.
Kernig s.
Kerr s.
Klippel-Feil s.
Lachman s.
lamp cord s.
Langoria s.
Lasègue s.
lateral capsular s.
lateral femoral notch s.
lateral gap s.
Laugier s.
Leichtenstern s.
Leri s.
Lhermitte s.
Light V s.
Linder s.
long tract s.
Lorenz s.
Ludington s.
Ludloff s.
Maisonneuve s.
Marie-Foix s.
Martel s.
masses s.
Matev s.
McMurray s.
Mendel-Bekhterev s.
Mennell s.
Meryon s.
milking s.
Minor s.
Morquio s.
Morton s.
movie s.
Mudder s.
Mulder s.
mute toe s.
Naffziger s.
Napoleon hat s.
Neer impingement s.
Nelson s.
neuroma s.
nonorganic physical s.
nutcracker s.
objective s.

obturator s.
ocular s.
Oppenheim s.
Oppenheimer s.
Ortolani s.
painful arc s.
patellar apprehension s.
patellar hesitation s.
pathognomonic s.
Patrick s.
Payr s.
pedestal s.
Pelken s.
percussion s.
peroneal s.
piano key s.
Piotrowski s.
piriformis s.
piston s.
pivot shift s.
plantar ecchymosis s.
Pollock s.
popliteal pressure s.
positive impingement s.
positive rim s.
posterior column s.
posterior drawer s.
posterior hiatal s.
posterior sag s.
posterolateral drawer s.
posteromedial drawer s.
pronation s.
pseudo-Babinski s.
pucker s.
Putti s.
Queckenstedt s.
rachitic rosary s.
radialis s.
Raimiste s.
Renee creak s.
reverse Hill-Sachs s.
ribbon s.
rim s.
ring s.
Riordan s.
Risser s. (grade 1-4)
Romberg s.
root tension s.
Roux s.
rugger jersey s.
Rust s.
Sarbo s.
Schlesinger s.

S

NOTES

sign *(continued)*
    sciatic tension s.
    scotty dog s.
    shift s.
    shoulder apprehension s.
    shoulder impingement s.
    shoulder-pad s.
    somatic s.
    Soto-Hall s.
    Speed s.
    spilled cup s.
    spilled teacup s.
    spine s.
    spur s.
    stair s.
    Stemmer s.
    stepladder s.
    stork s.
    Strümpell s.
    Strunsky s.
    suction s.
    sulcus s.
    Sullivan s.
    supinator fat pad s.
    swallow-tail s.
    teardrop s.
    terminal J s.
    Terry Thomas s.
    theater s.
    thermoregulatory s.
    thick patella s.
    Thomas s.
    Thompson s.
    thorn s.
    Thurston-Holland flag s.
    tibialis s.
    Tinel s.
    Tinel-Hoffmann s.
    toe spread s.
    toggle s.
    too-many-toes s.
    Trendelenburg s.
    tripod s.
    trolley-track s.
    trough s.
    tuck s.
    Turyn s.
    Uhthoff s.
    V s.
    vacant glenoid s.
    Valleix s.
    Vanzetti s.
    Voshell s.
    Waddell s.
    Waldenström s.
    Walker-Murdoch wrist s.
    Wartenberg s.
    Werenskiold s.
    wet leather s.
    Wilson s.
    Wimberger s.
    windshield wiper s.
    wink s.
    winking owl s.
    Yergason s.

SignaDRESS hydrocolloid dressing
signal
    hyperintense s.
    hypointense s.
    intervertebral disc nucleus s.
    s. void

Sigvaris stockings
Siladryl Oral
Silapap
silastic
    s. ball
    s. ball spacer prosthesis
    s. ball therapy
    s. button
    s. drain
    s. finger implant
    s. finger joint
    s. gel dressing
    s. lunate arthroplasty
    s. radial head prosthesis
    s. sheeting
    s. thumb prosthesis
    s. toe implant

silence
    electrical s.
silent
    s. fascicle
    s. hip stage
    myoelectrically s.
    s. period
    s. thrombosis
Silesian
    S. bandage
    S. bandage prosthetic support
    S. belt
Silflex intramedullary prosthesis
Silfverskiöld
    S. Achilles tendon lengthening
    S. Achilles tendon reconstruction
    S. disease
    S. procedure
    S. technique
    S. test
silhouette
    s. capsulectomy
    S. pedicle screw system
    S. spinal system
    S. therapeutic massage
silicone
    s. arthritis
    s. breast implant
    s. elastomer rubber ball implant
    s. gel

s. gel socket insert
s. implant arthroplasty
s. insole
s. material
s. MP implant
s. pad
s. rubber arthroplasty
s. rubber sphere
s. spacer
s. synovitis
s. thermoplastic splinting (STS)
s. trapezium prosthesis
Wonderflex s.
s. wrist arthroplasty
silicone-dacron tendon rod
silicone-only suspension (SOS)
Silicore foot pillow
Silipos
S. digital pad
S. Distal Dip prosthetic sheath/liner
S. gel
S. mesh cap
S. mesh tubing
S. Silicone Wonder Cup
S. suspension sleeve
silk
s. mesh gauze dressing
Owens s.
s. suture
SilkTouch CO₂ laser
Sillence osteogenesis imperfecta classification
SiloLiner gel liner
Silon silicone thermoplastic splinting material
Silopad
S. body sleeve
S. toe sleeve
Silosheath
S. gel
S. sock
silver
S. bunionectomy
s. dollar technique
s. nitrate
S. osteotome
S. procedure
s. sulfadiazine
silver-fork
s.-f. deformity
s.-f. fracture
Silverskiöld syndrome

Silver-Thera
S.-T. stocking electrode
S.-T. stockings
Simmonds-Menelaus
S.-M. metatarsal osteotomy
S.-M. proximal phalangeal osteotomy
Simmonds test
Simmons
S. cervical spine fusion
S. chisel
S. crimper
S. double-hole spinal screw
S. Multi-Matic orthopaedic bed
S. osteotome
S. osteotomy
S. plate
S. plating system
S. and Segil classification system
S. spinal arthrodesis
S. Vari-Hite orthopaedic bed
Simmons-Martin screw
Simonart band
simple
s. bone cyst
s. button patellar implant
S. Calculated Osteoporosis Risk Estimation (SCORE)
s. dislocation
s. fracture
s. joint
s. knee test (SKT)
s. metatarsus adductus
S. Shoulder Test patient questionnaire
s. shoulder test thermal alteration Thomas traction
s. suture
s. syndactyly
s. synovitis
simplex
S. cement adhesive
herpes s.
hidroacanthoma s.
S. P bone cement
SimplyStable trace
Simpson
S. arthrectomy catheter
S. sugar-tong splint
Simpulse
S. pulsing lavage
S. S/I lavage

S

NOTES

Sims
> S. position
> S. retractor

simulator
> Baltimore Therapeutic Equipment
> Work S.
> Ergos work s.
> Lido WorkSET work s.
> Spinal Physiotherapy S.
> Work Seat driving s.

simultaneous
> S. Interview Technique (SIT)
> s. remodeling

S incision

Sinding-Larsen-Johansson
> S.-L.-J. disease
> S.-L.-J. lesion
> S.-L.-J. syndrome

Sine-Aid IB

Singh
> S. index of osteoporosis
> S. osteoporosis classification
> S. osteoporosis index
> trabecular index of S.

single
> s. axis
> s. clamp
> s. cross-slot screwdriver
> s. heel rise
> s. pearl-face hip joint
> s. photon emission computed
> tomography (SPECT)
> s. plantar verruca
> s. proximal portal technique
> s. ray pattern
> s. reference point
> s. reference point instrument
> s. smooth-face hip joint

single-action rongeur

single-axis
> s.-a. ankle joint
> s.-a. ankle prosthesis
> s.-a. friction knee (SAFK)
> s.-a. knee unit
> s.-a. locking knee (SALK)
> s.-a. Syme DYCOR foot

single-blade saw

single-cannula system

single-channel
> MyoTrac s.-c.
> s.-c. surface EMG

single-column fracture

single-condylar graft

single-contrast arthrogram

single-fiber
> s.-f. electromyography (SFEMG)
> s.-f. EMG
> s.-f. needle electrode

single-heel rise test

single-incision fasciotomy

single-leg
> s.-l. spica cast
> s.-l. toe raise

single-level spinal fusion

single-limb stance

single-lobed skin flap

single-onlay cortical bone graft

single-organ athlete

single-panel knee immobilizer

single-photon electrospinal orthosis

single-point cane

single-prong broad acetabular retractor

single-rod construct

single-row exercise

single-sided bone saw

single-slot screwdriver

single-stage
> s.-s. tendon graft
> s.-s. tissue transfer

single-stemmed
> s.-s. silicone hemiprosthesis
> s.-s. toe implant

single-unit pattern

single-use device

sink
> counter s.

sinogram

sinography

sintered
> s. implant prosthesis
> s. titanium mesh

sintering
> s. of cobalt-chrome powder coating
> cobalt-chrome power s.

Sinterlock
> S. implant
> S. implant metal
> S. implant metal prosthesis

sinus
> air s.
> cervical ligament of tarsal s.
> coccygeal s.
> dermal s.
> s. histiocytosis
> lunate s.
> osteomyelitic s.
> peroneal s.
> talar s.
> tarsal s.
> s. tarsi
> s. tarsi region
> s. tarsi syndrome
> tentorial s.
> s. tract
> traumatic s.

sinusoidal

sinuvertebral nerve

SIO
    sacroiliac orthosis
SIPT
    Sensory Integration and Praxis test
Sir Henry Platt transverse approach
sirolimus
SIS
    Social Interaction Scale
sismotherapy
sisomicin
Sisson fracture reducing elevator
Sistron scissors
Sistrunk scissors
SIT
    Simultaneous Interview Technique
sit-and-reach
    s.-a.-r. box
    s.-a.-r. test
site
    donor s.
    Evans calcaneal lengthening
      osteotomy s.
    fracture s.
    harvest s.
    hook s.
    nerve entrapment s.
    nonunion of fracture s.
    operative s.
    pin s.
    recipient s.
    tibial insertion s.
sit/stand chair
Sit-Straight wheelchair cushion
sitter
    floor s.
sitting
    s. duct stretch test
    s. flexion
    s. flexion test
    s. knee extension
    s. position
    s. root test
    s. side bend
sit-to-stand
    s.-t.-s. test
    s.-t.-s. training parallel bar unit
sit-up test
Sivash hip prosthesis
size
    crosslink plate s.
sized orthotics for children (SOCS)
sizer
    Brannock Device shoe s.

SJA
    subtalar joint axis
SJF
    subtalar joint function
SJK
    Scheuermann juvenile kyphosis
Sjögren syndrome
S-K
    S-K reconstruction
    S-K reconstruction of distal
      radioulnar joint
skate
    arm s.
skateboard
skater's gait
skeletal
    s. age (SA)
    s. amyloidosis
    s. bed
    s. defect
    s. deformity
    s. disruption
    s. dysplasia
    s. extension
    s. growth factor
    s. hyperostosis syndrome
    s. hypoplasia
    s. hypoplasia disease
    idiopathic s.
    s. injury score
    s. limb deficiency
    s. maturation
    s. maturity
    s. muscle
    s. muscle fiber
    s. muscle relaxant
    s. pin
    s. repair system (SRS)
    s. stabilization
    s. tissue
    s. traction
    s. tuberculosis
    s. wry neck
skeletal-extraskeletal angiomatosis
skeletally immature
skeleton
    appendicular s.
    articulated s.
    bony s.
    s. hand
    s. shortening
    spidering s.
skeletonize

NOTES

S

skew
>   s. flap
>   s. foot

skewer

skewering

skewfoot
>   complex s.
>   s. deformity

ski
>   impact-release binding on s.
>   walker s.'s

skid
>   bone s.
>   hip s.
>   s. humeral head retractor
>   Meyerding bone s.
>   Murphy s.
>   Murphy-Lane bone s.

skier's
>   s. fracture
>   s. injury
>   s. thumb

skijump view

Skil-Care
>   S.-C. cushion
>   S.-C. cushion grip
>   S.-C. reclining wheelchair

skill
>   ambulation s.'s
>   articulatory s.
>   Assessment of Communication and
>   Interaction s.'s (ACIS)
>   S.'s Assessment Module (SAM)
>   Assessment of Motor and
>   Process s.'s (AMPS)
>   bed mobility s.
>   donning-doffing s.
>   Kohlman Evaluation of Living s.'s
>   (KELS)
>   Milwaukee Evaluation of Daily
>   Living s.'s (MEDLS)
>   palpatory s.
>   Performance Assessment of Self-
>   Care S.'s
>   physical daily living s.'s (PDLS)
>   Test of Visual-Motor s.'s (TVMS)
>   Test of Visual-Perception s.'s
>   (TVPS)

Skillbuilder half roll

Skillern fracture

Skil Saw

skin
>   s. adherence
>   s. blood flow determination
>   s. breakdown
>   s. bridge
>   S. Care kit
>   s. closure
>   s. coverage

>   s. creaking
>   s. crease
>   dorsal s.
>   s. flap
>   s. glue
>   s. graft
>   s. hook
>   hypertrophic s.
>   s. incision
>   s. marker
>   s. necrosis
>   necrotic s.
>   nonglabrous s.
>   s. pencil
>   perianal s.
>   s. plasty
>   s. preparation
>   s. resistance test
>   s. restriction
>   s. rolling
>   s. slapping
>   s. slough
>   s. staple
>   s. stroker
>   s. tag
>   s. tape
>   s. temperature monitoring probe
>   s. tension line
>   s. traction
>   undermined s.

skin-contact instrumentation

skinfold
>   s. caliper
>   s. measurement

skin-gliding test

Skinner line

skin-slough
>   incisional s.-s.

SkinTemp collagen skin dressing

skin-tight cast

skive

skived incision

skiving knife

Sklar
>   S. bone drill
>   S. bone saw
>   S. ligature needle
>   S. pin cutter
>   S. wire tightener

Skoog
>   S. procedure
>   S. procedure for release of
>   Dupuytren contracture
>   S. technique

SKT
>   simple knee test

skull
>   base of s. (BOS)
>   hot-cross-bun s.

s. plate screwdriver
s. tongs
skull-occiput-mandibular immobilization orthosis
skyline
s. radiograph
s. view
s. x-ray view of patella
Skytron
S. bed
S. operating room table
SL
scapholunate
stereolithography
SL cage
SLAC
scapholunate advanced collapse
scapholunate arthritis collapse
slack
motion s.
tissue s.
s. wrist
Slam'r wheelchair
slant
foam s.
OPTP S.
SLAP
superior labrum anterior and posterior
SLAP lesion
slap
foot s.
s. foot gait
s. hammer
slapping
s. gait
skin s.
Slatis
S. fixation
S. pelvic fracture frame
slatted plinth table
SLC
short leg cast
SLE
systemic lupus erythematosus
SLE arthropathy
sled
Penco Walker S.'s
walker s.'s
Sleeper Gripper prosthetic device
Sleep-eze 3 Oral
Sleepwell 2-nite

sleeve
arthroscopic monopolar thermal
stabilization forefoot
compression s.
BioCompression Pneumatic S.
circumferential ligamentous s.
cylindrical s.
drill s.
Edwards-Levine s.
Edwards modular system spinal s.
Edwards polyethylene s.
elbow s.
Electro-Mesh s.
epX suspension s.
excursion amplifier s.
forefoot compression s.
s. fracture
gel suspension s.
heel s.
Iceflex Endurance suction
suspension s.
knee s.
Knit-Rite suspension s.
malleolar gel s.
Mica 3x s.
neoprene elbow s.
neoprene knee s.
obturator s.
Pedifix forefoot compression s.
periosteal s.
pin s.
pneumatic compression s.
polyethylene s.
rod s.
Silipos suspension s.
Silopad body s.
Silopad toe s.
Super Grip s.
2-s. technique
s. type
slide
flexor pronator s.
Glassman-Engh-Bobyn
trochanteric s.
head-first s.
muscle s.
s. plate
trochanteric s.
slideboard
Activ s.
slider crank mechanism
sliding
s. AFO

S

NOTES

sliding *(continued)*
 s. arthrodesis
 s. barrel hook
 s. bone graft
 s. compression hip screw
 s. compression screw with sideplate
 s. fixation device
 s. flap
 s. hammer
 s. knot
 s. mat
 s. nail
 s. nail device
 s. plane osteotomy of Samilson
 s. tenotomy
 s. Z-plasty
slightly movable articulation
SlimLine cast boot
Slim Option shoe orthosis
Slimrest
 Core S.
Slimthetics orthotic
sling
 Action thumb s.
 AliMed hemi arm s.
 Ampoxen s.
 arm elevator s.
 Barton s.
 Böhler-Braun leg s.
 collar-and-cuff s.
 cradle arm s.
 CVA S.
 s. dressing
 envelope arm s.
 finger s.
 Fits-All s.
 FoamWrap finger s.
 foot s.
 s. frame
 Glisson s.
 hanging cast s.
 Harris Hemi Arm S.
 Harris splint s.
 s. immobilization
 s. immobilizer
 Jacksonville s.
 Kenny-Howard shoulder s.
 knee s.
 Kodel knee s.
 leg s.
 Legg-Perthes s.
 lymphedema s.
 Mersilene s.
 Murphy s.
 muslin s.
 Nada-Chair Back-Up portable
  back s.
 Pavlik s.
 pelvic s.

Posey s.
 pouch-type s.
 s. procedure
 Rauchfuss s.
 s. and reef technique
 resting foot s.
 rubber s.
 Salter s.
 s. seat sag
 s. seat wheelchair
 shoulder saddle s.
 sling-and-swathe s.
 Slingers arm s.
 slinger-style envelope s.
 soft tissue coaptation s.
 stockinette s.
 strap s.
 subcutaneous fat s.
 s. suspension range of motion
 s. suture
 swathe and s.
 Teare s.
 Thomas buckle s.
 Thomas Kodel s.
 thumb s.
 triangular arm s.
 universal s.
 Uni-Versatil s.
 Velpeau shoulder s.
 Vogue arm s.
 volar ulnar s.
 Weil pelvic s.
 Westfield-style envelope s.
sling-and-swathe
 s.-a.-s. bandage
 s.-a.-s. sling
sling-dressing
 Velpeau s.-d.
Slingers arm sling
slinger-style envelope sling
Slingshot shoulder immobilizer
slip
 s. angle
 s. angle spondylolisthesis
 central s.
 conjoined gastrocnemius soleus
  fascial s.
 flexor digitorum s.
 s. joint
 lateral s.
 s. of tendon
slip-joint pliers
Slip-N-Snip scissors
slip-on finger splint
slipped
 s. capital femoral epiphysis (SCFE)
 s. disc
 s. elbow

S

s. under femoral epiphysis (SUFE)
s. vertebral apophysis

slipper
Acu-Pressure s.
s. cast
Kite s.
PPCID s.'s
WalkCare s.'s

slipping
s. patella
s. rib
s. rib cartilage

slit catheter technique

sliver of bone

Slocum
S. ALRI test
S. anterior rotary drawer test
S. fusion technique
S. knee procedure
S. lateral pivot-shift test
S. maneuver
S. meniscal clamp
S. nail
S. pes anserinus transplant
S. rotary instability test
S. splint

Slo-Mo ball

slope
dorsal radial s.
sacral s.
tibial s.

slot
acetabular s.
S. distraction device
glenoid s.
s. table

slot-graft

slotted
s. acetabular augmentation
s. bolt
s. femur plate
s. mallet
s. nail
s. obturator-cannula system
s. tendon stripper

slough
skin s.

slow
s. axoplasmic transport (SAXT)
s. cautery
s. distraction
s. muscle
s. stretch

s. stretch reflex
s. union

slow-acting antirheumatic drug (SAARD)

SL-Plus stem

SLR
straight leg raising
SLR with Bragard test
SLR with external rotation test
SLR with Kernig test

SLRT
straight leg raising test

slump test

slurry
autogenous bone s.
bone s.
matrix-bone marrow s.

SLWC
short leg walking cast

Sly syndrome

SMA
spinal muscular atrophy (type I–III)
SMA prosthesis

SMALL
same-day microsurgical arthroscopic lateral-approach laser-assisted
SMALL fluoroscopic discectomy

small
s. cell osteogenic sarcoma
s. egress cannula
s. fracture
s. fragment screw
s. lamina spreader
s. nail spicule bur
s. patella syndrome
s. plate forceps
s. step distraction

small-base quad cane

small-diameter wire

small-headed screw

small-joint stiffness

Smart
S. Balance Master
S. Pin
S. Screw bioabsorbable implant

SmartBrace
S. brace
S. wrist splint

SmartKnit seamless diabetic sock

SmartPin instrument set

SmartPin/PLLA pin

SmartPReP PRP system

SmartTack fixation

NOTES

SmartWrap elbow brace
Smedberg
    S. brace
    S. hand drill
    S. twist drill
Smedley dynamometer
SMFA
    Short Musculoskeletal Function
    Assessment
SMI 3000, 5000 bed
smile
    inverted s.
Smillie
    S. cartilage chisel
    S. cartilage knife
    S. knee retractor
    S. meniscal knife
    S. meniscal scissors
    S. meniscectomy chisel
    S. meniscus hook retractor
    S. nail
    S. pin
Smillie-Beaver
    S.-B. blade
    S.-B. knife
Smith
    S. ankle fracture
    S. ankle prosthesis
    S. automatic perforated drill
    S. bone clamp
    S. cartilage knife
    S. dislocation
    S. flexor pollicis longus abductor-
    plasty
    S. maneuver
    S. & Nephew bracing and support
    system
    S. & Nephew medium barbed
    staple
    S. & Nephew reflection acetabular
    cup implant component
    S. & Nephew small barbed staple
    S. physical capacities evaluation
    S. and Ross test
    S. scissors
    S. STA-peg
    S. technique
Smith-Davis Converta-Hite orthopaedic
bed
Smith-Lemli-Opitz syndrome
Smith-Petersen
    S.-P. approach
    S.-P. chisel
    S.-P. cup
    S.-P. cup arthroplasty
    S.-P. curved gouge
    S.-P. curved osteotome
    S.-P. femoral neck nail
    S.-P. fracture pin

    S.-P. gooseneck gouge
    S.-P. hemiarthroplasty
    S.-P. hip cup prosthesis
    S.-P. impactor
    S.-P. intertrochanteric plate
    S.-P. nail with Lloyd adapter
    S.-P. osteotomy
    S.-P. reamer
    S.-P. rongeur
    S.-P. sacroiliac joint fusion
    S.-P. straight gouge
    S.-P. straight osteotome
    S.-P. synovectomy
    S.-P. technique
    S.-P. transarticular nail
Smith-Richards instrumentation
Smith-Robinson
    S.-R. anterior cervical discectomy
    S.-R. anterior fusion
    S.-R. cervical disc approach
    S.-R. cervical interbody fusion
    S.-R. interbody arthrodesis
    S.-R. operation
    S.-R. technique
Smithwick clip-applying forceps
SMO
    stainless steel and molybdenum
    supramalleolar orthosis
    SMO Moore pin
    SMO plate
    SMO prosthesis
smooth
    s. broach
    s. cobalt-chromium
    s. endoprosthesis
    s. muscle
    s. muscle hypertrophy
    s. Steinmann pin
    s. transfixion wire
smoother
    Gore s.
smoothie junior bur
smooth-tipped jeweler's forceps
SMPS
    sympathetic maintained pain syndrome
SMT
    spinal manipulative therapy
SNAGS
    sustained natural apophysial glides
SNAP
    sensory nerve action potential
    soluble *N*-eythyl-maleimide sensitive
    factor attachment protein
    SNAP receptor
snap
    s. finger
    s. fit
    S. fixation pin
    S. Lock wire/pin extractor

snap-fit
    s.-f. apparatus
    s.-f. device
snap-lock brace
snap-off compression (SOC)
Snap-Pak
    Mitek GII S.-P.
snapping
    s. hip
    s. hip syndrome
    s. knee syndrome
    s. scapula
    s. scapula syndrome
    tendon s.
    s. tendon
    s. thumb flexor
SNARE
    sensory nerve action potential receptor
    SNARE complex
snare
    Zimmer s.
Sneppen talar fracture
sniffer's position
snooze pillow
snowboarder's
    s. ankle
    s. fracture
snowboarding injury
Snow-Littler release
snowstorm knee
SNS
    sympathetic nervous system
snuffbox
    anatomic s.
snug
    S. seat
    s. traction
    S.'s wrap
SO
    shoulder orthosis
    spinal orthosis
soak
    Betadine s.
    Epsom salts s.
soap
    Betadine s.
SOC
    snap-off compression
social
    S. Integration World Health Organization Handicap Scale
    S. Interaction Scale (SIS)

society
    American Knee S.
    American Orthopaedic Foot and Ankle s. (AOFAS)
    Musculoskeletal Tumor S.
    National Academy on Aging S.
    National Down Syndrome S.
sock
    active s.
    AFO brace s.
    s. aid
    ankle-foot orthosis brace s.
    arthritis s.
    Bio-Wick s.
    Carolon AFO s.
    cast s.
    Comfort Ag prosthetic s.
    Comfort n' Care Seamfree s.'s
    Creative diabetic s.'s
    diabetic s.
    edema s.
    electrode s.
    gel stump s.
    molding s.
    Orlon with Lycra stump s.
    prosthetic s.
    Regal Acrylic/Stretch prosthetic s.
    Rx Comfort s.
    Silosheath s.
    SmartKnit seamless diabetic s.
    Soft Walk gel s.
    Spandex Lycra 3-ply stump s.
    Strassburg s.
    STS molding s.
    stump s.
    Thorlo s.'s
    Venosan support s.
Sock-Assist device
socket
    adjustable postoperative protective prosthetic s. (APOPPS)
    all-alumina s.
    all-polyethylene s.
    AML s.
    Arthropor II porous s.
    check s.
    Clearpro suction s.
    concave loading s.
    endoskeletal s.
    flexible s.
    Flo-Tech prosthetic s.
    s. gauge
    hard s.

S

NOTES

671

socket *(continued)*
    Icex s.
    intermediate s.
    ischial containment s.
    ischial-gluteal weightbearing s.
    metal-backed s.
    modular s.
    patellar tendon s. (PTS)
    s. pin
    Poly-Dial s.
    polyethylene s.
    preassembled metal-backed s.
    prosthetic s.
    s. purchase
    quadrilateral ischial weightbearing s.
    standard s.
    supracondylar s.
    suspension-type s.
    temporary s.
    total contact s.
    universal frame outer s. (UFOS)
    University of California cuff
      suspension PTB s.
    variable circumference
      suprapatellar s. (VCSPS)
    s. wrench
Socon spinal system
SOC pin
SOCS
    sized orthotics for children
    SOCS AFO system
    SOCS pad system
Sof
    S. Airr insole
    S. Matt pressure relieving mattress
    S. Sole motion control orthotic
    S. Sole Sof Gel heel pad
Sofamor spinal device
Sofflex
    S. mattress
    S. mattress system
Sof-Gel palm shield
Sofield
    S. femoral deficiency operation
    S. femoral deficiency technique
    S. osteotomy
    S. pinning
    S. retractor
SofPulse device
Sof-Rol
    S.-R. cast pad
    S.-R. dressing
SofSole Airr insole
Soft
    S. Silicones Wonderzorb
    S. Super Sport orthotic
    S. Support Preforms orthotic
    S. Touch stockings
    S. Walk gel sock

soft
    s. bone
    s. bulky dressing
    s. callus stage
    s. collar
    s. collar cervical orthosis
    s. copolymer foam
    s. corn
    s. corset
    s. cosmetic cover
    s. fibroma
    s. socket insert
    s. tissue
    s. tissue abnormality
    s. tissue abscess
    s. tissue biomechanics
    s. tissue blade retractor
    s. tissue calcification
    s. tissue coaptation sling
    s. tissue compromise
    s. tissue contracture
    s. tissue coverage
    s. tissue envelope
    s. tissue flap
    s. tissue graft
    s. tissue healing
    s. tissue hinge
    s. tissue injury
    s. tissue integrity
    s. tissue interface
    s. tissue interposition
    s. tissue irritability
    s. tissue lesion
    s. tissue maladaptation
    s. tissue manipulation
    s. tissue mass
    s. tissue massage
    s. tissue mobilization
    s. tissue myxoma
    s. tissue plication
    s. tissue release
    s. tissue restriction
    s. tissue sarcoma
    s. tissue stretching
    s. tissue tumor
    s. touch hand exerciser
softball sliding injury
SofTec rigid brace
Softeze water pillow
SoftFlex
    S. computer glove
    S. Wrist Wear
Softie shoe
Softip monofilament
Softouch Cold/Hot Pack
Softsplint foot splint
soft-vamp shoe
software
    Achieve s.

Image-I analysis s.
osteotomy analysis simulation s.
  (OASIS)
Stat Graphics s.
Yochum chiropractic s.
Sof-Wick dressing
Sofwire cable system
Solarcaine Aloe Extra Burn Relief
Solcotrans
S. autotransfusion system
S. orthopaedic drainage-refusion
  system
sole
Ambulator Bio-Rocker s.
s. of foot
s. insert
plaster s.
PodiAxis orthopaedic s.
Poro-in-between s.
s. reflex
rockerbottom s.
shock-absorbent s.
shoe s.
Texon s.
Vibram s.
sole-tap reflex
soleus
accessory s.
s. complex
gastrocnemius s.
s. muscle
s. syndrome
SOLEutions
S. custom orthosis
S. custom orthotic device
S. Prefab orthotic device
S. soft plus orthotic
S. sport shell orthotic
solid
s. ankle, cushioned heel (SACH)
s. ankle, cushioned heel foot
s. ankle, cushioned heel orthotic
s. ankle, cushioned heel prosthesis
s. ankle flexible endoskeletal
  (SAFE)
s. ankle joint
s. buckling implant material
s. hex bolt
s. silicone exoplant implant
  material
solitary
s. bone cyst
s. enchondroma

s. fibromatosis
s. myeloma
s. osteoma
Solitens transcutaneous electrical nerve
  stimulation unit
soluble *N*-eythyl-maleimide sensitive
  factor attachment protein (SNAP)
Solu-Medrol Injection
Solurex L.A.
Soluspan
solution
antibiotic and saline s.
antiseptic s.
bacitracin s.
Betadine scrub s.
Bunnell s.
colloid s.
crystalloid s.
dextrose s.
extravasation irrigation s.
ferumoxide injectable s.
heparinized Ringer lactate s.
Hibiclens s.
iodophor s.
irrigating s.
irrigation s.
Penlac Nail Lacquer topical s.
S. prosthesis
Rotaglide lubricating s.
saline s.
sterile saline s.
somatectomy
subtotal s.
somatic
s. dysfunction
s. innervation
s. muscle
s. nerve
s. sign
s. therapy
s. visceral disease mimicry
somatization
somatoautonomic
s. reflex (SAR)
s. reflex hypothesis
somatoprosthetics
somatosensory
s. deficit
s. evoked potential (SEP, SSEP)
s. evoked potential monitoring
s. test
somatosomatic reflex
somatovisceral correction

NOTES

Somerville
    S. anterior approach
    S. procedure
    S. technique
SOMI
    sternal-occipital-mandibular
      immobilization
    SOMI brace
    SOMI orthosis
Sominex Oral
Songer cable
sonic accelerated fracture healing system (SAFHS)
SonoAce PICO portable digital color ultrasound system
Sonocut ultrasonic aspirator
sonographic abnormality
sonography
sonometer
    clinical bone s.
    Omnisense 7000S bone s.
    Sahara clinical bone s.
    SoundScan 2000 bone s.
    SoundScan Compact bone s.
    UBIS 5000 quantitative ultrasound bone s.
    UBIS 5000 ultrasound bone s.
    ultrasound bone imaging s. (UBIS)
Sontec pliers
Sony CCD/RGB DXC-151 color video camera
Sorbie calcaneal fracture classification
Sorbie-Questor
    S.-Q. elbow
    S.-Q. total elbow prosthesis system
sorbitol level
Sorbothane
    S. antivibration glove
    S. heel cushion
    S. II heel cup
    S. insole
    S. orthotic device
    S. recoil pad
    S. rice sheller roller
    S. wrap
sore
    plaster s.
    pressure s.
    saddle s.
Soren
    S. ankle fusion
    S. arthrodesis
soreness
    delayed-onset muscle s.
Sorrells hip arthroplasty retractor system
Sorrel-type snowboard boot
SOS
    silicone-only suspension

    SOS total hip system
    SOS total knee system
SOT
    sacrooccipital technique
    Sensory Organization test
SOTO
    step out, turn out
    SOTO technique
Soto-Hall
    S.-H. bone graft
    S.-H. maneuver
    S.-H. sign
    S.-H. test
Soudre autogéné
sound
    flexible s.
    radiolucent s.
    rigid s.
    tearing s.
sounder
    pedicle s.
SoundScan
    S. 2000 bone sonometer
    S. Compact bone sonometer
source
    fiberoptic light s.
    light s.
    Wolf light s.
sourcil fracture
Souter
    S. hip operation
    S. hip procedure
    S. Strathclyde total elbow system
    S. unconstrained elbow prosthesis
Souter-Strathclyde elbow prosthesis
southern
    s. access
    S. California Orthopaedic Institute (SCOI)
Southwick
    S. biplane trochanteric osteotomy
    S. clamp
    S. lateral slip angle
    S. pin-holding apparatus
    S. pin-holding device
    S. screw extractor
    S. slide procedure
    S. two-tined retractor
Southwick-Robinson anterior cervical approach
Sox
    Champion Power S.
SP
    suprapatellar
    SP Walker cast
SpA
    spondyloarthropathy
Spa Bed

space
s. available for cord (SAC)
Barouk button s.
cartilage s.
costoclavicular s.
dead s.
disc s.
epidural s.
fascial s.
first web s.
haversian s.
hypoplastic disc s.
increased lateral joint s.
intercondylar s.
intercostal s. (ICS)
intermetatarsal s.
interpeduncular s.
interphalangeal joint s.
joint s.
lateral joint s.
medial clear s.
midpalmar s.
narrowed joint s.
palm s.
paraphysiological s.
Parona s.
s. of Poirier
popliteal s.
position in s.
prevertebral s.
properitoneal s.
retroperitoneal s.
retropharyngeal s.
s. shoe
subacromial s.
subcoracoid s.
suprasternal s.
thenar s.
tibiocalcaneal s.
tibiofibular clear s.
tibiotalar clear s.
spacer
acetabular s.
AlloCraft PL allograft s.
s. bar
Barouk s.
bayonet s.
s. between toes
bone s.
Button S.
ceramic vertebral s.
Graftech structural allograft
   cervical s.

Hourglass vertebral body s.
s. inserter
InterSpace hip s.
InterSpace knee s.
joint s.
Kinemax s.
passive s.
Plexiglas s.
prosthetic s.
proximal cement s.
rubber s.
silicone s.
Telescopic Plate Spacer implantable
   titanium s.
temporary articulating
   methylmethacrylate antibiotic s.
   (TAMMAS)
tibial s.
toe s.
TraXis Ti alloy s.
TraXis Vue alloy s.
trial s.
true s.
spacer-tensor jig
spade
s. finger
s. hand
Spahr metaphysial dysostosis
Spälteholz
S. bone-clearing technique
S. preparation
Spandex Lycra 3-ply stump sock
spanner gauge
spanning external fixator
sparing
glycogen s.
sacral nerve root s.
Spark handheld dynamometer
Spartan jaw wire cutter
spasm
arterial s.
carpal pedal s.
muscle s.
paraspinal muscle s.
paraspinous muscular s.
paravertebral muscle s.
peroneal muscle s.
spasmodic torticollis
spastic
s. cerebral palsy
s. diparesis
s. diplegia
s. disorder

S

NOTES

675

spastic *(continued)*
    s. equinovalgus
    s. equinus
    s. equinus gait
    s. flatfoot
    s. gait
    s. hand
    s. hemiplegia
    s. hindfoot valgus deformity
    s. intrinsic contracture
    s. paralysis
    s. paraplegia
    s. quadriplegia
    s. thumb-in-palm deformity
    s. varus hindfoot
spasticity
    Ashworth score of muscle s.
    s. measurement
    muscle s.
    s. treatment
    wrist s.
spatula
    cement s.
    s. foot
    s. forceps
spatulate thumb
SPC
    suprapatellar cuff
spear
    s. tackle
    s. tackler's spine
spearing
    injurious energy input s.
special
    s. Colles splint
    Heel Spur S.
    S. Seat
specialized nail
specific
    s. adaptation to imposed demand (SAID)
    s. adjustment
    s. curve
    s. thrust manipulation
specimen
    cadaveric s.
SPECT
    single photon emission computed tomography
Spectron
    S. EF total hip system
    S. hip prosthesis
spectroscopy
    Fourier transform infrared s.
    magnetic resonance s.
Spectrum tissue repair system
speech aid
speed
    S. arthroplasty

    S. brace
    S. hand splint
    S. osteotomy
    s. play training
    S. radial head fracture classification
    S. radius cap prosthesis
    S. sign
    S. sternoclavicular repair
    S. test
    S. V-Y muscle-plasty
speed-lock clamp
Spelcast car seat
Spence rongeur forceps
Spencer tendon lengthening
Spenco
    S. arch support
    S. boot
    S. insole
    S. liner
    S. orthotic device
    S. Second Skin dressing
    S. shoe insert
Spetzler anterior transoral approach
SpF spinal fusion stimulator
SPG
    stereophotogrammetry
sphenoid
    wing of s.
sphenoidal fossa
sphenoiditis
sphenoidostomy
sphenoidotomy
sphenopalatine ganglion block
sphere
    silicone rubber s.
spherical
    s. bur
    s. gliding principle
    s. reamer
spherical-headed screw
spherocentric
    s. fully constrained tricompartmental knee prosthesis
    s. knee system
spheroidal joint
sphincter
    s. muscle
    s. tone
sphygmomanometer
spica
    s. bandage
    s. cast
    Freedom thumb s.
    hip s.
    Schmeisser s.
    s. splint
    thumb s.
spicule
    bone s.

spider finger
spidering skeleton
Spiegleman acromioclavicular splint
Spier elbow arthrodesis
Spiessel internal screw fixation
spike
    ball-tip s.
    s. of bone
    endplate s.
    Gaenslen s.
    Gissane s.
    heel s.
    metaphysial s.
    s. osteotomy
    supracollicular s.
    s. washer implant
spiked
    s. Darrach-type elevator
    s. ligament washer
spilled
    s. cup sign
    s. teacup sign
spina
    s. bifida
    s. bifida aperta
    s. bifida occulta (SBO)
spinae
    erector s.
    thoracolumbar erector s.
spinal
    s. abscess
    s. accessory nerve
    s. accessory nerve injury
    s. analysis
    s. analysis machine (SAM)
    s. anesthesia
    s. angulation
    s. arteriography
    s. artery
    s. arthritis
    s. arthrodesis
    s. axial load
    s. axis
    s. brucellosis
    s. canal
    s. canal stenosis (SCS)
    s. column
    s. contour
    s. cord
    s. cord angiography
    s. cord atrophy
    s. cord block
    s. cord canal

s. cord compression
s. cord function intraoperative monitoring
s. cord injury (SCI)
s. cord injury without radiographic abnormality (SCIWORA)
s. cord-meningeal complex
S. Cord Motor Index and Sensory Indices
s. cord stimulator (SCS)
s. cord syndrome
s. cord tract
s. coronal plane deformity
s. curvature
s. decompression
s. deformity instability
s. degeneration
s. distraction
s. dysarthria
s. dysraphism
s. evoked potential
s. fascial release
s. fixation
s. fixation rigidity
s. fixation rod
s. fracture
s. fusion
s. fusion device
s. fusion pathomechanics
s. fusion position
s. fusion procedure
s. fusion stimulator
s. fusion system
s. fusion technique
s. hitch
s. implant
s. implant design
s. implant load to failure
s. infection
s. infection biopsy
s. injection therapy
s. injury operative stabilization
s. instability
s. instrumentation
s. joint mobilization
s. learning
s. level
s. load bearing
s. locking procedure
s. malignancy
s. manipulation
s. manipulative therapy (SMT)
s. manual therapy

NOTES

S

spinal *(continued)*
   s. membrane
   s. metastasis
   s. mobilization technique
   s. muscular atrophy (type I–III)
    (SMA)
   s. myoclonus
   s. needle
   s. orthosis (SO)
   s. osteoblastoma
   s. osteomyelitis
   s. osteosarcoma
   s. osteotomy
   s. osteotomy stabilization
   S. Physiotherapy Simulator
   s. posterior ligament
   s. process apophysis
   s. puncture
   s. rod cross-bracing
   s. segment
   s. shock
   s. stenotic myelopathy
   S. Technology bivalve TLSO brace
   s. transverse ligament
   s. tuberculosis
   s. tumor
   s. turning frame
SpinalPak
   S. bone growth stimulator
   S. spine fusion stimulator
spindle
   anulospiral ending of muscle s.
   s. cell lipoma
   s. effect
   muscle s.
   s. neuroma
spine
   adjustment of s.
   alar s.
   angular s.
   anterior column of s.
   anterior inferior iliac s. (AIIS)
   anterior maxillary s.
   anterior occipitocervical s.
   anterior superior iliac s. (ASIS)
   anterior tibial s.
   anterior upper s.
   s. apparatus
   axial loading of s.
   bamboo s.
   s. board
   cervical s. (C-spine)
   Chance fracture thoracolumbar s.
   Charcot s.
   chiropractic manual manipulation
    of s.
   Civinini s.
   cleft s.
   coccygeal s.

3-column s.
convexity of s.
s. deformity
fixation dysfunction of lumbar s.
s. flexion
s. frame
full cervical s. (FCS)
Gait, Arms, Legs, and S. (GALS)
gibbus deformity of s.
iliac s.
ischial s.
kinetic cervical s.
kissing s.'s
laminectomized s.
lower cervical s.
lower lumbar s.
lower thoracic s.
lumbar s. (L-spine)
lumbosacral s.
mandibular s.
maxillary s.
nasal s.
osteoporotic s.
palpation of anterior superior
  iliac s.
palpation of posterior superior
  iliac s.
poker s.
posterior-inferior s.
posterior sacroiliac s. (PSIS)
posterior superior iliac s. (PSIS)
posterior tibial s.
s. Power pelvic stabilizer belt
s. rotation
rugger jersey s.
sacral s.
s. sign
spear tackler's s.
thoracic s. (T-spine)
thoracolumbar s.
thoracolumbosacral s.
trochanteric s.
upper thoracic s.
variable screw placement system-
  instrumented lumbar s.
SpineCor
   S. nonrigid brace
   S. system
SpineScope
   Clarus S.
spinning probe
spinocerebellar
   s. ataxia
   s. degeneration
   s. tract
spinoglenoid
   s. ligament
   s. notch
spinographic angle

spinography
spinolaminar line
spinomuscular paralysis
spinopelvic
    s. transiliac fixation (STIF)
    s. transiliac fixation system
    s. transiliac fixation technique
Spinoscope noninvasive imaging system
spinothalamic tract
spinous
    s. plane
    s. process
    s. process fracture
    s. process plate
    s. process wire
    s. process wiring
    s. pull
    s. push
spiral
    s. bandage
    s. cortical reamer
    s. drill
    s. groove syndrome
    s. humeral groove
    s. joint
    s. line of femur
    s. oblique fracture
    s. oblique retinacular ligament
    s. oblique retinacular ligament
      reconstruction splint
    s. stay
    s. sulcus
    s. technique
    s. trochanteric reamer
Spira procedure
Spirec drill
spiritual healing
spirometer
    Buhl s.
Spittler procedure
Spitz-Holter valve implant material
Spitz nevus
SPL
    short plantar ligament
SPLATT
    split anterior tibialis tendon transfer
      SPLATT procedure
splayfoot deformity
splaying
    forefoot s.
    s. of toe
splint
    Abbott s.

    abduction finger s.
    abduction humeral s.
    abduction pillow cover s.
    abduction thumb s.
    Abouna s.
    abutment s.
    acrylic cap s.
    acrylic template s.
    active s.
    Adam and Eve rib belt s.
    Adams s.
    adjustable s.
    Adjusta-Wrist s.
    aeroplane s.
    A-Force dorsal night s.
    Agnew s.
    Ainslie acrylic s.
    air s.
    AirFlex carpal tunnel s.
    Airfoam s.
    airplane s.
    air pressure s.
    Air-Soft S.
    AliMed diabetic night s.
    AliMed turnbuckle elbow s.
    Alumafoam s.
    aluminum bridge s.
    aluminum fence s.
    aluminum finger cot s.
    aluminum foam s.
    aluminum hand s.
    aluminum wire s.
    anchor s.
    Anderson s.
    angle s.
    ankle-foot orthotic s.
    anterior acute flexion elbow s.
    anterior shin s.
    any-angle s.
    Aquaplast s.
    armchair s.
    Asch s.
    Ashhurst leg s.
    s. attachment
    backboard s.
    balanced s.
    Balkan femoral s.
    ball-peen s.
    banana finger extension s.
    Banana Split S.
    banjo s.
    Barlow cruciform infant s.
    baseball finger s.

S

NOTES

splint (*continued*)
basic hand s.
Basswood s.
Bavarian s.
Baylor adjustable cross s.
Baylor metatarsal s.
Bend-A-Boot foot s.
Bennett basic hand s.
birdcage s.
Bloom s.
Blount s.
Blue Line ThumbStay s.
Blue Line UNO s.
Blue Line Wrist Control s.
board s.
Böhler-Braun s.
Böhler wire s.
Bond arm s.
s. bone
Boston thoracic s.
Bosworth s.
boutonnière s.
Bowlby arm s.
bracketed s.
Brady balanced-suspension s.
Brady leg s.
Brant aluminum s.
Brooke Army Hospital s.
Browne s.
Buck extension s.
Buck traction s.
buddy s.
Budin hammertoe s.
Budin toe s.
Bunnell active hand and finger s.
Bunnell finger extension s.
Bunnell gutter s.
Bunnell outrigger s.
Bunnell reverse knuckle-bender s.
Bunnell safety-pin s.
Bunny boot foot s.
Burnham finger s.
Burnham thumb s.
Cabot leg s.
Cabot posterior s.
calibrated clubfoot s.
Campbell traction s.
cap s.
Capener coil s.
Capener finger s.
Carl P. Jones traction s.
Carpal Lock cock-up s.
Carpal Lock wrist s.
Carter s.
cartilage elastic pullover kneecap s.
Chandler felt collar s.
clavicular cross s.
Clayton greenstick s.
clubfoot s.

CMC s.
coaptation s.
cock-up arm s.
cock-up hand s.
cock-up wrist s.
Colles s.
Comforfoam s.
Comforter S.
Comfy elbow s.
composite spring elastic s.
compression sleeve shin s.
Comprifix ankle s.
Cone s.
constant tension s.
Converse s.
cool Irom s.
Cordon-Colles fracture s.
Cosmolon closure for s.
counterrotational s.
countertraction s.
Craig abduction s.
Cramer wire s.
CTS Gripfit s.
cubital tunnel s.
Culley ulnar s.
Curry walking s.
Darco foot s.
Darco Medical-Surgical shoe and
  toe alignment s.
Davis metacarpal s.
Delbet s.
Denis Browne s. (DBS)
Denis Browne clubfoot s.
Denis Browne hip s.
Denis Browne talipes hobble s.
DePuy aeroplane s.
DePuy any-angle s.
DePuy coaptation s.
DePuy open-spindle s.
DePuy open-thimble s.
DePuy-Pott s.
DePuy rocking leg s.
DePuy rolled Colles s.
dermal interposition s.
derotator s.
DeRoyal LMB finger s.
digit s.
Digit-Aide fifth toe s.
DonJoy knee s.
DonJoy wrist s.
dorsal extension block s.
dorsal wrist s.
dorsiflexion foot s.
Dorsiwedge night s.
double-occlusal s.
double sugar-tong s.
dropfoot s.
drop wrist s.
Dupuytren s.

Duran-Houser wrist s.
Dyna knee s.
dynamic s.
Early Fit night s.
Easton cock-up s.
Easy Access foot s.
Eaton s.
Eggers contact s.
Elastomull s.
elbow extension s.
elbow flexion s.
elephant-ear clavicular s.
Engelmann thigh s.
Engen palmar wrist s.
Erich s.
Extend-It finger s.
extension block s.
Ezeform s.
felt collar s.
fence s.
Ferciot tiptoe s.
fiberglass s.
Fillauer night s.
finger cot s.
finger extension clockspring s.
finger flexion s.
Finger-Hugger s.
finger sled s.
Firm D-Ring wrist support s.
flat s.
flexor hinge s.
fold-over finger s.
footdrop night s.
forearm s.
Formatray mandibular s.
Forrester s.
Foster s.
Fox clavicular s.
Fractomed s.
fracture s.
Framer s.
Freedom neutral position s.
Freedom omni progressive s.
Freedom Progressive Resting s.
Freedom sportsfit s.
Freedom ultimate grip s.
Frejka pillow s.
Friedman s.
frog-leg s.
Froimson s.
full-hand s.
full-occlusal s.
functional s.

Funsten supination s.
Futuro s.
gait lock s. (GLS)
Gallows s.
Galveston s.
Ganley s.
Gibson s.
Gilchrist s.
Gilmer s.
Gordon s.
Gunning s.
gutter s.
hairpin s.
half ring leg s.
half-shell s.
hallux valgus night s.
Hammond s.
hand cock-up s.
Hanna night s.
Hare compact traction s.
Harrington outrigger s.
Harris s.
Hart extension finger s.
Heal Well night s.
Heel Free s.
Hexcelite sheet s.
hinged cylinder s.
hinged Thomas s.
HIPciser abduction s.
Hirschtick utility shoulder s.
Hodgen hip s.
Hodgen leg s.
humeral fracture abduction s.
HV NightSplint s.
HV SoftSplint s.
Ilfeld s.
Ilfeld-Gustafson s.
infant abduction s.
inflatable elbow s.
Innoboot s.
Irom bilateral s.
Irom Regal s.
Isoprene plastic s.
Jacoby bunion s.
Jacoby heel s.
James s.
Jet-Air s.
Joint-Jack finger s.
Jonell countertraction finger s.
Jonell thumb s.
Jones arm s.
Jones metacarpal s.
Jones traction s.

NOTES

splint *(continued)*
Joseph s.
Kanavel cock-up s.
Karfoil s.
Kazanjian s.
Keller-Blake half-ring s.
Keller-Blake leg s.
Kenny-Howard s.
Kerr abduction s.
Keystone s.
kinetic s.
Kleinert s.
Klenzak double-upright s.
knee brace s.
knee immobilizer s.
knuckle-bender s.
lace-lock ankle s.
ladder s.
Lambrinudi s.
leaf s.
Levis arm s.
Lewin finger s.
Lewin-Stern finger s.
Lewin-Stern thumb s.
Liberty One s.
s. liner
Link Stack Split S.
Link toe s.
Liston s.
live s.
LMB finger s.
LMB wire-foam economical
    resting s.
Lockhart toe s.
long arm s.
long leg s. (LLS)
loop-lock cock-up s.
Love s.
Lynx wrist, hand, finger orthosis
    arm positioner s.
Lytle metacarpal s.
magnet s.
Magnuson abduction humeral s.
malleable metal finger s.
Malmö hip s.
Mason s.
Mason-Allen Universal hand s.
Mayer s.
McGee s.
McIntire s.
McLeod padded clavicular s.
memory s.
metal s.
Middeldorpf s.
Moberg s.
modified Oppenheimer s.
Mohr finger s.
molded posterior plaster s.
Murphy s.

Murray-Jones arm s.
Murray-Thomas arm s.
neutral position s.
New Mind Set toe s.
N'ice Stretch night s.
night s.
occlusal s.
OCL volar s.
O'Donoghue knee s.
O'Donoghue stirrup s.
OEC s.
O'Malley jaw fracture s.
open-air s.
Oppenheimer spring wire s.
Oppenheimer with reverse knuckle-
    bender s.
opponens s.
Orfit s.
Ortho-Glass s.
Ortho-last s.
Orthomedics Stretch and Heel s.
Ortho-Mold s.
orthopaedic strap clavicular s.
Orthoplast isoprene s.
outrigger s.
Oval-8 ring s.
padded aluminum s.
padded board s.
padded plywood s.
padded tongue blade s.
s. padding
palmar cock-up s.
palmar wrist s.
pan s.
s. pan netting
passive night stretch s.
Pavlik harness s.
Peabody s.
Pearson attachment to Thomas s.
pelvic s.
PF Night Splint II s.
PFO night s.
Phelps s.
Phillips s.
Phoenix Outrigger s.
pillow s.
Pil-O-Splint wrist s.
plantar fasciitis night s.
Plastalume bulb-ended s.
Plastalume straight s.
plaster of Paris s.
plaster slab s.
pneumatic s.
4-point IROM s.
Polycentric Hinged Ulnar
    Deviation S.
Polyform s.
polyvinyl alcohol s.
Pond adjustable s.

Ponseti s.
poroplastic s.
Porzett s.
Postalume finger s.
posterior mold s.
Potts s.
Pro-glide s.
Progress s.
4-prong finger s.
Protecto s.
Pucci s.
Puth abduction s.
Putti s.
QualCraft s.
QuickCast s.
Quik s.
Radial Hinged Ulnar Deviation S.
radial slab s.
radiolucent s.
ratchet flexor tenodesis s.
Redi-Around finger s.
resting pan s.
reverse knuckle-bender s.
Robert Jones s.
Roger Anderson s.
Rolyan AquaForm wrist and thumb
  spica s.
Rolyan Gel Shell spica s.
Rosen s.
Rumel aluminum bridge s.
Russell s.
safety pin s.
Sager traction s.
SAM s.
Sam s.
Saturn carpal tunnel s.
Sayre s.
Scott ankle s.
Scott humeral s.
Scottish Rite s.
Scott Uniform tennis elbow s.
Seattle s.
shin s.
short arm s. (SAS)
short arm sugar-tong s.
short leg s.
shoulder spica s.
Simpson sugar-tong s.
slip-on finger s.
Slocum s.
SmartBrace wrist s.
Softsplint foot s.
special Colles s.

Speed hand s.
spica s.
Spiegleman acromioclavicular s.
spiral oblique retinacular ligament
  reconstruction s.
spreading hand s.
spring cock-up s.
spring-wire safety pin s.
Stack s.
Stader s.
static s.
Stax fingertip s.
stirrup plaster s.
Stock finger s.
strap clavicular s.
Stretch and Heel night s.
Stromeyer s.
Stuart Gordon hand s.
Stubbs acromioclavicular s.
sugar-tong plaster s.
surgical s.
suspension s.
swan-neck s.
Swanson dynamic toe s.
Swanson hand s.
synergistic wrist motion s.
Synergy s.
Taylor s.
Teare arm s.
tennis elbow s.
tension night s. (TNS)
T-finger s.
therapeutic s.
thermoplastic s.
Thomas full-ring s.
Thomas hinged s.
Thomas knee s.
Thomas leg s.
Thomas posterior s.
Thomas suspension s.
Thompson modification of Denis
  Browne s.
Thumbkeeper s.
thumb spica s.
thumb web s.
ThumSaver CMC Long s.
ThumSaver CMC Short s.
ThumSaver MP s.
ThumZ'Up thumb s.
Ticonium s.
Titus forearm s.
Titus wrist s.
Toad finger s.

S

NOTES

splint *(continued)*
  Tobruk s.
  toe alignment s.
  Tomberlin-Alemdaroglu s.
  Toronto s.
  torsion bar s.
  traction s.
  triangular pillow s.
  turnbuckle elbow s.
  type 501, 502, 504, 602 finger s.
  ulnar gutter s.
  Universal acromioclavicular s.
  Universal gutter s.
  Universal support s.
  Urias air s.
  Urias pressure s.
  U-splint s.
  U-stirrup s.
  Valentine s.
  Van Arsdale triangular s.
  Van Rosen s.
  Velcro extenders s.
  VersaWrist wrist s.
  Vesely-Street s.
  volar plaster s.
  Volkmann s.
  von Rosen abduction s.
  von Rosen cruciform s.
  Wanchik neutral position s.
  Weil s.
  well-leg s.
  well-padded s.
  Wertheim s.
  Wheaton bunion s.
  Wilson s.
  Winter s.
  wire grip finger s.
  wire grip toe s.
  wraparound s.
  WristJack wrist s.
  wrist motion s.
  Wrist Resist s.
  wrist rest s.
  yucca wood s.
  Zimfoam s.
  Zimmer airplane s.
  Zimmer clavicular cross s.
  Zim-Trac traction s.
  Zim-Zip rib belt s.
  Zollinger s.
  Zucker s.
splintage
splinted in position of function
splintered fracture
splinting
  dynamic s.
  s. material
  s. method
  night s.

  pelvic s.
  silicone thermoplastic s. (STS)
  Strong dorsal extension block s.
  s. therapy
splintlike pain
split
  s. anterior tibialis tendon transfer
    (SPLATT)
  s. anterior tibial tendon
  s. anterior tibial tendon procedure
  s. calvarial bone graft
  s. foot
  s. fracture
  s. hand
  s. heel approach
  s. heel fracture
  s. heel incision
  s. incision
  longitudinal tendon s.
  s. patellar approach
  s. pelvis
  peroneus brevis s. (PBS)
  s. Russell skeletal traction
  s. screen
  s. stirrup
split-depression fracture
split-finger hook
split-hand deformity
split-nail deformity
split-thickness
  s.-t. skin excision (STSE)
  s.-t. skin graft (STSG)
spoke-wheel configuration
Sponastrine dysplasia
spondylalagia
spondylalgia
spondylarthritis
spondylectomy
spondylexarthrosis
spondylitis
  ankylosing s.
  Bekhterev rheumatoid s.
  Bekhterev-Strümpell s.
  s. deformans
  hypertrophic s.
  juvenile-onset ankylosing s.
  Kümmell s.
  Marie-Strümpell s.
  rheumatoid s.
  tuberculous s.
spondylizema
spondyloarthropathy (SpA)
  inflammatory s.
  sacroiliac joint inflammatory s.
spondyloarthrosis
spondylodesis
  ventral derotation s. (VDS)
spondylodiscitis
spondylodynia

spondyloepiphysial
  s. dysplasia
  s. dysplasia of Maroteaux
spondylogenic
spondylolisthesis
  anteroinferior s.
  5 classifications of s.
  congenital s.
  degenerative s.
  doweling s.
  dysplastic s.
  Gill-Manning-White s.
  high-grade s.
  isthmic s.
  lumbosacral s.
  Meyerding grading of s.
  pathologic s.
  postlaminectomy 2-level s.
  s. reduction
  s. reduction fixation
  sagittal roll s.
  slip angle s.
  symptomatic s.
  traumatic s.
  Winter s.
spondylolisthetic pelvis
spondyloloptosis
spondylolysis
  cervical s.
  contralateral s.
spondylomalacia
spondylometer
spondylopathy
spondylophyte
spondyloptosis
spondylopyosis
spondyloschisis
spondylosis
  central spine s.
  cervical s.
  s. deformans
  degenerative s.
  dystrophic s.
  hyperostotic s.
  lumbar s.
  Nurick classification of s.
  rhizomelic s.
  Scheuermann dystrophic s.
  thoracolumbar s.
spondylosyndesis
spondylotherapy

spondylotic
  s. bar
  s. spur
spondylotomy
sponge
  Adaptic s.
  bone wax gelatin s.
  buffing s.
  s. clamp
  EZ Bend s.
  gauze s.
  Helistat absorbable collagen
    hemostatic s.
  Instat collagen s.
  laparotomy s.
  Mikulicz s.
  Pedic s.
  Ray-Tec s.
  s. stick
  Telfa s.
  s. test
  Vistec x-ray detectable s.
sponge-holding forceps
spongialization
spongiosa
  primary s.
  s. screw
spongiosum
  osteoma s.
spongy
  s. appearance
  s. bone
Sponsel oblique osteotomy
spontaneous
  s. activity
  s. amputation
  s. fracture
  s. hyperemic dislocation
  s. median neuropathy
  s. postfracture epiphysiodesis
  s. rupture
  s. vacuum phenomenon
  s. wrist clunk
spoon
  maroon s.
  meniscal s.
  s. plate
Sporothrix schenckii
sporotrichosis
S'port
  S. Max back support
  S. Max sacroiliac belt
  S. Max stabilization pad

S

NOTES

S'port *(continued)*
>Posture S.
>Scully Hip S.

sport
>S.'s Activity Scale
>s.'s anemia
>s.'s anemia exercise
>s.'s chiropractic
>S. Cord
>s.'s injury
>lateral motion racket s.
>s.'s medicine
>s.'s medicine law
>s.'s participation
>pivoting s.'s
>S.'s Plus II back belt
>S. Preforms orthotic
>stop-and-go s.'s
>s.'s tape
>s.'s terminal device

SportCord exercise and rehabilitation system

Sportelli system collimator mounted contact shield

Sporthotics orthotic

Sportono
>cementless S. (CLS)

Sport-Rite
>S.-R. Olympian device
>S.-R. orthotics
>S.-R. Runner device

Sports-Caster I, II knee brace

Sports-Grip bar

sportsman's
>s. hernia
>s. toe

SportsRAC arm care system

sportstape
>Leukotape P s.

Sportstim
>S. muscle stimulation electrode
>S. stimulator

Sport-Stirrup orthosis

SporTX
>S. pulsed direct current stimulator
>S. stimulation device

spot
>café-au-lait s.
>Carleton s.
>de Morgan s.
>s. film
>s. radiograph
>s. view
>s. weld

spot-face reamer

Spotorno
>S. cementless hip arthroplasty stem
>S. hip prosthesis
>S. index

spotted bone disease

SPR
>selective posterior rhizotomy
>superior peroneal retinaculum

Sprague arthroscopic technique

sprain
>acromioclavicular s.
>ankle s.
>anterior cruciate s.
>anterior talofibular s.
>calcaneofibular s.
>chronic ankle s.
>chronic foot s.
>deltoid s.
>fibular collateral s.
>foot s.
>s. fracture
>inversion ankle s.
>joint s.
>lateral ankle s.
>lateral collateral s.
>ligament rupture s.
>medial collateral s.
>postacute s.
>posterior cruciate s.
>posterior oblique s.
>relapsing ankle s.
>rider's s.
>syndesmotic s.
>talocrural s.
>talonavicular s.
>tibiofibular s.

sprained ankle syndrome

Spratt
>S. bone curette
>S. mastoid curette

spray
>air plasma s. (APS)
>AliCool splint s.
>Aqua S.
>HandClens ultra antiseptic s.
>L'Aprina topical s.
>low-pressure plasma s. (LLPS)
>Proderm topical s.
>s. and stretch
>s. and stretch technique
>vasocoolant s.

spread
>s. foot
>Fowler s.
>s. hand

spreader
>Assistant Free calibrated femoral tibial s.
>Bailey rib s.
>s. bar
>Beeson cast s.
>Beeson plaster s.
>Blount bone s.

Blount laminar s.
Bobechko s.
bone s.
Burford-Finochietto rib s.
Burford rib s.
calcaneal s.
Cloward s.
Haglund-Stille plaster s.
Harrington s.
Henning cast s.
Henning plaster s.
Inge s.
laminar s.
Lilienthal rib s.
M-Pact cast s.
Nelson rib s.
small lamina s.
TSRH eyebolt s.
Weinraub joint and calcaneal s.

spreading
s. forceps
s. hand splint

Sprengel deformity
spring
S. angled adjustable barbell
s. cock-up splint
compression s.
s. finger
s. fixation
Gruca-Weiss s.
internal fixation s.
s. ligament
s. ligament complex
s. pin
s. plate
s. swivel thumb
s. test
Weiss s.

Springer fracture
Springlite
S. Advantage DP
S. G foot component
S. II foot component
S. lower limb prosthesis
S. low profile Symes II
S. polyolefin BK cover
S. polyurethane AK, BK conical cover
S. super low profile Symes II
S. toe filler

spring-loaded
s.-l. knee lock

s.-l. lock orthosis
s.-l. nail

spring-mounted electromagnet
spring-wire
s.-w. ankle-foot orthosis
s.-w. safety pin splint

sprint
S. Climber
S. cross trainer
S. Runner

sprinter's fracture
Spri Xercise board
sprung pelvis
S.P. 100 transcutaneous electrical neural stimulator
spur
acromial s.
anterior impingement s.
bone s.
calcaneal s.
calcific s.
cartilaginous s.
chondroosseous s.
degenerative s.
fibrous s.
s. formation
heel s.
impingement s.
inferior s.
osteophytic s.
s. pad
painful s.
plantar calcaneal s.
posterior s.
prominent s.
retrocalcaneal s.
s. sign
spondylotic s.
subacromial s.
traction s.
uncovertebral s.

spur-crushing clamp
spuria
pelvis s.

spurious
s. ankylosis
s. articular process
s. rib
s. torticollis

Spurling
S. maneuver
S. rongeur
S. test

S

NOTES

Spurling-Kerrison
 S.-K. rongeur forceps
 S.-K. upbiting and downbiting
  rongeur
spurring
 anterior s.
 bony s.
 degenerative s.
 inferior s.
spurt muscle
squamooccipital bone
squamous cell
squamous-type bone
square
 S. Module Seating System
 rocker balance s.
square-ended
 s.-e. distraction rod
 s.-e. hook
square-end pliers
square-hole broach
square-hollow chisel
square-shaped
 s.-s. awl
 s.-s. wrist test
squat
 s. jump
 s. lift
 s. test
squatting
 s. ability
 s. test
squeeze
 s. ball
 s. dynamometer
 s. exerciser
 Schaffer s.
 s. test
squinting patella
SR
 stabilizing reversal
SRF
 semirigid fiberglass cast
SRL
 short radiolunate
 SRL ligament
SRN
 superficial radial nerve
S-ROM
 S-ROM acetabular cup
 S-ROM Arthropor I–III prosthesis
 S-ROM Arthropor oblong prosthesis
 S-ROM contained shell
 S-ROM femoral stem prosthesis
 S-ROM hip prosthesis
 S-ROM hip replacement system
 S-ROM modular femoral
  component
 S-ROM modular stem

 S-ROM modular total knee system
 S-ROM Poly-Dial insert
 S-ROM proximally modular total
  hip system
 S-ROM Super Cup
 S-ROM super cup prosthesis
 S-ROM ZZT I, II prosthesis
SR-PLLA
 self-reinforcing polylevolactic acid
SRS
 skeletal repair system
 SRS injectable cement
SS
 suture system
SSCS
 segmental spinal correction system
SSEP
 somatosensory evoked potential
S-shaped
 S-s. deformity
 S-s. foot
 S-s. incision
SSHR
 steady state heart rate
SSI
 School Setting Interview
 segmental spinal instrumentation
 shoulder subluxation inhibitor
  anterior-posterior fusion with SSI
  SSI brace
S-Soles insole
SST
 stainless steel rod
St.
 St. Georg-Buchholz ankle prosthesis
 St. Georg fully constrained
  prosthesis
 St. Georg sledge unicompartment
  prosthesis
 St. John's Wort
 St. Jude prosthesis
stab
 s. incision
 s. wound
 s. wound arthroscopic entry portal
stabilimetry
stability
 ankle s.
 elbow s.
 glenohumeral joint s.
 immediate postoperative s. (IPS)
 knee s.
 lateral s.
 ligamentous s.
 Limits of S. (LOS)
 lumbar spine rotational s.
 posterior s.
 rotary s.

tibiotalar s.
S. total hip system

stabilization

anterior short-segment s.
s. approach
atlantoaxial s.
cervical spine s.
cervicothoracic junction s.
s. of chevron procedure
definitive s.
distal radioulnar joint s.
dynamic lumbar s.
flexion compression spine injury s.
foot s.
fracture s.
iliac crest bone graft s.
lower cervical spine posterior s.
myoplastic muscle s.
occipitocervical s.
odontoid fracture s.
open s.
patellar tendon s. (PTS)
s. plate
posterior lower cervical spine s.
prophylactic operative s.
provisional s.
rhythmic s.
sacral spine s.
screw s.
skeletal s.
spinal injury operative s.
spinal osteotomy s.
subluxation s.
thoracolumbar spine s.
s. training
TSRH crosslink s.
wire s.

stabilizer

ankle s.
Dynamic foot s.
foot s.
forearm s.
Freedom thumb s.
Heel Hugger therapeutic heel s.
kneecap s.
KT-1000 foot s.
Palumbo ankle s.
patellar s.
secondary s.
Verteflex arthrotonic s.

stabilizing

s. bar

s. hinge
s. reversal (SR)

stable

s. burst fracture
s. cervical spine injury
s. gait
s. hinge joint
s. to motion
s. reduction
s. vertebra

Stablecut sawblade

Stableloc

S. Colles fracture external fixator
S. external wrist fixation system
S. II external fixation
S. II external fixation system

stack

S. shoulder procedure
S. splint

stacking cone

Stader

S. pin
S. pin guide
S. splint

Stadol NS

stage

1-s. amputation
distraction-flexion s. (DFS)
Eichenholz s.
Enneking disease s.
Ficat and Arlet disease s.
Greulich-Pyle skeletal maturation s.
hard callus s.
implant s.
late s.
S. model of industrial rehabilitation
Risser s.
silent hip s.
soft callus s.

2-stage

2-s. hip fusion
2-s. Syme amputation
2-s. tendon grafting technique
2-s. tendon graft reconstruction

staged procedure

staggered procedure

staggering gait

staghorn calculus

staging

Enneking s.
Functional Assessment S. (FAST)
Lichtman s.

NOTES

staging *(continued)*
    Outerbridge degenerative arthritis s.
    Waldenström s.
Stagnara
    S. gouge
    S. wake-up test
stagnation
    foot s.
    qi s.
Staheli
    S. rotational profile
    S. shelf procedure
    S. technique
    S. test
Stahl
    S. classification (stage I-V)
    S. index
    S. Kienbock disease classification
    S. staging system
stain
    Elastichrome s.
    Gram s.
    port-wine s.
    reticulin s.
    Stevenel blue s.
    Verhoeff s.
stainless
    s. steel
    s. steel alloy
    s. steel clamp
    s. steel equipment
    s. steel implant metal prosthesis
    s. steel mesh
    s. steel and molybdenum (SMO)
    s. steel plate
    s. steel rod (SST)
    s. steel screw
    s. steel staple
    s. steel wire
stair
    s. running test
    s. sign
staircase phenomenon
StairClimber assist device
stairclimber's foot
stair-climbing exercise
StairMaster exercise system
stairstep
    cervical s.
    s. fracture
stall bar
Stamm
    S. metatarsal osteotomy
    S. method
    S. procedure
    S. procedure for intraarticular hip fusion
stamp
    Gelfoam s.

stamping gait
stance
    calcaneal s.
    double-leg s.
    frontside snowboard s.
    initial s.
    late s.
    s. phase
    s. phase of gait
    s. phase walking
    single-limb s.
    terminal s.
    through s.
stand
    Atlas adjustable s.
    Cherf cast s.
    Grand Stand support s.
    heel s.
    IMP turnstile casting s.
    stork s.
    turnstile casting s.
    Versa-Helper floor s.
standard
    s. deviation
    S. E-Z-On Vest
    s. goniometric measure
    s. imaging sequence
    s. 2-inch blade retractor
    s. 4-inch blade retractor
    s. medullary nail
    s. shell ankle-foot orthosis
    s. socket
    s. thoracotomy
    s. U patellar support
standardized growth curve
standing
    s. apprehension test
    s. dorsoplantar view
    s. flexion
    s. flexion test
    s. frame orthosis
    s. Gillet test
    s. knee bend PSIS-sacrum contact
    s. lateral view
    s. side bend
    s. stability walking component
    s. weightbearing view
Stanford Hypnotic Clinical Scale
Stanisavljevic technique
Stanmore
    S. knee replacement
    S. shoulder arthroplasty
    S. shoulder prosthesis
    S. total hip replacement
    S. totally constrained elbow prosthesis
Staodyne EMS+2 neurostimulator
stapedial tenotomy

STA-peg
    subtalar joint arthroereisis peg
    STA-peg implant
    STA-peg procedure
    Smith STA-peg
STA-Pen writer pen
Staph-Chek
    S.-C. pad
    S.-C. Synergy fabric
staphylococcal
    s. arthritis
    s. pyomyositis
staphylorrhaphy elevator
staple
    s. arthroereisis
    Arthrotek meniscus s.
    automatic s.
    barbed s.
    Biomet s.
    Blount fracture s.
    Bostick s.
    s. capsulorrhaphy
    capsulorrhaphy s.
    Coventry s.
    Day fixation s.
    DePalma s.
    Downing s.
    s. driver
    duToit shoulder s.
    Ellison fixation s.
    epiphysial s.
    s. extractor
    Fastlok implantable s.
    s. fixation
    GIA s.
    s. gun
    Hernandez-Ros bone s.
    s. holder
    Howmedica Vitallium s.
    s. inserter
    s. introducer
    Johannesberg s.
    Krackow HTO blade s.
    3M s.
    memory compression s.
    meniscal s.
    s. migration
    O'Brien s.
    osteoclast tension s.
    Richards fixation s.
    SD sorb s.
    skin s.

    Smith & Nephew medium
      barbed s.
    Smith & Nephew small barbed s.
    stainless steel s.
    Stone 4-point s.
    Stryker soft tissue s.
    s. suture
    tabletop Stone s.
    TA metallic s.
    TA Premium 30, 55, 90 s.
    Uni-Clip s.
    vitallium s.
    Wiberg fracture s.
    Zimaloy s.
stapler
    Auto Suture s.
    Biologically quiet s.
    Closer s.
    Dwyer spinal mechanical s.
    GIA s.
    Hall double-hole spinal s.
    metaphysial s.
    Oswestry-O'Brien spinal s.
    powered metaphysial s.
    Wiberg fracture s.
Staples
    S. elbow arthrodesis
    S. repair
    S. technique
stapling
    Blount s.
    epiphysial s.
    percutaneous s.
    physial s.
STAR
    Scandinavian total ankle replacement
    STAR ankle joint prosthesis
    STAR technique
star
    4-s. exercise program
    s. gait
starch
    s. bandage
    s. test
Stardox wrist brace
Stark
    S. arthrodesis
    S. graft
Starrett pin vise
starter
    nail s.
stasimorphia
stasis ulcer

S

NOTES

Statak
S. anchor system
S. curette
S. soft tissue attachment device
state
gradient-recalled acquisition in
steady s. (GRASS)
Middlesex Elderly Assessment of
Mental S. (MEAMS)
pathomechanical s.
proinflammatory s.
prothrombotic s.
Stat Graphics software
static
s. alignment
s. arthropathy
s. back
s. compression
s. compression plate
s. evaluation
s. fatigue
s. fixation
s. foot deformity
s. foot pain
s. footprint
s. listing
s. listing nomenclature
s. locking nail
s. lock nailing
s. orthosis
s. palpation
s. scoliosis
s. splint
s. stretch
s. stretching
s. tendon transfer
s. traction
statically
Staticin Topical
station
Aquatrend water workout s.
s. and gait
gait and s.
s. test
unsteadiness of gait and s.
stationary
s. angle guide
s. arthropathy
s. attachment flexible endoskeletal
(SAFE)
s. attachment flexible endoskeletal
orthotic
stature
short s.
status
ambulatory s.
hydration s.
intact neurovascular s.
s. loading

neurovascular s.
s. post
Repeatable Battery for the
Assessment of
Neuropsychological S. (RBANS)
Stauffer modification
Stax fingertip splint
stay
length of s. (LOS)
spiral s.
s. wire
StayFuse implant
stay-retractor
Freebody s.-r.
S-T Cort
STC 900-series travel chair
steady state heart rate (SSHR)
steal
s. effect
s. syndrome
stealth
S. anchor
S. frame
S. image-guided system
S. knee brace
steam sterilization
Stedman awl
steel
austenitic stainless s.
S. correction
S. maneuver
martensitic stainless s.
S. rule of thirds
S. shank
s. sole plate orthosis
stainless s.
S. triple innominate osteotomy
S. triradiate osteotomy
steering wheel injury
Steffee
S. instrument
S. instrumentation technique
S. pedicle plate
S. pedicle screw-plate system
S. plate and screw
S. screw plate
S. spinal instrumentation
S. thumb arthroplasty
S. variable spine plating system
Steichen neurovascular free flap
Steida
S. bony process
S. fracture
Steinbach mallet
Steinberg
S. infiltration block
S. rating scale
**Steinbrocker rheumatoid arthritis
classification**

Steindler
  S. effect
  S. elbow arthrodesis
  S. flexorplasty
  S. matricectomy
  S. procedure
  S. stripping
Steinert
  S. disease
  S. epiphysial fracture classification
Steinhauser bone clamp
Steinmann
  S. extension nail
  S. fixation pin
  S. pin fixation
  S. pin with ball bearing
  S. pin with Crowe pilot point
  S. pin with pin chuck
  S. tendon forceps
  S. test
  S. traction
stellate
  s. fracture
  s. nail bed laceration
  s. sympathetic ganglion block
Stellbrink fixation device
Stelling and Tucker polydactyly classification
stem
  Aequalis s.
  APR hip s.
  APR I femoral s.
  Aufranc-Turner s.
  s. base plate
  Biomet revision hip s.
  calcar replacement s.
  collarless s.
  s. component
  Continuum hip s.
  contoured femoral s. (CFS)
  Corail HA-coated s.
  CRM s.
  s. deformation
  Engh-Glassman femoral s.
  Exeter s.
  Extend s.
  s. extractor
  s. failure
  fenestrated s.
  F2L Multineck femoral s.
  Harris-Galante s.
  HG multilock hip s.
  hydroxyapatite-coated s.

implant s.
intramedullary s.
Iowa s.
Kirschner s.
KMP femoral s.
Linear hip s.
Link MP microporous hip s.
long s. (LS)
Mallory-Head femoral s.
Moore s.
Natural-Hip titanium hip s.
nonfenestrated s.
Omnifit s.
Omnifit-C s.
Opti-Fix hip s.
Osteonics Omnifit-C s.
Osteonics Omnifit-HA hip s.
PCA hip s.
Perfecta femoral s.
PFC hip s.
Precision hip s.
press-fit s.
primary s. (PS)
Profile hip s.
Profix metaphysial tibial s.
Ranawat-Burstein porous s.
regular s.
s. removal
Revision hip s.
Richards modular s.
roundback s.
SL-Plus s.
Spotorno cementless hip arthroplasty s.
S-ROM modular s.
straight femoral s.
Taperloc femoral s.
trial s.
Ultima calcar s.'s
Ultima Fx s.'s
Zimmer bone s.
stemmed tibial prosthesis
Stemmer sign
Stener-Gunterberg hip operation
Stener lesion
stenosans
  tenosynovitis serosa s.
stenosed
stenosing tenosynovitis
stenosis, pl. **stenoses**
  achondroplastic s.
  ankylosing spinal s.
  central canal s.

S

NOTES

stenosis *(continued)*
  cervical s.
  combined s.
  congenital s.
  constitutional s.
  degenerative s.
  foraminal s.
  lateral recess s. (LRS)
  multisegmental spinal s.
  neural foraminal s. (NFS)
  spinal canal s. (SCS)
stent
  Carcon s.
  Dacron s.
  s. dressing
  Omnifit HA hip s.
  synthetic s.
stenting
Stenver view
Stenzel
  S. rod
  S. rod prosthesis
step
  CUBEx multifunctional s.
  s. defect
  s. drill
  equinus s.
  s. exercise
  s. length
  s. osteotomy
  s. out, turn out (SOTO)
  s. screw
  s. time
  s. width
step-cut
  s.-c. lengthening
  s.-c. osteotomy
  s.-c. reamer
  s.-c. transection
step-down
  s.-d. drill
  s.-d. osteotomy
Stephen
  S. scissors
  S. spreader bar
stepladder sign
step-off
  s.-o. between bone fracture
    fragments
  s.-o. of fracture
steppage gait
stepper
  Diamondback 1100 recumbent s.
  Diamondback 1100 self-generated s.
  Diamondback 100 upright s.
  NuStep total body recumbent s.
step-up
  lateral s.-u.

stereoarthrolysis
stereognosis
stereolithography (SL)
  s. cage
stereophotogrammetry (SPG)
  optical s.
  roentgen s.
stereotactic arc
stereotaxic anterior capsulotomy
Steri-Clamp
  S.-C. clamp
  IMP S.-C.
  Innovative Medical Products S.-C.
Steri-Cuff
  S.-C. disposable tourniquet cuff
  S.-C. Plus
sterile
  s. condition
  s. dry dressing (SDD)
  s. loosening
  s. matrix
  s. pencil
  s. saline solution
  s. sheet
  s. sheeting
  s. towel
sterilization
  ethylene oxide s.
  gas s.
  steam s.
  tissue s.
Steri-Strip skin closure
Sterivap cement gun
sterna (*pl. of* sternum)
sternal
  s. approximator
  s. attachment component
  s. rib
sternal-occipital-mandibular
  s.-o.-m. immobilization (SOMI)
  s.-o.-m. immobilizer
  s.-o.-m. immobilizer orthosis
sternal-occipital-manubrial immobilizer
sternochondral articulation
sternoclavicular (SC)
  s. angle
  s. articulation
  s. disc
  s. joint (SCJ)
  s. joint dislocation
  s. joint injury
  s. joint reconstruction
  s. joint reduction
  s. joint separation
  s. ligament
sternocleidomastoid
  s. muscle
  s. muscle fibromatosis

sternocostal
  s. joint
  s. ligament
sternohyoid muscle
sternomastoid muscle
sternooccipital mandibular immobilizer orthosis
sternothyroid muscle
sternotomy
sternoxiphoid plane
sternum, pl. **sterna**
  duplicate s.
  s. fracture
sternum-splitting approach
steroid
  epidural s.
  s. injection
  s. myopathy
  performance-enhancing s.
  tapering dose s.
  s. therapy
steroid-induced
  s.-i. avascular necrosis
  s.-i. bone disease
  s.-i. osteonecrosis
Stevenel blue stain
Stevens-Street
  S.-S. elbow prosthesis
  S.-S. elbow prosthesis template
Steward-Milford fracture classification
Stewart
  S. arm operation
  S. distal clavicular excision
  S. styloidectomy
Stewart-Morel syndrome
Steytler-Van Der Walt procedure
STH-2 hip prosthesis
sthenometry
stick
  Back Revolution S.
  dressing s.
  FMS Intracell s.
  Intracell massage s.
  Intracell Sprinter s.
  sponge s.
  switching s.
  s. tie ligature
  weighted walking s.
Stickler syndrome
Stieda
  S. fracture
  S. tubercle

STIF
  spinopelvic transiliac fixation
  STIF system
stiff
  s. gait
  s. man syndrome
  s. ray
  s. ribbon retractor
  s. toe
stiff-knee gait
stiff-legged gait
stiffness
  axial s.
  fusion s.
  joint s.
  resting shear s.
  shear s.
  small-joint s.
  torsional s.
stiff-soled shoe
stifle joint
stigmatic electrode
Stiles-Bunnell transfer technique
Still disease
Stille
  S. bone biter
  S. bone chisel
  S. bone drill
  S. bone drill set
  S. bone gouge
  S. brace
  S. bur
  S. hand drill
  S. osteotome
  S. plaster shears
  S. rongeur
Stille-Horsley
  S.-H. bone forceps
  S.-H. bone rongeur
  S.-H. rib forceps
Stille-Liston bone-cutting forceps
Stille-Luer
  S.-L. bone rongeur
  S.-L. duckbill rongeur
  S.-L. rongeur forceps
Stille-Luer-Echlin rongeur
Stille-pattern trephine and bone drill set
Stiller rib
Stille-Ruskin bone rongeur
Stille-Sherman bone drill

S

NOTES

StIM
StIM neuromuscular stimulator system
StIM system
Stimoceiver implant material
Stimprene
S. electrotherapy brace
S. wrap
Stimson
S. anterior shoulder reduction technique
S. dressing
S. gravity method
gravity method of S.
S. maneuver
S. reduction
stimulated graciloplasty
stimulating
s. electrode
s. massage
stimulation
antidromic s.
continuous s.
cookbook s.
cranial electrical s. (CES)
cycled s.
direct electrical nerve s. (DENS)
double simultaneous sensory s.
electrical bone-growth s. (EBGS)
electrical nerve s.
electrical surface s.
electronic bone s. (EBI)
electrotherapeutic point s. (ETPS)
external-coil electrical s.
functional electrical s. (FES)
functional neuromuscular s.
galvanic s.
high-voltage pulsed s. (HVPS)
high-voltage pulsed galvanic s. (HVPGS)
interferential s. (IFC)
interferential electrical s.
lateral electrical surface s. (LESS)
magnetic s.
marrow s.
microamperage electrical nerve s. (MENS)
microamperage neural s. (MNS)
neuromuscular electrical s. (NMES)
OrthoLogic 1000 bone growth s.
OsteoGen bone growth s.
Osteo-Stim implantable bone growth s.
PEMF bone growth s.
pulsed electric magnetic field bone growth s.
reciprocal s.
repetitive nerve s.
rhythmic auditory s. (RAS)

transcutaneous electrical nerve s. (TENS)
stimulation-ultrasound
Amrex SynchroSonic muscle s.-u.
stimulator
Acupoint s.
AcuTENS transcutaneous nerve s.
AME bone growth s.
Amrex muscle s.
Back Hammer muscle s.
battery-pack Osteo-Stim bone s.
Biolectron bone growth s.
BioStim Digital NMS muscle s.
bone growth s.
constant direct current s.
dorsal column s. (DCS)
EBI Medical OsteoGen bone growth s.
EBI SpF-2 implantable bone s.
EBI SpF-T implantable bone s.
electrical bone-growth s. (EBGS)
Electro-Acuscope 85 s.
EMS 2000 neuromuscular s.
Endo Multi-Mode s.
Freedom Micro Pro s.
galvanic electrode s.
G5 Porta-Plus muscle s.
implanted bone growth s.
Intelect electric s.
Intelect Legend s.
Intelect 600MP microcurrent s.
interferential s.
Magnum 100 s.
Magnum 101 Plus s.
Master-Stim interferential s.
Maxima II transcutaneous electrical nerve s.
Medi-Stim s.
Mettler Trio neuromuscular electrical s.
Micro-Z neuromuscular s.
MS322 muscle s.
neuromuscular III s.
Nuwave transcutaneous electrical nerve s.
Ortho DX electromedical s.
Orthofix Cervical-Stim bone growth s.
Orthofuse implantable growth s.
OrthoGen bone growth s.
OrthoLogic 1000 bone growth s.
OrthoPak II bone growth s.
OsteoGen implantable bone growth s.
Osteo-Stim implantable bone growth s.
PGS-3000 pulsed galvanic s.
Physio-Stim Lite bone growth s.
Piezo electro-needleless s.

Precision spinal cord s.
prizm Electro-Mesh Z-Stim-II s.
pulsed galvanic s.
repetitive nerve s. (RNS)
Respond II muscle s.
SpF spinal fusion s.
spinal cord s. (SCS)
spinal fusion s.
SpinalPak bone growth s.
SpinalPak spine fusion s.
Sportstim s.
SporTX pulsed direct current s.
S.P. 100 transcutaneous electrical
  neural s.
Stimuplex-S nerve s.
Super Stimm MF s.
Surgi-Stim s.
SynchroSonic s.
SysStim 226 muscle s.
Theramini 1, 2 electrotherapy s.
Theratouch 4.7 s.
ThermaStim muscle s.
Trio-Stim neuromuscular s.
Zimmer Osteo Stim bone
  growth s.
Z-Stim IF 100, 250 microprocessor
  controlled s.
Z-Stim 100 microprocessor
  controlled s.
stimulator/ultrasound
Intelect Combo s./u.
Stimulite honeycomb mattress overlay
stimulus, pl. **stimuli**
s. artifact
conditioned s. (CS)
maximal s.
paired s.
submaximal s.
subthreshold s.
supramaximal s.
test s.
threshold s.
unconditional s. (US)
Stimuplex block needle
Stimuplex-S nerve stimulator
Stinchfield test
stinger injury
sting mat
stippled epiphysis
stippling
STIR
short time inversion recovery

stirrup
Aircast pneumatic air s.
Allen s.
Böhler s.
s. brace
Comfort Cast s.
s. plaster splint
split s.
Swivel-Strap ankle s.
traction s.
walking s.
stitch
Allgöwer s.
apical s.
baseball s.
Bunnell s.
Frost s.
intracuticular s.
Kessler s.
Mersilene Kessler s.
Pulvertaft fish-mouth s.
roll s.
Rousso s.
stitcher
Acufex meniscal s.
Stiwer
S. bone-holding forceps
S. hand drill
STJ
subtalar joint
St Joseph Adult Chewable Aspirin
STNP
subtalar joint neutral position
stock
bone s.
S. finger splint
osteopenic bone s.
poor bone s.
Stockholm hand arm vibration
  syndrome staging system
stockinette
s. bandage
basket s.
bias-cut s.
Buck traction s.
orthopaedic s.
s. sling
s. tube
tubular s.
Velpeau s.
stocking-glove distribution
stockings
antiembolic s.

S

NOTES

stockings *(continued)*
 CircAid elastic s.
 compression s.
 dropfoot redression s.
 elastic s.
 Jobst s.
 long leg s.
 Medi Plus compression s.
 Orthawear antiembolism s.
 Planostretch s.
 pneumatic compression s.
 SCD s.
 Sigvaris s.
 Silver-Thera s.
 Soft Touch s.
 TED s.
 thromboembolic s.
 Zimmer antiembolism s.
Stokes amputation
stone
 s. arthrodesis
 s. basket screw mounted handle
 S. bunionectomy
 S. clamp-locking device
 S. 4-point staple
 S. procedure
 pumice s.
Stookey reflex
stool
 foot s.
 nested step s.
 Swedish support s.
stop
 s. action brace
 Elite posterior adjustable s.
Stopain Spray topical analgesic spray
stop-and-go sports
stopwatch
storiform pattern
stork
 s. leg
 s. sign
 s. stand
Storz
 S. meniscotome
 S. Microsystems drill bit
 S. Microsystems plate cutter
 S. Microsystems pliers
 S. oblique arthroscope
 S. screw
stout-neck curette
stove-in pelvis
stovepipe leg
straddle
 s. fracture
 s. injury
StraddleSitter seating aid
straight
 s. basket forceps

 s. bone rongeur
 s. chisel
 s. curette
 s. femoral stem
 s. gouge
 s. hex screwdriver
 s. incision
 s. last shoe
 s. lateral instability
 s. leg raising (SLR)
 s. leg raising exercise
 s. leg raising test (SLRT)
 s. osteotome
 s. periosteal elevator
 s. pituitary rongeur
 s. posterior portal
 s. power reamer
 s. scissors
 s. spine syndrome
 s. stem femoral component
 s. threaded rod
 s. walker brace
strain
 acute foot s.
 articular s.
 back s.
 Brunhilde s.
 compression s.
 elastic s.
 s. energy
 foot s.
 s. fracture
 s. gauge
 muscle s.
 plastic s.
 postural s.
 shear s.
 tensile s.
 thoracolumbosacral s. (TLS)
 TLS s.
strain/counterstrain technique
strain-gauge extensometer
strain-sprain injury
strain-stress curve
strap
 Band-It tennis elbow s.
 Beta Pile II, III splint s.
 buddy s.
 Butterfly cushion with s.
 capsular s.
 Cho-pat Achilles tendon s.
 Cho-pat Dual Action Knee S.
 Cho-pat elbow s.
 Cho-pat ITB S.
 s. clavicular splint
 counterforce s.
 crotch s.
 D-ring s.
 Eclipse Gel elbow s.

elastic s.
external elastic s.
extremity mobilization s.
FoamWrap ThumDuction s.
foot drop s.
fork s.
Gel-Bank patellar s.
infrapatellar s.
Lema s.
Levine patellar tendon s.
S. Lok ankle brace
Meek clavicular s.
s. muscle
neoprene wrist s.
Nylatex s.
Partridge s.
Pebax fastening s.
PIP/DIP s.
Pro-Tec patellar tendon s.
QualCraft s.
Scott elastic ankle s.
s. sling
stretch-out s.
suprapatellar s.
suspension s.
Synergistic suspension s.
valgus corrective ankle s.
varus corrective ankle s.
Velcro s.

strapping
adhesive s.
AliStrap Velcro-type s.
garter s.
loop and hook s.
Low-Dye s.

Strassburg sock
Strata hip system
strategy
cuing s.
diagnostic s.

Stratis ST ACL reconstruction system
Stratos orthotic
stratum corneum
Stratus impact-reducing pylon
Straub technique
Strayer
S. Achilles lengthening procedure
S. gastrocnemius recession
S. gastrocnemius-soleus recession
S. lengthening
S. tendon technique

streaming potential
streblodactyly

street
S. forearm nail
S. medullary pin
Streeter dysplasia
Street-Stevens humeral prosthesis
strength
5/5 s.
s. against resistance
axial gripping s.
bending s.
bone s.
bone-screw interface s.
BUE s.
C-D instrumentation fixation s.
cervical extension s.
Cotrel pedicle screw fixation s.
s. curve
extensor hallucis longus s.
extrinsic muscle s.
fatigue s.
fixation s.
graft s.
grip s.
hand grasp s.
hand grip s.
intrinsic muscle s.
isometric cervical extension s.
Lovett clinical scale of s.
motor s.
pedicle screw pull-out s.
pinch s.
pull-out s.
tensile s.
s. test eccentric bilateral
s. testing
torsional gripping s.
s. training
ultimate s.
yield s.

strength-duration curve
strengthened
gas atomized dispersion s. (GADS)
strengthening
s. exerciser
rehabilitation muscle s.
wrist extensor s.
wrist flexor s.
streptococcal myositis
stress
arch s.
bending s.
biomechanical s.
contact s.

NOTES

stress *(continued)*
    s. distribution
    s. dorsiflexion projection
    s. examination
    fatigue s.
    s. film
    s. fracture
    heat s.
    hyperextension s.
    s. injury
    laxity to varus s.
    longitudinal arch s.
    low-contact s. (LCS)
    measured s.
    mediolateral s.
    principal s.
    s. radiograph
    s. radiography
    s. riser
    s. roentgenography
    s. rupture
    shear s.
    s. shielding
    tensile s.
    s. test
    s. testing
    torsional s.
    s. transfer
    transverse arch s.
    valgus s.
    varus-valgus s.
    s. view
    Von Mises s.
    s. x-ray
stress-corrosion cracking
stressor
Stress-Ray varus-valgus device
stress-relaxation
    intraoperative s.-r.
stress-strain curve
stress-testing arthrometer
stretch
    s. cable
    carpal tunnel s.
    crossed-leg pike down s.
    diagonal s.
    elastic s.
    general capsular s.
    heel cord s.
    S. and Heel night splint
    s. injury
    low-load prolonged s. (LLPS)
    passive s.
    s. pattern
    quick s.
    s. receptor
    s. reflex
    repeated quick s. (RQS)
    slow s.

    spray and s.
    static s.
    s. test
    triplane s.
    Vapo coolant spray and s.
    wrist extensor s.
    wrist and finger flexor s.
stretcher
    hamstring s.
    shoe s.
stretching
    bullet s.
    s. contraindication
    gastrocnemius-soleus s.
    nerve s.
    s. program
    range of motion therapeutic s.
    soft tissue s.
    static s.
    s. velocity
stretch-out strap
Stretch-Rite exerciser system
striata
    osteopathia s.
striatal
    s. lesion
    s. toe
striated
    s. muscle
    s. nail
Strickland
    S. modification
    S. technique
    S. tendon repair
stride
    S. Analyzer
    s. length
    s. length of gait
    s. time
strike
    heel s.
    knee s.
    s. phase of gait
striker
    forefoot s.
    forefoot-to-rearfoot s.
string drawing board
stringiness
stringing peg
strip
    corticocancellous bone s.
    Fas-Trac s.
    gastrocnemius-soleus fascial s.
    s. posting
    Thera-Band s.
stripe
    vertebral s.
striped muscle

stripout
    screw s.
stripper
    Acufex microsurgical tendon s.
    Brand tendon s.
    Bunnell tendon s.
    cartilage s.
    Fischer tendon s.
    orthopaedic surgical s.
    pigtail tendon s.
    slotted tendon s.
    tendon s.
stripping
    Steindler s.
stroke
    heat s.
    s. test
    s. volume
stroker
    skin s.
stroke-related deconditioning
stroking
    deep s.
stroller
    adapted s.
stroma, pl. **stromata**
    fibrovascular connective tissue s.
Stromeyer
    S. Achilles tenotomy procedure
    S. splint
Stromgren
    S. ankle brace
    S. support
Stromqvist hook pin system
Strong dorsal extension block splinting
Stronghands hand exerciser
strontium-85 resorption rate
Stroop test
structural
    s. aluminum malleable (SAM)
    s. bone graft
    s. component
    s. congenital myopathy
    s. curve
    s. derangement
    s. intersegmental distortion
    s. scoliosis
structure
    articular s.
    contiguous vertebral s.
    cordlike s.
    extraarticular s.
    graft s.

Hedrocel tantalum metal s.
intraarticular s.
keystone s.
ligamentous s.
neurovascular s.
osseous s.
posterolateral s.
ring s.
uniaxial s.
waist of anatomical s.
Wolff law of bone s.
structured bone
strumming
    perpendicular s.
Strümpell
    S. disease
    S. sign
Strümpell-Marie disease
Strunsky sign
strut
    s. bone graft
    fibrotic s.
    s. fusion technique
    Littig s.
    s. plate fixation
    2-s. tibial graft technique
Struthers
    arcade of S.
    ligament of S.
strut-type pin
Stryker
    S. bed
    S. camera
    S. cartilage knife
    S. CPM exerciser
    S. dermatome
    S. drill
    S. fracture frame
    S. Howmedica Osteonics
    S. Intracompartmental Pressure
      Monitor System
    S. knee joint laxity device
    S. knee laxity arthrometer
    S. lag screw
    S. leg exerciser
    S. power instrumentation
    S. saw
    S. screwdriver
    S. SE3 drive system
    S. soft tissue staple
    S. surgical hand table
    S. turning frame
    S. viewing arthroscope

S

NOTES

Stryker-Notch view
STS
> silicone thermoplastic splinting
>> STS molding sock

STSE
> split-thickness skin excision

STSG
> split-thickness skin graft

STT
> scaphotrapezoid-trapezial
> superficial tibiotalar
>> STT joint
>> STT ligament

Stuart Gordon hand splint
stubbed shoulder
Stubbs
> S. acromioclavicular splint
> S. elastic wrist support
> S. 4-way clavicle brace

stucco keratosis
stuck finger
student
> s. elbow
> National Alliance for Blind S.'s

studio cycling
study
> air-contrast s.
> anatomopathological s.
> bone density s.
> cinematographic gait s.
> cohort s.
> Copenhagen Stroke s.
> Cornwall hip fracture s.
> Doppler s.
> double-contrast s.
> electrophysiologic s.
> evoked potential s.
> fluorescein s.
> injection s.
> Johns Hopkins National Low Back Pain S.
> kinematic s.
> Michigan Bone Health S.
> nerve conduction s. (NCS)
> radiodiagnostic s.
> roentgen-stereophotogrammatic s.
> sudomotor s.
> in vivo s.

Stulberg
> S. hip classification
> S. hip positioner
> S. Mark II leg positioner
> S. method

stump
> amputation s.
> s. of bone
> s. edema
> foot s.
> s. hallucination

> s. neuralgia
> s. neuroma
> painful s.
> s. revision
> s. shrinker
> s. sock
> s. wrapping

stuttering of gait
STx
> STx lumbar traction device
> STx Saunders lumbar disc device

stylet
> blunt s.

stylohyoid
styloid
> s. fracture
> s. process

styloidectomy
> Stewart s.

styloideum
> os s.

stylus
> tibial s.

Styrofoam filler block
subacromial
> s. bursa
> s. bursa injection subacute rehabilitation sulindac
> s. bursal adhesion
> s. bursitis
> s. bursography
> s. decompression
> s. impingement syndrome
> s. portal
> s. space
> s. spur

subacromiodeltoid bursa
subacute
> s. hematogenous osteomyelitis
> s. subperiosteal hemorrhage

subadjacent segment
subaponeurotic abscess
subarachnoid block
subarticular
> s. cyst
> s. screw

subastragalar
> s. amputation
> s. dislocation
> s. fusion

subaxial
> s. posterior cervical spinal fusion
> s. subluxation

subcalcaneal bursitis
subcapital
> s. fracture
> s. osteotomy

subchondral
> s. bone

s. bone cyst
s. lesion
s. lucency
s. plate
s. sclerosis
subclavian
s. artery
s. artery injury
s. steal syndrome
s. vein
s. vein injury
subclavicular approach
subclavius
s. muscle
s. tendon graft
subcondylar
s. deformity
s. osteotomy
subcoracoid
s. bone
s. shoulder dislocation
s. space
subcortical defect
subcostal
s. muscle
s. plane
subcrural joint
subcutaneous
s. abscess
s. anterior transposition
s. calcaneal bursa
s. drain
s. fat sling
s. fracture
s. granuloma annulare
s. infrapatellar bursa
s. intracompartmental soft tissue
sarcoma
s. operation
s. palmar fasciotomy
s. patellar bursa
s. pseudosarcomatous fibromatosis
s. synovial bursa
s. tenotomy
s. tissue
s. trochanteric bursa
subcuticular suture
subdeltoid
s. bursa
s. bursal adhesion
s. bursitis
subdermal plexus
subdural button

subfascial
s. abscess
s. incision
s. transposition
subgaleal abscess
subglenoid shoulder dislocation
subgluteal
s. bursitis
s. hematoma
subjacent
**Subjective Shoulder Rating Scale
patient questionnaire**
sublaminar
s. fixation
s. wire
s. wiring
sublesional ulceration
subligamentous dissection
Sublimaze injection
sublimis
s. bridge syndrome
flexor digitorum s. (FDS)
s. tendon
s. tenodesis
subluxated metatarsophalangeal joint
subluxation
AS s.
ASEx s.
ASIn s.
atlantoaxial s. (AAS)
atlantoaxial rotatory s.
atlantooccipital s.
calcaneocuboid s.
compensatory structural s.
congenital hip s.
Crowe s.
facet s.
facilitated s.
fixation s.
foraminal encroachment s.
functional s.
glenohumeral joint s.
hip s.
joint s.
Madelung s.
manipulable s.
metatarsophalangeal s.
neuroarticular s.
neurofunctional s.
nonmanipulable s.
patellar s.
peroneal tendon s.
PIEx s.

NOTES

subluxation *(continued)*
> PIIn s.
> proximal tibiofibular s.
> radial head s.
> radiocapitellar s.
> radioulnar s.
> rotatory atlantoaxial s.
> sacroiliac s.
> shoulder s.
> s. stabilization
> subaxial s.
> talar s.
> tibiofibular s.
> unilateral facet s.
> unilateral interfacetal dislocation
>   or s. (UID/S)
> vertebral s.
> Volkmann s.
> wrist s.
> Yergason test of shoulder s.

subluxed vertebra
subluxing patella
submandibular
submaximal stimulus
subneural apparatus
suboccipital muscle
subperiosteal
> s. abscess
> s. amputation
> s. cortical defect
> s. dissection
> s. exposure
> s. fracture
> s. giant cell reparative granuloma
> s. new bone
> s. new bone formation

subperiosteal-paraarticular–type osteoid osteoma
subphrenic abscess
subplatysmal abscess
subsartorial tunnel
subscapular
> s. angle
> s. artery injury
> s. nerve injury
> s. tendinitis

subscapularis
> s. bursitis
> s. muscle
> s. rupture
> s. tendon
> s. tendon transfer

subscapularis-capsular lengthening
subsidence
> benign s.
> component s.
> prosthesis component s.
> vertical s.

subspinous dislocation

substance
> bone s.
> metachromatic mucoid s.

substitute
> AlloCraft bone spacer s.
> AlloMatrix injectable putty bone
>   graft s.
> Biocoral bone graft s.
> bone s.
> bone graft s. (BGS)
> Boplant Surgibone bovine bone s.
> dermal s.
> Healos bone graft s.
> OsteoSet bone graft s.
> OsteoSet-T medicated bone graft s.
> Pro Osteon 500 bone graft s.
> protein-based bone graft s.

substituting knee prosthesis
substitution
> arthroscopy-assisted patellar
>   tendon s.
> Carrell fibular s.
> creeping s.
> extensor s.
> Marshall patelloquadriceps tendon s.
> patellar tendon s.
> patelloquadriceps tendon s.
> tendon s.

subsulfate
subsurface white band
subtalar
> s. arthralgia
> s. arthrodesis
> s. arthroereisis
> s. arthrosis
> s. arthrotomy
> s. articulation
> s. capsulotomy
> s. coalition
> s. distraction bone block fusion
> s. interosseous ligament
> s. inversion test
> s. joint (STJ)
> s. joint arthritis
> s. joint arthroereisis peg (STA-peg)
> s. joint axis (SJA)
> s. joint dislocation
> s. joint function (SJF)
> s. joint incongruency
> s. joint instability
> s. joint neutral position (STNP)
> s. laxity
> s. MBA implant
> s. motion
> s. pronation
> s. supination
> s. tilt
> s. varus

subtendinous
    s. iliac bursa
    s. prepatellar bursa
subthreshold
    s. force
    s. stimulus
subtotal
    s. lateral meniscectomy
    s. maxillectomy
    s. plantar fasciectomy
    s. somatectomy
subtraction osteotomy
subtrochanteric
    s. femoral fracture
    s. osteotomy
subungual
    s. abscess
    s. exostosis
    s. fibroma
    s. granuloma
    s. hematoma
    s. onychomycosis
subvertebral muscle
succinate
    methylprednisolone sodium s.
sucker shaver
suction
    autotransfusion s.
    s. biter
    s. cannula
    s. drainage
    irrigation s.
    s. nozzle
    s. punch
    s. pyramid
    s. sign
    s. socket suspension
    s. suspension prosthesis
    s. tip
    s. tube
suction-bubble technique
suction-irrigation
    s.-i. system
    s.-i. technique
Sudeck
    S. atrophy
    S. disease
    S. syndrome
sudomotor
    s. activity
    s. activity test
    s. function

    s. startle reflex
    s. study
SUFE
    slipped under femoral epiphysis
Sufenta injection
sufentanil citrate
Sugarless C-Chews
sugar-tong
    s.-t. cast
    s.-t. plaster splint
    s.-t. traction
Sugioka transtrochanteric rotational osteotomy
suit
    body-exhaust s.
    G s.
Sukhtian-Hughes
    S.-H. fixation
    S.-H. fixation device
sulcus, pl. **sulci**
    s. angle
    bicipital s.
    calcaneal s.
    s. calcanei
    carpal s.
    cuboid s.
    gluteal s.
    humerus s.
    inferior costal s.
    interarticular s.
    intertubercular s.
    lateral bicipital s.
    malleolar s.
    medial bicipital s.
    obturator s.
    paraglenoid s.
    radial s.
    semicanal of humerus s.
    semilunar s.
    s. sign
    spiral s.
    supraacetabular s.
    talar s.
    s. of talus
    s. test
    s. of wrist
sulfadiazine
    silver s.
sulfate
    magnesium s.
sulfated mucopolysaccharide
sulfide
sulfoxide

S

NOTES

Sullivan sign
Sully shoulder stabilizer brace
Sulzer
S. Orthopaedics
S. Orthopaedics instrument
S. prosthesis
Sunday staphylorrhaphy elevator
Sunderland
S. classification of nerve injury
S. first-degree nerve injury
S. nerve injury classification
Sundt shunt
sunrise view
sunset view
Supartz joint fluid therapy
super
S. Cut laminectomy rongeur
S. Grip sleeve
S. Jock n' Jill store Superfeet
orthotic
S. Stimm MF stimulator
s. wedge
s. wrap
superabduction
Superblade blade
SuperCup acetabular cup prosthesis
superextension
Superfeet Custom Pre-Fabricated Orthotic
superficial
s. circumflex iliac artery
s. femoral artery (SFA)
s. heat modality
s. infection
s. medial ligament
s. necrosis
s. palmar arch
s. peroneal nerve
s. posterior compartment
s. posterior sacrococcygeal ligament
s. radial nerve (SRN)
s. temporal artery
s. temporal vein
s. tibiotalar (STT)
s. tibiotalar ligament
s. transverse ligament
s. TV metacarpal ligament
s. TV metatarsal ligament
s. varicosity
s. white onychomycosis (SWO)
superficialis
s. arcade
flexor digitorum s. (FDS)
s. tendon
superflexion
Superform Contours orthotic
Superglue adhesive
superincumbent

superior
s. border
s. costotransverse ligament
s. dislocation
s. endplate
s. extensor retinaculum
s. extensor retinaculum of foot
s. glide
s. gluteal nerve
s. gluteal neurovascular bundle
s. labrum anterior and posterior (SLAP)
s. labrum anterior and posterior lesion
s. laryngeal artery
s. laryngeal nerve
s. laryngeal nerve external branch
s. leaf
s. peroneal retinaculum (SPR)
s. pole of patella
s. portal
s. process
s. radioulnar joint
S. Sleeprite Hi-Lo orthopaedic bed
s. sulcus tumor
s. thoracic pedicle screw
s. thyroid artery
s. thyroid vein
s. tibial articulation
s. tibiofibular joint
s. vena cava
superman back exercise technique
supermarket elbow
supernumerary
s. bone
s. digit
s. lumbar segmentation
s. thumb
s. toe
superoinferior tilt
superolateral outflow portal
superomedial
s. calcaneonavicular ligament
s. fragment
s. portal
s. region
SuperQuad assistive device
supersensitivity
Cannon Law of Denervation S.
denervation s.
Super-Seven exercise
SuperSkin thin film dressing
Superstabilizer
S. cemented stem extender
S. press-fit stem extender
supertubercular wedge osteotomy/bunionectomy
supinate

supination
    s. contracture
    s. deformity
    s. of foot
    hindfoot s.
    s. injury
    pronation and s.
    subtalar s.
    s. torque
supination-adduction
    s.-a. fracture
    s.-a. injury
supination-eversion
    s.-e. fracture
    s.-e. injury
supination-external
    s.-e. rotation (SER)
    s.-e. rotation injury
    s.-e. rotation IV
    s.-e. rotation IV fracture
supination-inversion rotation injury
supination-outward rotation injury
supination-plantarflexion injury
supinator
    s. fat pad sign
    s. fossa
    s. fossa supraclavicular fossa
    Frenkel exercises
    s. jerk
    s. jerk reflex
    s. longus reflex
    s. muscle
    s. syndrome
supine
    s. chest press
    s. C-Trax traction
    s. C-Trax traction system
    s. iliac gapping test
    s. long sitting test
    s. position
    s. position driver
    s. straight leg raising test
Suppan foot operation
supplement
    oral nutritional s.
supplementation
    zinc s.
supple neck
supplier
    National Association of Medical
    Equipment S.'s
    National Registry of Rehabilitation
    Technology S.'s

supply
    blood s.
    longitudinal blood s.
    reanastomosis of blood s.
support
    Accommodator arch s.
    Accu-Back back s.
    Achillotrain active Achilles
    tendon s.
    Active Ankle s.
    Act joint s.
    Act knee s.
    AliMed-Freedom arthritis s.
    AliMed wrist/thumb s.
    ankle stabilizing orthosis s.
    Anna-Dote Positioning S.
    arch s.
    Arizona universal leg s.
    ASO s.
    Assistant Free foot/ankle s.
    back s.
    Back-Huggar lumbar s.
    BackThing lumbar s.
    Band-It magnetic elbow s.
    base of s.
    Bauerfeind s.
    BIOflex Magnet Back S.
    BioSkin DP wrist s.
    BioWrap lumbosacral/sacral s.
    Birkenstock Blue Footbed arch s.
    Birkenstock high-flange arch s.
    Body Gard neoprene s.
    boomerang wrist s.
    Carabelt lower back s.
    Carpal-Lock wrist s.
    Castech extremity s.
    cavus foot s.
    cervical s.
    ChinUpps cervicofacial s.
    Chiroflow adjustable back s.
    Cho-pat knitted compression s.
    cock-up wrist s.
    Comfort Cool neoprene s.
    Comprifix active ankle s.
    Compro Plus Knee s.
    Core Reflex wrist s.
    Core Universal elastic knee s.
    Core Universal elbow s.
    Core Universal rib s.
    Corfit System 7000 Series
    Lumbosacral S.
    Cryo/Cuff compression s.
    cutout knee s.

S

NOTES

support *(continued)*
    Cybertech 1000 back s.
    DayTimer carpal tunnel s.
    Deltoid-Aid arm s.
    DePuy s.
    Desk-rest arm s.
    Epi-Lock elbow s.
    Epipoint elbow s.
    Epitrain active elbow s.
    Epitrain knitted elbow s.
    Epitrain Viscoped s.
    Ergo Cush back s.
    Ergoflex Premiere back s.
    external s.
    Ezy Wrap lumbosacral s.
    Fits-All s.
    FlexLite hinged knee s.
    Foot Hugger foot s.
    fork strap prosthetic s.
    Freedom accommodator arch s.
    Freedom arthritis s.
    Freedom back s.
    Freedom elastic long wrist s.
    Friedman s.
    Futuro wrist s.
    s. garment
    Genutrain P3 knee s.
    geriatric chair trunk s.
    horizontal platform s. (HPS)
    Houston halo cervical s.
    IMP-Capello arm s.
    Innovation Sports bracing s.
    Juzo s.
    Kallassy ankle s.
    Kerr-Lagen abdominal s.
    Knee Sleeve knee s.
    Lo Bak spinal s.
    Loving Comfort maternity s.
    Loving Comfort postpartum s.
    Lumbotrain lumbosacral s.
    Malleoloc ankle s.
    Malleo-Med soft ankle s.
    Malleotrain ankle s.
    ManuTrain active wrist s.
    Markwort ankle s.
    MKG knee s.
    Mold-In-Place back s.
    Momma-Too Maternity S.
    Monitor Master monitor s.
    Morton toe s.
    Mother-To-Be abdominal s.
    Mother-To-Be Support Maternity S.
    neoprene ankle s.
    neoprene back s.
    Nightimer carpal tunnel s.
    Night Splint s.
    obese s.
    Obus back s.
    OEC wrist/forearm s.

    Omotrain active shoulder s.
    Ortho-Pal body s.
    OSI Well Leg S.
    Palumbo knee s.
    Parham s.
    PattStrap knee s.
    Pediatric Advanced Life S. (PALS)
    Performance Wrap knee s.
    peripatellar retinacular s.
    Philadelphia collar cervical s.
    Plastazote arch s.
    Playmaker s.
    Powerstep foot s.
    PPT gel stirrup ankle s.
    ProFlex wrist s.
    prosthetic s.
    QualCraft ankle s.
    QualCraft short elastic wrist s.
    Relax-A-Bac posture s.
    Rolyan foot s.
    sacral s.
    Scott double-strap ankle s.
    Scott hinged knee s.
    Sheffield s.
    ShiatsuBACK back s.
    Shoulder Ease abduction s.
    Sidekick foot s.
    Silesian bandage prosthetic s.
    Spenco arch s.
    S'port Max back s.
    standard U patellar s.
    Stromgren s.
    Stubbs elastic wrist s.
    SureStep ankle s.
    TakeOff elbow s.
    Taylor clavicle s.
    Thera-Back back s.
    therapeutic spinal s.
    Thermoskin 4-way elastic knee s.
    tibial fracture brace proximal s.
     (TFB-PS)
    Valeo back s.
    Viscoped S s.
    ViscoSpot s.
    walking with s.
    walking without s.
    well-leg s.
    Whitman arch s.
    WorkAbout Carpal Mate wrist s.
    WorkMod back s.
    wrist hand extension
     compression s. (WHECS)
    WrisTimer CTS s.
    WrisTimer PM carpal tunnel s.
    Wrist Pro wrist s.

supported extension exercise
supporting bone
suppression
    chemical selective s. (CHESS)

suppurative
- s. arthritis
- s. flexor tenosynovitis
- s. joint infection
- s. myositis
- s. osteitis
- s. osteomyelitis
- s. periostitis
- s. synovitis

supraacetabular sulcus

supraclavicular
- s. approach
- s. brachial block anesthesia
- s. fossa
- s. fossa artery

supracollicular spike

supracondylar (SC)
- s. amputation
- s. cuff
- s. femoral derotational osteotomy
- s. humeral fracture
- intramedullary s. (IMSC)
- s. medullary nail
- s. nonunion
- s. pad
- s. plate
- s. process
- s. process syndrome
- s. screw
- s. socket
- s. varus osteotomy
- s. Y-shaped fracture

supracondylar-suprapatellar (SCSP, SC-SP)

supraganglionic injury

supraglenoid tuberosity

suprahyoid

Supralen
- S. cradle orthotic
- S. Schaefer orthotic

supralevator abscess

supramalleolar
- s. derotational osteotomy
- s. flap
- s. open amputation
- s. orthosis (SMO)
- s. varus derotation osteotomy
- s. venous ulcer

supramaximal stimulus

supranaviculare

supraoccipital bone

suprapatellar (SP)
- s. cannula

- s. cuff (SPC)
- s. plica
- s. portal
- s. pouch
- s. reflex
- s. strap
- s. tendinitis

suprapubic

suprascapular
- s. nerve
- s. nerve entrapment test
- s. nerve injury
- s. nerve syndrome
- s. neuritis

suprasellar capsule

supraspinal ligament

supraspinatus
- s. calcification
- s. implant
- s. muscle
- s. outlet
- s. syndrome
- s. tendinitis
- s. tendon
- s. test

supraspinous
- s. ligament
- s. muscle

suprasternal
- s. bone
- s. notch
- s. plane
- s. space

suprasyndesmotic
- s. fracture
- s. membrane
- s. screw fixation

supratectal transverse fracture

supratubercular
- s. wedge osteotomy
- s. wedge osteotomy bunionectomy

sural
- s. island flap
- s. island flap for foot and ankle reconstruction
- s. nerve
- s. neuritis
- s. neuroma
- s. neuropathy

Surbaugh legholder

sure
- S. Sport pad
- S. Step ankle brace

S

NOTES

SureClosure
    S. closure
    S. device
    S. skin stretching system
Sure-Flex
    S.-F. III prosthetic foot
    S.-F. prosthesis
SureStep
    S. ankle support
    S. ankle support system
Suretac
    S. bioabsorbable shoulder fixation
      device
    S. drill
    S. guidewire
    S. shoulder fixation
surface
    apposing articular s.
    articular s.
    Bazooka support s.
    cancellous bone s.
    s. cement
    ceramic-on-ceramic bearing s.
    concave articular s.
    contiguous articular s.
    distal concave articular s.
    eburnated bone s.
    s. electrode
    s. electromyography (sEMG)
    endosteal s.
    erosion of articular s.
    facet s.
    freshen the s.
    irregular articular s.
    Micro-Aire débridement of bone s.
    s. profile
    radioulnar s.
    s. replacement
    s. replacement hip arthroplasty
    roughen the s.
    shearling s.
    s. shoe interaction
    volar s.
    wear-resistant s.
    weightbearing s.
surfer's knot
Surfit adhesive
Surgairtome air drill
SurgAssist
    S. leg positioner
    S. surgical legholder
surgeon
    American Academy of
      Orthopaedic S.'s (AAOS)
    s. thumb
surgery
    ablative s.
    adult scoliosis s.

American Association for Hand S.
    (AAHS)
anterior cervicothoracic junction s.
anterior lower cervical spine s.
anterior minimally invasive s.
    (AMIS)
arthroscopic laser s.
bypass s.
cervical disc s.
cervicothoracic junction s.
closed s.
computer-assisted orthopaedic s.
    (CAOS)
failed flatfoot s.
first ray s.
H-block nail s.
heel spur s.
Hospital for Special S. (HSS)
hypotensive s.
intradural tumor s.
joint-preservation s.
joint replacement s.
kyphosis correction s.
lateral column lengthening s.
limb-salvage s.
lower extremity bypass s.
lower posterior lumbar spine and
    sacrum s.
McCash hand s.
minimum incision s. (MIS)
MRI-directed s.
nerve transposition s.
open disc s.
orthopaedic s.
peripheral vascular s. (PVS)
posterior lower cervical spine s.
posterior lumbar interbody fusion s.
posterior lumbar spine and
    sacrum s.
posterior upper cervical spine s.
ProTrac system for knee s.
scoliosis s.
traumatic, unidirectional Bankart
    lesion s.
ulnar nerve transposition s.
Unilink system for hand s.
vascular s.
Surgibone
    Boplant S.
    S. implant
    Unilab S.
surgical
    s. ablation
    s. anastomosis
    s. approach
    s. autoimmunization
    s. corset
    s. dressing room (SDR)
    s. exposure

s. fixation
s. galvanism
s. glove
s. hand tray
s. knife handle
s. leg pedestal
s. loupe
s. neck
s. neck fracture
s. orthopaedic drill
s. pin driver
s. prosthesis
s. reconstruction
s. reduction
s. rod
S. Simplex P adhesive
S. Simplex P radiopaque bone cement
S. Simplex P radiopaque cement
s. splint
s. staple applier
s. technique
s. treatment

Surgicel
S. fibrillar hemostat
S. implant
S. Nu-Knit absorbable hemostat

Surgilase CO_2 laser
Surgilast tubular elastic dressing
SurgiLav machine
Surgi-Stim
S.,-S. postsurgical therapy system
S.,-S. stimulator
Surgitek prosthesis
Surgitube tubular gauze
Surgivac drain
survey
bone s.
metastatic bone s.
susceptibility testing
suspension
balanced s.
below-knee s.
corset s.
cuff s.
s. feeder
fingertrap s.
flexible hinge s.
hip disarticulation s.
hip hemipelvectomy s.
knee disarticulation s.
panmetatarsal tendon s.
patellar tendon-bearing s. (PTBS)

SC s.
silicone-only s. (SOS)
s. splint
s. strap
suction socket s.
s. traction
transfemoral s.
suspension-type socket
suspensory
sustained
s. ankle clonus
s. loading
s. natural apophysial glides (SNAGS)
s. pressure technique
sustentacular fragment
sustentaculum
s. tali
s. tali fracture
Sutherland
S. hip operation
S. hip procedure
S. lateral transfer
Sutherland-Greenfield osteotomy
Sutherland-Rowe incision
Sutter
S. device
S. double-stem silicone implant prosthesis
S. implant
S. MCP finger joint prosthesis
S. silicone metacarpophalangeal joint
S. silicone metacarpophalangeal joint arthroplasty
Sutter-CPM
S.-CPM knee apparatus
S.-CPM knee device
sutural bone
suture
s. abscess
Acufex bioabsorbable Suretac s.
Allgöwer-Donati s.
s. anchor
s. anchor shoulder repair
s. anchor technique
baseball s.
Bell s.
Bio-FASTak s.
BioSorb s.
Biosyn synthetic monofilament s.
Bondek s.
braided s.

S

NOTES

suture *(continued)*
  bregmatomastoid s.
  bulb s.
  bundle s.
  Bunnell crisscross s.
  Bunnell figure-of-8 s.
  Bunnell wire pull-out s.
  button s.
  caprolactam s.
  Caprosyn s.
  Carrel s.
  Chinese fingertrap s.
  core s.
  cotton s.
  Dacron s.
  Dafilon s.
  Dagrofil s.
  Dexon s.
  Donati s.
  double right-angle s.
  Dupuytren s.
  end-to-end s.
  epitenon s.
  Ethibond s.
  Ethicon s.
  Ethiflex s.
  Ethilon s.
  fascial s.
  fear-near, near-far s.
  figure-of-8 s.
  fingertrap s.
  fishmouth end-to-end s.
  s. fixation
  Gillis s.
  Gore-Tex nonabsorbable s.
  grasping s.
  guy s.
  s. hole drill
  horizontal mattress s.
  interrupted s.
  intradermal s.
  jugal s.
  Kessler grasping s.
  Kessler-Tajima s.
  Krackow s.
  s. of Krause
  lamboid s.
  lashing s.
  lateral trap s.
  Le Dentu s.
  linen s.
  locking horizontal mattress s.
  lockout s.
  Mason-Allen s.
  mattress s.
  Maxon s.
  McLaughlin modification of
    Bunnell pull-out s.
  Mersilene s.
  MicroMite anchor s.
  modified Kessler s.
  modified Kessler-Tajima s.
  monofilament s.
  muscle-to-bone s.
  nail s.
  Nicoladoni s.
  nonabsorbable s.
  Nurolon s.
  nylon s.
  Panacryl s.
  s. passer
  passing s.
  PDS s.
  Perma-Hand silk s.
  pin s.
  polybutester s.
  Polydek s.
  polydioxanone s. (PDS)
  polyester s.
  polyethylene s.
  polygalactic acid s.
  polyglactin s.
  polyglycolic acid s.
  polyglyconate s.
  polypropylene s.
  Polysorb s.
  popoff s.
  Prolene s.
  pull-out s.
  Pulvertaft end-to-end s.
  Pulvertaft interweave s.
  s. punch
  pursestring s.
  s. pusher
  s. pusher talofibular joint
  retention s.
  running s.
  safety-bolt s.
  s. scissors
  silk s.
  simple s.
  sling s.
  staple s.
  subcuticular s.
  s. system (SS)
  Tajima modified Kessler s.
  Teflon-coated s.
  tendon s.
  Tevdek s.
  transosseous s.
  Tycron s.
  UltraFix MicroMite anchor s.
  undyed s.
  USP#2 s.
  vertical mattress s.
  Vicryl s.
  violet monofilament s.
  wire s.

sutureless avascular meniscal repair
suture-loop technique
Suture-Self dressing
suturing
    Johnson medial meniscal s.
    meniscus s.
    Morgan-Casscells meniscus s.
Sven-Johansson
    S.-J. extractor
    S.-J. femoral neck nail
Swafford-Lichtman division
swaged needle
swallow-tail sign
swan-neck
    s.-n. chisel
    s.-n. deformity reduction
    s.-n. facies
    s.-n. finger deformity
    s.-n. gouge
    s.-n. splint
Swann-Morton surgical blade
Swanson
    S. carpal lunate implant
    S. carpal scaphoid implant
    S. classification
    S. convex condylar arthroplasty
    S. dynamic toe splint
    S. elevator
    S. finger joint
    S. finger joint implant
    S. finger joint prosthesis
    S. flexible hallux valgus prosthesis
    S. great toe implant
    S. great toe prosthesis
    S. Grip-X hand exerciser
    S. hand splint
    S. interpositional wrist arthroplasty
    S. lunate awl
    S. mallet
    S. metacarpal prosthesis
    S. metacarpophalangeal implant
    S. metatarsal broach
    S. metatarsal prosthesis
    S. metatarsophalangeal joint
    arthroplasty
    S. osteotome
    S. osteotomy
    S. PIP joint arthroplasty
    S. radial head implant
    S. radial head implant arthroplasty
    S. radiocarpal implant
    S. reamer
    S. reconstruction

    S. scaphoid awl
    S. silastic elbow prosthesis
    S. silicone wrist arthroplasty
    S. small joint implant
    S. technique
    S. trapezium implant
    S. T-shaped great toe silastic
    prosthesis
    S. ulnar head implant
    S. wrist joint implant
    S. wrist prosthesis
swathe, swath
    arm s.
    s. and sling
sway
    anteroposterior lateral s.
    s. back
    body s.
    lateral s.
    postural s.
swaying gait
SWD
    shortwave diathermy
sweating
    excessive s.
    plantar s.
sweat test
Swede-O
    S.-O Ankle Loc brace
    S.-O Arch-Lok
Swede-O-Universal
    S.-O-U. brace
    S.-O-U. orthosis
Swediauer disease
Swedish
    S. approach
    S. gymnastics
    S. Helparm
    S. knee cage
    S. knee cage orthosis
    S. massage
    S. movement
    S. portal
    S. support stool
swelling
    boggy s.
    fusiform soft tissue s.
    joint s.
    postfracture s.
SwimEx
    S. aquatic therapy
    S. aquatic therapy bodyCushion

S

NOTES

SwimEx (*continued*)
    S. hydrotherapy system
    S. pool
swimmer's
    s. shoulder
    s. view
swimming pool granuloma
swing
    s. phase
    s. phase of gait
    s. time
SwingAlong walker caddy
Swinger car bed
swing-phase
    s.-p. acceleration
    s.-p. control
swing-through gait
swing-to gait
Swiss
    S. Balance orthotic
    S. ball
    S. ball therapy
    S. cancellous screw
    S. MP joint implant
    S. pattern osteotome
switching stick
swivel
    s. clamp
    s. dislocation
    s. utensil
    s. walker
Swivel-Strap
    Aircast S.-S.
    S.-S. ankle brace
    S.-S. ankle stirrup
SWO
    superficial white onychomycosis
swollen disc
SWT
    shock-wave therapy
Sydney line
Syed-Neblett implant
Syed template implant
symbrachydactyly
Syme
    S. amputation prosthesis
    S. ankle disarticulation amputation
    S. Dycor prosthetic foot
    S. foot prosthesis
    S. operation
    S. procedure
symmetric
    s. sacral plate
    s. thumb duplication
    s. tonicity
    s. vertebral fusion
symmetrical thoracic vertebral plate
symmetry
    weightbearing s.

sympathectomy
    cervical s.
    chemical s.
    lumbar s.
    peripheral chemical s.
    preganglionic s.
sympathetic
    s. block
    s. blockade
    s. chain
    s. component
    s. dysfunction
    s. innervation
    s. maintained pain syndrome (SMPS)
    s. nerve
    s. nervous system (SNS)
    s. reflex dystrophy
    s. trunk
sympathetically mediated pain
sympathicotonia
symphalangism
symphysial mobility
symphysis, pl. **symphyses**
    amphiarthrodial s.
    pubic s.
    s. pubis
    s. pubis diastasis
symptom
    S.'s Checklist 90 Revised (SCL-90R)
    functionally debilitating s.
    irritable s.
    s. magnification syndrome
    Oehler s.
    Pratt s.
    S.'s and Sports Participation Rating Scale
symptomatic
    s. nonunion
    s. spondylolisthesis
    s. synovial plica
    s. torticollis
symptomatology
Syms traction
Synaptic 2000 pain management system
synarthrodial joint
synarthrophysis
synarthrosis
Synatomic total knee prosthesis
synchondritic fracture
synchondrosis, pl. **synchondroses**
    neurocentral s.
    tibiofibular s.
synchondrotomy
synchronized fibrillation
synchronous scapuloclavicular rotation
synchrony
    arm heel-strike s.

SynchroSonic
    S. stimulator
    S. U/HVG50 ultrasound/stimulator
syncope
    heat s.
syndactylism
syndactylization
syndactylized finger
syndactyly
    burn s.
    complete s.
    complex s.
    complicated complex s.
    incomplete s.
    pure s.
    reduction s.
    ring finger–small finger s.
    simple s.
syndesmectomy
syndesmectopia
syndesmitis
syndesmopexy
syndesmophyte
syndesmoplasty
syndesmorrhaphy
syndesmosis, pl. **syndesmoses**
    s. rupture
    s. screw lucency
    s. sprain of ankle
    tibiofibular s.
syndesmotic
    s. avulsion
    s. diastasis
    s. ligament
    s. screw
    s. sprain
syndesmotomy
syndrome
    Aarskog-Scott s.
    acetabular rim s.
    acute exertional compartment s.
      (AECS)
    acute locked-back s.
    acute low back s.
    Adair-Dighton s.
    Adamantiades-Behçet s.
    Albright s.
    Albright-McCune-Sternberg s.
    alcohol fat embolism s.
    algodystrophy s.
    Alpers s.
    altitude s.
    anterior cervical cord s.

anterior compartment s. (ACS)
anterior tibial compartment s.
anterolateral impingement s.
anteversion s.
anular constricting band s.
Apert s.
Arnold-Chiari s.
arthroonychodysplasia s.
athletic heart s.
Baastrup s.
Babinski-Fröhlich s.
Babinski-Nageotte s.
Bamberger-Marie s.
Barre-Lieou s.
Barsony-Polgar s.
Barsony-Teschendorf s.
Basser s.
Beals s.
Behavioral Assessment of the
  Dysexecutive S. (BADS)
Behçet s.
Behr s.
benign hypermobile joint s.
benign joint hypermobility s.
  (BJHS)
bent-knee s.
Bertolotti s.
bicipital s.
bilateral acute radicular s.
bilateral chronic radicular s.
Bing-Horton s.
bioenergy imbalance s. (BIS)
BK mole s.
black heel s.
Bloom s.
blue foot s.
blue toe s.
body cast s.
Brissaud s.
broad thumb–big toe s.
Brown-Séquard s. (BSS)
Bruns gait apraxia Bruns s.
burning-feet s.
Cacchione s.
Caffey s.
Caffey-Silverman s.
calcaneal spur s.
Calvé-Legg-Perthes s.
Caplan s.
carpal tunnel s. (CTS)
Carpenter s.
Carter-Wilkinson criteria for
  hypermobility s.

S

NOTES

syndrome *(continued)*

cast s.
cauda equina s.
central cord s.
central heel pad s.
central herniation s.
cervical acceleration/deceleration s.
cervical dorsal outlet s.
cervical rib s.
cervicoencephalic s.
cervicogenic s.
Cestan-Chenais s.
Charcot s.
Charles Bonnet s.
choke s.
chronic anterior exertional
  compartment s. (CAECS)
chronic compartment s. (CCS)
chronic heel pain s. (CHPS)
chronic intractable benign pain s.
  (CIBPS)
chronic musculoskeletal pain s.
  (CMPS)
Claude s.
clenched fist s.
clumsy hand s.
Cobb s.
Cockayne s.
Coffin-Lowry s.
common peroneal nerve s.
compartment s.
complex regional pain s. (CRPS)
complex regional pain s. type 2
  (CRPS-2)
compression s.
computer-assisted carpal tunnel s.
congenital band s.
Conradi s.
constriction band s.
conus medullaris s.
copper deficiency s.
coracoid impingement s.
cord-traction s.
Cornelia de Lange s.
Costen s.
costoclavicular s.
Cotton-Berg s.
Cowden s.
CREST s.
crossover s.
Crouzon s.
crush s.
cubital tunnel s.
cuboid s.
Cushing s.
cyclops s.
dancing bear s.
dead arm s.
de Barsy s.

deconditioning s.
Dejerine-Sottas s.
de Lange s.
de Quervain s.
derangement s.
diffuse idiopathic skeletal
  hyperostosis s.
DiGeorge s.
disc s.
DISH s.
DOOR s.
dorsi jam s.
double crush s.
Down s.
droopy shoulder s.
drug-related hydantoin s.
Duplay s.
Dyggve-Melchior-Clausen s.
Dyke-Davidoff-Masson s.
dysfunction s.
dysplastic nevus s.
Eagle-Barrett s.
Eaton-Lambert s.
Eddowes s.
Edwards s.
Ehlers-Danlos s. (EDS)
Ekbom restless leg s.
Ellis-van Creveld s.
empty can s.
entrapment s.
eosinophilia-myalgia s.
Erdheim s.
exercise-induced compartment s.
exertional anterior compartment s.
  (EACS)
exertional deep posterior
  compartment s. (EDPCS)
extraarticular pain s.
fabella s.
facet joint s.
failed back s. (FBS)
failed back surgery s. (FBSS)
failed surgery s.
Fanconi s.
Fanconi-Albertini-Zellweger s.
far-out s.
fat embolism s.
fat pad s.
FAV s.
Fazio-Londe s.
fetal alcohol s.
fibromyalgia s. (FMS)
filum terminale s.
flat back s.
flexor carpi ulnaris s.
flexor origin s.
floppy infant s.
forearm compartment s.
fragile X s.

Freeman-Sheldon s.
frozen shoulder s.
Funk tibialis posterior tendon
  dysfunction classification s.
Funston s.
GALOP s.
Gardner s.
Gardner-Diamond s.
General Adaption S. (GAS)
Goldenhar s.
Gowers s.
gracilis s.
Grisel s.
Guillain-Barré s.
Guyon tunnel s.
Haglund s.
Hajdu-Cheney s.
hammer digit s.
hammertoe s. (HTS)
hamstring s.
hand-arm vibration s.
hand-foot s.
hand-foot-uterus s.
Hand-Schüller-Christian s.
heart-and-hand s.
heel compression s.
heel pain s.
heel spur s.
heel spur/plantar fasciitis s.
Heerfort s.
hip joint s.
HLA B27-related
  spondyloarthropathy intersection s.
Hoffa s.
Hoffmann s.
hungry bone s.
Hurler s.
Hurler-Scheie s.
hyperflexed toe compartment s.
hypermobile joint s.
hypermobility s. (HMS)
hyperostosis s.
hypersensitivity s.
hypothenar hammertoe s.
idiopathic skeletal hyperostosis s.
iliacus s.
iliocostalis lumborum s.
ilioinguinal s.
iliotibial band friction s. (ITBFS)
impingement s.
infrapatellar contracture s. (IPCS)
inguinal ligament s.
internal snapping hip s.

interosseous nerve s.
intersection s.
Isaacs s.
Jaccoud s.
Jackson s.
Jackson-Gorham s.
Jackson-Weiss s.
Jadassohn-Lewandowsky s.
Jaffe-Campanacci s.
Jarcho-Levin s.
Johanson-Blizzard s.
Karsch-Neugebauer s.
Kast s.
Kearns-Sayre s.
Kenny-Caffey s.
Kinsbourne s.
Kleine-Levin s.
Klippel-Feil s. (KFS)
Klippel-Trenaunay s.
Klippel-Trenaunay-Weber s.
Klüver-Bucy s.
Kniest s.
Kocher-Debré-Semelaigne s.
Kretschmer s.
Kuskokwim s.
Lambert-Eaton myasthenic s.
  (LEMS)
Larsen s.
lateral column s.
lateral gutter s.
lateral hyperpressure s.
lateral patellar compression s.
Laurence-Biedl s.
Laurence-Moon s.
Laurence-Moon-Biedl s.
Lawrence-Seip s.
leg-foot-toe s.
Legg-Calvé-Perthes s.
Legg-Calvé-Waldenström s.
LEOPARD s.
Leri s.
Leriche s.
Leri-Weill s.
levator scapulae s.
Lhermitte s.
Linberg s.
Little s.
Lobstein s.
local adaptation s. (LAS)
Looser-Milkman s.
lumbago-mechanical instability s.
lumbar flat back s.
lumbar thecoperitoneal shunt s.

NOTES

S

syndrome *(continued)*
    lumbosacral mechanical s.
    Maffucci s.
    Marfan s.
    Maroteaux-Lamy s.
    Mazabraud s.
    McArdle s.
    McCune-Albright s.
    mechanical low back pain s.
    medial tibial s. (MTS)
    medial tibial stress s. (MTSS)
    Meige s.
    meningeal s.
    metabolic s. (MS)
    metatarsal overload s.
    Meyer-Betz s.
    microgeodic s.
    Milch fracture classification s.
    milkman's s.
    Milwaukee shoulder s.
    miserable misalignment s.
    mixed cord s.
    Morel s.
    Morquio s.
    Morquio-Brailsford s.
    Morquio-Ullrich s.
    Morton s.
    Mueller Weiss s.
    multifidus s.
    multiple pterygium s.
    multiple synostoses s.
    myofascial pain s. (MPF)
    Naffziger s.
    nail-patella s.
    naviculocapitate fracture s.
    neck pain s.
    nerve entrapment s.
    Neumann s.
    neuroarticular s.
    neurogenic s.
    Nievergelt-Pearlman s.
    occupational stress s. (OSS)
    Ollier s.
    Oppenheim s.
    Osebold-Remondini s.
    Osgood-Schlatter s.
    osteoporosis pseudoglioma s.
    Ostrum-Furst s.
    overtraining s.
    overuse s.
    Paget juvenile s.
    Paget-Schrötter s.
    pain-all-over s.
    pain dysfunction s.
    painful arc s.
    paraneoplastic neuromuscular s.
    Parsonage-Aldren-Turner s.
    Parsonage-Turner s.
    Patau s.

    patellar clunk s.
    patellar malalignment s.
    patellar pair s.
    patellofemoral pain s. (PPS)
    patellofemoral stress s.
    peroneal compartment s.
    pes anserinus s.
    Peterson s.
    Pfeiffer s.
    phalangeal microgeodic s.
    phantom limb s.
    piriformis s.
    plantar fasciitis s.
    plica s.
    Plummer-Vinson s.
    Poland s.
    popliteal entrapment s.
    popliteal pterygium s.
    postcasting s.
    postconcussive s.
    posterior cord s.
    posterior impingement s.
    posterior interosseous nerve
      compression s.
    posterior joint s.
    posterior knee pull s.
    postfracture s.
    postphlebitis s.
    postpolio s.
    postpyelomyelitis s.
    posttraumatic algodystrophic s.
    posttraumatic chronic cord s.
    postural s.
    Pouteau s.
    predislocation s.
    pronator teres s.
    Proteus s.
    prune-belly s.
    pseudoradicular s.
    psoas tendon s.
    punch drunk s.
    quadratus lumborum s.
    quadrilateral space s.
    radial sensory nerve entrapment s.
    radial tunnel s.
    Raynaud s.
    rectus adductor s.
    reflex sympathetic dystrophy s.
      (RSDS)
    Refsum s.
    Reiter s.
    repetitive stress s. (RSS)
    Rett s.
    Riley-Day s.
    ring s.
    rotator cuff impingement s.
    rotatores s.
    Rotter-Erb s.
    Roussy-Lévy s.

Rubinstein-Taybi s.
Rust s.
sacroiliac hypermobility s.
sacroiliac joint s.
Sanfilippo s.
SAPHO s.
scalenus anterior s.
scaphocapitate s.
scapulocostal s.
scapuloperoneal s.
Schanz s.
Scheie s.
Scheuermann s.
Schwartz s.
Schwartz-Jampel s.
secondary hip-spine s.
second impact s.
seronegative enthesopathy and
  arthropathy s.
serotonin s.
short leg s.
shoulder-girdle s.
shoulder-hand s.
shoulder-hand-finger s.
Shwachman s.
Shy-Drager s.
sick scapula s.
Silverskiöld s.
Sinding-Larsen-Johansson s.
sinus tarsi s.
Sjögren s.
skeletal hyperostosis s.
Sly s.
small patella s.
Smith-Lemli-Opitz s.
snapping hip s.
snapping knee s.
snapping scapula s.
soleus s.
spinal cord s.
spiral groove s.
sprained ankle s.
steal s.
Stewart-Morel s.
Stickler s.
stiff man s.
straight spine s.
subacromial impingement s.
subclavian steal s.
sublimis bridge s.
Sudeck s.
supinator s.
supracondylar process s.

suprascapular nerve s.
supraspinatus s.
sympathetic maintained pain s.
  (SMPS)
symptom magnification s.
synovial plica s.
TAR s.
tarsal tunnel s. (TTS)
temporomandibular joint s.
tension neck s.
tensor fascia lata s.
tethered cord s.
tethered patellar tendon s.
thoracic inlet s.
thoracic outlet s. (TOS)
thrombocytopenia-absent radius s.
Tietze s.
transient bone marrow edema s.
transversospinalis s.
traumatic compartment s.
trigger finger s.
trochanteric s.
Turner s.
Uhthoff s.
ulnar cubital tunnel s.
ulnar impaction s.
ulnar styloid impaction s.
ulnocarpal abutment s.
ulnocarpal impaction s.
ulnolunate abutment s.
unbalanced wrist s.
unilateral acute radicular s.
unilateral chronic radicular s.
valgus extension overload s.
VATER s.
vertebral steal s.
vertebral subluxation s.
vibration white finger s.
vibrator hand s.
viscerospinal s.
volar compartment s.
von Hippel-Lindau s.
Wallenberg s.
washboard s.
Weber s.
whiplash s.
whiplash-shaken infant s.
whistling face s.
Wilkie s.
windblown hand, whistling face s.
wrist pain s.
yellow nail s.

S

NOTES

synergia
> detrusor-sphincter s.

synergist

synergistic
> s. finger motion
> s. gangrene
> s. muscle
> S. suspension strap
> s. wrist motion
> s. wrist motion splint

synergy
> S. flexible splinting material
> S. hinge system
> S. joint rehabilitation
> limb s.
> S. spine rehab system
> S. splint
> S. Therapeutic System

syngraft

synosteosis

synostosis
> cervical s.
> congenital radioulnar s.
> fibula protibial s.
> phalangeal s.
> proximal tibiofibular s.
> radioulnar s. (type I, II)
> tibiofibular s.

synostotic

Synovator arthroscopic blade

synovectomy
> Albright s.
> arthroscopic s.
> arthroscopically assisted s.
> s. blade
> carpal s.
> dorsal s.
> palmar s.
> 6-portal s.
> Porter-Richardson-Vainio s.
> Smith-Petersen s.
> volar s.
> Wilkinson s.

synovia (*pl. of* synovium)

synovial
> s. biopsy
> s. bursa
> s. cavity
> s. cell sarcoma
> s. chondroma
> s. chondromatosis
> s. cyst
> s. disease
> s. fistula
> s. fluid
> s. fold
> s. fringe
> s. frond
> s. hernia

> s. herniation
> s. histopathology
> s. injury
> s. joint
> s. membrane
> s. nodule
> s. nonunion
> s. osteochondromatosis
> s. outpouching
> s. plica
> s. plica syndrome
> s. pseudarthrosis
> s. resector
> s. rongeur
> s. shaver
> s. sheath
> s. stromal cell
> s. tag
> s. tap
> s. tumor

synoviocyte

synoviogram

synovioma

synoviorthesis

synovitis
> boggy s.
> bursal s.
> chronic hemorrhagic villous s.
> chronic purulent s.
> crystal-induced s.
> dendritic s.
> diffuse pigmented villonodular s. (DPVNS)
> disseminated pigmented villonodular s.
> dry s.
> extraarticular pigmented villonodular s.
> filarial s.
> Finkelstein test for s.
> florid s.
> focal pigmented villonodular s.
> fungous s.
> hemorrhagic villous s.
> s. hyperplastica
> hypertrophic s.
> inflammatory s.
> lead s.
> localized nodular s. (LNS)
> metatarsophalangeal joint s.
> monarticular s.
> nontraumatic s.
> parapatellar s.
> particulate s.
> pigmented nodular s.
> pigmented villonodular s. (PVNS, PVS)
> postoperative s.
> proliferative s.

puerperal s.
purulent s.
reactive s.
recurrent s.
rheumatoid arthritis s.
scarlatinal s.
serous s.
s. sicca
silicone s.
simple s.
suppurative s.
tendinous s.
transient s.
traumatic s.
tuberculous s.
vaginal s.
vibration s.
villonodular s.
villous s.

synovitis-acne-pustulosis-hyperostosis osteomyelitis (SAPHO)
synovium, pl. **synovia**
cartilage s.
exuberant s.
opaque s.
pannus of s.

synpolydactyly
Synthaderm dressing
Synthes
S. CerviFix system
S. compression hip screw
S. dorsal distal radius plate
S. drill
S. fixation system
S. guidepin
S. ligament washer
S. Microsystems drill bit
S. Microsystems plate cutter
S. Microsystems plate-holding forceps
S. Microsystems pliers
S. mini L-plate
S. pie plate
S. Schuhli implant system
S. USS
S. wire guide

synthesis, pl. **syntheses**
activity s.
s. of continuity
muscle protein s.
proteoglycan s.

synthetic
s. augmentation

s. bone implant
s. cancellous bone void filler
s. cortical bone
s. cortical bone void filler
s. graft bypass to ankle
s. material
s. prosthesis
s. stent
s. testosterone

Synvisc injection therapy
syphilitic
s. abscess
s. amyotrophy
s. osteochondritis

Syracuse anterior I plate
syringe
cement s.
s. grip
Terumo s.

syringes (*pl. of* syrinx)
syringohydromyelia
syringoma
chondroid s.

syringometaplasia
syringomyelia
posttraumatic s.
secondary posttraumatic s.

syrinx, pl. **syringes**
SysStim 226 muscle stimulator
Systec irrigation
system
ABG cement-free hip s.
above-knee suction enhancement s.
Accu-Cut osteotomy guide s.
Accu-Flo ultrafiltration s.
Acculength arthroplasty measuring s.
Accu-SPINA s.
AccuSway balance measurement s.
Ace intramedullary femoral nail s.
ACET s.
acetabular cup s.
acetabular prosthesis s.
AcroContin drug delivery s.
AcroMed VSP fixation s.
Acryl-X-II bone cement removal s.
Acryl-X orthopaedic cement removal s.
Action traction s.
Acufex microsurgical rear-entry to front-entry femoral guide s.
AcuFix anterior cervical plate s.
AcuMatch integrated hip s.

NOTES

system *(continued)*
Acumed great toe s.
Acuson imaging s.
Acustar surgical navigation s.
Acutrak fusion s.
Acutrak screw s.
Acutrak small bone fixation s.
Adjustaback wheelchair backrest s.
Advance PS total knee s.
Advantim revision knee s.
Advantim total knee s.
Aequalis s.
Aesculap ABC cervical plating s.
Affinity Anterior Cervical Cage S.
AGC Biomet total knee s.
AGC knee replacement s.
Agee carpal tunnel release s.
Agee WristJack fracture
  reduction s.
Agility total ankle s.
AIM femoral nail s.
Air-Back spinal s.
Aircast Knee S.
air inflation s.
Airtrac ambulatory cervical/lumbar
  traction s.
Alcon Closure S.
AlgoMed infusion s.
Allen shoulder/wrist arthroscopy
  traction s.
Alliance rehabilitation s.
Allofit acetabular cup s.
Allo-Pro hip s.
All-Pro ScanX-12 digital
  imaging s.
Alphatec mini lag-screw s.
Alphatec small fragment s.
Alta modular trauma s.
Ambi compression hip screw s.
American Joint Commission on
  Cancer staging s.'s
American shoulder and elbow s.
  (ASES)
American Society of
  Anesthesiologists physical status
  classification s.
AMK fixed bearing knee s.
AMK total knee s.
AML total hip s.
Amplatz anchor s.
Amset ALPS anterior locking
  plate s.
Amset R-F fixation s.
Anametric total knee s.
anatomically based exercise s.
anatomic medullary locking hip s.
Anchorlok soft tissue suture
  anchor s.
Anderson s.

Andersson hip status s.
AnkleTough rehabilitation s.
Anspach 65K Universal
  instrument s.
anterior cervical plate fixation s.
  (ACFS)
anterior Kostuik-Harrington
  distraction s.
anterior locking plate s. (ALPS)
anterior plate s. (APS)
antimigration s. (AMS)
AOFAS hallux rating s.
Apex Universal Drive and
  Irrigation S.
Apollo DXA bone densitometry s.
Apollo hip s.
Apollo knee prosthesis s.
Apollo total knee s.
APR II hip s.
APR total hip s.
Aqua-Cel heating pad s.
Aquaciser hydrodynamic
  measurement s.
Aquaciser 100R underwater
  treadmill s.
Aquanex hydrodynamic
  measurement s.
AquaSens fluid monitoring s.
Aqua Spray wet nail
  débridement s.
Ariel computerized exercise s.
Arthrex instruments and s.'s
ArthroCare arthroscopic s.
Arthro-Flo arthroscopic irrigation s.
Arthro-Lock s.
ArthroProbe laser s.
articular-ligamentous s.
Artisan cement s.
Ascent total knee s.
Ashhurst fracture classification s.
ASIF s.
Asnis 3 cannulated screw s.
Asnis 2 guided-screw s.
Assistant Free self-retaining hip
  surgery retractor s.
Association Research Circulation
  Osseous classification s.
Atavi atraumatic spine fusion s.
Atavi atraumatic spine surgery s.
Atavi TiTLE rod fixation s.
Atlantis cervical plate s.
Atlas cable s.
AuRA cemented total hip s.
autonomic nervous s.
Autovac TC orthopaedic
  autotransfusion s.
A-V Impulse s.
AVS spinal s.
axial spinal s.

Axiom modular knee s.
Axiom total knee s.
Axis fixation s.
AxyaWeld bone anchor s.
AxyaWeld J-tip suture welding s.
BacFix s.
Back Bull lumbar support s.
Back Revolution S.
Back Trainer spinal exercise s.
Bad Wildungen Metz spine s.
BAK/C Cervical Interbody
  Fusion S.
BAK Interbody Fusion S.
BAK Interbody Fusion S.
BAK/T thoracic interbody fusion s.
Balance Master training and
  assessment s.
BAPS ankle s.
Bassett electrical stimulation s.
Bateman UPF II bipolar knee s.
Batson vertebral brain s.
Becker orthopaedic spinal s.
  (BOSS)
Becker orthopaedic thermoformable
  ankle s.
Bigliani/Flatow shoulder s.
bilateral variable screw
  placement s.
Biodex Balance S.
Biodex Unweighing Support S.
Biodynamic Molding S.
Biofix absorbable fixation s.
Bio Flote air flotation s.
Bio-1000 knee brace s.
Biomechanical Ankle Platform S.
  (BAPS)
Biomet M2A metal-on-metal
  articulation for hip replacement s.
Biomet Maxim knee s.
Biomet revision knee s.
Biomet Ultra-Drive ultrasonic
  revision s.
Bio-Modular total shoulder s.
Bionicare 1000 stimulator s.
bioresorbable drug delivery s.
Biosensor biomechanical testing s.
BMP cabling and plating s.
body logic rehabilitation s.
Body Masters MD 510 hi-lo
  pulley s.
Body Response s.
Bolin wedge filter s.
bone density and arthritis testing s.

bone staple s.
Boston Classification S.
Boston elbow s.
Bottoms-Up posture s.
Bowden cable suspension s.
Boyer degenerative joint disease
  grading s.
Bremer halo s.
Bridge Hip s.
Brighton electrical stimulation s.
Browlift bone bridge s.
Buechel-Pappas total ankle
  replacement s.
Cable-Ready cable grip s.
cable suspension s.
Calandruccio external fixation s.
California soft spinal s. (CASS)
cannula s.
cannulated guided hip screw s.
Cannulated Plus screw s.
capsuloligamentous s.
Carbon Monotube long bone
  fracture external fixation s.
Cascade Up and About s.
CC Rider closed-chain
  rehabilitation s.
CD Horizon Sextant S.
Cemex s.
central nervous s. (CNS)
Cervifix s.
Charnley-Howorth Exflow s.
Charnley-Merle d'Aubigné disability
  grading s.
Charnley total hip s.
Chiba spinal s.
C-2 hip s.
Chirotech x-ray s.
Chonstruct chondral repair s.
Cincinnati Knee Rating S.
CircPlus bandage/wrap s.
Circul'Air shoe process s.
Circulator boot s.
CKS knee s.
Clanton turf toe grading s.
closed drainage s.
CLS hip s.
Coblation spinal surgery s.
Codman ACP s.
Codman anterior cervical plating s.
Codman Ti-frame posterior
  fixation s.
Cofield total shoulder s.
Cohort anterior plate s.

NOTES

723

system *(continued)*

Combi Multi-Traction S.
combined magnetic field s.
ComfortWalk foot s.
Command hip instrumentation s.
Command joint replacement
  instrument s.
Compass stereotactic s.
compliant prestress s. (CPS)
Concept arthroscopy power s.
Concept beach chair shoulder
  positioning s.
Concept Precise ACL guide s.
Concept rotator cuff repair s.
Concept self-compressing cannulated
  screw s.
Concept Sterling arthroscopy
  blade s.
Concise compression hip screw s.
concurrent force s.
Conserve hip s.
Constant and Murley shoulder
  scoring s.
ConstaVac autoreinfusion s.
contact laser delivery s.
Contact SPH cups s.
Continuum knee s. (CKS)
Contour Meniscus Arrow
  bioresorbable repair s.
Coombs bone biopsy s.
Coordinate complete revision
  knee s.
coordinate s. (X, Y, Z)
CO_2 powered gun s.
Corail hip s.
Corin hip arthroplasty s.
Corkscrew rotator cuff repair s.
Counter Rotation S. (CRS)
CPT hip s.
CRM s.
Crowe congenital hip dysplasia
  classification s.
CRS Tibial Torsion S.
cruciate condylar knee s.
Cryo/Cuff Knee Compression
  Dressing S.
C-Tek anterior cervical plate s.
curved Küntscher nail s.
Cybex I, II+ exercise s.
Cybex 340 isokinetic rehabilitation
  and testing s.
Cybex training s.
Dallas grading s.
Dall-Miles cable/crimp cerclage s.
Dall-Miles cable grip s.
DataHand s.
d'Aubigné hip status s.
deep bonding s. (DBS)

Deknatel orthopaedic
  autotransfusion s.
DEPA s.
Diab-A-Foot protection s.
Digital Biofeedback S.
Dimension hip s.
Discovery elbow s.
double-cannula s.
double inflow cannula s.
DTT s.
dual-lock total hip replacement s.
Dual Range Limiter S.
Dupont distal humeral plate s.
Duraloc acetabular cup s.
Durasul head s.
Dwyer-Wickham electrical
  stimulation s.
DynaFix external fixation s.
DynaFlex multilayer compression s.
Dyna-Lok pedicle screw s.
Dyna-Lok plating s.
dynamic stabilizing innersole s.
  (DSIS)
Dynasplint shoulder s.
Easyspine pedicle screw and rod s.
EBI Medical Systems bone
  healing s.
EBI Medical Systems Orthofix
  fixation s.
EBI XFix DynaFix S.
ECT internal fracture fixation s.
EDG s.
Edintrak II s.
Edwards modular s.
ElastaTrac home lumbar traction s.
Electri-Cool cold therapy s.
electrotherapy s. (ES)
Elite hip s.
Emerald implantation s.
EMG biofeedback s.
Endius endoscopic access s.
Endius TriFix thoracolumbar
  pedicle screw s.
Endolite transtibial s.
endoscopic carpal tunnel release s.
endoskeletal alignment s. (EAS)
Endotrac blade s.
Endotrac carpal tunnel release s.
Envision anterior cervical plate s.
EPIC functional evaluation s.
E-Series hip s.
Eska modular hip s.
Evans fracture classification s.
Ewald elbow arthroplasty rating s.
Exact-Fit ATH hip replacement s.
Exeter total hip s.
EX-FI-RE external fixation s.
Exogen bone healing s.

Exogen 2000 sonic accelerated fracture healing s.
Extend total hip s.
facet screw s.
facilitated spinal s.
FASTak suture anchor s.
FAST 1 intraosseous infusion s.
felt apron Bowden cable suspension s.
Fenlin total shoulder s.
Fernandez point-score wrist assessment s.
Fernandez scale posttraumatic wrist assessment s.
Ferno AquaCiser underwater treadmill s.
Fillauer endoskeletal alignment s.
Fillauer modular shuttle lock s.
filtration s.
FIN s.
Finn knee s.
Fitnet joint testing s.
Fixateur Interne fixation s.
FlexiTherm Thermographic S.
Flowtron pneumatic compression system BioCryo s.
FluoroNav virtual fluoroscopy s.
FluoroScan imaging s.
FMP acetabular s.
Foamart foot impression s.
Foot screw s.
Foot-Station 3-D foot imaging s.
Foundation total knee and hip s.
Fowler knee s.
FP5000 pump s.
Freehand prosthesis s.
Freeman-Swanson knee s.
F-Scan foot force and gait analysis s.
F-Scan in-shoe s.
F-Scan pressure measurement s.
fusimotor s.
fusion and reconstruction s. (FRS)
GDLH posterior spinal s.
GD Regainer S.
Gem total knee s.
Genesis II foot s.
Genesis II foot/ankle s.
Genesis II total knee s.
genital s.
Genucom ACL laxity analysis s.
Genucom knee flexion analysis s.
Geomedic s.

Gillette double-flexure ankle joint s.
Glider II patient transfer s.
Global Fx shoulder fracture s.
Global total shoulder arthroplasty s.
Golden mean testing s.
Golf Exercise S.
Gonstead pelvic marking s.
GPS s.
Graf stabilization s.
graft containment s.
Granberg cervical traction s.
gravitational platelet separation s.
gravity extension locking s. (GELS)
Gray revision instrument s.
Green-O'Brien evaluation s.
GTS 2-piece implant s.
Guardian limb salvage s.
Guldmann Overhead Trac S.
Haid UBP s.
Hajdu staging s.
Hall mandibular implant s.
Hall modular acetabular reamer s.
halo cervical traction s.
Hannover scoring s.
Harrington rod and hook s.
Harris hip status s.
Hausmann Work-Well work hardening s.
haversian s.
HBS bone screw s.
HCMI Chiropractic S.
headless bone screw s.
Herbert bone screw s.
Heritage hip s.
Hermes Evolution tricompartmental knee s.
Hermes total knee s.
Hexcel total condylar knee s.
Hipokrat bimodular shoulder s.
Histofreezer cryosurgical s.
HJD total hip s.
Hoffmann external fixation s.
hook probe s.
Hot/Ice S. III
Howmedica knee s.
Howmedica total ankle s.
Howmedica VSF fixation s.
HybridFit total hip s.
HybridFit total knee s.
hydraulic test s.
HydroFlex arthroscopy irrigating s.

NOTES

system *(continued)*
HydroTrack underwater treadmill s.
Hypobaric transfemoral s.
Hypobaric transtibial s.
ICRS arthroscopic staging s.
Ilizarov limb-lengthening s.
immune s.
Impact modular total hip s.
Impact total hip s.
Impingement-Free Tibial Guide S.
implantable internal s.
Index Chemicus Registry S. (ICRS)
Indiana tome carpal tunnel
  syndrome release s.
In-Fast bone screw s.
Infinity hip s.
InFix interbody fusion s.
Inglis-Pellicci elbow arthroplasty
  rating s.
Innomed arthroplasty measuring s.
Innovative COR/T implant s.
Insall-Burstein II modular total
  knee s.
Insight knee positioning and
  alignment s.
Instratek titanium cannulated small
  bone screw s.
instrumentation s.
In-Tac bone-anchoring s.
Integral hip s.
integrated shape and imaging s.
  (ISIS)
InteliJET fluid management s.
Inteq small joint suturing s.
Interax total knee s.
interbody fusion cage s.
Intermedics natural hip s.
internal fixation plate-screw s.
International 10-20 s.
International Listing S.
Iowa hip status rating s.
ipos arch support s.
IPS total hip s.
irrigation s.
ISKD s.
Isola fixation s.
Isola spinal instrumentation s.
Itrel II, III spinal cord
  stimulation s.
Jacobson s.
Joint Activate S.'s (JAS)
joint coordinate s. (JCS)
Judet hip status s.
Julstro Self-Treatment s.
Jurgan pin ball s.
J-Vac closed drainage s.
Kaltenborn joint mobilization s.
Kaneda anterior spinal/scoliosis s.
  (KASS)

Kellgren-Lawrence grading s.
Kendall A-V impulse s.
Keramos ceramic/ceramic total
  hip s.
K-Fix Fixator s.
K2 hemi toe implant s.
Kinamed Exact-Fit ATH s.
Kin-Con isokinetic exercise s.
Kinematic II condylar and
  stabilizer total knee s.
Kinematic II rotating hinge knee s.
Kinemax modular condylar and
  stabilizer total knee s.
Kinemax Plus total knee s.
Kinemetric guide s.
KineTec ECT s.
Kinetik great toe implant s.
Kirschner II-C shoulder s.
Kirschner integrated shoulder s.
knee extensor s.
knee signature s.
KobyGard s.
Koby Isogard surgical treatment s.
Kofoed scoring s.
Kostuik-Harrington distraction s.
Kurtzke functional s.
Kyle fracture classification s.
Langenskiöld grading s.
Larson hip status s.
LCR s.
LCS mobile bearing knee s.
LCS total knee s.
Leibinger Profyle hand s.
Liberty spinal s.
Lido Active Multijoint S.
Lidoback isokinetic dynamometry s.
Lido Passive Multijoint S.
Lifeline Wall Gym 2000 fitness s.
Linear total hip s.
Link custom partial pelvis
  replacement s.
Link Endo-Model rotational knee s.
Link Lubinus SP II hip
  replacement s.
Link Saddle Prosthesis Endo-Model
  hip replacement s.
LiteNest portable seating s.
locomotor s.
LoCon-T distal radial plating s.
Lone Star retractor s.
Lordex lumbar spine s.
Lorenz osteosynthesis s.
Lubinus AP hip s.
Lubinus SP II anatomically adapted
  hip s.
Luhr fixation s.
Lumbo 90 home care traction s.
lumbosacral cartilaginous s.
Luque II fixation s.

Lynco biomechanical orthotic s.
Mackinnon-Dellon staging s.
MacroPore OS spinal s.
Madajet XL jet-injection
  anesthesia s.
Magerl hook-plate s.
Magerl plate-screw s.
Magna-FX cannulated screw s.
Malcolm-Lynn radiolucent spinal
  retraction s.
Malcolm-Rand radiolucent headrest
  and retraction s.
Mallory-Head modular calcar s.
manual gun s.
Maramed Miami fracture brace s.
Mark III halo s.
Mark II Sorrells hip arthroplasty
  retractor s.
Mason fracture classification s.
matrix seating s.
Mattrix spinal cord stimulation s.
Maxim Modular Knee S.
Mayo Clinic hip scoring s.
McCain TMJ arthroscopic s.
Medical Examination and
  Diagnostic Coding S. (MEDICS)
Medical Research Council s.
Medtronic spinal cord
  stimulation s.
Meniscus Mender II s.
Mephisto speed lacing s.
Metasul metal-on-metal hip
  prosthesis s.
MG II total knee s.
Microloc knee s.
Micro-Mill knee instrument s.
MicroPhor iontophoretic drug
  delivery s.
Midas Rex instrumentation s.
Miller-Galante I condylar total
  knee s.
Miller-Galante revision knee s.
Mimix bone replacement s.
Minaar classification s.
Mini-Acutrak small bone fixation s.
mini lag screw s. (MLS)
Mirage Spinal S.
Mitek anchor s.
Mitek GII suture anchor s.
Mitek VAPR tissue removal s.
modified Wagner classification s.
Modular Acetabular Revision S.
  (MARS)

modular S-ROM total hip s.
Moe s.
Monotube external fixator s.
Monticelli-Spinelli circular external
  fixation s.
Moore hip endoprosthesis s.
Morrey elbow arthroplasty rating s.
MosaicPlasty s.
Moss fixation s.
motorized shaving s.
Mouradian humeral fixation s.
MRI-compatible plate and screw s.
Multi Balance S. (MBS)
Multidex chronic wound
  treatment s.
Multi Podus boot s.
Multi Podus foot s.
Multitak SS s.
Multitak suture snap s.
musculotendinous s.
Musgrave Footprint S.
M3-X extremity fixation s.
Myobock s.
Natural-Hip s.
Natural-Knee II s.
Navitrack computer-assisted
  surgery s.
Neer II shoulder s.
Neer II total knee s.
Neff femorotibial nail s.
Newport hip s.
NexGen complete knee s.
NexGen complete knee
  replacement s.
Nex-Link spinal fixation s.
Nexus wheelchair seating s.
NoHands Mouse-Foot-Operated
  Computer Mouse S.
NordiCare Back Therapy S.
Norm testing and rehabilitation s.
Nucleotome s.
OctaFix occipital fixation s.
OEC Mini 6600 imaging s.
Ogden fracture classification s.
Ogden plate s.
Ogden tissue reattachment mini s.
Oklahoma cable s.
Olerud pedicle fixation s.
Olerud PSF fixation s.
Omega compression hip screw s.
Omega Plus compression hip s.
Omnifit Plus hip s.
Omnifit total knee s.

NOTES

system *(continued)*

OnTrack s.
open double-decked hook
cervical s.
Optetrak comprehensive knee s.
Optetrak total knee replacement s.
Opti-Fix total hip s.
Option hip s.
optoelectric measuring s.
Optotrak motion measurement s.
Orth-evac autotransfusion s.
Orth-evac postoperative
transfusion s.
Orthodoc presurgical planning s.
Orthogenesis LPS limb preservation
prosthesis s.
Ortholoc Advantim revision knee s.
Ortholoc Advantim total knee s.
Orthomerica TC AFO s.
Orthomet Axiom total knee s.
Orthomet Perfecta total hip s.
OrthoPak bone growth stimulator s.
OrthoPAT s.
Osada portable electric
handpiece s.
Osada portable handpiece s.
Oscar ultrasonic bone cement
removal s.
OSI modular table s.
OssaTron shock wave therapy s.
osteochondral autograft transfer s.
(OATS)
Osteo-clage cable s.
Osteonics Scorpio posterior cruciate
retaining total knee s.
Osteopower modular handpiece s.
OsteoView 2000 imaging s.
Otto Bock MOBIS mobility s.
Oxford meniscal unicompartmental
knee s.
Panoview arthroscopic s.
ParaMax ACL guide s.
parasympathetic nervous s. (PNS)
Partnership s.
PCA primary total knee s.
PCA Universal total knee
instrument s.
Peak anterior compression plate s.
Peak Fixation S.
Peak Motus Motion
Measurement S.
PEC modular total knee s.
PEC total hip s.
Pedar in-shoe measurement s.
Pedar pressure insole s.
Pedar pressure measurement s.
pediatric s.
pedicle screw s.
Perfecta total hip s.

PerFixation s.
Performance modular total knee s.
Performance unicompartmental
knee s.
perioperative autotransfusion s.
peripheral nervous s. (PNS)
peripheral vascular s. (PVS)
PFC modular total knee s.
PFC Sigma knee s.
PFC TC3 modular knee s.
PFC total hip replacement s.
PGP flexible nail s.
Phoenix foot s.
Phoresor II iontophoretic drug
delivery s.
Phoresor PM900 iontophoresis s.
pin ball s.
Pinch Gauge and Jackson Strength
Evaluation S.
Pinnacle acetabular cup s.
Pinn-ACL guide s.
Pinn anterior cruciate ligament
guide s.
Pinwheel S.
Pipkin fracture classification s.
PlastiCast adjustable joint cast s.
plate-screw s.
PlexiPulse DVT prophylaxis s.
PMT halo s.
Podospray nail drill s.
point and pressure s.'s
3-point pressure s.
Polarus Plus humeral fixation s.
Polarus positional humeral
fixation s.
polyaxial s.
Polycentric and Wide-Track knee s.
Pop Rivet fixation s.
4-in-1 positioning block s.
Postel hip status s.
posterior cruciate condylar knee s.
posterior rod s.
Powerbelt exercise s.
PPT insole s.
PPT soft tissue orthotic s.
Precision Osteolock femoral
component s.
Precision Strata hip s.
press-fit total condylar knee s.
pressure transducer-monitor s.
pretarget filtration s.
Profile total hip s.
Profix total knee replacement s.
Profore Four-Layer bandage s.
programmable VariGrip II
prosthetic control s.
Promos modular shoulder s.
prospective payment s. (PPS)
Protector meniscus suturing s.

ProTrac cruciate reconstruction s.
Providence Scoliosis S.
Provisional Fixation TC-100
  plating s.
Proxiderm wound closure s.
Puddu osteotomy s.
Pulsavac III wound débridement s.
Pump It Up pneumatic socket
  volume management s.
Puno-Winter-Byrd s.
PWB transpedicular spine
  fixation s.
Pylon intramedullary nail s.
Quick-Sil silicone s.
QuickTack periosteal fixation s.
radiolucent wrist fixation s.
Rancho Cube S.
rearfoot stability s. (RSS)
ReCap femoral resurfacing s.
Reebok Slide S.
Reebok Step S.
Reese osteotomy guide s.
Reflection ceramic acetabular s.
Reflex anterior cervical plate s.
ReFlexion first MPJ implant s.
Replica total hip replacement s.
resorbable graft containment s.
Restoration acetabular s.
Restoration-HA hip s.
Restore ACL guide s.
reticuloendothelial s.
ReUnite resorbable orthopaedic
  fixation s.
Revelation hip s.
Revo rotator cuff repair s.
rHead implant s.
Richards fixator s.
Richards hip endoprosthesis s.
Richards modular hip s.
Richards Solcotrans orthopaedic
  drainage-reinfusion s.
right-handed orthogonal
  coordinate s. (RHOCS)
Riseborough-Radin fracture
  classification s.
Rochester compression s.
Rod TAG suture anchor s.
Roger Anderson s.
Rogozinski screw s.
Rogozinski spinal fixation s.
Rogozinski spinal rod s.
Roho pediatric seating s.
Rolyan Reach N Range Pulley S.

Romano curved drilling s.
Rotaglide total knee s.
Russell-Taylor femoral interlocking
  nail s.
Sabolich above-knee socket s.
SC-AcuFix anterior cervical
  plate s.
Schatzker fracture classification s.
Scorpio total knee s.
Scotchcast length splinting s.
Secure Yet Gentle surgical
  dressing s.
segmental spinal correction s.
  (SSCS)
segmented orthopaedic system total
  hip and knee s.
Selby I, II fixation s.
Select shoulder s.
Severin radiographic classification s.
Shadow-Line ACF spine
  retractor s.
SharpShooter tissue repair s.
shaving s.
Sherman remote podiatric
  vacuum s.
shoulder arm s. (SAS)
Shuttle MiniClinic resistance s.
Siemens Sonocur Basic
  extracorporeal shockwave
  therapy s.
Silhouette pedicle screw s.
Silhouette spinal s.
Simmons plating s.
Simmons and Segil classification s.
single-cannula s.
skeletal repair s. (SRS)
slotted obturator-cannula s.
SmartPReP PRP s.
Smith & Nephew bracing and
  support s.
Socon spinal s.
SOCS AFO s.
SOCS pad s.
Sofflex mattress s.
Sofwire cable s.
Solcotrans autotransfusion s.
Solcotrans orthopaedic drainage-
  refusion s.
Soma Gonio s.
Soma pulley s.
sonic accelerated fracture healing s.
  (SAFHS)

S

NOTES

system *(continued)*

SonoAce PICO portable digital color ultrasound s.
Sorbie-Questor total elbow prosthesis s.
Sorrells hip arthroplasty retractor s.
SOS total hip s.
SOS total knee s.
Souter Strathclyde total elbow s.
Spectron EF total hip s.
Spectrum tissue repair s.
spherocentric knee s.
spinal fusion s.
SpineCor s.
spinopelvic transiliac fixation s.
Spinoscope noninvasive imaging s.
SportCord exercise and rehabilitation s.
SportsRAC arm care s.
Square Module Seating S.
S-ROM hip replacement s.
S-ROM modular total knee s.
S-ROM proximally modular total hip s.
Stability total hip s.
Stableloc external wrist fixation s.
Stableloc II external fixation s.
Stahl staging s.
StairMaster exercise s.
Statak anchor s.
Stealth image-guided s.
Steffee pedicle screw-plate s.
Steffee variable spine plating s.
STIF s.
StIM s.
StIM neuromuscular stimulator s.
Stockholm hand arm vibration syndrome staging s.
Strata hip s.
Stratis ST ACL reconstruction s.
Stretch-Rite exerciser s.
Stromqvist hook pin s.
Stryker Intracompartmental Pressure Monitor S.
Stryker SE3 drive s.
suction-irrigation s.
supine C-Trax traction s.
SureClosure skin stretching s.
SureStep ankle support s.
Surgi-Stim postsurgical therapy s.
suture s. (SS)
SwimEx hydrotherapy s.
sympathetic nervous s. (SNS)
Synaptic 2000 pain management s.
Synergy hinge s.
Synergy spine rehab s.
Synergy Therapeutic S.
Synthes CerviFix s.
Synthes fixation s.

Synthes Schuhli implant s.
System Alloclassic hip s.
TAG anchor s.
Talar-Fit implant s.
Tamarack flexure joint s.
Taperloc hip s.
TEC interface s.
The Healthy Back S.
Thera-Band resistive therapy s.
Therabath paraffin heat therapy s.
Thera-Ciser light exercise s.
Thera-Ciser therapeutic exercise s.
Thera-Wedge s.
Thompson hip endoprosthesis s.
Thompson leg check s.
THORP s.
tibia coordinate s.
tibial torsion s.
Ti-Fit total hip s.
titanium hollow screw plate s.
top-loading screw and rod s.
Torus external fixation s.
Total Condylar Knee s.
Total Gym rehabilitation s.
Townley anatomic knee s.
TransFix ACL s.
TransFix femoral fixation s.
TraumaJet wound debridement s.
triangle blade s.
Triax monotube external fixation s.
Trilogy acetabular cup s.
Trim-It screw s.
Tri-Motion Knee S.
Trio medialized rod s.
triple envelope s.
Tri-Wedge total hip s.
True/Fit femoral intramedullary rod s.
True/Flex intramedullary rod s.
True-Lok external fixator s.
Trunkey fracture classification s.
TSRH crosslink s.
TSRH fixation s.
TSRH spinal implant s.
TSRH Universal spinal instrumentation s.
TurnAide therapeutic s.
Turning Board Exercise S.
Tylok high-tension cable s.
UBP s.
Ulson fixator s.
Ultima hip replacement s.
Ultima total hip s.
Ultimax distal femoral intramedullary rod s.
Ultra-Drive bone cement removal s.
Ultra-Drive ultrasonic revision s.
UltraFix RC suture anchor s.

Ultra-Guard FS hip bracing s.
Ultra-Guard hip orthosis s.
UltraPower drill s.
Ultra-X external fixation s.
unicompartmental knee s.
Unicondylar Geomedic hemi-knee s.
Uniflex nailing s.
unilateral variable screw
  placement s.
Uniportal fascial release s.
UniSyn modular hip s.
Universal bone plate s.
Up and About s.
VAC Freedom s.
Vanguard complete knee s.
Vapr s.
variable axis knee s.
variable screw placement s.
Vector low back analysis s.
Vermont pedicle fixation s.
Versaback back s.
Versa-Fx femoral hip fixation s.
Versalok low back fixation s.
VerSys hip s.
VertAlign spinal support s.
Vertetrac ambulatory traction s.
Vicon 3-dimensional gait
  analysis s.
Vilex cannulated screw s.
Vilex screw s.
VSF fixation s.
VSP s.
Wagner revision hip s.
WalkAide s.
WarmTouch patient warming s.
Warm-Up active wound therapy s.
Wedge TAG suture anchor s.
West Point Ankle Grading S.
Wiltse pedicle screw fixation s.
Wisconsin spinal fracture s.
Wit portable TENS s.

woodpecker s.
wound closure s.
Wrightlock posterior fixation s.
Wrightlock spinal fixation s.
WrisTimer carpal tunnel support s.
Xact ACL graft-fixation s.
Xia hook s.
Xia hook/spinal s.
Xia spinal s.
X-Y sensor s.
Y-knot tying s.
ZAAG Bone Anchoring S.
Zenith Electrotherapy ultrasound s.
Zephir anterior cervical plate s.
Zest Anchor Advanced Generation
  Bone Anchoring S.
Zickel fracture classification s.
Zimmer anatomic hip s.
Zimmer collarless polished taper
  hip s.
Zimmer CPT 12/14 hip s.
Zimmer crossover instrumentation s.
Zimmer-Hall drive s.
Zimmer hip implant s.
Zimmer Pulsavac wound
  débridement s.
Zimmer THARIES surface
  arthroplasty s.
Zimmer unicompartmental high-flex
  knee s.
ZMR hip s.
ZMS intramedullary fixation s.
Zone Specific II meniscal repair s.
Zuni exercise s.
Zweymuller hip s.

systemic
  s. lupus erythematosus (SLE)
  s. sclerosis
systolic blood pressure
systremma

NOTES

T

T buttress plate
T condylar fracture
T fracture
T score

T28

Trapezoidal-28
T28 hip prosthesis

T2-weighted dual-echo sequence

TA

TA metallic staple
TA Premium 30, 55, 90 staple

TAA

total ankle arthroplasty

tab

T.'s Elite mobility monitor
T. Grabber

tabes dorsalis

tabetic

t. arthropathy
t. foot
t. gait
t. osteoarthropathy

table

Adapta physical therapy t.
adjusting t.
Advocate electric flexion
distraction t.
Air-Drop chiropractic t.
Air-Flex chiropractic t.
Albee orthopaedic t.
Allen hand/arm surgery t.
AlphaStar t.
American Chiropractic College of
Radiology adjusting t.
AMIS extension t.
AM-MI orthopaedic t.
Anatomotor traction/massage t.
Andrews SST-3000 spinal
surgery t.
anteroposterior t. (ATPC)
Apollo TM electric flexion t.
APS Hi-Lo electric lift t.
ATT-300 LAT traction t.
Back Specialist chiropractic t.
Back Specialist electric t.
Back Specialist manual t.
bariatric mat t.
Bell t.
Berstein cast t.
cast t.
Chick CLT operating t.
Chick fracture t.
Chick-Langren orthopaedic t.
Chiro-Manis chiropractic t.

circumductor t.
Cobb attachment for Albee-
Compere fracture t.
craniosacral t.
crank t.
Crystal adjusting t.
cutout t.
DC-101 chiropractic t.
DDP t.
DePuy graft preparation t.
Diamond biomechanical t.
Ergo style flexion t.
Eurotech Diamond t.
Eurotech Emerald t.
Eurotech Platinum t.
Eurotech Sapphire t.
EZ-Up inversion t.
flexion-distraction chiropractic t.
fluoroscopic t.
fracture t.
friction-reduced examination t.
friction-reduced segmented t.
Galaxy 900HS adjusting t.
Galaxy McManis hylo t.
Gemini chiropractic t.
Green-Anderson growth t.
Hercules TM drop-adjusting t.
Hessco 300, 500 series
hydrotherapy t.
Hill Air-Drop HA90C t.
hi-lo t.
HLT-405 instrument adjusting t.
horseshoe therapy t.
hydromassage t.
inner t.
intersegmental traction
chiropractic t.
Jackson spinal surgery and
imaging t.
knavel t.
knee-chest t.
Leander chiropractic t.
Leander motorized flexion t.
Legend Hy-Lo adjusting t.
Legend stationary adjusting t.
Lloyd chiropractic t.
long axis traction chiropractic t.
Magnum 101 Plus t.
Marquet fracture t.
Massage Time Pro hydromassage t.
mat t.
McKenzie Repex t.
Med-Fit cranial-sacral t.
Meridian Intersegmental t.
Midland tilt t.

T

table *(continued)*
        Multi-Lock hand operating t.
        orthopaedic t.
        over-bed t.
        Paris manual therapy t.
        passive traction t.
        PET/Eurotech Generation 2000 t.
        physical therapy t.
        Platinum stationary t.
        Powermatic t.
        Protege manual flexion
          distraction t.
        PT tilt t.
        Rath treatment t.
        Re-Lax-O chiropractic t.
        resistive exercise t.
        Roger Anderson t.
        Sapphire t.
        t. short leg
        Skytron operating room t.
        slatted plinth t.
        slot t.
        Stryker surgical hand t.
        Telos fracture t.
        t. tie
        tilt t.
        Titan Apollo electric flexion t.
        Titan Meridian Intersegmental
          Traction t.
        Titan Nova manual flexion-
          extension multi flex t.
        Topaz manual flexion t.
        Tri W-G t.
        TX-1, TX-7 traction t.
        VAX-D therapy t.
        Verteflex Intersegmental Traction T.
        Williams Advantage t.
        Williams Model 170 t.
        Winco Folding Treatment T.
        Zenith ACS t.
        Zenith chiropractic t.
        Zenith-Cox flexion/distraction t.
        Zenith Hylos t.
        Zenith stationary t.
        Zenith Thompson t.
        Zenith Verti-Lift t.
        Zodiac TM Manual Flexion-
          Distraction t.
tablet
        bonemeal t.
tabletop Stone staple
taboparesis
Tab-Strap knee immobilizer
Tachdjian
        T. classification
        T. fractional lengthening
        T. hamstring lengthening
        T. orthosis

        T. pin
        T. procedure
Tacit threaded anchor
tack
        biodegradable surgical t.
        t. breakage
        membrane t.
        T. test
tack-and-pin forceps
tackle
        spear t.
tackler's
        t. arm
        t. exostosis
Tacoma sacral plate
tacrine HCl
Tacticon
        T. peripheral neuropathy kit
        T. peripheral neuropathy screening
          device
        T. quantitative sensory testing
tactile
        t. anesthesia
        t. discrimination
Tae Bo
TAG
        tissue anchor guide
        TAG anchor system
tag
        skin t.
        synovial t.
tai
        t. chi
        t. chi chuan exercise
tailbone
tailor's
        t. ankle
        t. bunion
        t. bunionectomy
        t. bunionette
Tait graft
Tajima
        T. method
        T. modified Kessler suture
        T. suture technique
Takakura index
Take-apart forceps
TakeOff elbow support
Take-Out Extractor
TAL
        tendo Achillis lengthening
talalgia
talar
        t. avulsion fracture
        t. axis–first metatarsal base angle
          (TAMBA)
        t. beak
        t. beaking
        t. body

t. body fusion
t. body nonunion
t. canal
t. declination angle
t. dislocation
t. dome
t. head
t. malunion
t. neck
t. neck class injury (I–III)
t. neck exostosis
t. neck fracture
t. neck osteotomy
t. neck tunnel
t. osteochondral fracture
t. process
t. ridge
t. shift
t. sinus
t. subluxation
t. sulcus
t. tilt (TT)
t. tilt angle
t. triple arthrodesis

Talar-Fit implant system
talectomy
Trumble t.
tali
sustentaculum t.
talipes
t. calcaneocavus
t. calcaneovalgus
t. calcaneovarus
t. calcaneus
t. cavovalgus
t. cavovarus
t. cavus
t. cavus deformity
t. convex pes valgus
t. equinovalgus
t. equinovarus (TEV)
t. equinus
flexible t.
t. planovalgus
t. planus
t. tendinoplasty
t. transversoplanus
t. varus

Tall-ette toilet seat
Talma disease
talocalcaneal
t. angle
anteroposterior t.

t. coalition
t. fusion
t. index
t. index classification
t. joint
t. ligament
t. ligament disruption
t. osteotomy
talocalcaneonavicular
t. complex
t. joint
t. ligament articulation
talocrural
t. alignment
t. angle
t. fusion
t. joint
t. restriction
t. sprain
talocruralis
talofibular
t. articulation
t. joint
t. ligament
talometatarsal angle
talonavicular (TN)
t. angle
t. arthrodesis
t. articulation
t. bone
t. capsule
t. capsulotomy
t. dislocation
t. fusion
t. joint
t. ligament
t. ossicle
t. ossicle of Pirie
t. sprain
Talon compression hip screw
talotibial exostosis
talus
t. alignment
beaking of head of t.
t. body fracture
congenital vertical t. (CVT)
flattop t.
t. foot deformity
t. lateral posterior process
t. lateral tubercle
osteochondral fracture of dome
of t.
sulcus of t.

NOTES

talus *(continued)*
    Tricodur T. compression dressing
    truncated wedge tarsometatarsal
      arthrodesis vertical t.
    valgus tilt of t.
    vertical t.

TAM
    total active motion

Tamae harvesting

Tamarack
    T. flexure joint
    T. flexure joint system

TAMBA
    talar axis–first metatarsal base angle

TAMMAS
    temporary articulating
      methylmethacrylate antibiotic spacer

tamp
    bone t.
    inflatable bone t. (IBT)
    tension band wire t.

tandem
    t. connector
    t. gait
    t. gait test

tangential
    t. hand
    t. incision
    t. layer
    t. standing radiograph
    t. x-ray view

Tang retractor

**Tanita Professional Body Composition
Analyzer**

tank
    Hubbard t. (HT)
    Hubbard physical therapy t.
    therapy t.

Tanner developmental model

**Tanner-Whitehouse bone-age reference
value**

tantalum-ball marker

tantalum mesh

tap
    AO t.
    t. drill
    dynamic condylar screw t.
    screw t.
    4-t. screw
    Screw-Lok t.
    synovial t.

tape
    anthropometric measuring t.
    benzoin adherent t.
    bias-cut t.
    cast t.
    Delta-Lite casting t.
    DynaSport athletic t.
    Elastikon elastic t.

    EnduraFIX t.
    EnduraSPORTS t.
    EnduraTape t.
    Expandover athletic t.
    fiberglass-free cast t.
    foam t.
    graded Gore-Tex t.
    Gulick II t.
    Leukotape sports t.
    Lightplast athletic t.
    Medipore H surgical t.
    Mersilene t.
    moleskin traction t.
    Powerflex t.
    Scotchcast 2 cast t.
    skin t.
    sports t.
    t. traction
    TufStuf II cast t.
    Ultra-Light athletic t.
    umbilical t.
    Zonas porous t.

taper
    t. cut needle
    Eurotaper 12/14 t.
    fiber metal t.
    Morse t.
    VerSys fiber metal t.

tapered
    collarless, polished, t. (CPT)
    t. hand reamer
    t. needle
    t. pin
    t. reamer

tapering dose steroid

taper-jaw forceps

Taperloc
    T. femoral component
    T. femoral prosthesis
    T. femoral stem
    T. hip system

taping
    basket-weave ankle t.
    buddy t.
    figure-of-8 t.
    Gibney t.
    Low-Dye t.
    patellar t.
    plantar fasciitis t.
    prophylactic t.
    t. technique

tapir
    bouche de t.

tapotement

tapping test of arm disability

TAR
    thrombocytopenia-absent radius
    total ankle replacement
    TAR syndrome

TARA
total articular replacement arthroplasty
total articular resurfacing arthroplasty
TARA total hip prosthesis
Taratynov disease
tarda
osteogenesis imperfecta t. (OIT)
Tardieu spasticity measurement scale
tardive muscular dystrophy
tardy ulnar palsy
target
t. of manipulation
T. prosthesis
t. ulcer
targeter
bone screw t.
IMP bone screw t.
targeting
t. bead
distal t.
t. drill guide
nail-mounted t.
Tarlov cyst
tarsal
t. amputation
t. arthrodesis
t. bar
t. bone
t. bone fracture
t. bridge
t. canal
t. canal artery
t. coalition
t. dislocation
t. joint
t. joint infection
t. medullostomy
t. navicular
t. navicular bursitis
t. plate
t. pronator shoe
t. sinus
t. sinus artery
t. tunnel
t. tunnel release (TTR)
t. tunnel syndrome (TTS)
t. wedge osteotomy
tarsalgia
tarsectomy
tarsectopia
tarsi (*pl. of* tarsus)
tarsitis
tarsoclasia

tarsoepiphysial aclasis
tarsometatarsal (TMT)
t. amputation
t. angle
t. articulation
t. dislocation
t. fracture-dislocation
t. joint
t. joint injury
t. junction
t. ligament
t. osteoarthritis
t. truncated-wedge arthrodesis
tarsophalangeal reflex
tarsotibial amputation
tarsotomy
tarsus, pl. **tarsi**
ligament of t.
ossa tarsi
sinus tarsi
tartrate resistant acid phosphatase (TRAP)
task
T. Force on Standards of Physical Therapy
metabolic equivalent of t. (MET)
walking t.
taut
t. band
t. foot
Tavernetti-Tennant knee prosthesis
Taylor
T. apparatus
T. back brace
T. clavicle support
T. percussion hammer
T. procedure
T. retractor
T. spinal frame
T. spinal retractor blade
T. spine brace
T. splint
T. technique
T. thoracolumbosacral orthosis
Taylor-Knight brace
T-Bar
T-B. guide
T-B. trigger point massager
TBI
traumatic brain injury
TBM
total bone matrix

NOTES

T

TCA
transcondylar axis
TCAT
Toglia Category Assessment Test
TCC
total contact casting
TCCK unconstrained knee prosthesis
T-cell
T-c. depletion
T-c. receptor antibody
TCFO
Therapy Carrot Finger Orthosis
TCFO placement wand
TCL
tibial collateral ligament
T-clamp
Pratt T-c.
Presbyterian Hospital T-c.
Tc-99m
technetium-99m
TCO
total contact orthosis
TCO$_2$
transcutaneous oxygen level
TCOM
transcutaneous oxygen monitor
TCP III
total condylar prosthesis III
TD
temperature differential
terminal device
TEA
Test of Everyday Attention
tea-and-toast diet
TEA-Ch
Test of Everyday Attention for Children
teacup fracture
Teale amputation
team
donor t.
t. handball
recipient t.
tear
acute meniscal t.
anterior horn meniscal t.
anterior oblique meniscal t.
bowstring t.
bucket-handle t.
cleavage t.
complex meniscal t.
degenerative meniscal t.
deltoid ligament t.
flap meniscal t.
full-thickness cuff t.
horizontal meniscal t.
horse-tail Achilles tendon t.
iatrogenic dural t.
incomplete t.
interstitial meniscal t.

intraoperative dural t.
Johnson-Jahss classification of
posterior tibial tendon t.
labral t.
lateral t.
longitudinal displaced complete t.
longitudinal incomplete
intrameniscal t.
longitudinal meniscal t.
longitudinal split t.
L-shaped rotator cuff t.
meniscal lateral t.
meniscal radial t.
meniscal transverse t.
meniscocapsular t.
midsubstance t.
mop-end Achilles tendon t.
mop-end mid-substance t.
Neer acromioplasty for rotator
cuff t.
oblique meniscal t.
parrot-beak t.
posterior cruciate ligament t.
posterior horn meniscal t.
posterior oblique meniscal t.
radial meniscal t.
rotator cuff t.
TFC t.
through-and-through t.
transverse t.
triangular fibrocartilage complex t.
vertical longitudinal t.
V-shaped rotator cuff t.
teardrop
t. fracture
t. line
t. sign
teardrop-shaped flexion-compression fracture
Teare
T. arm splint
T. sling
tearing sound
teaspoon
nylon t.
TEC
Total Environment Control
TEC interface system
TEC liner
Techmedica implant
technetium
t. labeled methylene diphosphonate
t. stannous pyrophosphate
technetium-99 methylene diphosphonate
technetium-99m-labeled monoclonal antigranulocyte antibody
technetium-99m (Tc-99m)
t.-99m diphosphonate scan

t.-99m methylene diphosphate bone
scan
t.-99m phosphate
t.-99m pyrophosphate
t.-99m pyrophosphate scan
t.-99m sulfur colloid scan
**Techni-Care surgical scrub
technique**
abduction traction t.
abductor slide t.
Abumi t.
accessory movement t.
Ace-Colles frame t.
Achilles tendon taping t.
active-release t. (ART)
adduction traction t.
Albizzia t.
Alexander t.
Allgöwer suture t.
Amstutz resurfacing t.
Anderson screw placement t.
Andrews t.
anterior iliofemoral t.
anterior quadriceps
musculocutaneous flap t.
AO-ASIF compression t.
AO surgical t.
Armistead t.
arthrographic capsular distension
and rupture t.
Asher physical build assessment t.
ASIF screw fixation t.
Asnis t.
Atasoy V-Y t.
Avila t.
avulsion t.
axial pin t.
Badgley t.
bag-of-bones t.
Bailey-Badgley t.
Bailey-Dubow t.
Baker t.
Barbour t.
barrier t.
Barsky t.
basic t.
Basmajian t.
Batch-Spittler-McFaddin t.
Baumgaertel and Gotzen calcaneal
fracture reduction t.
Baumgard-Schwartz tennis elbow t.
Beckenbaugh t.
Becker t.

Becton t.
Bell-Tawse open reduction t.
biframed distraction t.
bilateral arm raise back exercise t.
Black t.
Blackburn t.
Blair t.
Bleck recession t.
Blount tracing t.
Bobath t.
Böhler calcaneal fracture
reduction t.
Bohlman cervical fusion t.
Bohlman triple-wire t.
bone marrow stimulating t.
Bonfiglio modification of
Phemister t.
Bonola t.
Bora t.
Borggreve-Hall t.
Bosworth t.
Bowers t.
Boyd-Anderson t.
Boyd-McLeod tennis elbow t.
Boyes brachioradialis transfer t.
Brady-Jewett t.
Brand tendon transfer t.
bridge back exercise t.
Brooks t.
Brooks-Jenkins atlantoaxial fusion t.
Broström injection t.
Brown t.
Bruser t.
Bryan-Morrey t.
Buck-Gramcko t.
Bugg-Boyd t.
Buncke t.
Bunnell atraumatic t.
Bunnell tendon suturing t.
Bunnell tendon transfer t.
bur-down t.
Burgess t.
Burkhalter modification of Stiles-
Bunnell t.
Burkhalter transfer t.
Burow skin flap t.
Burrows t.
Calandruccio t.
Callahan fusion t.
Camino catheter t.
Camitz t.
Campbell t.
Canale t.

T

NOTES

technique *(continued)*

cannulated reaming t.
Capello t.
Carnesale t.
Carrell fibular substitution t.
Caspar anterior cervical plating t.
CBP t.
cementless t.
central semi suture-loop meniscal
repair t.
central slip sparing t.
central splitting t.
cerclage t.
cervical screw insertion t.
cervical spondylotic myelopathy
fusion t.
chevron t.
Chiari t.
Childress ankle fixation t.
chiropractic manipulative reflex t.
(CMRT)
Cho tendon t.
Chow transbursal carpal tunnel
release t.
Chrisman-Snook ankle t.
Cierny-Mader t.
Cincinnati t.
Clancy ligament t.
Clark transfer t.
Cloward t.
t. of Cobb
Cobb scoliosis measuring t.
Codivilla tendon lengthening t.
Cofield t.
Cole t.
Coleman flatfoot t.
Collis broken femoral stem t.
Coltart fracture t.
combination of isotonics t.
compression t.
Connolly t.
contoured anterior spinal plate t.
contract-relax t.
conventional t.
Conyers t.
Coonse-Adams t.
coracoclavicular t.
costotransversectomy t.
cotyloplasty t.
counterstrain t.
Cox flexion-distraction t.
Craig Handicap Assessment and
Reporting T. (CHART)
craniosacral therapy t.
Crego tendon transfer t.
Cubbins shoulder dislocation t.
Cuniard and Campell t.
Curtis t.
Cyriax t.

Davis drainage t.
DeBastiani t.
decompression t.
decortication t.
DePalma modified patellar t.
Dewar-Barrington clavicular
dislocation t.
Dewar-Harris shoulder t.
Dewar posterior cervical fusion t.
Deyerle femoral fracture t.
Dickinson calcaneal bursitis t.
Dickson transplant t.
Dimon-Hughston t.
distraction t.
distraction osteogenesis t.
Doll trochanteric reattachment t.
Doppler t.
double-looped semitendinous and
gracilis hamstring graft knee
reconstruction t.
double portal t.
double-rod t.
dowel graft t.
doweling spondylolisthesis t.
DREZ modification of Eriksson t.
drilling t.
Drummond spinous wiring t.
Dunn t.
DuVries deltoid ligament
reconstruction t.
Eastwood t.
Eaton-Littler t.
Eberle contracture release t.
Eftekhar broken femoral stem t.
Eggers tendon transfer t.
Ellis-Jones peroneal tendon t.
Ellison t.
Ellis skin traction t.
Ender femoral fracture t.
Eriksson brachial block t.
Eriksson ligament t.
Essex-Lopresti axial fixation t.
Essex-Lopresti calcaneal fracture t.
European compression t. (ECT)
Evans ankle reconstruction t.
excision-curettage t.
extraarticular t.
extremity mobilization t.
facet excision t.
facilitatory t.
Fahey t.
Fairbanks t.
Farmer t.
fear-near, near-far suture t.
Ferkel torticollis t.
FHL release t.
Fielding modification of Gallie t.
finger t.
Fish cuneiform osteotomy t.

fixation t.
flat-cut t.
Flatt t.
flexor hallucis longus release t.
Flynn t.
Forbes modification of Phemister
  graft t.
Ford triangulation t.
Fowler t.
Fowles dislocation t.
freehand suturing t.
French fracture t.
Froimson t.
Frost posterior tibialis t.
functional squats back exercise t.
funnel t.
fusion t.
Gaenslen split-heel t.
Gallie atlantoaxial fusion t.
Gallie wire fixation t.
Gallie wiring t.
Galveston t.
Ganley t.
Garceau tendon t.
Ger t.
Giannestras modification of
  Lapidus t.
Gill sliding graft t.
gliding-hole-first t.
gluteal/hamstring raise back
  exercise t.
Goldberg t.
Goldner-Clippinger t.
Goldstein spinal fusion t.
Gonstead t.
Gordon joint injection t.
great toe arthroplasty implant t.
  (GAIT)
Green-Banks t.
Greulich-Pyle t.
Grice-Green t.
Grosse-Kempf tibial t.
Guhl t.
Guttmann t.
Hackethal stacked nailing t.
Hall t.
Hamas t.
hamstring fixation t.
Hardinge t.
Harmon transfer t.
Harriluque t.
Harrington-Luque t.
Hauser patellar realignment t.

Hendler unitunnel t.
Henning inside-to-outside t.
Henry acromioclavicular t.
Hermodsson internal rotation t.
Hey Groves fascia lata t.
Hey Groves-Kirk t.
Hey Groves ligament
  reconstruction t.
Heyman t.
high-velocity, low-amplitude
  thrust t.
HIO t.
hip hinge back exercise t.
Hirschhorn compression t.
Hitchcock tendon t.
Hodgson t.
Hohl-Moore t.
Hoke-Kite t.
hold-relax t.
hole-in-one t.
Hollywood roll t.
Hori t.
hot dog t.
Howard t.
Hungerford t.
Huntington tibial t.
Ilizarov ankle fusion t.
Ilizarov limb-lengthening t.
inferior capsular split t.
injection t.
Insall-Hood reconstruction t.
Insall ligament reconstruction t.
inside-out tissue repair t.
inside-to-outside t.
interference screw t.
interspinous segmental spinal
  instrumentation t. (ISSI)
intrafocal reduction t.
inverting knot t.
ischemic tourniquet t.
Isobaric epidural/spinal anesthesia t.
isometric t.
Jacobs locking hook spinal rod t.
Jansey t.
Jeffery t.
Johnson pelvic fracture t.
Johnson staple t.
Kapandji pinning t.
Kapandji-Sauvé t.
Kapel elbow dislocation t.
Kaplan t.
Kashiwagi t.
Kaufer tendon t.

NOTES

technique *(continued)*
    Kaufmann t.
    Kennedy ligament t.
    Kessler suture t.
    keyhole tenodesis t.
    King t.
    King-Richards dislocation t.
    Kite and Lovell t.
    Klein t.
    Kloehn craniofacial remodeling t.
    kneeling reciprocal back exercise t.
    Krackow locking loop t.
    Krackow locking suture t.
    Krackow-Thomas-Jones t.
    Kumar spica cast t.
    Küntscher t.
    Lambrinudi t.
    Lapidus hammertoe t.
    Larson t.
    Leadbetter t.
    Lee t.
    Lehman t.
    Leibolt t.
    Lewit stretch t.
    Lichtman t.
    Liebolt radioulnar t.
    Lindholm t.
    line-to-line reaming t.
    Lippman-Cobb t.
    Lipscomb t.
    Lister t.
    Little t.
    Littler t.
    Littler-Cooley t.
    Lloyd-Roberts fracture t.
    local standby anesthesia t.
    locking-suture t.
    Losee modification of MacIntosh t.
    Losee sling and reef t.
    Louisiana ankle wrap t.
    Low-Dye taping t.
    Ludloff t.
    lumbar accessory movement t.
    Luque instrumentation concave t.
    Luque instrumentation convex t.
    Luque sublaminar wiring t.
    Lyden t.
    Lynn Achilles tendon repair t.
    MacIntosh t.
    Magerl screw placement t.
    Magerl translaminar facet screw fixation t.
    Magilligan measuring t.
    Magnuson t.
    Ma-Griffith t.
    Maitland t.
    Majestro-Ruda-Frost tendon t.
    Malawer excision t.
    Mallory t.

    manipulative t.
    Mankin t.
    Mann t.
    Manske t.
    manual push-pull t.
    Marks-Bayne t.
    Marshall ligament repair t.
    Marshall-McIntosh t.
    Martin patellar wiring t.
    Matti-Russe t.
    Mazet t.
    McConnell t.
    McElvenny t.
    McFarland-Osborne t.
    McReynolds open fracture reduction t.
    medial cortical overlap t.
    medial heel skive t.
    Mendelsohn modification of matricectomy suture t.
    Mensor-Scheck t.
    microneurosurgical t.
    Milch cuff resection of ulna t.
    Milch elbow t.
    Milford mallet finger t.
    mille pattes t.
    Millesi modified t.
    Mital elbow release t.
    miter t.
    Mizuno t.
    modified Crawford Campbell inlaid bone-grafting t.
    Moe scoliosis t.
    Mohs t.
    Monticelli-Spinelli distraction t.
    Moore t.
    Morrison t.
    mosaicplasty t.
    Moss t.
    muscle energy t.
    Nalebuff-Millender lateral band mobilization t.
    neural arch resection t.
    Neviaser acromioclavicular t.
    Nicholas ligament t.
    Nicholas 5-in-1 reconstruction t.
    Niebauer-King t.
    Nimmo receptor-tonus t.
    Nirschl t.
    noninvasive t.
    no-touch t.
    OATS t.
    Ober tendon t.
    Obwegeser sagittal mandibular osteotomy t.
    Ogata t.
    Ollier t.
    open-bowl cement t.
    open palm t.

O'Phelan t.
Osborne-Cotterill elbow t.
Osgood modified t.
Osmond-Clarke t.
Ostrup harvesting t.
outside-in t.
outside-to-outside arthroscopy t.
Pack t.
Palmer t.
palpatory t.
pants-over-vest t.
Papineau t.
Parachute t.
Parrish-Mann hammertoe t.
partial sit-ups back exercise t.
Parvin gravity t.
passive gliding t.
Paterson t.
Paulos ligament t.
Pauwels t.
Peacock transposing t.
peg-and-socket t.
Perry t.
Pheasant elbow t.
Phemister-Bonfiglio t.
Phemister onlay bone graft t.
PNF t.
3-point pressure t.
Ponseti t.
2-portal t.
3-portal t.
Porter-Richardson-Vainio t.
posterior flap t.
posterior iliofemoral t.
posterolateral costotransversectomy t.
postganglionic t.
postisometric relaxation traction t.
postisometric stretch t.
Pratt t.
preemptive blockade t.
preganglionic t.
press-fit acetabular implant
  insertion t.
prone blocking t.
proximal-to-distal dissection t.
Puddu tendon t.
Pulvertaft weave tendon repair t.
quadruped back exercise t.
Quénu nail plate removal t.
Rayhack t.
reciprocal arm raise back
  exercise t.
reduction t.

Reichenheim t.
reverse lunge back exercise t.
reverse wedge t.
rhythmic initiation t.
Rideau t.
Riordan tendon transfer t.
Risser t.
Risser-Ferguson t.
Roberts t.
Robinson-Southwick fusion t.
Rockwood-Green t.
Rogers cervical fusion t.
Rood t.
Royle-Thompson transfer t.
Russe t.
Ryerson t.
sacral bar t.
sacrooccipital t. (SOT)
Saha transfer t.
Salter t.
Sarmiento trochanteric fracture t.
Scaglietti closed reduction t.
Schauwecker patellar wiring t.
Schnute wedge resection t.
Schober t.
Scott glenoplasty t.
screw insertion t.
Scuderi t.
second-generation cementing t.
Seddon t.
Sell-Frank-Johnson extensor shift t.
semi-suture-loop t.
semitendinosus t.
Serafin t.
Sever modification of Fairbank t.
SharpShooter tissue repair t.
Sharrard transfer t.
shish kebab t.
short lever accessory movement t.
side lunge back exercise t.
side-lying back exercise t.
Silfverskiöld t.
silver dollar t.
Simultaneous Interview T. (SIT)
single proximal portal t.
Skoog t.
2-sleeve t.
sling and reef t.
slit catheter t.
Slocum fusion t.
Smith t.
Smith-Petersen t.
Smith-Robinson t.

T

NOTES

technique *(continued)*
 Sofield femoral deficiency t.
 Somerville t.
 SOTO t.
 Spälteholz bone-clearing t.
 spinal fusion t.
 spinal mobilization t.
 spinopelvic transiliac fixation t.
 spiral t.
 Sprague arthroscopic t.
 spray and stretch t.
 2-stage tendon grafting t.
 Staheli t.
 Stanisavljevic t.
 Staples t.
 STAR t.
 Steffee instrumentation t.
 Stiles-Bunnell transfer t.
 Stimson anterior shoulder
  reduction t.
 strain/counterstrain t.
 Straub t.
 Strayer tendon t.
 Strickland t.
 strut fusion t.
 2-strut tibial graft t.
 suction-bubble t.
 suction-irrigation t.
 superman back exercise t.
 surgical t.
 sustained pressure t.
 suture anchor t.
 suture-loop t.
 Swanson t.
 Tajima suture t.
 taping t.
 Taylor t.
 tension band wiring t.
 Teuffer t.
 third-generation cementing t.
 Thomas-Thompson-Straub transfer t.
 Thompson-Henry t.
 thoracic lymphatic pump t.
 thoracolumbar spondylosis
  surgical t.
 threaded-hole-first t.
 Tohen tendon t.
 Torg t.
 transiliac bar t.
 triangulation t.
 triple bundle t.
 triple-wire t.
 Tullos t.
 Turco clubfoot release t.
 unassisted locking-suture t.
 unitunnel t.
 unlocking spiral t.
 vacuum cement mix t.
 vasomotor t.

 Vastamäki t.
 Veleanu-Rosianu-Ionescu t.
 Verdan t.
 vertical loop suture t.
 Vidal-Adrey fracture t.
 Viladot surgical t.
 Wadsworth t.
 Wagner open reduction t.
 Wagoner cervical t.
 Warner-Farber ankle fixation t.
 Watkins fusion t.
 Watson t.
 Watson-Cheyne t.
 Weaver-Dunn acromioclavicular t.
 Weber-Vasey traction-absorption
  wiring t.
 Weinstein-Ponseti t.
 Wellmerling t.
 Wertheim-Bohlman t.
 Whitesides t.
 Whitesides-Kelly cervical t.
 wick t.
 wick catheter t.
 Williams flexion back exercise t.
 Williams-Haddad t.
 Wilson t.
 Wilson-Jacobs tibial fracture
  fixation t.
 Windson-Insall-Vince grafting t.
 Winograd ingrown nail t.
 Winter spondylolisthesis t.
 wire removal t.
 Woodward t.
 Zancolli rerouting t.
 Zarins-Rowe ligament t.
 Zeier transfer t.
 Zielke t.

TechnoGel insole
technology
 Cascading Tower T.
 Footwear Integration T. (FIT)
 GADS t.
 professional protective t. (PPT)
 segmentally demineralized bone t.
 VSL t.
 work evaluation systems t.
tectal plate
Tectonic magnet
tectoral ligament
TED
 thromboembolic disease
 TED hose
 TED stockings
teeth *(pl. of* tooth)
Teflon
 T. cannula
 T. implant
 T. tri-leaflet prosthesis

Teflon-coated
T.-c. driver
T.-c. suture
Tegaderm dressing
Tegner
T. activity rating scale
T. knee reconstruction activity
score
Tei-Shin
Tekscan in-shoe monitoring device
telangiectasia
calcinosis, Raynaud, esophageal
motility disorders, sclerodactyly, t.
(CREST)
telangiectasia-ataxia
telangiectatic osteosarcoma
Telectronics
T. electrical stimulation apparatus
T. electrical stimulation device
Teledyne Water Pik misting massage
teleroentgenography
telescopic
T. Plate Spacer implantable
titanium spacer
t. view guide
telescoping
t. brace
t. medullary rod
t. nail
t. tubular device
telethermometer
Telfa
T. bolster
T. gauze
T. gauze dressing
T. sponge
Telos fracture table
TELS
The Experience of Leisure Scale
TEM
terminal extensor mechanism
temper
T. Foam
T. Foam cube
T. Foam cushion
t. tantrum elbow
temperature
capillary refill, sensation, motor
function, t. (CSMT)
t. differential (TD)
optimal cutting t. (OCT)
wet globe t.
Temperlite saw blade

template
acetabular cup t.
Charnley t.
femoral condylar t.
malleable t.
Moore t.
Mueller t.
Pedrialle t.
prosthesis t.
rod t.
Stevens-Street elbow prosthesis t.
thermoplastic t.
tibial track t.
transparent t.
templating roentgenogram
Temple
T. University nail
T. University plate
temporal
t. bone
t. bone fracture
t. dispersion
t. fascia graft
temporalis fascia flap
temporary
t. articulating methylmethacrylate
antibiotic spacer (TAMMAS)
t. callus
t. cavity phenomenon
t. cerclage wire
t. external fixator
t. prosthetic fitting
t. socket
temporomandibular
t. joint (TMJ)
t. joint arthralgia
t. joint dislocation
t. joint syndrome
Tempur-Pedic
T.-P. pressure relieving Swedish
mattress
T.-P. pressure relieving Swedish
pillow
tenaculum-reducing forceps
tenalgia crepitans
tender
t. point (TeP)
t. point examination
Tenderlett device
tenderness
bony t.
costovertebral angle t. (CVAT)
CVA t.

T

NOTES

tenderness *(continued)*
    joint line t.
    myofascial t.
    percussion t.
    pillar t.
    point t.
    rebound t.
tender point (TeP)
tendinitis, tendonitis
    Achilles t.
    acute calcific t.
    anterior tarsal t.
    biceps t.
    bicipital t.
    birefringent lipid crystals in t.
    calcific t.
    chronic Achilles t.
    de Quervain t.
    digital flexor t.
    infrapatella t.
    infrapatellar t.
    infraspinatus t.
    patellar t.
    peripatellar t.
    peroneal t.
    popliteus t.
    posterior tibial t. (PTT)
    radial wrist extensor t.
    rotator cuff calcific t.
    semimembranosus t.
    subscapular t.
    suprapatellar t.
    supraspinatus t.
    ulnar wrist extensor t.
    wrist extensor t.
    wrist flexor t.
tendinopathy
    Achilles t.
    Blazina t.
    insertion t.
    peroneus longus t. (PLT)
    posterior tibial t.
    primary peroneus longus t.
    rotator cuff t.
tendinoplasty
    talipes t.
tendinosis
    angiofibroblastic hyperplasia t.
    calcific t.
    insertional Achilles t.
    medial tennis elbow t.
tendinosuture
tendinotrochanteric ligament
tendinous
    t. attachment
    t. fiber
    t. sheath
    t. synovitis
tendinum

tendo
    t. Achillis
    t. Achillis lengthening (TAL)
    t. Achillis mechanism
    t. calcaneous lengthening
    t. calcaneus
    t. calcaneus lengthening
tendolysis
tendon
    abductor digiti quinti t.
    abductor hallucis t.
    abductor pollicis brevis t.
    abductor pollicis longus t.
    accessory communicating t.
    Achilles t. (AT)
    adductor hallucis t.
    adductor pollicis brevis t.
    adherent profundus t.
    t. advancement
    anchoring t.
    anterior tibial t.
    aponeurosis of t.
    attenuation of t.
    attrition of t.
    attrition rupture of t.
    biceps brachialis t.
    biceps brachii t.
    biceps femoris t.
    bicipital t.
    t. bowing
    t. bowing in arthritis
    brachialis t.
    brachial plexus t.
    brachioradialis t.
    calcaneal t.
    carpi radialis brevis t.
    carpi radialis longus t.
    t. cartilage
    t. centralization
    t. checkrein procedure
    common extensor t.
    conjoined t.
    digital extensor t.
    digital flexor t.
    digiti quinti proprius t.
    digitorum communis t.
    t. disorder
    t. displacement
    ECRB t.
    ECRL t.
    ECU t.
    EDB t.
    EHL t.
    EIP t.
    elbow extensor t.
    evertor t.
    t. excursion
    extensor carpi radialis brevis t.
    extensor carpi radialis longus t.

extensor carpi ulnaris t.
extensor digiti minimi t.
extensor digiti quinti t.
extensor digitorum brevis t.
extensor digitorum communis t.
extensor digitorum longus t.
extensor hallucis longus t.
extensor indicis proprius t.
extensor pollicis brevis t.
extensor pollicis longus t.
extensor quinti t.
t. fixation
flexor carpi radialis t.
flexor carpi ulnaris t.
flexor digitorum communis t.
flexor digitorum longus t.
flexor digitorum profundus t.
flexor digitorum sublimis t.
flexor digitorum superficialis t.
flexor hallucis brevis t.
flexor hallucis longus t.
flexor pollicis brevis t.
flexor pollicis longus t.
flexor profundus t.
flexor sublimis t.
t. forceps
gastrocnemius t.
gastrocnemius-soleus t.
G-lengthening of semitendinosus t.
Golgi t.
t. gouge
t. grabber
gracilis t.
t. graft (TG)
hamstring t.
t. harvester
t. healing
Hector t.
hilus of t.
iliopsoas t.
t. inflammation
infrapatellar t.
infraspinatus t.
interosseous t.
t. interposition
t. interposition arthroplasty
t. irregularity
t. jerk
t. leader
t. lengthening
t. lengthening osteotomy
long head biceps t.
lumbrical t.

midpatellar t.
t. needle
t. nodularity
t. nodule
obturator internus t.
palmaris longus t.
t. passer
patellar t.
patelloquadriceps t.
peroneal t.
peroneus brevis t.
peroneus longus t.
peroneus tertius t.
plantaris t.
t. plate
t. plica
popliteal t.
popliteus t.
posterior tibial t. (PTT)
postoperative flexor t. (PFT)
ProCol bovine bioprosthesis t.
profundus t.
pronator teres t.
proprius t.
t. prosthesis
quadriceps t.
rectus femoris t.
t. reflex
t. release
t. repair
rerouted t.
rider's t.
t. rod
rotator cuff t.
t. rupture
sartorius t.
semimembranosus t.
semitendinosus t.
t. sheath
t. sheath endoscopy
slip of t.
snapping t.
t. snapping
split anterior tibial t.
t. stripper
sublimis t.
subscapularis t.
t. substitution
superficialis t.
supraspinatus t.
t. suture
t. thickening
thumb extensor t.

T

NOTES

tendon *(continued)*
    thumb flexor t.
    tibial t.
    tibialis anterior t.
    tibialis posterior t.
    toe extensor t.
    t. transfer
    t. transplantation
    t. transposition
    t. trapping
    triceps brachii t.
    tropocollagen t.
    t. tucker
    t. tunneler
    wrist extensor t.
    t. Z-lengthening around knee and ankle
    Z-lengthening of biceps t.
tendon-bearing-supracondylar
    patellar t.-b.-s.
tendon-bearing-supracondylar
    patellar t.-b.-s. (PTB)
tendon-bone
    t.-b. allograft
    t.-b. attachment
    bone-patellar t.-b. (BPB, BPTB)
    t.-b. bridge
tendon-braiding forceps
tendon-holding forceps
tendonitis *(var. of* tendinitis)
tendon-passing forceps
tendon-pulling forceps
tendon-retrieving forceps
tendon-seizing forceps
tendon-to-bone attachment
tendon-tunneling forceps
tendopathy
    plantar t.
tendoscopy
tendosuspension
    Hibbs t.
    Jones t.
tendosynovitis
tendotomy
tendovaginitis
tenectomy
tennis
    t. elbow
    t. elbow arm band
    t. elbow splint
    t. elbow test
    t. fracture
    t. heel
    t. leg
    t. shoulder
    t. thumb
    t. toe
tenocyte

tenodesis
    Andrews iliotibial band t.
    Andrews lateral t.
    anterolateral femorotibial ligament t.
    band t.
    biceps t.
    calcaneal t.
    Chrisman-Snook t.
    Darrach ulnar t.
    t. effect
    Eggers t.
    Ellison iliotibial band t.
    Evans t.
    extensor hallucis longus t.
    femorotibial ligament t.
    Fowler t.
    hallucis brevis t.
    t. of heel cord
    iliotibial band t.
    interphalangeal t.
    key-grip t.
    keyhole t.
    MacIntosh extraarticular t.
    MacIntosh iliotibial band t.
    Moberg key-grip t.
    modified Watson-Jones ankle t.
    Mueller anterolateral femorotibial ligament t.
    Norwood iliotibial band t.
    t. orthosis
    SCOI arthroscopic t.
    semitendinosus t.
    sublimis t.
    t. test
    triple t.
    Watson-Jones ankle t.
    Westin t.
tenodynia
tenography
tenolysis
    flexor t.
    peroneal t.
tenomyoplasty
tenomyotomy
tenonectomy
tenonitis
tenontodynia
tenontomyoplasty
tenontomyotomy
tenontophyma
tenontoplastic
tenontoplasty
tenontothecitis
tenoperiostitis
tenophyte
tenoplastic reconstruction
tenoplasty
tenorrhaphy
tenositis

tenostosis
tenosuspension
tenosuture
tenosynography
tenosynovectomy
    dorsal t.
    flexor t.
tenosynovial
    t. giant cell tumor
    t. injection
    t. sheath
tenosynovitis
    adhesive t.
    bicipital t.
    t. crepitans
    de Quervain stenosing t.
    flexor hallucis longus t.
    gonococcic t.
    gonorrheal t.
    granulomatous t.
    t. hypertrophica
    infectious t.
    localized nodular t.
    nodular t.
    peroneal t.
    t. serosa stenosans
    stenosing t.
    suppurative flexor t.
    tuberculous peroneal t.
    villonodular t.
    villous t.
tenotomized
tenotomy
    Achilles t.
    adductor t.
    Braun shoulder t.
    curb t.
    extensor t.
    fenestrated t.
    flexor t.
    Fowler central slip t.
    graduated t.
    inverted-Y Achilles t.
    t. knife
    Lichtblau t.
    open t.
    percutaneous t.
    semiopen sliding t.
    sliding t.
    stapedial t.
    subcutaneous t.
    transverse t.

    Veleanu-Rosianu-Ionescu adductor t.
    Z-plasty t.
tenovaginitis
    inflammatory t.
TENS
    transcutaneous electrical nerve
    stimulation
    TENS therapy
    TENS unit
tensegrity
tensile
    t. force
    t. strain
    t. strength
    t. stress
Tensilon
    T. test
    T. test for myasthenia gravis
tensing test
tensiometer
    Acufex t.
tensiometry
tension
    t. band
    t. band fixation
    t. band of knee
    t. band plate
    t. band wire
    t. band wire tamp
    t. band wiring technique
    capsular-ligamentous t.
    t. curve
    t. force
    t. fracture
    graft t.
    heel t.
    t. isometer
    t. loading
    t. myositis
    t. neck syndrome
    neural t.
    t. neuralgia
    t. night splint (TNS)
    oxygen t.
    residual t.
tension-band wiring
tensioner
    cable t.
    Dwyer t.
    Kirschner wire t.
tension-free Millesi nerve graft
tensor
    t. fasciae latae anchovy

T

NOTES

tensor (*continued*)
t. fascia femoris flap
t. fascia lata (TFL)
t. fascia lata muscle flap
t. fascia lata syndrome
tent frame
tentorial sinus
tenuous vascularity
Tenzel elevator
TeP
tender point
TEPP
total extraperitoneal repair
Teq-Trode electrode
teratologic dislocation
terbinafine
t. HCl
t., hydrochloride cream
t., oral
t., topical
teres
anterior pronator t.
t. major muscle
t. minor muscle
pronator t. (PT)
terminal
t. device (TD)
t. extensor mechanism (TEM)
t. head
t. J sign
t. knee extension
t. latency
t. overgrowth
t. stance
t. Syme procedure
terrible triad of shoulder
Terrmocork diabetic shoe
Terry
T. nail
T. Thomas sign
TERT
total end-range time
tertiary amputation
Terumo syringe
TES belt
test
abduction external rotation t.
abduction load and shift t.
abduction stress t.
accordion t.
Achilles squeeze t.
Achilles tendon t.
active bending t.
active knee extension t.
actual leg length t.
Adams forward-bending t.
Adams position t.
Adams scoliosis t.
adduction load and shift t.

adduction stress t.
Adson t.
AKE t.
Alcohol Use Disorders Identification t.
Allen t.
Allis t.
ALRI t.
Anderson medial-lateral grind t.
Andrews anterior instability t.
ankle clonus t.
ankle dorsiflexion t.
anterior drawer t. (ADT)
anteroposterior stress t.
antinuclear antibody t.
anvil t.
AO pseudoisochromatic color plate t.
Apley compression t.
Apley distraction t.
Apley grinding t.
Apley knee t.
Apley scratch t.
apprehension t.
ARA T.
arch-up t.
arm fossa t.
arthrometer t.
axial compression t.
axial load t.
axial manual traction t.
axon reflex t.
Babinski t.
ballottement t.
Barlow hip instability t.
Barlow provocative t.
Beals t.
Beckhterev t.
Beery Visual Motor Integration T.
Behavioral Inattention T. (BIT)
Bekhterev sitting t.
belly-press t.
bench t.
Bennett Hand Tool Dexterity T.
Benton Constructional Praxis T.
Berg balance t.
biceps jerk reflex t.
Bielschowsky head tilt t.
big toe t.
Biodex t.
block t.
blot t.
Booth t.
bounce home t.
bowstring t.
Boyes t.
bracelet t.
brachial plexus tension t.
Bragard t.

break t.
British t.
brush t.
Bunnell t.
Bunnell-Littler t.
Burke t.
Burn bench t.
calcidiol t.
calf squeeze t.
Callaway t.
Caplan Indented Paragraph T.
carpal compression t.
Carroll t.
catch and clunk t.
Centinela supraspinatus t.
cerebellar function t.
cervical compaction t.
cervical sidegliding t.
Chaddock t.
Charpy impact t.
chest expansion t.
Chiene t.
Children's Paced Auditory Serial
  Addition T. (CHIPASAT)
Childress duck waddle t.
chin-to-chest t.
circle draw t.
Clarke patellar compression t.
clock balance t.
clunk t.
Cognitive Performance T. (CPT)
cold pressor t.
Coleman lateral block t.
Combat Task t.
compression t.
concealed straight leg raising t.
conduction velocity t.
confrontational t.
Contextual Memory T. (CMT)
contralateral straight leg raising t.
costoclavicular syndrome t.
Cotton ankle instability t.
Cotton fibular bone hook t.
cough t.
Cozen t.
Cram t.
crank t.
crossed straight leg raise t.
crossover t.
Cybex isokinetic t.
d'Ambrosia t.
Deerfield t.
de Kleyn t.

Derifield-Thompson t.
Deyerle sciatic tension t.
dial t.
digital response t.
dipyridamole handgrip t.
disc diffusion t.
disc space saline acceptance t.
distal compression t.
distraction t.
dorsal drawer t.
dorsiflexion-eversion t.
double leg raise t.
Downey texture discrimination t.
drawer t.
drop-arm t.
dual photon densitometry t.
duck-waddle t.
Dugas t.
Duncan prone rectus t.
Dunn multiple comparison t.
Durkan carpal compression t.
Dvorak t.
Dynatron 2000 muscle t.
Eden t.
elbow flexion t.
elbow jerk reflex t.
Elithorn Maze T.
Elson middle slip t.
Ely heel-to-buttock t.
empty can t.
endpoint of orthopaedic t.
eversion stress t.
T. of Everyday Attention (TEA)
T. of Everyday Attention for
  Children (TEA-Ch)
excessive laxity t.
external rotation-abduction stress t.
  (EAST)
external rotation stress t.
extrinsic entrapment t.
extrinsic tightness t.
FABER t.
FABERE t.
FADIR t.
Fastex proprioceptive and agility t.
Feagin shoulder dislocation t.
femoral nerve stretch t.
femoral nerve traction t.
fibular bone hook t.
fibular compression t.
figure-of-4 t.
figure-of-8 t.
fingertips-to-floor t.

NOTES

T

test (continued)
finger-to-finger t.
finger-to-nose t.
Finkelstein t.
first metatarsus rise t.
FirstSTEP Developmental
Screening T.
Fisher Protected Least Significant
Difference t.
Fist-Palm-Side T.
Fist-Ring T.
flat-hand t.
flexion-rotation-drawer knee
instability t.
flexion spinal radiography t.
flip t.
fluctuation t.
foot placement t.
foraminal compression t.
forced adduction t.
forearm supination t.
forefoot adduction correction t.
forefoot block t.
Fortin finger t.
Fournier t.
Fowler t.
FRD t.
Froment ulnar nerve function t.
fulcrum t.
Gaenslen t.
Galant t.
Galeazzi t.
Galveston Orientation and
Amnesia T. (GOAT)
Garrick t.
George t.
Gerber t.
Gilchrist t.
Gillet marching t.
gluteus maximus tensing t.
Goldman-Fristoe t.
golfer's elbow t.
Gordon squeeze t.
gracilis t.
gravity drawer t.
gravity stress t.
grimace t.
grinding t.
grip strength t.
Grooved Pegboard T.
Hamilton ruler t.
Harris Infant Neuromotor T.
(HINT)
Hautant t.
Hawkins t.
heel-palm t.
heel-rise t.
heel tap t.
heel-tip t.

heel-to-knee t.
heel-to-shin t.
Helfet t.
hip abduction stress t.
Hoffa t.
9-hole peg t.
Homans t.
Hoover t.
hop t.
Hughston external rotation
recurvatum t.
Hughston knee jerk t.
Hughston-Losee jerk t.
Hughston plica t.
Hughston posterolateral drawer t.
Hughston posteromedial drawer t.
hyperabduction syndrome t.
hyperextension t.
iliac compression t.
iliacus t.
iliopsoas t.
impingement t.
T. of Infant Motor Performance
(TIMP)
inhibition t.
intrinsic tightness t.
inversion stress t.
ischemic forearm exercise t.
Jack t.
jackknife t.
Jackson compression t.
Jacob shift t.
Jakob t.
Jamar t.
Jansen t.
Jebsen Hand Function T.
Jebsen-Taylor hand function t.
jerk t.
Jobe t.
jogging in place t.
Jolly t.
Kelikian push-up t.
Kemp t.
Kernig t.
Kleiger t.
Kleinman shear t.
knee-drop t.
knee flexion stress t.
knee instability t.
knee jerk reflex t.
knee laxity t.
kneeling bench t.
Knox Cube T.
Kolmogorov-Smirnov t.
Kruskal-Wallis t.
Lachman t.
Lam inversion t.
Lasègue rebound t.
lateral block t.

lateral pivot shift t.
lateral squeeze t.
leaning hop t.
LEAP monofilament t.
1-leg hop for distance t.
1-leg stance t.
Lewin-Gaenslen t.
Lewin punch t.
Lewin reverse Lasègue t.
Lewin snuff t.
Lewin standing t.
Lewin supine t.
Lewis-Prusik t.
Lichtman t.
lift-off t.
ligamentous instability t.
light touch t.
Lippman t.
load shift t.
load and shift t.
locking-position t.
Losee knee instability t.
Lovett t.
Ludington t.
lumbar extension t.
lumbar lateral flexion t.
lumbar protective mechanism t.
lumbar rotation t.
lunotriquetral ballottement t.
lunotriquetral shear t.
Lysholm knee t.
MacIntosh lateral pivot shift t.
Maddox rod t.
Maigne t.
Maitland slump t.
manual muscle t.
matchstick t.
Maudsley t.
Maximum Voluntary Efforts T.
McMurray t.
Mennell t.
Michele t.
MicroFET2 muscle t.
middle finger t.
military posture t.
milk t.
Mills t.
Minnesota Manual Dexterity T.
Minnesota Rate of Manipulation t.
  (MRMT)
Minnesota Rate of Manipulation t.
  (MRMT)
Minnesota Spatial Relations T.

6-minute walk t.
Moberg Picking Up T.
monofilament pressure t.
Morton t.
Murphy punch t.
Naffziger t.
navicular drop t.
Neer impingement t.
nerve compression t. (NCT)
nerve conduction velocity t.
nerve function t.
Neviaser t.
89-newton t.
Nobel t.
Noyes flexion rotation drawer t.
Ober t.
oblique retinacular ligament
  tightness t.
O'Connor finger dexterity t.
O'Connor tweezer dexterity t.
O'Donoghue t.
O'Driscoll posterolateral pivot t.
opposition t.
T. of Oral and Limb Apraxia
  (TOLA)
T. of Orientation for Rehabilitation
  Patients (TORP)
OsteoGram bone density t.
Osteomark bone-loss urine t.
Osteopatch bone density t.
overhead exercise t.
Paced Auditory Serial Addition t.
  (PASAT)
Paget t.
pain, asymmetry, range, tone,
  special t. (PARTS)
pain provocation t.
palm-up t.
parachute t.
2-part Apley t.
passive accessory motion t.
passive patellar glide t.
passive patellar tilt t.
passive physiological t.
patellar apprehension t.
patellar glide t.
patellar inhibition t.
patellar retraction t.
patellar tap t.
Patrick t.
Patrick/FABERE t.
peak torque t.
pelvic rock t.

NOTES

T

test (*continued*)

Perkins t.
peroneal tunnel compression t.
Perthes tourniquet t.
Phalen wrist flexion t.
Physical Ability T. (PAT)
pick-up t.
pinprick hyperalgesia t.
pivot shift t.
plantarflexion-inversion t.
T. of Playfulness (ToP)
plica t.
2-point discrimination t.
posterior apprehension t.
posterior drawer t.
posterior stress t.
posterior subluxation t.
posterolateral drawer t.
posterolateral pivot t.
posteromedial pivot-shift t.
probe t.
probe-to-bone t.
prone extension t.
prone external rotation t.
prone knee-bend t.
prone knee flexion t.
prone rectus t.
proximal compression t.
pseudostability t.
pulse status-pull t.
push-pull t.
push-up t.
quadrant t.
quadriceps active t.
quadriceps contraction t.
quantitative sudomotor axon
  reflex t. (QSART)
Queckenstedt t.
Queckenstedt-Stookey t.
Quick Neurological Screening T.
  (QNST)
RA t.
recurvatum t.
rekindling t.
relocation t.
resisted straight leg raise t.
reverse Lachman t.
reverse Lasègue t.
reverse pivot shift t.
Rivermead Behavioral Memory T.
  (RBMT)
Romberg t.
Roos overhead exercise t.
rotary drawer t.
rotary instability t.
rotation drawer t.
rotation recurvatum t.
sag t.
sagittal stress t.

saline acceptance t.
scaphoid lift t.
scaphoid shift t.
scapular approximation t.
scapular elevation t.
Scheffé t.
Schober t.
scratch t.
seated flexion t.
seated root t.
Seddon coin t.
Semmes-Weinstein monofilament
  pressure t.
Sensory Integration and Praxis t.
  (SIPT)
Sensory Organization t. (SOT)
Sharp-Purser T.
shear t.
Sherman block t.
shift t.
shoulder abduction t.
shoulder depression t.
shuck t.
side-glide t.
side-jump t.
side-lying iliac compression t.
Silfverskiöld t.
Simmonds t.
simple knee t. (SKT)
single-heel rise t.
sit-and-reach t.
sitting duct stretch t.
sitting flexion t.
sitting root t.
sit-to-stand t.
sit-up t.
skin-gliding t.
skin resistance t.
Slocum ALRI t.
Slocum anterior rotary drawer t.
Slocum lateral pivot-shift t.
Slocum rotary instability t.
SLR with Bragard t.
SLR with external rotation t.
SLR with Kernig t.
slump t.
Smith and Ross t.
somatosensory t.
Soto-Hall t.
Speed t.
sponge t.
spring t.
Spurling t.
square-shaped wrist t.
squat t.
squatting t.
squeeze t.
Stagnara wake-up t.
Staheli t.

stair running t.
standing apprehension t.
standing flexion t.
standing Gillet t.
starch t.
station t.
Steinmann t.
t. stimulus
Stinchfield t.
straight leg raising t. (SLRT)
stress t.
stretch t.
stroke t.
Stroop t.
subtalar inversion t.
sudomotor activity t.
sulcus t.
supine iliac gapping t.
supine long sitting t.
supine straight leg raising t.
suprascapular nerve entrapment t.
supraspinatus t.
sweat t.
Tack T.
tandem gait t.
tennis elbow t.
tenodesis t.
Tensilon t.
tensing t.
thenar weakness t.
Thomas t.
Thomasen t.
Thompson t.
thumbnail t.
thumb-to-forearm t.
tibiotalar shuck t.
tight retinacular ligament t.
tilt-up t.
timed Allen t.
tissue compression t.
Toglia Category Assessment T.
  (TCAT)
tourniquet t.
transverse humeral ligament t.
treadmill t.
Trendelenburg t.
triangular fibrocartilage complex
  stability t.
triceps jerk reflex t.
triceps skinfold t.
triple-jump t.
Trömner t.
trunk incurvation t.

Tukey t.
ulnar grind t.
Underburger t.
unilateral standing t.
upper limb tension t. (ULTT)
valgus stress t.
Valpar Whole Body Range of
  Motion T.
Valsalva t.
varus stress t.
vertebral artery t.
vertical compression t.
vibration threshold t.
vibrometer t.
T. of Visual-Motor Skills (TVMS)
T. of Visual-Motor Skills: Upper
  Level Adolescents and Adults
  (TVMS:UL)
T. of Visual-Perception Skills
  (TVPS)
T. of Visual-Perceptual Skills:
  Upper Level Adolescents and
  Adults (TVPS:UL)
volitional muscle action t.
Voshell t.
wake-up t.
Waldron t.
walk t.
Wallenberg t.
water acceptance t.
Watson t.
Weber t.
Weinstein enhanced sensory t.
well leg straight leg raising t.
Wilson t.
Wingate aerobic t.
wipe t.
Wolf motor function t.
Wright t.
Wright-Adson t.
wrinkle t.
wrist flexion t.
Wu sole opposition t.
Yeager t.
Yeoman t.
Yergason shoulder subluxation t.

tester

Artscan 200 arthroscopic cartilage
  stiffness t.
Cybex t.
grip t.
GripTrack Commander strength t.
Jamar grip t.

T

NOTES

tester *(continued)*
>
> Nicholas manual muscle t.
> OSI laxity t.
> West nerve t.

testing
>
> active motion t. (AMT)
> active movement t.
> angle isometric t.
> aquatic cardiac evaluation and t.
>   (ACET)
> arthrometer t.
> biomechanical t.
> biothesiometer t.
> blunt pressure t.
> brush-evoked pain t.
> compression t.
> confirmatory t.
> Cybex t.
> Disk-Criminator sensory t.
> dynametric t.
> enzyme-based lactic acid blood t.
> exercise t.
> face validity of rehabilitation t.
> isokinetic t.
> isometric motor t.
> isometric strength t.
> isotonic motor t.
> manual muscle t. (MMT)
> mobility t.
> Model 810 axial closed-loop
>   hydraulic mechanical t.
> motion t.
> motor neglect t.
> MRI t.
> muscle t. (MT)
> nerve involvement t.
> neurological t.
> Omnitron exercise t.
> palpation t.
> passive mobility t.
> pincer t.
> PIVM t.
> premanipulative t.
> quantitative mechanical pain t.
> quantitative sensory t. (QST)
> range of motion t.
> ratio scale in rehabilitation t.
> reciprocal isokinetic t.
> rotation t.
> segmental mobility t.
> segmental motion t.
> shear t.
> strength t.
> stress t.
> susceptibility t.
> Tacticon quantitative sensory t.
> vertebral motion t.

tetanic contraction

tetanolysin

tetanospasmin

tetanus
>
> t. immune globulin
> t. prophylaxis

tetany

tethered
>
> t. cord syndrome
> t. patellar tendon syndrome
> t. spinal cord

tethering effect

tetracaine and dextrose

tetracalcium phosphate

tetraphasic action potential

tetraplegia
>
> International Classification for
>   Surgery of the Hand in T.
> traumatic t.

tetrapolar
>
> Electro-Diagnostic Instruments
>   Model 720 Bilateral T.

Teufel cervical brace

Teuffer
>
> T. technique
> T. tendo calcaneus repair

Teurlings wrist brace

TEV
>
> talipes equinovarus

Tevdek suture

Texas
>
> T. Scottish Rite Hospital (TSRH)
> T. T incision

Texon sole

textured allograft bone graft

TFA
>
> thigh-foot angle
> tibiofemoral angle

TFB-PS
>
> tibial fracture brace proximal support

TFC
>
> threaded fusion cage
> triangular fibrocartilage complex
>   TFC tear

TFCC
>
> triangular fibrocartilage complex

T-finger splint

T-Fix absorbable meniscal repair device

TFL
>
> tensor fascia lata

T-Foam
>
> T-F. bed pad
> T-F. cushion
> T-F. mattress
> T-F. pillow

TG
>
> tendon graft

T-Gel cushion

TGF
>
> transforming growth factor

THA
total hip arthroplasty
Thackray
T. hip prosthesis
T. low friction arthroplasty
thalamic
t. fracture
t. fragment
thalamotomy
thalassemia
thallium
radioisotope t.
t. scan
Than anaerobic threshold
T-handle
T-h. curette
T-h. elevator
ratcheting T-h.
T-h. Zimmer chuck
T-handled
T-h. awl
T-h. hook
T-h. nut wrench
T-h. reamer
T-h. screw wrench
T-h. trocar
THARIES
total hip articular replacement by internal eccentric shells
Tharies
T. femoral resurfacing component
T. hip component
T. hip replacement
T. hip replacement operation
T. hip replacement prosthesis
Thatcher
T. nail
T. screw
the
T. Backstroke
T. Beachcomber prosthetic foot
T. Experience of Leisure Scale (TELS)
T. Healthy Back System
T. Heeler inflatable heel protector
T. Institute for Rehabilitation Research (TIRR)
T. Knee Society clinical-rating scale
T. Painless One acupuncture needle
T. Rope stretch-and-traction device
T. Rope stretching device
T. Unloader

T. Wedge bioresorbable interference-fit implant
theater
t. ache
t. sign
theca
digital t.
thecal
t. abscess
t. injection
t. sac
t. whitlow
themoplastic ankle-foot orthosis
thenar
t. area
t. atrophy
t. branch
t. creaking
t. eminence
t. fascia
t. flap
t. muscle
t. palmar crease (TPC)
t. palsy
t. space
t. weakness test
theory, pl. **theories**
beam t.
Burnet clonal selection t.
closed-form bar t.
3-column spine t.
craniosacral t.
Denis Browne 3-column spine t.
kinetic energy t.
Maisel suppression t.
Marshall Hall t.
Neviaser t.
QLV t.
Thera
T. cane
T. Cane massager
T. Cane shoulder exerciser
Thera-Back back support
Thera-Band
T.-B. Aqua Belt
T.-B. assist
T.-B. ASSIST exerciser
T.-B. exercise ball
T.-B. Exercise System for Golfers
T.-B. hand exerciser
T.-B. handle
T.-B. Max
T.-B. Max resistive exercise

NOTES

757

Thera-Band *(continued)*
    T.-B. progressive weight
    T.-B. resistive exerciser
    T.-B. resistive therapy system
    T.-B. strip
    T.-B. System of Progressive
      Resistance
    T.-B. tubing
Therabath paraffin heat therapy system
TheraBeads microwaveable moist heat pack
Thera-Boot bandage
Thera-Ciser
    T.-C. light exercise system
    T.-C. therapeutic exercise system
Theracloud pillow
TheraCool cold therapy
Thera-Fit
Theraflex wrist exerciser
Therafoam padding
Theraform Selectives
Thera-Gesic cream
Theragloves
Theragym ball
Ther-A-Hoop exerciser
TheraKnit electrode glove
Thera-Loop exerciser
Thera-Med cold pack
Thera-Medic shoe
Theramini 1, 2 electrotherapy stimulator
therapeutic
    t. appliance
    t. conservatism
    t. exercise
    t. lifestyle change (TLC)
    t. light
    t. orthosis
    t. requirement
    t. shoe
    t. spinal support
    t. splint
    t. ultrasound
    t. ultrasound for tendon healing
Therapeutica Sleeping Pillow
therapeutics
    Journal of Manipulative and
      Physiological T. (JMPT)
Thera-P exercise bar
therapies (*pl. of* therapy)
Thera-Plast putty
Therap-Loop
    T.-L. door anchor
    T.-L. door handle
Thera-Pos elbow orthosis
Therapress pressure point release tool
TheraPulse bed
Thera-Putty CTS exerciser
therapy, pl. **therapies**

ablative laser t.
active-assistive motion t.
Acu-Magnet t.
amplitude-summation interferential
  current t. (ASICT)
animal-assisted t. (AAT)
anticoagulant t.
anticonvulsant t.
antisense gene t.
antithrombotic t.
aquatic t.
bee venom t.
Biodex Unweighing System partial
  weight t.
Bragg-peak photon-beam t.
brisement t.
carpal tunnel syndrome injection t.
T. Carrot Finger Orthosis (TCFO)
cell t.
chelation t.
chiropractic manipulative t. (CMT)
cold t.
Coldflo cold t.
compression t.
conservative t.
Cool-Aid continuous controlled
  cold t.
corrective t.
corticosteroid t.
craniosacral t. (CST)
deep muscle t.
diet t.
Diversified chiropractic
  manipulative t.
dry heat t.
edema heat t.
electrical stimulation t.
electric differential t. (EDit)
Electri-Cool continuous controlled
  cold t.
electron beam t.
EROS t.
ETPS t.
Exogen 2000+ noninvasive
  ultrasound t.
extended code t. (ECT)
extracorporeal shock wave t.
fad t.
flexion-distraction t.
fomentation t.
frequency-difference interferential
  current t. (FDICT)
geriatric physical t.
HBO t.
heat t.
herbal t.
high-voltage t. (HVT)
hot fomentation t.
hyperbaric oxygen t.

hypnotic t.
immunosuppressive t.
inferential t.
infrared t.
injection t.
interferential t.
intradiscal electrothermal t. (IDET)
intraosseous t.
intravenous t.
Kelsey unloading exercise t.
LaserPen laser t.
Livingstone t.
magnetic t.
manipulative t.
manual t.
massage t.
meridian t.
microcurrent t.
mind-body t.
moist heat t.
motion t.
moxa heat t.
moxibustion heat t.
neurological physical t.
neuromuscular electrical
  stimulation t.
NMES t.
occupational t. (OT)
orthomolecular
  medicine/megavitamin t.
ortho physical t.
osteomanipulative t. (OMT)
osteopathic manipulative t. (OMT)
outpatient physical t.
oxygen t.
pancreatic enzyme t.
parachute t.
paraffin heat t.
pediatric physical t.
perioperative antibiotic t.
physical t. (PT)
piperacillin/tazobactam t.
pneumatic compression t.
Polar Wrap cold t.
pool t.
positional release t.
postoperative t.
pressure t.
ProFlo vascular compression t.
proliferation t.
prophylactic antibiotic t.
pulsed short-wave t.
T. Putty

qi gong t.
radiation t.
range of motion t., ROM t.
recreational t. (RT)
reflex t.
Rolfing t.
sedation t.
shock-wave t. (SWT)
silastic ball t.
somatic t.
spinal injection t.
spinal manipulative t. (SMT)
spinal manual t.
splinting t.
steroid t.
Supartz joint fluid t.
SwimEx aquatic t.
Swiss ball t.
t. tank
Task Force on Standards of
  Physical T.
TENS t.
TheraCool cold t.
therapy electroconvulsive t.
tonification t.
transfusion t.
transverse friction t.
trial of conservative t.
trigger point t. (TPT)
tumor t.
ultrasound t.
vasoconstrictive t.
whirlpool t.
TheraSeed implant
Ther-A-Shapes positioner
Therasleep Cervical Pillow
Therasound transducer
Theratouch 4.7 stimulator
Thera-Wedge system
TheriLok bone void filler
thermal
  t. agent
  t. anesthesia
  t. capsulorrhaphy
  t. energy
  t. modality
thermalator
  T. heating unit
  Whitehall t.
Thermal Pack
ThermalSoft hot & cold packs
Thermapad pad
Thermasonic gel warmer

NOTES

Thermassage
> Aqua T.

ThermaStim
> T. muscle stimulator
> T. muscle warming device

Thermo
> T. Fusion
> T. hand comforter
> T. HK/Rohadur orthotic
> T. HK/Tepefom orthotic
> T. knee comforter

thermocoagulate
thermocoagulation
ThermoCork orthotic
thermocouple
> t. instrument
> low impedance t.
> t. skin temperature device

ThermoFlex
> Maramed T.

thermogram
thermographic
> t. examination
> t. finding
> t. scanner

thermography
> chiropractic t.
> infrared t.
> liquid crystal t. (LCT)

thermolabile plastic
Thermold heat moldable shoe lining
thermomassage
thermomechanical implant metal prosthesis
thermomoldable
> t. insert
> t. material

Thermophore
> T. hot pack
> T. moist heat pad

thermoplastic
> DynaPrene splinting t.
> t. elastomer (TPE)
> t. heating unit
> t. splint
> t. template

thermoregulate
thermoregulation
> localized t.

thermoregulatory sign
Thermoskin
> T. arthritic knee wrap
> T. brace
> T. heat retainer
> T. U wrist wrap
> T. 4-way elastic knee support

ThermoSKY orthotic material
Thermosport hot/cold wrap
thermotherapy

Thero-Skin gel padding
thickened synovial membrane
thickening
> cortical t.
> heel pad t.
> lamellar t.
> ligamentous t.
> tendon t.

thickness
> cortical t.
> t. of heel pad

thick patella sign
Thiemann disease
Thiersch
> T. medium split free graft
> T. thin split free graft
> T. wire

thigh
> t. atrophy
> t. corset
> t. cuff
> t. holder
> t. shell
> t. tourniquet

thigh-foot angle (TFA)
thigh-shank plane
thin
> t. disc
> t. glenoid retractor
> t. osteotome
> t. pin fixation

Thinline uncovered orthotic
THINSite dressing
thin-wire Ilizarov fixator
thiomalate
thiopental sodium
thiosulfate
thiotepa
> busulfan, melphalan, t. (BuMelTT)

third
> distal t. (D/3, distal/3)
> t. fibular muscle
> t. metacarpal
> middle t. (M/3)
> proximal t. (P/3)
> Steel rule of t.'s

third-generation cementing technique
THKAFO
> trunk-hip-knee-ankle-foot orthosis

Thomas
> T. buckle sling
> T. cervical collar brace
> T. classification
> T. collar
> T. collar cervical orthosis
> T. extrapolated bar graft
> T. fixator
> T. frame
> T. full-ring splint

T. heel
T. heel orthosis
T. hinged splint
T. knee splint
T. Kodel sling
T. leg splint
T. needle
T. posterior splint
T. procedure
T. rigid collar
T. sign
T. splint with Pearson attachment
T. suspension splint
T. test
T. traction
T. walking brace
T. walking caliper
T. wrench
Thomasen test
Thomas-Thompson procedure
Thomas-Thompson-Straub transfer technique
Thompson
T. anterolateral approach
T. anteromedial approach
T. arthroplasty
T. excision
T. femoral neck prosthesis
T. frame
T. hemiarthroplasty hip prosthesis
T. hip endoprosthesis system
T. hip prosthesis forceps
T. leg check system
T. modification
T. modification of Denis Browne splint
T. nail
T. posterior radial approach
T. quadricepsplasty
T. rasp
T. resection
T. sign
T. telescoping V osteotomy
T. test
Thompson-Epstein classification
Thompson-Henry
T.-H. approach
T.-H. technique
Thompson-Parkridge-Richards (TPR)
Thompson-Terwilliger procedure
Thomsen disease
thoraces (*pl. of* thorax)

thoracic
t. approach
t. bone
t. curve
t. curve scoliosis
t. duct
t. duct injury
t. epidural injection
t. extension component
t. facet fusion
t. hemivertebrae
t. hypokyphosis
t. inclination
t. inlet syndrome
t. kyphosis
t. lymphatic pump technique
t. manual traction
t. microtrauma
t. nerve
t. nerve injury
t. nerve palsy
t. orthosis (TO)
t. outlet syndrome (TOS)
t. pedicle
t. pedicle marker
t. plane
t. spinal fusion
t. spine (T-spine)
t. spine biopsy
t. spine decompression
t. spine fracture
t. spine kyphotic deformity
t. spine lordosis
t. spine orthosis
t. spine pedicle diameter
t. spine scoliotic deformity
t. spine vertebral osteosynthesis
t. vertebra
thoracoabdominal
t. approach
t. artery injury
t. incision
thoracoacromial artery
thoracodorsal
t. artery transfer
t. nerve
t. nerve injury
thoracoepigastric flap
thoracogenic scoliosis
thoracolumbar
t. burst fracture
t. corset
t. curve

NOTES

thoracolumbar *(continued)*
- t. erector spinae
- t. idiopathic scoliosis
- t. junction
- t. junction surgical exposure
- t. kyphoscoliosis
- t. kyphosis
- t. orthosis
- t. pedicle screw
- t. retroperitoneal approach
- t. spinal injury
- t. spine
- t. spine anterior exposure
- t. spine decompression
- t. spine flexion-distraction injury
- t. spine fracture-dislocation
- t. spine scoliosis
- t. spine stabilization
- t. spine vertebral osteosynthesis
- t. spondylosis
- t. spondylosis surgical technique
- t. standing orthosis brace
- t. trauma

thoracolumbosacral
- t. orthosis (TLSO)
- t. orthosis—flexion, extension, lateral bending, and transverse rotation (TLSO-FELR)
- t. plate
- t. spine
- t. strain (TLS)

thoracoscapular arthrodesis
thoracotomy
- t. approach
- left-sided t.
- right-sided t.
- standard t.

thorax, pl. **thoraces**
Thorlo socks
thorn sign
Thornton
- T. bar
- T. nail
- T. nail plate
- T. screw

thorny radiation
THORP
- titanium hollow screw osseointegrating reconstruction plate
- THORP system

THR
- total hip replacement

thread
- cancellous screw t.

threaded
- t. cancellous screw
- t. cortical dowel
- t. fusion cage (TFC)
- t. guidepin
- t. rod
- t. spinal fusion cage
- t. Steinmann pin
- t. suture anchor
- t. titanium acetabular prosthesis
- t. wire

threaded-hole-first technique
Three Color Concept of Wound classification
three-quarters prone position
threshold
- anaerobic t. (AT)
- bone conduction t.
- cutaneous pressure t.
- experimental t.
- lactate t. (LT)
- lactic acidosis t.
- mechanical pain t. (MPTh)
- pressure t.
- reflex t.
- t. stimulus
- Than anaerobic t.
- vibration perception t. (VPT)

thrombectomy
thrombin powder
thrombin-soaked Gelfoam
thrombocytopenia
thrombocytopenia-absent
- t.-a. radius (TAR)
- t.-a. radius syndrome

thromboembolic
- t. disease (TED)
- t. stockings

thromboembolism
thromboembolus
thrombogenesis
thrombophilia
thrombophlebitis
- femoroiliac t.

thrombosed
thrombosis, pl. **thromboses**
- deep venous t. (DVT)
- effort t.
- effort-induced t.
- iliofemoral t.
- t. radial artery
- silent t.
- venous t.

Thrombostat topical hemostatic
through-and-through
- t.-a.-t. fracture
- t.-a.-t. tear
- t.-a.-t. V-shaped horizontal osteotomy

through-range feel
through stance
through-the-knee amputation

thrower's
    t. elbow
    t. fracture
throwing
    t. function
    t. injury
thrust
    adjustive t.
    double-thumb t.
    lateral-to-medial t.
    t. manipulation
    pattern of t.
    t. plate prosthesis (TPP)
thumb
    abducted t.
    adducted t.
    adductor sweep of t.
    Bennett fracture of t.
    bifid t.
    bowler's t.
    breakdancer's t.
    clasped t.
    congenital clasped t.
    cortical t.
    t. deformity
    duplicate t.
    t. duplication
    t. extensor tendon
    t. flexor tendon
    floating t.
    Flotan t.
    t. forceps
    gamekeeper's t.
    hitch-hikers t.
    hypoplastic t.
    t. instability
    t. interphalangeal extension assist
    jeweler's t.
    laparoscopic surgeon's t.
    t. loop
    low-set t.
    mallet t.
    t. metacarpal
    t. metacarpophalangeal joint
     approach
    t. opposition
    t. pinch power
    t. polydactyly
    t. post
    pouce flottant t.
    proximal anular pulley of t.
    t. reconstruction
    t. screw

    short t.
    skier's t.
    t. sling
    spatulate t.
    t. spica
    t. spica cast
    t. spica splint
    spring swivel t.
    supernumerary t.
    surgeon's t.
    tennis t.
    trigger t.
    triphalangeal t.
    t. web
    t. web splint
thumb-in-palm deformity
Thumbkeeper
    Freedom T.
    T. splint
thumbnail test
thumb-pinch grasp
thumb-to-forearm test
thumb-wrist immobilizer
Thumper device
ThumSaver
    T. CMC Long splint
    T. CMC Short splint
    T. MP splint
ThumSling
    Action T.
ThumWrap
    FoamWrap T.
ThumZ'Up thumb splint
Thurston-Holland
    T.-H. flag sign
    T.-H. fracture
    T.-H. fragment
thyroid
    t. cartilage
    t. gland
thyrotropin-releasing hormone
Ti-Bac
    T.-B. acetabular component
    T.-B. II hip prosthesis
tibia, pl. **tibiae**
    absent t.
    t. bone
    t. coordinate system
    corticotomy of proximal t.
    distal t.
    dysplastic t.
    groove distal t.
    lip of t.

NOTES

tibia *(continued)*
malleolus medialis tibiae
medial malleolus of t.
osteochondrosis deformans tibiae
Phemister medial approach to t.
proximal t.
saber t.
transmetaphysial amputation of t.
t. valga
t. vara
tibial
t. acceleration
t. adamantinoma
t. aimer
t. aligner
t. artery
t. axial load injury
t. base plate
t. bolt
t. bone defect regeneration
t. bone graft
t. bowing
t. channel
t. collateral ligament (TCL)
t. collateral ligament bursitis
t. Collet
t. component
t. condyle
t. crest
t. cutting block
t. cutting guide
t. defect
t. deformity
t. diaphysial shortening
t. drill guide
t. driver
t. eminence
t. endoprosthesis
t. epiphysis
t. footprint
t. fracture brace proximal support
(TFB-PS)
t. guidepin
t. hallux sesamoid
t. head screw
t. hemimelia
t. hindfoot osteomusculocutaneous
rotationplasty
t. insert
t. insertion site
t. jig
t. lengthening
t. lift-off
t. longitudinal deficiency
t. malleolus
t. medullary canal
t. metaphysis
t. mortise
t. muscle

t. nerve
t. nerve injury
t. phenomenon
t. pin
t. plafond
t. plafond fracture
t. plateau
t. plateau fracture
t. plateau fracture-dislocation
t. plateau prosthesis
t. pseudarthrosis
t. punch
t. resector
t. retractor
t. retroflexion
t. retrotorsion
t. retroversion
t. rim
t. sag
t. sesamoid
t. sesamoid ligament
t. sesamoid position (TSP)
t. slope
t. spacer
t. stylus
t. talar tilt/tibiotalar tilt (TTT)
t. tendon
t. torsion
t. torsion system
t. track holder
t. track template
t. tray
t. tubercle
t. tubercle avulsion
t. tubercle prominence
t. tuberosity
t. tuberosity fractures in children
classification
t. tuberosity osteotomy
t. tunnel
t. tunnel enlargement
t. tunnel widening
t. varus
t. vein
t. wedge
tibialis
t. anterior
t. anterior muscle
t. anterior tendon
apophysitis t.
t. posterior dislocation
t. posterior function
t. posterior muscle
t. posterior tendon
t. sign
tibia-pro-fibula screw
tibioadductor reflex
tibiocalcaneal
t. arthrodesis

t. fusion
t. joint complex
t. ligament
t. medullary nailing
t. space
tibiofemoral
t. alignment
t. angle (TFA)
t. articulation
t. interaction
t. joint
tibiofibular
t. articulation
t. clear space
t. cyst
t. diastasis
t. fracture
t. fusion
t. joint
t. joint dislocation
t. joint instability
t. joint reduction
t. ligament
t. line
t. overlap
t. overlap measurement
t. rotation
t. sprain
t. subluxation
t. synchondrosis
t. syndesmosis
t. synostosis
tibionavicular ligament
tibiospring ligament
tibiotalar
t. angle
t. arthritis
t. clear space
deep anterior t. (DATT)
deep posterior t. (DPTT)
t. diastasis
t. fusion
t. impingement
t. instability
t. joint
t. joint primary arthrodesis
t. shuck test
t. stability
superficial t. (STT)
tibiotalocalcaneal
t. ankle fusion
t. arthrodesis
Tibone posterior capsulorrhaphy

Tib-Transformer orthosis
tic
articulatory t.
ticarcillin and clavulanate potassium
ticlike pain
Ti/CoCr hip prosthesis
Ticonium splint
Ti-Con prosthesis
tidemark
tie
free t.
table t.
Tiemann nail
tie-over bolster
tier
Harris wire t.
Tietze syndrome
Ti-Fit total hip system
Tiger blade
tight
t. retinacular ligament test
t. spinal canal trefoil canal
tightener
Charnley wire t.
Kirschner t.
Sklar wire t.
wire t.
tightness
adductor hamstring t.
hamstring t.
Tikhoff-Linberg
T.-L. radical arm procedure
T.-L. shoulder girdle resection
Tilastin hip prosthesis
tile
T. classification
t. plate facet replacement
T. polytrauma algorithm
T. view
Tillaux-Chaput
T.-C. fracture
T.-C. tubercle
Tillaux fracture
Tillman prosthesis
tilt
angular t.
anterior pelvic t.
anteroposterior t.
cock-robin head t.
innominate t.
manual talar t.
mediolateral t.
palmar t.

NOTES

T

tilt (*continued*)
  pelvic lateral t.
  posterior pelvic t.
  sacral t.
  subtalar t.
  superoinferior t.
  t. table
  talar t. (TT)
  tibial talar tilt/tibiotalar t. (TTT)
  T. and Turn Paragon bed
  varus t.
  t. wrist
  4XP T. System wheelchair
tilting
  coronal t.
  t. frame wheelchair
  t. reflex
Tilt-In-Space wheelchair conversion
tilt-up test
TIME
  Toddler and Infant Motor Evaluation
time
  activated partial thromboplastin t.
    (APTT)
  capillary filling t. (CFT)
  capillary refill t.
  conduction t.
  cycle t.
  double support t.
  echo t.
  floating t.
  intercritical t.
  loading t.
  operating t.
  partial thromboplastin t. (PTT)
  procedure t.
  prothrombin t. (PT)
  reaction t.
  repetition t. (TR)
  rise t.
  1-t. sharp débridement tray
  step t.
  stride t.
  swing t.
  tincture of t. (TOT)
  total end-range t. (TERT)
  total tourniquet t.
  tourniquet t.
  warm ischemic t.
timed Allen test
TiMesh implantable hardware fixation
timing
  right/left t.
TIMP
  Test of Infant Motor Performance
  tissue inhibitor of metalloproteinase
tincture
  t. of belladonna

  t. of benzoin
  t. of time (TOT)
tinea
  t. cruris
  t. gladiatorum
  t. pedis
  t. versicolor
Tinel-Hoffmann sign
Tinel sign
Tinetti
  T. Assessment tool
  T. gait assessment
Tiobi transfer
tip
  acromionizer t.
  Cloward cervical drill t.
  Fragmatome t.
  Frazier suction t.
  t. of medial malleolus
  t. pinch
  sacral bone t.
  screw t.
  suction t.
  Woodruff t.
tip-pinch dynamometry
tiptoe gait
tip-to-tip pinch
TIRR
  The Institute for Rehabilitation Research
  TIRR foot-ankle orthosis
Tisseel fibrin glue
tissue
  adipose t.
  t. anchor guide (TAG)
  bursal t.
  capsular support t.
  capsuloligamentous t.
  cartilaginous t.
  t. closure
  t. compression test
  connective t.
  Conrad-Bugg trapping of soft t.
  t. debris
  devitalized t.
  t. elongation
  t. expander
  exuberant granulation t.
  fatty t.
  fibroadipose t.
  fibrocartilaginous t.
  fibroconnective t.
  fibrofatty t.
  fibrous scar t.
  t. forceps
  granulation t.
  hypertrophic granulation t.
  t. inhibitor
  t. inhibitor of metalloproteinase
    (TIMP)

intervening connective t.
ligamentous support t.
t. mandrel implant material
muscular t.
necrotic t.
neural t.
t. nutrition
osseous t.
periarticular t.
perineural t.
periosteal t.
pharyngeal t.
t. pressure
t. pressure measurement
pressure-sensitive t.
pressure-tolerant t.
t. protector
t. repair
replacement t.
revascularized t.
scar t.
t. scissors
skeletal t.
t. slack
soft t.
t. sterilization
subcutaneous t.
t. texture abnormality (TTA)
tissue-engineered meniscal t.
t. transfer
t. transplant
t. transplantation
vascular t.
viable t.
viscoelastic t.
weak bony t.

tissue-engineered meniscal tissue
tissue-level response
TissueTak corkscrew implant
tissue-type plasminogen activator
Titan

T. Apollo electric flexion table
T. cemented hip prosthesis
T. Meridian Intersegmental Traction
table
T. Nova manual flexion-extension
multi flex table

titanium

t. alloy
t. cable
t. circumferential grommet
t. geometric device
t. half pin
t. hip prosthesis
t. hollow screw osseointegrating
reconstruction plate (THORP)
t. hollow screw plate system
t. implant
t. implant material
t. implant prosthesis
t. mandibular plate
t. microsurgical bipolar forceps
t. nail
plasma-sprayed t.
t. screw

titanium-alloy implant
titer

antistreptolysin-O t. (ASOT)

Ti-Thread prosthesis
Titian hip prosthesis
Titus

T. forearm splint
T. wrist splint

tivanium

t. cancellous bone screw
t. hip prosthesis
t. implant metal
t. implant metal prosthesis

TJ

triceps jerk

TJA

total joint arthroplasty

TJR

total joint replacement

TKA

total knee arthroplasty
trochanter-knee-ankle

TKR

total knee replacement

TLC

therapeutic lifestyle change

TLS

thoracolumbosacral strain
TLS strain

TLSO

thoracolumbosacral orthosis
TLSO brace

TLSO-FELR

thoracolumbosacral orthosis—flexion,
extension, lateral bending, and
transverse rotation

TMA

transmalleolar axis
transmetatarsal amputation
true metatarsus adductus
TMA prosthesis

T

NOTES

TMB
    IsoTis Orthobiologics Accell TMB
TMJ
    temporomandibular joint
TMT
    tarsometatarsal
TN
    talonavicular
        TN joint
T-nail
TNS
    tension night splint
TO
    thoracic orthosis
Toad finger splint
tobramycin-impregnated PMMA implant
Tobruk splint
Todd gait
toddler
    t. fracture
    T. and Infant Motor Evaluation
        (TIME)
Todd-Wells guide
toe
    t. alignment
    t. alignment splint
    t. amputation
    Astroturf t.
    t. block anesthesia
    t. box
    Butler procedure to correct
        overlapping t.'s
    t. cap
    Clanton turf t.
    claw t.
    t. clawing
    clubbed t.
    cock-up deformity of t.
    t. comb
    t. crest
    crossover second t.
    curly t.
    t. disarticulation tolcapone
    distal tuberosity of t.
    downgoing t.'s
    DuVries technique for
        overlapping t.
    t. extensor
    t. extensor muscle
    t. extensor tendon
    extra t.
    flail t.
    t. flexion
    t. flexor
    t. flexor muscle
    floating t.
    floppy t.
    t. gait
    great t.

    t. gripping exercise
    t. implant
    t. index
    jogger's t.
    lesser t.
    t. loop
    mallet t.
    marathoner's t.
    medial crossover t.
    medial deviation of second t.
    Morton t.
    overlapping fifth t.
    overriding fifth t.
    over-straight t.
    painful t.
    t. phenomenon
    t. plate
    t. plate extension
    t. pressure
    Primus flexible great t.
    t. prosthesis
    push-off by great t.
    t. raise exercise
    t. range of motion
    t. reflex
    runner's t.
    sand t.
    sausage t.
    searching big t.
    t. separator
    set angle of t.
    t. spacer
    spacer between t.'s
    t. spica cast
    splaying of t.
    sportsman's t.
    t. spread sign
    stiff t.
    striatal t.
    supernumerary t.
    tennis t.
    turf t.
    underlapping t.
    unilaterally upgoing t.
    upgoing t.'s
    varus t.
    V-Y plasty correction of varus t.
    t. walk
    t. walking
    webbed t.
    t. wedge
Toe-Aid dressing
toe-drop brace
toe-ground purchase
toe-heel gait
toeing-in gait
toeing out
toeing-out gait

toenail
>dystrophic t.
>gryphotic t.
>ingrowing t.
>ingrown t.
>onychomycotic t.

Toennis tumor forceps
toe-off
>t.-o. phase
>t.-o. phase of gait

ToeOFF orthosis
toe-out angle
toe-phalanx transplantation
toe-straight device
toe-toe gait
toe-to-groin
>t.-t.-g. cast
>t.-t.-g. modified Jones dressing

toe-to-hand transfer
toe-to-midthigh cast
toe-touch weightbearing
toe-walker
>idiopathic t.-w. (ITW)

toe-walking gait
toggle
>screw t.
>t. sign

toggle-recoil adjustment
Toglia
>T. Category Assessment
>T. Category Assessment Test
>(TCAT)

Tohen tendon technique
TOLA
>Test of Oral and Limb Apraxia

Tolectin DS
tolerance
>fatigue t.
>pressure t.

tolerated
>weightbearing as t. (WBAT)

tolerogenic immunosuppression
Tomasini brace
Tomberlin-Alemdaroglu splint
Tommy trapeze bar
tomogram
tomography
>computed t. (CT)
>computerized axial t. (CAT)
>conventional t.
>emission t.
>helical computed t.
>hypocycloidal ankle t.

>positron emission t. (PET)
>preoperative t.
>quantitative computed t. (QCT)
>single photon emission computed t.
>(SPECT)
>transpiral t.
>trispiral t.

Tom Smith arthritis
tone
>muscle t.
>sphincter t.

tone-inhibiting leg cast
tone-reducing ankle-foot orthosis
(TRAFO)
tongs
>Barton t.
>Barton-Cone t.
>Böhler t.
>cervical fracture t.
>Cherry traction t.
>cranial t.
>Crutchfield-Raney t.
>Gardner-Wells t.
>Raney-Crutchfield t.
>skull t.
>traction t.
>Trippi-Wells traction t.
>Vinke skull traction t.

tongue fracture
tongue-in-groove
>t.-i.-g. advancement
>t.-i.-g. recession

tonic
>t. muscle
>t. neck reflex

tonicity
>symmetric t.

tonification therapy
tonus
>myogenic t.

tool
>Acuforce 7.0 therapy t.
>AcuPressor myotherapy t.
>Adolescent and Pediatric Pain T.
>(APPT)
>ArthroWand t.
>Backnobber II massage t.
>Gore smoother crucial t.
>1-handed kitchen t.
>Index Knobber II massage t.
>Magnassager massage t.
>Original Backnobber massage t.

NOTES

T

tool (*continued*)

Original Index Knobber II massage t.

OsteoStat disposable power t.

Therapress pressure point release t.

Tinetti Assessment T.

too-many-toes sign

tooth, pl. **teeth**

Hutchinson teeth

toothed

t. cutter

t. tissue forceps

t. washer

ToP

Test of Playfulness

top

circular laminar hook with offset t.

topaz

T. manual flexion table

T. MicroDebrider

top-entry (open body) hook

tophaceous

t. deposit

t. disease

t. gout

tophectomy

tophus, pl. **tophi**

t. formation

gouty t.

topical

Topicycline Topical

top-loading screw and rod system

topography

internal t.

Toposar Injection

Toradol

T. Injection

T. Oral

Torg

T. classification

T. knee reconstruction

T. technique

torn

t. ligament

t. meniscus

tornado injury

Tornwaldt bursitis

Toronto

T. brace

T. Medical CPM exerciser

T. parapodium orthosis

T. pelvic fracture classification

T. splint

TORP

Test of Orientation for Rehabilitation Patients

total ossicular replacement prosthesis

Plastiport TORP

TORP prosthesis

torque

t. curve

t. force

frictional t.

t. heel shoe

t. load

peak t.

peak dorsiflexion t.

plantarflexion t.

t. production

rotatory t.

screw t.

t. screwdriver

supination t.

t. wrench

torque-meter

Compudriver digital t.-m.

torsion

angle of t.

t. bar

t. bar splint

t. dystonia

external tibial t.

femoral t.

femorotibial t.

internal tibial t. (ITT)

internal tibiofibular t.

medial t.

t. neurosis

tibial t.

t. unit

t. wedge fracture nonunion

torsional

t. abnormality

t. alignment

t. deformity

t. fracture

t. gripping strength

t. load

t. overload

t. rigidity

t. stiffness

t. stress

torsionometer

torticollis

acquired t.

congenital t.

dermatogenic t.

fixed t.

intermittent t.

mental t.

muscular t.

myogenic t.

neurogenic t.

nonspasmodic t.

spasmodic t.

spurious t.

symptomatic t.

tortipelvis

torus
- T. external fixation system
- t. fracture
- regeneration t.

TOS
- thoracic outlet syndrome

TOT
- tincture of time

total
- t. active motion (TAM)
- t. anatomical hinge knee brace
- t. ankle arthroplasty (TAA)
- t. ankle replacement (TAR)
- t. arthrodesis of wrist
- t. articular replacement arthroplasty (TARA)
- t. articular replacement arthroplasty prosthesis
- t. articular resurfacing arthroplasty (TARA)
- t. body movement
- t. body water
- t. bone matrix (TBM)
- T. Concept ankle/foot prosthesis
- t. condylar III fully constrained prosthesis
- t. condylar knee
- t. condylar knee prosthesis
- T. Condylar Knee system
- t. condylar prosthesis III (TCP III)
- t. condylar semiconstrained tricompartmental prosthesis
- t. contact bivalve ankle-foot orthosis
- t. contact cast
- t. contact casting (TCC)
- t. contact orthosis (TCO)
- t. contact shell ankle-foot orthotic
- t. contact socket
- t. elbow arthroplasty
- t. end-range time (TERT)
- T. Environment Control (TEC)
- t. eversion range of motion
- t. extraperitoneal repair (TEPP)
- T. Gym
- T. Gym rehabilitation system
- t. hip arthroplasty (THA)
- t. hip articular replacement by internal eccentric shells (THARIES)
- t. hip replacement (THR)
- t. hip replacement prosthesis
- t. hip revision

- t. hip stabilization orthosis
- t. joint arthroplasty (TJA)
- t. joint replacement (TJR)
- t. joint replacement prosthesis
- t. knee arthroplasty (TKA)
- T. Knee for Children
- t. knee implant
- t. knee instrumentation
- T. Knee 2100 prosthetic knee
- t. knee replacement (TKR)
- t. knee replacement prosthesis
- t. matricectomy
- t. maxillary osteotomy
- t. meniscectomy
- t. mesenteric apron method
- t. necrosis
- t. ossicular reconstruction
- t. ossicular reconstruction implant
- t. ossicular replacement prosthesis (TORP)
- t. parenteral nutrition (TPN)
- t. passive motion (TPM)
- t. patellectomy
- t. patellofemoral joint arthroplasty
- t. range of motion (TROM)
- t. replacement joint
- t. rotating knee (TRK)
- T. Shock prosthesis
- t. shoulder arthroplasty
- t. talus fracture
- t. tourniquet time
- t. transfer (TT)
- t. wrist arthroplasty

TotalGym Exercise Program

totally implantable lengthening device

Toti trephine drill

toto
- in t.

tottering gait

touchdown weightbearing

touch sensation

Touch-Test
- T.-T. sensory evaluation
- T.-T. sensory evaluator

Tourni-cot exsanguinating tourniquet

tourniquet
- Accuflate t.
- arthroscopic t.
- Bodenstab t.
- t. control
- Digikit finger t.
- digital t.
- double t.

NOTES

tourniquet *(continued)*
    Esmarch t.
    finger t.
    forearm t.
    t. gauge
    t. ischemia
    t. palsy
    t. paralysis
    pneumatic t.
    pneumatic ankle t.
    t. pressure
    Profex arthroscopic t.
    t. test
    thigh t.
    t. time
    Tourni-cot exsanguinating t.
    upper arm t.
towel
    Charnley t.
    t. clamp
    t. clip
    t. exercise
    t. roll
    sterile t.
Townley
    T. anatomic knee system
    T. bone graft screw
    T. femur caliper
    T. TARA prosthesis
    T. tibial plateau plate
    T. total knee prosthesis
Townley-horizontal platform prosthesis
Townsend-Gilfillan
    T.-G. plate
    T.-G. screw
Townsend Rebel convertible brace
toxemia
toxicity
    aluminum t.
    methotrexate t.
Toygar angle
TPC
    thenar palmar crease
TPE
    thermoplastic elastomer
    TPE ankle-foot orthosis
    TPE biomechanical foot orthosis
T-pin
    Delitala T-p.
    T-p. handle
T-plasty modification of Bankart shoulder operation
T-plate
    dorsal T-p.
    palmar T-p.
TPM
    total passive motion
TPN
    total parenteral nutrition

TPP
    thrust plate prosthesis
    TPP hip endoprosthesis
TPR
    Thompson-Parkridge-Richards
    TPR ankle prosthesis
TPT
    trigger point therapy
TR
    repetition time
TR-28
    TR-28 hip prosthesis
    TR-28 total hip replacement
trabecula, pl. **trabeculae**
    naked trabeculae
    osseous t.
    partially necrotic osseous t.
trabecular
    t. bone
    t. index of Singh
    t. traction
trabeculation
Trac
    T. II knee implant
    T. II knee prosthesis
trace
    SimplyStable t.
tracer catheter
tracheal injury
trachelomastoid muscle
tracheostomy
tracheotomy tube
tracing
    nerve t.
track
    Frenkel t.
    pin t.
track-bound joint
tracker
    T. knee brace
    Palumbo patella t.
    patella t.
tracking
    patellar t.
Trackmaster treadmill
tract
    anterior spinocerebellar t.
    anterior spinothalamic t.
    corticospinal t.
    gastrointestinal t.
    iliotibial t.
    lateral corticospinal t.
    pyramidal t.
    sinus t.
    spinal cord t.
    spinocerebellar t.
    spinothalamic t.
    urinary t.
    vestibulospinal t.

traction
ambulatory t.
t. anchor
Anderson t.
AOA halo cervical t.
Apley t.
t. application
t. atrophy
autologous t.
axial t.
axis t.
Baker trabecular t.
balanced skeletal t.
balanced suspension t.
banjo t.
t. bar
bidirectional t.
bipolar vertebral t.
Blackburn t.
Böhler tong t.
Borchgrevin t.
t. bow
t. bow nut
Bremer halo cervical t.
Bryant t.
Buck t.
calcaneal pin t.
Carpal Trac t.
t. cast
cervical AOA halo t.
cervical halter t.
cervical manual t.
C-Flex supine cervical t.
Chattanooga t.
Cherry tong t.
Cotrel t.
Crile head t.
Crutchfield skeletal tong t.
t. device
device for transverse t. (DTT)
Dunlop t.
Econo-Cerv supine cervical t.
Econo 90 lumbar home t.
ElastaTrac lumbar t.
elastic t.
t. epiphysis
t. epiphysitis
Exo-Static t.
t. exostosis
external t.
fingertrap t.
floating t.
t. footpiece

t. fracture
Freiberg t.
Frejka t.
Gallo t.
Gardner-Wells tong t.
gentle t.
Georgiade visor cervical t.
Graham t.
Granberry t.
halo cervical t.
halo-dependent t.
halo-femoral t.
halo-pelvic t.
halo-wheelchair t.
halter t.
Hamilton t.
Hamilton-Russell t.
t. handle
Handy-Buck t.
Hare t.
head-halter t.
Hoke-Martin t.
Holter t.
HomeStretch lumbar t.
t. hook
Houston halo cervical t.
Hoyer t.
Ingebrightsen t.
inhibitive t.
intermittent cervical t. (ICT)
isometric t.
isotonic t.
Jones suspension t.
Kessler t.
King cervical t.
Kirschner skeletal t.
Kuhlman t.
leg t.
Logan t.
longitudinal t.
low-profile halo t.
lumbar t.
lumbosacral t.
Lyman-Smith t.
lymphapress t.
manual t.
McBride tripod pin t.
metatarsal t.
Miami Acute collar cervical t.
Miami J collar cervical t.
Necktrac t.
Neufeld roller t.
t. neurapraxia

T

NOTES

traction *(continued)*
    Ortho-Vent t.
    overhead olecranon t.
    Pease-Thomson t.
    pelvic hyperextension t.
    Perkins t.
    Peterson t.
    Philadelphia collar cervical t.
    t. pin
    3-point skeletal t.
    pounds of t.
    Pronex home t.
    Pronex pneumatic cervical t.
    Pugh t.
    pulp t.
    Quantum 400 t.
    Quigley t.
    Raney-Crutchfield tong t.
    Roger Anderson t.
    rubber band t.
    Russell skeletal t.
    Saunders t.
    Sayre suspension t.
    sequential pneumatic pump t.
    simple shoulder test thermal
      alteration Thomas t.
    skeletal t.
    skin t.
    snug t.
    t. splint
    split Russell skeletal t.
    t. spur
    static t.
    Steinmann t.
    t. stirrup
    sugar-tong t.
    supine C-Trax t.
    suspension t.
    Syms t.
    tape t.
    Thomas t.
    thoracic manual t.
    t. tongs
    t. tongs screw
    trabecular t.
    transverse t.
    vertical t.
    Vinke tong t.
    Watson-Jones t.
    weight t.
    well-leg t.
    Wells t.
    Whitman t.
    Zimfoam splint t.
tractograph
    MOM t.
Tracto-Halter training

tractor
    Hamilton pelvic traction screw t.
    Zim-Trac traction splint t.
tractotomy
TRAFO
    tone-reducing ankle-foot orthosis
    TRAFO orthosis
Trager method
Tragerwork
trailer
    leaders and t.'s
train
    near-constant frequency t.'s
trainer
    athletic t.
    Biodex Gait T.
    Biodex target balance t.
    dynamic stabilization t.
    impulse inertial exercise t.
    Kinesthetic Ability T. (KAT)
    Monark Rehab T.
    Posture Pump Spine T.
    Shuttle Balance t.
    Sprint cross t.
training
    activity t. (AT)
    ankle disc t.
    balance board t.
    bowel t.
    DAPRE strength t.
    t. diet
    eccentric muscle t.
    endurance t.
    Fartlek t.
    flexibility t.
    functional t.
    gait t.
    hypertrophic strength t.
    interval t.
    isometric t.
    isotonic t.
    light intensity t.
    neural strength t.
    neurodevelopmental t.
    periodization of t.
    physical t. (PT)
    progression of t.
    progressive resistance t.
    proprioceptive t.
    propriosensory t.
    prosthetic t.
    prosthetic gait t.
    relaxation t.
    resistance t.
    t. room
    sensory-motor t.
    speed play t.
    stabilization t.
    strength t.

Tracto-Halter t.
variable resistance t.
weight t.

TRAM
transverse rectus abdominis
myocutaneous
TRAM flap
trampoline injury
tranexamic acid
trans
t. fat elaidic acid
t. unsaturated fatty acid
transacromial
t. approach
t. coracoacromial ligament repair
transaminase
glutamic-oxaloacetic t.
glutamic-pyruvic t.
transarticular
t. pin
t. screw
t. screw fixation
t. wire fixation
transaxillary approach
trans-bone plasty
transbrachioradialis approach
transcalcaneal approach
transcapitate
t. fracture
t. fracture-dislocation
transcapitellar
t. pin
t. wire fixation
transcarpal amputation
transcervical femoral fracture
transchondral fracture
transclavicular approach
transcondylar
t. amputation
t. axis (TCA)
t. fracture
transcutaneous
t. crush injury
t. electrical nerve stimulation
(TENS)
t. oxygen
t. oxygen level (TCO$_2$)
t. oxygen monitor (TCOM)
t. oxygen tension determination
transducer
differential variable reluctance t.
(DVRT)
ergonomically designed t.

force t.
FT03C t.
Hall-effect strain t.
in-shoe t.
linear-variable-differential t.
magnetic motion t.
multifrequency t.
pressure t.
rotatory-variable-differential t.
Therasound t.
transection
step-cut t.
transepicondylar axis
transepiphysial
t. fracture
t. separation
transfemoral
t. alignment
t. amputation
t. amputee
t. modular prosthesis
t. suspension
transfer
t. aid
anterior t.
anteromedial tubercle t.
autogenous osteocartilage t.
Baker lateral semitendinosus t.
Barr anterior t.
bed-to-chair t.
biceps brachialis muscle t.
t. board
bone t.
Boyes t.
brachioradialis t.
Brown fibular t.
Buncke t.
Bunnell posterior tibial tendon t.
Camitz tendon t.
Campbell t.
Chandler tendon t.
Chaves muscle t.
Clark pectoralis major t.
Columbus McKinnon assist for
lifting or t.
composite free tissue t.
coracoacromial ligament t.
crossed intrinsic t.
Dickson muscle t.
distal t.
double tendon t.
Drennan posterior t.
dynamic muscle t.

NOTES

T

775

transfer *(continued)*
    Eggers t.
    extensor digitorum t.
    extensor hallucis longus t.
    extensor tendon t.
    fibular t.
    Flatt tendon t.
    flexor digitorum longus tendon t.
    flexor to extensor tendon t.
    flexor-to-extensor tendon t.
    Fowler tendon t.
    free flap t.
    free gracilis muscle t.
    free tissue t.
    free toe t.
    Gage distal t.
    Ganley tendon t.
    gastrocnemius tendon t.
    Girdlestone tendon t.
    Green t.
    T. Handle support handle
    Harmon t.
    Henry muscle t.
    Hiroshim t.
    His-Haas muscle t.
    Hoffer split t.
    Huber abductor digiti quinti t.
    Ikuta pectoralis major t.
    iliopsoas t.
    iliotibial band t.
    independent t.
    ion t.
    Johnson-Spiegl tendon t.
    Jones t.
    Kessler posterior tibial tendon t.
    Lamb muscle t.
    lateral t.
    t. lesion
    Littler-Cooley abductor digiti
     quinti t.
    Littler-Cooley muscle t.
    load t.
    magnetization t.
    Manktelow pectoralis major t.
    McLaughlin subscapularis t.
    Menelaus triceps t.
    t. metatarsalgia
    microvascular osseous t.
    Moberg deltoid muscle t.
    Moberg deltoid-to-triceps t.
    muscle t.
    Mustard iliopsoas t.
    neuromuscular t.
    Ober anterior t.
    opponens t.
    patellar tendon t. (PTT)
    pedicled fibular t.
    peroneus brevis t.
    posterior deltoid-to-triceps t.

    posterior tibial tendon t.
    semitendinosus tendon t.
    Sharrard posterior t.
    single-stage tissue t.
    split anterior tibialis tendon t.
     (SPLATT)
    static tendon t.
    stress t.
    subscapularis tendon t.
    Sutherland lateral t.
    tendon t.
    thoracodorsal artery t.
    Tiobi t.
    tissue t.
    toe-to-hand t.
    total t. (TT)
    vascularized osseous t.
    Vastamäki muscle t.
    Whitman muscle t.
    wraparound neurovascular composite
     free tissue t.
    wraparound toe t.
transfer/augmentation
    FHL tendon t./a.
transfibular
    t. approach
    t. arthrodesis
    t. fusion
TransFix
    T. ACL system
    T. ACL system fixation
    T. femoral fixation system
transfixation amputation
transfixing pin
transfixion
    t. bolt
    t. screw
transformation
transforming
    t. growth factor (TGF)
    t. growth factor beta
transforming growth factor (TGF)
transfusion
    autologous blood t.
    blood t.
    t. therapy
transglenoid suture repair
transhamate
    t. fracture
    t. fracture-dislocation
transhumeral amputation
transient
    t. bone marrow edema
    t. bone marrow edema syndrome
    bone remodeling t.
    t. clonus
    t. compressive creep
    t. epiphysitis
    t. lesion

t. neurapraxia
t. osteopenia
t. osteoporosis
t. quadriplegia
t. synovitis
transiliac
t. amputation
t. bar technique
t. fracture
t. lengthening
t. rod fixation
transition
cervicothoracic t.
transitional vertebra
translaminar facet screw
Translating and Congruent Mobile-Bearing Knee
translation
anterior t.
anterior talar t. (ATT)
anteroposterior t.
caudal t.
cephalad t.
coronal plane deformity sagittal t.
dorsal t.
t. injury
t. mobility
t. motion
obligate t.
posterior t.
ulnar t.
vertical t.
translational
t. displacement
t. osteotomy
t. parameter
t. position
translatory
t. force
t. motion
translocation
ulnar t.
translumbar amputation
transmalleolar
t. ankle
t. ankle arthrodesis
t. axis (TMA)
t. drilling
t. portal
transmetacarpal amputation
transmetaphysial
t. amputation
t. amputation of tibia

transmetatarsal
t. amputation (TMA)
t. capsulotomy
transmission
t. electron microscopy
impulse-based nerve t.
nerve t.
nociceptive t.
nonimpulsed base nerve t.
transmitter
chest-band t.
transmitter-receiver
Itrel programmed t.-r.
transolecranon approach
transoral odontoid resection
transosseous suture
transparent
t. adhesive dressing
t. template
transpatellar tendon portal
transpedal
t. multiplanar wedge fusion
t. multiplanar wedge osteotomy
transpedicular
t. approach
t. fixation
t. fixation effective pedicle diameter
t. fixation system design
t. screw
transpedicularly implanted anterior spinal support device
transpelvic amputation
transperitoneal
t. approach
t. exposure
transphalangeal amputation
transpiral tomography
Transpire wrist orthosis
transplant
Bosworth femoroischial t.
d'Aubigné patellar t.
Elmslie-Trillat t.
fibular t.
free vascularized bone t.
one-half patellar tendon t.
patellar t.
pedicled t.
pes anserinus t.
Slocum pes anserinus t.
tissue t.
vascularized bone t.

NOTES

T

transplant *(continued)*
    whole bone t.
    whole fibular t.
transplantation
    allograft t.
    t. antigen
    autogenous cartilage t.
    autologous osteochondral t.
    Bosworth femoroischial t.
    femoroischial t.
    meniscal autograft t.
    muscle-tendon t.
    osteoarticular allograft t.
    tendon t.
    tissue t.
    toe-phalanx t.
transport
    axoplasmic t. (AXT)
    bulk flow axoplasmic t.
    fast axoplasmic t. (FAXT)
    slow axoplasmic t. (SAXT)
transposing index ray
transposition
    Dellon ulnar nerve t.
    dorsal subcutaneous nerve t.
    t. flap
    intermuscular neuroma t.
    intramuscular nerve t.
    intraosseous nerve t.
    MacKinnon modification of Dellon
      ulnar nerve t.
    nerve t.
    plantar t.
    subcutaneous anterior t.
    subfascial t.
    tendon t.
    ulnar nerve t.
transpositional
transsacral
    t. block
    t. fracture
transscaphoid
    t. dislocation fracture
    t. perilunate dislocation
transsphenoidal dissector
transsternal approach
transsyndesmotic screw fixation
transtendocalcaneus portal
transtentorial brainstem
transthoracic
    t. approach
    t. lateral view
transtibial
    t. amputation
    t. immediate postoperative
      prosthesis
transtriquetral
    t. fracture
    t. fracture-dislocation

transtrochanteric
    t. approach
    t. rotational osteotomy
    t. valgus osteotomy (TVO)
transversalis fascia
transversarium
    foramen t.
transverse (TV)
    t. acetabular ligament
    t. amputation
    t. approach
    t. arch stress
    t. atlantal ligament
    t. axis
    t. axis knee flexion
    t. capsulotomy
    t. carpal ligament
    t. chevron osteotomy
    t. connector
    t. deficiency
    t. diaphysial osteotomy
    t. disc
    t. fixation
    t. fixator application
    t. friction massage
    t. friction therapy
    t. humeral ligament test
    t. incision
    t. intertarsal ligament
    t. ligament of knee
    t. ligament rupture
    t. line of Park
    t. loading device
    t. metatarsal ligament
    t. metatarsal osteotomy
    t. myelopathy
    t. pedicle angle
    t. pedicle diameter
    t. plane
    t. plane alignment
    t. plane motion insufficiency
    t. process
    t. process fracture
    t. process of sacrum
    t. process of vertebra
    t. rectus abdominis myocutaneous
      (TRAM)
    t. retinacular ligament
    t. scapular ligament
    t. screw
    t. spinal ligament
    t. supracondylar osteotomy
    t. tarsal articulation
    t. tarsal joint
    t. tear
    t. tenotomy
    t. tibiofibular ligament
    t. traction
transversectomy

transversely
transversoplanus
    talipes t.
transversospinalis syndrome
transversum
transversus abdominis muscle
TRAP
    tartrate resistant acid phosphatase
trapdoor
trapeze bar
trapezia (*pl. of* trapezium)
trapezial
    t. area
    t. arthrosis
    t. prosthesis
    t. ridge
trapeziectomy
trapeziodeltoid interval
trapeziometacarpal
    t. capsule
    t. fusion
    t. joint
    t. joint replacement prosthesis
trapeziotrapezoidal joint
trapezium, pl. trapezia
    t. bone
    Burton-Pelligrini excising t.
    t. fracture
    t. implant prosthesis
    t. ossification
trapezius
    t. fiber analysis
    t. muscle
trapezoid
    t. bone
    t. bone of Henle
    t. bone of Lyser
    t. ligament
    t. line
    t. ossification
Trapezoidal-28 (T28)
    T.-28 hip prosthesis
    T.-28 internal prosthesis
trapezoidal
    t. imaging
    t. resection osteotomy
trapped meniscus
trapper
    FoamWrap finger t.
trapping
    Conrad-Bugg t.
    optical t.
    tendon t.

trauma
    arterial t.
    awakening t.
    birth t.
    cervical spine t.
    craniospinal t.
    geriatric t.
    high-energy t.
    hyperextension t.
    hyperflexion t.
    lumbar spine t.
    multiple t.
    musculoskeletal t.
    nonosseous tissue t.
    nonunion fracture t.
    repetitive t.
    t. score
    thoracolumbar t.
    t. view
trauma-induced membrane
TraumaJet wound debridement system
traumatic
    t. abscess
    t. amputation
    t. anterior instability
    t. anterior shoulder instability
    t. arthritis
    t. bone cyst
    t. brain injury (TBI)
    t. brain injury-related ataxia
    t. brain injury-related neglect
    t. burn injury
    t. cervical disc herniation
    t. cervical discopathy
    t. compartment syndrome
    t. dislocation
    t. displacement
    t. heel wound
    t. hemarthrosis
    t. hemiplegia
    t. neuroma
    t. osteoarthritis
    t. paraplegia
    t. prepatellar neuralgia
    t. sinus
    t. spondylolisthesis
    t. synovitis
    t. tetraplegia
    t., unidirectional Bankart lesion surgery
    t., unidirectional instability and Bankart lesion
traumatized ligament

T

NOTES

Trautman Locktite prosthetic hook
Trautmann chisel
traverse amputation
TraXis
> T. Ti alloy spacer
> T. Vue alloy spacer

tray
> Alcon Instrument Delivery
> System t.
> Bucky x-ray t.
> Denis Browne t.
> glenoid metal t.
> PFC offset tibial t.
> surgical hand t.
> tibial t.
> 1-time sharp débridement t.
> x-ray t.

Treace stapes drill
treatment
> acid t.
> active t.
> adjustive t.
> bone cyst t.
> Boyd-Ingram-Bourkhard t.
> Carrel t.
> Chapman point t.
> closed t.
> cold laser t.
> compression rod t.
> distraction-compression scoliosis t.
> dual compression scoliosis t.
> extracorporeal shock wave t.
> intradiscal electrothermal t. (IDET)
> IonGuard orthopaedic surface t.
> Kenny t.
> low-friction ion t. (LFIT)
> manual t.
> neurodevelopmental t.
> neuromuscular reflex t.
> neuromuscular scoliosis orthotic t.
> nonoperative t.
> osteopathic manipulative t.
> Parabath paraffin heat t.
> paraffin t.
> poliomyelitis t.
> rehabilitation t.
> ReJuveness scar t.
> SB+ testing and t.
> SB− testing and t.
> shock t.
> spasticity t.
> surgical t.
> ulcer t.
> viscosupplementation t.

Tredex
> Universal T.

tree
> BTE Assembly T.
> Finger Blocking T.

> pinch t.
> pipe t.

trellis formation
tremor
> action t.
> contraction t.
> essential t.
> intention t.
> pill rolling t.
> postural t.
> resting t.

tremulor
tremulousness
trench foot
Trendelenburg
> T. gait
> T. limp
> T. lurch
> T. position
> T. sign
> T. test

trephine
> bone t.
> Castroviejo t.
> t. drill
> hollow bone t.
> Michele vertebral t.
> t. needle biopsy
> Phemister biopsy t.

Trevor disease
Trevor-Fairbank disease
triad
> Charcot t.
> female athletic t.
> t. knee repair
> t. of O'Donoghue
> Virchow t.
> Waddell t.

Triad prosthesis
triage
> sidelines t.

trial
> t. acetabular cup
> t. base plate
> clinical t.
> component t.
> t. of conservative therapy
> t. driver
> t. femoral component
> t. fit
> Fracture Intervention T. (FIT)
> t. implant
> lower hook t.
> t. prosthesis
> radial t.
> t. range of motion
> t. reduction
> t. seating
> t. spacer

t. stem
ulnar t.
upper hook t.
trialkylphosphine gold complex
Triam Forte
triangle
Achilles t.
Alsberg t.
anal t.
anterior t.
aponeurotic t.
t. blade system
Bryant t.
Burow t.
cervical t.
clavipectoral t.
Codman t.
iliofemoral t.
IMP knee positioning t.
infraclavicular t.
intern's t.
Kager t.
Kanavel t.
knee positioning t.
Langenbeck t.
metal measuring t.
Middeldorpf t.
neutral t.
Petit t.
posterior t.
Rauchfuss t.
sacral t.
Volkmann t.
von Weber t.
Ward t.
Weber t.
Tri-angle shoulder abduction brace
triangular
t. advancement flap
t. ankle fusion frame
t. arm sling
t. bandage
t. base transverse bar configuration
t. bone reamer
t. compression device
t. defect
t. disc of wrist
t. external ankle fixation
t. fibrocartilage
t. fibrocartilage complex (TFC, TFCC)
t. fibrocartilage complex stability test

t. fibrocartilage complex tear
t. ligament
t. medullary nail
t. muscle
t. pillow splint
t. rasp
t. working zone
t. wrist bone
triangulated pedicle screw
triangulate triple frame
triangulating
triangulation
indirect t.
t. technique
t. technique for arthroscope
triaxial
t. motion
t. semiconstrained elbow prosthesis
t. total elbow arthroplasty
Tri-Axial prosthesis
Triax monotube external fixation system
tribology
tricalcium phosphate
triceps
t. brachii tendon
t. jerk (TJ)
t. jerk reflex test
t. skinfold test
t. surae jerk
t. surae muscle
t. surae reflex
t. surae release
tricepsplasty
triceps-splitting approach
Trichophyton
T. mentagrophytes
T. rubrum
trichterbrust
tricipital muscle
trick
t. knee
t. movement
Tricodur
T. compression support bandage
T. Epi compression bandage
T. Epi compression dressing
T. Talus compression bandage
T. Talus compression dressing
tricompartmental
t. implant
t. knee prosthesis
t. replacement

NOTES

Tri-Con component
Tricon-M
    T.-M component
    T.-M cruciate-sparing prosthesis
    T.-M patellar prosthesis
Tri-Core cervical support pillow
tricorrectional bunionectomy
tricortical
    t. iliac crest bone graft
    t. ilial strip graft
tricyclic antidepressant
trident hand
triethanolamine salicylate
triethiodide
triflanged
    t. Lottes nail
    t. medullary nail
Tri-Flex auxiliary suspension belt
Tri-Float pressure reduction mattress
trifurcation
trigeminal neuralgia
trigger
    t. digit
    t. finger
    t. finger release
    t. finger syndrome
    t. point
    t. point injection
    t. point therapy (TPT)
    t. thumb
    t. thumb release
TriggerWheel
    T. device
    T. Wand
trigonum
trilaminate cushion
trilateral knee-ankle-foot orthosis
trileaflet prosthesis
Trillat
    T. arthroplasty
    T. osteotomy
    T. procedure
Tri-Lock
    T.-L. press-fit prosthesis
    T.-L. total hip prosthesis with
    Porocoat
trilogy
    T. acetabular cup system
    T. prosthesis
Trilon multilayered material
trimalleolar ankle fracture
Trimedyne Omnipulse holmium laser
trimethoprim sulfamethoxazole
Trim-It screw system
Trimline knee immobilizer
trimmer
    motorized t.
Tri-Motion Knee System
Trinion meniscus screw

Trinkle
    T. bone drill
    T. brace
    T. brace and adapter
    T. chuck adapter
    T. power drill
    T. screwdriver
    T. Super-Cut twist drill
trio
    T. arthroscope
    T. medialized rod system
triode
Trio-Stim neuromuscular stimulator
tri-panel knee immobilizer
tripartite
    t. bone
    t. muscle origin
triphalangeal
    t. thumb
    t. thumb deformity
triphase technetium scintigraphy
triphasic action potential
Tripier amputation
triplanar
    t. protractor
    t. protractor apparatus
triplane
    t. construct
    t. motion
    t. osteotomy
    t. stretch
    t. tibial fracture
triple
    T. Antibiotic Topical
    t. arthrodesis
    t. bundle technique
    t. discharge
    t. envelope system
    t. frame
    t. hemisection
    t. innominate osteotomy
    t. ligamentous repair
    t. reamer
    t. tarsal fusion
    t. tenodesis
triple-frequency probe
triplegia
triple-injection cinearthrography
triple-jump test
triple-phase isotope bone scan
triple-wire
    t.-w. fusion
    t.-w. procedure
    t.-w. technique
triploscope
tripod
    t. cane
    t. foot

McBride t.
t. sign
tripoding gait
Trippi-Wells traction tongs
tripsis
triquetral fracture
triquetrolunate
    t. dislocation
    t. instability
triquetrum
    t. bone
    t. ossification
triquetrum-lunate arthrodesis
triradial
    t. cartilage
    t. resector blade
triradiate
    t. acetabular extensile approach
    t. cartilage
    t. incision
    t. transtrochanteric approach
trisalicylate
triscaphe
    t. arthrodesis
    t. fusion
    t. joint
trismus
trispiked
trispiral tomography
TriStander
triton tumor
trivector retaining approach
Tri-Wedge total hip system
Tri W-G table
TRK
    total rotating knee
trocar
    blunt t.
    sharp t.
    T-handled t.
trochanter
    greater t.
    t. holder
    lesser t.
trochanter-holding clamp
trochanteric
    t. advancement
    t. band
    t. bolt
    t. bursa
    t. bursitis
    t. migration
    t. osteotomy

t. pin
t. reamer
t. shift
t. slide
t. spine
t. syndrome
t. wire
trochanter-knee-ankle (TKA)
trochanterplasty
trochlea peronealis
trochlear
    t. defect
    t. groove
    t. notch
trochoid
    t. articulation
    t. joint
Troemner percussion hammer
troika
    aponeurotic t.
trolley
    Bolero lift bath t.
    Tupper t.
trolley-track sign
TROM
    total range of motion
    TROM knee brace
Trömner
    T. percussion
    T. test
Tronzo
    T. elevator
    T. intertrochanteric fracture
    classification
    T. prosthesis
trophic
    t. change
    t. fracture
    t. joint disorder
    t. ulcer
    t. ulceration
trophoneurosis
    muscular t.
tropism
    facet t.
tropocollagen tendon
tropometer
trough
    bone t.
    t. line
    t. sign
trousers
    military antishock t. (MAST)

NOTES

Trousseau point
Trow
    T. Bridge Terra-Round all-terrain
        prosthesis
    T. Bridge TerraRound foot
    T. Bridge TerraRound sports limb
    T. Bridge triple-speed drill
Trowbridge-Campau bone drill
true
    t. acetabular region
    t. acetabulum
    t. ankylosis
    T. Blue exercise band
    t. lateral view
    t. metatarsus adductus (TMA)
    t. rib
    t. spacer
    t. vertebra
**True/Fit femoral intramedullary rod
    system**
True/Flex
    T./F. intramedullary nail
    T./F. intramedullary rod system
True-Lok
    T.-L. external fixation
    T.-L. external fixator system
Tru-Fit
    T.-F. brace
    T.-F. custom-molded shoe
Trumble
    T. arthrodesis
    T. talectomy
Trümmerfeld
    T. line
    T. zone
Tru-Mold shoe
truncal dysmetria
truncated
    t. tarsometatarsal wedge arthrodesis
    t. wedge tarsometatarsal arthrodesis
        vertical talus
trunk
    anatomic nerve t.
    t. control
    t. curl
    t. incurvation test
    t. righting
    t. shift
    t. stabilization rehabilitation
        program
    sympathetic t.
Trunkey
    T. fracture classification
    T. fracture classification system
**trunk-hip-knee-ankle-foot orthosis
    (THKAFO)**
trunnion-bearing hip prosthesis
TruStep foot prosthesis

Tru-Support
    T.-S. EW bandage
    T.-S. SA bandage
Truswell-Hansen disease
TruWedge BGS osteotomy wedge
Trypanosoma gambiense
trypsin, balsam peru, and castor oil
Tsai-Stillwell procedure
Tscherne classification
T-shaped
    T-s. AO plate
    T-s. capsulotomy
    T-s. fracture
    T-s. incision
    T-s. inserter
TSP
    tibial sesamoid position
T-spine
    thoracic spine
TSRH
    Texas Scottish Rite Hospital
    TSRH buttressed laminar hook
    TSRH circular laminar hook
    TSRH corkscrew device
    TSRH crosslink
    TSRH crosslink stabilization
    TSRH crosslink system
    TSRH double-rod construct
    TSRH eyebolt spreader
    TSRH fixation system
    TSRH hook holder
    TSRH hook inserter
    TSRH hook-rod
    TSRH implant
    TSRH instrumentation
    TSRH L-bolt
    TSRH mini-corkscrew device
    TSRH pedicle hook
    TSRH pedicle screw
    TSRH plate
    TSRH rod fixation
    TSRH spinal implant system
    TSRH trial hook
    TSRH Universal spinal
        instrumentation system
    TSRH wrench
T-Stat Topical
T-Stick adhesive
T-strap
    medial T-s.
Tsuge
    T. debulking
    T. tendon repair
Tsuji laminaplasty
TT
    talar tilt
    total transfer
    TT Pylon prosthesis

TTA
    tissue texture abnormality
TTAP prosthesis
TTAP-ST acetabular prosthesis
TTR
    tarsal tunnel release
TTS
    tarsal tunnel syndrome
TTT
    tibial talar tilt/tibiotalar tilt
tube
        Adson suction t.
        Baron suction t.
        chest t.
        Chinese fingertrap t.
        Dawson-Yuhl suction t.
        digit t.
        Dynamic digit extensor t.
        endoneural t.
        Esmarch t.
        Exerband Pak bilateral t.
        Exerband Pak unilateral t.
        Ferguson-Frazier suction t.
        fingertrap t.
        t. flap graft
        t. foam
        Gillquist suction t.
        t. guide
        Hemovac suction t.
        irrigation t.
        Jergesen t.
        stockinette t.
        suction t.
        tracheotomy t.
        vent t.
TubeGauz bandage
tuber angle
tubercle
        adductor t.
        anterior tibial t.
        articular bone t.
        t. avulsion
        Chaput t.
        Chassaignac t.
        conoid t.
        Gerdy t.
        Ghon t.
        lateral tibial t.
        Lisfranc t.
        Lister t.
        medial calcaneal t.
        t. osteotomy
        Stieda t.

        talus lateral t.
        tibial t.
        Tillaux-Chaput t.
        Wagstaff t.
tubercular granuloma
tuberculoma
        bone t.
tuberculosis
        diaphysial t.
        extraarticular t.
        t. of hip
        metaphysial t.
        osteoarticular t.
        skeletal t.
        spinal t.
tuberculous
        t. arthritis
        t. dactylitis
        t. lesion
        t. peroneal tenosynovitis
        t. rheumatism
        t. sequestrum
        t. spinal osteomyelitis
        t. spondylitis
        t. synovitis
        t. trochanteric bursitis
        t. vertebral osteomyelitis
tuber-joint angle
tuberosity
        adductor t.
        t. avulsion fracture
        bicipital t.
        calcaneal t.
        t. of calcaneus
        t. of carpal bone
        t. of clavicle
        coracoid t.
        cuboidal t.
        t. of cuboid bone
        distal t.
        femoral t.
        t. fragment
        greater t.
        iliac t.
        infraglenoid t.
        ischial t.
        t. joint angle
        lateral t.
        lesser t.
        navicular t.
        parietal t.
        patellar t.
        posterior t.

T

NOTES

tuberosity *(continued)*
    radial t.
    sacral t.
    supraglenoid t.
    tibial t.
    ulnar t.
    ungual t.
    ununited tibial t.
tuberous xanthoma
Tubex gauze dressing
Tubigrip
    T. bandage
    T. dressing
    T. glove
tubing
    Dakin t.
    elastic t.
    Exerband t.
    Fit-Lastic therapy t.
    foam t.
    gel t.
    medullary vent t.
    PVC t.
    Silipos mesh t.
    Thera-Band t.
Tubsider Kneeling Seat
TUBS procedure
tubular
    t. bone plate
    t. elastic bandage
    t. punch
    t. stockinette
tubularization of graft
tubulization
tucker
    tendon t.
tuck sign
Tudor-Edwards bone-cutting forceps
Tuf Nex neck exerciser
Tuf-Skin tape adherent
TufStuf II cast tape
tuft
    distal t.
    finger t.
    t. fracture
tuftal resorption
tufted phalanx
Tuke saw
Tukey test
Tuli
    T. Pro Heel Cup
    T. rubber heel cup
TuliGel heel cup
tulip pedicle screw
Tullos technique
tumble
    T. Forms feeder
    T. Forms roll
tumbler graft

tumefaction
tumor
    Abrikossoff t.
    aggressive t.
    ball-valve t.
    Bednar t.
    benign t.
    blood vessel t.
    bone-forming t.
    bone marrow t.
    brown fat t.
    cartilaginous t.
    cerebellopontine angle t.
    Codman t.
    cortical desmoid t.
    cystic t.
    desmoid t.
    dumbbell t.
    Enneking staging of malignant soft tissue t.
    epidermal cell t.
    epiphysial chondromatous giant cell t.
    Ewing t.
    extraabdominal desmoid t.
    fatty tissue t.
    fibroblastic t.
    fibroid t.
    fibrous t.
    giant cell t. (GCT)
    glomus t.
    Gubler t.
    histiocytic t.
    hyperparathyroidism t.
    intraosseous t.
    lipid t.
    lumbar t.
    malignant soft tissue t.
    mesenchymal t.
    metastatic spinal t.
    nerve sheath t.
    neural t.
    neuroectodermal t.
    occult primary malignant t.
    plexiform fibrohistiocytic t.
    pluripotential mesenchymal t.
    Pott puffy t.
    primary t.
    t. resection
    Schwann t.
    soft tissue t.
    spinal t.
    superior sulcus t.
    synovial t.
    tenosynovial giant cell t.
    t. therapy
    triton t.
    vascular t.
    vertebral body t.

t. vessel
xanthomatous giant cell t.
tumoral calcinosis
tumor-bearing bone
tumor-grasping forceps
tumorous
t. condition
t. involvement
t. mass
tumor-replacement endoprosthesis
tunnel
bone t.
bottleneck femoral t.
carpal t. (CT)
cubital t.
t. drill guide
femoral t.
femoral drill t.
fibroosseous t.
Gaynor-Hart x-ray position of
carpal t.
t. locator guide
osseous t.
peroneal t.
radial t.
subsartorial t.
talar neck t.
tarsal t.
tibial t.
ulnar t.
t. view
tunnel-and-sling fixation
tunneler
tendon t.
Tunneloc bone mulch screw
Tunturi hand exerciser
Tuohy lumbar puncture needle
Tupman plate
Tupper
T. arthroplasty
T. hand-holder and retractor
T. trolley
turbinated bone
Turco
T. clubfoot release
T. clubfoot release technique
T. oblique posteromedial incision
T. posteromedial release
T. repair of talipes equinovarus
turf
t. toe
t. toe grading
t. toe injury

turgor
Turkel bone biopsy
TurnAide therapeutic system
turnbuckle
t. ankle brace
t. cast
t. distractor
t. elbow splint
t. jack
t. knee brace
t. wrist orthosis
turn-down tendon flap
Turn-Easy transfer aid
turned-up pulp deformity
turner
T. pin
T. prosthesis
rotating t.
T. syndrome
Turning Board Exercise System
turnover
bone t.
turnstile casting stand
turret exostosis
turtle neck nail
Turvy internal screw fixation
Turyn sign
Tutofix cortical pin
Tutoplast process
Tuxedo collar
TV
transverse
TVMS
Test of Visual-Motor Skills
TVMS:UL
Test of Visual-Motor Skills: Upper Level
Adolescents and Adults
TVO
transtrochanteric valgus osteotomy
TVPS
Test of Visual-Perception Skills
TVPS:UL
Test of Visual-Perceptual Skills: Upper
Level Adolescents and Adults
tweezers
Kaprelian easy-access t. (KEAT)
Twilite Oral
twin-blade oscillating saw
Twin Cities Lo-Profile halo
twist
t. drill
t. drill point

NOTES

twist *(continued)*
    t. hook
    t. maneuver
twisted plate
twister
    Axel wire t.
    Batzdorf cervical wire t.
    t. cable
    cerclage wire t.
    Cooley-Baumgarten wire t.
    DMP wire t.
    Miltex wire t.
    orthotic coiled spring t.
    Shifrin wire t.
    wire t.
Twist-Off Screw
twitch muscle
Tworek screw guide

TX-1, TX-7 traction table
Tycron suture
tying forceps
Tylok high-tension cable system
tyloma
tympanic bone
type
    T. C-50, C-90 AFO
    contraction t.
    t. 501, 502, 504, 602 finger splint
    foot t.
    frequency, intensity, time, t. (FITT)
    t. 1, 2 neurofibromatosis
    rectus foot t.
    Sanders t.
    sleeve t.
typhoid osteomyelitis
Tyrell hook

U

U Luque vertebral rod
U osteotomy
U wrench

UBC

UBC brace

UBE

uniaxial balance evaluation
upper body ergometer

UBIS

ultrasound bone imaging sonometer
UBIS 5000 quantitative ultrasound bone sonometer
UBIS 5000 ultrasound bone sonometer

UBP

universal bone plate
UBP system

UCB

unilateral calcaneal brace
University of California, Berkeley
UCB foot orthosis
UCB shoe insert

UCBL

University of California, Berkeley Laboratory
UCBL foot plate
UCBL orthosis

UCI

University of California, Irvine
UCI ankle prosthesis
UCI unconstrained prosthesis

UCL

ulnar collateral ligament

UCLA

University of California, Los Angeles
UCLA anatomic shoulder arthroplasty
UCLA functional long leg brace
UCLA Shoulder Rating scale

UCLC

ulnar collateral ligament complex

UCOheal orthotic
UCOlite orthosis
UE

upper extremity

Ueba release
Uematsu shoulder arthrodesis
UFO

Universal plantar fasciitis orthotic
Orthomerica UFO

UFOS

universal frame outer socket

UHMWPE

ultrahigh molecular weight polyethylene
UHMWPE prosthesis

UHR

universal head replacement
UHR locking ring mechanism

Uhthoff

U. sign
U. syndrome

UID

unilateral interfacetal dislocation

UID/S

unilateral interfacetal dislocation or subluxation

UKA

unicompartmental knee arthroplasty

ulcer

decubitus u.
diabetic neurotrophic u.
diabetic plantar hallux u.
u. dressing
high-grade u.
ischemic u.
low-grade u.
mal perforans u.
moderate-grade u.
neuropathic u.
neurotrophic food u.
peptic u.
plantar u.
pressure u. (grade I-IV)
recalcitrant neuropathic u.
stasis u.
supramalleolar venous u.
target u.
u. treatment
trophic u.
Wagoner u.

ulceration

neuropathic forefoot u.
neurotrophic u.
pinpoint u.
sublesional u.
trophic u.

ulcerative mutilating acropathy
Ullmann line
Ullrich

U. drill
U. drill guard

ulna

absent u.
u. bone
distal u.
Monteggia fracture-dislocation of u.
proximal u.

ulnar

u. anlage
u. antebrachial region
u. artery
u. artery injury
u. bearing
u. brace
u. bursa
u. carpal collateral ligament
u. clubhand
u. collateral ligament (UCL)
u. collateral ligament complex (UCLC)
u. collateral ligament injury
u. collateral ligament rupture
u. collateral nerve of Krause
u. column
u. convexity
u. creaking
u. cubital tunnel syndrome
u. deviation
u. deviation deformity
u. dimelia
u. drift
u. drift deformity
u. extensor
u. grind test
u. gutter splint
u. head
u. head excision
u. head implant prosthesis
u. hemiresection interposition arthroplasty
u. impaction syndrome
u. lengthening
u. malleolus
midcarpal u. (MCU)
u. minus variance
u. motor neurectomy
u. nerve (UN)
u. nerve block
u. nerve entrapment
u. nerve injury
u. nerve motor/sensory electromyogram
u. nerve palsy
u. nerve paralysis
u. nerve release
u. nerve transposition
u. nerve transposition surgery
u. neuropathy
u. notch
u. rasp
u. recession
u. reflex
u. ruler
u. sesamoid bone
u. side grip
u. styloid bone

u. styloid fracture
u. styloid impaction syndrome
u. synovial recess
u. translation
u. translocation
u. trial
u. tuberosity
u. tunnel
u. wrist extensor tendinitis

ulnaris

extensor carpi u. (ECU)
flexor carpi u. (FCU)
malleolus u.

ulnarward

ulnocarpal

u. abutment
u. abutment syndrome
u. arthrodesis
u. impaction syndrome
u. impingement
u. joint
u. ligament

ulnohumeral

u. angle
u. joint

ulnolunate

u. abutment syndrome
u. articulation
u. ligament

ulnomeniscotriquetral joint
ulnotriquetral ligament
ulnotriquetrum articulation
ULO

upper limb orthosis

ULP

upper limb prosthesis

Ulrich

U. bone-holding clamp
U. bone-holding forceps

Ulrich-St. Gallen forceps
Ulson fixator system
Ultec thin dressing
Ultima

U. calcar stems
U. C femoral component
U. Fx stems
U. hip replacement system
U. total hip system

ultimate

U. Cold N' Hot Pack
U. Hand Helper strengthening program
U. knee prosthesis
u. strength

Ultimax distal femoral intramedullary rod system
Ultrabrace

U. brace
U. knee orthosis

Ultra-Cut instrument
Ultra-Drive
  U.-D. bone cement removal system
  U.-D. plug puller
  U.-D. ultrasonic revision system
ultraendurance
UltraFix
  U. MicroMite anchor suture
  U. MicroMite suture anchor
  U. RC implant
  U. RC suture anchor
  U. RC suture anchor system
  U. rotator cuff repair implant
Ultraflex
  U. dynamic joint
  U. orthopaedic bed
Ultra-Guard
  U.-G. FS hip bracing system
  U.-G. hip orthosis system
**ultrahigh molecular weight polyethylene
  (UHMWPE)**
Ultra-Light athletic tape
UltraPower drill system
UltraSling
ultrasonic
  u. aspirator
  u. mobility aid
  u. probe
ultrasonography
  compression u.
  duplex Doppler u.
ultrasonometer
  QUS-2 calcaneal u.
UltraSorb suture anchor
ultrasound (US)
  Amrex therapeutic u.
  u. bone imaging sonometer (UBIS)
  compression u.
  Doppler u.
  duplex u.
  u. electrotherapy
  Exogen 2000+ noninvasive u.
  Mysono 201 portable u.
  u. phonophoresis
  pulsed u.
  quantitative u. (QUS)
  therapeutic u.
  u. therapy
ultrasound-guided
  u.-g. echo biopsy
  u.-g. stereotactic biopsy
ultrasound/stimulator
  SynchroSonic U/HVG50 u./s.

UltraStep orthotic
ultraviolet (UV)
  u. light
  u. light pressure
Ultra-X external fixation system
ULTT
  upper limb tension test
umbau zone
umbilical tape
UMS
  upper fossa active, medial knee pain, and
  short leg on the side ipsilateral to the
  weak fossa
UN
  ulnar nerve
unassisted locking-suture technique
unbalanced
  u. depolymerization
  u. hemivertebra
  u. wrist syndrome
uncemented femoral component
unciform
  u. bone
  u. fracture
  u. process
uncinate
  u. bone
  u. hypertrophy
  u. process fracture
uncommitted metaphysial lesion
uncompensated rotary scoliosis
unconditional stimulus (US)
unconstrained
  u. shoulder arthroplasty
  u. tricompartmental knee prosthesis
uncoordinated gait
uncovertebral
  u. arthrosis
  u. joint
  u. spur
undecylenic
  u. acid
  u. acid and derivatives
underarm
  u. body jacket
  u. brace
  u. cast
  u. orthosis
Underburger test
under direct vision
undergrowth
underlapping toe
undermined skin

NOTES

underscoring
undersurface of patella
underwater Bovie
underwear
>HipSaver protective u.

undetermined
>etiology u.

undifferentiated oligoarthritis
undisplaced fracture
undyed suture
ungual
>u. process
>u. tuberosity

unguarded osteotome
unguis incarnatus
unhappy triad of O'Donoghue
uniarticular
uniaxial
>u. balance evaluation (UBE)
>u. joint
>u. strain gauge
>u. structure

unicameral bone cyst
Uni-Clip staple
unicompartmental
>u. knee arthroplasty (UKA)
>u. knee implant
>u. knee prosthesis
>u. knee replacement
>u. knee system

unicondylar
>u. fracture
>U. Geomedic hemi-knee system
>u. prosthesis

unicortical screw
Uniflex
>U. calibrated step drill
>U. dressing
>U. drill bushing
>U. humeral nail
>U. intramedullary nail
>U. nailing system

Unigraft bone graft material
Unilab
>U. Surgibone
>U. Surgibone bone replacement
>material
>U. Surgibone surgical implant

unilateral
>u. acute radicular syndrome
>u. calcaneal brace (UCB)
>u. chronic radicular syndrome
>u. facet subluxation
>u. interfacetal dislocation (UID)
>u. interfacetal dislocation or
>subluxation (UID/S)
>u. pedicle cannulation
>u. posterior-anterior movement
>u. sacroiliac approach

>u. spastic leg
>u. standing test
>u. variable screw placement system

unilaterally upgoing toe
Unilink system for hand surgery
unilocular joint
uninhibited
>u. ankle motion
>u. flexion

union
>bony u.
>u. broach retention drill
>u. broach retention pin
>callous bone u.
>delayed fracture u.
>European Chiropractic U.
>faulty u.
>fibrous u.
>osteonal bone u.
>Osteotron stimulator for bone u.
>primary bone u.
>secondary bone u.
>slow u.
>vicious u.

Uni-Patch electrode gel
Unipen
>U. Injection
>U. Oral

unipennate muscle
Uniplane rocker
unipolar
>u. bearing
>u. cauterization
>u. cautery
>u. needle electrode
>u. release

uniportal
>u. arthroscopic microdiskectomy
>U. fascial release system
>u. plantar fasciotomy

Unique Vitamin E
unisegmental mobility
UniSyn modular hip system
unit
>AME microcurrent TENS u.
>Autoflex II, III CPM u.
>Back Bubble gravity traction u.
>Back Revolution traction/exercise u.
>basic multicellular remodeling u.
>BioMed TENS u.
>bone metabolic u.
>bone remodeling u.
>Bovie coagulating u.
>C-arm fluoroscopy u.
>Cybex Torso Rotation Testing and
>Rehabilitation U.
>Cybex Trunk Extension Flexion u.
>Dynasplint knee extension u.
>Eclipse TENS u.

Econo 90 traction u.
E-2 hydrocollator heating u.
ElastaTrac home lumbar traction u.
EMG retrainer biofeedback u.
Exo-Bed traction u.
Exo-Overhead traction u.
functional spinal u. (FSU)
G5 Fleximatic
 massage/percussion u.
G5 Vibramatic
 massage/percussion u.
Gymmy exercise u.
home cervical traction u. (HCTU)
Hydra-Cadence gait-control u.
hydraulic knee u.
Hydrocollator heating u.
intervertebral motor u.
Jace hand continuous passive
 motion u.
Magnatherm SSP electromagnetic
 therapy u.
MENS u.
motor u.
musculotendinous u.
myofascial u.
myotatic u.
Orthodyne Enhancer u.
Orthotic Research and Locomotor
 Assessment U. (ORLAU)
over-the-door traction u.
Pebax counter u.
postanesthesia care u. (PACU)
rotator u.
single-axis knee u.
sit-to-stand training parallel bar u.
Solitens transcutaneous electrical
 nerve stimulation u.
u. spinal rod
TENS u.
Thermalator heating u.
thermoplastic heating u.
torsion u.
vertebral motion u. (VMU)
wrist flexion u.
unitary plastic
United States (U.S.)
 U. S. Manufacturing Company
 (USMC)
Unitek steel crown
unitunnel technique
univalve cast
univalved

universal
 U. acromioclavicular splint
 U. AerobiCycle
 U. bone grafting/impacting forceps
 u. bone plate (UBP)
 U. bone plate system
 u. canvas body restraint
 u. coronal movement
 U. distal radius fracture
 classification
 U. drill point
 U. femoral head prosthesis
 u. Fitstep
 U. fixation screw
 u. frame outer socket (UFOS)
 u. full-circle manual goniometer
 U. gutter splint
 u. head replacement (UHR)
 U. hex screwdriver
 U. hip prosthesis
 U. I, II prosthesis
 u. incision
 U. knee positioner
 U. lateral positioner
 U. Minimally Invasive Assistant
 Free hip surgery instruments
 U. modular femoral hip component
 extractor
 u. nail
 U. plantar fasciitis orthotic (UFO)
 u. precautions
 U. radial component
 U. sacral spine instrumentation
 u. sling
 U. sling and swathe shoulder
 immobilizer
 U. 2-speed hand drill
 U. spine classification (type A-C)
 U. support splint
 U. Tredex
 u. tri-panel knee immobilizer
 U. wire clamp
Uni-Versatil sling
university
 U. of British Columbia brace
 U. of California, Berkeley (UCB)
 U. of California, Berkeley
 Laboratory (UCBL)
 U. of California Berkeley
 Laboratory orthosis
 U. of California Biomechanics
 Laboratory heel cup

NOTES

U

793

university *(continued)*
  U. of California cuff suspension
   PTB socket
  U. of California, Irvine (UCI)
  u. of California, Los Angeles
   (UCLA)
  U. of Florida LINAC
  Louisiana State U. (LSU)
unknown
  etiology u.
unleveling
  pelvic u.
unloader
  U. ADJ Unloader brace
  U. Bi-ComPF knee brace
  U. Express Unloader brace
  U. Select Unloader brace
  U. Spirit knee brace
  The U.
unlocking spiral technique
unmineralized osteoid
unmyelinated
Unna
  U. boot cast
  U. boot wrap
  U. paste
  U. paste boot
  U. paste shell
Unna-Flex Plus venous ulcer kit
unopposed
unplanned valgus osteotomy
unreduced dislocation
unremodeled defect
unrestricted closed and open chain
 knee extension exercise
unsegmented vertebral bar
unsound ankylosis
unstable
  u. cervical spine injury
  u. fracture
  u. fracture-dislocation
  u. joint
unsteadiness of gait and station
unsteady gait
unstriated muscle
unsustained clonus
unthreaded wire
ununited
  u. fracture
  u. tibial tuberosity
unwinding
  myofascial u.
up
  U. and About system
  press u.
up-angle hook
upbiting
  u. basket forceps
  u. rongeur

upcurved punch forceps
upcut rongeur
upgoing toes
6U portal
upper
  u. arm tourniquet
  u. body cycle
  u. body ergometer (UBE)
  u. cervical spine anterior construct
  u. cervical spine anterior exposure
  u. cervical spine fusion
  u. cervical spine posterior construct
  u. cervical spine procedure
  u. extremity (UE)
  u. extremity myoelectric prosthesis
  u. fossa active, medial knee pain,
   and short leg on the side
   ipsilateral to the weak fossa
   (UMS)
  u. hand retractor
  U. 7 head halter
  u. hook trial
  u. limb orthosis (ULO)
  u. limb prosthesis (ULP)
  u. limb tension test (ULTT)
  u. limits of normal
  u. motor neuron disease
  u. motor neuron lesion
  u. thoracic spine
Uppsala screw
upright
  orthosis overlapped u.
  u. skeletal radiography
  u. view
upright-Y incision
uptake
  maximal oxygen u.
  maximum oxygen u.
upward-cutting triangular knife
urarthritis
Urbaniak
  U. neurovascular free flap
  U. scapular flap
Urban Walkers shoe
Ureacin-20
  U.-20 cream
  U.-20 creme
Ureacin-10 lotion
urethane
  Poron cellular u.
Urias
  U. air splint
  U. pressure splint
uric acid crystal
uricosuric agent
urinary
  u. incontinence
  u. nitrogen

u. output
u. tract
urine culture
urogenital diaphragm
urologic complication
US
ultrasound
unconditional stimulus
U.S.
United States
U.S. Army bone chisel
U.S. Army gouge
U.S. Army osteotome
U.S. Manufacturing Company
U-shaped
U-s. incision
U-s. retractor
Uslenghi
U. drill guide
U. plate
USMC
United States Manufacturing Company

USMC luxury liner
USMC multiaxis ankle
USMC stance locking safety knee
USP#2 suture
U-splint splint
USS
Synthes USS
ustilaginea
necrosis u.
U-stirrup splint
Utah
U. artificial arm
U. artificial limb
utensil
Good Grips u.
swivel u.
Utrata forceps
UV
ultraviolet

NOTES

U

V

V blade plate
V capsulotomy
V nail plate
V osteotomy
V sign

V40

V40 femoral head implant
component
V40 forged femoral head

V1 halo ring
V-A alignment rod
VABS

Vineland Adaptive Behavior Scales,
Revised

VAC

vacuum-assisted closure
VAC Freedom system
VAC GranuFoam heel dressing
Wound VAC

Vac

Sani V.

vacant glenoid sign
Vac-Lok immobilization cushion
Vac-Pac

V.-P. pad
V.-P. positioner

Vacumix vacuum pump
vacuolar myelopathy
vacuum

v. cement mix technique
v. disc
facet joint v.
M-Pact cast v.
v. phenomenon
v. pump

vacuum-assisted closure (VAC)
vagal reaction
vaginal

v. hand ligament
v. ligament of hand
v. pack
v. synovitis

vagoglossopharyngeal neuralgia
vagus nerve
Vainio arthroplasty
Valenti

V. arthroereisis device
V. arthroplasty
V. procedure

Valentine splint
Valeo back support
valga

coxa v.

manus v.
tibia v.

valgoid
valgum

genu v.
idiopathic genu v. (IGV)

valgus

v. angle
v. angulation
v. bar
calcaneal v.
congenital convex pes plano v.
v. contracture
convex pes v.
v. corrective ankle strap
cubitus v.
digitus v.
v. extension osteotomy
v. extension overload syndrome
flexible pes v.
v. foot
forefoot v.
genu v.
hallux v. (HV)
heel v.
v. heel deformity
v. high tibial osteotomy
hindfoot v.
idiopathic hallux v.
v. instability
v. intertrochanteric-wedge osteotomy
juvenile hallux v.
v. knee
v. knee control pad
v. knee motion
Mayday distal first metatarsal
osteotomy for hallux v.
McBride bunion hallux v.
metatarsus v.
pes plano v.
physiologic v.
rearfoot v.
senile hallux v.
v. stress
v. stress test
v. subtrochanteric osteotomy
talipes convex pes v.
v. tilt of talus
v. wedge-prop osteotomy
v. Y-shaped prop osteotomy

Valium Oral
Valleix

V. phenomenon
V. sign

Valls hip prosthesis

Valls-Ottolenghim-Schajowicz needle biopsy

Valpar

> V. Component Work Samples
> V. component work sample series
> V. Whole Body Range of Motion Test

valproic acid

Valsalva

> V. maneuver
> V. test

value

> mean v.
> Tanner-Whitehouse bone-age reference v.
> V. Walker brace

valve

> bulb and thumb screw v.
> Heyer-Schulte bur hole v.
> Quadtro cushion with Isoflap v.

vamp of shoe

van

> V. Arsdale triangular splint
> V. Beek nerve approximator
> V. Buchem disease
> V. Buren sequestrum forceps
> V. der Hoeve disease
> V. Neck disease
> V. Ness procedure
> v. Ness rotational arthroplasty
> v. Ness rotationplasty
> v. Rosen splint

vanadium

Vanderbilt Pain Management Inventory

Vanghetti limb prosthesis

Vanguard

> V. complete knee system
> V. Uni unicompartmental knew replacement

Vanore osteotomy

Vantage Performance monitor (VPM)

Vanzetti sign

VAPC

> Veterans Administration Prosthetic Center
> VAPC dorsiflexion assist orthosis

Vapo coolant spray and stretch

Vapr

> V. coagulation and cautery device
> V. system

vara

> adolescent tibia v.
> coxa v.
> developmental coxa v.
> false coxa v.
> infantile tibia v. (ITV)
> manus v.
> tibia v.

variable

> v. axis knee system
> v. circumference suprapatellar socket (VCSPS)
> metabolic v.
> v. resistance training
> v. screw placement (VSP)
> v. screw placement system
> v. screw placement system instrumentation
> v. screw placement system-instrumented lumbar spine
> v. screw plate (VSP)
> v. spinal plating (VSP)

variance

> negative ulnar v. (NUV)
> positive ulnar v. (PUV)
> ulnar minus v.

Vari-Angle

> V.-A. clip applier
> V.-A. screw

variant

> Becker v.
> Neuhauser v.
> 4-part v.

variation

> hindfoot anatomic v.
> postural v.

vari-balance board set

varices (*pl. of* varix)

varicosity

> superficial v.

Vari-Duct hip and knee orthosis

Vari-Firm Medicine Ball

VariFix spinal implant device

Vari-Flex prosthetic foot

VariGrip spinal implant device

Varikopf hip prosthesis

VariLock socket lock

varix, pl. **varices**

Varney

> V. acromioclavicular brace
> V. pin

Varni-Thompson Pediatric Pain Questionnaire

varum

> genu v.

varus

> calcaneal v.
> v. contracture
> v. corrective ankle strap
> cubitus v.
> v. derotational osteotomy
> digitus v.
> dynamic hallux v.
> forefoot v.
> genu v.
> v. habitus
> hallux v.

heel v.
v. hindfoot
v. hindfoot deformity
v. knee
v. knee control pad
v. malalignment
v. malunion
metatarsus v. (MTV)
metatarsus primus v. (MPV)
metatarsus primus adductus (MPA)
v. MTP angle
pes v.
v. plafond
rearfoot v.
v. rotational osteotomy (VRO)
v. rotation shortening osteotomy
v. stress test
subtalar v.
v. supramalleolar osteotomy
talipes v.
tibial v.
v. tilt
v. toe

varus-valgus
v.-v. adjustment screw
v.-v. angulation
v.-v. instability
knee v.-v.
v.-v. lift-off
v.-v. plane
v.-v. stress
v.-v. stress of elbow

vascular
v. accident
v. assessment
v. bundle implantation
v. bundle implantation into bone
v. endothelium
v. forceps
v. gangrene
v. inflow
v. injury
v. invasion
v. metaphysial bone
v. nonunion
v. surgery
v. tissue
v. tumor

vasculare
heloma v.

vascularity
femoral head v.
tenuous v.

vascularized
v. bone graft
v. bone transplant
v. fibular graft
v. free flap
v. osseous transfer
v. osteoseptocutaneous fibular
autogenous graft
v. rib strut graft

vasculature

vasculitis
mesenteric v.
rheumatoid v.

vasculopathy

vasoconstriction

vasoconstrictive therapy

vasocoolant spray

vasodilation
flow-mediated v. (FMD)

vasodilator

vasodilatory effect

vasogenic shock

vasomotor
v. disorder
v. technique

vasopneumatic intermittent compression

vasopressor

vasospasm

vasospastic ischemia

Vastamäki
V. muscle transfer
V. paralysis
V. technique

vastus
v. intermedius
v. intermedius muscle
v. lateralis (VL)
v. lateralis muscle
v. lateralis ridge
v. medialis
v. medialis advancement (VMA)
v. medialis muscle
v. medialis obliquus (VMO)
v. medialis obliquus:vastus lateralis
(VMO:VL)

VATER
vertebral abnormality, anal imperforation,
tracheoesophageal fistula, and radial,
ray, or renal anomalies
vertebral (defects), (imperforate) anus,
tracheoesophageal (fistula), radial and
renal (dysplasia) anomalies
VATER syndrome

NOTES

vault
> plantar v.

VAX-D
> vertebra axial decompression
>> VAX-D therapy table

VBI
> vertebrobasilar insufficiency

VC
> voluntary closing
> voluntary control

VCSPS
> variable circumference suprapatellar
> socket

VD
> video densitometry

VDA
> video-dimensional analysis

VDDR
> vitamin D-dependent rickets

VDRR
> vitamin D-resistant rickets

VDS
> ventral derotation spondylodesis
>> VDS compression rod
>> VDS hex nut
>> VDS screw
>> VDS screwdriver
>> VDS wrench

VE
> vocational evaluation

vector
> V. intertrochanteric nail
> V. low back analysis system
> major injury v. (MIV)
> v. point
> v. quantity

vectored adjustment
Vectra Genisys laser system device
vehicle
vein
> anterior jugular v.
> axillary v.
> v. of Batson
> Boyd communicating perforation v.
> brachiocephalic v.
> carotid v.
> cephalic v.
> Cockett communicating
> perforating v.'s
> common iliac v.
> grafting v.
> iliac v.
> iliolumbar v.
> innominate v.
> intercostal v.
> intermetatarsal v.
> internal iliac v.
> internal jugular v.
> lingual v.

> lumbar v.
> middle sacral v.
> middle thyroid v.
> peroneal v.
> popliteal v.
> saphenous v.
> subclavian v.
> superficial temporal v.
> superior thyroid v.
> tibial v.
> vertebral v.

vela (*pl. of* velum)
velar
> fronting of v.

Velcro
> V. closure
> V. extenders splint
> V. fitting
> V. Hand Exerboard
> V. immobilization
> V. immobilizer
> V. strap

Velcro-Lock mat platform
Veleanu-Rosianu-Ionescu
> V.-R.-I. adductor tenotomy
> V.-R.-I. technique

velocity
> angular v.
> conduction v.
> free-walking v.
> maximum conduction v.
> maximum eversion v.
> maximum inversion v.
> mean flow v.
> motion v.
> motor conduction v.
> motor nerve conduction v.
> (MNCV)
> muscle fiber conduction v.
> nerve conduction v. (NCV)
> orthodromic v.
> peak height v. (PHV)
> propagation v.
> push-off v.
> sensory nerve conduction v.
> stretching v.

Velocor footbed
Velpeau
> V. axillary lateral view
> V. axillary radiograph
> V. bandage
> V. cast
> V. deformity
> V. dressing
> V. plaster
> V. shoulder immobilizer
> V. shoulder sling
> V. sling-dressing

V. stockinette
V. wrap
velum, pl. **vela**
Venable
V. plate
V. screw
Venable-Stuck nail
vena cava
Venn-Watson classification
Venodyne boot
venography
epidural v.
intraosseous v.
magnetic resonance v.
Venosan
V. support hose
V. support sock
venous
v. cleft
v. compression
v. foot pump
v. stasis dermatitis
v. thromboembolic disease (VTED)
v. thrombosis
ventral
v. derotating spinal wrench
v. derotation spondylodesis (VDS)
ventriculography
ventriculoperitoneal shunt
ventroflexion
vent tube
VePesid
V. Injection
V. Oral
Verbrugge
V. bone clamp
V. bone-holding forceps
V. needle
Verbrugge-Hohmann bone retractor
Verdan
V. osteoplastic thumb reconstruction
V. technique
Verebelyi-Ogston decancellation procedure
Veress needle
Verhoeff stain
Verlow brace
Vermont
V. Interdependent Services Team Approach (VISTA)
V. pedicle fixation system
V. spinal fixator (VSF)

V. spinal fixator articulation
V. spinal fixator clamp
Vernier
V. caliber gauge
V. caliper
Verocay body
verruca, pl. **verrucae**
v. cryotherapy
mosaic plantar v.
single plantar v.
v. vulgaris
verruciformis
epidermodysplasia v.
verrucous lesion
Versaback back system
VersaBond medium-viscosity bone cement
VersaClimber RX exercise machine
VersaFlex tubing kit
Versa-Fx
V.-F. femoral fixation
V.-F. femoral hip fixation system
Versa-Helper floor stand
Versalok low back fixation system
VersaPulse holmium laser
Versa-Stim self-adhering electrode
versatility
attachment v.
Versa-Trainer exerciser
VersaWrist wrist splint
versicolor
tinea v.
version
external v.
femoral neck v.
Gait Abnormality Rating Scale Modified V. (GARS-M)
internal v.
Occupational Performance History Interview - Second V. (OPHI-II)
Rivermead Behavioral Memory Test-Extended V. (RBMT-E)
Versi-Splint carry bag
VerSys
V. fiber metal taper
V. hip system
V. prosthesis
VertAlign spinal support system
vertebra, pl. **vertebrae**
apex v.
apical v.
v. axial decompression (VAX-D)
basilar v.

V

NOTES

vertebra *(continued)*
    biconcave v.
    block v.
    body of v.
    butterfly v.
    caudal v.
    cervical v.
    cleft v.
    coccygeal v.
    codfish v.
    displaced v.
    dorsal v.
    end v.
    false v.
    first cervical v.
    fish v.
    fractured v.
    fused v.
    hourglass v.
    last normal v. (LNV)
    lumbar v.
    lumbosacral v.
    malposed v.
    midbody of v.
    neural tube defect-related anomaly
      of v.
    olisthetic v.
    pear-shaped v.
    v. plana
    v. prominens reflex
    sacral v.
    scalloping of v.
    second cervical v.
    stable v.
    subluxed v.
    thoracic v.
    transitional v.
    transverse process of v.
    true v.
    wasp-waist v.
    wedge-shaped v.
    wedging of olisthetic v.

vertebral
    v. abnormality, anal imperforation,
      tracheoesophageal fistula, and
      radial, ray, or renal anomalies
      (VATER)
    v. adjustment
    v. angiography
    v. ankylosis
    v. arch
    v. arteriography
    v. artery
    v. artery test
    v. arthritis
    v. bar
    v. block
    v. body
    v. body anterior cortex

v. body collapse
v. body corpectomy
v. body decompression
v. body endplate
v. body fracture
v. body impactor
v. body stapling wedge resection
v. body tumor
v. bone
v. border
v. canal
v. column
v. column cleft
v. compression
v. (defects), (imperforate) anus,
    tracheoesophageal (fistula), radial
    and renal (dysplasia) anomalies
    (VATER)
v. derangement
v. end plate
v. exposure
v. fascia
v. formula
v. fusion
v. instability
v. lesion
v. level
v. medicine
v. motion segment
v. motion testing
v. motion unit (VMU)
v. nerve
v. neural reflection
v. notch
v. osteomyelitis
v. osteosynthesis
v. osteosynthesis fusion rate
v. plana fracture
v. polyarthritis
v. rib
v. ring apophysis
v. rotation
v. scalloping
v. segmentation anomaly
v. stable burst fracture
v. steal phenomenon
v. steal syndrome
v. stripe
v. subluxation
v. subluxation complex (VSC)
v. subluxation syndrome
v. vein
v. wedge compression fracture
v. wedging

vertebrectomy
Bohlman anterior cervical v.
cervical v.
cervical spondylotic myelopathy v.

microsurgical thoracoscopic v.
partial cervical v.
vertebrobasilar
v. injury
v. insufficiency (VBI)
vertebrocostal rib
vertebrogenic interference
vertebropelvic ligament
vertebroplasty
vertebrosternal rib
Verteflex
V. arthrotonic stabilizer
V. Intersegmental Traction Table
Vertetrac ambulatory traction system
vertical
anatomical v.
v. axis
v. capsulotomy
v. compression
v. compression test
v. foot board
v. loading
v. longitudinal tear
v. loop suture technique
v. loop suture technique for
meniscus repair
v. mattress suture
v. pedicle diameter
v. plane
v. sacral compaction
v. sagittal split osteotomy (VSO)
v. septum
v. shear (VS)
v. shear fracture
v. shock pylon
v. subsidence
v. suspension reflex
v. symphysial mobility
v. talus
v. talus foot deformity
v. traction
v. translation
verticality control
VertiGraft textured allograft bone graft
VertiLok 2-stage closure procedure
Vertstreken closed medullary nailing
very low calorie diet (VLCD)
vesalian bone
vesalianum
Vesalius bone
Vesely-Street
V.-S. splint
V.-S. split nail

vesicocutaneous fistula
vesicostomy
Vess chair
vessel
v. clamp
v. dilator
endosteal v.
great v.
haversian v.
v. hook
humeral circumflex v.
lymph v.
milking of v.
periosteal v.
popliteal v.
v. shifting
tumor v.
vest
Bremer AirFlo halo v.
halo v.
Little cargo v.
Minerva v.
Ortho-Trac pneumatic v.
Standard E-Z-On V.
Vitrathene v.
weighted v.
vestibular ball
Vestibulator positioning tumble form
vestibulocerebellar ataxia
vestibulospinal
v. reflex
v. tract
vestigial muscle
**Veterans Administration Prosthetic
Center (VAPC)**
**V-groove hollow-ground connection
design**
viability
viable tissue
Vibram
V. rockerbottom shoe
V. sole
Vibramat
vibration
v. glove
v. perception threshold (VPT)
v. sensation
v. sense
v. sensitivity
v. synovitis
v. threshold test
v. white finger syndrome
whole-body v.

V

NOTES

vibrative
vibrator
    v. hand syndrome
    Magic Wand v.
vibratory massage
vibrogram
    digital v.
vibromasseur
vibrometer test
vibrotherapeutics
vicious union
**Vicon 3-dimensional gait analysis
system**
Vicryl suture
Victorian brace
Vidal-Adrey
    V.-A. fracture technique
    V.-A. modified Hoffman external
      fixation device apparatus
    V.-A. modified Hoffmann external
      fixation device
    V.-A. modified Hoffmann fixation
video densitometry (VD)
video-dimensional analysis (VDA)
videofluoroscopy
video-gate analysis
videoradiography
vidian neuralgia
**Vidicon vacuum chamber pickup tube
for video camera**
Vi-Drape
    V.-D. dressing
    Ioban V.-D.
view
    abdominal v.
    abduction and external rotation v.
    ABER v.
    Adams v.
    Alexander v.
    Allstate v.
    anterior v.
    anterior-draw stress v.
    anteroposterior v.
    apical lordotic v.
    AP supine v.
    Arcelin v.
    axial calcaneus v.
    axial sesamoid v.
    axillary lateral v.
    ball-cathers v.
    baseline v.
    Beath v.
    bicipital tuberosity v.
    Böhler calcaneal v.
    Böhler lumbosacral v.
    Breuerton v.
    Broden v.
    Bucky v.
    Burnham v.

calcaneal axial v.
Canale v.
Canale-Kelly v.
carpal tunnel v.
Carter-Rowe v.
charger v.
cine v.
clenched fist v.
coalition v.
coned-down v.
cross-table lateral v. (CTLV)
dens x-ray v.
Didiee v.
dorsiflexion v.
dorsoplantar radiographic v.
dynamic stress x-ray v.
erect v.
false profile v.
FCS v.
Ferguson v.
Ficat v.
frog-leg lateral v.
Garth v.
Grashey v.
Harris v.
Harris-Beath axial calcaneus v.
Hermodsson tangential v.
Hill-Sachs v.
hip-to-ankle v.
Hobb v.
Hughston v.
iliac oblique v.
infrapatellar v.
inlet v.
intraoperative v.
inversion ankle stress v.
Jones v.
Judet pelvic x-ray v.
lateral bending v.
lateral monopodal stance v.
lateral oblique v.
lateral tilt stress ankle v.
Lauren v.
Lawrence v.
Lowell v.
Löwenstein v.
magnification v.
Merchant v.
mortise v.
Neer lateral v.
Neer transscapular v.
nonstanding lateral oblique v.
nonweightbearing v.
Norgaard v.
notch v.
oblique v.
obturator oblique v.
odontoid x-ray v.
outlet v.

patellar skyline v.
plantar axial v.
plantarflexion stress v.
prayer v.
push-pull ankle stress v.
push-pull hip v.
radial head-capitellum v.
Robert v.
Rosenberg v.
scapulolateral v.
semisupinated oblique v.
serendipity v.
skijump v.
skyline v.
spot v.
standing dorsoplantar v.
standing lateral v.
standing weightbearing v.
Stenver v.
stress v.
Stryker-Notch v.
sunrise v.
sunset v.
swimmer's v.
tangential x-ray v.
Tile v.
transthoracic lateral v.
trauma v.
true lateral v.
tunnel v.
upright v.
Velpeau axillary lateral v.
von Rosen v.
weightbearing dorsoplantar v.
West Point axillary lateral v.
White leg length v.
x-ray v.
Y scapular v.
Zanca v.
Vigilon dressing
vigorimeter
Viking postoperative shoe
Viladot
V. arthroereisis device
V. implant
V. prosthesis
V. surgical technique
Vilex
V. cannulated screw system
V. F-Series dual-thread screw
V. Ouchless Hook
V. screw system

villonodular
v. synovitis
v. tenosynovitis
villous
v. lipomatous proliferation
v. synovitis
v. tenosynovitis
villusectomy
vinblastine
Vincasar PFS Injection
vinculum, pl. **vincula**
v. breve
intertendinous v.
vincula longa connection
Vineland Adaptive Behavior Scales, Revised (VABS)
Vinertia
V. implant metal
V. implant metal prosthesis
Vinke
V. skull traction tongs
V. tong traction
violet monofilament suture
viral
v. monarthritis
v. myositis
viral-associated arthritis
Virchow triad
Virgin hip screw
Virtual hip joint
Virtullene brace material
visceral tendon sheath
visceroptosis
viscerosomatic reflex
viscerospinal syndrome
viscoelastic
v. creep
v. heel insert
v. insole
v. material
v. polymer
quasilinear v. (QLV)
v. tissue
viscoelasticity
Viscoheel
V. K heel cushion
V. K, N orthosis
V. N cushion
V. SofSpot viscoelastic heel cushion
Viscolas
V. heel cushion

NOTES

Viscolas *(continued)*
  V. heel pain and disability benefit
  V. orthosis
Viscoped
  V. S insole
  V. S support
viscosity
  blood v.
ViscoSpot
  V. heel cushion
  V. support
viscosupplementation treatment
viscous
vise
  allograft bone v.
  AlloGrip bone v.
  v. like pain
  pin v.
  Starrett pin v.
VISI
  volar flexed intercalated segment
  instability
vision
  V. Epic wheelchair
  under direct v.
visor
  v. halo fixation device
  v. osteotomy
visor/sandwich osteotomy
VISTA
  Vermont Interdependent Services Team
  Approach
Vistec x-ray detectable sponge
visual
  v. analog scale
  V. Analog Scale of Handicap
  v. closure
  v. evoked potential
  v. evoked response
  v. neglect
  v. orientation
  v. perception
visual-motor integration (VMI)
visual-spatial ability impairment
Vita ADE cream
vitalism
vitallium
  v. cup arthroplasty
  v. humeral replacement prosthesis
  v. implant
  v. implant material
  v. implant metal
  v. Küntscher nail
  v. Luhr plate
  v. screw
  v. staple
Vitalock
  V. cluster acetabular component
  V. solid-back acetabular component

vitamin
  v. C, D, K deficiency
  v. D-dependent rickets (VDDR)
  v. D receptor gene serum assay
  v. D-resistant rickets (VDRR)
  v. E emollient
Vitoss
  V. Scaffold synthetic cancellous
  bone void filler
  V. synthetic bone
Vitox
  V. alumina ceramic material
  V. femoral head
Vitrathene
  V. jacket
  V. vest
Viva shoe
Vivatek ultimate healing machine
Vivelle Transdermal
VL
  vastus lateralis
Vladimiroff-Mikulicz amputation
VLCD
  very low calorie diet
VMA
  vastus medialis advancement
VMC
  void metal composite
V-medullary nail
VMI
  visual-motor integration
VMO
  vastus medialis obliquus
  VMO exercise
  VMO retraining
VMO:VL
  vastus medialis obliquus:vastus lateralis
  VMO:VL EMG ratio
VMU
  vertebral motion unit
VO
  voluntary opening
vocal cord
vocational
  v. assessment
  v. evaluation (VE)
  v. feasibility
  v. rehabilitation (VR)
Vogue arm sling
void
  v. metal composite (VMC)
  signal v.
volar
  v. angulation deformity
  v. antebrachial region
  v. approach
  v. aspect
  v. beak ligament
  v. capsule

v. carpal ligament
v. compartment syndrome
v. condyle
v. digital artery
v. epineurolysis
v. flexed intercalated segment instability (VISI)
v. glide
v. intercalary wrist instability
v. midline oblique incision
v. plaster splint
v. plate arthroplasty
v. plate repair
v. semilunar wrist dislocation
v. shear fracture
v. surface
v. synovectomy
v. T plate
v. ulnar sling
v. wrist
v. zigzag finger incision

volarly
volarward approach
volitional

v. activation
v. activity
v. contraction
v. exercise
v. fatigue
v. muscle action test
v. resisted flexion
v. resisted flexion and extension

volitionally
Volkmann

V. bone curette
V. bone hook
V. canal
V. claw hand
V. clawhand deformity
V. contracture
V. disease
V. fracture
V. ischemia
V. ischemic paralysis
V. rake retractor
V. splint
V. subluxation
V. triangle

Volkov-Oganesian

V.-O. elbow distraction device
V.-O. external fixation
V.-O. external fixation apparatus
V.-O. external fixation device

Volkov-Oganesian-Povarov hinged distraction apparatus
volley of pain
Volpicelli functional ambulation scale
Voltaren-XR Oral
volume

cartilage v.
v. conduction
stroke v.

volumeter

Ableware V.
foot v.
hand v.
v. set

volumetric wear rate
voluntary

v. activity
v. closing (VC)
v. closing terminal device
v. control (VC)
v. control 4-bar knee
v. muscle
v. opening (VO)
v. opening terminal device

Volz

V. total wrist arthroplasty
V. wrist
V. wrist prosthesis

vomer bone
von

v. Bekhterev reflex
v. Gies joint
v. Hippel-Lindau syndrome
v. Lackum transection shift jacket
v. Lackum transection shift jacket brace
v. Langenbeck periosteal elevator
V. Mises stress
v. Recklinghausen disease
v. Rosen abduction splint
v. Rosen cruciform splint
v. Rosen splint hip orthosis
v. Rosen view
v. Saal medullary pin
v. Schwann law
v. Weber triangle

Voorhoeve disease
Voshell

V. bursa
V. sign
V. test

V

NOTES

Vostal
>V. classification of radial fracture
>V. radial fracture classification

V-osteotomy
>Japas V-o.

VPM
>Vantage Performance monitor

VPT
>vibration perception threshold

VR
>vocational rehabilitation

VRO
>varus rotational osteotomy

Vrolik disease

VS
>vertical shear

VSC
>vertebral subluxation complex

VSF
>Vermont spinal fixator
>>VSF clamp
>>VSF fixation system
>>VSF rod
>>VSF screw

V-shaped
>V-s. fracture
>V-s. incision
>V-s. osteotomy
>V-s. rotator cuff tear

VSL technology

VSO
>vertical sagittal split osteotomy

VSP
>variable screw placement
>variable screw plate
>variable spinal plating
>>VSP fixation
>>VSP plate
>>VSP plate instrumentation
>>VSP system

VTED
>venous thromboembolic disease

vulgaris
>verruca v.

Vulpian atrophy

Vulpian-Bernhardt spinal muscular atrophy

Vulpius
>V. Achilles tendon reconstruction
>V. equinus deformity operation
>V. lengthening
>V. procedure

Vulpius-Stoffel procedure

VuRyser monitor lift

V-Y
>V-Y advancement flap
>V-Y Kutler flap
>V-Y plasty
>V-Y plasty correction
>V-Y plasty correction of varus toe
>V-Y quadricepsplasty

WACH
wedge adjustable cushioned heel
WACH orthopaedic shoe
wad
flexor w.
mobile w.
Waddell
W. Chronic Back Pain Disability
index
W. sign
W. triad
wadding
cotton sheet w.
shot w.
waddle
duck w.
waddling gait
Wadsworth
W. elbow approach
W. posterolateral approach
W. technique
W. unconstrained elbow prosthesis
wafer
w. distal ulna resection
w. procedure
Wagdy double-V osteotomy
Wagner
W. acetabular reamer
W. approach
W. classification
W. closed pinning
W. device external fixator
W. disease
W. distraction device
W. distractor
W. external fixation apparatus
W. external fixation device
W. femoral lengthening
W. femoral metaphysial shortening
W. fixation
W. fixer
W. frame
W. grade
W. leg-lengthening apparatus
W. limb lengthening method
W. line
W. modification of Syme
amputation
W. multiple K-wire osteosynthesis
W. open reduction technique
W. profundus advancement
W. prosthesis
W. retractor
W. revision hip system
W. skin incision

W. 2-stage Syme amputation
W. tibial lengthening
W. trochanteric advancement
Wagner-Schanz
W.-S. screw
W.-S. screw apparatus
W.-S. screw device
wagon
dumbbell w.
w. wheel fracture
Wagoner
W. cervical technique
W. posterior approach
W. ulcer
Wagstaffe fracture
Wagstaffe-Le Fort fracture
Wagstaff tubercle
Wainwright plate
waist
w. of anatomical structure
w. fracture
w. of phalanx
w. of scaphoid
w. suspension belt
waist-to-hip ratio
wakeboarding
wake-up test
Waldenström
W. classification
W. disease
W. sign
W. staging
Waldron test
WALK
weight-activated locking knee
walk
heel w.
heel-and-toe w.
lift-off of heel in w.
nonweightbearing crutch w.
w. test
toe w.
Walkabout walker
WalkAide system
Walk-A-Matic walker
walkaway
WalkCare slippers
walker
air w.
Aircast pneumatic w.
ATO w.
w. basket
Body Armor short leg w.
CAM W. II
CAM Walker ankle w.

walker *(continued)*
cast w.
Castaway ankle w.
Castaway leg w.
Charcot restraint orthotic w.
(CROW)
Comfy w.
controlled ankle w.
Darco Body Armor short leg w.
Delta w.
DH pressure relief w.
EasyStep pressure relief w.
Equalizer air w.
Guardian Red Dot w.
Hi-Top II adjustable w.
Hi-Top foot/ankle w.
W. hollow quill pin
Lumex w.
Maddacrawler prone support w.
Merry W.
Moon W.
obese w.
ORLAU swivel w.
4-point w.
Roll-A-Bout 4-wheel w.
Rollator Nova w.
rubber sole cast w.
rubber wedge w.
W. ruptured disc curette
Sabel cast w.
short leg w.
w. skis
w. sleds
swivel w.
Walkabout w.
Walk-A-Matic w.
3-wheel w.
Zimmer w.
Walker-Murdoch wrist sign
walking
w. adjunct
aerobic w.
w. aid
w. biomechanics
bipedal w.
w. boot cast
w. brace
crutch w.
w. cycle
w. footprints classification
w. heel
heel-and-toe w.
idiopathic toe w.
w. mechanics
nonweightbearing crutch w.
w. pole
w. program
stance phase w.
w. stirrup

w. task
toe w.
w. without support
w. with support
Walk-'n-Tone exerciser
Walk-Rite device
wall
medial w.
Walldius Vitallium mechanical knee prosthesis
Wallenberg
W. procedure
W. syndrome
W. test
wallerian degeneration
wallet neuritis
wall-slide exercise
Wal-Pil-O neck pillow
Walsh
protocol of W.
Walter-Liston forceps
Walther fracture
Walton
W. cartilage clamp
W. maneuver
W. meniscal clamp
W. scissors
W. wire-pulling forceps
Walton-Ruskin forceps
Wanchik
W. neutral position splint
W. writer
wand
ArthroCare w.
ArthroWand disposable surgical w.
Essential Energy Whole House W.
extensor w.
TCFO placement w.
TriggerWheel W.
Wangensteen
W. needle
W. needle holder
Wanger leg lengthening device
waning discharge
ward
W. periosteal elevator
W. triangle
warfarin sodium
warm
w. ischemia
w. ischemic time
W. 'n' Form lumbosacral corset
W. Springs brace
warm-and-form
w.-a.-f. cast
w.-a.-f. insert
warmer
gel w.
Thermasonic gel w.

warmth
    joint w.
WarmTouch patient warming system
Warm-Up active wound therapy system
Warner-Farber ankle fixation technique
Warren-Mack rotating drill
Warren-White Achilles tendon
  lengthening
Warsaw hip prosthesis
wart
    mosaic w.
    plantar w. (PW)
    W. stick wart remover
Wartenberg
    W. pinwheel
    W. sign
washboard syndrome
washer
    C w.
    contoured w.
    w. crimper
    female w.
    w. holder
    male w.
    oval w.
    plate spacer w.
    spiked ligament w.
    Synthes ligament w.
    toothed w.
WasherLoc device
wash mitt
wasp-waist vertebra
Wassel
    W. classification of thumb
      polydactyly
    W. thumb duplication classification
    W. thumb duplication (type IV)
Wasserstein
    W. fixation
    W. fixation device
wasting
    quadriceps w.
Watanabe
    W. discoid meniscus classification
    W. pin
    W. pin holder
    W. retractor
watch crystal nail
Watco
    W. brace
    W. knee immobilizer
water
    w. acceptance test

    Essential Energy W.
    total body w.
water-cooled power bur
Waterman osteotomy
WaterPik irrigation
Waterpillow
    Mediflow W.
water-soluble contrast agent
Watkins
    W. fusion
    W. fusion technique
Watson
    W. maneuver
    W. scaphotrapeziotrapezoidal fusion
    W. technique
    W. test
Watson-Cheyne technique
Watson-Jones
    W.-J. ankle tenodesis
    W.-J. anterior approach
    W.-J. arthrodesis
    W.-J. bone gouge
    W.-J. fracture repair
    W.-J. frame
    W.-J. guidepin
    W.-J. incision
    W.-J. lateral approach
    W.-J. nail
    W.-J. navicular fracture
    W.-J. navicular fracture
      classification
    W.-J. procedure
    W.-J. reconstruction
    W.-J. spinal fracture classification
    W.-J. tibial fracture classification
    W.-J. traction
Watson-Williams intervertebral disc
  rongeur
Waugh
    W. knee prosthesis
    W. total ankle replacement
      prosthesis
wave
    A w.
    double flexion w.
    Epos Ultra orthopaedic shock w.
    F w.
    H w.
    w. keyboard
    M w.
    OssaTron shock w.
    positive sharp w.
    W. Web

W

NOTES

waveform
>biphasic w.
>bipolar IF w.
>electrical stimulator w.
>micro w.
>monophasic w.
>Russian w.

wax
>bone w.
>Horsley bone w.

way
>W.'s of Coping checklist
>giving w.

Wayfarer modifiable foot prosthesis
Wayne County reduction
WBAT
>weightbearing as tolerated

WC, W/C, WCh
>wheelchair

WD
>wrist disarticulation

WDWN, WD WN
>well developed, well nourished

weak
>w. bony tissue
>w. foot

weakness
>breakaway w.
>give-way w.
>motor w.
>overstretch w.
>ratchety w.

wear
>abnormal shoe w.
>accelerated chondral w.
>asymmetric w.
>backside w.
>3-body w.
>w. debris
>eccentric w.
>shoe w.
>SoftFlex Wrist W.

wear-and-tear degeneration
wear-resistant surface
weather-ache
weave
>bob and w.

weaver
>w, bottom
>w, rockerbottom shoe

Weaver-Dunn
>W.-D. acromioclavicular operation
>W.-D. acromioclavicular technique
>W.-D. procedure
>W.-D. resection

web
>w. area
>w. area of hand
>w. border

>w. border of hand
>w. contracture
>w. corn
>finger w.
>thumb w.
>Wave W.

Webb
>W. bolt nail
>W. fixation
>W. pin
>W. procedure
>W. stove bolt

webbed
>w. finger
>w. toe

Weber
>W. antiglide plate
>W. B, C fracture
>W. classification of physial injury
>W. fracture classification
>W. frame
>W. hip implant
>W. humeral osteotomy
>W. Permalock
>W. procedure
>W. static 2-point discrimination
>W. subcapital osteotomy
>W. syndrome
>W. test
>W. triangle
>W. zone

Weber-Danis ankle injury classification
Weber-Vasey traction-absorption wiring
>**technique**

Webril
>W. bandage
>W. cotton padding
>W. dressing
>W. immobilization

webspace
>w. creep
>w. flap
>w. incision
>w. infection
>interdigital w.

Webster
>W. meniscectomy scissors
>W. needle
>W. needle holder

Wechsler
>W. Adult Intelligence scale
>W. Memory scale

Weck
>W. clip
>W. knife
>W. microsuture cutting scissors
>W. osteotome

Wedeen wire passer

wedge
    abduction w.
    w. adjustable cushioned heel (WACH)
    w. adjustable cushioned heel shoe
    bed w.
    bone w.
    bumper w.
    cast w.
    closing base w.
    compensatory w.
    w. compression fracture
    Duo-Cline Dual Support contoured bed w.
    w. fixation
    w. flexion-compression fracture
    Good 'N Bed w.
    w. graft
    Hapad heel w.
    heel w.
    heel-to-toe medial shoe w.
    inner heel w. (IHW)
    lateral w.
    w. matrix resection (WMR)
    medial heel w. (MHW)
    medial heel-and-sole w.
    medial sole w.
    metaphysial w.
    w. nonunion
    open w. (OW)
    w. osteotomy
    Positex knee w.
    w. posting
    w. resection
    roof w.
    Saunders mobilization w.
    seating w.
    self-adhering varus/valgus w.
    shoe w.
    super w.
    W. TAG suture anchor system
    tibial w.
    toe w.
    TruWedge BGS osteotomy w.
    Yancy cast w.
wedge-and-groove joint
wedged shoe
wedge-shaped
    w.-s. uncomminuted fragment
    w.-s. uncomminuted tibial plateau fracture
    w.-s. vertebra

wedging
    w. cast
    navicular w.
    w. of olisthetic vertebra
    vertebral w.
    w. of vertebral interspace
WeeFIM
    Functional Independence Measure for Children
    WeeFIM instrument
weekend athlete
Wegener granulomatosis
Wegner
    W. disease
    W. line
weight
    w. acceptance
    ankle w.
    body w.
    w. boot
    cutting w.
    distal segment w.
    handheld w. (HHW)
    lean body w. (LBW)
    progressive w.
    w.'s and pulleys
    Thera-Band progressive w.
    w. traction
    w. training
weight-activated locking knee (WALK)
weightbearing
    w. acetabular dome
    w. as tolerated (WBAT)
    w. axis
    w. brace
    w. crutch
    w. dorsoplantar radiograph
    w. dorsoplantar view
    full w. (FWB)
    w. ground reaction force
    w. joint
    pain with w.
    partial w. (PWB)
    progression to full w.
    progressive w.
    protective w.
    w. rotational injury
    w. surface
    w. symmetry
    w. tangential radiograph
    toe-touch w.
    touchdown w.
    w. x-ray

W

NOTES

weight/composition
> body w./c.

weighted
> w. glove
> w. pen
> w. vest
> w. walking stick

weightlifter's
> w. clavicle
> w. shoulder

weightlifting
weight-relieving
> w.-r. caliper
> w.-r. Forte harness
> w.-r. orthosis

weight-training program
Weil
> W. implant
> W. osteotomy
> W. pelvic sling
> W. splint

Weiland
> W. classification
> W. harvesting
> W. iliac crest bone graft

Weil-Blakesley intervertebral disc rongeur
Weil-modified Swanson implant
Weil-type Swanson-design hammertoe implant
Weinraub joint and calcaneal spreader
Weinstein enhanced sensory test
Weinstein-Ponseti technique
Weinstock desyndactylization
wei qi
WEIS
> Work Environment Impact Scale

Weise jack screw
Weiss
> W. amputation saw
> W. spring

Weissman classification
Weit-Arner retractor
Weitbrecht
> W. foramen
> W. ligament
> W. retinaculum

Weitlaner retractor
3-2 Weitlaner self-retaining retractor
Welander distal myopathy
weld
> callus w.
> cold w.
> hot w.
> spot w.

well
> w. developed, well nourished (WDWN, WD WN)
> w. leg straight leg raising test

well-differentiated myxoid liposarcoma
Weller
> W. cartilage forceps
> W. cartilage scissors
> W. total hip joint prosthesis

well-leg
> w.-l. cast
> w.-l. holder
> w.-l. raising
> w.-l. splint
> w.-l. support
> w.-l. traction

Wellmerling technique
well-padded splint
Wells
> W. pedicle clamp
> W. traction

well-seated prosthesis
Wenger plate
Werdnig-Hoffmann
> W.-H. disease
> W.-H. spinal muscular atrophy

Werenskiold sign
Wernicke aphasia
Wertheim-Bohlman technique
Wertheim splint
west
> W. bone chisel
> W. bone gouge
> W. hand dissector
> W. nerve tester
> W. osteotome
> W. Point Ankle Grading System
> W. Point axillary lateral radiograph
> W. Point axillary lateral view
> W. and Soto-Hall patella operation

Westcott Pyramid Program
Westergren sedimentation rate
Wester meniscal clamp
western
> W. Ontario Instability Index (WOSI)
> W. Ontario and McMaster University osteoarthritis index
> W. Ontario Rotator Cuff (WORC)
> W. Ontario Rotator Cuff Index

Westfield acromioclavicular immobilizer
Westfield-style envelope sling
Westhaven Yale Multidimensional Pain Inventory (WHYMPI)
Westin-Hall incision
Westin tenodesis
Westin-Turco category
Weston shelf procedure
Westphal phenomenon
West-Soto-Hall patellectomy
wet
> w. gangrene

w. globe temperature
w. leather sign

wet-to-dry dressing

WFE

Williams flexion exercise

WFL

within functional limits

Wheaton

W. bunion splint
W. Pavlik harness
W. Pavlik Harness brace

WHECS

wrist hand extension compression support

wheel

Carborundum grinding w.
w. chair seating component
pin w.
shoulder w.
3-w. walker

wheelchair (WC, W/C, WCh)

Action Jr. w.
Amigo mechanical w.
antitipper w.
Applause Super-Hemi w.
AquaTrek W.
w. chain
w. confinement
w. cushion
electric w.
Epic w.
folding frame w.
Gendron bariatric w.
Invacare manual w.
Jay J2 w.
Kuschkin Ace w.
Landeez all-terrain w.
Lumex lightweight w.
manual w.
Navigator power w.
Nitro w.
power w.
Quickie Carbon w.
Quickie EX w.
Quickie GPS w.
Quickie GP Swing-Away w.
Quickie GPV w.
Quickie Kidz w.
Quickie Recliner w.
Quickie Ti w.
reclining frame w.
rigid frame w.
self-propelling w.
Shark pediatric w.

Skil-Care reclining w.
Slam'r w.
sling seat w.
tilting frame w.
W. User's Shoulder Pain Index (WUSPI)
Vision Epic w.
4XP Tilt System w.
Zippie 2 w.
Zippie P500 w.

whettle bone

whiplash

acute w.
chronic w.
w. injury
reflex rebound component of w.
w. syndrome

whiplash-shaken infant syndrome

whirlpool

w. bath (WPB)
w. therapy

whiskering

whistling face syndrome

white

w. band on degenerated implant
w. blood cell count
w. blood cell scan
W. chisel
W. epiphysiodesis
w. fixation
W. leg length view
w. matter
w. muscle
W. and Panjabi cervical spine criteria
W. posterior ankle fusion
W. posterior arthrodesis
W. screwdriver
W. slide procedure
W. tendo calcaneus lengthening

Whitecloud-LaRocca

W.-L. cervical arthrodesis
W.-L. fibular strut graft

Whitehall

W. Glacier Pack
W. thermalator

Whitesides

W. line
W. Ortholoc II condylar femoral prosthesis
W. technique
W. tissue pressure determination
W. total knee prosthesis

NOTES

W

Whitesides-Kelly cervical technique
Whitfield's Ointment
whitlow
>   herpetic w.
>   thecal w.

Whitman
>   W. arch support
>   W. femoral neck reconstruction
>   W. frame
>   W. maneuver
>   W. muscle transfer
>   W. osteotomy
>   W. paralysis
>   W. plate
>   W. talectomy procedure
>   W. traction

Whitney single-use plastic curette
WHO
>   wrist-hand orthosis

WHO/LAR
>   World Health Organization/International
>   League Against Rheumatism
>   WHO/LAR Response Criteria
>   WHO/LAR Response Criteria for
>   Rheumatoid Arthritis
>   WHO/LAR Response Criteria for
>   Rheumatoid Arthritis growth plate
>   widening

whole
>   w. bone fresh-frozen allograft
>   w. bone transplant
>   w. fibular transplant
>   w. fresh-frozen calcaneal allograft

whole-body vibration
whorled pattern
WHYMPI
>   Westhaven Yale Multidimensional Pain
>   Inventory

Wiberg
>   angle of W.
>   center-edge angle of W.
>   W. center-edge angle
>   W. fracture angle
>   W. fracture staple
>   W. fracture stapler
>   W. patellar classification
>   W. periosteal elevator
>   W. type II patellar contour

Wichman retractor
wick
>   w. catheter technique
>   w. technique

wicking catheter
wide
>   w. excision
>   w. periosteal elevator
>   w. toe box
>   w. toebox shoe

wide-based gait

wide-mesh petroleum gauze dressing
widening
>   ankle mortise w.
>   interpedicular distance widening
>   joint w.
>   tibial tunnel w.
>   WHO/LAR Response Criteria for
>   Rheumatoid Arthritis growth
>   plate w.

width
>   step w.

Wiet
>   W. cup forceps
>   W. graft-measuring instrument

Wikco ankle machine
Wilco ankle exerciser
Wilde
>   W. ethmoid forceps
>   W. intervertebral disc rongeur
>   W. rongeur forceps

Wiley-Galey classification
Wilke
>   W. boot
>   W. boot brace

Wilkie syndrome
Wilkinson synovectomy
William
>   W. Harris hip prosthesis
>   W. microlumbar disc excision

Williams
>   W. Advantage table
>   W. brace
>   W. discectomy
>   W. discography
>   W. exercise program
>   W. flexion back exercise technique
>   W. flexion exercise (WFE)
>   W. interlocking Y-nail
>   W. Model 170 table
>   W. nail
>   W. orthosis
>   W. procedure
>   W. rod
>   W. screwdriver
>   W. self-retaining retractor

Williams-Haddad technique
Williger
>   W. bone curette
>   W. bone mallet
>   W. periosteal elevator

willow fracture
Wilmington
>   W. arthroscopic portal
>   W. plastic jacket
>   W. scoliosis brace

Wilson
>   W. ankle fusion
>   W. approach
>   W. bolt

W. bone graft
W. bunionectomy
W. cone arthrodesis
W. convex frame
W. disease
W. double oblique osteotomy
W. fracture
W. gonad retractor
W. muscle
W. oblique displacement osteotomy
W. plate
W. procedure
W. procedure for extraarticular
  fusion of elbow
W. sign
W. splint
W. technique
W. test
Wilson-Burstein hip internal prosthesis
Wilson-Cook prosthesis repositioner
Wilson-Jacobs
W.-J. tibial fixation
W.-J. tibial fracture fixation
  technique
Wiltberger anterior cervical approach
Wiltse
W. ankle osteotomy
W. approach
W. bilateral lateral fusion
W. discectomy
W. fixator
W. osteotomy of ankle
W. pedicle screw
W. pedicle screw fixation system
W. screw-rod
W. system aluminum master rod
W. system cross-bracing
W. system double-rod construct
W. system H construct
W. system single-rod construct
W. system spinal rod
W. varus supramalleolar osteotomy
Wiltze angle
Wimberger sign
Winco
W. adjusting bench
W. Folding Treatment Table
windblown
w. deformity
w. hand, whistling face syndrome
w. hip
w. knee

wind-cold
wind-heat
windlass
W. mechanism
reverse w.
window
cast w.
cortical w.
femoral cortical w.
windowed cast
windowing
cortical w.
windshield
w. wiper effect
w. wiper sign
Windson-Insall-Vince grafting technique
windswept
w. deformity
w. hip
wind-up
w.-u. injury
w.-u. phenomenon
wing
angel w.
Badgley resection of iliac w.
dorsal w.
w. excision of Littler
iliac w.
w. of ilium
keel and w.
w. plate
w. of sphenoid
Wingate aerobic test
winging
w. motion
w. of scapula
scapular w.
wink
anal w.
W. retractor
w. sign
Winkelmann rotationplasty
winking
Gunn jaw w.
w. owl sign
Winograd
W. ingrown nail technique
W. nail plate removal
W. partial matricectomy
W. technique for ingrown nail
**Winquist femoral shaft fracture
classification**

W

NOTES

Winquist-Hansen
 W.-H. classification of femoral
  fracture
 W.-H. femoral fracture classification
 W.-H. fracture comminution
  classification
winter
 W. convex fusion
 W. splint
 W. spondylolisthesis
 W. spondylolisthesis technique
winterize body
Winter-King-Moe scoliosis
wipe test
wire
 Babcock stainless steel w.
 band w.
 bayonet-point w.
 beaded transfixion w.
 bead-loaded w.
 w. bending pliers
 bind w.
 bone suturing wire chisel-tip w.
 Brooker w.
 Bunnell pullout w.
 calibrated guide w.
 cerclage w.
 chisel-tip w.
 circular w.
 circumferential w.
 Compere fixation w.
 compression w.
 conical-point w.
 w. contour preparation
 w. crimper
 crossed Kirschner w.
 w. cutter
 Dall-Miles cerclage w.
 definitive cerclage w.
 diamond-point wire double-
  strand w.
 diamond tip w.
 double-looped cerclage w.
 double-stranded wire double-
  twisted w.
 w. drill
 w. and drill guide
 w. driver
 Drummond w.
 encircling w.
 figure-of-8 w.
 w. fixation bolt
 w. frame collar
 w. grip finger splint
 w. grip toe splint
 Ilizarov w.
 interfragmentary w.
 intraosseous w.

90-90 intraosseous wire Nitinol
 flexible w.
Isola w.
Kirschner w. (K-wire)
w. knot
Lengemann w.
w. loop
loop circumferential w.
w. loop fixation
Luque cerclage w.
Magnuson w.
Martin loop circumferential w.
monofilament w.
nonthreaded w.
oblique w.
olive w.
Oppenheimer spring w.
Outrigger w.
over-tying w.
w. passage
w. passer
w. penetration depth
w. prosthesis-crimping forceps
w. removal technique
RotaWire guide w.
Schauwecker patellar tension
 band w.
sharp-pointed w.
small-diameter w.
smooth transfixion w.
spinous process w.
w. stabilization
stainless steel w.
stay w.
sublaminar w.
w. suture
temporary cerclage w.
tension band w.
Thiersch w.
threaded w.
w. tightener
w. traction bow
trochanteric w.
4-w. trochanter reattachment
w. twister
unthreaded w.
Wisconsin button w.
Wisconsin interspinous w.
Wisconsin spinous w.
wire-cutting
 w.-c. forceps
 w.-c. scissors
wire-extracting forceps
wire-fixation buckle
Wire-Foam Orthotic
wire-holding forceps
wire-pulling forceps

wire-tightening
    w.-t. clamp
    w.-t. forceps
wire-twisting forceps
wiring
    cervical oblique facet w.
    circumferential w.
    compression w.
    facet fracture stabilization w.
    facet subluxation stabilization w.
    figure-of-8 w.
    interfacet w.
    interspinous w.
    intraosseous w.
    Luque w.
    oblique facet w.
    posterior interspinous w.
    Schauwecker patellar w.
    spinous process w.
    sublaminar w.
    tension-band w.
    Wisconsin w.
Wisconsin
    W. button
    W. button wire
    W. interspinous segmental spinal instrumentation
    W. interspinous wire
    W. spinal fracture system
    W. spinous wire
    W. wire fixation
    W. wiring
Wissinger rod
Wister wire/pin cutter
within functional limits (WFL)
Wit portable TENS system
Wixson hip positioner
WMR
    wedge matrix resection
wobble
    w. board
    Wooden W.
Wohlfart-Kugelberg-Welander disease
wolf
    W. arthroscope
    W. blade plate ankle arthrodesis
    W. full-thickness free graft
    W. light source
    W. motor function test
Wolfe-Böhler cast breaker
Wolfe hand surgery graft
Wolferman drill

Wolff
    W. law
    W. law of bone structure
Wolfson frame
Wolin meniscoid lesion
Wolvek sternal approximation fixation
Wonder-Cup heel cup
Wonderflex silicone
Wonder-Spur heel cup
Wonderzorb
    Soft Silicones W.
wood
    w. probe reflexology device
    w. screw
wooden
    w. postoperative clogs
    w. shoe
    W. Wobble
wooden-soled shoe
woodpecker system
Woodruff
    W. screw
    W. screwdriver
    W. tip
Woodson
    W. elevator
    W. probe
Woodward
    W. arthroplasty
    W. operation wound
    W. procedure
    W. technique
Woodway treadmill
Woofry-Chandler
    W.-C. classification
    W.-C. classification of Osgood-Schlatter lesion
wool
    lamb's w.
WORC
    Western Ontario Rotator Cuff
Woringer-Kolopp disease
work
    concentric w.
    w. conditioning
    eccentric w.
    W. Environment Impact Scale (WEIS)
    w. evaluation systems technology
    w. hardening
    w. hardening exercise
    w. hardening program
    manual w.

W

NOTES

work *(continued)*
  negative w.
  physical w.
  rhythmic handgrip w.
  W. Seat driving simulator
  sedentary w.
WorkAbout Carpal Mate wrist support
Worker Role Interview (WRI)
workgroup
  National Arthritis Data W.
working
  w. orthopaedic surgery film
  w. zone
WorkMod back support
work-of-fracture
**World Health Organization/International
  League Against Rheumatism
  (WHO/LAR)**
worm drive
wormian bone
Worth disease
WOSI
  Western Ontario Instability Index
wound
  chronic heel w.
  w. cleanser
  closed w.
  w. closure
  w. closure system
  w. culture
  w. dehiscence
  w. dressing
  foot puncture w.
  w. gel
  gunshot w.
  Gustilo classification of
    puncture w.
  incised w.
  w. irrigation
  joint w.
  w. measuring guide
  open w.
  w. packing
  puncture w.
  stab w.
  traumatic heel w.
  W. VAC
  Woodward operation w.
Wound-Evac drain
woven
  w. bone
  w. gastrocnemius aponeurosis
WPB
  whirlpool bath
W-plasty
wrap
  Ace w.
  Action elbow w.
  Action wrist w.

ankleRAP postsurgical wound w.
backRAP postsurgical wound w.
BodyIce cold pack w.
boot w.
Champ CTS cold therapy w.
Circulon w.
Coban elastic w.
Co-Flex adherent w.
Coopercare Lastrap support w.
digit w.
DK 201 cryotherapy w.
Dura-Kold reusable compression
  ice w.
Dura-Soft soft-compression reusable
  ice or heat w.
Elasto-Gel hot/cold w.
Elasto-Gel shoulder therapy w.
Elasto-Link joint w.
Electro-Link joint w.
FoamWrap Final Flexion w.
gauze w.
gel w.
Gelocast Unna boot
  compression w.
Goode w.
Heat Plus Massage lower body w.
hipRAP postsurgical wound w.
Ice Wedge hot/cold therapy w.
joint w.
Kerlix w.
kneeRAP w.
Kold W.
loop-over w.
neck w.
Nylatex w.
orthoRaps postsurgical wound w.
PneuGel ankle w.
PneuGel shoulder w.
Scott wrist w.
shoulderRAP postsurgical wound w.
Snugs w.
Sorbothane w.
Stimprene w.
super w.
Thermoskin arthritic knee w.
Thermoskin U wrist w.
Thermosport hot/cold w.
Unna boot w.
Velpeau w.
wristRAP postsurgical wound w.
wraparound
  w. flap bone graft
  w. neurovascular composite free
    tissue transfer
  w. neurovascular free flap
  w. splint
  w. toe transfer
wrapping
  compressive centripetal w.

nerve w.
stump w.

wrench
Allen w.
beaded-pin w.
box-end w.
cannulated w.
conical nut w.
Fox w.
Harrington flat w.
hex w.
Key-loc w.
locknut w.
Mueller w.
open-end w.
w. pin
socket w.
T-handled nut w.
T-handled screw w.
Thomas w.
torque w.
TSRH w.
U w.
VDS w.
ventral derotating spinal w.

wrenched knee
wrestler's elbow
WRI
Worker Role Interview
Wright
W. knee prosthesis
W. maneuver
W. Medical bone anchor
W. monoblock titanium implant
W. plate
W. test
W. titanium prosthesis
W. Universal brace
Wright-Adson test
Wrightlock
W. posterior fixation system
W. spinal fixation system
wringer
w. arm
w. injury
wrinkle test
Wrisberg
W. lesion
ligament of W.
wrist
w. arthroscopy
w. bone

w. brace
w. capsule
w. contracture
w. creaking
w. curl
w. deformity
w. disarticulation (WD)
dorsal arch of w.
w. drop
w. extension
w. extensor
w. extensor strengthening
w. extensor stretch
w. extensor tendinitis
w. extensor tendon
w. and finger flexor stretch
w. first
w. flexion reflex
w. flexion test
w. flexion unit
w. flexor strengthening
w. flexor tendinitis
w. gauntlet
golfer's w.
gymnast's w.
w. hand extension compression support (WHECS)
w. immobilizer
w. instability
w. joint implant prosthesis
w. motion
w. motion splint
oarsman's w.
w. pain syndrome
palmar w.
W. Pro wrist support
W. Pro wrist support device
W. Resist splint
w. rest splint
slack w.
w. spasticity
w. speed profile
w. stretch exercise
w. subluxation
sulcus of w.
tilt w.
total arthrodesis of w.
triangular disc of w.
volar w.
Volz w.
wrist-driven
w.-d. flexor hinge orthosis

NOTES

W

wrist-driven *(continued)*
    w.-d. lateral prehension orthosis
    w.-d. wrist-hand orthosis
wrist-hand orthosis (WHO)
Wristiciser exerciser
WrisTimer
    W. carpal tunnel support system
    W. CTS support
    W. PM carpal tunnel support
WristJack wrist splint
wristlet
    elastic w.
    Freedom USA w.
wristRAP postsurgical wound wrap
writer
    w. paralysis
    Wanchik w.

writing
    Children's Handwriting Evaluation Scale for Manuscript W. (CHES-M)
    w. hand
wry neck, wryneck
Wu
    Wu bunionectomy
    Wu sole opposition test
Wurzburg
    W. plate
    W. screw
WUSPI
    Wheelchair User's Shoulder Pain Index
Wylie lumbar bulldog clamp

X

X clamp
X plate
X-10 Crosslink plate
Xact ACL graft-fixation system
X-Act podiatric marker
xanthogranuloma
juvenile x.
xanthoma
Achilles tendon x.
fibrous x.
malignant fibrous x.
tuberous x.
xanthomatous giant cell tumor
Xenophor femoral prosthesis
Xercise
X. band
X. Band exercise device
X. tube resistive device
Xeroform gauze dressing
xerography
xeroradiography
xerotic
Xertube
Xia
X. hook/spinal system
X. hook system
X. spinal system
XIP
x-ray in plaster
xiphisternal joint
xiphoid
x. bone
x. process
XiScan
X. fluoroscope
X. fluoroscopy
X. mini-C-arm
X-long cement forceps
XLS
Polysorb meniscal stapler XLS
Xomed drill

XOP
x-ray out of plaster
XO-soft-sole orthotic
XPE foot orthosis
x-ray
artifact on x-r.
Cedell-Magnusson classification of arthritis on x-r.
dorsal planar x-r.
dorsiflexion stress ankle x-r.
dynamic motion x-r.
FCS x-r.
Harris-Beath axial hindfoot x-r.
hip-to-ankle x-r.
intraoperative x-r.
lateral tilt stress ankle x-r.
nonweightbearing x-r.
x-r. out of plaster (XOP)
x-r. overlay
penciling of ribs on x-r.
x-r. photogrammetry
plantar stress ankle x-r.
x-r. in plaster (XIP)
x-r. position
postreduction x-r.
sagittal stress x-r.
stress x-r.
x-r. tray
x-r. view
weightbearing x-r.
Xsensibles shoe
X-shaped plate
X-Static silver fiber shoe lining fiber
XTB knee extension device
Xtra Depth shoe
X-Y
X-Y plotter
X-Y sensor system
XY
frontal plane XY
X, Y, Z axis

X

Y

Y bone plate
Y fracture
Y incision
Y line
Y osteotomy
Y scapular view

Yale brace
Yamanda myelotomy knife
Yancey osteotomy
Yancy cast wedge
Yankauer periosteal elevator
Yasargil

Y. elevator
Y. Leyla retractor arm
Y. ligature carrier
Y. ligature guide
Y. micro rasp
Y. needle holder
Y. spring hook

Y-axis translatory displacement
Yeager test
year

disability adjusted life y. (DALY)

Yee posterior shoulder approach
yellow

y. cartilage
y. ligament
y. marrow
y. nail syndrome

Yeoman test
Yergason

Y. shoulder subluxation test
Y. sign
Y. test of shoulder subluxation

yield strength
Y-knot tying system
Y-nail

Williams interlocking Y-n.

Yochum chiropractic software
yoga
yoked muscle
Yoke transposition procedure
Y-osteotomy
young

Y. hinged knee prosthesis
Y. medial approach
Y. modulus
Y. pelvic fracture classification
Y. procedure

Youngswick

Y. osteotomy
Y. procedure

Youngswick-Austin metatarsal head procedure
Yount

Y. fasciotomy
Y. procedure

Y-shaped

Y-s. incision
Y-s. plate

Y-strap knee immobilizer
Y-T fracture
Yuan screw
yucca wood splint
Yu osteotomy
Y-V

Y-V plasty
Y-V plasty incision

Y

Z

Z band
Z bunionectomy
Z disc
Z fixation nail
Z foot
Z foot deformity
Z line
Z pin
Z retractor
Z score

ZAAG

Zest Anchor Advanced Generation
ZAAG Bone Anchoring System

Zachary sensory grade

Zadik

Z. foot operation
Z. foot procedure
Z. total matricectomy
Z. total nail bed ablation

Zahn

line of Z.

Zaias nail biopsy

Zanca view

Zancolli

Z. biceps tendon rerouting
Z. capsuloplasty
Z. clawhand deformity procedure
Z. flexion capsulodesis
Z. lasso procedure
Z. procedure for clawhand
deformity
Z. reconstruction
Z. rerouting technique
Z. static lock procedure

Zang

Z. metatarsal cap
Z. metatarsal cap implant

Zarins-Rowe

Z.-R. ligament technique
Z.-R. procedure

Zeasorb-AF Powder

zebra body myopathy

Zeichner implant

Zeier transfer technique

Zelicof orthopaedic awl

zenith

Z. ACS table
Z. chiropractic table
Z. Electrotherapy ultrasound system
Z. Hylos table
Z. stationary table
Z. Thompson table
Z. Verti-Lift table

Zenith-Cox flexion/distraction table

Zenker

Z. degeneration
Z. necrosis

Zephir anterior cervical plate system

zest

Z. Anchor Advanced Generation
(ZAAG)
Z. Anchor Advanced Generation
Bone Anchoring System

Zickel

Z. classification
Z. fracture
Z. fracture classification system
Z. medullary apparatus
Z. nail fixation
Z. nailing
Z. rod
Z. subcondylar nail
Z. subtrochanteric fracture fixation
Z. subtrochanteric fracture operation
Z. subtrochanteric nail
Z. supracondylar device
Z. supracondylar fixation apparatus
Z. supracondylar medullary nail

zidovudine-induced myopathy

Ziehen-Oppenheim disease

Zielke

Z. bifid hook
Z. derotator bar
Z. distraction device
Z. gouge
Z. instrumentation for scoliosis
spinal fusion
Z. pedicular instrumentation
Z. rod
Z. technique

zigzag

z. approach
z. compensatory deformity
z. finger incision

Zimaloy

Z. femoral head prosthesis
Z. implant metal
Z. implant metal prosthesis
Z. staple

Zimfoam

Z. head halter
Z. pad
Z. pin
Z. splint
Z. splint traction

Zimmer

Z. airplane splint
Z. anatomic hip system
Z. antiembolism stockings

Z

Zimmer *(continued)*
Z. bone cement
Z. bone stem
Z. cartilage clamp
Z. Cebotome bone cement drill
Z. Centralign Precoat hip prosthesis
Z. chuck
Z. Cibatome cement eater
Z. clavicular cross splint
Z. collarless polished taper hip system
Z. compression hip screw
Z. continuous anatomical passive exerciser
Z. CPT 12/14 hip system
Z. crossover instrumentation system
Z. dermatome
Z. electrical stimulation apparatus
Z. electrical stimulation device
Z. extractor
Z. femoral canal broach
Z. femoral condyle blade-plate
Z. fracture frame
Z. goniometer
Z. gouge
Z. hand drill
Z. head halter
Z. hip implant system
Z. hip prosthesis
Z. impaction screw-plate
Z. knee immobilizer
Z. laminectomy frame
Z. low-viscosity adhesive
Z. low-viscosity cement
Z. microsaw
Z. NexGen LPS knee femoral component
Z. Orthair ream driver
Z. orthopaedic device
Z. oscillating saw
Z. Osteo Stim bone growth stimulator
Z. pin
Z. PMMA precoat process
Z. postoperative shoe
Z. protractor
Z. Pulsavac wound débridement system
Z. reamer brace
Z. rotary bur
Z. screwdriver
Z. shoulder prosthesis
Z. side plate
Z. skin graft mesher
Z. snare
Z. telescoping nail
Z. THARIES surface arthroplasty system
Z. tibial bolt

Z. tibial nail cap
Z. tibial prosthesis
Z. unicompartmental high-flex knee system
Z. Universal drill
Z. walker
Z. Y plate
Zimmer CPT 12/14 hip system
Zimmer-Gigli saw blade
Zimmer-Hall drive system
Zimmer-Hoen forceps
Zimmer-Hudson shank
Zimmer-Kirschner hand drill
Zimmerlin atrophy
Zimmerman pericyte
Zimmer-Schlesinger forceps
Zimmer-Statak anchor
Zim-Trac
Z.-T. traction splint
Z.-T. traction splint tractor
Zim-Zip rib belt splint
Zinacef Injection
Zinco
Z. Air Cam brace
Z. Airprene brace
Z. ankle orthosis
Z. Cam Walker brace
Z. Castaway D brace
Z. Hi-Top brace
Z. Minerva cervical brace
Z. Multi-Lig knee brace
Z. Pin Cam Walker brace
Z. thumb-wrist immobilizer
zipper
Z. antidisconnect device
z. cast
Zippie
Z. P500 wheelchair
Z. 2 wheelchair
Ziramic femoral head
zirconia
z. femoral head prosthesis
z. orthopaedic prosthesis
z. orthopaedic prosthetic head
zirconium
z. oxide arthroplasty material
z. oxide ceramic prosthesis
oxidized z.
Z-lengthening
Achilles tendon Z-l.
Z-l. of biceps tendon
ZMC
zygomatic-malar complex
ZMC fracture
ZMR hip system
ZMS intramedullary fixation system
Zodiac TM Manual Flexion-Distraction table
Zohar shoe

Zollinger
    Z. legholder
    Z. splint
Zollner rasp
zonal sclerosis
Zonas porous tape
Zone
    Z. Specific II meniscal repair
    Z. Specific II meniscal repair
      system
zone
    autonomous z.
    cornuradicular z.
    cut-back z.
    dorsal root entry z. (DREZ)
    elastic z.
    endplate z.
    fracture z.
    growth z.
    Gruen z.
    hyperintense z.
    hypertrophic z.
    isolated z.
    Kambin triangular working z.
    Lissauer z.
    Looser z.
    maturation z.
    neutral z. (NZ)
    orbicular z.
    paraphysiologic z.
    peripolar z.
    polar z.
    proliferating z.
    z. of Ranvier
    red-red meniscal z.
    red-white meniscal z.
    resting z.
    triangular working z.
    Trümmerfeld z.
    umbau z.
    Weber z.
    working z.
zone-specific cannula
zonography
Zorbacel shock-absorbing material
Zoroc plaster
Z-osteotomy
    inverted scarf Z-o.
Z-plasty
    Z-p. approach
    Broadbent-Woolf 4-limb Z-p.
    Cozen-Brockway Z-p.
    double-opposing Z-p.

    4-flap Z-p.
    frontal plane Z-p.
    Gudas scarf Z-p.
    Z-p. incision
    4-limb Z-p.
    Z-p. local flap graft
    Peet Z-p.
    Z-p. release
    scarf Z-p.
    sliding Z-p.
    Z-p. tenotomy
Z-shaped plate
Z-slide
    Z-s. lengthening
    Z-s. lengthening in hallux limitus
Z-stent prosthesis
Z-step cut
Z-Stim
    Z-S. IF 100, 250 microprocessor
      controlled stimulator
    Z-S. 100 microprocessor controlled
      stimulator
ZTT
    ZTT acetabular cup
    ZTT I, II acetabular cup prosthesis
    ZTT I, II cup
Zuckerkandl dehiscence
Zucker splint
Zuelzer
    Z. awl
    Z. hook
    Z. hook plate
    Z. screw
Zuni
    Z. exercise system
    Z. gym
    Z. harness
Zweymuller
    Z. cementless hip prosthesis
    Z. hip system
Zwipp
    Z. classification
    Z. method
    Z. subtalar joint instability
      measurement
zygapophysial, zygapophyseal
    z. arthrology
    z. articulation
    z. joint
    z. joint injection
zygodactyly
zygomatic bone
zygomatic-malar complex (ZMC)

NOTES

Z

Zymderm collagen implant

Zyranox femoral head

Contents: The Appendices

Appendix 1
Anatomical Illustrations

anatomic planes

frontal (coronal) plane: a vertical plane at right angles to a sagittal plane, dividing the body into anterior and posterior portions, or any plane parallel to the central coronal plane.

longitudinal plane: running lengthwise; in the direction of the long axis of the body or any of its parts.

median (midsagittal) plane: a plane vertical in the anatomic position, through the midline of the body that divides the body into right and left halves.

sagittal plane: plane parallel to the median plane; sagittal planes are vertical planes in the anatomic position.

subcostal plane: a transverse plane passing through the inferior limits of the costal margin, i.e., the tenth costal cartilages; it marks the boundary between the hypochondriac and epigastric regions superiorly and the lateral and umbilical regions inferiorly.

transpyloric plane: a transverse plane midway between the superior margins of the manubrium sterni and the symphysis pubis; the pylorus may be located on this plane in the supine or prone positions, but in the erect (anatomic) position it descends to a lower level.

transverse plane: a plane across the body at right angles to the coronal and sagittal planes; transverse planes are perpendicular to the long axis of the body or limbs, regardless of the position of the body or limb; in the anatomic position, transverse planes are horizontal planes; otherwise the two terms are not synonymous.

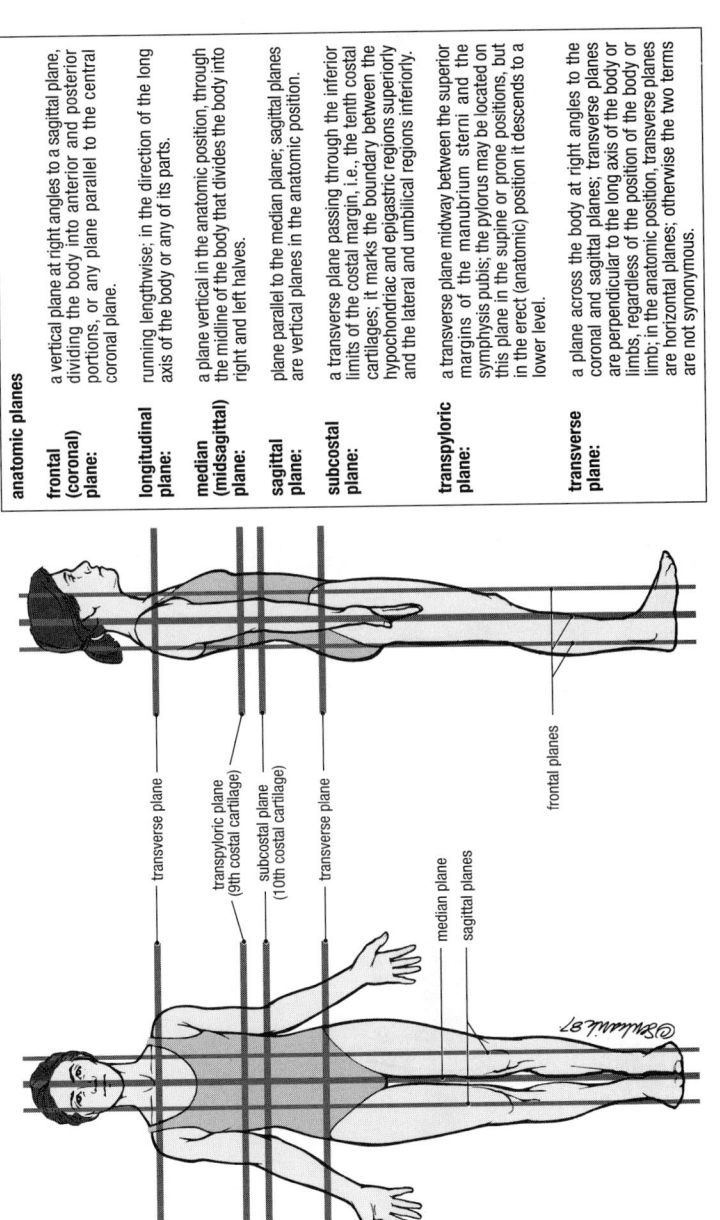

transverse plane

transpyloric plane (9th costal cartilage)

subcostal plane (10th costal cartilage)

transverse plane

median plane

sagittal planes

frontal planes

terms of relationship: anatomic planes

terms of relationship: body part terminology

medial: relating to the middle or center; nearer to the median or midsagittal plane.

lateral: farther from the median or midsagittal plane.

superior: situated nearer the vertex of the head in relation to a specific reference point.

inferior: situated nearer the soles of the feet in relation to a specific reference point.

anterior: the front surface of the body; often used to indicate the position of one structure relative to another, i.e., situated nearer the front part of the body.

posterior: the back surface of the body; often used to indicate the position of one structure relative to another, i.e., nearer the back of the body.

proximal: nearest the trunk or the point of origin, said of part of a limb, of an artery or a nerve, etc., so situated.

distal: situated away from the center of the body, or from the point of origin; specifically applied to the extremity or distant part of a limb or organ.

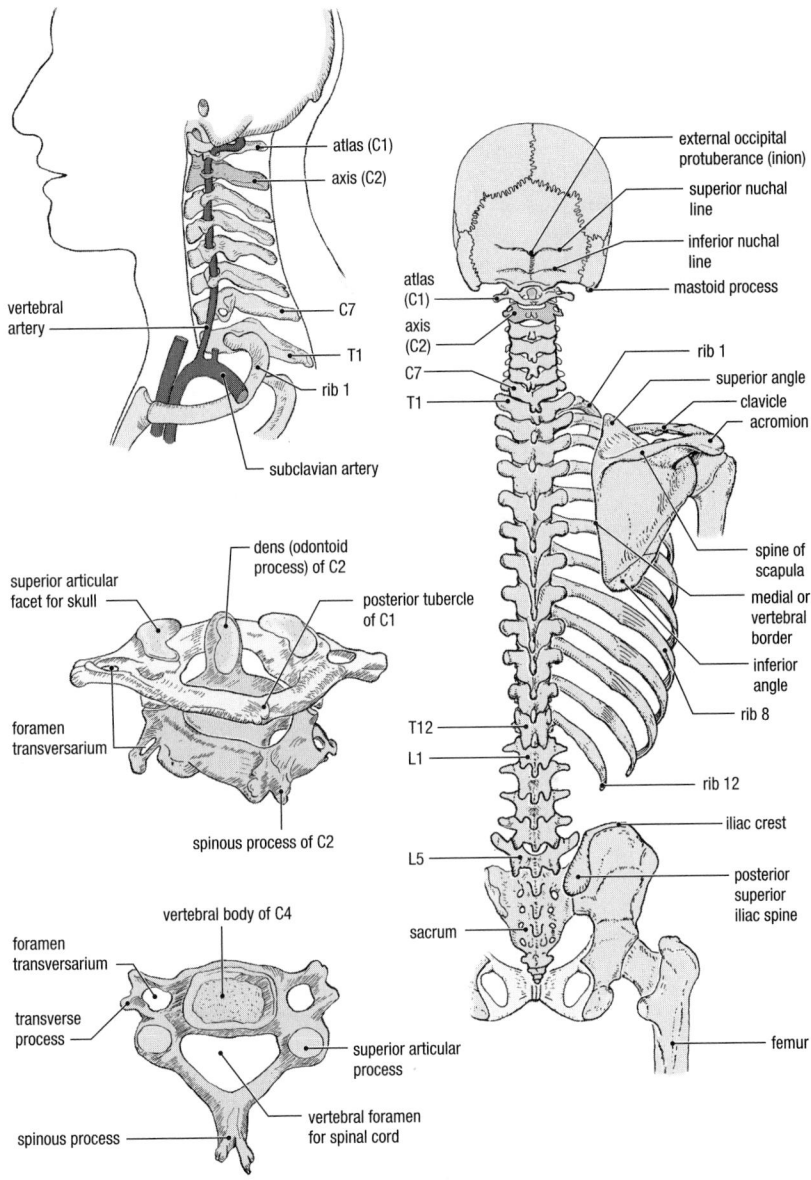

atlas (C1)
axis (C2)
vertebral artery
C7
T1
rib 1
subclavian artery

external occipital protuberance (inion)
superior nuchal line
inferior nuchal line
mastoid process
atlas (C1)
axis (C2)
C7
T1
rib 1
superior angle
clavicle
acromion
spine of scapula
medial or vertebral border
inferior angle
rib 8
T12
L1
rib 12
iliac crest
L5
posterior superior iliac spine
sacrum
femur

dens (odontoid process) of C2
superior articular facet for skull
posterior tubercle of C1
foramen transversarium
spinous process of C2

vertebral body of C4
foramen transversarium
transverse process
superior articular process
spinous process
vertebral foramen for spinal cord

bony landmarks of the back and vertebral column

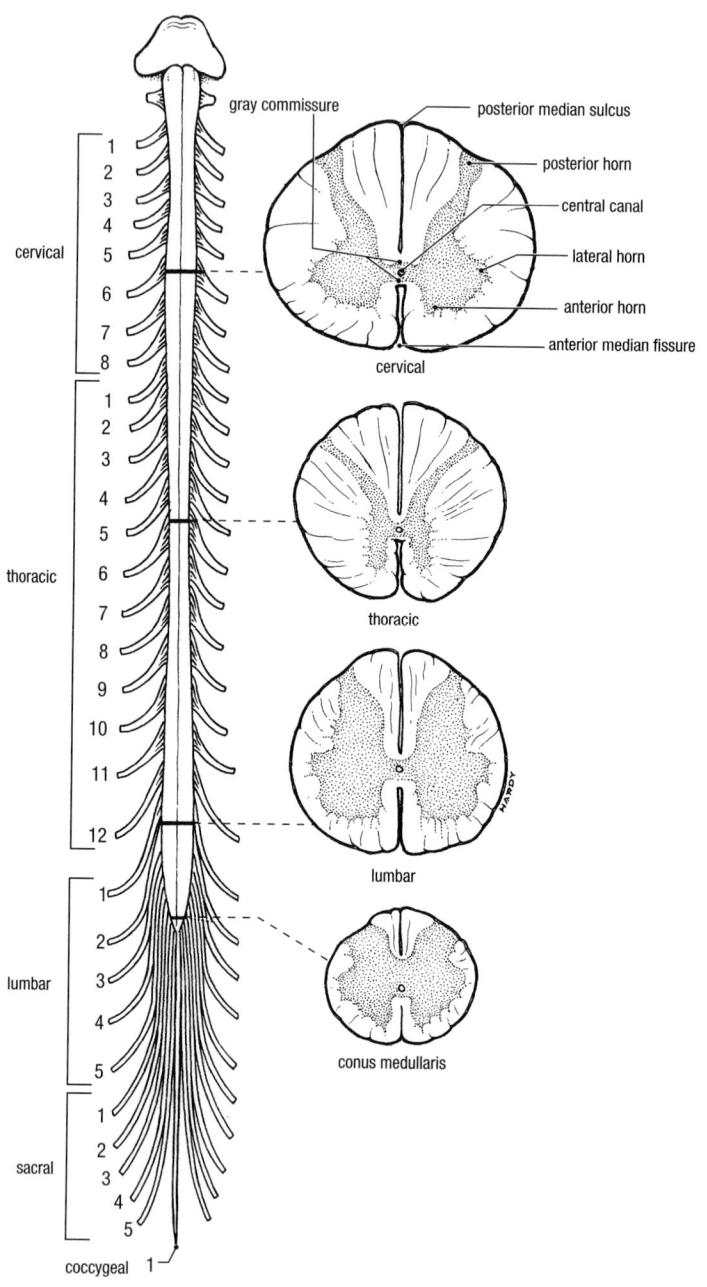

spinal cord showing cross-sections at various levels

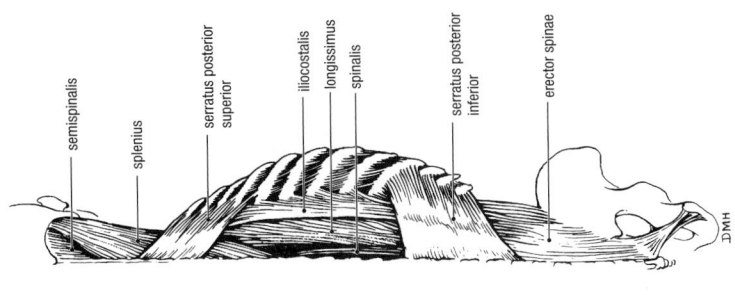

semispinalis

splenius

serratus posterior superior

iliocostalis

longissimus

spinalis

serratus posterior inferior

erector spinae

DMH

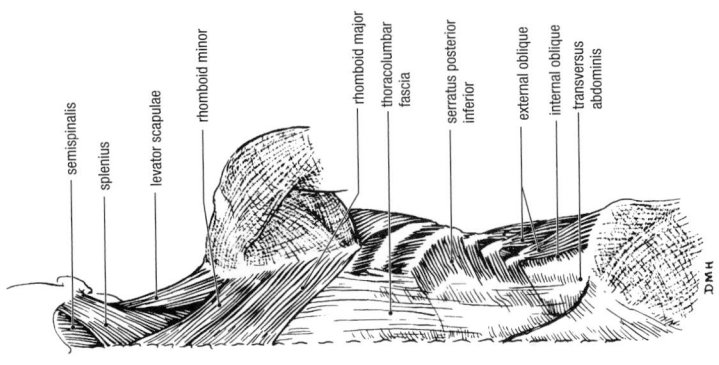

semispinalis

splenius

levator scapulae

rhomboid minor

rhomboid major

thoracolumbar fascia

serratus posterior inferior

external oblique

internal oblique

transversus abdominis

DMH

extrinsic and intrinsic muscles of the back

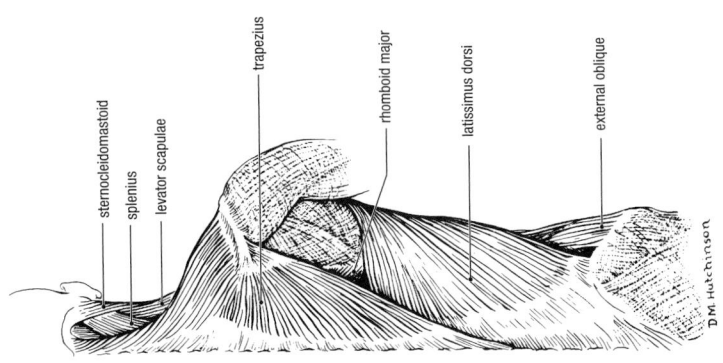

sternocleidomastoid

splenius

levator scapulae

trapezius

rhomboid major

latissimus dorsi

external oblique

DM Hutchinson

A5

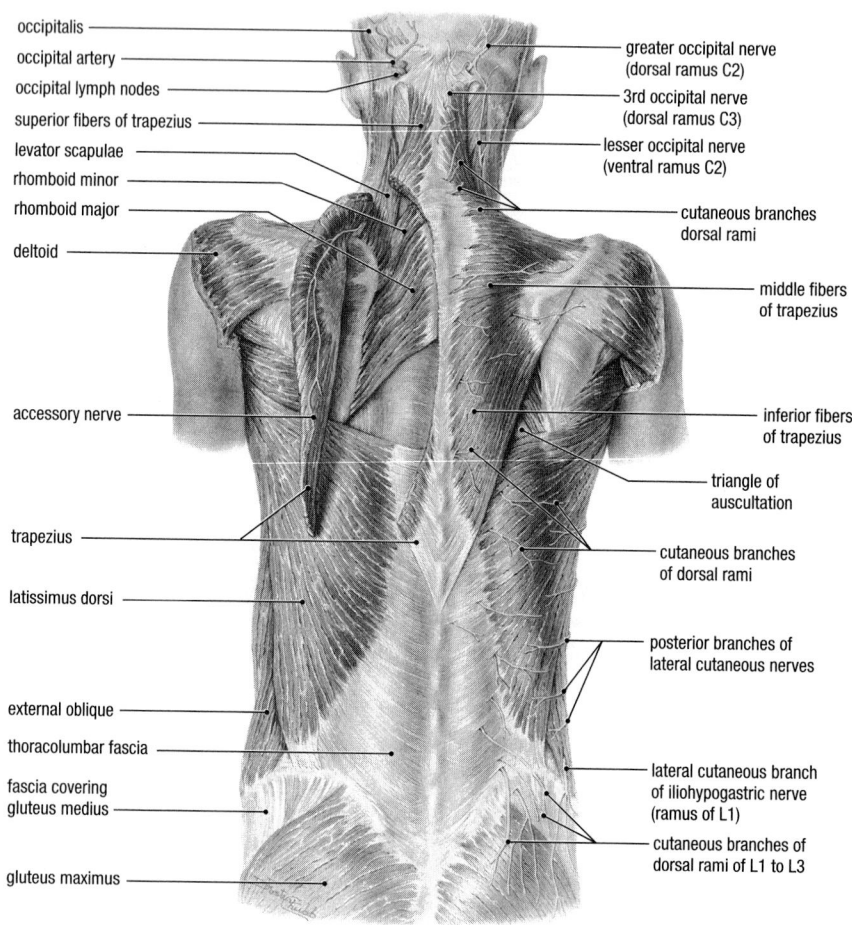

occipitalis

occipital artery

occipital lymph nodes

superior fibers of trapezius

levator scapulae

rhomboid minor

rhomboid major

deltoid

accessory nerve

trapezius

latissimus dorsi

external oblique

thoracolumbar fascia

fascia covering
gluteus medius

gluteus maximus

greater occipital nerve
(dorsal ramus C2)

3rd occipital nerve
(dorsal ramus C3)

lesser occipital nerve
(ventral ramus C2)

cutaneous branches
dorsal rami

middle fibers
of trapezius

inferior fibers
of trapezius

triangle of
auscultation

cutaneous branches
of dorsal rami

posterior branches of
lateral cutaneous nerves

lateral cutaneous branch
of iliohypogastric nerve
(ramus of L1)

cutaneous branches of
dorsal rami of L1 to L3

superficial muscles of the back, posterior view

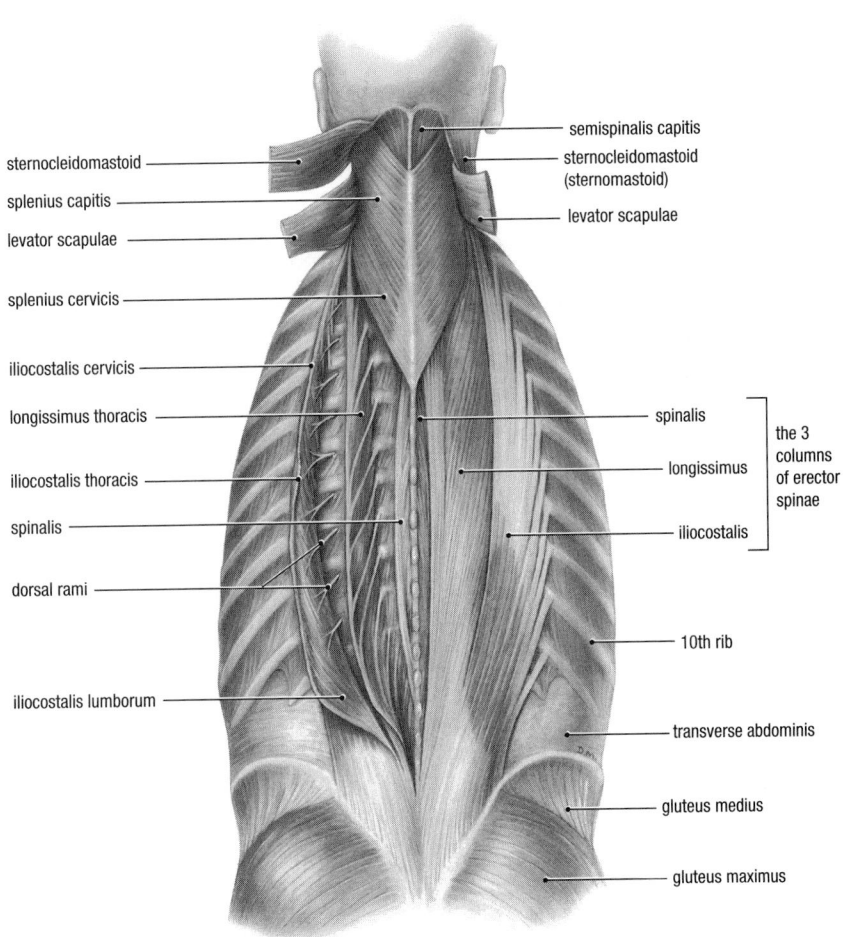

semispinalis capitis

sternocleidomastoid

sternocleidomastoid (sternomastoid)

splenius capitis

levator scapulae

levator scapulae

splenius cervicis

iliocostalis cervicis

longissimus thoracis

spinalis

longissimus

the 3 columns of erector spinae

iliocostalis thoracis

spinalis

iliocostalis

dorsal rami

10th rib

iliocostalis lumborum

transverse abdominis

gluteus medius

gluteus maximus

deep muscles of the back, posterior view

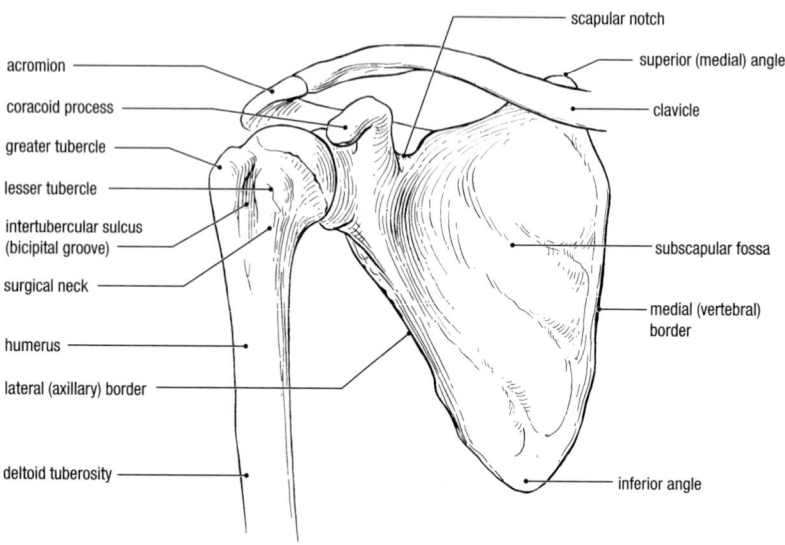

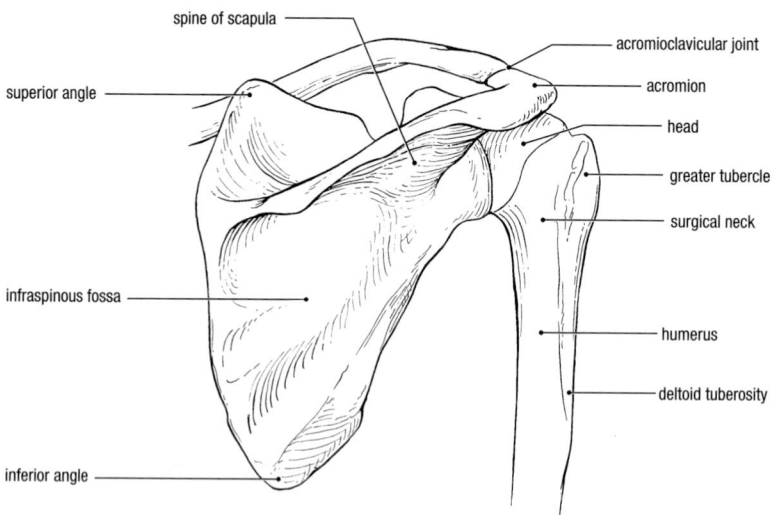

pectoral girdle and humerus: (top) anterior view; (bottom) posterior view

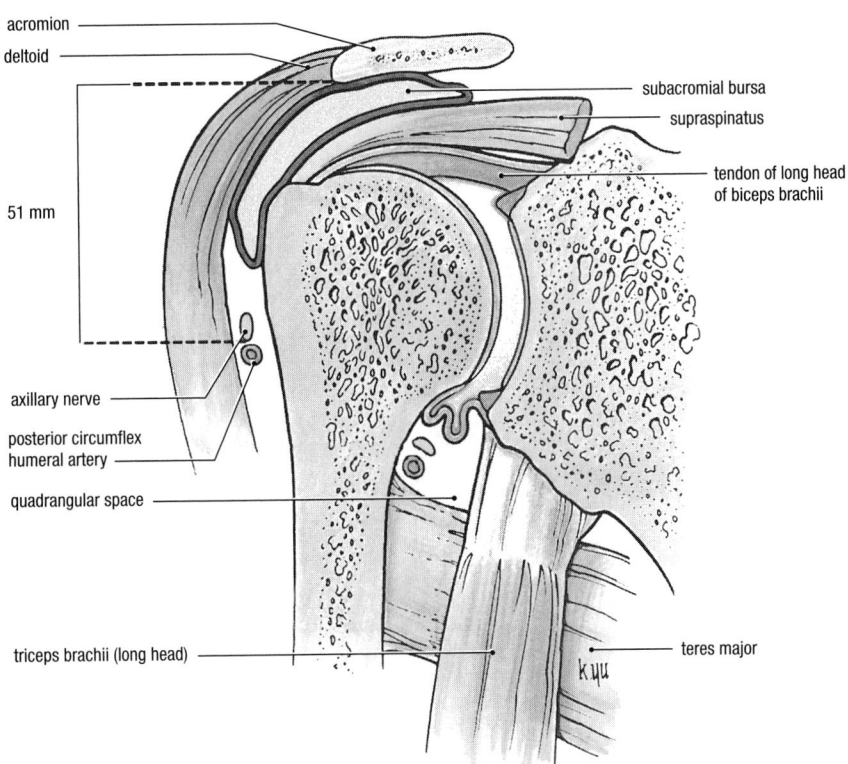

acromion

deltoid

subacromial bursa

supraspinatus

tendon of long head
of biceps brachii

51 mm

axillary nerve

posterior circumflex
humeral artery

quadrangular space

triceps brachii (long head)

teres major

coronal section of the shoulder joint, posterior view

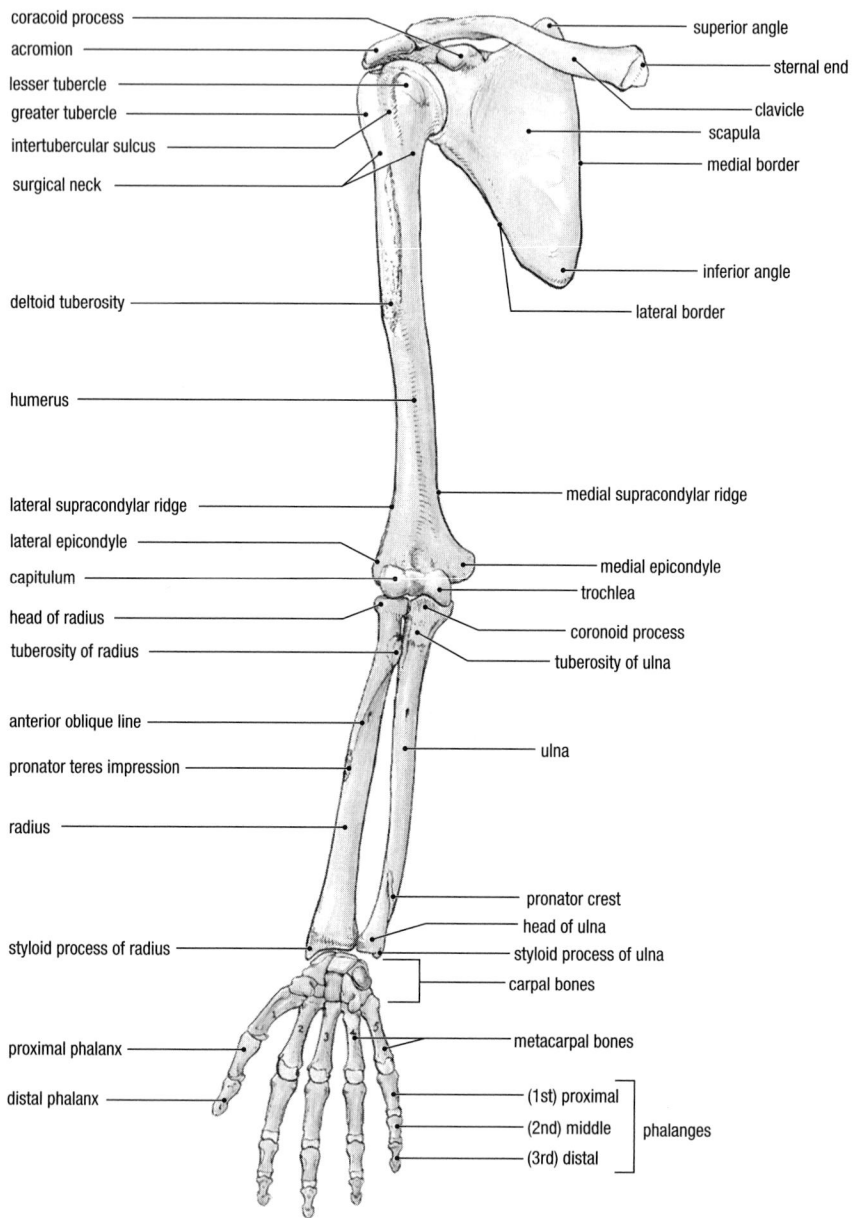

coracoid process — superior angle
acromion — sternal end
lesser tubercle — clavicle
greater tubercle — scapula
intertubercular sulcus — medial border
surgical neck

deltoid tuberosity — inferior angle
— lateral border

humerus

lateral supracondylar ridge — medial supracondylar ridge
lateral epicondyle — medial epicondyle
capitulum — trochlea
head of radius — coronoid process
tuberosity of radius — tuberosity of ulna

anterior oblique line — ulna
pronator teres impression

radius

— pronator crest
— head of ulna
styloid process of radius — styloid process of ulna
— carpal bones

— metacarpal bones
proximal phalanx

distal phalanx — (1st) proximal
— (2nd) middle   phalanges
— (3rd) distal

bones of the upper limb, anterior view

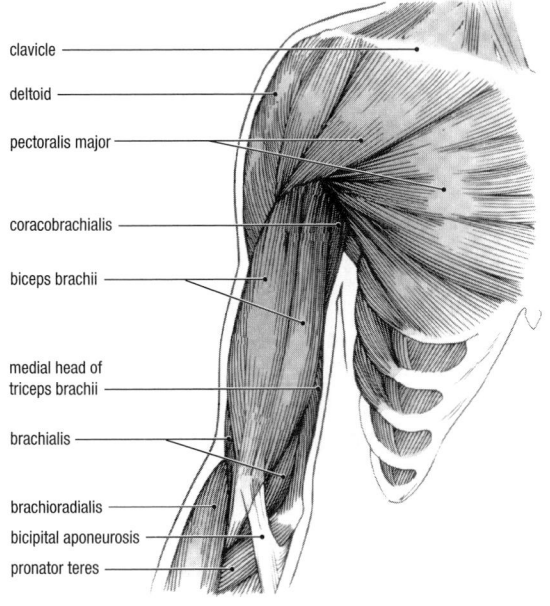

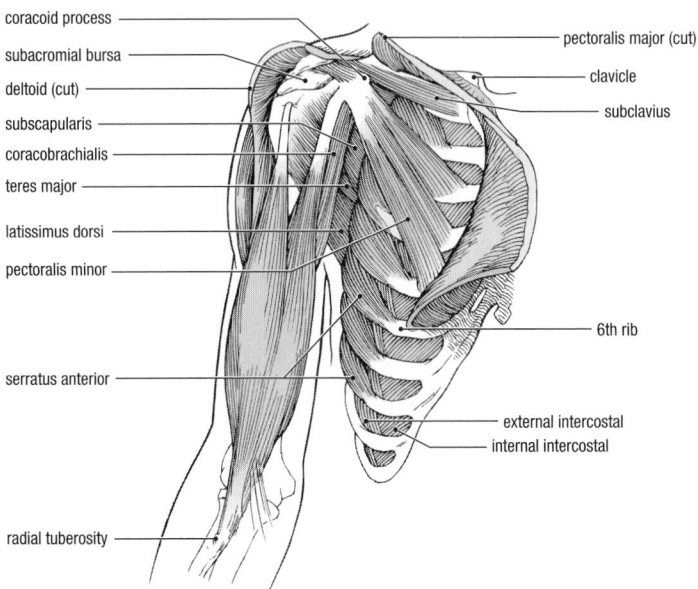

superficial (top) and deep (bottom) muscles of the shoulder and chest

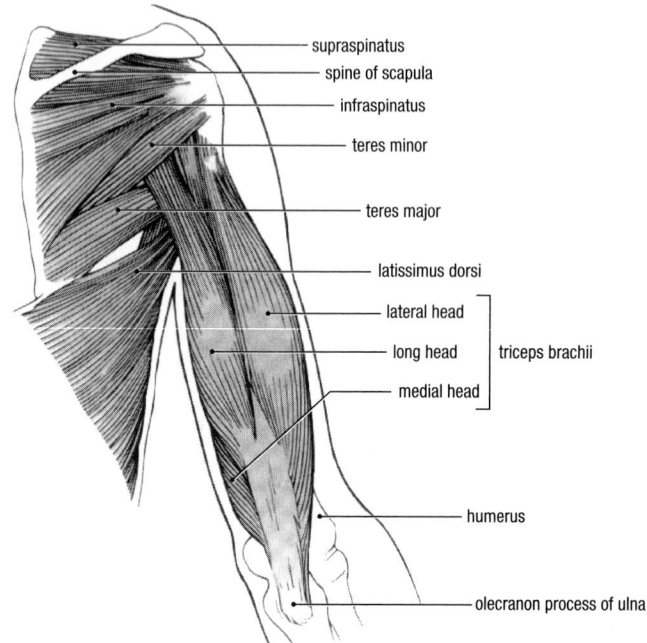

muscles of the arm, posterior view

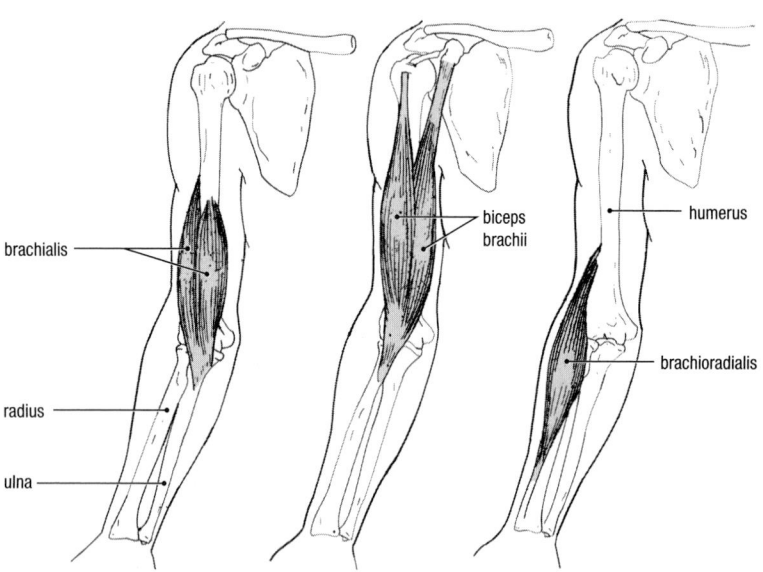

muscles of the arm, anterior view

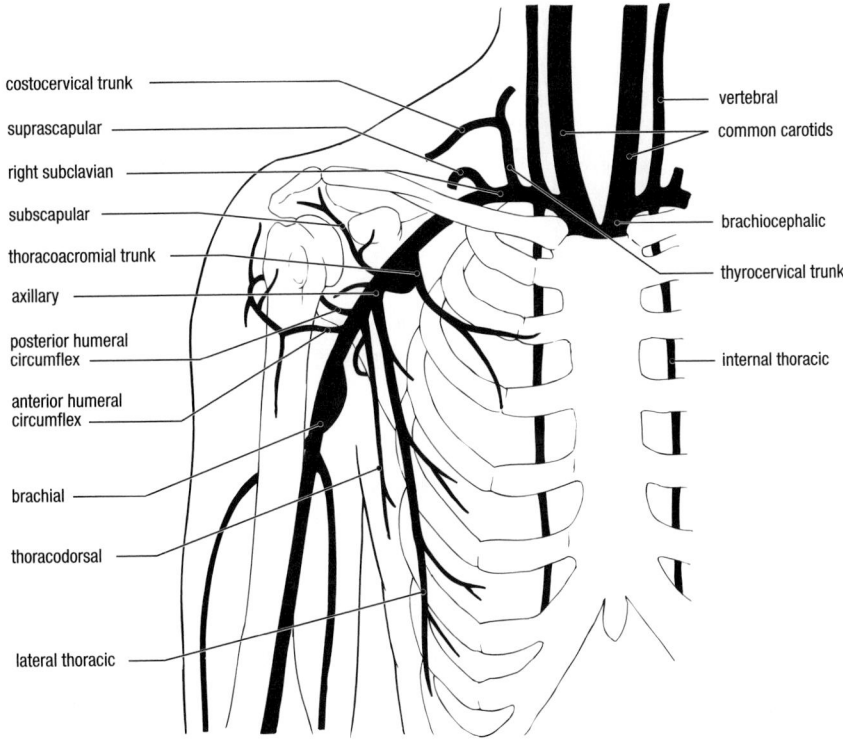

costocervical trunk

suprascapular

right subclavian

subscapular

thoracoacromial trunk

axillary

posterior humeral circumflex

anterior humeral circumflex

brachial

thoracodorsal

lateral thoracic

vertebral

common carotids

brachiocephalic

thyrocervical trunk

internal thoracic

blood supply to the shoulder

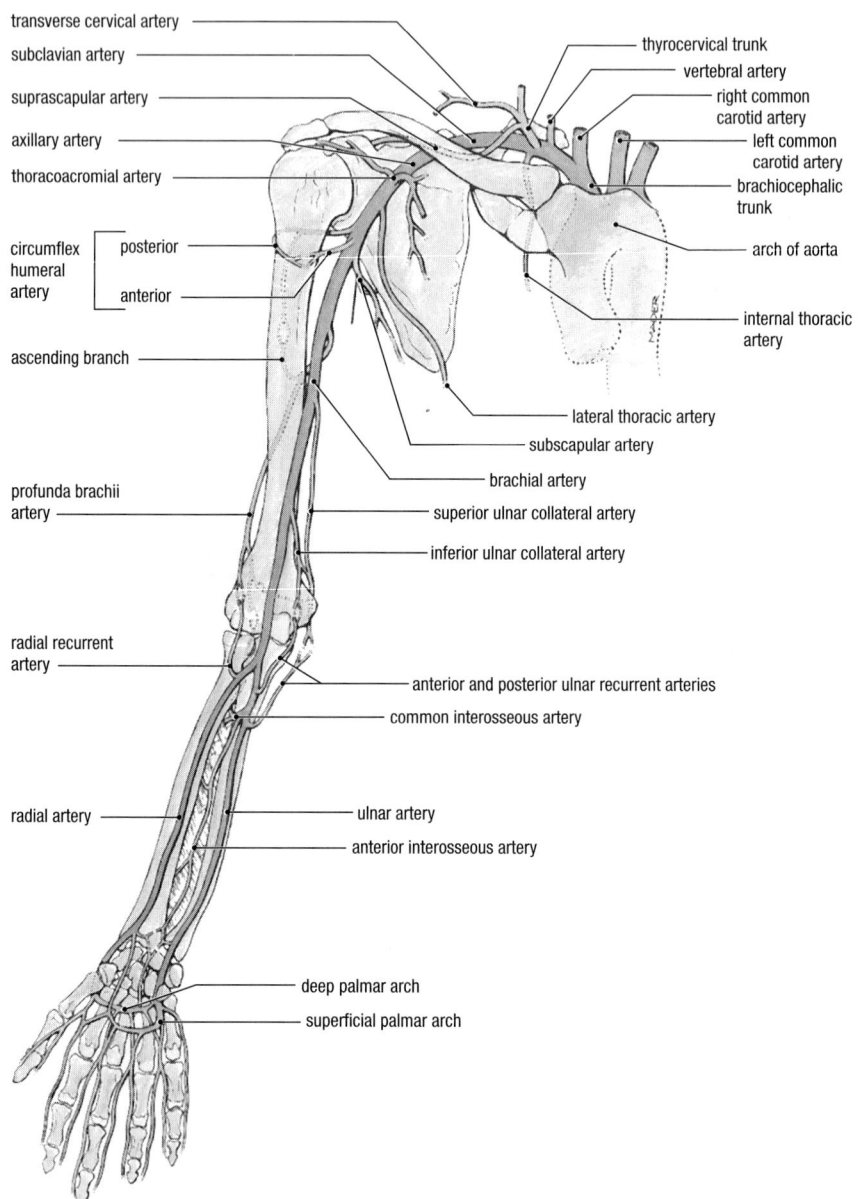

transverse cervical artery

subclavian artery

suprascapular artery

axillary artery

thoracoacromial artery

circumflex humeral artery — posterior

circumflex humeral artery — anterior

ascending branch

profunda brachii artery

radial recurrent artery

radial artery

thyrocervical trunk

vertebral artery

right common carotid artery

left common carotid artery

brachiocephalic trunk

arch of aorta

internal thoracic artery

lateral thoracic artery

subscapular artery

brachial artery

superior ulnar collateral artery

inferior ulnar collateral artery

anterior and posterior ulnar recurrent arteries

common interosseous artery

ulnar artery

anterior interosseous artery

deep palmar arch

superficial palmar arch

arteries of the upper limb, anterior view

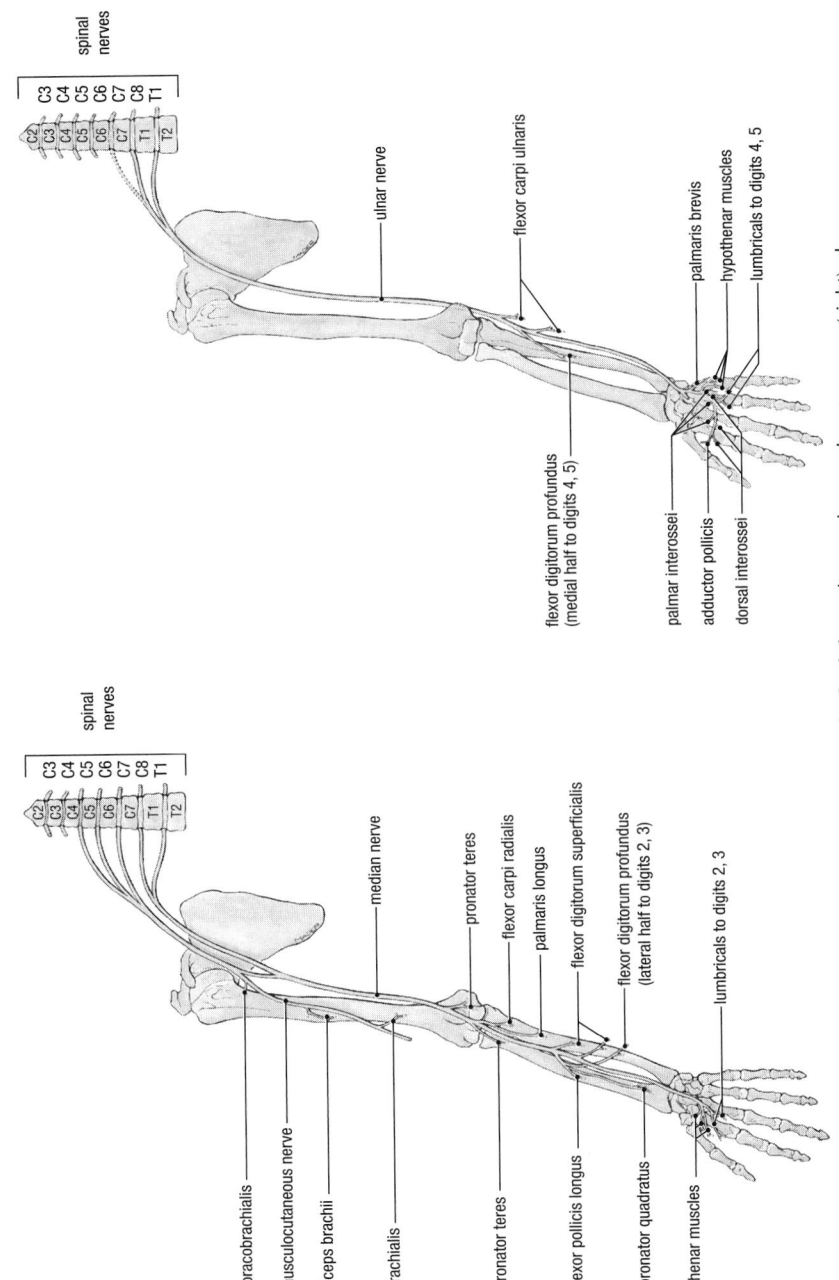

nerves that innervate the muscles of the upper limb: (left) median and musculocutaneous; (right) ulnar nerve

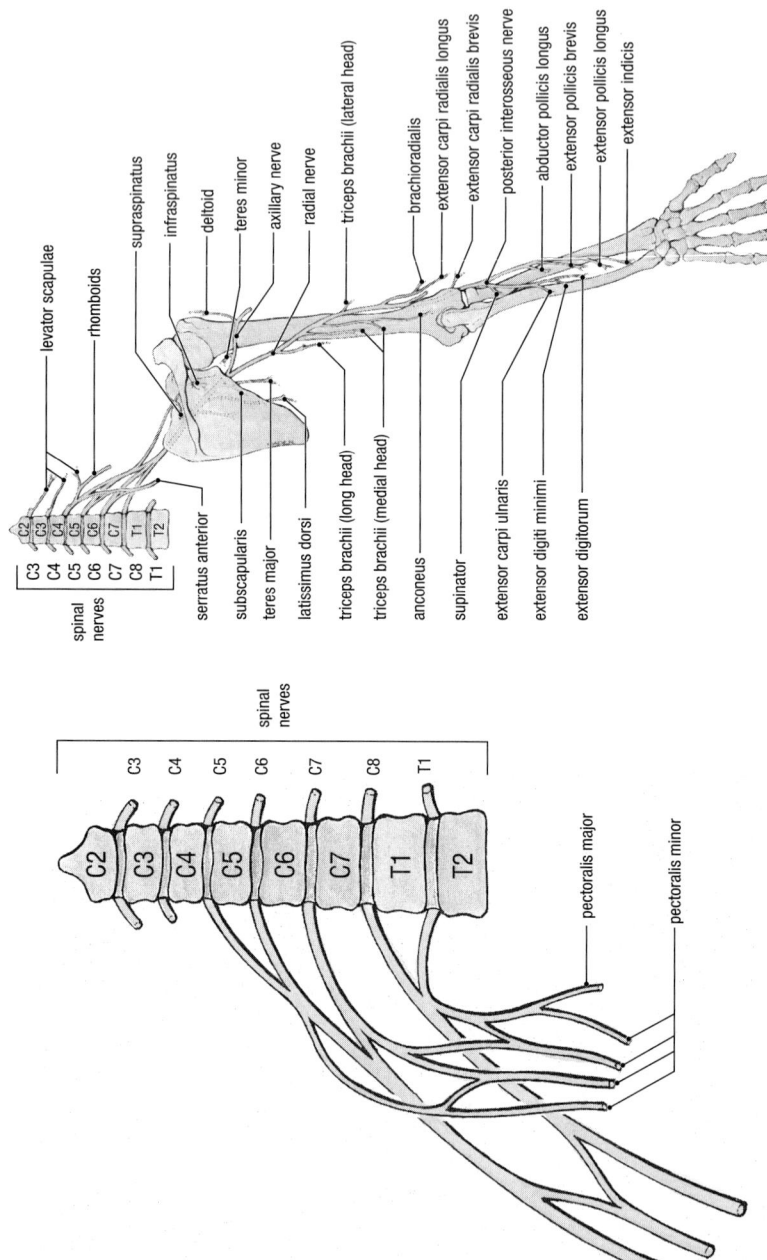

nerves that innervate the muscles of the upper limb: (left) medial and lateral pectoral nerves; (right) radial nerve

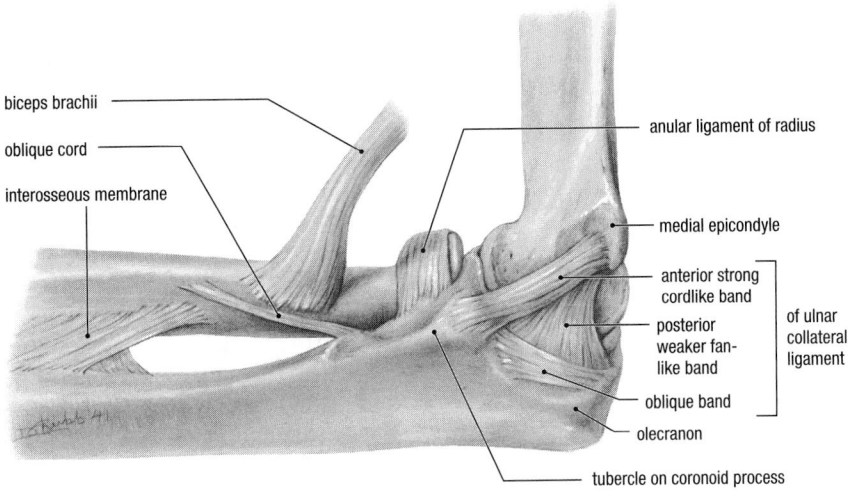

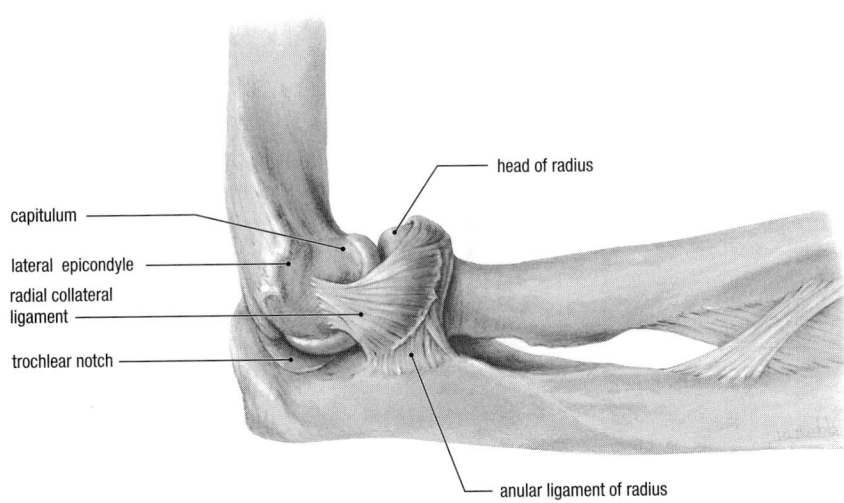

collateral ligaments of the elbow: (top) medial view; (bottom) lateral view

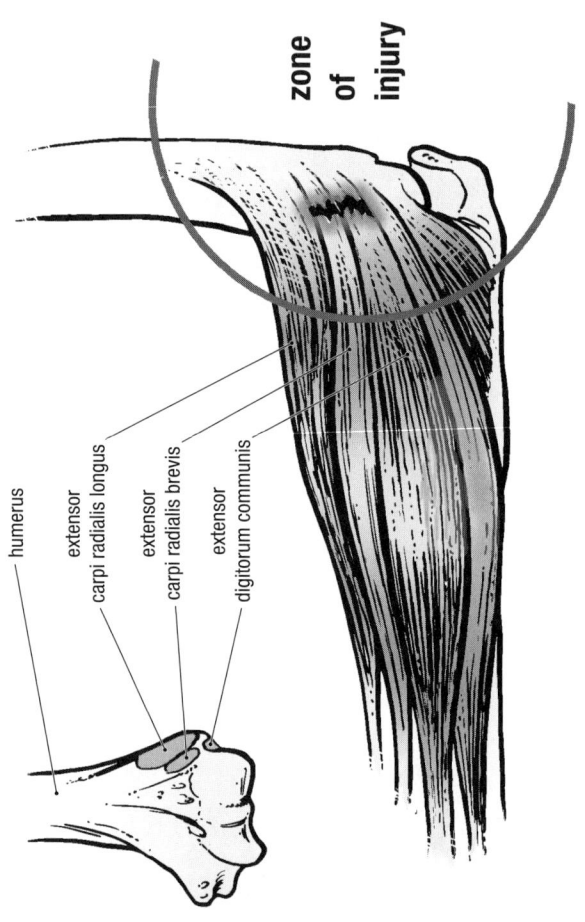

humerus

extensor
carpi radialis longus

extensor
carpi radialis brevis

extensor
digitorum communis

zone
of
injury

tennis elbow release: the forearm extensor muscles originate as a conjoined tendon from the lateral epicondyle of the elbow; note critical zone of injury

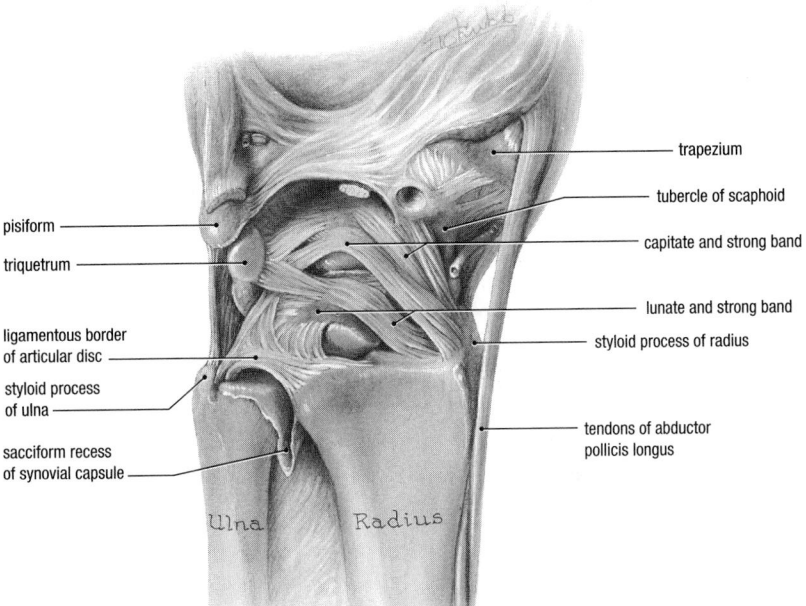

trapezium

tubercle of scaphoid

capitate and strong band

lunate and strong band

styloid process of radius

tendons of abductor pollicis longus

pisiform

triquetrum

ligamentous border of articular disc

styloid process of ulna

sacciform recess of synovial capsule

Ulna

Radius

ligaments of the distal radioulnar, radiocarpal, and intercarpal joints

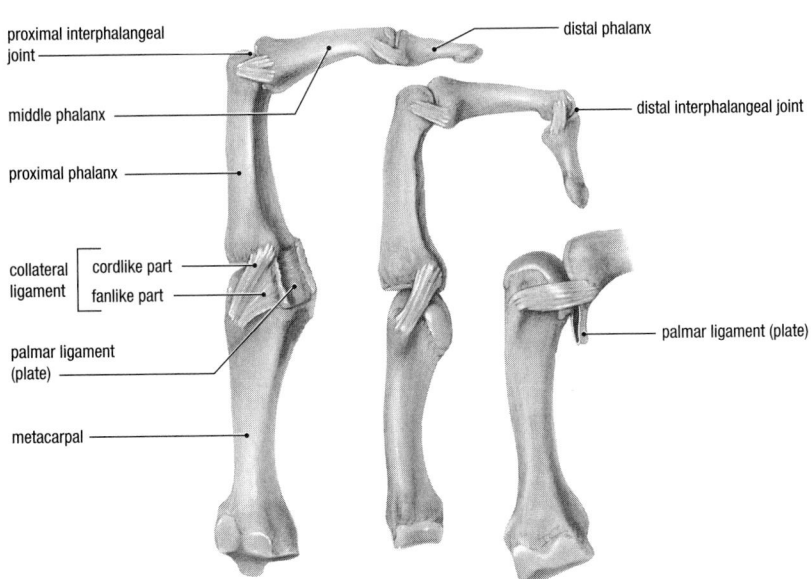

proximal interphalangeal joint

distal phalanx

middle phalanx

distal interphalangeal joint

proximal phalanx

collateral ligament

cordlike part

fanlike part

palmar ligament (plate)

palmar ligament (plate)

metacarpal

ligaments of metacarpophalangeal and interphalangeal joints

A19

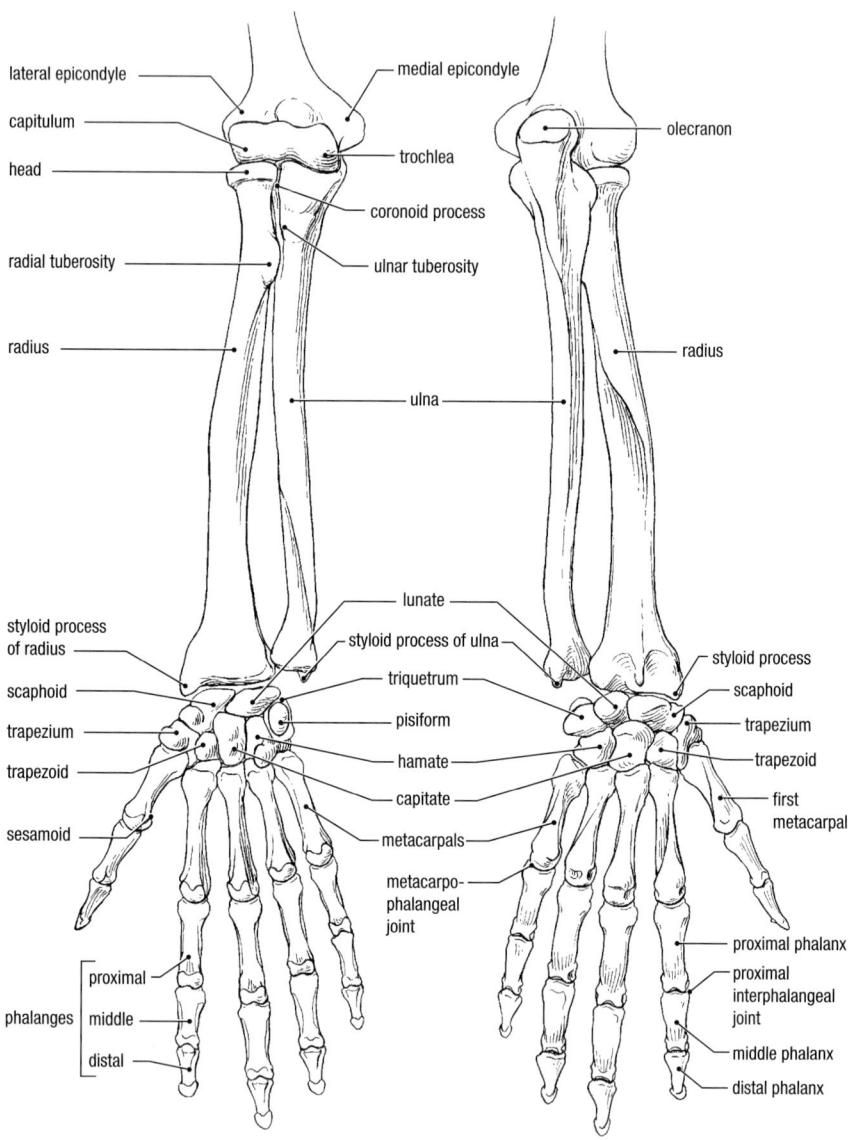

lateral epicondyle

medial epicondyle

capitulum

olecranon

head

trochlea

coronoid process

radial tuberosity

ulnar tuberosity

radius

radius

ulna

lunate

styloid process
of radius

styloid process of ulna

styloid process

scaphoid

triquetrum

scaphoid

trapezium

pisiform

trapezium

trapezoid

hamate

trapezoid

capitate

first
metacarpal

sesamoid

metacarpals

metacarpo-
phalangeal
joint

proximal phalanx

proximal

proximal
interphalangeal
joint

phalanges middle

middle phalanx

distal

distal phalanx

bones of the forearm and hand: (left) anterior view; (right) posterior view

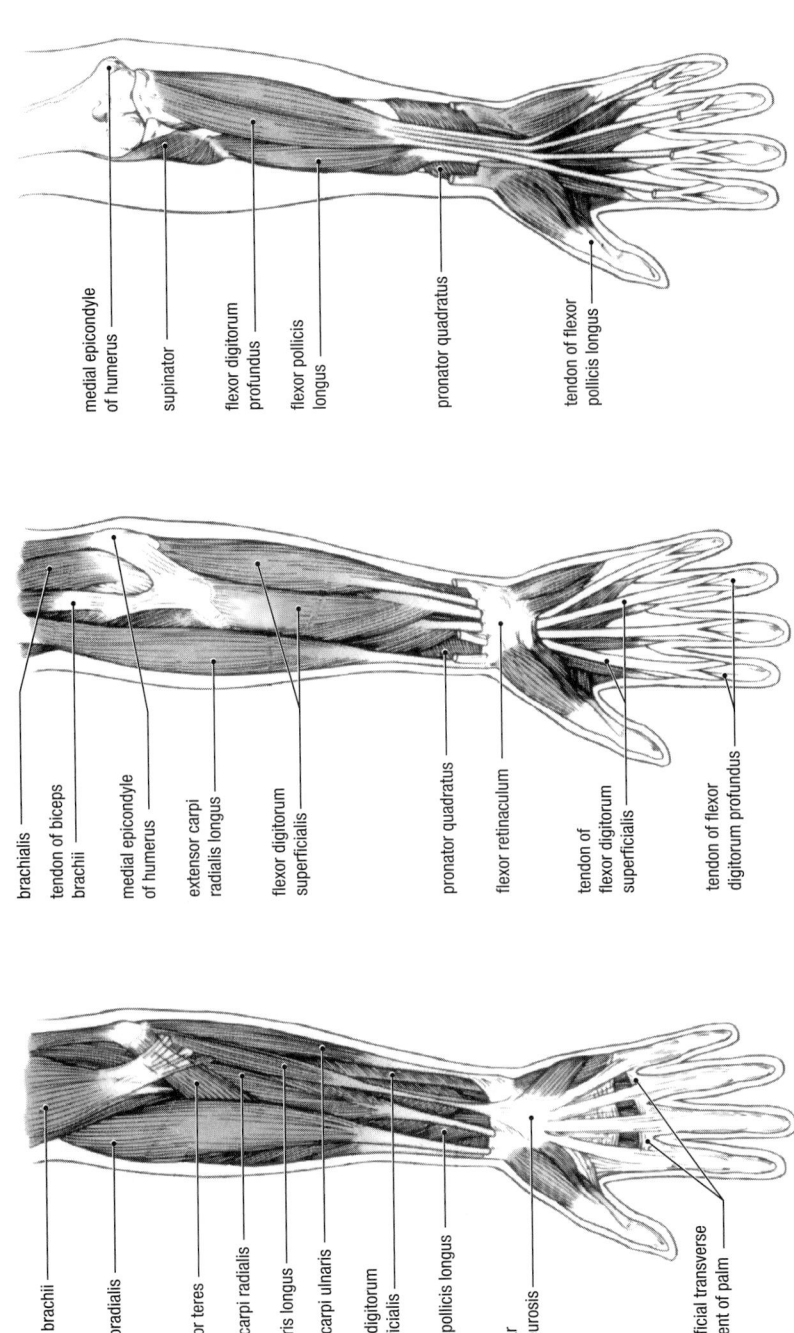

medial epicondyle
of humerus

supinator

flexor digitorum
profundus

flexor pollicis
longus

pronator quadratus

tendon of flexor
pollicis longus

brachialis

tendon of biceps
brachii

medial epicondyle
of humerus

extensor carpi
radialis longus

flexor digitorum
superficialis

pronator quadratus

flexor retinaculum

tendon of
flexor digitorum
superficialis

tendon of flexor
digitorum profundus

biceps brachii

brachioradialis

pronator teres

flexor carpi radialis

palmaris longus

flexor carpi ulnaris

flexor digitorum
superficialis

flexor pollicis longus

palmar
aponeurosis

superficial transverse
ligament of palm

muscles of the wrist and hand, anterior view: (left) superficial; (middle) midlevel; (right) deep

A21

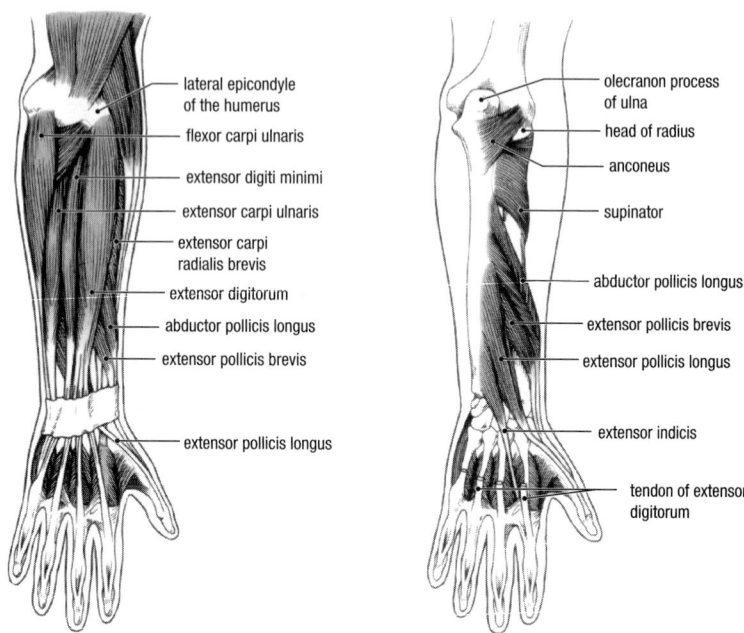

muscles of the wrist and hand, posterior view: (left) superficial; (right) deep

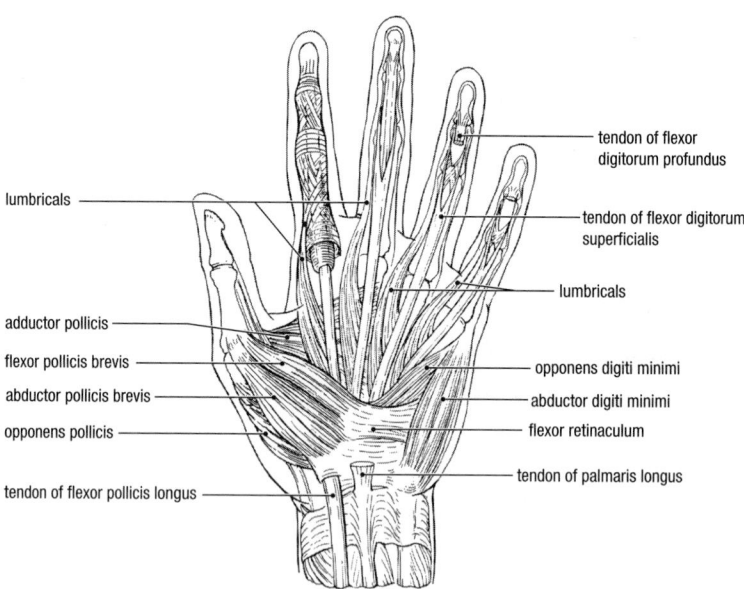

muscles of the hand, anterior (palmar) view

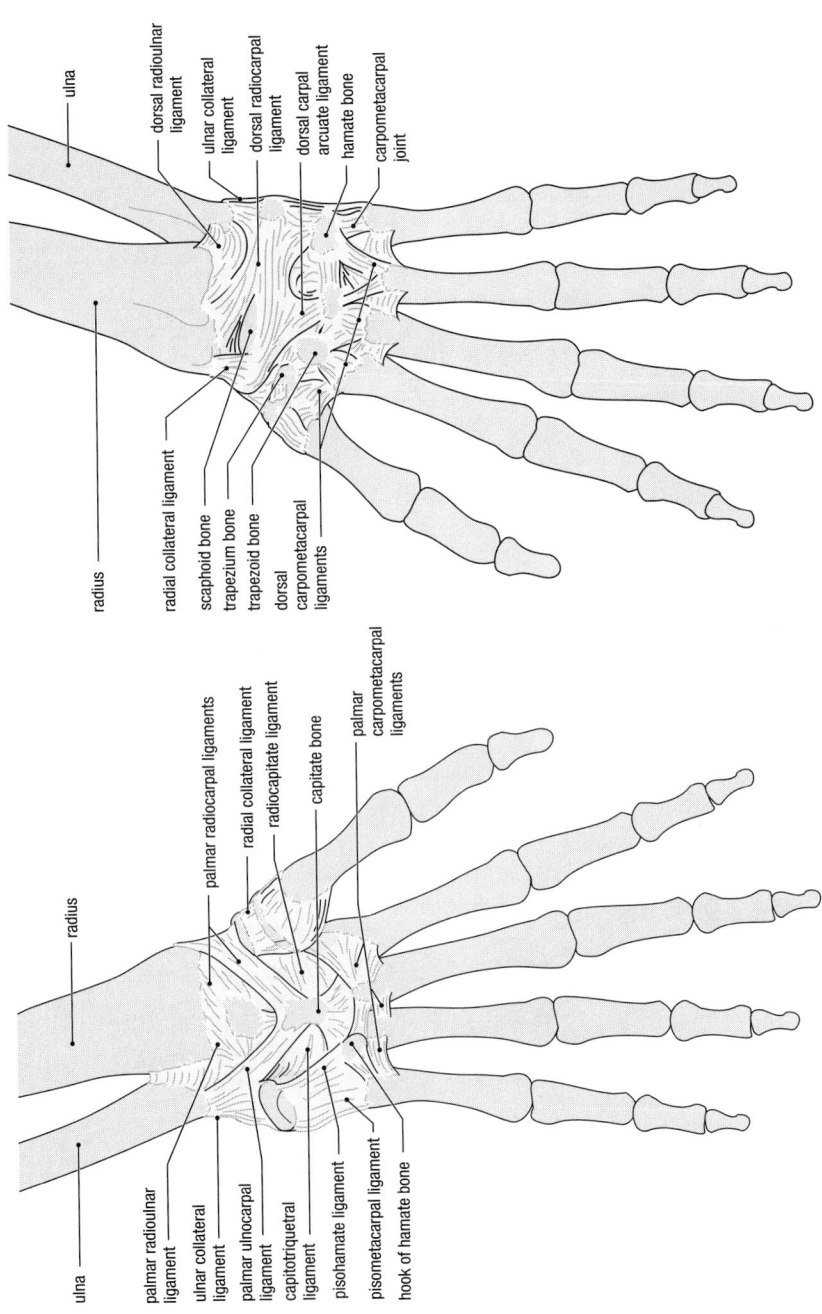

wrist showing relative positions of skeletal structures and ligaments: (left) anterior (palmar) view of left hand; (right) posterior (dorsal) view of left hand

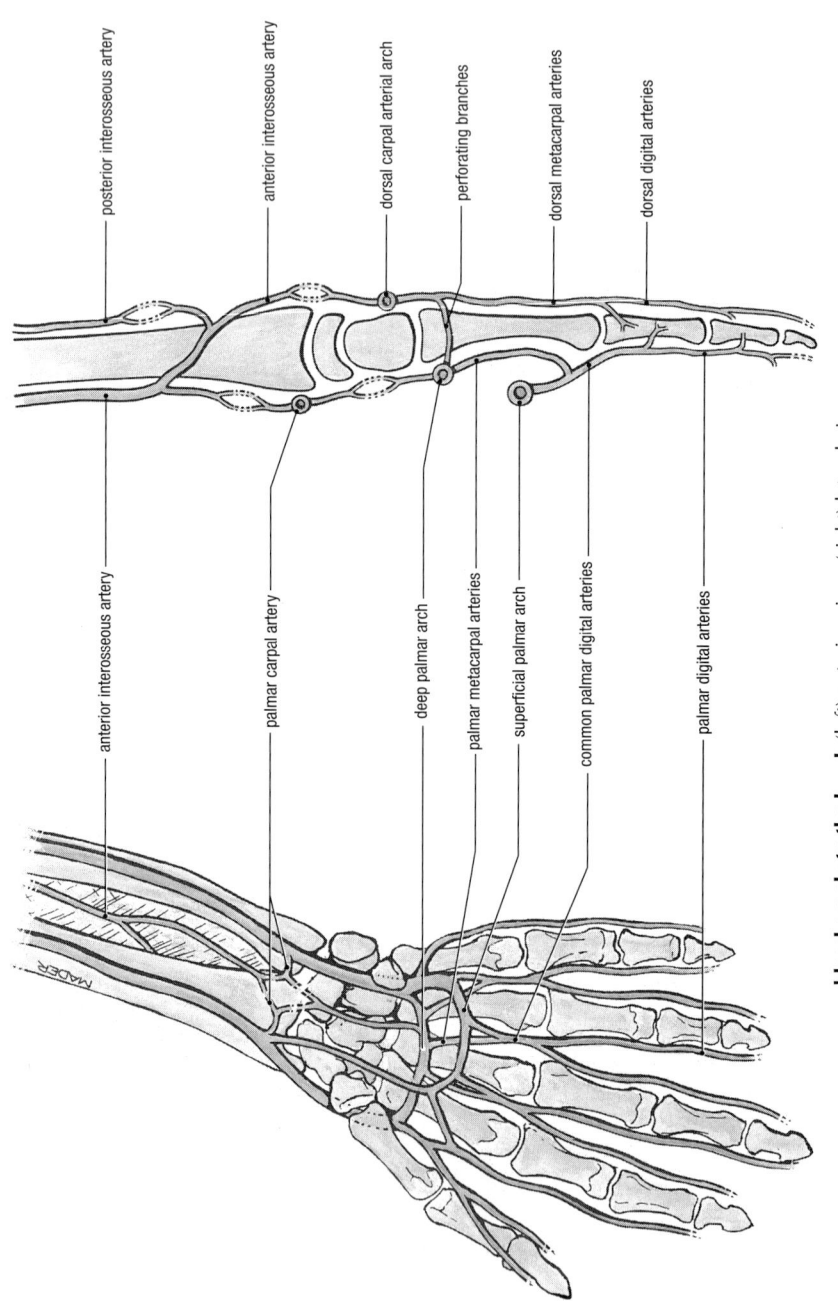

blood supply to the hand: (left) anterior view; (right) lateral view

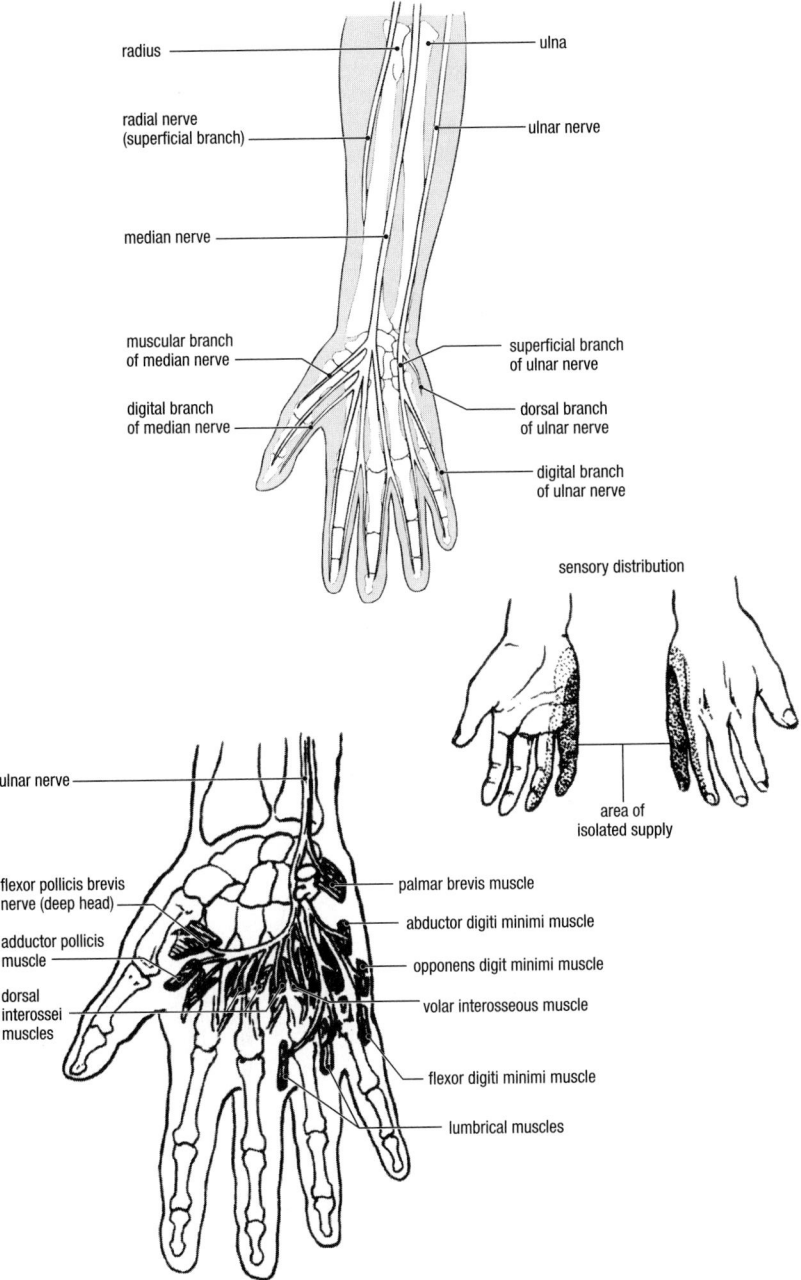

nerves of the hand, sensory distribution

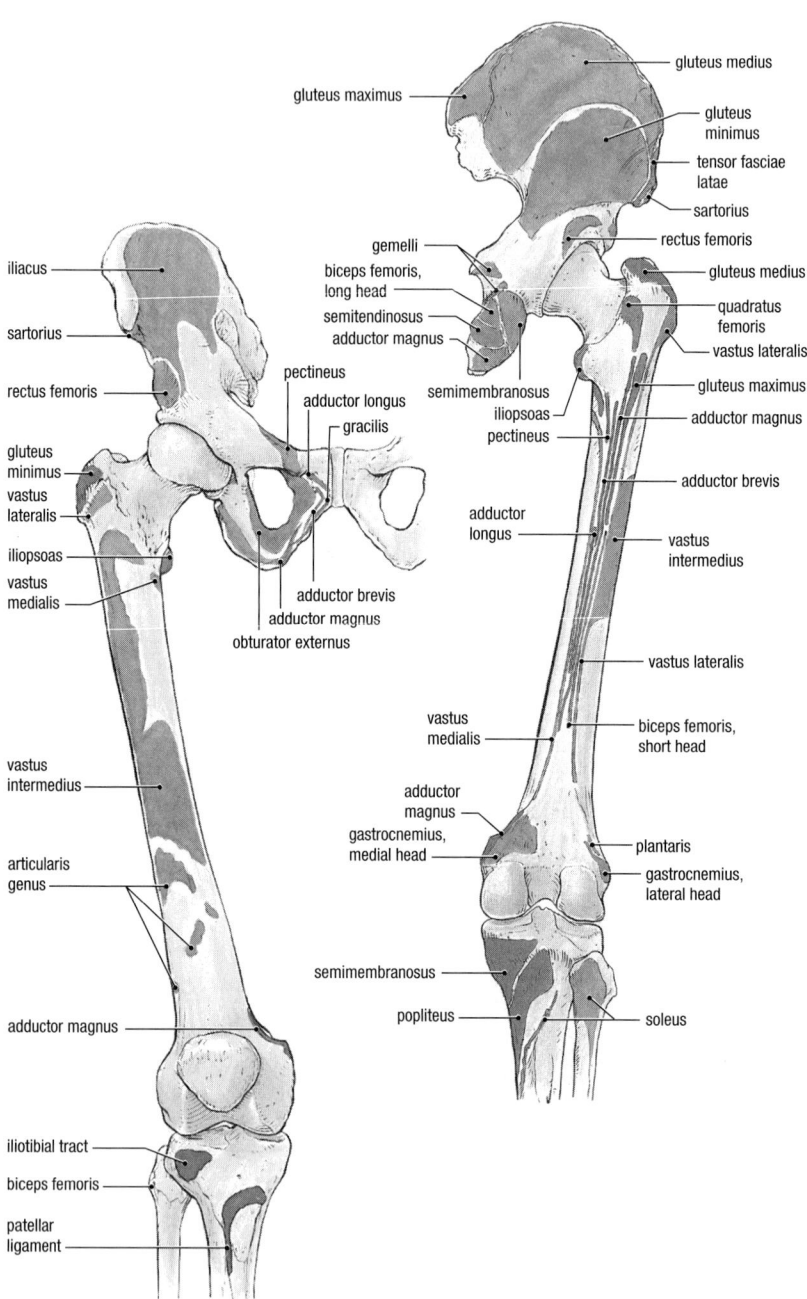

bones of the lower limbs showing muscle attachments: (left) anterior view; (right) posterior view

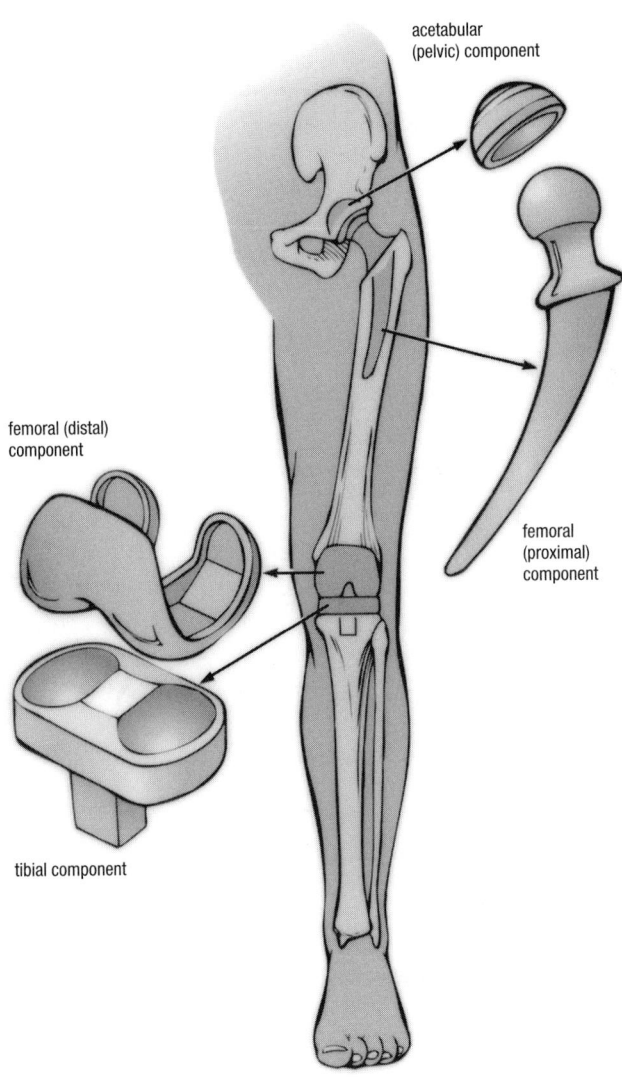

acetabular
(pelvic) component

femoral (distal)
component

femoral
(proximal)
component

tibial component

hip and knee replacement

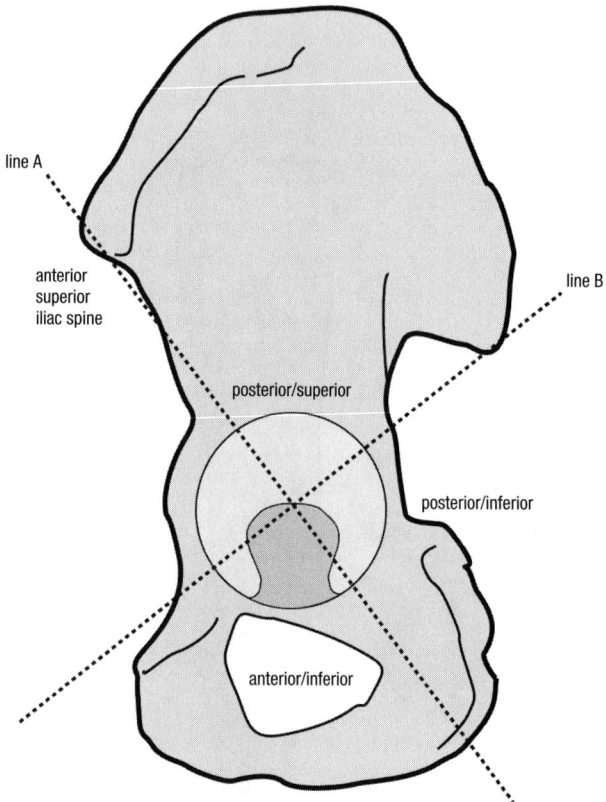

hybrid total hip arthroplasty: quadrant system for safe placement of acetabular screws

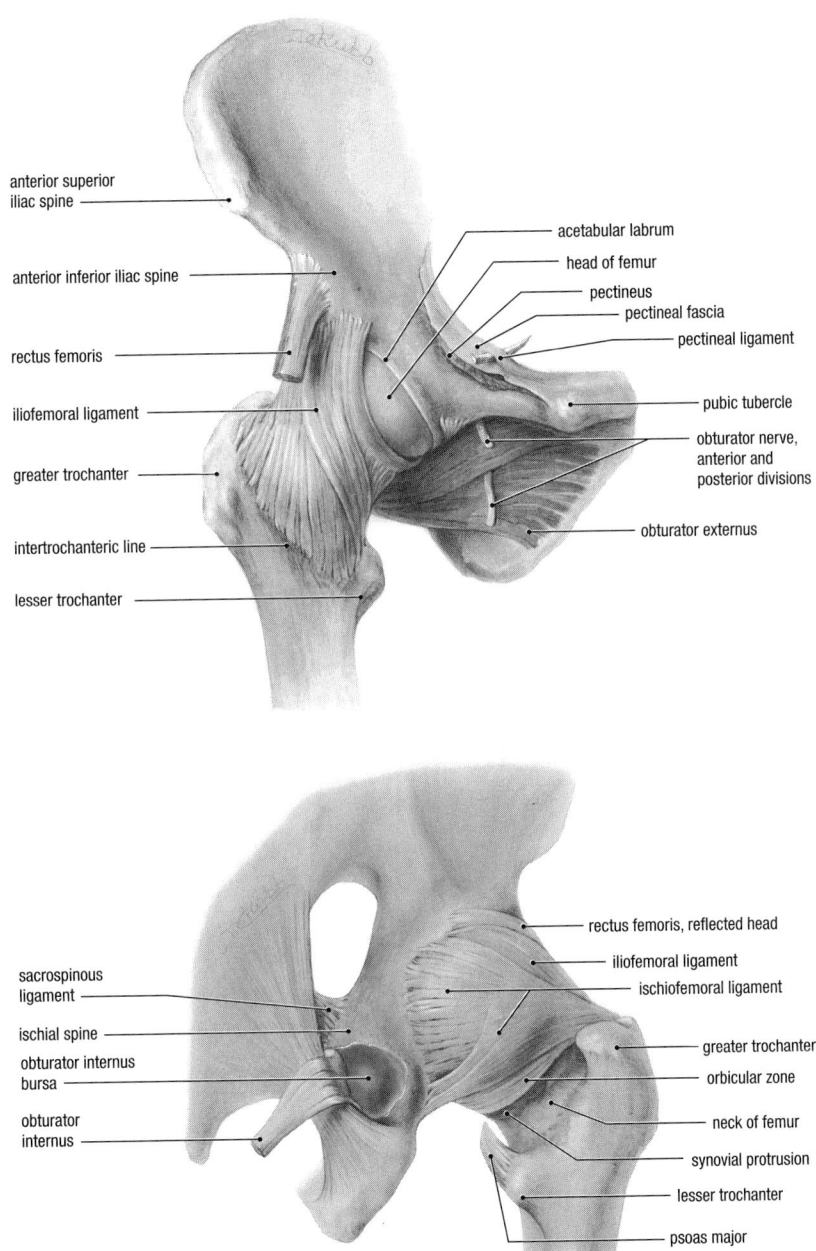

anterior superior iliac spine

anterior inferior iliac spine

rectus femoris

iliofemoral ligament

greater trochanter

intertrochanteric line

lesser trochanter

acetabular labrum

head of femur

pectineus

pectineal fascia

pectineal ligament

pubic tubercle

obturator nerve, anterior and posterior divisions

obturator externus

sacrospinous ligament

ischial spine

obturator internus bursa

obturator internus

rectus femoris, reflected head

iliofemoral ligament

ischiofemoral ligament

greater trochanter

orbicular zone

neck of femur

synovial protrusion

lesser trochanter

psoas major

hip joint: (top) anterior view; (bottom) posterior view

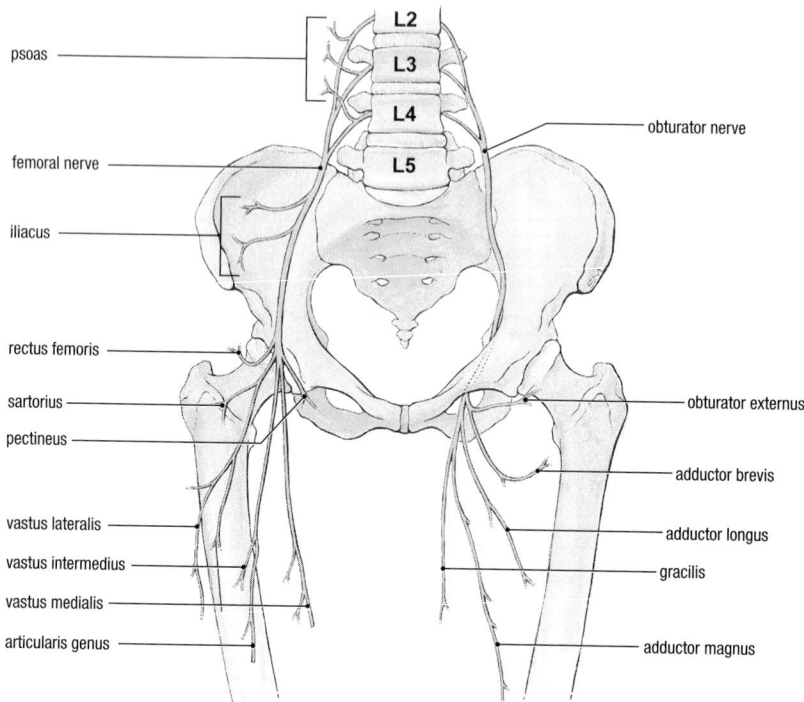

psoas

femoral nerve

iliacus

rectus femoris

sartorius

pectineus

vastus lateralis

vastus intermedius

vastus medialis

articularis genus

L2

L3

L4

L5

obturator nerve

obturator externus

adductor brevis

adductor longus

gracilis

adductor magnus

femoral and obturator nerves

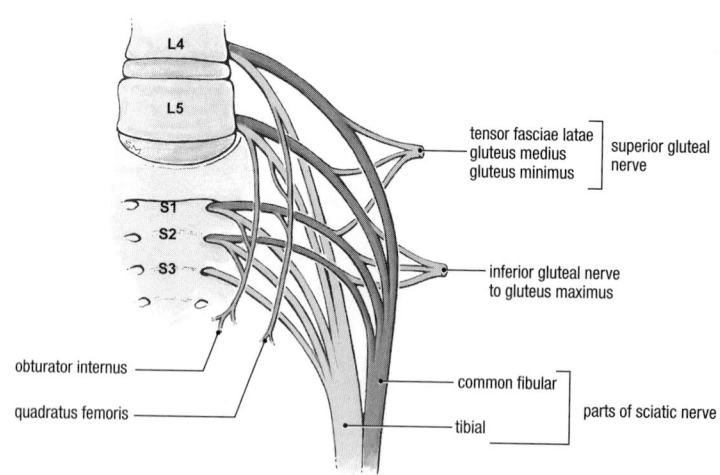

L4

L5

S1

S2

S3

tensor fasciae latae
gluteus medius
gluteus minimus

superior gluteal nerve

inferior gluteal nerve
to gluteus maximus

obturator internus

quadratus femoris

common fibular

tibial

parts of sciatic nerve

formation of the sciatic nerve in the pelvis

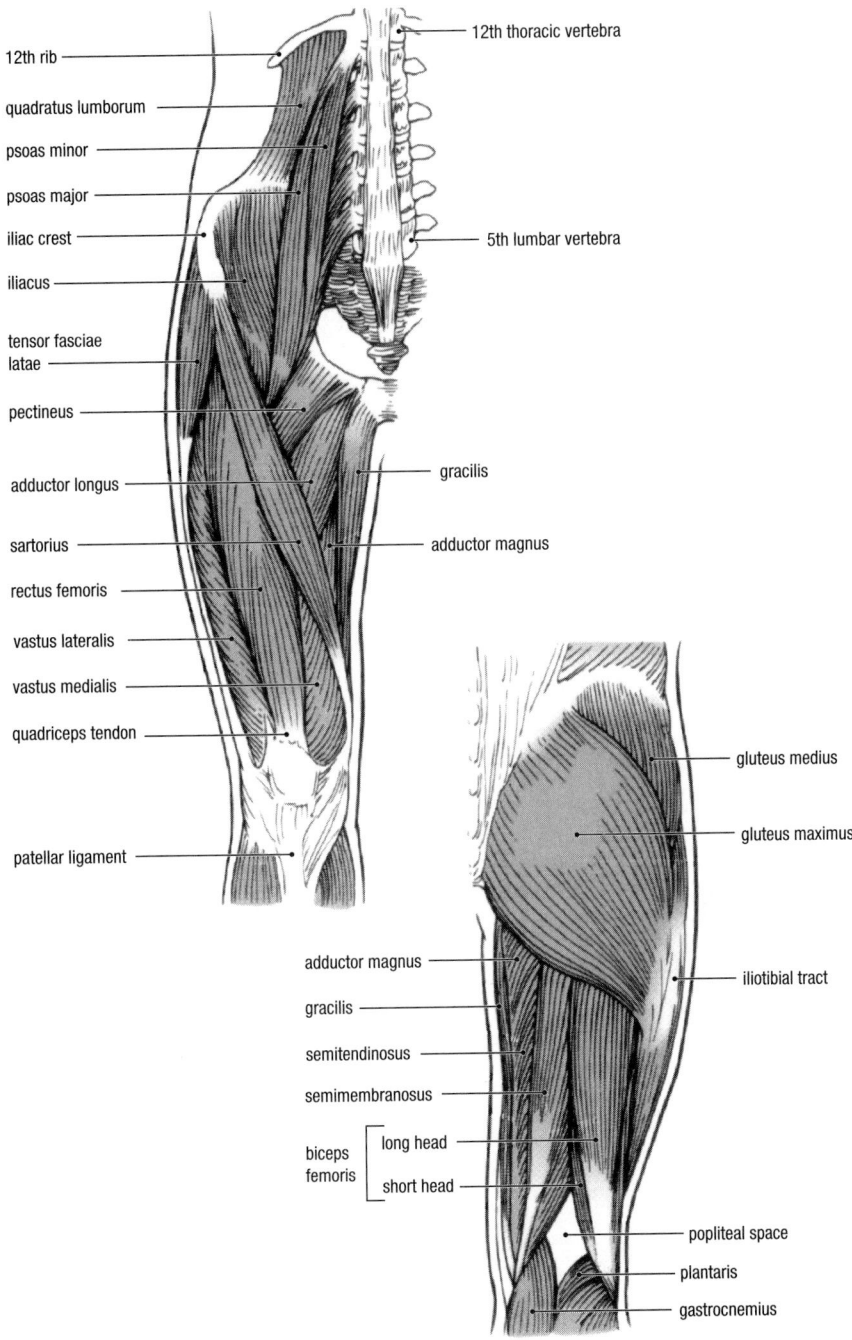

superficial muscles of the hip and thigh: (left) anterior view; (right) posterior view

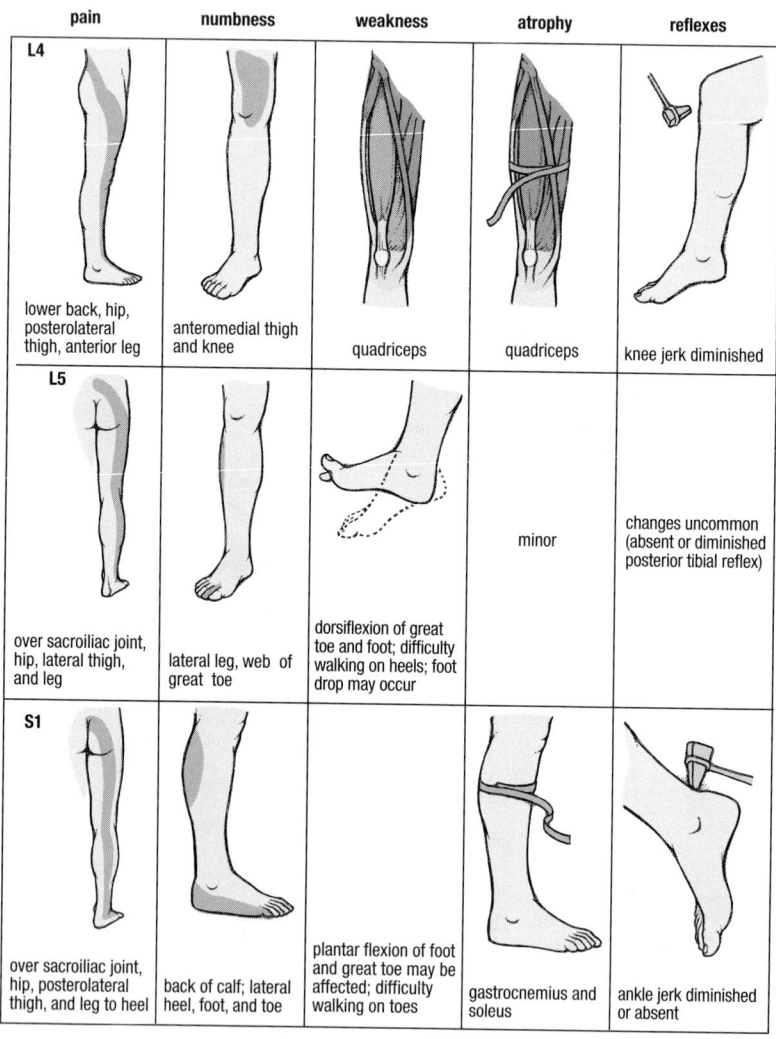

pain	numbness	weakness	atrophy	reflexes
L4				
lower back, hip, posterolateral thigh, anterior leg	anteromedial thigh and knee	quadriceps	quadriceps	knee jerk diminished
L5				
over sacroiliac joint, hip, lateral thigh, and leg	lateral leg, web of great toe	dorsiflexion of great toe and foot; difficulty walking on heels; foot drop may occur	minor	changes uncommon (absent or diminished posterior tibial reflex)
S1				
over sacroiliac joint, hip, posterolateral thigh, and leg to heel	back of calf; lateral heel, foot, and toe	plantar flexion of foot and great toe may be affected; difficulty walking on toes	gastrocnemius and soleus	ankle jerk diminished or absent

intervertebral disc herniation (nerves compressed: L4, L5, and S1)

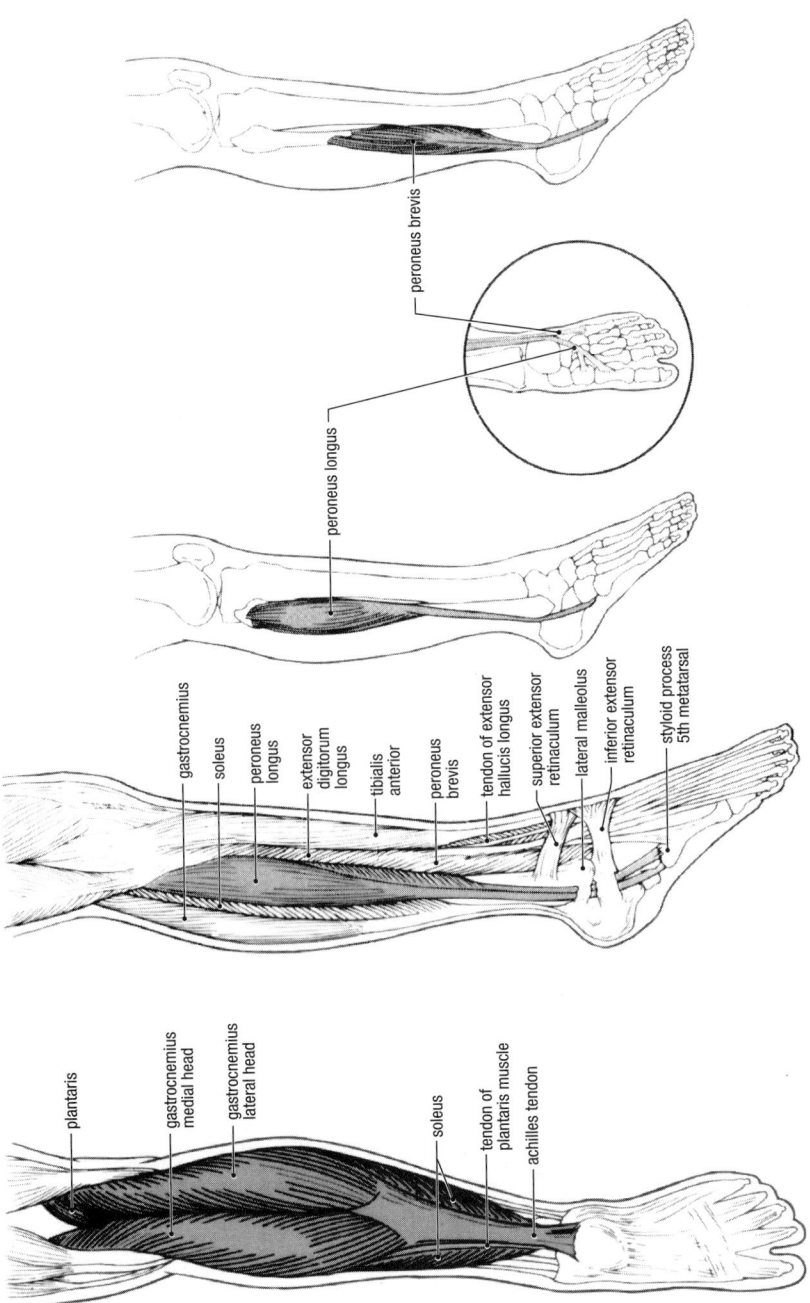

muscles of the lower leg: (left) superficial compartment, posterior view; (middle and right) lateral compartment

peroneus brevis

peroneus longus

gastrocnemius
soleus
peroneus longus
extensor digitorum longus
tibialis anterior
peroneus brevis
tendon of extensor hallucis longus
superior extensor retinaculum
lateral malleolus
inferior extensor retinaculum
styloid process 5th metatarsal

plantaris
gastrocnemius medial head
gastrocnemius lateral head
soleus
tendon of plantaris muscle
achilles tendon

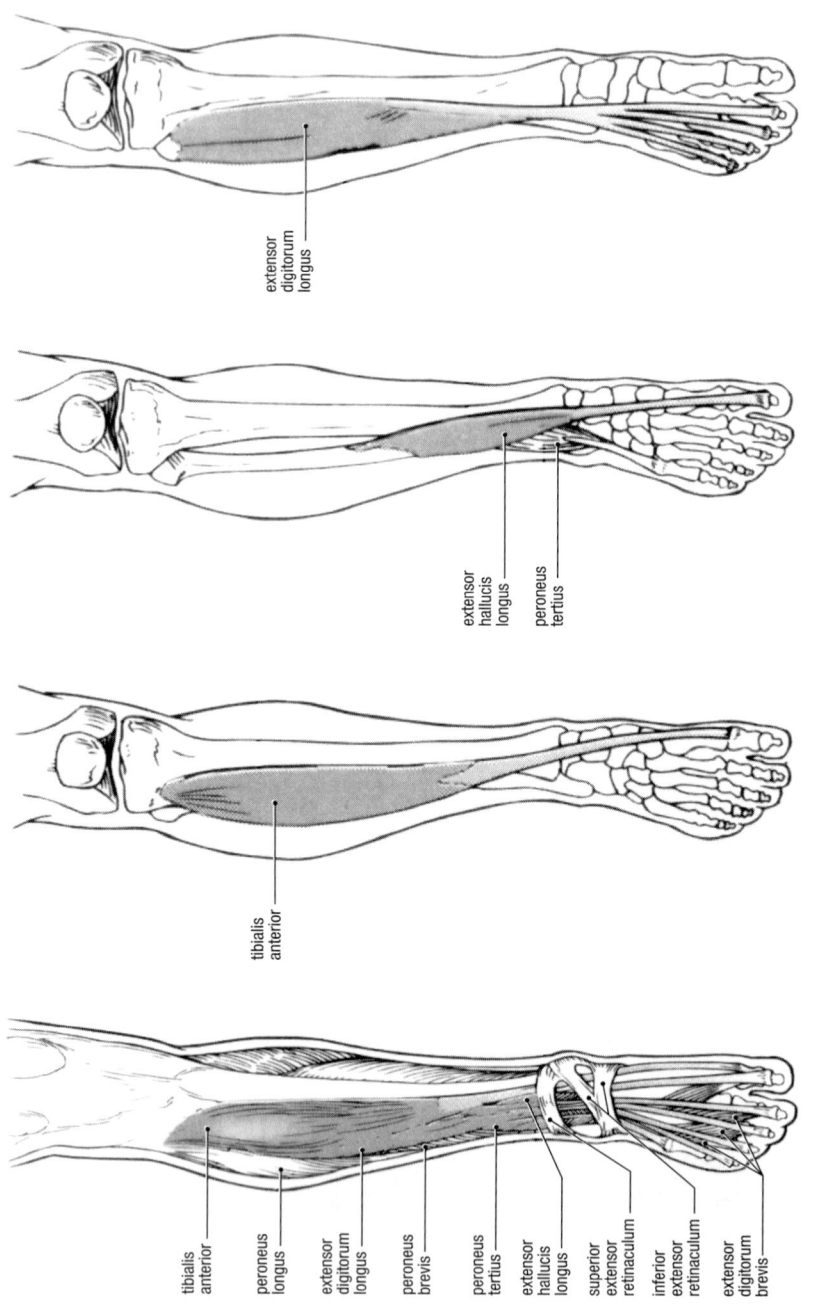

muscles of the lower leg, anterior compartment

extensor digitorum longus

extensor hallucis longus

peroneus tertius

tibialis anterior

tibialis anterior
peroneus longus
extensor digitorum longus
peroneus brevis
peroneus tertius
extensor hallucis longus
superior extensor retinaculum
inferior extensor retinaculum
extensor digitorum brevis

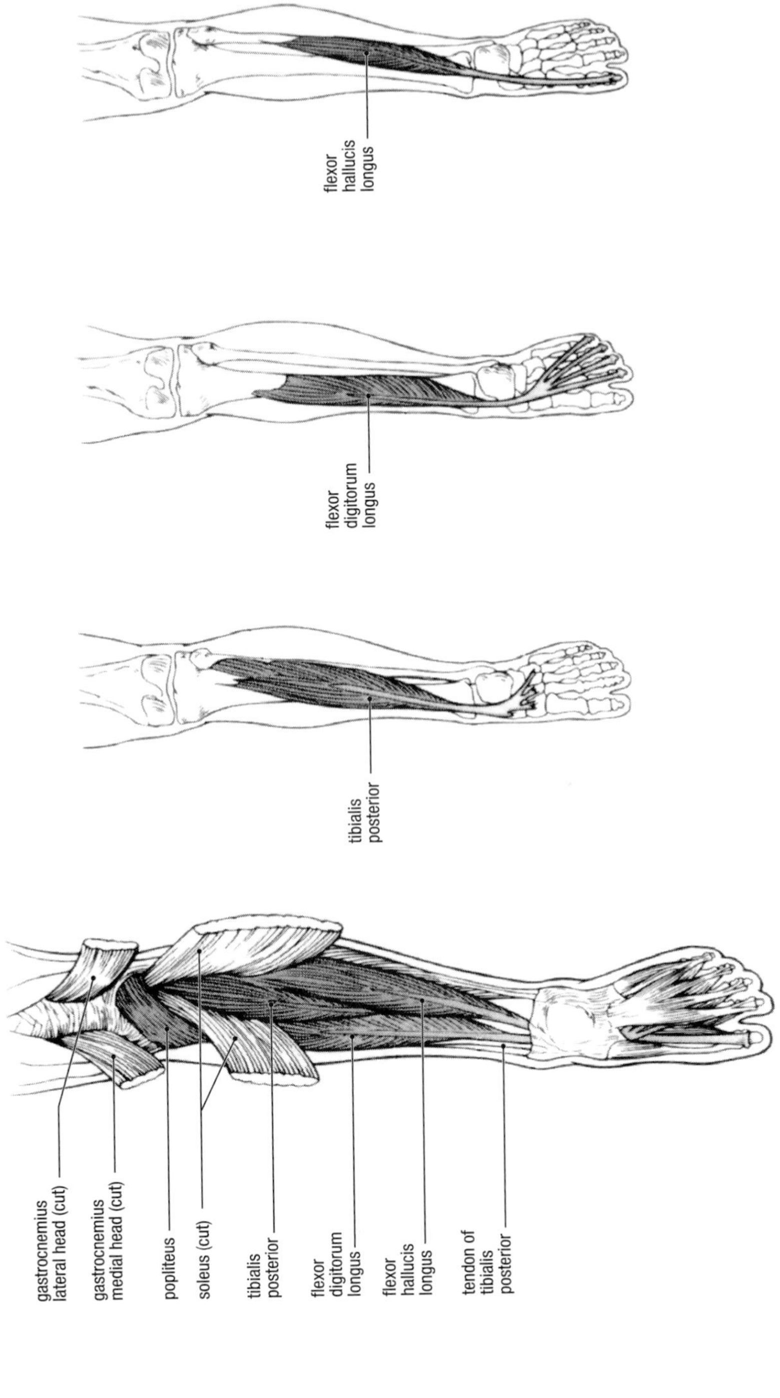

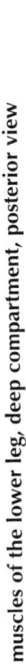

flexor
hallucis
longus

flexor
digitorum
longus

tibialis
posterior

gastrocnemius
lateral head (cut)

gastrocnemius
medial head (cut)

popliteus

soleus (cut)

tibialis
posterior

flexor
digitorum
longus

flexor
hallucis
longus

tendon of
tibialis
posterior

muscles of the lower leg, deep compartment, posterior view

A35

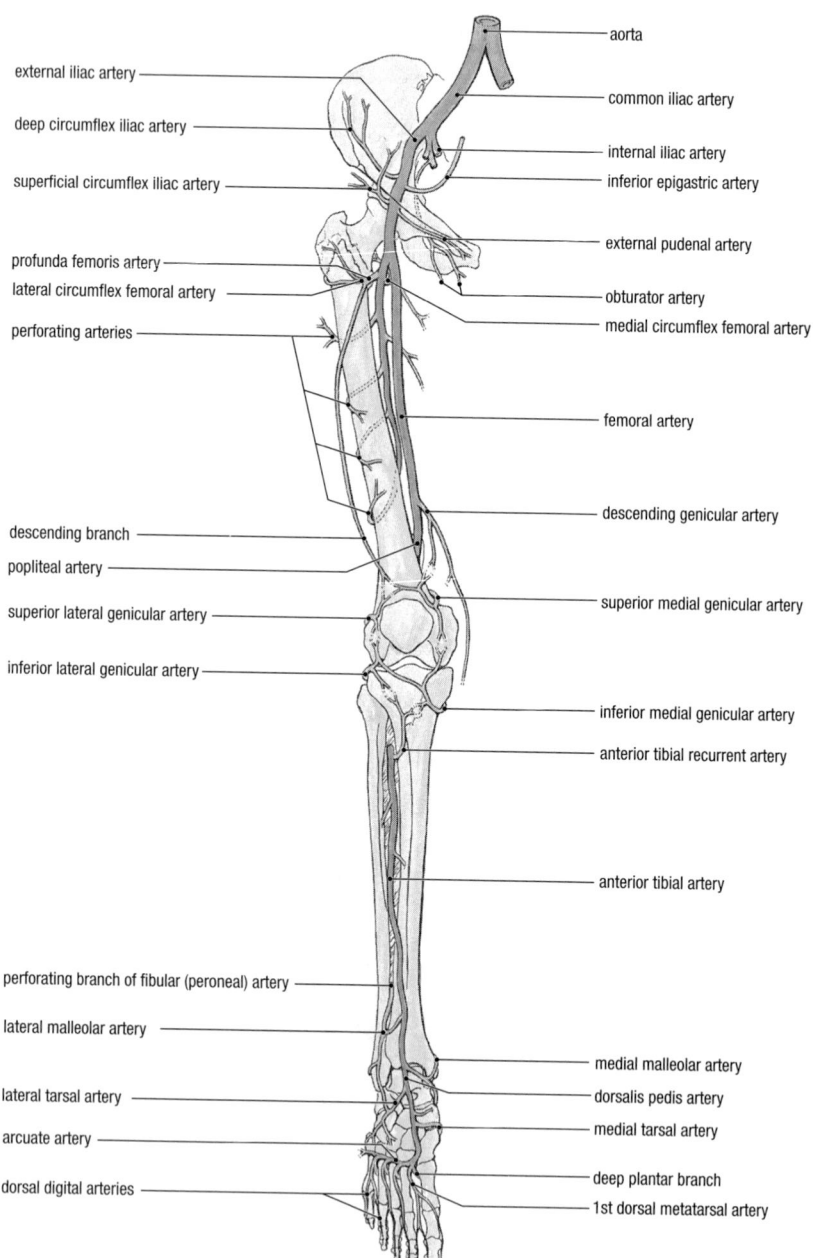

external iliac artery

deep circumflex iliac artery

superficial circumflex iliac artery

profunda femoris artery

lateral circumflex femoral artery

perforating arteries

descending branch

popliteal artery

superior lateral genicular artery

inferior lateral genicular artery

perforating branch of fibular (peroneal) artery

lateral malleolar artery

lateral tarsal artery

arcuate artery

dorsal digital arteries

aorta

common iliac artery

internal iliac artery

inferior epigastric artery

external pudenal artery

obturator artery

medial circumflex femoral artery

femoral artery

descending genicular artery

superior medial genicular artery

inferior medial genicular artery

anterior tibial recurrent artery

anterior tibial artery

medial malleolar artery

dorsalis pedis artery

medial tarsal artery

deep plantar branch

1st dorsal metatarsal artery

arteries of the lower limb, anterior view

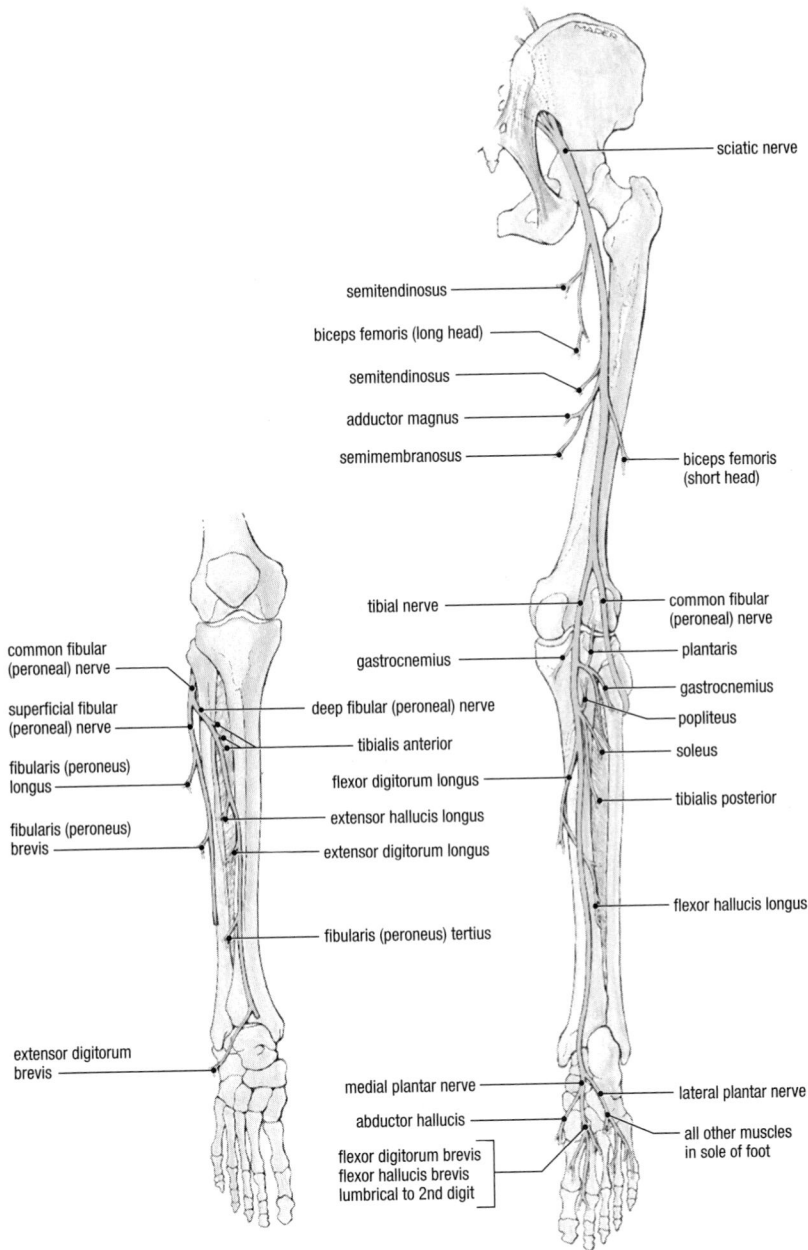

motor distribution of the nerves of the lower limb: (left) common fibular (peroneal) nerve; (right) sciatic nerve

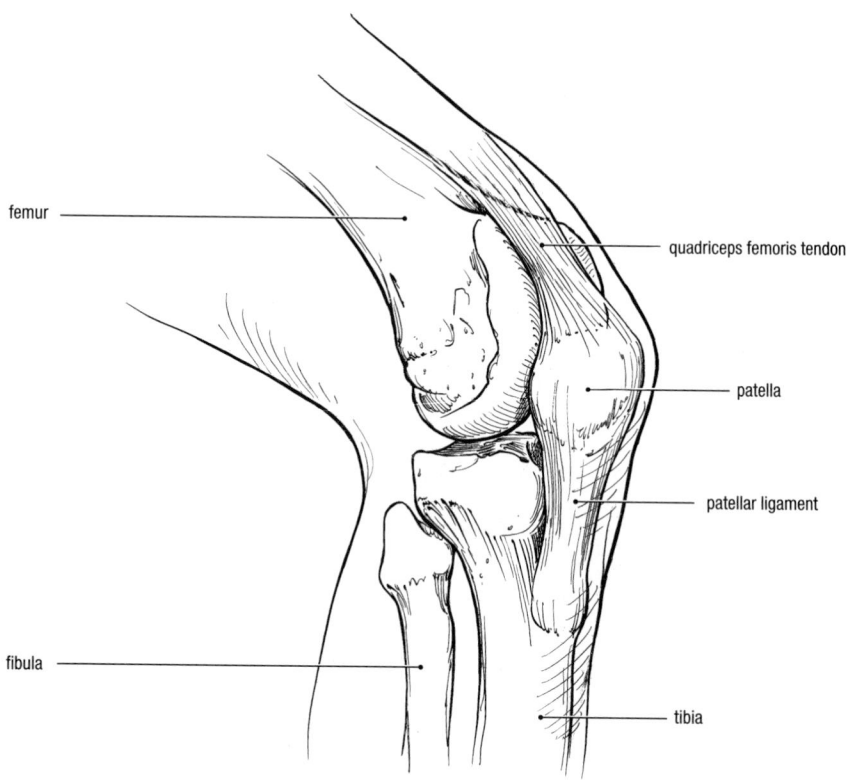

femur

quadriceps femoris tendon

patella

patellar ligament

fibula

tibia

the bones of the knee joint

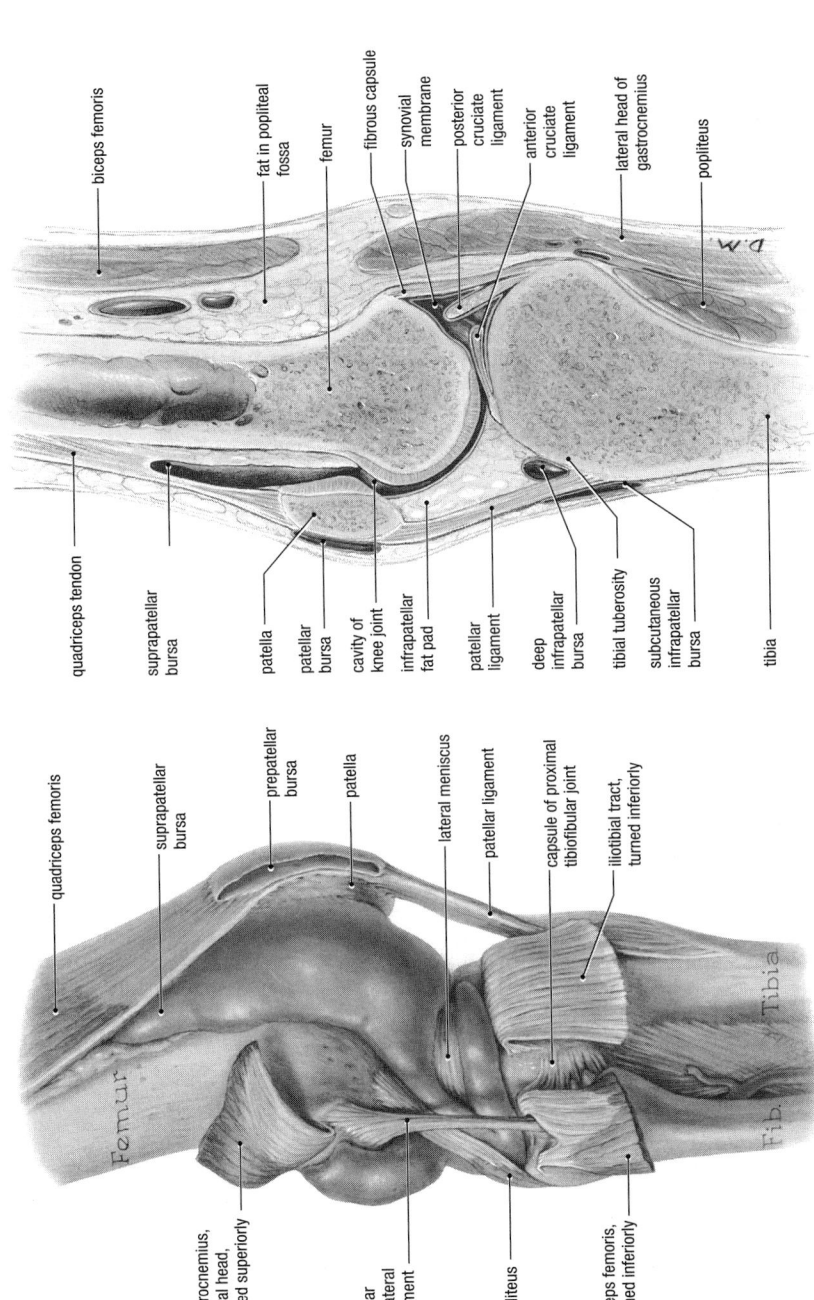

biceps femoris

fat in popliteal fossa

femur

fibrous capsule

synovial membrane

posterior cruciate ligament

anterior cruciate ligament

lateral head of gastrocnemius

popliteus

quadriceps tendon

suprapatellar bursa

patella

patellar bursa

cavity of knee joint

infrapatellar fat pad

patellar ligament

deep infrapatellar bursa

tibial tuberosity

subcutaneous infrapatellar bursa

tibia

sagittal section through lateral aspect of intercondylar notch of femur

quadriceps femoris

suprapatellar bursa

prepatellar bursa

patella

lateral meniscus

patellar ligament

capsule of proximal tibiofibular joint

iliotibial tract, turned inferiorly

gastrocnemius, lateral head, turned superiorly

fibular collateral ligament

popliteus

biceps femoris, turned inferiorly

distended knee joint, lateral view

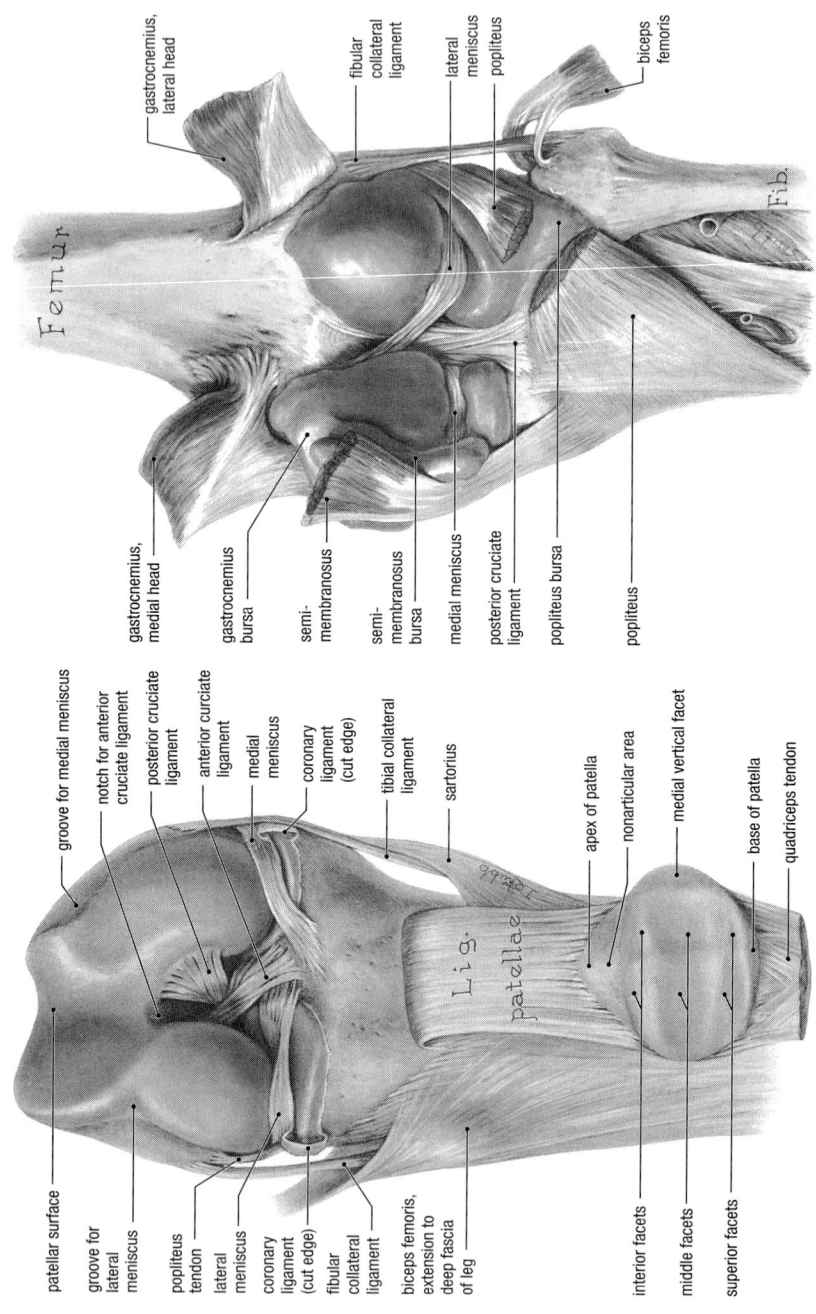

articular surfaces and ligaments of the knew joint: (left) anterior view; (right) posterior view

Posterior view labels (top illustration):

gastrocnemius, lateral head
fibular collateral ligament
lateral meniscus
popliteus
biceps femoris
Femur
Fib.
gastrocnemius, medial head
gastrocnemius bursa
semi-membranosus
semi-membranosus bursa
medial meniscus
posterior cruciate ligament
popliteus bursa
popliteus

Anterior view labels (bottom illustration):

groove for medial meniscus
notch for anterior cruciate ligament
posterior cruciate ligament
anterior curciate ligament
medial meniscus
coronary ligament (cut edge)
tibial collateral ligament
sartorius
apex of patella
nonarticular area
medial vertical facet
base of patella
quadriceps tendon
Lig. patellae
patellar surface
groove for lateral meniscus
popliteus tendon
lateral meniscus
coronary ligament (cut edge)
fibular collateral ligament
biceps femoris, extension to deep fascia of leg
interior facets
middle facets
superior facets

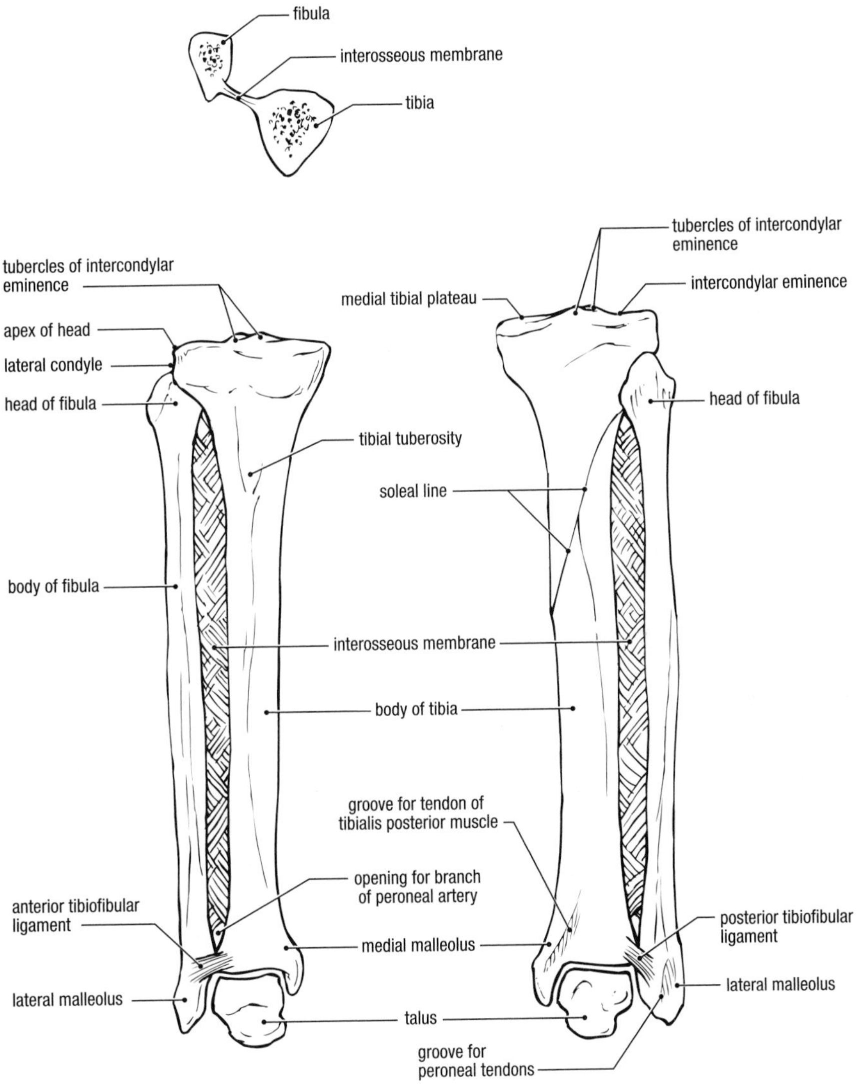

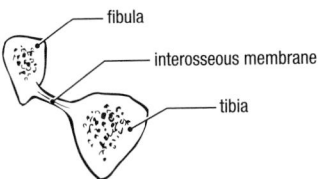

fibula

interosseous membrane

tibia

tubercles of intercondylar eminence

tubercles of intercondylar eminence

medial tibial plateau

intercondylar eminence

apex of head

lateral condyle

head of fibula

head of fibula

tibial tuberosity

soleal line

body of fibula

interosseous membrane

body of tibia

groove for tendon of tibialis posterior muscle

opening for branch of peroneal artery

anterior tibiofibular ligament

posterior tibiofibular ligament

medial malleolus

lateral malleolus

lateral malleolus

talus

groove for peroneal tendons

bones of lower leg: (left) anterior view; (right) posterior view; (top) cross-section

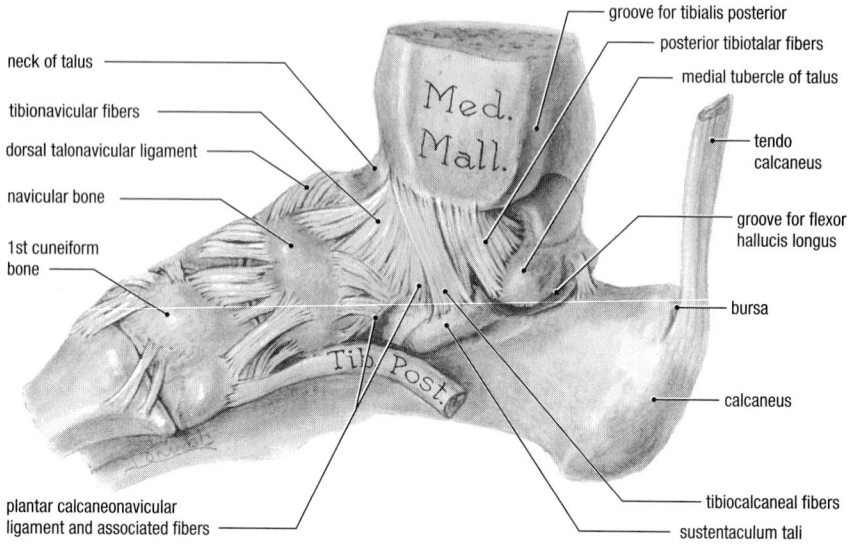

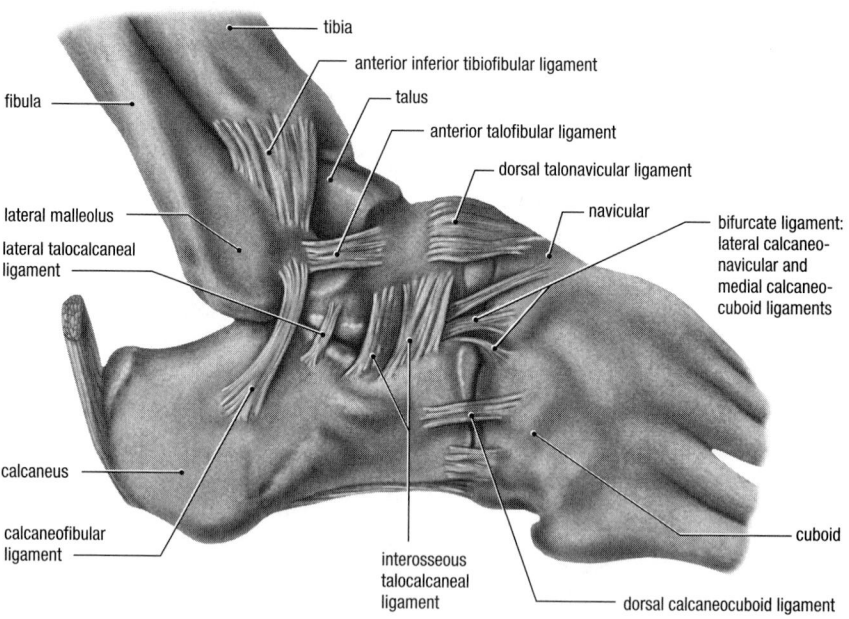

ligaments of the ankle: (top) medial view; (bottom) lateral view

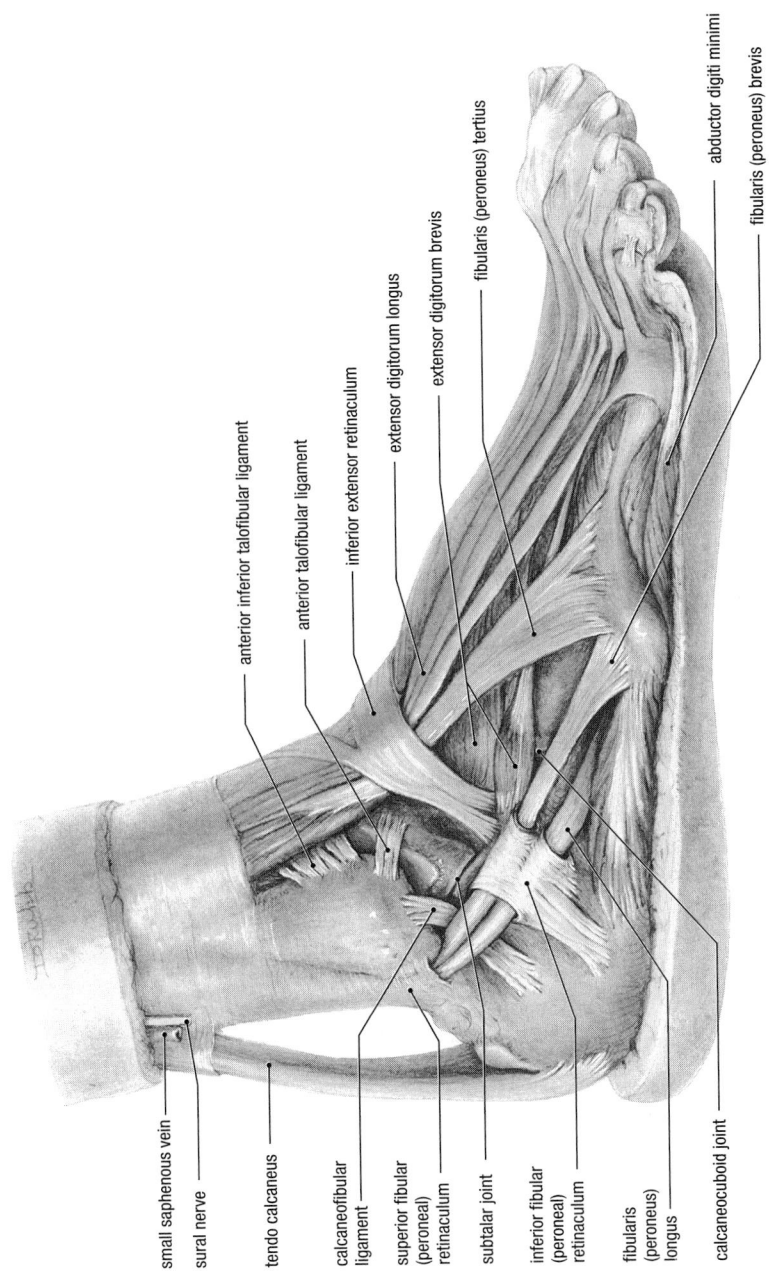

tendons of the ankle, lateral view

abductor digiti minimi

fibularis (peroneus) brevis

fibularis (peroneus) tertius

extensor digitorum brevis

extensor digitorum longus

inferior extensor retinaculum

anterior talofibular ligament

anterior inferior talofibular ligament

small saphenous vein

sural nerve

tendo calcaneus

calcaneofibular ligament

superior fibular (peroneal) retinaculum

subtalar joint

inferior fibular (peroneal) retinaculum

fibularis (peroneus) longus

calcaneocuboid joint

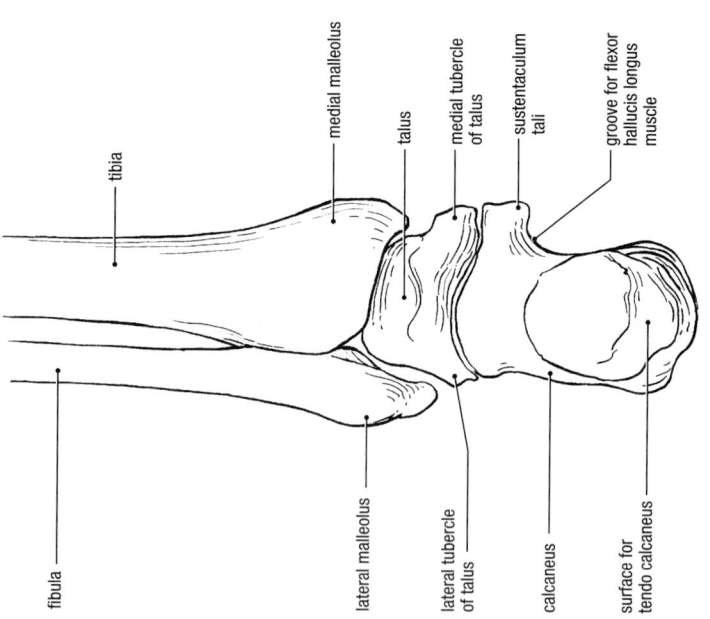

bones of the ankle and foot: (left) posterior view; (right) dorsal view

forefoot

midfoot

hindfoot

distal
middle
proximal
phalanges

head
shaft
base
metatarsals

medial
intermediate
lateral
cuneiforms

navicular
cuboid
talus
medial tubercle
lateral tubercle
calcaneus

tibia

medial malleolus

talus

medial tubercle of talus

sustentaculum tali

groove for flexor hallucis longus muscle

fibula

lateral malleolus

lateral tubercle of talus

calcaneus

surface for tendo calcaneus

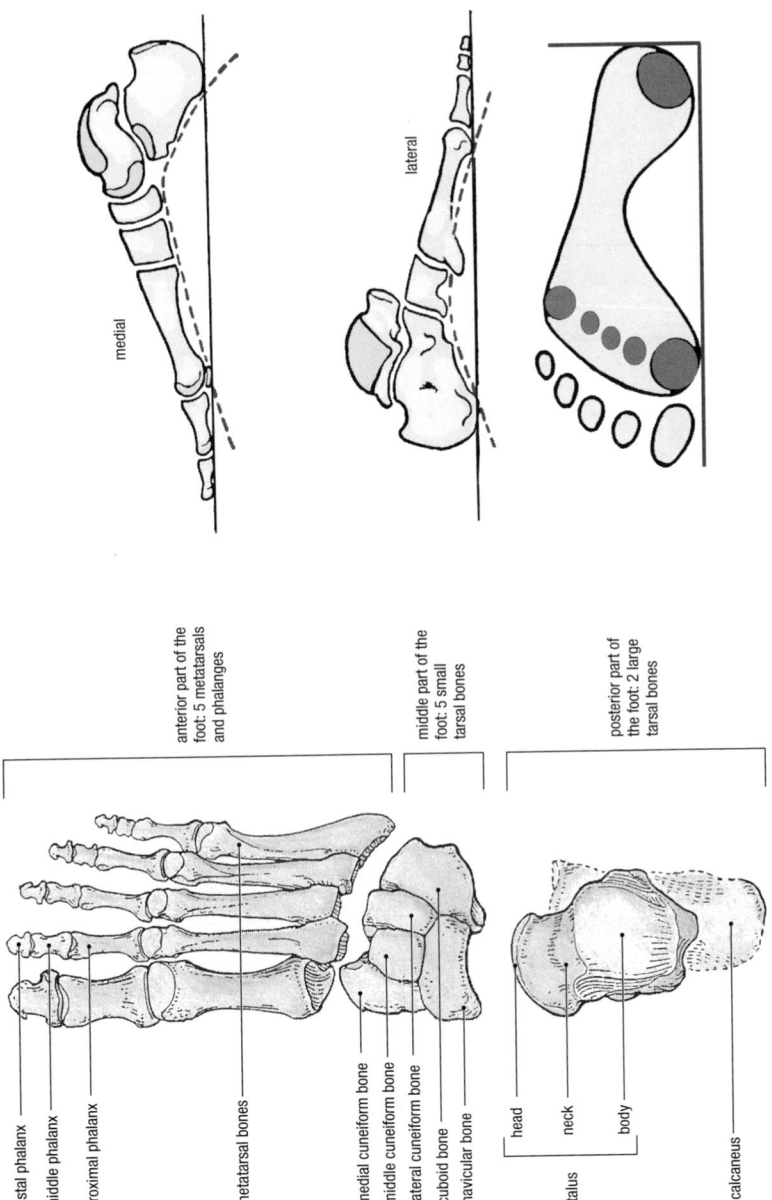

medial

lateral

(top) **medial and lateral longitudinal arches of the foot;** (bottom) **bearing points of the foot**

anterior part of the foot: 5 metatarsals and phalanges

middle part of the foot: 5 small tarsal bones

posterior part of the foot: 2 large tarsal bones

distal phalanx

middle phalanx

proximal phalanx

metatarsal bones

medial cuneiform bone

middle cuneiform bone

lateral cuneiform bone

cuboid bone

navicular bone

head

neck

body

talus

calcaneus

bones of the foot, dorsal view

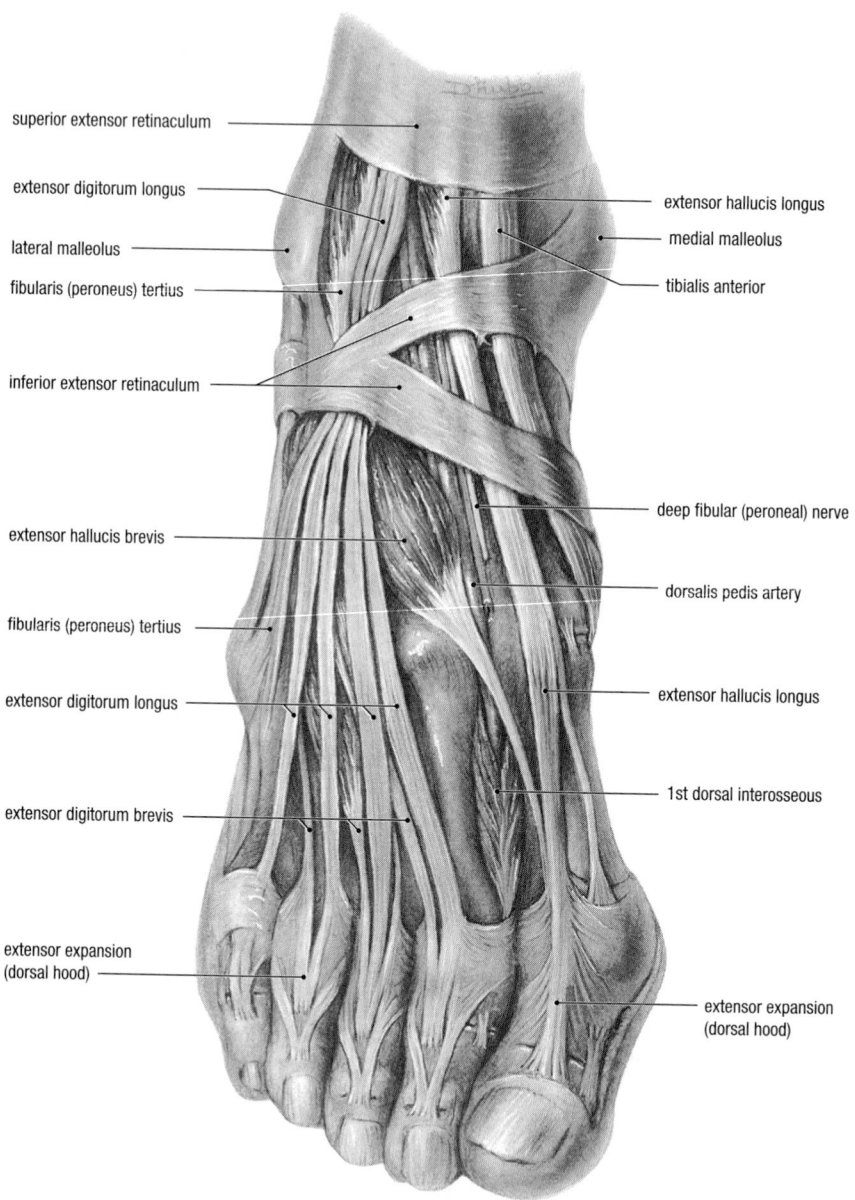

superior extensor retinaculum

extensor digitorum longus

lateral malleolus

fibularis (peroneus) tertius

inferior extensor retinaculum

extensor hallucis brevis

fibularis (peroneus) tertius

extensor digitorum longus

extensor digitorum brevis

extensor expansion
(dorsal hood)

extensor hallucis longus

medial malleolus

tibialis anterior

deep fibular (peroneal) nerve

dorsalis pedis artery

extensor hallucis longus

1st dorsal interosseous

extensor expansion
(dorsal hood)

muscles of the dorsum of the foot

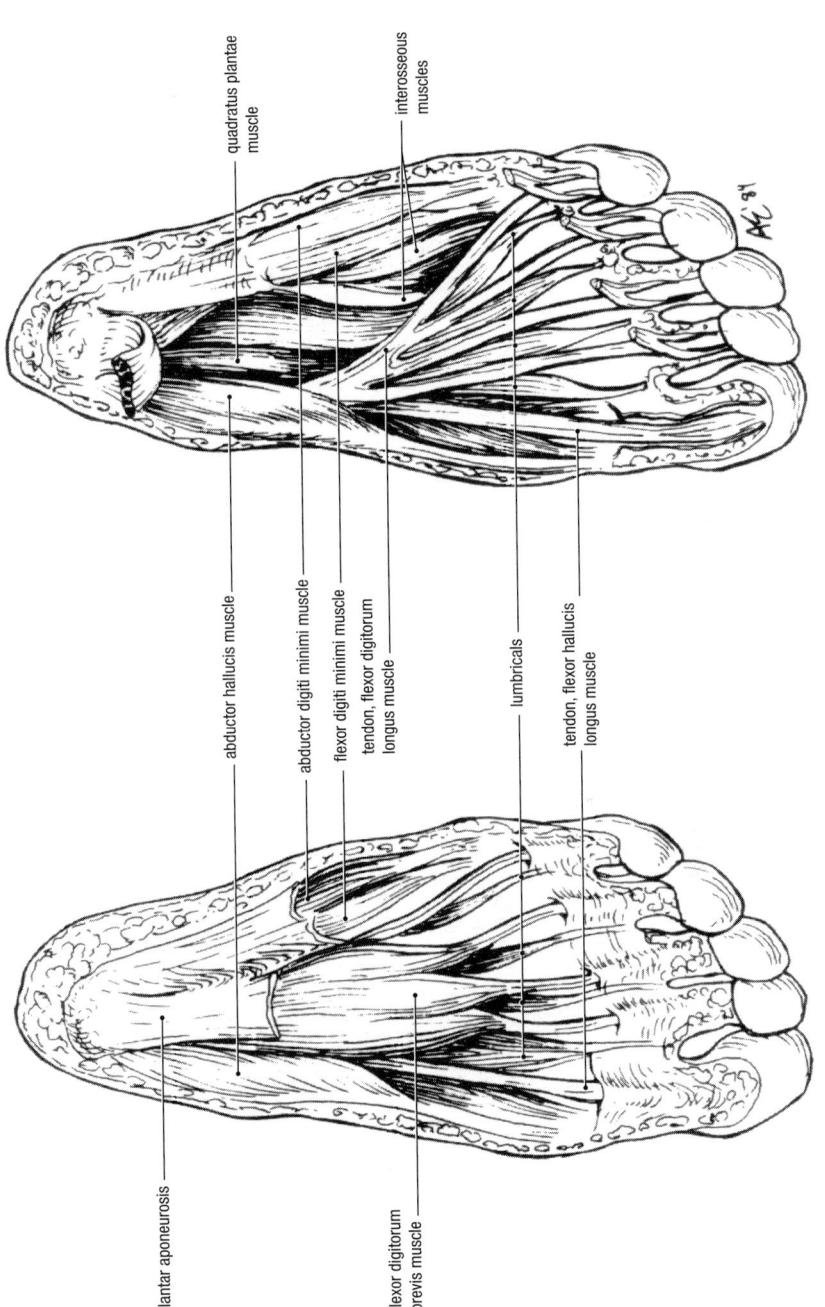

quadratus plantae muscle

interosseous muscles

abductor hallucis muscle

abductor digiti minimi muscle

flexor digiti minimi muscle

tendon, flexor digitorum longus muscle

lumbricals

tendon, flexor hallucis longus muscle

plantar aponeurosis

flexor digitorum brevis muscle

superficial muscles of the plantar foot: (left) 1st layer; (right) 2nd layer

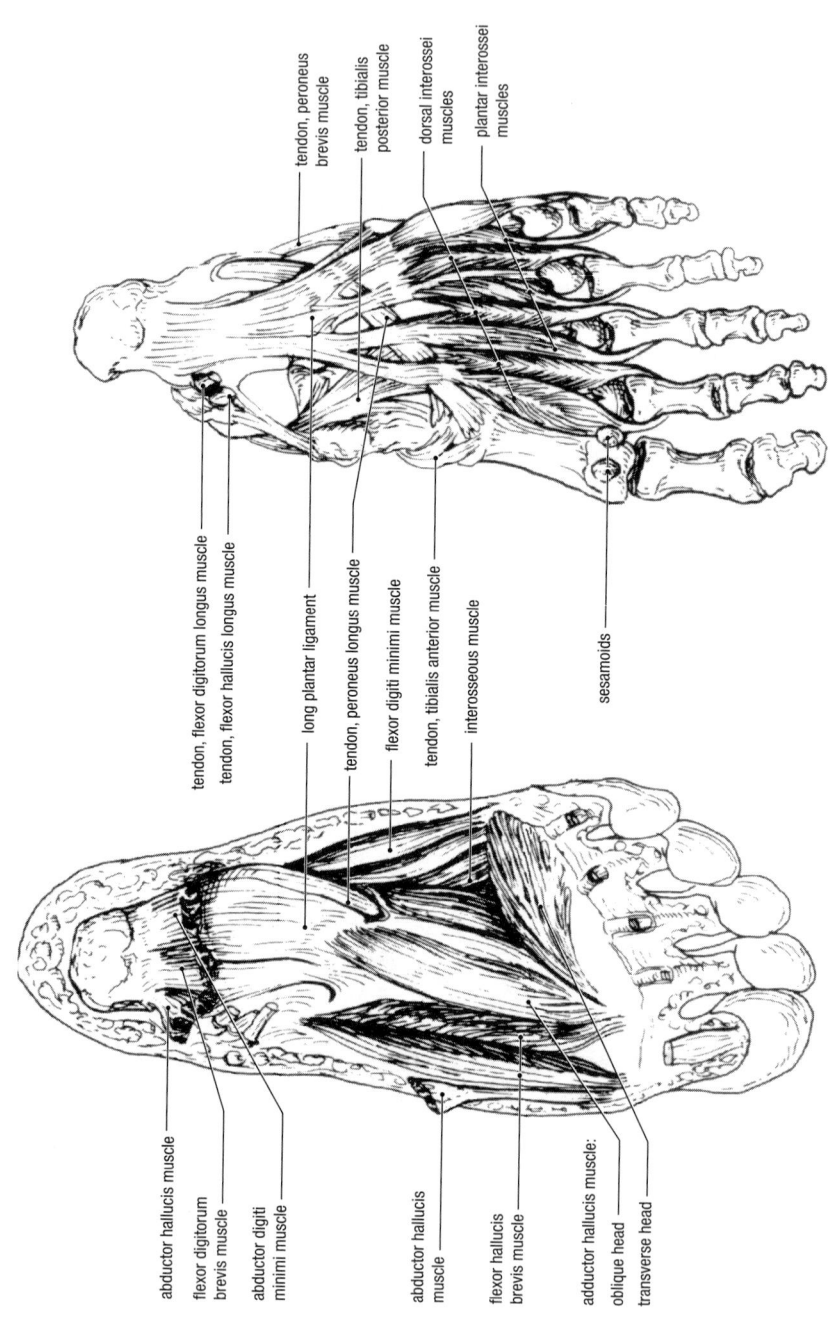

deep muscles of the plantar foot: (left) 3rd layer; (right) 4th layer with deep ligaments

tendon, peroneus brevis muscle

tendon, tibialis posterior muscle

dorsal interossei muscles

plantar interossei muscles

tendon, flexor digitorum longus muscle

tendon, flexor hallucis longus muscle

long plantar ligament

tendon, peroneus longus muscle

flexor digiti minimi muscle

tendon, tibialis anterior muscle

interosseous muscle

sesamoids

abductor hallucis muscle

flexor digitorum brevis muscle

abductor digiti minimi muscle

abductor hallucis muscle

flexor hallucis brevis muscle

adductor hallucis muscle:

oblique head

transverse head

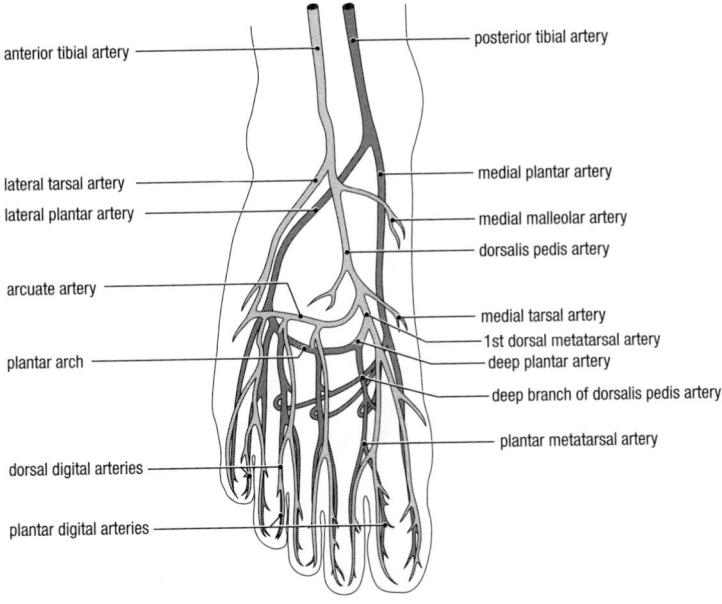

dorsum of the foot showing the arterial circulation

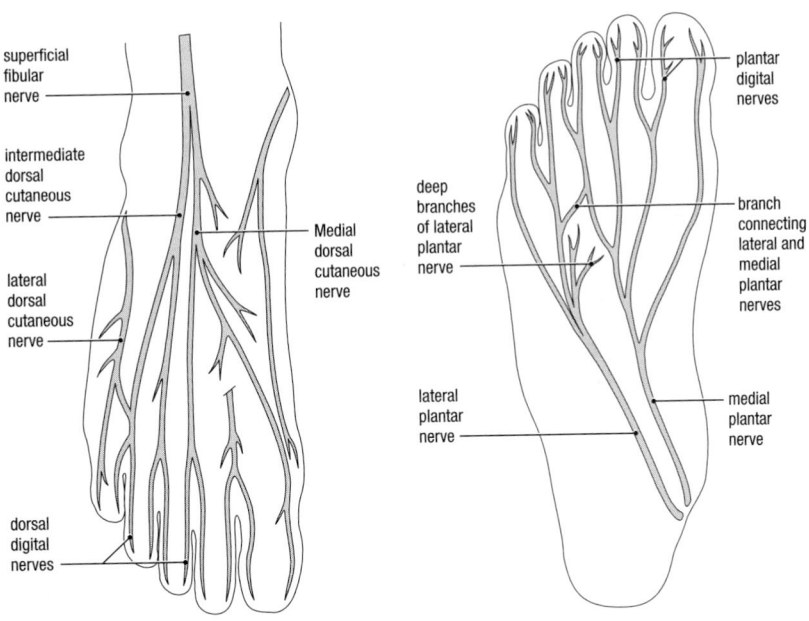

innervation of the foot: (left) dorsal view; (right) plantar view

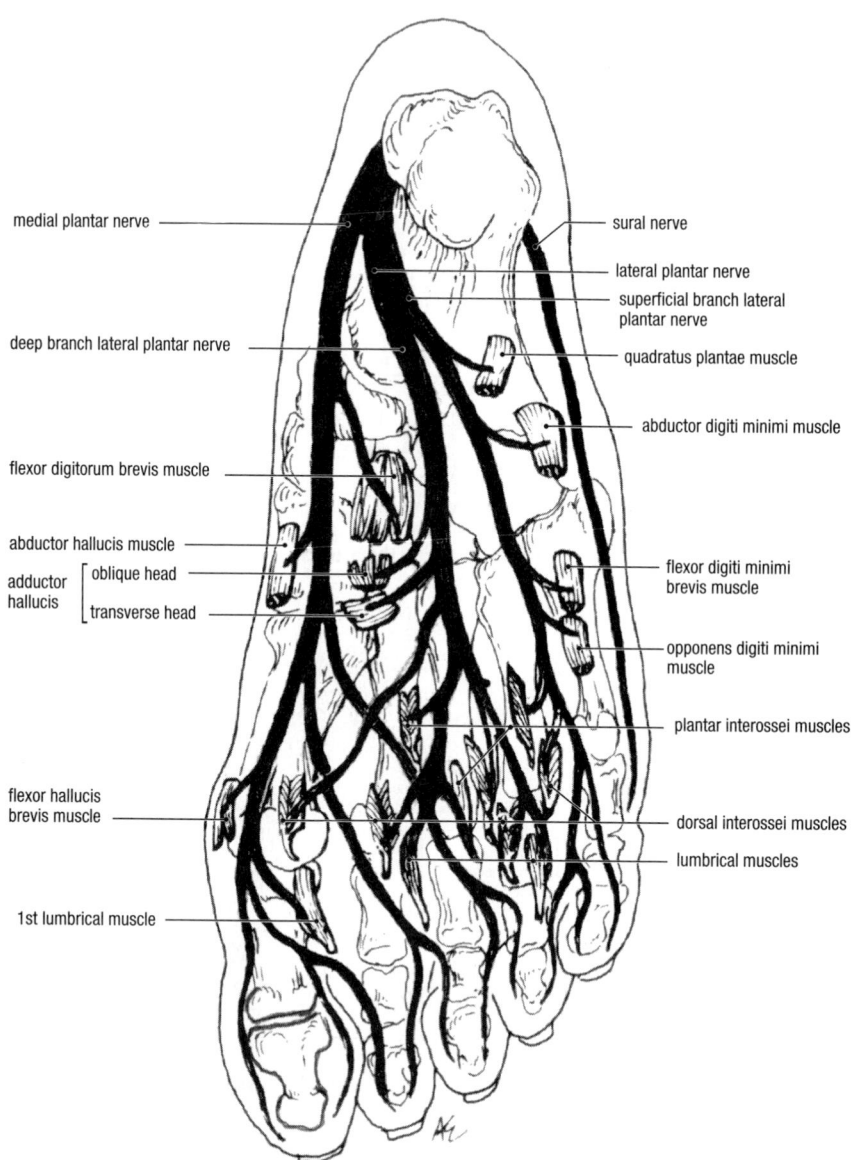

medial plantar nerve

sural nerve

lateral plantar nerve

superficial branch lateral
plantar nerve

deep branch lateral plantar nerve

quadratus plantae muscle

abductor digiti minimi muscle

flexor digitorum brevis muscle

abductor hallucis muscle

flexor digiti minimi
brevis muscle

adductor
hallucis ⎡ oblique head

opponens digiti minimi
muscle

⎣ transverse head

plantar interossei muscles

flexor hallucis
brevis muscle

dorsal interossei muscles

lumbrical muscles

1st lumbrical muscle

distribution of the tibial nerve in the foot

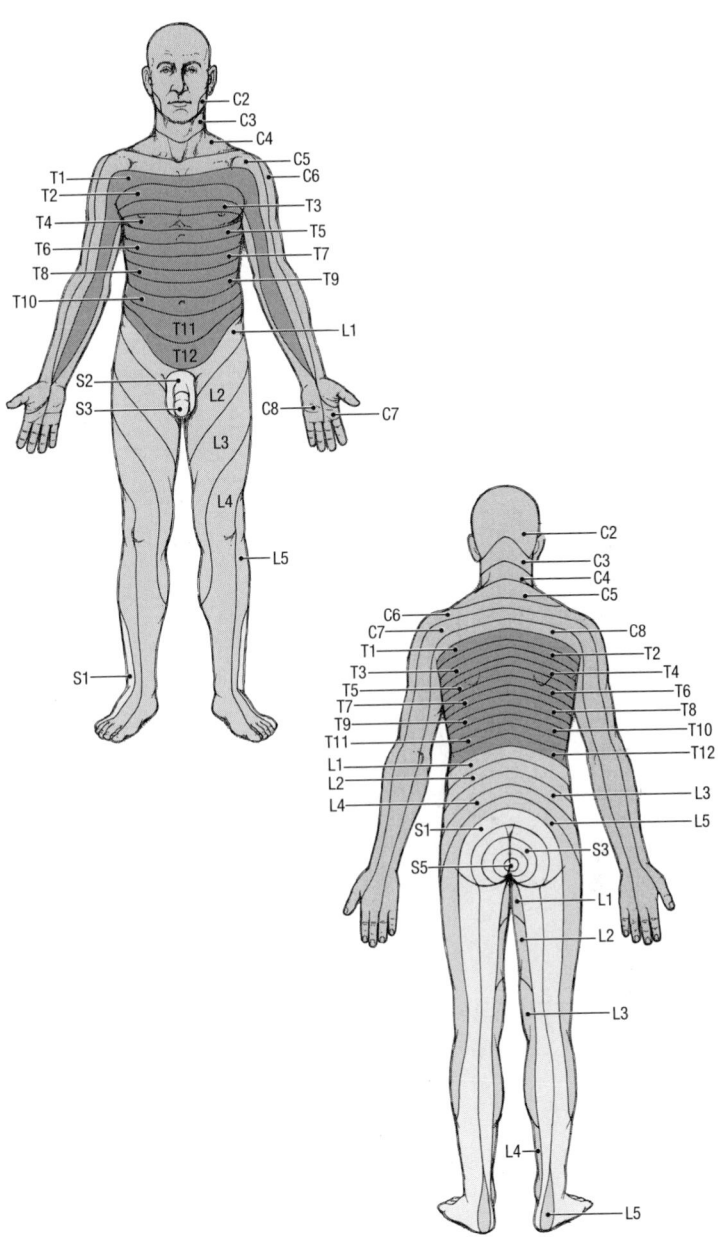

dermatomes

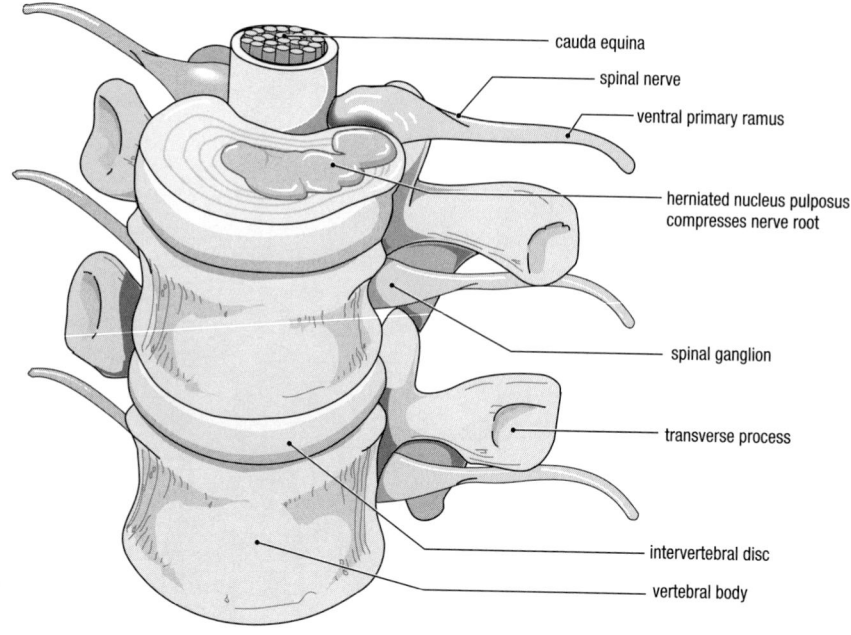

cauda equina

spinal nerve

ventral primary ramus

herniated nucleus pulposus
compresses nerve root

spinal ganglion

transverse process

intervertebral disc

vertebral body

anterosuperior view of portion of spinal column showing a herniation of the intervertebral disc

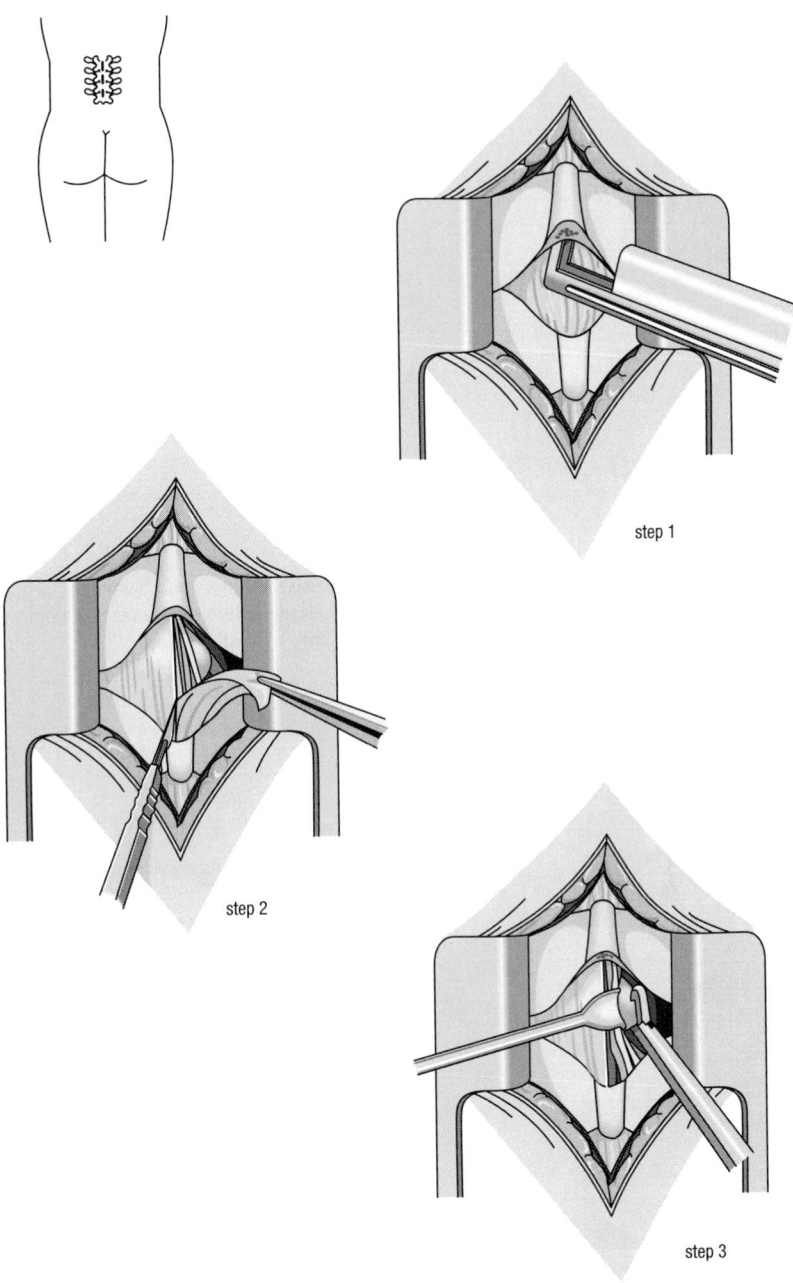

step 1

step 2

step 3

surgical procedure, shown in 3 steps, of the excision of an intervertebral disc during discectomy

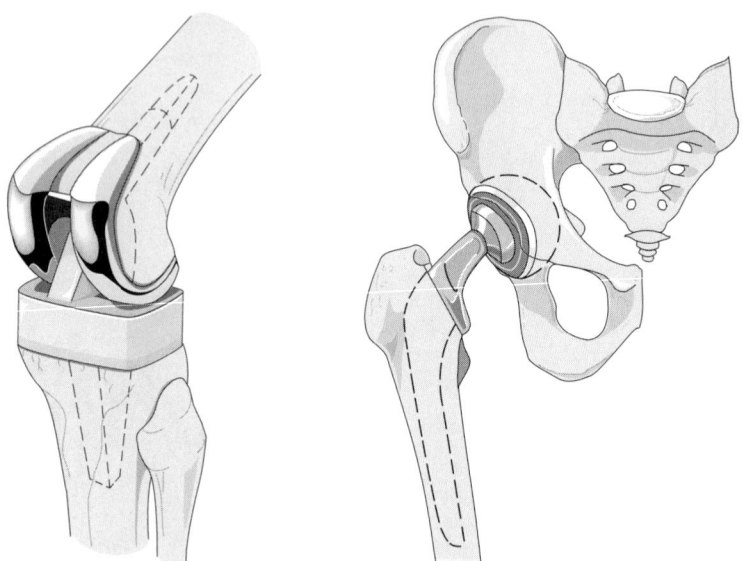

(left) anterolateral view of knee where bones that comprise the hinge joint have been replaced with a prosthetic knee; (right) anterior view of pelvic skeleton where the bones that comprise the ball and socket joint of the hip have been replaced with a prosthetic hip

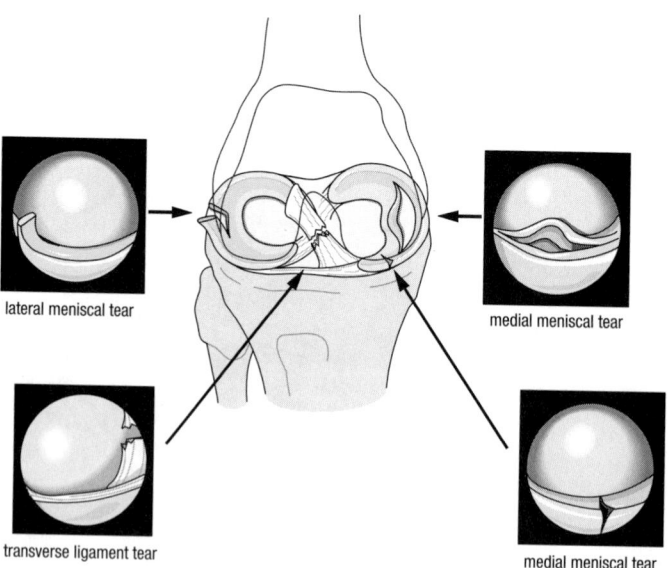

lateral meniscal tear

medial meniscal tear

transverse ligament tear

medial meniscal tear

anterior view of knee joint surrounded by arthroscopic views of tears

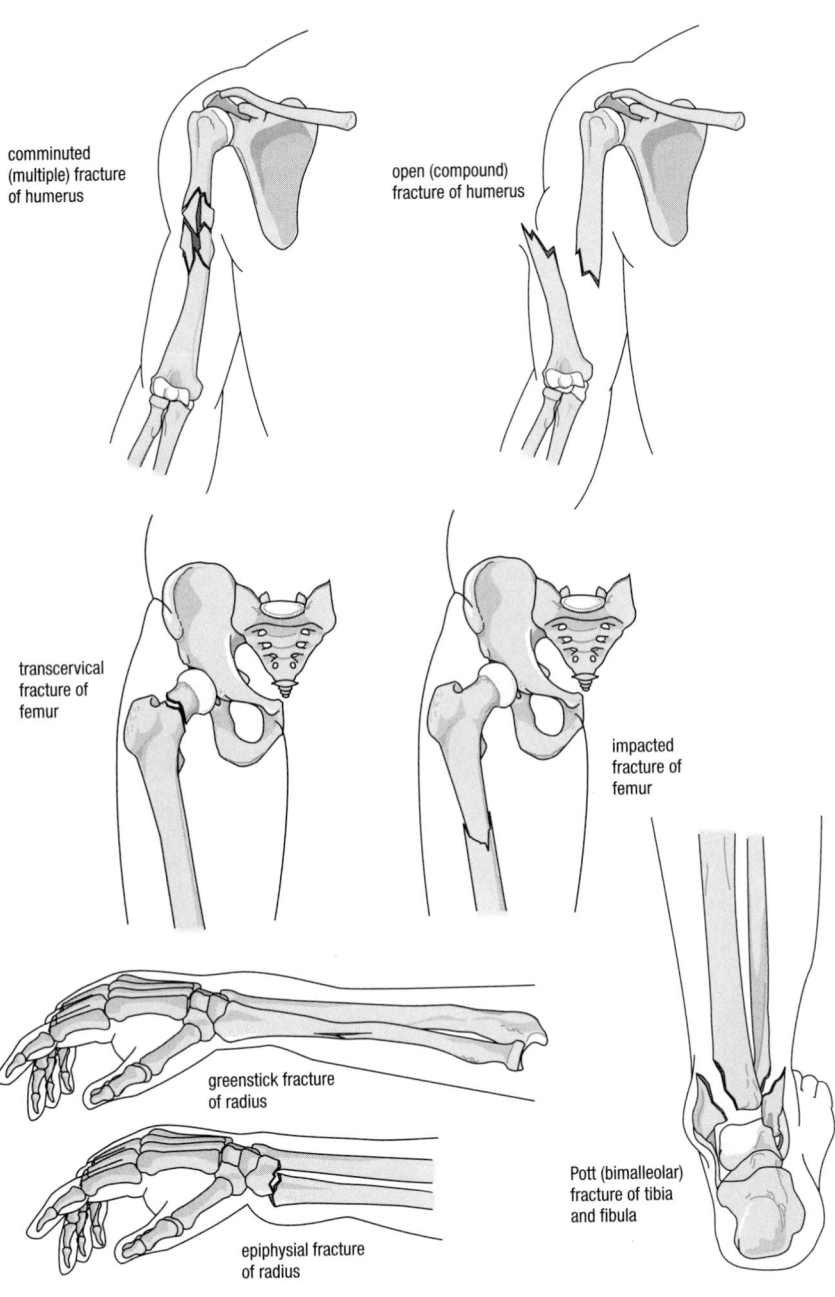

comminuted (multiple) fracture of humerus

open (compound) fracture of humerus

transcervical fracture of femur

impacted fracture of femur

greenstick fracture of radius

epiphysial fracture of radius

Pott (bimalleolar) fracture of tibia and fibula

types of fractures

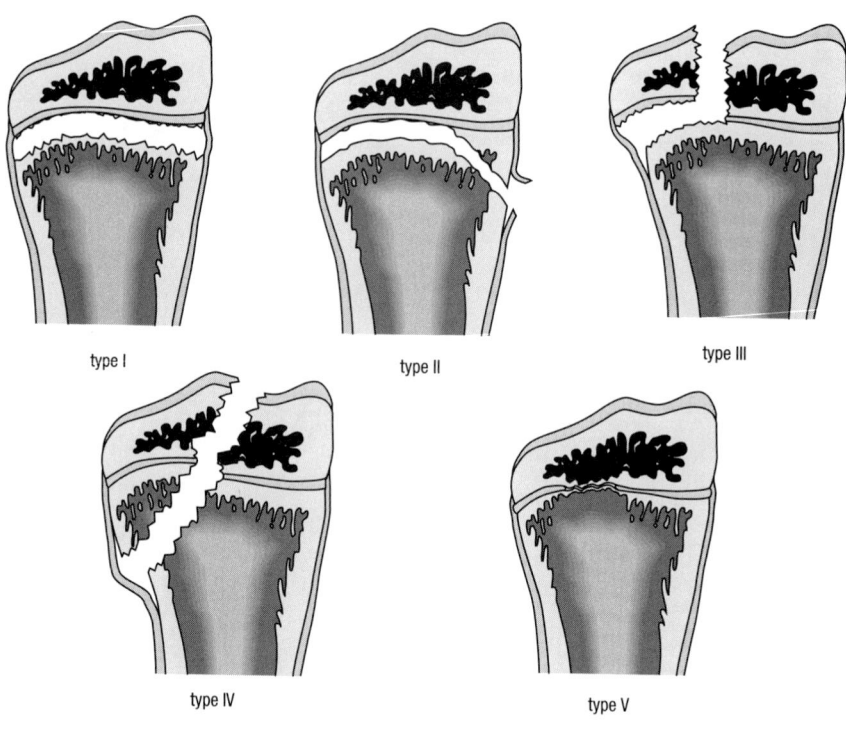

type I

type II

type III

type IV

type V

5 groups of the Salter-Harris classification of epiphysial plate injuries

direction of fracture lines

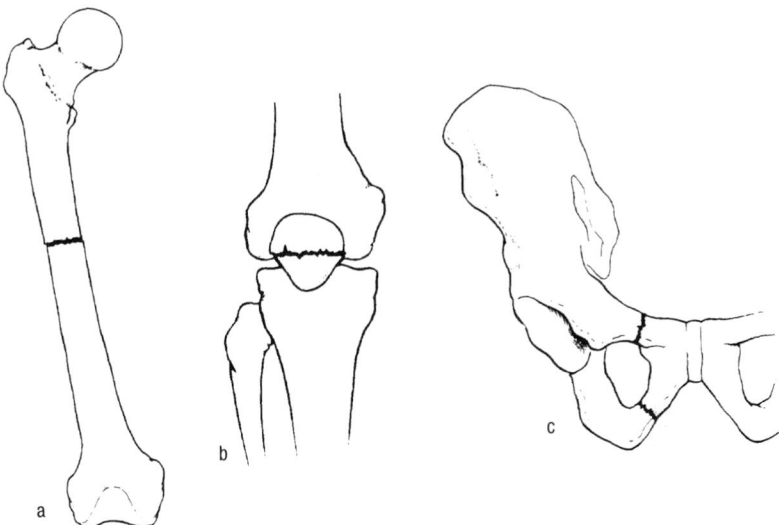

transverse fractures: (a) transverse fracture of the middle 3rd of femur; (b) transverse fracture of midpatella; (c) transverse fracture of superior and inferior pubic rami

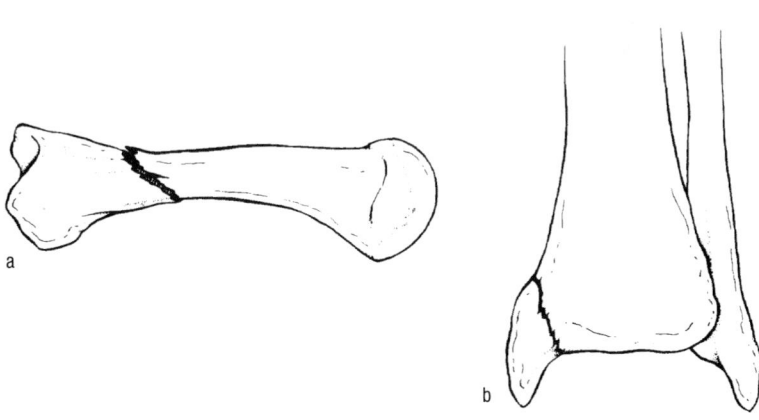

oblique fractures: (a) oblique fracture of proximal 3rd of metacarpal; (b) oblique fracture of medial malleolus

A57

spinal fractures

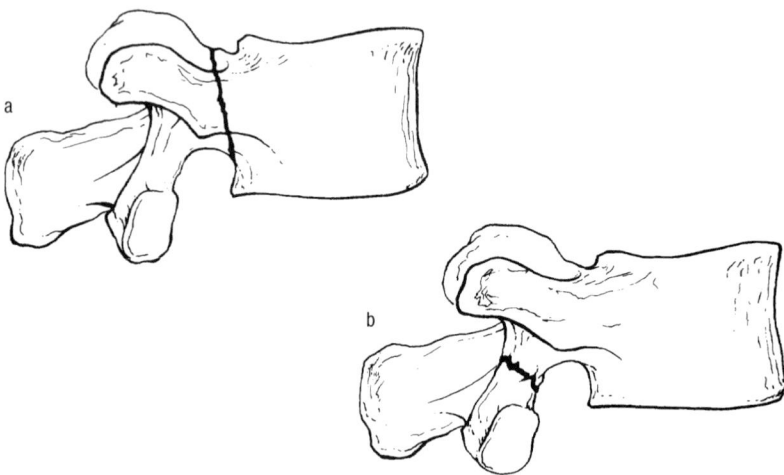

(a) fracture through the pedicle; (b) fracture through the pars interarticularis

shoulder fractures

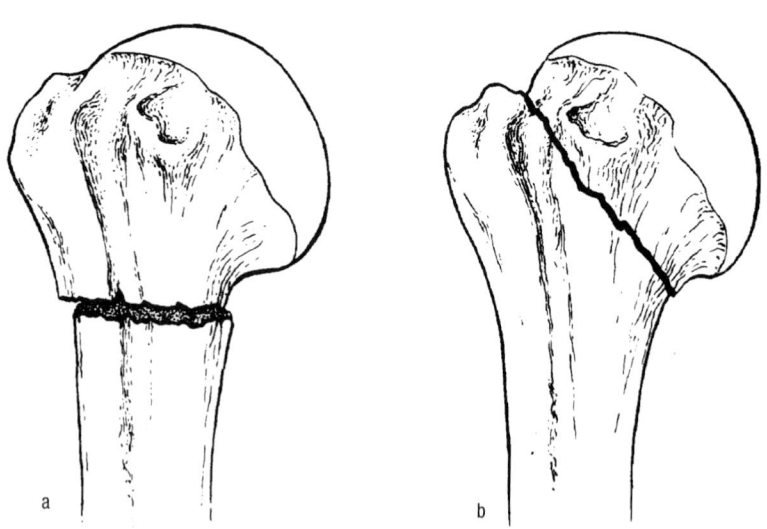

(a) transverse fracture of the surgical neck of the humerus; (b) fracture of the anatomic neck of the humerus

elbow fractures

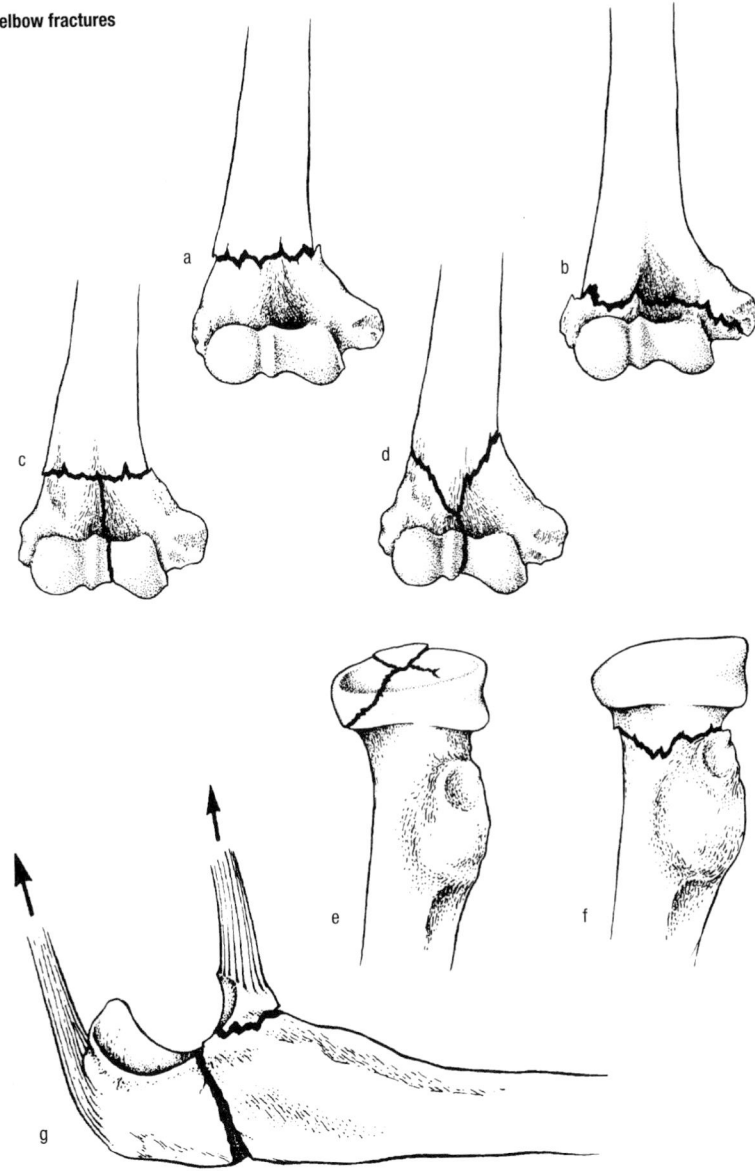

(a) supracondylar fractures are fractures that occur above the level of the condyles; (b) transcondylar fracture; note that the fracture extends through both condyles; (c) T-shaped fracture; (d) Y-shaped fracture; (e) comminuted fracture of the head of the radius; (f) transverse nondisplaced fracture of the neck of the radius; (g) fracture of the olecranon and coronoid process; muscle contraction can cause distraction of fracture fragments

pelvic fractures

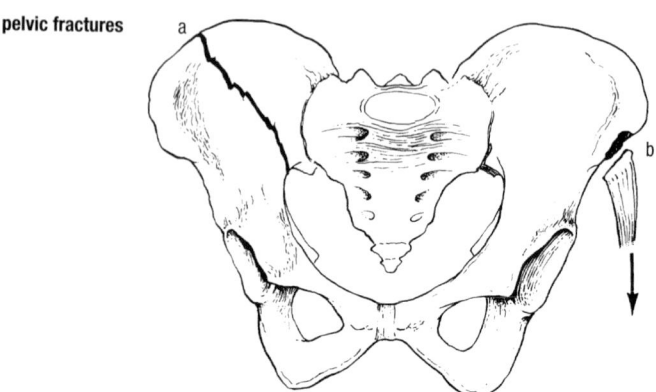

fractures of the ilium: (a) oblique fracture through the wing of the ilium; (b) avulsion fracture of the anteroinferior iliac spine

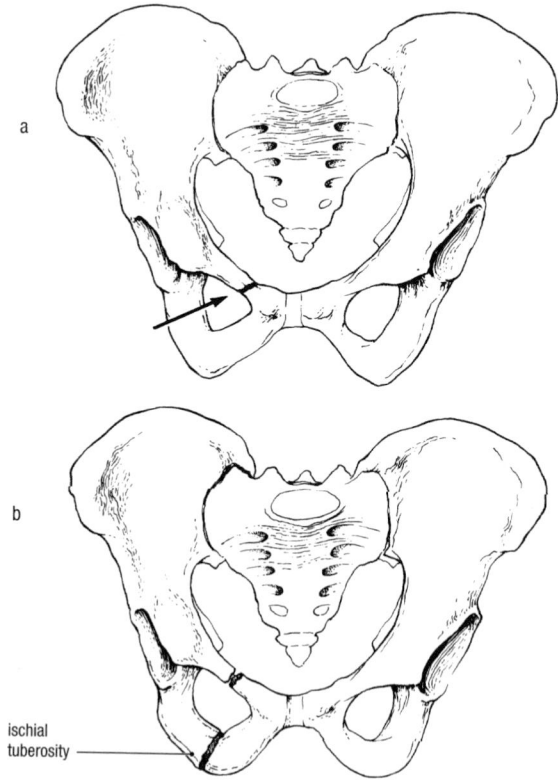

ischial
tuberosity

(a) oblique fracture of the superior pubic ramus; (b) transverse fractures of the inferior ischial ramus and superior pubic ramus

hip fractures

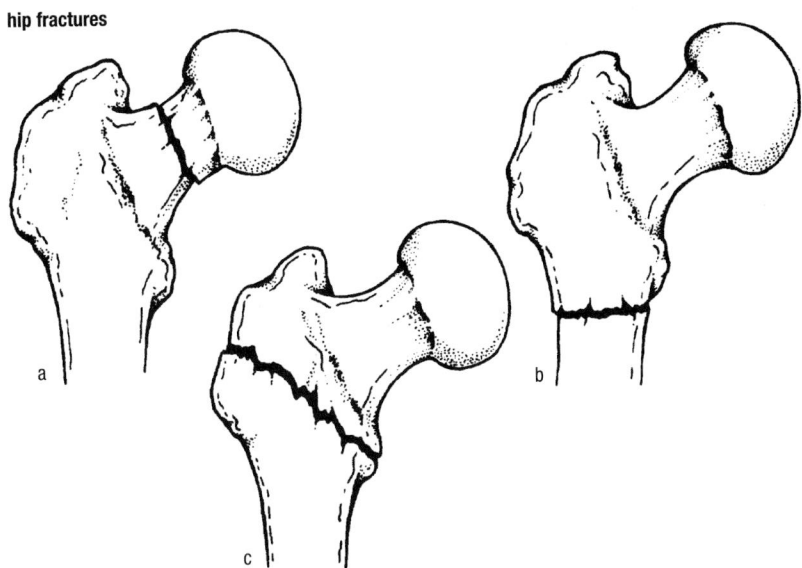

fractures of the hip are described by the location in which they occur: (a) transverse intracapsular fracture; (b) oblique intertrochanteric fracture; (c) transverse subtrochanteric fracture

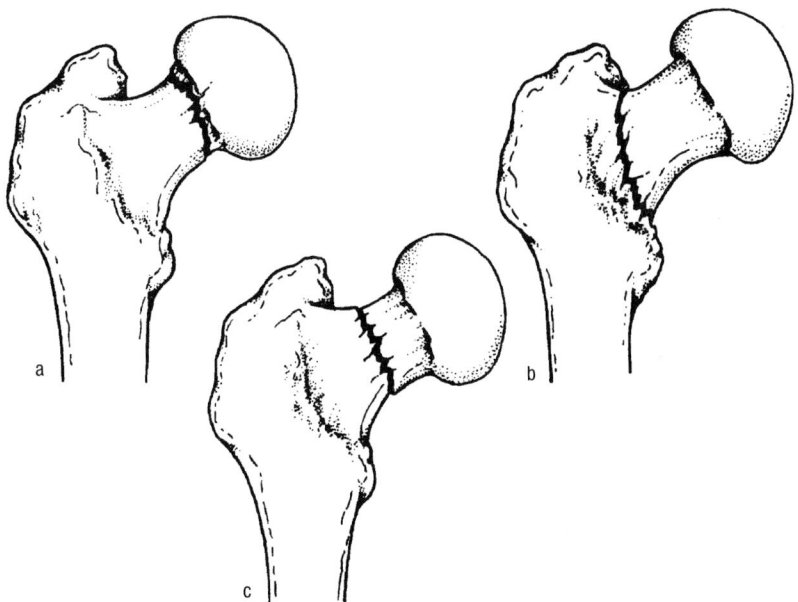

subclassification of intracapsular fractures: (a) subcapital fracture; (b) transcervical fracture; (c) base of neck fracture

knee fractures

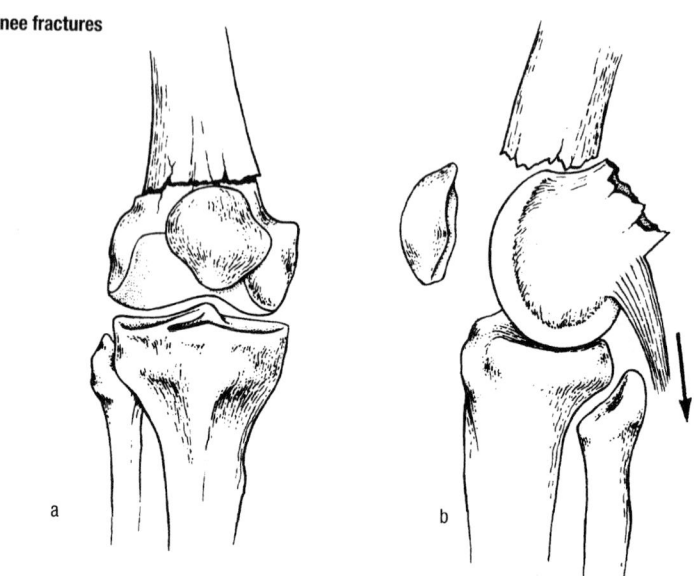

a   b

supracondylar fracture: transverse supracondylar fracture of the femur (note the pull of the gastrocnemius muscle, causing the distal fragment to be rotated posteriorly)

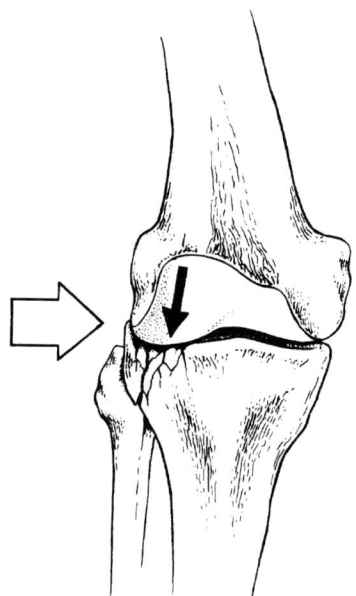

a valgus force applied to the knee causes the hard femoral condyle to be driven into the softer tibial plateau, resulting in depression of the tibial plateau

ankle fractures

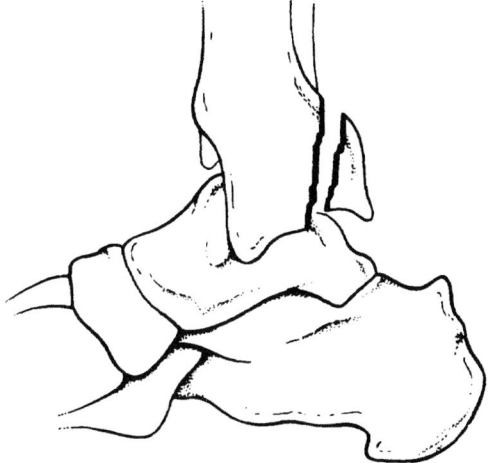

fracture of the posterior malleolus

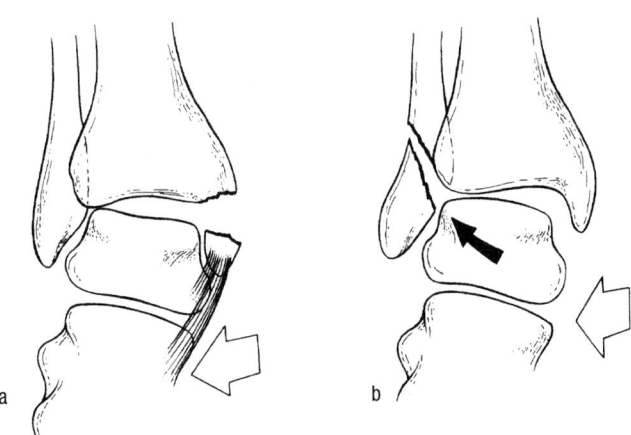

(a) avulsion fracture of the medial malleolus; (b) oblique fracture of the lateral malleolus

ankle fractures

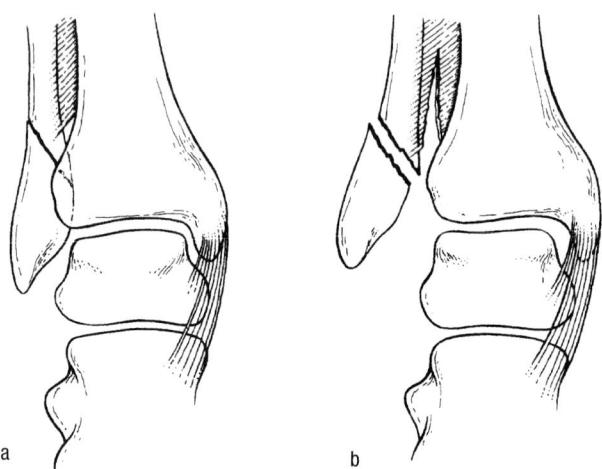

a   b

(a) fractures of the lateral malleolus occurring above its articular surface; thus, the ankle mortise is not involved; (b) similar fracture as in (a), above the articular surface with disturbance of the mortise due to separation of the syndesmosis

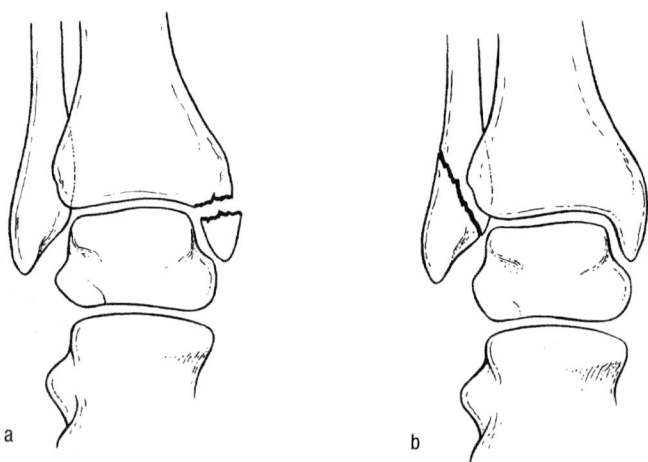

a   b

fractures of the malleoli: (a) transverse fracture of the medial malleolus; (b) oblique fracture of the lateral malleolus

ankle fractures

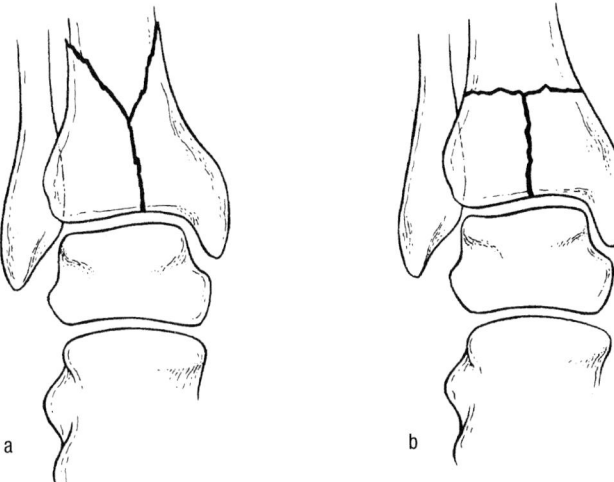

(a) Y-shaped comminuted intraarticular fracture of the distal tibia; (b) T-shaped comminuted intraarticular fracture of the distal tibia

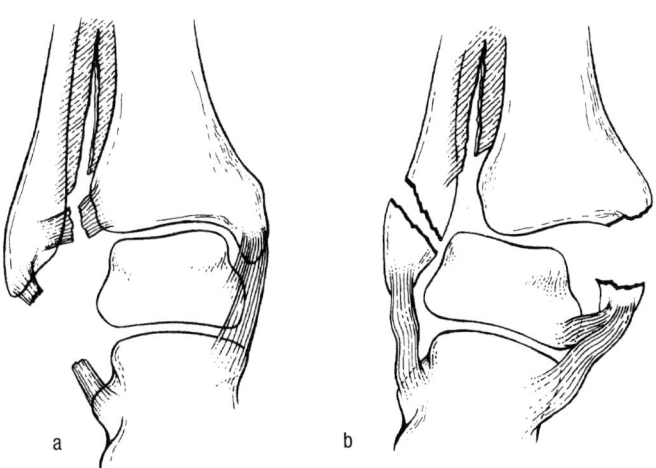

separation of the distal tibiofibular syndesmosis: (a) separation of the tibiofibular syndesmosis without an accompanying fracture; (b) separation of the syndesmosis associated with fracture of the medial and lateral malleoli

leg fractures

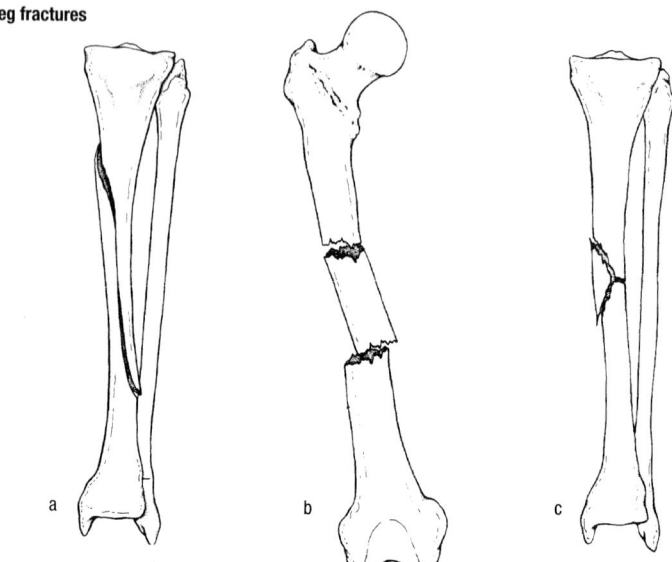

(a) spiral fractures of the middle third of the tibia; (b) segmental fracture of the femur; (c) butterfly fragment

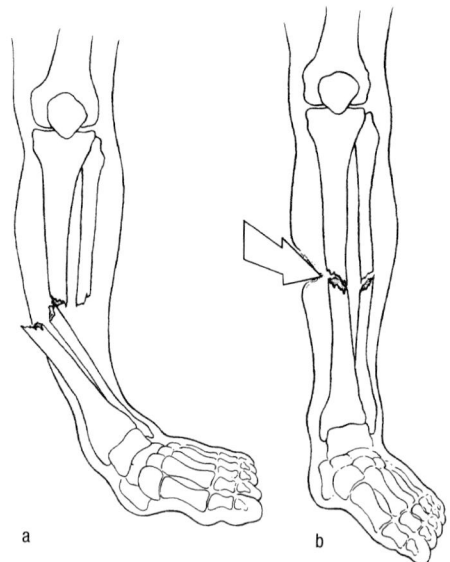

(a) compound fracture caused by an inside-out injury where the skin defect is caused, following the fracture, by the bone perforating the skin from within; (b) outside-in compound fracture where the skin defect is produced by the fracturing agent entering from without

foot fractures

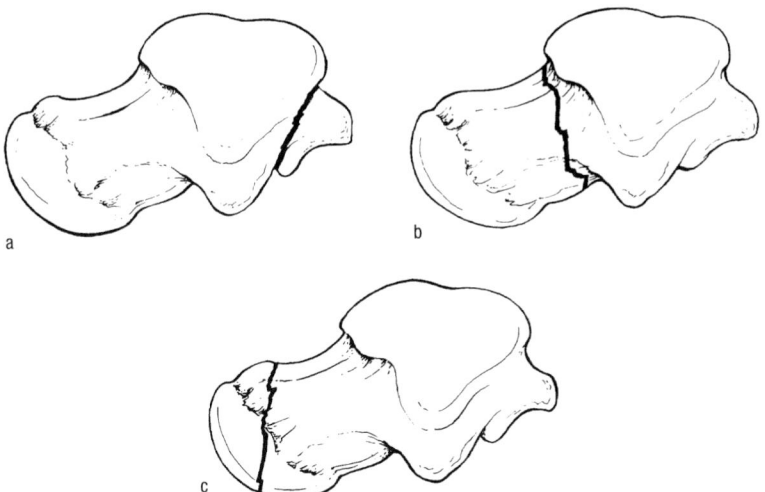

(a) fractures of the talus can be described by the anatomic area involved: (a) fracture of the posterior process; (b) fracture of the body; (c) fracture of the head

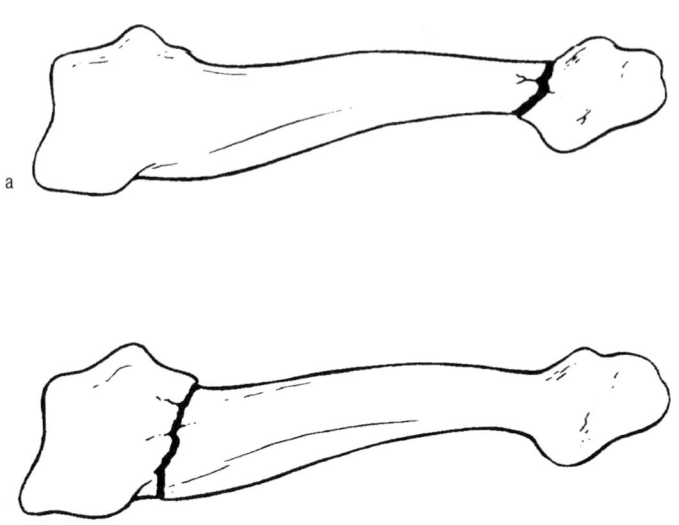

(a) fracture of the head of a metatarsal; (b) fracture of the base of a metatarsal

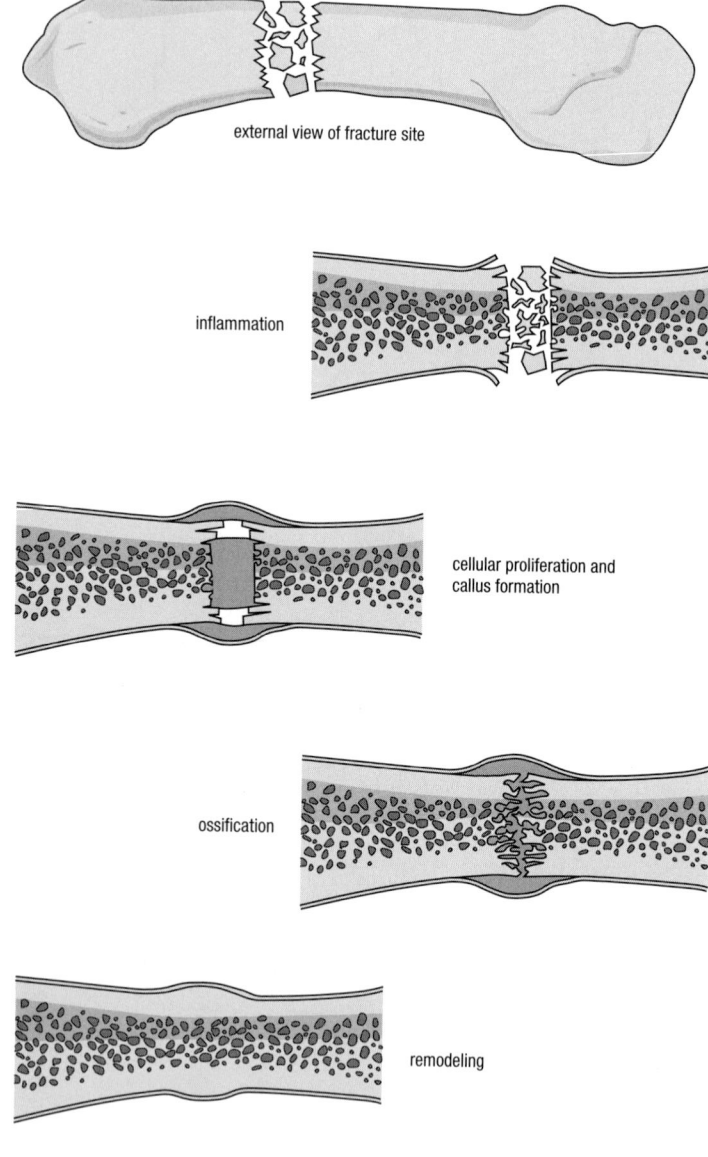

external view of fracture site

inflammation

cellular proliferation and
callus formation

ossification

remodeling

the process by which a bone fracture heals

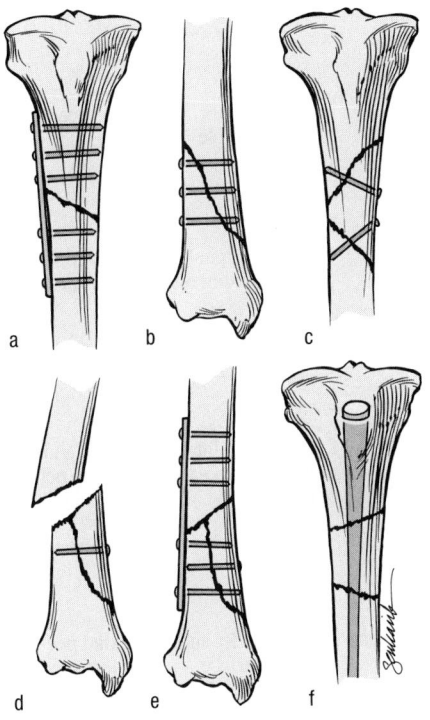

internal fixation: (a) plate and 6 screws for a transverse or short oblique fracture; (b) screws for a long oblique or spiral fracture; (c) screws for a long butterfly fragment; (d, e) plate and 6 screws for a short butterfly fragment; (f) medullary nail for a segmental fracture

Appendix 2
Muscles

Muscle	Origin	Insertion	Nerve	Action

1. Muscles of the Shoulder

Muscle	Origin	Insertion	Nerve	Action
Deltoid	Lateral one-third of clavicle, acromion, and spine of scapula	Deltoid tuberosity of humerus	Axillary, C5, C6	Abducts, adducts, flexes, extends, and rotates arm medially
Infra-spinatus	Infraspinous fossa of scapula	Middle facet of greater tubercle of humerus	Suprascapular, C5, C6	Rotates arm laterally; helps to hold humeral head in glenoid cavity of scapula
Latissimus dorsi	Spines of T7-T12 thoracolumbar fascia, iliac crest, ribs 9-12	Floor of bicipital groove of humerus	Thoracodorsal, C6, C7, C8	Extends, adducts, and medially rotates humerus; raises body towards arms during climbing
Pectoralis major	Clavicular head: anterior surface of medial half of clavicle	Lateral lip of inter-tubercular groove of humerus	Lateral and medial pectoral nerves; clavicular head C5 and C6, sternocostal head C7, C8, and T1	Abducts, medially rotates humerus; draws scapula anteriorly and inferiorly
Pectoralis minor	3rd to 5th ribs near the costal cartilages	Medial border and superior surface coracoid process of scapula	Medial pectoral nerve C8 and T1	Stabilizes scapula against thoracic wall
Subscapularis	Subscapular fossa	Lesser tubercle of humerus	Upper and lower subscapular, C5, C6, C7	Medially rotates arm and adducts it; helps to hold humeral head in glenoid cavity
Supraspinatus	Supraspinous fossa of scapula	Superior facet of greater tubercle of humerus	Suprascapular, C4, C5, C6	Initiates and assists deltoid in abduction of arm and acts with rotator cuff muscles

Muscle	Origin	Insertion	Nerve	Action
Teres minor	Superior portion of lateral border of scapula	Inferior facet of greater tubercle of humerus	Axillary, C5, C6	Laterally rotates arm; helps to hold humeral head in glenoid cavity of scapula
Teres major	Dorsal surface of inferior angle of scapula	Medial lip of intertubercular groove of humerus	Lower subscapular, C6, C7	Adducts and rotates arm medially

2. Muscles of the Arm

Muscle	Origin	Insertion	Nerve	Action
Anconeus	Lateral epicondyle of humerus	Lateral surface of olecranon and superior part of posterior surface of ulna	Radial, C7, C8, and T1	Assists triceps in extending forearm abducts ulna during pronation
Biceps brachii	Long head, supraglenoid tubercle; short head, coracoid process	Radial tuberosity of radius	Musculocutaneous, C5, C6	Flexes arm and forearm, supinates forearm
Brachialis	Distal anterior surface of humerus	Coronoid process of ulna and ulnar tuberosity	Musculocutaneous, C5, C6	Flexes forearm in all positions
Coraco-brachialis	Tip of coracoid process of scapula	Middle one-third of medial surface of humerus	Musculocutaneous, C5, C6, C7	Flexes and adducts arm
Triceps	Long head, infraglenoid tubercle; lateral head, superior to radial groove of humerus; medial head to radial groove	Posterior surface of olecranon process of ulna	Radial, C6, C7, C8	Chief extensor of forearm at elbow

3. Muscles of the Anterior Forearm

Muscle	Origin	Insertion	Nerve	Action
Flexor carpi radialis	Medial epicondyle of humerus	Bases of 2nd and 3rd metacarpals	Median, C6, C7	Flexes forearm; flexes and abducts hand
Flexor digitorum profundus	Anteromedial surface of ulna, interosseous membrane	Base of distal phalanges of medial 4 fingers	Ulnar and median, C8, T1	Flexes distal interphalangeal joints and hand
Flexor carpi ulnaris	Humeral head medial epicondyle of humerus; ulnar head; olecranon and posterior border of ulna	Pisiform bone, hook of hamate, and base of 5th metacarpal	Ulnar, C7, C8	Flexes and adducts hand, flexes forearm

Muscle	Origin	Insertion	Nerve	Action
Flexor digitorum superficialis	Medial epicondyle, coronoid process of ulna, superior anterior border of radius	Middle phalanges of finger	Median, C7, C8, T1	Flexes proximal interphalangeal joints; flexes hand at wrist
Flexor pollicis longus	Anterior surface of radius, interosseous membrane, and coracoid process	Base of distal phalanx of thumb	Median, C8, T1	Flexes thumb
Palmaris longus	Medial epicondyle of humerus	Distal half of flexor retinaculum, palmar aponeurosis	Median, C7, C8	Flexes hand at wrist and forearm
Pronator quadratus	Anterior surface of distal ulna	Anterior surface of distal radius	Anterior interosseous nerve from median, C8, and T1	Pronates forearm; helps hold radius and ulna together
Pronator teres	Medial epicondyle of humerus and coracoid process of ulna	Middle of lateral surface of radius	Median, C6, C7	Pronates and flexes arm at elbow

4. Muscles of the Posterior Forearm

Muscle	Origin	Insertion	Nerve	Action
Abductor pollicis longus	Interosseous membrane, middle 3rd of posterior surface of radius and ulna	Lateral surface of base of 1st metacarpal	Radial, deep branch, posterior interosseous nerve C7, C8	Abducts thumb and hand
Articularis cubiti	Distal portion of posterior aspect of shaft of humerus	Posterior fibrous capsule of elbow joint	Radial, C7, C8	Retracts posterior joint capsule during extension of elbow
Brachioradialis	Lateral supracondylar ridge of humerus	Base of radial styloid process	Radial, C5, C6, C7	Flexes forearm
Extensor digitorum	Lateral epicondyle of humerus	Extensor expansion, base of middle and digital phalanges	Radial, deep branch, posterior interosseous nerve C7, C8	Extends fingers and hand at wrist
Extensor digiti minimi	Common extensor tendon and interosseous membrane	Extensor expansion, base of middle and distal phalanges	Radial, deep branch, posterior interosseous nerve C7, C8	Extends little finger
Extensor carpi radialis brevis	Lateral epicondyle of humerus	Posterior base of 3rd metacarpal	Radial, deep branch, C7, C8	Extends fingers and abducts hands at wrist

Muscle	Origin	Insertion	Nerve	Action
Extensor carpi radialis longus	Lateral supracon-dylar ridge of humerus	Dorsum of base of 2nd metacarpal	Radial, C6, C7	Extends and abducts hand at wrist and joint
Extensor carpi ulnaris	Lateral epicondyle and posterior surface of ulna	Base of 5th metacarpal	Radial, deep branch, posterior interosseous nerve C7, C8	Extends and adducts hand at wrist joint
Extensor pollicis longus	Interosseous membrane, middle one-third of posterior surface of ulna	Base of distal phalanx of thumb	Radial, deep branch, posterior interosseous nerve C7, C8	Extends distal phalanx of thumb and abducts hand
Extensor pollicis brevis	Interosseous membrane and posterior surface of middle 3rd of radius	Base of proximal phalanx of thumb	Radial, deep branch, posterior interosseous nerve C7, C8	Extends proximal phalanx of thumb and abducts hand
Extensor indicis	Posterior surface of ulna and inter-osseous membrane	Extensor expansion of index finger	Radial, deep branch, posterior interosseous nerve C7	Extends index finger, helps extend hand
Supinator	Lateral epicondyle of humerus, radial collateral and annular ligaments, crest of ulna	Lateral side of upper part of radius	Radial, deep branch, C5, C6	Supinates forearm

5. Muscles of the Hand

Muscle	Origin	Insertion	Nerve	Action
Abductor digiti minimi	Pisiform, piso-hamate ligament, flexor retinaculum	Medial side of base of proximal phalanx of little finger	Ulnar, deep, branch C8, T1	Abducts little finger
Abductor pollicis brevis	Flexor retinaculum, scaphoid, and trapezium	Lateral side of base of proximal phalanx of thumb	Median, recurrent branch, C8, T1	Abducts thumb
Adductor pollicis	Capitate and bases of 2nd and 3rd metacarpals, (oblique head); palmar surface of 3rd metacarpal (transverse head)	Medial side of base of proximal phalanx of the thumb	Ulnar, deep branch, C8, T1	Adducts thumb towards middle digit
Dorsal interossei (4)	Adjacent sides of metacarpal bones	Extensor expansions and bases of pha-langes of digits 2-4	Ulnar, deep branch, C8, T1	Abducts fingers; flexes metacarpo-phalangeal joints; extends interpha langeal joints

Muscle	Origin	Insertion	Nerve	Action
Flexor digiti minimi brevis	Flexor retinaculumand hook of hamate	Medial side of base of proximal phalanx of little finger	Ulnar, deep branch, C8, T1	Flexes proximal phalanx of little finger
Flexor pollicis brevis	Flexor retinaculum and trapezium	Base of proximal phalanx of thumb	Median, recurrent branch, C8, T1	Flexes thumb
Lumbricals (4)	1-2 lateral, 3-4 medial side of tendons of flexor digitorum profundus	Lateral side of extensor expansion	Median (two lateral), ulnar (two medial)	Flexes metacarpophalangeal joints, extends interphalangeal joints
Opponens digiti minimi	Flexor retinaculum and hook of hamate	Medial side of 5th metacarpal	Ulnar, deep branch, C8, T1	Opposes little finger with thumb
Opponents pollicis	Flexor retinaculum and tubercles of scaphoid and trapezium	Lateral side of 1st metacarpal	Median, recurrent branch, C8, T1	Opposes thumb to other digits
Palmar interossei (3)	Palmar surfaces of 2nd, 4th, and 5th metacarpals (unipennate muscles)	Bases of proximal phalanges in same sides as their origins; extensor expansion	Ulnar, deep branch, C8, T1	Adducts fingers; flexes metacarpophalangeal joints; extends interphalangeal joints
Palmaris brevis	Ulnar side of flexor retinaculum, palmar aponeurosis	Skin of ulnar side of hand	Ulnar, superficial, T1	Wrinkles skin on palmar side of hand

6. Anterior Muscles of the Thigh

Muscle	Origin	Insertion	Nerve	Action
Abductor brevis/minimus	Inferior pubic ramus	Pectineal line; uppermost linea aspera of femur	Obturator, L2, L3, L4	Adducts, flexes, rotates thigh
Abductor longus	Body of pubis below its crest	Middle one-third of linea aspera of femur	Obturator, branch of anterior division, L2, L3, L4	Adducts, flexes, rotates thigh laterally
Adductor magnus	Ischiopubic ramus; ischial tuberosity	Linea aspera; medial supra-condylar line; adductor tubercle	Obturator, L2, L3, L4; sciatic L4	Adducts, flexes, rotates, and extends thigh
Gracilis	Body and inferior ramus of pubis	Superior part of medial surface of tibia	Obturator, L2, L3	Adducts and flexes thigh; flexes and rotates leg medially

Muscle	Origin	Insertion	Nerve	Action
Iliacus	Iliac crest, iliac fossa; ala of sacrum	Lesser trochanter, psoas major tendon	Femoral, L2, L4	Flexes and rotates thigh medially with psoas major
Obturator externus	Margin of obturator foramen and obturator membrane	Trochanteric fossa of femur	Obturator, L3, L4	Rotates thigh laterally
Pectineus	Pectineal line of pubis	Pectineal line of femur	Femoral, L3, L4; obturator	Adducts and flexes thigh; helps with rotation
Rectus femoris	Anterior-inferior iliac spine; ilium rim of acetabulum	Base of patella; tibial tuberosity	Femoral, L2, L3, L4	Extends leg at knee joint; stabilizes hip; helps iliopsoas flex thigh
Sartorius	Anterior-superior iliac spine, superior part of notch inferior to it	Upper medial side of tibia	Femoral, L2, L3	Flexes, abducts, rotates thigh at hip laterally; flexes, rotates leg at knee joint
Vastus intermedius	Upper shaft of femur; lower lateral intermuscular septum	Base of patella; by patellar ligament to tibial tuberosity	Femoral	Extends leg at knee joint
Vastus lateralis	Intertrochanteric line; greater trochanter; linea aspera; gluteal tuberosity; lateral intermuscular septum	Lateral side of patella; tibial tuberosity	Femoral, L2, L3, L4	Extends leg at knee joint
Vastus medialis	Intertrochanteric line; linea aspera; medial intermuscular septum	Medial side of patella; tibial tuberosity	Femoral, L2, L3, L4	Extends leg at knee joint

7. Medial Muscles of the Thigh

Muscle	Origin	Insertion	Nerve	Action
Abductor brevis	Body and inferior ramus of pubis	Pectineal line and proximal part of linea aspera of femur	Obturator, L2, L3, L4	Adducts thigh; aids in flexion
Adductor longus	Body of pubis inferior to pubic crest	Middle one third of linea aspera of femur	Obturator, L2, L3, L4	Adducts thigh
Adductor magnus	Ischiopubic ramus; ischial tuberosity	Linea aspera; medial supra-condylar line; adductor tubercle	Obturator and sciatic	Adducts, flexes, and extends thigh

Muscle	Origin	Insertion	Nerve	Action
Gracilis	Body of inferior pubic of ramus	Superior part of medial surface of tibia	Obturator, L2, L3	Adducts thigh; flexes leg; helps rotate thigh medially
Obturator externus	Margin of obturator foramen and obturator membrane	Trochanteric fossa of femur	Obturator, L3, L4	Laterally rotates thigh; steadies head of femur in acetabulum
Pectineus	Pectineal line of pubis	Pectineal line of femur	Femoral, L2 and L3; branch of obturator	Adducts and flexes thigh; aids in medial rotation of thigh

8. Muscles of the Gluteal Region

Muscle	Origin	Insertion	Nerve	Action
Coccygeus (ischio-coccygeus)	Ischial spine	Inferior end of spine	Branches of S4 and S5 nerves	Forms small part of pelvic diaphragm that supports pelvic viscera and flexes coccyx
Gluteus maximus	Ilium; sacrum; coccyx; sacro-tuberous ligament	Gluteal tuberosity; iliotibial tract	Inferior gluteal, L5, S1, S2	Extends and rotates thigh laterally
Gluteus medius	Ilium between iliac crest and anterior and posterior gluteal lines	Greater trochanter	Superior gluteal, L5, S1	Abducts and rotates thigh medially; helps keep pelvis level
Gluteus minimus	Ilium between anterior and posterior gluteal lines	Greater trochanter	Superior gluteal, L5, S1	Abducts and rotates thigh medially; helps keep pelvis level
Inferior gemellus	Ischial tuberosity	Obturator internus tendon	Nerve to quadratus femoris	Rotates thigh laterally
Obturator internus	Ischiopubic rami; obturator membrane	Greater trochanter	Nerve to obturator internus, L5, S1	Abducts and rotates thigh laterally
Piriformis	Pelvic surface of sacrum; sacrotub-erous ligament	Superior border of greater trochanter	Sacral, S1, S2	Rotates thigh medially
Quadratus femoris	Ischial tuberosity crest	Inter-trochanteric	Nerve to quadratus femoral, L5, S1	Rotates thigh laterally

Muscle	Origin	Insertion	Nerve	Action

9. Posterior Muscles of the Thigh *

Biceps femoris	Long head from ischial tuberosity; short head from linea aspera and upper supra-condylar line	Lateral side of head of fibula; tendon split here by fibular collateral ligament of knee	Tibial (long head), common peroneal; division of sciatic nerve, L5, S1, S2	Flexes leg medially; extends thigh
Semimembra-nosus	Ischial tuberosity	Medial condyle of tibia	Tibial portion of sciatic, L5, S1, S2	Extends thigh; rotates leg medially; helps raise trunk of body against gravity
Semitendinosus	Ischial tuberosity	Medial surface of superior part of tibia	Tibial division of sciatic nerve, L5, S1, S2	Extends thigh; flexes leg; rotates knee medially when flexed

* These 3 muscles collectively are called hamstrings.

10. Muscles of the Anterior and Lateral Leg

Anterior				
Articularis genus	Distal portion of anterior aspect of shaft of femur	Synovial membrane of supra-patellar bursa of knee joint	Femoral, L2-L4	Retracts synovial membrane during extension of the knee
Tibialis anterior	Lateral tibial condyle; inter-osseous membrane	1st cuneiform; 1st metatarsal	Deep peroneal, L4, L5	Dorsiflexes and inverts foot
Extensor hallucis longus	Middle one-half of anterior surface of fibula; interosseous membrane	Base of distal phalanx of great toe	Deep peroneal, L5, S1	Extends great toe; dorsiflexes and inverts foot
Extensor digitorum longus	Lateral tibial condyle; upper two thirds of fibula	Bases of middle and distal phalanges	Deep peroneal, L5, S1	Extends great toe and dorsiflexes ankle
Peroneus tertius	Distal one third of fibula; interosseous membrane	Base of 5th metatarsal	Deep peroneal	Dorsiflexes and inverts foot
Lateral				
Peroneus brevis	Lower lateral side of fibula; inter-osseous membrane	Base of 5th metatarsal	Superficial peroneal	Everts and plantar flexes foot

Muscles

A77

Muscle	Origin	Insertion	Nerve	Action
Peroneus longus	Lateral tibial condyle; head and upper lateral side of fibula	Base of 1st metatarsal; medial cuneiform	Superficial peroneal	Everts and plantar flexes foot

11. Posterior Muscles of the Leg

Superficial group

Muscle	Origin	Insertion	Nerve	Action
Gastrocnemius	Lateral (head) and medial (head) femoral condyle	Posterior aspect of alcaneus via tendo calcaneus	Tibial, S2, S2	Flexes knee; plantar flexes ankle when knee extended
Soleus	Upper fibular head; soleal line on tibia	Posterior aspect of calcaneus via tendo calcaneus	Tibial, S1, S2	Plantar flexes foot and ankle
Plantaris	Lower lateral supracondylar lineand oblique popliteal ligament	Posterior surface of calcaneus	Tibial, S1, S2	Assist gastrocnemius in plantar flexing ankle and flexing knee

Deep group

Muscle	Origin	Insertion	Nerve	Action
Popliteus	Lateral surface of lateral condyle of femur and lateral meniscus	Posterior surface of tibia, superior to soleal line	Tibial, L4, L5, S1	Weakly flexes knee and unlocks knee
Flexor hallucis longus	Inferior two thirds of posterior surface of fibula and interior part of interosseous membrane	Base of distal phalanx of great toe	Tibial, S2, S3	Flexes great toe at all joints; weakly plantar flexes ankle supports medial longitudinal arches of foot
Flexor digitorum longus	Medial portion of posterior surface of tibia inferior to soleal line	Base of distal phalanges of lateral 4 digits	Tibial, S2, S3	Flexes lateral 4 digits; plantar flexes ankle; supports arches of foot
Tibialis posterior	Interosseous membrane; posterior surface of tibia inferior to soleal line; posterior surface of fibula	Tuberosity of navicular cuneiform and cuboid; base of 2-4 metatarsals	Tibial, L4, L5	Plantar flexes ankle; inverts foot

Muscle	Origin	Insertion	Nerve	Action

12. Muscles of the Foot

Dorsum of foot

Muscle	Origin	Insertion	Nerve	Action
Extensor digitorum brevis	Dorsal surface of calcaneus	Lateral side of long extensor tendons with slips to proximal phalanges 2-4 toes	Deep peroneal, L5, S1	Assist in extending middle 3 toes
Extensor hallucis brevis	Dorsal surface of calcaneus	Base of proximal phalanx of great toe	Deep peroneal, L5, S1	Extends great toe

Sole of foot

Muscle	Origin	Insertion	Nerve	Action
Abductor digit minimi	Medial and lateral tubercles of calcaneus, plantar aponeurosis and intermuscular septa	Lateral side of base of proximal phalanx of 5th digit	Lateral plantar, S2, S3	Abducts and flexes 5th digit
Abductor hallucis	Medial tubercle of calcaneus; flexor retinaculum and plantar aponeurosis	Medial side of base of proximal phalanx of 1st digit	Medial plantar, S2, S3	Abducts and flexes great toe
Adductor hallucis; oblique head	Base of metatarsals 2-4	Proximal phalanx of great toe	Deep branch of lateral plantar, S2, S3	Adducts great toe; assists in maintaining transverse arch
Adductor hallucis; transverse head	Capsule of lateral 4 metatarsophalangeal joints	Tendon of head attached to lateral sides of base of proximal phalanx of 1st digit	Deep branch of plantar, S2, S3	Adducts great toe; assists in maintaining transverse arch
Dorsal interossei (4)	Adjacent shafts of metatarsals	Proximal phalanges of 2nd toe medial and lateral sides; 3rd and 4th toes lateral sides	Lateral plantar, S2, S3	Abducts toes; flexes and extends proximal and distal phalanges
Flexor digitorum brevis	Medial tubercle of calcaneus, plantar aponeurosis and intermuscular septa	Middle phalanges of lateral 4 toes	Medial plantar, S2, S3	Flexes middle phalanges of lateral 4 toes
Flexor digiti minimi brevis	Base of 5th metatarsal	Proximal phalanx of 5th toe	Lateral plantar, S2, S3	Flexes 5th toe
Flexor hallucis brevis	Cuboid; 3rd cuneiform	Proximal phalanx of great toe	Medial plantar, S2, S3	Flexes great toe

Muscle	Origin	Insertion	Nerve	Action
Lumbricals (4)	Tendons of flexor digitorum longus	Proximal phalanges; extensor expansion	1st by medial plantar nerve; lateral 3 by lateral plantar nerve, S2, S3	Flexes metatarso-phalangeal joints and extends inter-phalangeal joints
Plantar inter-ossei (3)	Medial sides of metatarsals 3-5	Medial side of base of proximal phalanges 3-5	Lateral plantar, S2, S3	Adducts toes; flexes proximal and extends distal phalanges
Quadratus plantae	Medial and lateral side of calcaneus	Tendons of flexor digitorum longus	Lateral plantar, S2, S3	Assists in flexing toes

13. Muscles of the Thoracic Wall

Muscle	Origin	Insertion	Nerve	Action
External intercostals	Lower border of ribs	Upper border of rib below	Intercostal	Elevates rib in inspiration
Internal intercostals	Lower border of ribs	Upper border of rib below	Intercostal	Depresses ribs; interchondral part elevates ribs
Transverse thoracic	Posterior surface of lower sternum and xiphoid	Inner surface of costal cartilages 2-6	Intercostal	Depresses ribs
Subcostals	Inner surface of lower ribs near their angles	Upper borders of ribs 2 or 3 below	Intercostal	Elevates ribs
Levator costarum	Tips of transverse processes of C7 and T7-T11 vertebrae	Subjacent ribs between tubercle and angle	Dorsal primary rami of C8-T11	Elevates ribs; assists with lateral bending

14. Muscles of the Anterior Abdominal Wall

Muscle	Origin	Insertion	Nerve	Action
External oblique	External surface of lower 8 ribs, 5-12	Anterior one-half of iliac crest; anterior-superior iliac spine; pubic tubercle; linea alba	Intercostal T7-T11; subcostal T12	Compresses ab-domen; flexes trunk; assists in forced expiration
Internal oblique	Lateral two thirds of inguinal liga-ment; iliac crest; thoracolumbar fascia	Lower 4 costal cartilages; lineal alba; pubic crest; pectineal line	Intercostal T7-T11;subcostal ; T12 iliohypo-gastric and ilioinguinal L1	Compresses ab-domen; flexes trunk; assists in forced expiration

Muscle	Origin	Insertion	Nerve	Action
Transverse abdominis	Lateral one-third of inguinal ligament; iliac crest; thoraco-lumbar fascia; lower 6 costal cartilages	Linea alba; pubic crest; pectineal line	Intercostal T7-T12; subcostal T12; iliohypogastric and ilioinguinal L1	Compresses abdomen; depresses ribs
Rectus abdominis	Pubic crest and pubic symphysis	Xiphoid process and costal cartilages 5-7	Intercostal T7-T12	Depresses ribs; flexes trunk
Pyramidalis	Pubic body	Linea alba	Subcostal T12	Tenses linea alba

15. Muscles of the Posterior Abdominal Wall

Muscle	Origin	Insertion	Nerve	Action
Quadratus lumborum	Medial one-half of inferior border of twelfth rib and tips of lumbar transverse processes	Iliolumbar ligament and internal tip of iliac crest	Ventral branches of T12, L1-L4	Extends, laterally flexes vertebral column; flexes 12th rib during inspiration
Psoas major	Sides of T12-L5 vertebra and disc; transverse processes	Lesser trochanter of femur	Anterior rami of L1, L2, and L3	Flexes and rotates thigh laterally at hip; flexes lumbar vertebral anteriorly and laterally
Psoas minor	Sides of T12-L1 vertebra and inter-vertebral disc	Pectineal line, ilio-pectineal eminence via iliopectineal arch	Anterior rami of L1, L2	Works conjointly with psoas major to flex thigh at hip; stabilizes joint

16. Superficial Muscles of the Back

Muscle	Origin	Insertion	Nerve	Action
Erector spinae	Arises by a broad tendon from post-erior part of iliac crest, posterior surface of sacrum, sacral and inferior lumbar spinous processes and supraspinous ligament	Iliocostalis lumborum, thoracis and cervicis; Longissimusthora-cis, cervicis and capitis; spinalis: thoracis, cervicis and capitis	Posterior rami of spinal nerves	Extend vertebral column and head
Interspinales	Superior surface of spinous processes of cervical and lumbar vertebrae	Inferior surface of spinous process of vertebrae superior to vertebrae of origin	Posterior rami of spinal nerves	Assist in extension and rotation of vertebral column

Muscle	Origin	Insertion	Nerve	Action
Intertrans-versarii	Transverse process of cervical and lumbar vertebrae	Transverse process of adjacent vertebrae	Posterior and anterior rami of spinal nerves	Assists in lateral bending of vertebral column; stabilizes vertebral column
Latissimus dorsi	Spines of T5-T12	Floor of bicipital groove	Thoracodorsal	Adducts, extends, and rotates arm medially
Levator scapulae	Transverse process of C1-C4	Superior part of medial border of scapula	Dorsal scapular C5; cervical C3-C4	Elevates scapula
Rhomboid major	Spines of T2-T5	Medial border of scapula	Dorsal scapular, C4, C5	Adducts scapula
Rhomboid minor	Spines of C7-T1	Root of spine of scapula	Dorsal scapular, C4, C5	Adducts scapula
Serratus anterior	External surface oflateral parts of 1-8 ribs	Anterior surface of medial border of scapula	Long thoracic nerve, C5, C6, C7	Protracts and rotates scapula
Serratus posterior-superior	Ligamentum nuchae, supraspinal ligament and spines of C7-T3	Superior borders of 2-4 ribs	Intercostal, 2-5	Elevates ribs
Serratus posterior-inferior	Spinal processes of T11 to L2 vertebrae	Inferior border of 8-12 ribs near their angles	Anterior thoracic spinal 9-12	Depresses ribs
Transverso-spinal	Transverse process of C4-T12 vertebrae; multifidus arises from sacrum, ilium, transverse process of T1-T3 and articular process of C4-C7	Thoracis, cervicis, and capitis	Spinal, posterior rami	Extends and rotates vertebral column; stabilizes vertebrae during movement
Trapezius	External occipital protuberance, superior nuchal line, ligamentum nuchae, spines of C7-T12	Lateral one-third of clavicle, acromion, and spine of scapula	Spinal accessory, C3-C4	Adducts, rotates, elevates, and depresses scapula

Muscle	Origin	Insertion	Nerve	Action

17. Suboccipital Muscles

Muscle	Origin	Insertion	Nerve	Action
Obliquus capitis inferior	Spine of axis C2	Transverse process of atlas, C1	Suboccipital	Extends and laterally rotates head
Obliquus capitis superior	Transverse process of atlas, C1	Occipital bone above inferior nuchal line	Suboccipital	Extends, rotates, and laterally flexes head
Rectus capitis posterior major	Spine of axis, C2 inferior nuchal line	Lateral portion of	Suboccipital and laterally flexes head	Extends, rotates,
Rectus capitis posterior minor	Posterior tubercle of atlas, C1	Occipital bone below inferior nuchal line	Suboccipital	Extends, rotates, and laterally flexes head

18. Muscles of the Neck

Cervical muscles

Muscle	Origin	Insertion	Nerve	Action
Platysma	Superficial fascia over upper part of deltoid and pectoralis major	Mandible; skin and muscles over the mandible and angle of mouth	Facial, CN VII	Depresses lower jaw and lip and angle of mouth; wrinkles skin of neck
Sternocleido-mastoid	Lateral surface of mastoid process of temporal bone and lateral half of superior nuchal line	Mastoid process and lateral one half of superior nuchal line	Spinal accessory, C2-C3	Tilts head; laterally flexes and rotates face to opposite side, raises thorax

Suprahyoid muscles

Muscle	Origin	Insertion	Nerve	Action
Digastric	Anterior belly from digastric fossa of mandible posterior belly from mastoid notch	Intermediate tendon attached to body of hyoid	Anterior belly: mylohyoid nerve, branch of alveolar nerve; Posterior belly: facial nerve CN 7	Depresses mandible and elevates hyoid and tongue
Mylohyoid	Mylohyoid line of mandible	Median raphe and body of hyoid bone	Mylohyoid and trigeminal, CN 3	Elevates hyoid and tongue; depresses mandible
Styloid	Styloid process	Body of hyoid	Facial, CN 7	Elevates and retracts hyoid
Geniohyoid	Genial tubercle of mandible	Body of hyoid	C1 via the hypoglossal nerve	Pulls hyoid bone anterosuperiorly, shortens floor of mouth; widens pharynx

Muscle	Origin	Insertion	Nerve	Action
Infrahyoid muscles				
Omohyoid	Inferior belly from medial lip of suprascapular notch and supra-scapular ligament; superior belly from intermediate tendon	Inferior belly to intermediate tendon: superior belly to body of hyoid	Ansa cervicalis, C1-C3	Depresses and retracts hyoid and larynx
Sternohyoid	Manubrium sterni and medial end of clavicle	Body of hyoid	Ansa cervicalis, C1-C3	Depresses hyoid and larynx
Sternothyroid	Manubrium sterni; 1st costal cartilage	Oblique line of thyroid cartilage	Ansa cervicalis, C1-C3	Depresses thyroid cartilage and larynx
Thyrohyoid	Oblique line of thyroid cartilage	Body and greater horn of hyoid	C1 via hypo-glossal nerve	Depresses and retracts hyoid and larynx

19. Prevertebral Muscles

Muscle	Origin	Insertion	Nerve	Action
Lateral vertebral				
Anterior scalene	Transverse process of C4-C6 vertebrae	1st rib	Cervical, C4, C5, C6	Elevates 1st rib; laterally flexes and rotates neck
Middle scalene	Posterior tubercles of transverse processes of C4-C5 vertebrae	Superior surface of 1st rib, posterior groove for subclavian artery	Cervical spine, anterior rami	Elevates 1st rib during forced inspiration; flexes neck laterally
Posterior scalene	Posterior tubercles of transverse processes of C4-C5 vertebrae	External border of 2nd rib	Anterior rami of cervical spine, C7, C8	Elevates 2nd rib during forced inspiration; flexes neck laterally
Anterior vertebral				
Longus capitis	Basilar part of occipital bone processes	Anterior tubercles of C3-C6 transverse	Spinal, anterior rami, C1-C3	Flexes and twists head anteriorly
Longus colli	Anterior tubercle of C2 vertebra; bodies of C1-C3 and transverse processes of C3-C6 vertebrae	Bodies of C5-T3 vertebrae, transverse processes of C3-C5 vertebrae	Spinal, anterior rami, C2-C6	Flexes and rotates head to opposite side
Rectus capitis anterior	Anterior surface of lateral mass of atlas, C1	Base of skull, anterior to occipital condyle	C1 and C2	Flexes head

Muscle	Origin	Insertion	Nerve	Action
Rectus capitis lateralis	Transverse processes of C1	Jugular process of occipital bone	C1 and C2	Flexes head; helps stabilize head
Rectus capitis posterior	Spinous processes of C2 vertebra	Middle of inferior nuchal line of occipital bone	Suboccipital	Extends head
Splenic capitis, et cervicis	Inferior one-half of ligamentum nuchae, spinous processes of C7-T3 of T4 vertebrae line of occipital bone	Splenius capitis: superolaterally to mastoid process of temporal bone, lateral 3rd of superior nuchal Splenius cervicis: posterior tubercles of transverse C1-C3 or C4 vertebrae		

20. Muscles of Facial Expression

Muscle	Origin	Insertion	Nerve	Action
Auricularis anterior, posterior, and superior	Epicranial aponeurosis and mastoid part of temporal bone	Auricle (external ear)	Facial	Protraction, retraction, and elevation of external ear
Buccinator	Mandible; pterygo-mandibular raphe; alveolar processes	Angle of mouth	Facial, CN 7	Presses cheek against molar teeth to aid in chewing
Corrugator supercilii	Medial supra-orbital margin	Skin of medial eyebrow	Facial, CN 7	Draws eyebrow medially and inferiorly producing vertical wrinkles above nose
Depressor anguli oris	Oblique line of mandible	Angle of mouth	Facial, CN 7	Depresses angle of mouth
Depressor labii inferioris	Mandible below mental foramen	Orbicularis oris and skin of lower lip	Facial, CN 7	Depresses lower lip
Depressor septi	Incisor fossa of maxilla	Mobile part of nasal septum	Facial	Helps dilate nostril during inspiration; depresses nasal septum
Levator anguli oris	Canine fossa of maxilla	Angle of mouth	Facial, CN 7	Elevates angle of mouth medially
Levator labii superioris	Maxilla above infraorbital foramen	Skin of upper lip and alar cartilage of nose	Facial, CN 7	Elevates upper lip, dilates nose

Muscles

Muscle	Origin	Insertion	Nerve	Action
Levator labii superioris alaeque nasi	Frontal process of maxilla	Skin of upper lip	Facial	Elevates ala of nose and upper lip
Mentalis	Incisor fossa of mandible	Skin of chin	Facial, CN 7	Elevates and protrudes lower lip
Nasalis	Maxilla lateral to incisor fossa	Nasal cartilages	Facial, CN 7	Draws ala (side) of nose toward nasal septum
Occipito-frontalis	Superior nuchal line; upper orbital margin	Epicranial aponeurosis	Facial, CN 7	Elevates eyebrows; wrinkles forehead
Orbicularis oculi	Medial orbital margin; medial palpebral ligament; lacrimal bone	Skin and rim of orbit; tarsal plate; lateral palpebral raphe	Facial, CN 7	Closes and/or squints eyelids
Procerus	Nasal bone and cartilage	Skin between eyebrows	Facial, CN 7	Depresses medial end of eyebrow; produces wrinkles over nose
Zygomaticus major	Zygomatic arch	Angle of mouth	Facial, CN 7	Draws angle of mouth backwards and upwards
Zygomaticus minor	Zygomatic arch	Angle of mouth	Facial, CN 7	Elevates upper lip

21. Muscles of Mastication

Muscle	Origin	Insertion	Nerve	Action
Lateral pterygoid	Superior head from infratemporal surface of sphenoid; inferior head from lateral surface of lateral pterygoid plate	Neck of mandible; articular disc and capsule of temporomandibular joint	Trigeminal, CN V3	Protracts and depresses mandible; produces side-to-side movements of mandible
Masseter	Lower border and medial surface of zygomatic arch of mandible	Lateral surface of coronoid process, ramus and angle	Trigeminal, CN V3	Elevates mandible
Medial pterygoid	Tuber of maxillary; medial surface of lateral pterygoid plate; pyramidal process of palatine bone	Medial surface of angle and ramus of mandible	Trigeminal, CN V3	Protracts, protrudes and elevates mandible, closes jaw; produces grinding motion

Muscle	Origin	Insertion	Nerve	Action
22. Muscles of Eye Movement				
Ciliary	Scleral spur	Meridional, radial, and circular fibers are intrinsic to ciliary body	Para-sympathetic fibers of oculo-motor nerve and ciliary ganglion	Relieve tension on lens of eye, allowing it to become more convex for near vision
Inferior rectus	Common tendinous ring	Sclera just behind cornea	Oculomotor, CN 3	Depresses, adducts, and rotates eyeball medially
Lateral rectus	Common tendinous ring	Sclera just behind cornea	Abducens, CN 6	Abducts eyeball
Medial rectus	Common tendinous ring	Sclera just behind cornea	Oculomotor, CN 3	Adducts eyeball
Superior rectus	Common tendinous ring	Sclera just behind cornea	Oculomotor, CN 3	Elevates, adducts, and rotates eye medially
Inferior oblique	Floor of orbit lateral to lacrimal groove	Sclera beneath lateral rectus	Oculomotor, CN 3	Rotates eyeball upward and laterally, elevates adducted eye
Superior oblique	Body of sphenoid bone above optic canal	Sclera beneath superior rectus	Trochlear, CN 4	Abducts, depresses and medially rotates eyeball
Levator palpebrae superioris	Lesser wing of sphenoid above and anterior to optic canal	Tarsal plate and skin of upper eyelid	Oculomotor, CN 3	Elevates upper eyelid

23. Muscles of the Palate

Muscle	Origin	Insertion	Nerve	Action
Levator veli palatini	Petrous part of temporal bone; cartilage of auditory tube	Aponeurosis of soft palate	Vagus via pharyngeal plexus, CN 10, 11	Elevates soft palate
Musculus uvulae	Posterior nasal spine of palatine bone; palatine aponeurosis	Mucous membrane of uvula	Vagus nerve via pharyngeal plexus, CN 10, 11	Elevates uvula
Palato-pharyngeus	Hard palate and palatine aponeurosis	Lateral wall of pharynx	Cranial part of accessory nerve CN 11 through pharyngeal branch of vagus nerve CN 10 via pharyngeal plexus	Tenses soft palate; moves walls of pharynx superiorly, anteriorly, and medially during swallowing

Muscle	Origin	Insertion	Nerve	Action
Tensor veli palatini	Scaphoid fossa; spine of sphenoid; cartilage of auditory tube	Palatine aponeurosis	Mandibular branch nerve, CN V3, via otic ganglion	Tenses soft palate and opens auditory tube during swallowing and yawning

24. Muscles of the Tongue

Muscle	Origin	Insertion	Nerve	Action
Genioglossus	Superior part of mental spine of mandible	Dorsum of tongue and body of hyoid bone	Hypoglossal, CN 12	Depresses tongue; pulls tongue anteriorly for protrusion
Hyoglossus	Body of greater horn of hyoid bone	Side and inferior aspect of tongue	Hypoglossal, CN 12	Depresses and retracts tongue
Inferior long muscle of tongue	Root of tongue and body of hyoid bone	Apex of tongue	Hypoglossal, CN 12	Curls tip of tongue inferiorly and shortens tongue
Palatoglossus	Palatine aponeurosis	Side of tongue	Cranial part of accessory nerve CN 12 through pharyngeal branch of vagus nerve CN 10 via pharyngeal plexus	Elevates posterior tongue and draws soft palate onto tongue
Superior long muscle of tongue	Submucous fibrous layer and median fibrous septum	Margins of tongue and mucous membrane	Hypoglossal, CN 12	Curls tip and sides of tongue superiorly and shortens tongue
Transverse muscle of tongue	Median fibrous septum	Fibrous tissue at margins of tongue	Hypoglossal, CN 12	Narrows and elongates tongue; aids in protrusion of tongue
Vertical muscle of tongue	Superior surface of borders of tongue	Inferior surface of borders of tongue	Hypoglossal, CN 12	Flattens tongue; aids in protrusion of tongue

25. Muscles of the Pharynx

Circular muscles

Muscle	Origin	Insertion	Nerve	Action
Crico-pharyngeus	Posterolateral cricoid cartilage on 1 side	Posterolateral cricoid cartilage of other side	Vagus, CN 10	Serves as upper esophageal sphincter
Geniohyoid	Inferior mental spine of mandible	Body of hyoid bone	C1 via hypo-glossal	Pulls hyoid bone superiorly; shortens floor of mouth; widens pharynx

Muscle	Origin	Insertion	Nerve	Action
Inferior constrictor	Arch of cricoid and oblique line of thyroid cartilage	Median raphe of pharynx	Vagus via pharyngeal plexus; recurrent and external laryngeal, CN 10, 11	Constricts lower pharynx
Middle constrictor	Greater and lesser horns of hyoid; stylohyoid ligament	Median raphe	Vagus via pharyngeal plexus, CN 10, 11	Constricts lower pharynx
Superior constrictor	Medial pterygoid plate; pterygoid hamulus; pterygo-mandibular raphe; mylohyoid line of mandible; side of tongue	Median raphe and pharyngeal tubercle of skull	Vagus via pharyngeal plexus	Constricts upper pharynx

Longitudinal muscles

Muscle	Origin	Insertion	Nerve	Action
Palato-pharyngeus	Hard palate; aponeurosis of soft palate	Thyroid cartilage and muscles of the pharynx	Vagus via pharyngeal plexus, CN 10, 11	Elevates pharynx and closes nasopharynx
Salpingo-pharyngeus	Cartilage of auditory tube	Muscles of the pharynx	Vagus via pharyngeal plexus	Elevates naso-pharynx; opens auditory tube
Stylo-pharyngeus	Styloid process	Thyroid cartilage and muscles of the pharynx	Glossopharyngeal, CN 9	Elevates pharynx and larynx

26. Muscles of the Larynx

Muscle	Origin	Insertion	Nerve	Action
Aryepiglottic	Apex of arytenoid cartilage	Side of epiglottic cartilage	Recurrent laryngeal	Adducts
Cricothyroid	Arch of cricoid cartilage	Inferior horn and lower lamina of thyroid cartilage	External laryngeal	Tenses and stretches vocal fold
Lateral crico-arytenoid	Arch of cricoid cartilage	Muscular process of arytenoid cartilage	Recurrent laryngeal, CN 10	Adducts
Oblique arytenoid	Muscular process of arytenoid cartilage	Apex of opposite arytenoid	Recurrent laryngeal, CN 10	Closes inter-cartilaginous portion of rima glottidis
Posterior crico-arytenoid	Posterior surface of lamina of cricoid cartilage	Muscular process of arytenoid cartilage	Recurrent laryngeal, CN 10	Abducts

Muscle	Origin	Insertion	Nerve	Action
Thyro-arytenoid	Inner surface of thyroid lamina cartilage	Anterolateral surface of arytenoid	Recurrent laryngeal, CN 10	Adducts; relaxes vocal fold
Thyroepi-glottic	Anteromedial surface of lamina of thyroid cartilage	Lateral margin of epiglottic cartilage	Recurrent laryngeal, CN 10	Adducts
Transverse arytenoid	Posterior surface of arytenoid cartilage	Opposite arytenoid cartilage	Recurrent laryngeal, CN 10	Adducts
Vocalis	Anteromedial surface of lamina of thyroid cartilage	Vocal process	Recurrent laryngeal, CN 10	Relaxes posterior vocal ligaments; maintains tension of anterior part of ligament

27. Summary of Autonomic Ganglia of the Head and Neck

Ganglion	Location	Parasympathetic Fibers	Sympathetic Fibers	Chief Distribution
Ciliary	Behind eyeball between optic nerve and lateral rectus muscle	Inferior division oculomotor nerve via short ciliary nerves	Internal carotid artery, long ciliary nerve	Ciliary muscle and sphincter pupillae (para-sympathetic); dilator pupillae and tarsal muscle (sympathetic)
Pterygo-palatine	In pterygopalatine fossa below maxillary nerve, lateral to the sphenopalatine foramen and anterior pterygoid canal	Facial nerve, greater petrosal nerve, and pterygoid nerve	Internal carotid plexus	Nasal, palatine, and lacrimal glands via maxillary, zygo-matic, and lacrimal nerves
Submandibular	Lateral surface of hyoglossus muscle, deep to the mylohyoid muscle, suspended from the lingual nerve	Facial nerve, chorda tympani and lingual nerve	Plexus on facial artery	Submandibular and sublingual glands
Otic	Below foramen ovale	Glossopharyngeal nerve, its tympanic branch, lesser petrosal nerve	Plexus on middle meningeal	Parotid gland

Muscle	Origin	Insertion	Nerve	Action

28. Muscles of the Ears

Muscle	Origin	Insertion	Nerve	Action
Stapedius	Internal walls of pyramidal eminence of posterior wall of tympanic cavity	Neck of the stapes	Facial, cranial nerve V2	Dampens vibrations of stapes reflexively in response to loud nose
Tensor tympani	Canal for tensor tympani of petrous part of temporal bone and cartilage of pharyngo-tympanic (auditory) tube	Handle of malleus	Branch of mandibular nerve, cranialnerve V3 via otic ganglion	Tenses tympanic membrane to dampen excessive vibration

29. Cranial Nerves

Nerve	Cranial Exit	Cell Bodies	Components	Chief Function
I: Olfactory	Cribriform plate	Nasal mucosa	SVA	Smell
II: Optic	Optic canal	Ganglion cells of retina	SSA	Vision
III: Oculomotor	Superior orbital fissure	Nucleus CN III (midbrain)	GSE	Eye movements (superior, inferior, and medial recti, inferior oblique, and levator palpebrae superioris muscles)
		Edinger-Westphal nucleus (midbrain)	GVE	Constriction of pupil (sphincter pupillae muscle) and accommodation (ciliary muscle)
IV: Trochlear	Superior orbital fissure	Nucleus CN IV (midbrain)	GSE	Eye movements (superior oblique muscle)
V: Trigeminal	Superior orbital fissure; foramen rotundum and foramen ovale	Motor nucleus CN V (pons)	SVE	Muscles of mastication, (mylohyoid, anterior belly of digastric, tensor veli palatini, and tensor tympani muscles)
		Trigeminal ganglion	GSA	Sensation in head (skin and mucous membranes of face and head)

Nerve	Cranial Exit	Cell Bodies	Components	Chief Function
VI: Abducens	Superior orbital fissure	Nucleus CN VI (pons)	GSE	Eye movement (lateral rectus muscle)
VII: Facial	Stylomastoid foramen	Motor nucleus CN VII (pons)	SVE	Muscle of facial expression (posterior belly of digastric stylohyoid and stapedius muscles)
		Salivatory nucleus (pons)	GVE	Lacrimal and salivary secretion
		Geniculate ganglion	SVA	Taste from anterior two thirds of tongue and palate
		Geniculate ganglion	GVA	Sensation from palate
		Geniculate ganglion	GSA	Sensation from external acoustic means
VIII: Vestibulo-cochlear	Does not leave skull	Vestibular ganglion	SSA	Equilibrium, hearing
IX: Glosso-pharyngeal	Jugular foramen	Nucleus ambiguus (medulla)	SVE	Elevation of pharynx (stylopharyn-geus muscle)
		Dorsal nucleus (medulla)	GVE	Secretion of saliva (parotid gland)
		Inferior ganglion	GVA	Sensation in carotid sinus and body, tongue, and pharynx
		Inferior ganglion	SVA	Taste from posterior one third of tongue
		Inferior ganglion	GSA	Sensation in external and middle ear
X: Vagus	Jugular foramen	Nucleus ambiguus	SVE	Muscles of movements of pharynx, larynx, and palate
		Dorsal nucleus (medulla)	GVE	Involuntary muscle and gland control in thoracic and abdominal viscerae

Nerve	Cranial Exit	Cell Bodies	Components	Chief Function
		Inferior ganglion	GVA	Sensation in pharynx, larynx, and other viscera
		Inferior ganglion	SVA	Taste from root of tongue and epiglottis
X. Vagus		Superior ganglion	GSA	Sensation in external ear and external acoustic meatus
XI: Accessory	Jugular foramen	Spinal cord (foramen)	SVE	Movement of head and shoulder (sternocleido-mastoid and trapezius muscles)
XII: Hypo-glossal	Hypoglossal canal	Nucleus CN XII (medulla)	GSE	Muscles of movements of tongue

Appendix 3
Ligaments and Tendons

Latin name	English name	Articulation

Shoulder/Upper Arm

Latin name	English name	Articulation
Lm. acromioclaviculare	Acromioclavicular l.	Connects acromion to clavicle; strengthens articular capsule
Lm. anulare radii	Anular l. of radius	Connects head of radius in radial notch
Lm. collaterale ulnare	Collateral ulnar l.	Connects medial epicondyle to humerus and coronoid process of ulna and olecranon
Lm. conoideum	Conoid l.	Connects coracoid process of scapula to clavicle
Lm. coracoacromiale	Coracoacromial l.	Connects coracoid process to acromion
Lm. coracoclaviculare	Coracoclavicular l.	Connects coracoid process of scapula to clavicle
Lm. coracohumerale	Coracohumeral l.	Connects coracoid process of scapula to humerus
Lm. costoclaviculare	Costoclavicular l.	Connects 1st costal cartilage to clavicle
La. glenohumeralia	Glenohumeral ligs.	Connects articular capsule of humerus to glenoid cavity and anatomical neck of humerus
Lm. interclaviculare	Interclavicular l.	Connects clavicle to opposite clavicle
Lm. Orbiculare radii	Anular l. of radius	L. that encircles and holds head of radius in radial notch of ulna
La. sternoclaviculare anterius	Anterior sternoclavicular l.	Fibrous band that reinforces sternoclavicular joints anteriorly
La. sternoclavicular posterius	Posterior sternoclavicular l.	Fibrous band that reinforces sternoclavicular joints posteriorly
Lm. suspensorium axillae	Suspensory l.	Connects between clavipectoral fascia downward to axillary fascia
Lm. transversum humeri	Transverse humeral l.	Connects obliquely from greater to lesser tuberosity of humerus
Lm. transversum scapulae inferius	Inferior transverse l.	Connects scapula to glenoid cavity; creates foramen of scapula for vessels/nerves

Latin name	English name	Articulation
Lm. transversum scapulae superius	Superior transverse l	Connects coracoid process to scapular notch of scapula
Lm. trapezoideum	Trapezoid l.	Connects coracoid process to clavicle

Hand/Forearm

Latin name	English name	Articulation
Lm. anulare radii	Anular l. of radius	Connects radius to ulna
Lm. carpi radiatum	Radiate l. of wrist	Multiple fibrous bands on palmar surface of metacarpal joints
Lm. carpi transversum	Transverse carpal l.	Continuous with antebrachial fascia
Lm. carpi volare	Transverse carpal l.	Reinforcing fibers in antebrachial fascia, palmar surface of wrist
La. carpometacarpalia dorsalia	Dorsal carpometacarpal ligs.	Joins carpal bones to bases of metacarpals
La. carpometacarpalia palmaria	Palmar carpometacarpal ligs.	Joins carpal bones to metacarpals ligs.
Lm. collateralia articulationum interphalangealium manus	Collateral ligs. of of interphalangeal articulations	Fibrous bands on each side of interphalangeal joints of fingers
Lm. collateralia articulationum metacarpophalangealium	Collateral ligs. of metacarpophalangeal articulations	Fibrous bands on sides of each metacarpophalangeal joints
Lm. collaterale carpi radiale	Radial carpal collateral l.	Connects styloid process of radius to scaphoid
Lm. collaterale carpi ulnare	Ulnar carpal collateral l.	Connects styloid process of ulna to triquetral and pisiform bones
Lm. collaterale radiale	Collateral radial l.	Connects lateral epicondyle of humerus to anular l. of radius
Lm. intercarpalia dorsalia	Dorsal intercarpal ligs.	Connects carpal bones together
Lm. intercarpalia interossea	Interosseous intercarpal ligs.	Connects various carpal bones
Lm. intercarpalia palmaria	Palmar intercarpal ligs.	Connects various carpal bones
La. metacarpalia dorsalia	Dorsal metacarpal ligs.	Interconnects bases of metacarpal bones
La. metacarpalia interossea	Interosseous metacarpal ligs.	Interconnects bases of metacarpal bones
La. metacarpalia palmaria	Palmar metacarpal ligs.	Interconnects bases of metacarpals

Latin name	English name	Articulation
Lm. metacarpeum transversum profundum	Deep transverse metacarpal l.	Interconnects heads of metacarpals
Lm. metacarpale transversum superficiale	Superficial transverse metacarpal l.	Between longitudinal bands of palmar aponeurosis
Lm. natatorium	Superficial transverse metacarpal l.	Thickening of deep fascia in most distal part of base of triangular palmar aponeurosis
La. palmaria	Palmar l.	Connects anterior aspect of each metacarpophalangeal and interphalangeal joints of hand
La. palmaria articulationis interphalangeae manus	Palmar ligs. of interphalangeal joints of hand	Interphalangeal articulations of hand between collateral articulations
La. palmaria articulationis metacarpophalangeae	Palmar ligs. of metacarpal joints	Connects metacarpophalangeal joints to collateral ligs.
Lm. pisohamatum	Pisohamate l.	Connects pisiform bone to hook of hamate bone
Lm. pisometacarpeum	Pisometacarpal l.	Connects pisiform bone to bases of metacarpals
Lm. quadratum	Quadrate l.	Connects radial notch of ulna to neck of radius
Lm. radiocarpale dorsale	Dorsal radiocarpal l.	Connects radius to carpal bones
Lm. radiocarpale palmare	Palmar radiocarpal l.	Connects radius to lunate, triquetral, capitate, and hamate bones
Lm. ulnocarpale palmare	Palmar ulnocarpal l.	Connects styloid process of ulna to carpal bones

Head/Neck

Latin name	English name	Articulation
Lm. anulare stapedis	Anular l. of stapes	Connects stapes to fenestra vestibuli
La. anularia	Anular l. of trachea	Connects adjacent tracheal cartilages
Lm. articulare anterius	Anterior l. of auricle	Connects zygomatic process to helix
Lm. articulare posterius	Anterior l. of auricle	Connects mastoid process to conchal eminence
Lm. articulare superius	Superior l. of auricle	Connects osseous external acoustic meatus to helix
Lm. ceratocricoideum	Ceratocricoid l.	1 of 3 ligs. reinforcing cricothyroid articulation capsule
Lm. corniculopharyngeal	Cricopharyngeal l.	Connects corniculate cartilage and cricoid cartilage

Latin name	English name	Articulation
Lm. cricoarytenoideum posterius	Cricoarytenoid l.	Connects arytenoid cartilage to lamina of cricoid cartilage
Lm. cricopharyngeum	Cricopharyngeal l.	Connects tip of corniculate cartilage and lamina of cricoid cartilage
Lm. cricotracheale	Cricotracheal l.	Connects cricoid cartilage with 1st ring of trachea
Lm. hyaloideocapsulare	Hyalocapsular l.	Connects vitreous body to posterior surface of lens of eye
Lm. hyoepiglotticum	Hyoepiglottic l.	Connects epiglottis to upper border of hyoid bone
Lm. hyothyroideum laterale	Lateral thyroid l.	Connects superior horn of thyroid cartilage to tip of greater horn of hyoid cartilage
Lm. hyothyroideum medium	Median thyroid l.	Central portion of thyroid membrane
Lm. incudis posterius	Posterior l. of incus	Ligamentous band extending from short crus of incus
Lm. incudis superius	Superior l. of incus	Connects body of incus with root at tympanic recess
La. intracapsularia	Intrascapular l.	Ligs. located within and separate from articular capsule of synovial joints
Lm. jugale	Cricopharyngeal l.	Connects tip at corniculate cartilage and lamina at cricoid cartilage and pharyngeal mucosa
Lm. laterale articulationis temporomandibularis	Lateral l. of temporomandibular joints	Capsular l. that passes down and backward across lateral surface of temporomandibular joints
Lm. mallei anterius	Anterior l. of malleus	Connects base of anterior process to spine of sphenoid
Lm. mallei laterale	Lateral l. of malleus	Connects posterior half of tympanic notch to neck of malleus
Lm. mallei superius	Superior l. of malleus	Connects from head of malleus to epitympanic recess
Lm. mediale articulationis temporomandibularis	Medial l. of temporomandibular joints	Strengthens medial part of articular capsule
La. ossiculorum auditus	L. of auditory ossicles	Connects ear bones with each other and with walls of tympanic cavity
Lm. palpebrale externum	Lateral palpebral l.	Connects tarsal plates to orbital eminence of zygomatic bone

Ligaments and Tendons

Appendix 3

Latin name	English name	Articulation
Lm. palpebrale laterale	Lateral palpebral l.	Connects tarsal plates to orbital eminence of zygomatic bone
Lm. palpebral mediale	Medial palpebral l.	Connects medial ends of tarsal plates to maxilla at medial orbital margin
Lm. sphenomandibulare	Sphenomandibular l.	Connects from spine to sphenoid bone to lingula of mandible
Lm. spirale cochleae	Spiral l. of cochlear duct	Forms outer wall of cochlear duct to which basal lamina attaches
Lm. spirale ductus cochlearis	Spiral l. of cochlear duct	Forms outer wall of cochlear duct to which basal lamina attaches
Lm. stylohyoideum	Stylohyoid l.	Connects from tip of styloid process to lesser cornu of hyoid bone
Lm. stylomandibulare	Stylomandibular l.	Connects from tip of styloid process to temporal bone
Lm. suspensorium bulb	Suspensory l.	Connects between lateral and medial orbital margins
Lm. suspensorium glandulae thyroideae	Suspensory l.	Connects from sheath of thyroid gland to thyroid and cricoid cartilages
Lm. tarsale externum	Lateral palpebral l.	Connects tarsal plates to orbital eminence of zygomatic bone
Lm. tarsale internum	Medial palpebral l.	Connects between medial ends of tarsal plates to maxilla at medial orbital margin
Lm. temporomandibular	Lateral temporo-mandibular l.	Capsular l. that passes obliquely down and backward across lateral surface of temporomandibular joints
Lm. thyroepiglotticum	Thyroepiglottic l.	Connects petiole of epiglottis to interior of thyroid cartilage
Lm. thyrohyoideum laterale	Lateral thyroid l.	Connects superior horn of thyroid cartilage to tip of greater horn of hyoid cartilage
Lm. thyrohyoideum medium	Median thyrohyoid l.	Central thickened portion of thyroid membrane
La. trachealia	Anular l.	Connects adjacent tracheal cartilages
Lm. ventriculare	Vestibular l.	Inferior border of quadrangular membrane that underlies ventricular fold of larynx
Lm. vestibulare	Vestibular l.	Inferior border of quadrangular membrane that underlies ventricular fold of larynx

Latin name	English name	Articulation
Lm. vocale	Vocal l.	Connects on either side from thyroid cartilages to vocal process of arytenoid cartilages

Thorax/upper abdomen

Lm. colli costae	Costotransverse l.	Connects neck of rib to corresponding transverse process
Lm. costotransversarium anterius	Superior costotransverse l.	Connects transverse rib to next highest vertebra
Lm. costotransversarium laterale	Lateral costotransverse l.	Connects tip of transverse process to neck of rib
Lm. costotransversarium posterius	Lateral costotransverse l.	Connects tip of process to neck of ribs
Lm. costotrans-versarium superius	Superior costotransverse l.	Connects neck of ribs to transverse process of next higher vertebrae
Lm. costoxiphoideum	Costoxiphoid l.	Connects xiphoid process to 7th and often 6th cartilages
Lm. pulmonale	Pulmonary l.	2-layered fold formed as pleura of mediastinum is reflected onto lung inferior to root of lung
Lm. sternocostale intraarticulare	Intraarticular sternocostal l.	Connects between a costal cartilage and cartilage and sternum within articular capsule
La. sternocostalia radiata	Radiate sternocostal l.	Fibers of articular capsule that radiate from costal cartilage to anterior surface of sternum
La. sternopericardiaca	Sternopericardial l.	Connects from pericardium to sternum
La. suspensoria mammaria	Suspensory l. of breast	Connects from fibrous stroma of mammary gland to overlying skin
Lm. tuberculi costae	Lateral costotransverse l.	Connects tip of transverse process to posterior surface of neck and rib
Lm. vena cava sinistrae	Left vena caval l.	Connects from left brachiocephalic vein to oblique vein of left atrium

Spine

Lm. alaria	Alar l.	Connects axis to occiput; limits rotation of head
Lm. apicis dentis axis	Apical dental l.	Connects axis to occiput

Latin name	English name	Articulation
Lm. atlantooccipitale laterale	Lateral atlantooccipital l.	Connects occiput to atlas
Lm. capitis costae intraarticulare	Interarticular l. of head of rib	Connects crest of rib to intervertebral disc
Lm. capitis costae radiatum	Radiate l. of head of rib	Connects head of rib to adjacent vertebrae/discs
Lm. caudale integumenti communis	Caudal retinaculum	Forms coccygeal foveola
Lm. costotransversarium	Costotransverse l.	Connects neck of rib to transverse process of corresponding vertebra
Lm. costotransversarium laterale	Lateral costotransverse l.	Connects transverse process of vertebra to corresponding rib
Lm. costotransversarium superius	Superior costotransverse l.	Connects neck of rib to transverse process of vertebra above
Lm. cruciforme atlantis	Cruciform l. of atlas	Connects transverse l. of atlas to longitudinal fascicles
La. flava	Yellow ligs.	Joins laminae of 2 adjacent vertebrae
Lm. iliofemorale	Iliofemoral l.	Connects anterior/inferior iliac spine and intertrochanteric femur
Lm. iliolumbale	Iliolumbar l.	Connects L4-L5 to iliac crest
Lm. interspinalia	Interspinal ligs.	Interconnects spinous processes
Lm. intertransversaria	Intertransverse ligs.	Interconnects vertebral transverse processes
Lm. longitudinale anterius	Anterior longitudinal l.	Extends from occiput/atlas to sacrum
Lm. longitudinale posterius	Posterior longitudinal l.	Extends from occiput to coccyx
Lm. lumbocostale	Lumbocostal l.	Connects 12th rib to transverse processes of L1-L2
Lm. nuchae	Radiate l.	Connects head of each rib to bodies of 2 vertebrae with which it articulates
Lm. sacrococcygeum anterius	Anterior sacrococcygeal l.	Connects sacrum to coccyx
Lm. sacrococcygeum laterale	Lateral sacrococcygeal l.	Connects 1st coccygeal vertebra to sacrum; completes foramen of S5
Lm. sacrococcygeum posterius profundum	Deep posterior sacrococcygeal l.	Terminal portion of posterior longitudinal l.; unites S5 and profundum coccyx

Latin name	English name	Articulation
Lm. sacrococcygeum posterius	Superficial posterior sacrococcygeal l.	Connects sacral hiatus to coccyx superficiale
La. sacroiliaca anteriora	Anterior sacroiliac ligs.	Connects sacrum to ilium
La. sacroiliaca interossea	Interosseous sacroiliac ligs.	Numerous bundles connecting tuberosities of sacrum to those of ilium
La. sacroiliaca posteriora	Posterior sacroiliac ligs.	Connects ilium and iliac spines to sacrum
Lm. sacrospinalum	Sacrospinal l.	Connects ischium to lateral margins of sacrum
Lm. sacrotuberale	Sacrotuberal l.	Connects ischial tuberosity to sacrum and coccyx and iliac spine
Lm. supraspinale	Supraspinal l.	Interconnects tips of spinous processes of vertebrae
Lm. transversum atlantis	Transverse l. of atlas	Horizontal portion of cruciform l. of atlas

Abdominal/Pelvic

Lm. arcuatum laterale	Lateral arcuate l.	Connects 1st lumbar vertebrae and 12th rib to diaphragm
Lm. arcuatum mediale	Medial arcuate l.	Connects body of 1st lumbar vertebra to transverse process
Lm. arcuatum medianum	Median arcuate l.	Connects crura of diaphragm that arches over aorta
Lm. arcuatum pubis	Inferior pubic l.	Arches across pubic symphysis
Lm. cardinale	Cardinale l.	Connects uterine l., cervix and vault of lateral fornix of vagina
Lm. coronarium hepatis	Coronary l. of liver	Connects peritoneal reflections to diaphragm at margins of bare area of liver
Lm. duodenorenale	Duodenorenal l.	Connects termination of hepatoduodenal to front of right kidney
Lm. falciforme	Falciform process of rotuberous l.	Passes from ischial tuberosity to ilium, sacrum, and coccyx
Lm. falciforme hepatis	Falciform l. of liver	Connects liver to diaphragm and anterior abdominal wall
Lm. fundiforme clitoris	Fundiform l. of clitoris	Connects linea alba with fascia of clitoris

Latin name	English name	Articulation
Lm. fundiforme penis	Fundiform l. of penis	Connects linea alba with fascia of penis
Lm. gastrophrenicum	Gastrocolic l.	Connects stomach with transverse colon
Lm. gastrophrenicum	Gastrophrenic l.	Connects greater curvature of stomach with inferior surface of diaphragm
Lm. gastrosplenicum	Gastrosplenic l.	Connects greater curvature of stomach with ilium of spleen
Lm. genitoinguinale	Genitoinguinal l.	In a fetus, a fold of mesorchium containing gubernaculum testis
Lm. hepatocolicum	Hepatocolic l.	Connects hepatoduodenal l. to transverse colon
Lm. hepatoesophageum	Hepatoesophageal l.	Connects between liver and part of esophagus
Lm. hepatogastricum	Hepatogastric l.	Connects liver to lesser curvature of stomach
Lm. hepatorenale	Hepatorenal l.	A prolongation of coronary ligs. downward over right kidney
Lm. ischiocapsulare	Ischiofemoral l.	Connects from ischium upward and laterally over femoral neck
Lm. lacunare	Lacunar l.	Connects from medial end of inguinal l. to pectineal line
Lm. laterale vesicae	Lateral bladder l.	Passes from 1 side of bladder to blend with pelvic fascia
Lm. pectineale	Pectineal l.	Strong fibrous band that passes laterally from lacunar l. along pectineal line of pubis
Lm. phrenicocolicum	Phrenicocolic l.	Connects from left flexure of colon to diaphragm
Lm. phrenicolienal	Phrenosplenic l.	Connects between diaphragm and spleen
Lm. phrenicosplenicum	Phrenicosplenic l.	Connects between diaphragm and spleen
Lm. pubicum inferius	Inferior pubic l.	Arches across inferior aspect of pubic symphysis
Lm. pubicum superius	Superior pubic l.	Passes transversely above pubic symphysis
Lm. pubofemorale	Pubofemoral l.	Connects from superior ramus of pubis to intertrochanteric femur

Latin name	English name	Articulation
Lm. puboprostaticum	Puboprostatic l.	Anchors prostate and neck of bladder to pubis on each side
Lm. puboprostaticum mediale	Puboprostatic l.	Anchors prostate and neck of bladder to pubis on each side
Lm. pubovesicale	Pubovesical l. (female)	Fascial thickening comparable with puboprostatic l.
Lm. pubovesicale	Pubovesical l. (male)	Connects between lower part of pubic symphysis and prostate and bladder
Lm. sacrodurale	Sacrodural l.	Connects between midline of inferior part of dorsal sac to posterior longitudinal l. of sacrum
Lm. sacroiliacum posterius	Posterior sacroiliac l.	Connects from ilium to sacrum posterior to sacroiliac joints
Lm. sacrospinale	Sacrospinal l.	Connects between ischial spine and sacrum and coccyx
Lm. serosum	Serous l.	Connects certain viscera to abdominal wall or to each other
Lm. splenorenale	Suspensory l.	Connects from pubic symphysis to deep fascia of clitoris
Lm. suspensorium ovarii	Suspensory l.	Extends upward from upper pole of ovary
Lm. suspensorius penis	Suspensory l.	Connects from pubic symphysis to deep fascia of penis
Lm. teres hepatis	Round l.	Connects from umbilicus to liver where it continues to origins of left portal vein
Lm. teres uteri	Round l.	Attached to uterus on either side of front and below opening of uterine tube and connects to labium majus
Lm. transversale cervicis	Cardinal l.	Connects uterine cervix and vault of lateral fornix of vagina
Lm. transversum pelvis	Transverse perineal l.	Thickened anterior border of perineal membrane
Lm. triangulare dextrum hepatis	Right triangular l.	Connects from right lobe of liver to diaphragm
Lm. triangulare sinistrum hepatis	Left triangular l.	Connects from left lobe of liver to diaphragm

Ligaments and Tendons

A103

Latin name	English name	Articulation
Hip/Thigh		
Lm. capitis femoris	L. of head of femur	Connects femur, acetabular notch, and transverse l. of acetabulum
Lm. inguinale	Inguinal l.	Connects ilium to pubis
Lm. ischiofemorale	Ischiofemoral l.	Connects ischium to femur
Lm. transversum acetabuli	Transverse l. of acetabulum	Connects acetabular lip of hip joints to acetabular notch
Knee/Calf		
Lm. capitis fibulae anterius	Anterior l. of head of fibula	Connects head of fibula to lateral condyle of tibia
Lm. capitis fibulae posterius	Posterior l. of head of fibula	Connects head of fibula to lateral condyle of tibia
Lm. collaterale fibulare	Collateral fibular l.	Connects lateral epicondyle of femur to head of fibula
Lm. collateral tibiale	Collateral tibial l.	Connects medial epicondyle of femur to medial meniscus and tibia
Lm. cruciatum anterius genus	Anterior cruciate l. of knee	Connects lateral condyle of femur to condylar eminence of tibia
La. cruciata genus	Cruciate ligs. of knee	Bundles in knee joints between condyles of femur
Lm. cruciatum posterius genus	Posterior cruciate l. of knee	Connects medial condyle of femur to intercondylar area of tibia
Lm. menisci lateralis	Posterior meniscofemoral l.	Connects between medial condyle of femur to posterior crus of lateral meniscus
Lm. meniscofemorale anterius	Anterior meniscofemoral l.	Connects lateral meniscus to posterior cruciate l.
Lm. meniscofemorale posterius	Posterior meniscofemoral l.	Connects lateral meniscus to medial condyle of femur
Lm. patellae	Patellar l.	Connects patella to tibial tuberosity
Lm. popliteum arcuatum	Arcuate popliteal l.	Connects fibula to articular capsule
Lm. popliteum obliquum	Oblique popliteal l.	Connects medial condyle of tibia to lateral epicondyle of femur
Lm. teres femoris	Head of femur l.	Connects from fovea in head of femur to borders of acetabular notch

Latin name	English name	Articulation
Lm. tibiofibulare anterius	Anterior tibiofibular l.	Connects tibia to fibula
Lm. tibiofibulare medium	Interosseous membrane	
Lm. tibiofibulare posterius	Posterior tibiofibular l.	Connects tibia to distal fibula
Lm. tibionaviculare	Medial l.	Connects from medial malleolus of tibial downward to tarsal bones
Lm. transversum genus	Transverse l. of knee	Connects lateral meniscus to medial meniscus

Foot and Ankle

Latin name	English name	Articulation
Lm. bifurcatum	Bifurcate l.	Dorsum of foot; comprises calcaneonavicular and calcaneocuboid ligs.
Lm. calcaneocuboideum	Calcaneocuboid l.	Connects calcaneus to cuboid
Lm. calcaneocuboideum plantare	Plantar calcaneocuboid l. short plantar l.	Connects calcaneus to cuboid
Lm. calcaneofibulare	Calcaneofibular l.	Connects fibula to calcaneus
Lm. calcaneonaviculare	Calcaneonavicular l.	Connects calcaneus to navicular bone
Lm. calcaneonaviculare dorsale	Dorsal calcaneonavicular l.	Connects calcaneus to navicular bone
Lm. calcaneonaviculare plantare	Plantar calcaneonavicular l.	Connects sustentaculum tali to navicular; supports talus
Lm. calcaneotibiale	Calcaneotibial l.	Connects medial malleolus to sustentaculum tali of calcaneus
Lm. collateralia articulationum	Collateral ligs. of metatarsophalangeal articulations	Fibrous bands on sides of each metatarsophalangeal joints
Lm. cruciatum cruris	Inferior extensor of foot	Joins malleolus to dorsum of foot
La. cuboideonaviculare dorsale	Dorsal cuboideonavicular l.	Connects cuboid and navicular bones
La. cuboideonaviculare plantare	Plantar cuboideonavicular l.	Connects cuboid and navicular bones
Lm. cuneocuboideum dorsale	Dorsal cuneocuboid l.	Connects cuboid and lateral cuneiform bones
Lm. cuneocuboideum interosseum	Interosseus cuneocuboid l.	Connects cuboid and lateral cuneiform bones
Lm. cuneocuboideum plantare	Plantar cuneocuboid l.	Connects cuboid and lateral cuneiform bones

Latin name	English name	Articulation
La. cuneometatarsalia interossea	Interosseous cuneometatarsal ligs.	Connects cuneiform and metatarsal bones
La. cuneonavicularia dorsalia	Dorsal cuneonavicular ligs.	Connects navicular and cuneiform bones
La. cuneonavicularia plantaria	Plantar cuneonavicular ligs.	Connects navicular to cuneiform bones
La. intercuneiformia dorsalia	Dorsal intercuneiform ligs.	Connects dorsal surfaces of cuneiform bones
La. intercuneiformia interossea	Interosseous intercuneiform ligs.	Connects adjacent cuneiform bones
La. intercuneiformia plantaria	Plantar intercuneiform ligs.	Joins plantar surfaces of cuneiform bones
Lm. laterale articulationis talocruralis	Lateral l. of ankle joints	Lateral side of ankle joints
Lm. mediale articulationis talocruralis	Medial l. of ankle	Connects medial malleolus of tibia to tarsal bones
La. meniscofemoralia	Meniscofemoral ligs.	Connects from posterior part of lateral meniscus to lateral surface of medial meniscus
Lm. metatarsale transversum profundum	Deep transverse metatarsal l.	Joins heads of metatarsals
Lm. metatarsale transversum superficiale	Superficial transverse metatarsal l.	Lies on sole of foot beneath heads of metatarsals
La. metatarsalia dorsalia	Dorsal metatarsal ligs.	Interconnects bases of metatarsal bones
La. metatarsalia interossea	Interosseous metatarsal ligs.	Interconnects bases of metatarsal bones
La. metatarsalia plantaria	Plantar metatarsal ligs.	Plantar surface of metatarsal bones
La. plantaria articulationum interphalangealium pedis	Plantar ligs. of interphalangeal articulations	Interphalangeal articulations of foot between collateral ligs.
La. plantaria articulationum metatarsophalangeal	Plantar ligs. of metatarsophalangeal articulations	Plantar surface of metatarsophalangeal articulations between collateral ligs.
Lm. plantare longum	Long plantar l.	Connects calcaneus to bases of metatarsal bones
Lm. talocalcaneare laterale	Lateral talocalcaneal l.	Connects talus to calcaneus
Lm. talocalcaneare mediale	Medial talocalcaneal l.	Connects tubercle of talus to sustentaculum tali of calcaneus

Latin name	English name	Articulation
Lm. talocalcaneum	Talocalcaneal l.	Connects talus and calcaneus
Lm. talocalcaneum interosseum	Interosseous talo-calcaneal l.	Connects calcaneus to talus
Lm. talofibulare anterius	Anterior talofibular l.	Connects lateral malleolus of fibula to posterior process of talus.
Lm. talonaviculare	Talonavicular l.	Connects neck of talus to navicular bone
Lm. talotibiale	Medial tibiotalar l.	Connects downward from medial malleolus of tibia of tarsal bones.
La. tarsi	Ligs. of tarsus	Connects bones of tarsus
La. tarsi dorsalia	Dorsal ligs. of tarsus	Collectively, bifurcate, dorsal cuboideonavicular, cuneocuboid, cuneonavicular, intercuneiform, and talonavicular ligs.
La. tarsi interossea	Interosseous ligs. of tarsus	Collectively, interosseous, cuneocuboid, intercuneiform, and talocalcaneal ligs.
La. tarsi plantaria	Plantar ligs. of tarsus	Inferior ligs. of foot (long plantar, plantar calcaneocuboid, calcaneo-navicular, cuneonavicular, cuboideo-navicular, intercuneiform, cuneocuboid)
La. tarsometatarsalia dorsalia	Dorsal tarsometatarsal ligs.	Connects bases of metatarsals to dorsal cuboid and cuneiform bones
La. tarsometatarsalia plantaria	Plantar tarsometatarsal ligs.	Connects metatarsal bones to cuboid and cuneiform bones
Lm. transversum cruris	Superior extensor retinaculum of foot	Connects tibia to fibula; holds extensor tendons in place
Tendo calcaneus	Achilles tendon calcaneal tendon	Connects triceps surae muscle to tuberosity of calcaneus

Abbreviations used: l., ligament; La. ligamenta; ligs., ligaments; Lm., ligamentum

Ligaments and Tendons

Professional Organizations, Associations, and Titles

Professional Organizations and Associations

Academy of Forensic and Industrial Chiropractic Consultants (AFICC)

American Academy of Neurological and Orthopaedic Surgeons (AANOS)

American Academy of Orthopaedic Surgeons (AAOS)

American Academy of Orthotists and Prosthetists (AAOP)

American Academy of Physical Medicine and Rehabilitation (AAPMR)

American Academy of Podiatric Sports Medicine (AAPSM)

American Association of Hand Surgery (AAHS)

American Association of Hip and Knee Surgeons (AAHKS)

American Association of Orthopaedic Foot and Ankle Surgeons (AAOFAS)

American Association of Tissue Banks (AATB)

American Back Society (ABS)

American Board of Certification of Orthotics and Prosthetics (ABC)

American Board of Orthopaedic Surgery (ABOS)

American Board of Physical Therapy Specialists (ABPTS)

American Chiropractic Association (ACA)

American Chiropractic Association Council on Sports Injuries and Physical Fitness

American College of Chiropractic Consultants (ACCC)

American College of Chiropractic Orthopedists (ACCO)

American College of Foot & Ankle Orthopedics & Medicine (ACFAOM)

American College of Foot and Ankle Surgeons (ACFAS)

American College of Occupational and Environmental Medicine (ACOEM)

American College of Rheumatology (ACR)

American College of Sports Medicine (ACSM)

American Congress of Rehabilitation Medicine (ACRM)

American Health Care Association (AHCA)

American Institute of Orthopaedic and Sports Medicine (AIOSM)

American Medical Society for Sports Medicine (AMSSM)

American Occupational Therapy Association (AOTA)

American Orthopaedic Foot and Ankle Society (AOFAS)

American Orthopaedic Society (AOS)

American Orthopaedic Society for Sports Medicine (AOSSM)

American Orthotic and Prosthetic Association (AOPA)

American Osteopathic Academy of Orthopaedics (AOAO)

American Osteopathic Academy for Sports Medicine (AOASM)

American Osteopathic Association (AOA)

American Osteopathic Board of Orthopedic Surgery (AOBOS)

American Osteopathic College of Occupational & Preventive Medicine (AOCOPM)

American Physical Therapy Association (APTA)
American Podiatric Medical Association (APMA)
American Rheumatism Association (ARA)
American Shoulder and Elbow Surgeons (ASES)
American Society of Orthopaedic Physician's Assistants (ASOPA)
American Society for Testing and Materials (ASTM)
American Spinal Injury Association (ASIA)
Americans with Disabilities Act (ADA)
Arthroscopy Association of North America (AANA)
Association of Rehabilitation Nurses (ARN)
Association for the Study of Internal Fixation (ASIF)
Association of Bone and Joint Surgeons (ABJS)
Association of Chiropractic Colleges (ACC)
Board of Certification in Orthopedic Surgery
British Orthopaedic Association (BOA)
Canadian Academy of Sport Medicine (CASM)
Canadian Association of Physical Medicine and Rehabilitation (CAPMR)
Canadian Athletic Therapists Association (CATA)
Canadian Orthopaedic Nurses Association (CONA)
Canadian Physiotherapy Association (CPA)
Chiropractic Rehabilitation Association (CRA)
Commission on Accreditation of Rehabilitation Facilities (CARF)
Council on Chiropractic Education (CCE)
Council on Chiropractic Education International (CCEI)
European Society of Foot and Ankle Surgeons (ESFAS)
Federation of Chiropractic Licensing Boards (FCLB)
Fellow of the American College of Sports Medicine (FACSM)
Fellow of the American Occupational Therapy Association (FAOTA)
Fellow of the American Physical Therapy Association (FAPTA)
Fitness Safety Standards Committee (FSSC)
Foundation for Chiropractic Education and Research (FCER)
International Cartilage Repair Society (ICRS)
International Chiropractors Association (ICA)
International Headache Society (IHS)
International Knee Documentation Committee (IKDC)
International Society of Arthroscopy, Knee Surgery, and Orthopaedic Sports
  (ISAKOS)
International Society for Prosthetics and Orthotics (ISPO)
Medical Research Council (MRC)
Musculoskeletal Transplant Foundation (MTF)
National Academy of Sports Medicine (NASM)
National Association of Medical Equipment Suppliers (NAMES)
National Association of Orthopaedic Nurses (NAON)

National Association of Orthopaedic Technologists (NAOT)
National Board of Chiropractic Examiners (NBCE)
National Rehabilitation Association (NRA)
North American Spine Society (NASS)
Occupational Injury Prevention Rehabilitation Society (OIPRS)
Occupational Safety and Health Administration (OSHA)
Orthopaedic Trauma Association (OTA)
Policy and Review Committee for Human Research
Visiting Nurse Association (VNA)

Professional Titles
Certified Orthotist (CO)
Certified Pedorthist (CPed)
Certified Prosthetist (CP)
Certified Prosthetist/Orthotist (CPO)
Doctor of Chiropractic (DC)
Doctor of Occupational Therapy (OTD)
Doctor of Physical Therapy (DPT)
Doctor of Podiatric Medicine (DPM)
Doctor of Podiatry (DP)
Industrial Physical Therapist (IPT)
Master of Physical Therapy (MPT)
Occupational Therapist (OT)
Occupational Therapist (Canada) (OT-C)
Occupational Therapist, Licensed (OT-L)
Occupational Therapist, Registered (OT-R)
Orthopedic Certified Specialist (OCS)
Physical Therapist (PT)
Physical Therapy Assistant (PTA)
Sports Certified Specialist (SCS)

Sample Reports and Dictation

ARTHROSCOPY RIGHT KNEE

PREOPERATIVE DIAGNOSIS: Loose body, right knee.

POSTOPERATIVE DIAGNOSES
1. Advanced medial compartmental osteoarthritis with mild patellofemoral arthritis, right knee.
2. Two loose bodies, right knee.
3. Complex large tear medial meniscus, right knee.
4. Incompetent anterior cruciate ligament with fibers intact.
5. Mild degenerative tear, lateral meniscus.

PROCEDURES PERFORMED
1. Arthroscopic débridement, osteoarthritic right knee.
2. Arthroscopic partial medial meniscectomy, right knee.
3. Removal of 2 loose bodies, right knee.

DESCRIPTION OF PROCEDURE: The patient was brought to the operating room and a general anesthetic was applied in the supine position. Sterile prep and free drape were performed on the right knee. Under tourniquet control, an anterolateral portal was made and the scope was introduced in the knee. Diagnostic arthroscopy revealed grade 2 changes in the patella; however, the trochlear groove looked normal. The medial gutter was clear. The medial compartment revealed a complex tear of the entire medial meniscus as well as a small loose body in the medial and anterior compartment. The ACL appeared to be damaged but there were some fibers in appropriate orientation. The lateral compartment showed some degenerative changes to the meniscus, but was overall intact. There was a large loose body in the lateral compartment.

An anteromedial portal was made. We proceeded to do a partial medial meniscectomy all the way from the anterior horn around to the posterior horn. This was a very complex tear, and it was débrided back to stable tissue. There was a full-thickness lesion on the tibial plateau and on the distal femoral condyle. Overall, the cartilage was quite thin. The ACL was probed, and it was somewhat incompetent but the fibers did appear to be in appropriate alignment. We suspect it was a nonfunctioning ACL.

There was a loose body approximately 8 x 5 mm in the anterior compartment. This was removed through an anteromedial portal.

We then moved to the lateral gutter and palpated the large loose body. We made a small incision and could grasp the loose body with a snap. This was quite large, and we had to make a small arthrotomy to remove this piece, which was probably about 2 x 1 cm in size. It was oval in nature. We then proceeded to close the arthrotomy using 2-0 Polysorb and then we closed the portals and the skin wound using 2-0 nylon. The knee was infiltrated with local anesthetic. The tourniquet was let down. The wound was dressed with gauze and a tensor wrap.

The patient was reversed from anesthetic and transferred to the postanesthetic recovery room without difficulty. He will be discharged home today for followup in 1 week's time.

BLATT PROCEDURE OF WRIST

PREOPERATIVE DIAGNOSIS: Old scaphoid fracture with scapholunate widening and osteoarthritis.

POSTOPERATIVE DIAGNOSIS: Old scaphoid fracture with scapholunate widening and osteoarthritis.

PROCEDURES PERFORMED
1. Blatt procedure, right wrist.
2. Local flap advancement, right wrist.

INDICATIONS: This pleasant 55-year-old gentleman presents with painful right wrist after repeated injuries and chronic use of his hands bilaterally. We have discussed the possibility of management with ligamentous tightening attempt in the right wrist according to Blatt, to which the patient agreed. He understands that he may have persistent discomfort in the right wrist despite our best attempts at soft tissue reconstruction with consideration for a possible proximal row carpectomy or fusion in the future.

DESCRIPTION OF PROCEDURE: Under general anesthesia, the patient was prepped and draped in the usual manner. The incision line was made to access the scapholunate region, and intraoperative microscopy was utilized throughout the procedure to ensure alignment of the scapholunate bones, as well as location of the capitate. The scaphoid bone itself was noted to have a distal intercalated segment instability (DISI) deformity, and Kirschner wire was placed in both the lunate and the scaphoid for rotation after the capsule had been elevated from the radius for suturing and placement post reduction. Two 0.045 Kirschner wires were used to maintain the reduction of the scapholunate alignment followed by using a 4-0 Ti-Cron for suturing of the capsule to the softened scaphoid. The scapholunate bones were also noted to be significantly softened and a cyst was noted within the scaphoid bone itself.

No obvious separation was noted within the scapholunate junction, and this appeared to be reduced on intraoperative fluoroscopy. Hemostasis was maintained with electrocautery.

The wound edges were undermined and closed with 4-0 Prolene suture. The hand was placed in a resting splint. Jurgan pin balls were placed over the Kirschner wires for postoperative comfort. A total of 10 mL of 0.5% Marcaine without epinephrine was infiltrated for postoperative comfort. The patient tolerated the procedure well. There were no complications.

CEMENTED TOTAL KNEE REPLACEMENT

PREOPERATIVE DIAGNOSIS: Right knee posttraumatic arthritis with varus deformity and flexure contracture.

POSTOPERATIVE DIAGNOSIS: Right knee posttraumatic arthritis with varus deformity and flexure contracture.

PROCEDURE PERFORMED: Cemented right total knee replacement.

ANESTHESIA: Spinal.

ESTIMATED BLOOD LOSS: 100 mL.

SPECIMENS: Soft tissues, synovium, articular cartilage, bone, and osteophyte.

DESCRIPTION OF PROCEDURE: The patient was taken to the operating room and placed on the operating room table in a sitting position. Spinal anesthesia was administered, antibiotics given, and a Foley catheter placed. Her left knee was injected with 1 mL of Depo-Medrol 40 mg for comfort. Her right leg was prepped and draped in the usual sterile fashion after a tourniquet was placed on her thigh and set to 325 mmHg. The leg was exsanguinated and the tourniquet inflated, the knee flexed at 90 degrees, and a midline incision made.

A standard median parapatellar arthrotomy was performed and the patellar everted. Full thickness articular cartilage loss of the medial compartment with bone-on-bone articulation, marginal osteophytes, and a meniscal tear was seen. The remnant of the posterior horn and the medial meniscus was subluxed and removed. A medial sleeve release was performed off the medial shelf osteophyte on the tibia for balancing and

A113

exposure. The lateral meniscus was removed; the anterior cruciate ligament was incompetent and its stump removed. The posterior cruciate ligament would be resected later in the case as per surgeon's protocol in this posttraumatic arthritic knee.

A synovectomy was performed. A drill hole was made in the distal femur, cannulating the intramedullary canal in line with the shaft. The Centerpulse Natural-Knee II System was utilized as the 1st cutting block was applied to the anterior aspect of the distal femur. An 11-mm resection in 5 degrees of valgus was made based on preoperative templating. Sizing was performed and a size 3 condylar cutting block was applied to the cut surface of the distal femur in external rotation using the posterior condylar and epicondylar axes as references. Anterior and posterior condylar cuts were made protecting the collateral ligament structures. The chamfer guide was exchanged for the condylar guide. Anterior and posterior chamfer cuts were made in sequence along with the notch cut as per protocol. A large osteophyte was removed from the posterior medial aspect of the femur and release of the capsule there performed. No osteophyte on the tibia was removed for fear of medial collateral insufficiency after release.

Next, the intramedullary tibial cutting guide was applied with the leg in hyperflexion. The center of the ankle mortise was used as a reference. The lateral tibial plateau was used for a reference of depth of cut as well as posterior inclination. An 11-mm resection perpendicular to the axis of the tibia was then created. This did not completely bottom the defect posteromedially about the osteophyte. A size 2 tibial preparation tray was then fixed to the cut surface of the proximal tibia. It was lateralized and externally rotated so the center of the tray was just medial to the tibial tubercle. This allowed for osteophyte posteromedially and did not involve the defect of the sloping posterior medial tibia. Peg drill holes were created and keyhole punching performed as per protocol. Trial was performed with the size 2 tibial trial and a size 3 femoral trial component along with an 11-mm ultracongruent insert. Full extension was achieved; no collateral instability with varus or valgus stress testing and extension was noted; 1+ excursion with varus and valgus stress testing in flexion was accepted. The tourniquet was deflated at 29 minutes.

The patella everted circumferentially, exposed caliper measurement made and a 7-mm resection of articular patella performed. A size 2 template was placed along the horizontal axis of the patella and peg drill holes were created. The entire cut surface of the patella was encompassed with the template. Trial was performed and no lateral release was necessary.

All trial components were removed, pulse lavage irrigation solution was used to clean all cut surfaces of bone of bloody and bony remnant. It was then packed dry as 2 bags of Concert PMMA bone cement were mixed under vacuum pressure utilizing the twister system. The cement was allowed to cure for 2 minutes under suction. Manual pressurization technique was utilized as the following components were cemented in sequence, being a size 2 tibial component, size 3 standard femoral component, and a size 2, 3-pegged all-polyethylene Durasul patella component. Excessive cement was cleaned from all interfaces as cement cured within 10 minutes. Irrigation was performed and cleaning of the tibial component completed as an 11-mm Durasul ultracongruent liner was engaged and secured. The knee was reduced; stability check and range of motion deemed acceptable. At this point pulse lavage irrigation solution was used.

Medium Hemovac drains were brought through the anterior, medial, and lateral fascial and skin flaps. The extensor mechanism was closed using #1 figure-of-8 and horizontal Vicryl sutures. The subcutaneous tissues were closed with the tourniquet deflated at 43 minutes using #1 Vicryl and 0 Vicryl sutures. Skin staples were placed. A sterile compression dressing, reinfusion system, and knee immobilizer were applied. The patient was moved to the gurney and to the recovery room in stable condition under regional anesthesia. Neurologic checks could not be performed for this reason.

Closed Reduction of Radial Head Fracture

Preoperative Diagnosis: Fracture of radial head, left elbow.

Postoperative Diagnosis: Fracture of radial head, left elbow.

Procedure Performed: Closed reduction of radial head, left elbow.

Anesthesia: General.

Indications: This very pleasant young lad fell on an outstretched hand. He was seen in the emergency room and x-rays demonstrated a type II radial neck fracture, likely a Salter-Harris II variant. He had loss of pronation and supination and x-rays demonstrated approximately 5 mm of lateral displacement. For that reason, we discussed closed reduction, possible open reduction, and the parents consented.

Description of Procedure: The patient was brought to the operating suite and administered a general anesthetic without complication. The patient was placed in the supine position. Under fluoroscopic guidance, the fractured neck was reduced to anatomic position. This was held at 90 degrees and repeat x-rays were performed. A posterior splint at 90 degrees and neutral pronation/supination was utilized and x-rays were utilized once again to ensure that loss of reduction had not occurred. The fracture was stable.

The patient was transferred to the recovery room in stable condition.

4-CORNER PARTIAL CARPAL FUSION

PREOPERATIVE DIAGNOSIS: Osteoarthritis, right wrist, secondary to scapholunate ligament disruption.

POSTOPERATIVE DIAGNOSIS: Stage 3 to stage 4 osteoarthritis of right wrist secondary to scapholunate ligament disruption.

PROCEDURE PERFORMED: A 4-corner partial carpal fusion, right wrist, with excision of proximal pole of scaphoid.

INDICATIONS: This is a 50-year-old man with a past history of carcinoma of the prostate who has had a long history of right greater than left wrist arthritis. He has had 2 previous arthroscopies of the right wrist which provided temporary relief. X-rays show stage 3 to stage 4 ostearthritis of the right wrist secondary to scapholunate ligament disruption. There is some contact of the capitate on the distal radius, but there is still a fairly good lunate facet on the distal radius. The plan is for a 4-corner fusion to unload the wrist radially.

DESCRIPTION OF PROCEDURE: The patient was brought to the operating room and administered a spinal anesthetic. A pneumatic tourniquet was elevated to 250 mmHg. A standard, 8-cm dorsal approach to the right wrist was used. The interval between the 2nd and 4th extensor compartments was used, removing the extensor pollicis longus tendon from harm's way. A direct dorsal arthrotomy was performed. The joint was completely filled with noninflammatory synovial tissue, and the anatomy was quite distorted. The wrist was shortened and radially deviated.

The patient had complete splaying between the scaphoid and the lunate, and the capitate was almost touching the distal radius and had migrated proximally. The scaphoid was very unstable. We removed the part that was impinging on the radial styloid with a small osteotome. We removed a portion of bone measuring about 1 x 1 x 5 mm. This dealt with the radial carpal impingement, particularly with radial deviation of the wrist.

With distraction, we removed the articular cartilage from the joints between the capitate and the lunate, between the lunate and the hamate, and between the triquetrum and the hamate in particular. The articulation between the hamate and the capitate seemed quite good, as well as the articulation between the triquetrum and the lunate; we did not specifically take these joints apart since they seemed to be so strong ligamentously. We felt he had enough instability in the wrist without me causing the wrist to be more unstable.

We morselized a portion of the proximal scaphoid that we had excised and packed it between the bony surfaces and then supplemented this with 1 mL of AlloMatrix bone putty. Then, in compression, we inserted 4 K-wires, 2 in a retrograde fashion from the capitate and hamate into the lunate and triquetrum bones, 1 from the radial side and 1 from the ulnar side, and transversely across the proximal carpal row. Good overall stability was achieved clinically. X-rays confirmed good position of the K-wires and good overall position of the wrist. In particular, we tried to correct the DISI deformity and correct the radial deviation.

The K-wires were all bent 1 cm from the skin and left protruding. They were manipulated around the extensor tendons so that there was no impingement, and the EPL tendon was spared the K-wire impingement.

The wound was closed with interrupted 2-0 Vicryl suture for the capsule of the wrist, interrupted 2-0 Vicryl for the fascia around the tendon sheaths, interrupted 3-0 Vicryl for subcutaneous, and the skin was closed with staples. The wound was dressed with Sofra-Tulle gauze, sterile toppers, and then a below-elbow volar thumb spica splint applied and held with Kling wrap. Tourniquet time was 105 minutes.

FEMUR FRACTURE DISCHARGE SUMMARY

ADMITTING DIAGNOSIS: Fracture right distal femur.

PROCEDURES PERFORMED: Closed reduction and percutaneous screw fixation, right distal femur fracture.

HOSPITAL COURSE: The patient is an 11-year-old boy who was admitted to the hospital after injuring his knee playing volleyball. He had a Salter II fracture of the distal femur on the right side. Care was transferred to me due to the on-call schedule. He was taken to the operating room the day after admission and had an uncomplicated closed reduction and percutaneous screw fixation. On postoperative day 1 he was doing very well. His pain was controlled with Tylenol No. 3. He was mobilized with crutches. He seemed to be doing quite well. We will mobilize him tomorrow and discharge him home on postoperative day 3, if he was getting around safely on crutches. He will be seen in followup 1 week after discharge. He will go home using Tylenol No. 3 for pain control. He did have a reaction to Toradol and this has been discontinued. The reaction was in the form of hallucinations and diaphoresis.

GANGLION EXCISION, RIGHT KNEE

PREOPERATIVE DIAGNOSIS: Ganglion, right knee.

POSTOPERATIVE DIAGNOSIS: Two ganglia, anterior aspect of right knee.

PROCEDURE PERFORMED: Excision of 2 ganglia, right knee.

DESCRIPTION OF PROCEDURE: The patient was anesthetized and then the right knee was prepped and free draped. An incision was made over the lump on the anterior aspect of the right knee and dissection was carried down to the lump. This was in 2 separate pockets with 2 separate attachments. A ganglion of the pes anserinus bursa was identified. The 2 areas were thoroughly excised and their bases sutured. Vicryl sutures were placed, and the skin was closed with staples. A sterile bandage was applied, and the patient was sent to the recovery room with a pressure bandage on the right knee. Arrangements were made for followup in the outpatient clinic.

HIP HEMIARTHROPLASTY

PREOPERATIVE DIAGNOSES
1. Infected right total hip arthroplasty.
2. Acute fracture of left hip.

POSTOPERATIVE DIAGNOSES
1. Infected right total hip arthroplasty.
2. Acute fracture of left hip.

PROCEDURE PERFORMED: Left hip hemiarthroplasty.

ANESTHESIA: Spinal.

ESTIMATED BLOOD LOSS: 500 mL.

INDICATIONS: This pleasant and most unfortunate gentleman was admitted to the hospital early yesterday in preparation for revision total hip arthroplasty on the right side. Our plan was to remove the components and apply an antibiotic-laden cement spacer. Unfortunately, on his travels to the hospital he slipped and fell, fracturing his left hip.

We discussed this case with numerous colleagues and we felt the safest plan would be to stage the procedures with hemiarthroplasty of the left hip first. Ideally, a cemented hemiarthroplasty would have been the best choice; however, infection of a cemented hemiarthroplasty is a difficult revision. Thus, we elected to perform an uncemented modular Moore hemiarthroplasty on the left hip.

We discussed this with the family numerous times, and they understood and consented.

The patient arrived to the operating room after seeing internal medicine and anesthesia preoperatively in consultation.

DESCRIPTION OF PROCEDURE: The patient was brought to the operating room and was administered a spinal anesthetic without complication. The patient was placed in right lateral decubitus position and latex precautions were followed. He was placed in the lateral decubitus position and held in place with the Montreal frame.

Utilizing a curvilinear incision slightly posterior (We will utilize the posterolateral approach if revision is required), the skin and subcutaneous tissue were dissected. The iliotibial band was dissected and it was necessary to "T" the iliotibial band because it was very tight. The anterior one–third of the gluteus medius and minimus muscles was reflected as per Hardinge approach. The fracture was identified, and the saw was taken to the femoral neck. The femoral head was retrieved and sized. It was felt to be appropriately sized at 55.

Once this was performed, the leg was placed in the bag. Using box osteotome, followed by starter reamer, followed by a rasp, the calcar was reamed appropriately and a 55-mm uncemented modular Moore prosthesis was inserted without complication. This was reduced and it was, in fact, very stable.

Thorough irrigation was placed into the wound. Closure consisted of 1-0 Polysorb for the gluteus medius, minimus, and iliotibial band layers, and 2-0 Polysorb subcutaneously. Staples were applied to the skin. Instrument, needle, and sponge counts were correct.

POSTOPERATIVE PLAN: This gentleman will be made weightbearing as tolerated. Once he recovers from this surgery, we will plan to forge ahead with revision right total hip arthroplasty and removal of the components. We will keep him on intravenous antibiotics to protect his left hemiarthroplasty and likely send him back to the hospital near his home for rehabilitation.

Sample Reports

Hybrid Total Hip Replacement

Preoperative Diagnosis: Posttraumatic osteonecrosis of the right hip, status post intramedullary nailing of right femur with malunion.

Preoperative Diagnosis: Posttraumatic osteonecrosis of the right hip, status post intramedullary nailing of right femur with malunion.

Procedure Performed: Hybrid right total hip replacement.

Anesthesia: Spinal.

Estimated Blood Loss: 100 mL.

Specimens: Femoral head, soft tissue, and bone.

Description of Procedure: The patient was taken to the operating room and placed on the operating room table in a sitting position. Spinal anesthesia was administered. Antibiotics were given. A Foley catheter placed. The patient was moved into the left lateral decubitus position. The right hip and thigh were prepped and draped in the usual sterile fashion. Longitudinal oblique incisional scars from the previous surgery were seen. These were not traditional nailing scars and would be avoided, as the posterior mini-incisional total hip replacement exposure would be utilized.

A short oblique incision on the posterior lateral hip trochanter was made to use the mini-incisional posterior approach. The subcutaneous tissues were dissected down to the fascia lata, which was split throughout the length of the wound. Scar tissue was seen from the previous procedure. The sciatic nerve was identified and protected throughout the case. The gluteus minimus and medius muscles were reflected anteriorly off the posterolateral hip capsule. The piriformis muscle had been previously bisected and was scarred in the bursa. The bursa was incised and the external rotators stripped from the flare of the trochanter to the top of the lesser trochanter. Heterotopic ossification posterosuperiorly was seen and chiseled. A curvilinear capsulotomy was performed protecting the sciatic nerve, identifying the hip joint. A Charnley pin was placed in the ilium above the acetabulum and positioned at 10 o'clock at 60 degrees for retraction. A mark was made in the greater trochanter and a measurement recorded. This patient had at least a 6-mm leg length discrepancy preoperatively.

The hip was dislocated and the femoral head was dislocated into the mini-incisional wound. Cleaning of the intersection of the femoral neck and trochanter was performed as a femoral neck osteotomy was made 5 mm above the lesser trochanter based on preoperative templating. The head was removed and degenerative and not collapsed. Circumferential exposure of the acetabulum ensued. Scar tissue was removed along with synovium. Circumferential removal of the labrum was performed.

The Centerpulse Natural-Hip System was utilized as a 44-mm reamer was used to obtain medialization of the true floor of the acetabulum. Thereafter, acetabular reamers in 2-mm increments in even sizes were utilized to prepare the acetabular bed at this level. Reaming to 48 mm was performed in a position of 45 degrees of abduction and 25 degrees of flexion mimicking the patient's anatomy. Excellent bone support was seen as the reamer was engaged circumferentially. A trial was performed with the 48-mm trial component. It was engaged but not easily seated to the floor. For this reason, a 49-mm component would be chosen which would allow for a 1.5-mm press-fit as per protocol.

A Centerpulse Converge cluster-hole sealed porous acetabular component was then opened and prepared. It was engaged into an irrigated acetabular bed into a position of 45 degrees of abduction and 25 degrees of flexion and malleted securely. Excellent fixation was seen; no need for screws.

A 28-mm inner diameter liner was engaged with the elevation in the posterosuperior position and secured. The acetabulum was protected. The leg was placed in maximum adduction, 90 degrees internal rotation, and flexion as a minimally invasive retractor was used to protect the sciatic nerve. Lateralization of the greater trochanter was performed deliberately to prevent malposition of instrumentation into the femoral canal due to previous malunion.

A box chisel was used to remove bone from the osteotomy site. The T-handled awl was used to cannulate the intramedullary canal. The cortical reamers from the Centerpulse Natural-Hip System were utilized starting with size 0 and ending with size 2 as cortical chatter was felt. Valgus instrumentation of the canal was performed to prevent varus malpositioning. Next, broaching was performed with size 0, size 1, and a final size 2 broach in slight anteversion matching the anteversion of the femoral neck with the leg in 90 degrees internal rotation. A size 2 broach was seated just below the osteotomy level and calcar planing was performed. Trial was performed with an offset trunnion and a 28 x +4-mm trial femoral head was used. The hip was reduced. Excellent stability and range of motion was seen without impingement. Lengthening of 5 to 6 mm was achieved, correlating with preoperative templating.

All trial components were removed. The acetabulum was again exposed. An apical screw plug was placed. Irrigation was performed and a dorsal 28-mm inner diameter liner for a 49-mm Converge acetabular component with a 10-degree elevation was engaged with the elevation in the posterosuperior position and malleted securely. The acetabulum was again protected. The proximal femur was again exposed. A large, 25.5 mm Richards cement hook was placed down the canal to 150 mm. Pulse lavage irrigation solution was used to clean the canal of bloody and bony remnant. Upon completion of irrigation, the femoral canal was packed dry as 2 bags of Simplex P bone cement mixed under vacuum pressure utilizing a twisted system. The cement was allowed to cure for 2 minutes under suction. Retrograde filling of the canal was performed utilizing the twisted system, and 5 seconds of pressurization was utilized.

A size 2 offset cemented Natural-Hip stem with a 10-mm centralizer was then engaged with cement mantle in proper anteversion, malleted until there was collar-to-calcar contact. Excess cement was cleaned from the interface as cement cured for 10 minutes. The trunnion was cleaned, and a 28 x +4-mm cobalt chrome femoral head was engaged and the hip reduced. Excellent stability and range of motion was seen. The hip was abducted.

The capsule was closed with a running #1 Vicryl suture. Medium Hemovac drains were brought through the anterolateral fascial flap and skin flap. The abductor mechanism was closed with a #1 figure-of-8 Vicryl suture running. The subcutaneous tissues were closed using #1 Vicryl and 0 Vicryl sutures. Skin staples were placed. A sterile compression dressing, reinfusion system, and hip abduction pillow were applied. The patient was placed in a supine position and moved to the gurney, where an x-ray was taken and confirmed position of components and cement fixation of the stem. Neurologic checks could not be performed in the recovery room due to spinal anesthetic on board.

NANCY NAIL STABILIZATION OF FOREARM FRACTURE

PREOPERATIVE DIAGNOSIS: Fractured radius and ulna, left.

POSTOPERATIVE DIAGNOSIS: Fractured radius and ulna, left.

PROCEDURE PERFORMED: Nancy nail stabilization, left forearm fracture.

ANESTHESIA: General.

IMPLANTS USED: Two 2.5-cm titanium Nancy nails.

DESCRIPTION OF PROCEDURE: The patient was brought to the operating room, and a general anesthetic was applied in the supine position. Sterile prep and drape was performed on the left arm. Under radiolucent guidance, we made a small hole in the bone just proximal to the radial growth plate and introduced a 2.5-cm molded titanium Nancy nail. It was advanced to the level of the fracture, and with some manipulation we were able to get across the fracture and extended it up to the radial tuberosity. We manipulated the wire to get optimal position of the fracture. We moved to the proximal ulna, made a small drill hole distal to the growth plate, introduced another 2.5-cm molded wire, and advanced it down to the level of the fracture, across the fracture, and to the distal ulna. We then manipulated both wires so that we had good reduction of the fracture.

We then bent and cut the wires outside the skin and closed the wounds with 3-0 PDS suture followed by Steri-Strips, Sofra-Tulle dressing, Betadine gauze, and a well-padded above-elbow circumferential cast with the arm in neutral rotation. The patient was reversed from anesthetic without difficulty and transferred to the postanesthetic recovery room.

OPEN FEMUR FRACTURE FIXATION

PREOPERATIVE DIAGNOSIS: Grade 3B femur fracture, segmental.

POSTOPERATIVE DIAGNOSIS: Grade 3B open femur fracture.

PROCEDURE PERFORMED: Irrigation and debridement right femur, intramedullary nailing of right femur.

ANESTHESIA: General.

FLUIDS: Crystalloid and 3 units of packed red blood cells.

PROGNOSIS: Guarded.

CONDITION: Guarded.

ESTIMATED BLOOD LOSS: 800 mL.

SPECIMEN: None.

INDICATIONS: The patient is a 78-year-old male who was a restrained driver involved in a motor vehicle accident. He was brought to an outside emergency room where he was diagnosed with a right open femur fracture and an aortic leak. He was transferred to our institution because we had bypass capability. The cardiothoracic and trauma surgery team agreed that the femur should be stabilized as soon as possible. This would allow them access to his aorta. An external fixator was not preferred because they would have to turn him in multiple positions and the external fixator would get in the way. He was cleared for intramedullary nailing of his right femur.

DESCRIPTION OF PROCEDURE: The patient was taken to the operating room where he was placed under general anesthesia. His right thigh and lower extremity were prepped and draped in the usual sterile fashion. The 1-cm wound on the lateral thigh was extended 7 cm on both sides and the vastus lateralis muscle was split, exposing the bone ends. The bone ends were irrigated with 9 liters of saline; the middle 3 bags had antibiotic irrigation. Once this was completed, attention was turned to the knee.

A 4-cm incision was made at the level of the knee. The patellar tendon was split. A guidewire was placed centered on the anteroposterior and lateral views at the top of Blumensaat line. The guidewire was placed. Once this was acceptable on AP and lateral planes, it was over-reamed. A guidewire was then placed and cannulated through the segmental femur and into the distal femur. This was performed open, as there was an open wound. Successive reaming began from 9 to 13. It was sized as a 360 nail. A 360 nail was placed down the canal. It was proximally locked with locking screws on the jig. First they were drilled, measured, and the appropriate size was placed. The first was an 85 and the second was a 70. The jig was removed and a locking-head screw was placed. AP and lateral views of the femur showed the nail to be within the bone and in place.

Traction was put on the femur and x-rays of the contralateral femur and hip were used to estimate rotation. This was locked under C-arm guidance.

First, a knife was used to make an incision and then, under fluoroscopic guidance, the proximal locking screws were placed. They were first drilled. C-arm imaging confirmed AP and lateral planes. A 40-mm and then a 42-mm screw were placed distal and proximal, respectively. AP and lateral views confirmed good reduction of the fracture with screws in place. Final C-arm images were taken.

All wounds were vigorously irrigated. The lateral wound of the vastus lateralis was closed with 0 Vicryl suture. The tensor fascia was closed with 1-0 Vicryl suture. The subcutaneous tissue was closed with 2-0 Vicryl. Skin was closed with staples. All wounds were closed with 2-0 Vicryl suture and staples except the knee wound. The patellar tendon was closed with 0 Vicryl suture. A sterile dressing was applied.

He was taken to the intensive care unit intubated and in guarded condition.

OPEN REDUCTION OF WRIST WITH ACUMED VOLAR PLATING

PREOPERATIVE DIAGNOSIS: Recent malunion from open Galeazzi fracture, left wrist.

POSTOPERATIVE DIAGNOSIS: Recent malunion from open Galeazzi fracture, left wrist.

PROCEDURE PERFORMED: Open reduction, volar plating with Acumed volar plating system.

ANESTHESIA: General.

INDICATIONS: This is a generally healthy, 31-year-old man who was involved in a serious motor vehicle accident 1 month ago. He sustained a grade II open Galeazzi fracture-dislocation of left wrist, sprain of his low back through a previous L5-S1 spondylolisthesis, and injury to the right knee. He initially had a débridement and K-wire fixation within 8 hours of the injury. This initially did reasonably well, but it has started to become unstable, particularly with persistent malposition of the distal radius at the radiocarpal joint.

DESCRIPTION OF PROCEDURE: The patient was given a general anesthetic. We examined his knee under anesthetic. It showed stable collateral ligaments and good range of motion. Anterior cruciate ligament was unstable on Lachman test compared to the normal left knee.

Under tourniquet control at 250 mmHg on the left upper arm, the old incision was utilized. We used the Z portion of the incision. The radial wound was very well healed. The ulnar wound was still weeping a little bit. This was débrided to a minor degree. We went down through the fascia. We opened up the fascia just ulnar to the flexor carpi radialis tendon. There was no sign of any deep infection. The dissection proximally was easy; distally it was extremely stuck down. The 2 K-wires were removed. There was significant shortening of the distal radius. Unfortunately, this was a 4-part intraarticular fracture with the radial styloid process and the lunate facet fracture being hopelessly displaced and a small intraarticular piece between the distal radius and the scaphoid. Ultimately, we were able to lever it into position and place the contoured Acumed plate on the volar surface. We fixed it proximally with 1 screw, distally with 2 K-wires, and then supplemented it with 4 threaded, locked 2.3-mm screws and 1 radial styloid screw.

The C-arm was brought in. It showed good reduction of the fracture in the lateral view. In the AP view there was still some residual shortening. There appeared to be about 1 cm in loss of radial inclination. The screws on AP appeared to be too distal and on the lateral it appeared that the screws matched the distal articular surface fairly well and were not intraarticular.

The fracture complex was quite stable with passive pronation and supination which was almost full. There was some crepitus. We think this was because the mechanics of his distal radioulnar joint were abnormal from the dislocation and not from an intraarticular screw. We removed a screw that was the most ulnar and this did not seem to help the crepitus with pronation and supination.

The fracture was extremely comminuted. We really did not think that repositioning the ulnar screws would help much since there was only a sliver of bone to work with distally. We are hoping the fracture construct will heal as is. We can go back and remove the fixation at a later date, if necessary, and do a distal radioulnar joint arthroplasty.

The wound was closed with interrupted 2-0 Vicryl suture in 2 layers and then staples for skin. It was dressed with Sofra-Tulle gauze, sterile toppers, and then a below-elbow posterior splint was applied and held with Kling wrap.

OPEN REDUCTION INTERNAL FIXATION AND BONE GRAFT OF TIBIAL PLATEAU FRACTURE

PREOPERATIVE DIAGNOSIS: Left lateral tibial plateau fracture.

POSTOPERATIVE DIAGNOSIS: Left lateral tibial plateau fracture.

PROCEDURES PERFORMED: Open reduction internal fixation and bone graft of depressed left lateral tibial plateau fracture.

ANESTHESIA: General.

INDICATIONS: This man sustained a fracture of his lateral tibial plateau about a week ago while at work. He also has a lot of bruising in his calf. Ultrasound today showed there was no clot.

DESCRIPTION OF PROCEDURE: The patient was anesthetized with general anesthetic. The left leg was prepped and draped.

Under tourniquet control, we made a lateral incision. We went through the tibial tract and down to the tibial plateau itself. This plateau was depressed by about 4 or 5 mm. We made a drill hole through the condyle and with this we were able to lever up the fracture. This came together well. We cracked some AlloMatrix and Osteoset pellets up into this area. We then inserted a screw across the plateau. There was a bit of an open-book character to this fracture, so we think the screw compression should help hold it in place. An intraoperative x-ray was done using a mini-C-arm, and we thought the position of the screw was satisfactory as well as the fracture fragment.

The wound was then closed in layers, being careful to repair the lateral meniscus. This came together well. A Jones dressing was applied. He was returned to the recovery room in good condition.

OPEN REDUCTION INTERNAL FIXATION OF MEDIAL MALLEOLUS

PREOPERATIVE DIAGNOSIS: Right medial malleolar fracture.

POSTOPERATIVE DIAGNOSIS: Right medial malleolar fracture.

PROCEDURE PERFORMED: Open reduction internal fixation of right medial malleolus.

ANESTHESIA: General endotracheal.

ESTIMATED BLOOD LOSS: Minimal.

TOURNIQUET TIME: 60 minutes.

INDICATIONS: The patient is a 22-year-old gentleman who was involved in a motor vehicle accident. He sustained a closed right medial malleolar fracture as well as closed fractures of the left 2nd, 3rd, and 4th metacarpals. The hand surgeon on call took responsibility for the hand injury. The right medial malleolar fracture was displaced and was indicated for surgery.

DESCRIPTION OF PROCEDURE: The patient was brought to the operating room and placed on the operating table in supine position. The anesthesiologist administered general endotracheal anesthesia, and preoperative antibiotics were given. The right lower extremity was prepped and draped in the usual sterile fashion. A thigh tourniquet was applied. The left upper extremity was prepped and draped in the usual sterile fashion and the hand surgeon performed the closed reduction and percutaneous pinning of the left 2nd, 3rd, and 4th metacarpals while the right ankle was being addressed.

Once the right ankle was prepped and draped, the right tourniquet was inflated. A longitudinal incision was made over the medial malleolus. Subcutaneous tissues were divided. The fracture site was identified. The fracture was thoroughly irrigated. A curette was used to remove a hematoma that had formed. The fracture edges were carefully dissected free from the surrounding tissues with a 15 blade. Once this was done, the fracture again was irrigated. With the fracture opened up, the medial dome of the talus was visualized. There was no evidence of any significant condylar injuries to the talus. Once this was done, with the aid of a bone reduction clamp the malleolus was reduced in an anatomic position. Two guidewires of the Synthes cannulated style were placed, 1 anterior and 1 posterior to the reduction clamp. The wires were checked fluoroscopically and shown to be in appropriate position. This revealed that the fracture was anatomically reduced. Once this was done, a 40-mm, 4.0 cannulated screw was placed over each of the 2 guidewires. Excellent purchase was achieved. Excellent compression of the fracture was achieved as well. Once this was done, AP, lateral and mortise views on fluoroscopy were checked and showed anatomic reduction of the fracture and proper placement of the hardware.

Once this was done, the wound was again thoroughly irrigated. Superficial tissues were closed with 4-0 Vicryl sutures and the skin was closed with interrupted 4-0 nylon sutures. Xeroform gauze dressing was applied with an AO splint incorporated into the bandage. The patient was awoken from anesthesia without complications and transferred to the recovery room in stable condition.

REDUCTION AND FIXATION OF METACARPAL FRACTURE

PREOPERATIVE DIAGNOSIS: Left 5th metacarpal fracture.

POSTOPERATIVE DIAGNOSIS: Left 5th metacarpal fracture.

PROCEDURE PERFORMED: Reduction and K-wire fixation of fracture, left 5th metacarpal.

ANESTHESIA: General endotracheal.

INDICATIONS: The patient was roughhousing with his father when he punched a window, sustaining a left 5th metacarpal fracture through the distal shaft with approximately 50 degrees of volar angulation. He was brought to the operating room for reduction and K-wire fixation.

DESCRIPTION OF PROCEDURE: In the operating room under general endotracheal anesthesia with the patient supine, the left hand was prepped and draped in the usual fashion. The fracture was reduced into what clinically appeared to be anatomic position, and a percutaneous, 0.035 nonthreaded Kirschner wire was passed distal to proximal through the metacarpal head and down the shaft. Position was then examined using C–arm and found to be anatomic. The wire was cut approximately 0.5 cm from the skin surface.

Bactigras dressing, followed by fluff gauze and Kling wrap was applied followed by a volar plaster splint padded with Webril bandage and secured in place with Kling wrap and a tensor bandage. The patient tolerated the procedure well and left the operating room in good condition.

REVISION TOTAL KNEE REPLACEMENT

PREOPERATIVE DIAGNOSIS: Light anterior knee pain for 4 years after right total knee replacement for patellofemoral arthritis.

POSTOPERATIVE DIAGNOSIS: Right anterior knee pain for 4 years after right total knee replacement for patellofemoral arthritis.

PROCEDURE PERFORMED: Revision right total knee replacement for a new patellar button right knee.

ANESTHESIA: General.

COMPONENT USED: Biomet size large single-hole patellar button. No change in other components.

TOURNIQUET TIME: 75 minutes.

INDICATIONS: The patient is a 74-year-old man with a past history of coronary artery disease. Four years ago he had a right total knee replacement performed. The femoral and tibial components were replaced but not the patellar component. Since the surgery the patient has had stiffness and anterior knee pain. Preoperative x-rays show no obvious loosening or problems. Preoperative workup showed no evidence of infection. He now presents for revision total knee replacement to redo the patella and resurface it.

DESCRIPTION OF PROCEDURE: The patient was brought to the operating room and administered a general anesthetic. The pneumatic tourniquet was elevated to 300 mmHg.

The old, 20-cm anterior approach to the right knee was used. Soft tissues were quite thickened. No sign of any infection. A median parapatellar arthrotomy was performed. We did some soft tissue releases and everted the patella. The patella was extensively eroded with arthritis. There were some large bone spurs, particularly superiorly, and a 2 x 2 x 1-cm loose body in the superior portion of the patella, which was completely excised.

We flexed the knee and looked for any obvious loosening of the femoral, tibial, or polyethylene components. Everything looked solid. There was no sign of any infection or abnormal wear.

We used sharp dissection to expose the patella and then applied the patellar clamp from the Osteonics set, cut off 10 mm of bone, sized it to a size large patella, and made a single drill hole as per the guide. We then irrigated the patella and suctioned dried it. One bag of Simplex cement was inserted in a vacuum chamber and, when it was doughy in consistency, we pressed it into the patella and applied the large Biomet patella with patellar clamp. After 15 minutes, we removed the clamp. A lateral retinacular release was required because the patella seemed a little bit tight in flexion, was above the scarring laterally, and we released the structures as much as we thought was safe. Ultimately patellar tracking was good. The range of motion was from 0 to about 120 degrees of flexion intraoperatively.

The arthrotomy was closed with interrupted figure-of-8 0 Vicryl sutures for a nice watertight closure, interrupted 2-0 for subcutaneous tissue, and the skin was closed with staples. The wound was dressed with Sofra-Tulle gauze, sterile toppers, and a Jones dressing. The patient tolerated procedure well.

SHOULDER DÉBRIDEMENT AND ARTHROTOMY FOR DRAINING SINUS

PREOPERATIVE DIAGNOSIS: Chronic draining sinus, left shoulder.

POSTOPERATIVE DIAGNOSIS: Chronic draining sinus, left shoulder.

PROCEDURE PERFORMED: Débridement and arthrotomy, left shoulder.

ESTIMATED BLOOD LOSS: 20 mL.

COMPLICATIONS: Nil.

INDICATIONS: This 45-year-old female with longstanding rheumatoid arthritis apparently had numerous bouts of septic arthritis in multiple joints in the summertime. She was seen at an outside hospital and débrided numerous times. Unfortunately, her left shoulder has never really gone on to complete resolution of drainage, despite 5 debridement procedures.

Apparently her orthopedic surgeon saw her for reassessment, and the decision was made to continue arthrotomies and serial débridement of the left shoulder, as needed.

We discussed the risks with this very pleasant patient, and she consented and understood.

DESCRIPTION OF PROCEDURE: The patient was brought to the operating suite and administered a general anesthetic. It should be noted that flexion and extension views were done preoperatively and did show approximately 3.5 mm of change with respect to the atlas-dens interval (ADI) on the flexion and extension views. A gentle intubation was performed, the patient was placed in the supine position, and the table was elevated about 45 degrees. The limb was prepped and draped in the usual fashion.

Utilizing the previous skin incision, which was centered on the anterior one third of the deltoid, the skin and subcutaneous tissue were dissected. The wound edges were débrided and blunt dissection was used to dissect down to the joint capsule. This previous incision was via the deltoid muscle. It should be noted that there was no frank intraarticular pus but rather the purulent material was seen superficially.

Nonetheless, the joint was thoroughly irrigated with 12 liters of saline. A soft drain was placed in an intraarticular fashion and stitched. Closure consisted of 2-0 Polysorb suture for the deltoid, 2-0 Polysorb subcutaneously, and Prolene stitch for the skin. Appropriate dressings were applied. Instrument, needle, and sponge count correct.

SHOULDER MANIPULATIOND AND ARTHROSCOPY

PREOPERATIVE DIAGNOSIS: Left frozen shoulder.

POSTOPERATIVE DIAGNOSIS: Left frozen shoulder.

PROCEDURE PERFORMED: Manipulation under anesthesia with arthroscopic débridement with release of the anterior capsule.

ANESTHESIA: General endotracheal.

ESTIMATED BLOOD LOSS: 10 mL.

PROPHYLAXIS: Ancef 1 g.

COMPLICATIONS: None.

SPECIMEN: None.

DESCRIPTION OF PROCEDURE: The patient gave informed consent and was brought to the operating room. The patient was given general anesthesia. Once adequate anesthesia was obtained, the patient was given IV antibiotics and manipulation was then performed. Manipulation at first had limited forward flexion to about 120 degrees, external rotation to 30 degrees, and internal rotation to 10 degrees. The patient had abduction to 110 degrees. These were the endpoints. Once manipulation was performed, the patient had full forward flexion, abduction and external rotation. Internal rotation was similar to the contralateral side, about 30 degrees in the abducted position. When range of motion was improved, breakage of adhesions was felt.

At this point, the patient was then positioned and pads were placed to protect the appropriate areas. The patient was then placed in the beachchair position and then prepped and draped in the usual sterile manner.

Two portals were made; posterior and anterior portals were made. Examination of the shoulder was performed. The glenohumeral joint showed significant synovitis, which was then débrided. The rotator cuff was intact. The biceps anchor was attached, and the biceps tendon was intact. There was significant synovitis, mostly anterior and superior. Once this was débrided, rotator cuff was checked once again and shown to be intact. At this point, once satisfactory débridement was performed and the rotator interval was cleared and opened, the instruments were brought to the subacromial space. The subacromial space showed no subacromial abnormalities. Rotator cuff was intact and there was good clearance noted. There was no inflammation noted in this region.

The shoulder was irrigated with copious amounts of irrigation fluid and the wounds were then closed with 4-0 nylon sutures. Duramorph was placed inside the joint and in the portals. Dressings were applied and shoulder was placed in an immobilizer. The patient tolerated the procedure well and was brought to the recovery area in satisfactory condition.

TOTAL HIP ARTHROPLASTY

PREOPERATIVE DIAGNOSIS: Advanced osteoarthritis of right hip secondary to likely avascular necrosis from an old hip fracture.

POSTOPERATIVE DIAGNOSIS: Advanced osteoarthritis of right hip secondary to likely avascular necrosis from an old hip fracture.

PROCEDURE PERFORMED: Right total hip arthroplasty.

ANESTHESIA: General.

IMPLANTS USED
1. Exeter #3 prosthesis.
2. A 44-mm offset cemented stem.
3. A 28-mm, +4 head.
4. A 56-mm HA Trident cluster cup.
5. Two screws.
6. Neutral polyethylene liner.

DESCRIPTION OF PROCEDURE: The patient was brought to the operating room and a general anesthetic was applied in the supine position. The patient was placed in the left lateral decubitus position and supported with a Montreal frame. All bony prominences were padded. Sterile prep and drape was performed on the right hip, leg, and buttock.

A lateral incision was made and dissection was carried down to the subcutaneous tissues and through the iliotibial band and vastus lateralis muscle, onto the existing plates and the previous fracture fixation. Five of the screws in the plate were removed; the 6th was stripped. We therefore used an osteotome to break the head of the screw off and removed the plate. We then used a screw remover device to remove the screw from the bone without difficulty. There were 2 screws placed deep to the plate and these were both removed without difficulty. We then placed some Gelfoam over the screw holes and closed the vastus lateralis muscle over top with a Gelfoam in a temporary fashion.

We then elevated the anterior one third of the abductors off the trochanter and then did a capsulectomy. The hip was dislocated and a femoral neck cut was made. We released a portion of the gluteus maximus insertion and did a thorough release posteriorly on the femoral neck and released a portion of the psoas muscle. We then débrided the periacetabular tissues, and they were quite thick. We had good visualization. We reamed down to the floor of the acetabulum to a size 56. We impacted a cluster 56 cup. This was secured with 2 screws with excellent purchase. The neutral liner was put into position. Nu Gauze was placed in the acetabulum after removing a posterior osteophyte and we then proceeded to approach the proximal femur.

We started with a box osteotome followed by a T-handled awl, followed by a rasp starting at 0 and 44, up to #3 and 44. Trial reduction with a standard head revealed reasonably good soft tissue tension but probably a little bit loose.

The hip was dislocated, the broach was removed and a medium bone cement plug was placed 18 cm from the tip of the trochanter. The canal was irrigated with cold saline and packed with gauze. Three packages of Simplex cement were mixed in a vacuum

Sample Reports

mixer. After approximately 4 minutes the cement was injected into the canal and pressurized. The pressure was placed laterally on the femur over top of the screw holes at the same time. We then placed the #3 prosthesis into the femur and seated it appropriately in appropriate version. It was held in position until the cement was hard. Excess cement was removed. We did a trial reduction with the +4 head and we had good soft tissue tension and stability. The hip was dislocated and the +4 head was tapped under the Morse taper. The hip was atraumatically reduced.

We then irrigated the hip thoroughly and then proceeded to appose the abductors back on the trochanter in an anatomic fashion using 1-0 Ti-Cron suture.

We then moved to the lateral aspect of the femur and opened up the vastus lateralis muscle once again. There was some extruded cement; this was all removed. We divided the lateral edge of the femur and then proceeded to close the vastus lateralis using a running stitch of 1-0 Polysorb suture. This came together anatomically.

We then injected the hip joint with 20 mg of 0.25% Marcaine with 30 mg of Toradol. We then proceeded to close the iliotibial band and tensor fasciae latae using 1-0 Polysorb in an anatomic fashion. The subcutaneous layer was closed with 2-0 Polysorb and the skin with staples. The wound was dressed with Bactigras gauze, abdominal laparotomy pads, and Cover-Roll bandage.

The patient was reversed from anesthetic and transferred to the postanesthetic recovery room without difficulty. He will be transferred back to the floor when stable. He will be mobilized, weightbearing as tolerated. He will be started on deep venous thrombosis prophylaxis. He will continue on infection prophylaxis, of which he received 1 dose preoperatively.

ULNAR SHAFT OPEN REDUCTION AND PLATING

PREOPERATIVE DIAGNOSIS: Displaced fracture, left ulnar shaft.

POSTOPERATIVE DIAGNOSIS: Displaced fracture, left ulnar shaft, work related.

PROCEDURE PERFORMED: Open reduction and plating, left ulnar shaft.

ANESTHESIA: General.

TOURNIQUET TIME: 42 minutes.

INDICATIONS: This is a healthy, 25-year-old, right-handed man who works on the drilling rigs. He was injured at work 2 days ago when a large pipe hit his left arm. He was seen in the emergency department and referred to my clinic. X-ray showed a displaced fracture of left ulnar shaft. He now presents for definitive fixation.

DESCRIPTION OF PROCEDURE: The patient was brought to the operating room and given a general anesthetic. Once asleep, a pneumatic tourniquet was elevated to 250 mmHg on the left upper arm. The elbow was flexed across his chest. A subcutaneous incision measuring about 10 cm was made over the ulna. Dissection was taken directly down onto bone. Care was taken to prevent injury to the superficial branch of the ulnar nerve, which was kept out of harm's way dorsally but not specifically identified and dissected.

The fracture was quite jagged. The soft tissue was removed and it was reduced anatomically and held with a 6-hole, 3.5-mm DCP plate. On the subcutaneous part of the ulna, anatomic reduction was achieved and maintained in 2 planes with good compression of the fracture site and good fixation hold for all screws.

The fixation position was checked with intraoperative C-arm and found to be very good in 2 planes.

The wound was closed with interrupted 2-0 Vicryl suture for the fascia and subcutaneous layer, and the skin with staples. The wound was dressed with soft gauze, sterile toppers, and a below-elbow posterior splint was applied and held with Kling wrap.

Common Terms by Procedure

Arthroscopy Right Knee
anterior cruciate ligament (ACL)
anteromedial portal
arthroscopic débridement
arthrotomy
degenerative tear
diagnostic arthroscopy
femoral condyle
full-thickness lesion
loose body
medial compartmental osteoarthritis
medial gutter
medial meniscectomy
medial meniscus
partial medial meniscectomy
patellofemoral arthritis
Polysorb
portal
sterile prep and free drape
supine position
tibial plateau
trochlear groove

Blatt Procedure of Wrist
Blatt procedure
capitate
distal intercalated segment instability (DISI)
DISI deformity
intraoperative microscopy
Jurgan pin balls
Kirschner wire
ligamentous tightening
local flap advancement
0.5% Marcaine without epinephrine
osteoarthritis
prepped and draped in the usual manner
Prolene suture
proximal row carpectomy

scaphoid fracture
scapholunate bone
scapholunate widening
Ti-Cron suture

Cemented Total Knee Replacement
all-polyethylene Durasul patella component
anterior cruciate ligament
articular cartilage loss
bone cement
bone-on-bone articulation
cemented right total knee replacement
Centerpulse Natural-Knee II System
chamfer cut
chamfer guide
collateral ligament
compression dressing
condylar guide
Concert PMMA bone cement
cutting block
Depo-Medrol
Durasul patella component
excursion
exsanguinated
extensor mechanism
femoral trial component
figure-of-8 suture
flexure contracture
Foley catheter
Hemovac drain
intramedullary canal
intramedullary tibial cutting guide
irrigation solution
keyhole punching
lateral meniscus
lateral tibial plateau
manual pressurization technique

marginal osteophyte
medial compartment
medial meniscus
medial sleeve release
midline incision
neurologic check
parapatellar arthrotomy
patella
peg drill hole
polymethylmethacrylate (PMMA)
posterior cruciate ligament
posterior horn
posttraumatic arthritis
pulse lavage irrigation solution
recovery room
regional anesthesia
skin staple
sleeve release
spinal anesthesia
stable condition
standard median parapatellar
  arthrotomy
sterile compression dressing
stress testing
synovectomy
templating
tibial tubercle
total knee replacement
trial component
tourniquet inflated
ultracongruent insert
varus deformity
Vicryl suture

Closed Reduction of Radial Head Fracture

anatomic position
closed reduction
fluoroscopic guidance
general anesthetic
radial head
radial neck fracture
supine position
type II radial neck fracture

4-Corner Partial Carpal Fusion

AlloMatrix bone putty
arthroscopy
capitate
4-corner partial carpal fusion
distal intercalated segment instability
  (DISI)
DISI deformity
dorsal approach
dorsal arthrotomy
extensor pollicis longus (EPL)
EPL tendon
extensor compartment
extensor pollicis longus tendon
hamate
Kling wrap
K-wire
lunate facet
osteoarthritis
pneumatic tourniquet
proximal pole of scaphoid
radial deviation
radial styloid
retrograde fashion
scaphoid
scapholunate ligament disruption
Sofra-Tulle gauze
spinal anesthetic
sterile topper
synovial tissue
thumb spica splint
triquetrum
Vicryl suture

Femur Fracure Discharge Summary

closed reduction
day of admission
distal femur fracture
mobilize
on-call schedule
operating room
pain control
percutaneous screw fixation

Common Terms

postoperative day
Salter II fracture
Toradol
Tylenol No. 3

Ganglion Excision, Right Knee
ganglion
pes anserinus bursa
recovery room
sterile bandage
Vicryl suture

Hip Hemiarthroplasty
antibiotic-laden cement spacer
box osteotome
calcar
curvilinear incision
femoral neck
gluteus medius muscle
gluteus minimus muscle
Hardinge approach
hemiarthroplasty
hip hemiarthroplasty
iliotibial band
instrument, needle, and sponge counts
lateral decubitus position
Montreal frame
Polysorb suture
rasp
spinal anesthetic
starter reamer
subcutaneous tissue
total hip arthroplasty
uncemented modular Moore
   hemiarthroplasty

Hybrid Total Hip Replacement
abduction pillow
acetabulum
box chisel
Centerpulse Natural-Hip System
Charnley pin

Centerpulse Converge cluster-hole
   sealed porous acetabular component
curvilinear capsulotomy
external rotator
fascial flap
femoral head
figure-of-8 suture
Foley catheter
gluteus medius muscle
gluteus minimus muscle
greater trochanter
Hemovac drain
heterotopic ossification
instrumentation
internal rotation
intramedullary canal
intramedullary nailing
left lateral decubitus position
lesser trochanter
malposition
malunion
neurologic check
operating room
osteotomy
piriformis muscle
posterolateral hip capsule
posttraumatic osteonecrosis
preoperative templating
prepped and draped
pulse lavage irrigation
proximal femur
recovery room
retrograde filling
scar tissue
sciatic nerve
Simplex P bone cement
skin flap
skin staple
spinal anesthesia
stability and range of motion
subcutaneous tissue
T-handled awl
total hip replacement

trial component
trunnion
usual sterile fashion
Vicryl suture

Nancy Nail Stabilization of Forearm Fracture

Betadine gauze
drill hole
general anesthetic
growth plate
molded wire
Nancy nail stabilization
PDS suture
postanesthetic recovery room
radial tuberosity
radiolucent guidance
Sofra-Tulle dressing
Steri-Strips

Open Femur Fracture Fixation

anteroposterior (AP)
AP plane
antibiotic irrigation
Blumensaat line
C-arm guidance
C-arm imaging
crystalloid
external fixator
femur fracture
general anesthesia
guidewire
intensive care unit
intramedullary nailing
irrigation and debridement
lateral plane
locking screw
360 nail
open femur fracture
packed red blood cells
patellar tendon
prepped and draped

sterile dressing
subcutaneous tissue
successive reaming
usual sterile fashion
vastus lateralis muscle
Vicryl suture

Open Reduction of Wrist with Acumed Volar Plating

Acumed volar plating system
anterior cruciate ligament
below-elbow posterior splint
collateral ligament
flexor carpi radialis tendon
fracture construct
Galeazzi fracture
Galeazzi fracture-dislocation
intraarticular fracture
Kling wrap
K-wire fixation
Lachman test
malposition
malunion
open Galeazzi fracture
radial styloid process
radiocarpal joint
radioulnar joint arthroplasty
radius
range of motion
scaphoid
Sofra-Tulle gauze
sterile topper
Vicryl suture

Open Reduction Internal Fixation and Bone Graft of Tibial Fracture

AlloMatrix
condyle
drill hole
fracture fragment
general anesthetic

intraoperative x-ray
Jones dressing
lateral meniscus
mini-C-arm
open reduction internal fixation
Osteoset pellet
recovery room
tibial plateau fracture
tourniquet control

Open Reduction Internal Fixation of Medial Malleolus

anatomic reduction
AO splint
cannulated screw
curette
dome of the talus
general endotracheal anesthesia
guidewire
medial malleolar fracture
metacarpal
nylon suture
open reduction internal fixation
operating room
prepped and draped
recovery room
stable condition
subcutaneous tissue
superficial tissue
supine position
Synthes cannulated guidewire
thigh tourniquet
usual sterile fashion
Vicryl suture
Xeroform gauze dressing

Reduction and Fixation of Metacarpal Fracture

Bactigras dressing
C-arm
fluff gauze
fracture reduction

general endotracheal anesthesia
Kirschner wire
Kling wrap
K-wire fixation
metacarpal fracture
metacarpal head
nonthreaded Kirschner wire
tensor bandage
Webril bandage

Revision Total Knee Replacement

anterior approach
anterior knee pain
arthrotomy
Biomet patella
Biomet size large single-hole patellar button
bone spur
Jones dressing
lateral retinacular release
median parapatellar arthrotomy
Osteonics patellar clamp
patellar button
patellar clamp
patellar component
patellar tracking
patellofemoral arthritis
pneumatic tourniquet
preoperative x-ray
range of motion
revision total knee replacement
Simplex cement
Sofra-Tulle gauze
soft tissue release
sterile topper
subcutaneous tissue
total knee replacement
watertight closure

Shoulder Débridement and Arthrotomy for Draining Sinus

arthrotomy
atlas-dens interval (ADI)
blunt dissection
chronic draining sinus
débrided
débridement procedure
deltoid muscle
draining sinus
flexion and extension views
general anesthetic
gentle intubation
intraarticular fashion
instrument, needle, and sponge count
intraarticular pus
joint capsule
operating suite
Polysorb suture
prepped and draped
Prolene stitch
rheumatoid arthritis
septic arthritis
serial debridement
soft drain
subcutaneous tissue
supine position
usual fashion
wound edge

Shoulder Manipulation and Arthroscopy

abducted position
abduction
anterior capsule
anterior portal
arthroscopic debridement
beach chair position
biceps anchor
biceps tendon
débrided
débridement

Duramorph
external rotation
forward flexion
frozen shoulder
general endotracheal anesthesia
glenohumeral joint
immobilizer
informed consent
internal rotation
manipulation under anesthesia
nylon suture
operating room
posterior portal
prepped and draped
range of motion
recovery area
rotator cuff
rotator interval
subacromial space
stable condition
synovitis
tolerated the procedure well
usual sterile fashion

Total Hip Arthroplasty

abdominal laparotomy pad
abductor
acetabulum
advanced osteoarthritis
anatomic fashion
avascular necrosis
Bactigras gauze
bone cement plug
bony prominence
box osteotome
cemented stem
cold saline
Cover-Roll bandage
débrided
deep venous thrombosis prophylaxis
excellent purchase
Exeter #3 prosthesis
fracture fixation

Gelfoam
general endotracheal anesthesia
gluteus maximus insertion
hip fracture
hip joint
iliotibial band
lateral decubitus position
lateral incision
0.25% Marcaine
Montreal frame
Morse taper
Nu Gauze
offset cemented stem
operating room
osteotome
periacetabular tissue
polyethylene liner
Polysorb suture
postanesthetic recovery room
posterior osteophyte
prophylaxis
proximal femur
psoas muscle
rasp
screw remover device
Simplex cement
soft tissue tension
standard head
sterile prep and drape
subcutaneous layer
subcutaneous tissue
supine position
tensor fasciae latae
T-handled awl
Ti-Cron suture

Toradol
total hip arthroplasty
trial reduction
Trident cluster cup
trochanter
vacuum mixer
vastus lateralis muscle
weightbearing as tolerated

Ulnar Shaft Open Reduction and Plating

anatomic reduction
below-elbow posterior splint
DCP plate
definitive fixation
displaced fracture
dynamic compression plate (DCP)
emergency department
fascia
fixation position
general anesthetic
intraoperative C-arm
Kling wrap
open reduction
operating room
plating
pneumatic tourniquet
soft gauze
soft tissue
sterile topper
subcutaneous layer
superficial branch of the ulnar nerve
ulnar shaft
Vicryl suture

Appendix 7
Drugs by Indication

ACROMEGALY
Ergot Alkaloid and Derivative
  Apo® Bromocriptine [Can]
  bromocriptine
  Parlodel® [US/Can]
  pergolide
  Permax® [US/Can]
  PMS-Bromocriptine [Can]
Growth Hormone Receptor Antagonist
  pegvisomant
  Somavert® [US]
Somatostatin Analog
  octreotide
  Sandostatin LAR® [US/Can]
  Sandostatin® [US/Can]

ANESTHESIA (GENERAL)
Barbiturate
  Brevital® Sodium [US/Can]
  methohexital
General Anesthetic
  Amidate® [US/Can]
  desflurane
  Diprivan® [US/Can]
  enflurane
  Ethrane® [US]
  etomidate
  Forane® [US]
  halothane
  isoflurane
  Ketalar® [US/Can]
  ketamine
  propofol
  sevoflurane
  Sevorane AF™ [Can]
  Suprane® [US/Can]
  Ultane® [US]

ANESTHESIA (LOCAL)
Local Anesthetic
  AK-T-Caine™ [US]
  Alcaine® [US/Can]
  Americaine® Anesthetic Lubricant [US]
  Americaine® [US-OTC]
  Ametop™ [Can]
  Anbesol® Baby [US/Can]
  Anbesol® Maximum Strength [US-OTC]
  Anbesol® [US-OTC]
  Anestacon® [US]
  Anusol® [US-OTC]
  Babee® Teething® [US-OTC]
  Band-Aid® Hurt-Free™ Antiseptic Wash [US-OTC]
  benzocaine
  benzocaine, butyl aminobenzoate, tetracaine, and benzalkonium chloride
  benzocaine, gelatin, pectin, and sodium carboxymethylcellulose
  Benzodent® [US-OTC]
  Betacaine® [Can]
  bupivacaine
  Burnamycin [US-OTC]
  Burn Jel [US-OTC]
  Burn-O-Jel [US-OTC]
  Carbocaine® [Can]
  Cepacol® Anesthetic Troches [US-OTC]
  Cepacol® Maximum Strength [US-OTC]
  Cepacol® Mouthwash/Gargle [US-OTC]
  Cepacol Viractin® [US-OTC]
  Cetacaine® [US]
  cetylpyridinium

cetylpyridinium and benzocaine
Chiggerex® [US-OTC]
Chiggertox® [US-OTC]
chloroprocaine
Citanest® Forte [Can]
Citanest®Plain [US/Can]
cocaine
Cylex® [US-OTC]
Detane® [US-OTC]
dibucaine
Diocaine® [Can]
dyclonine
ethyl chloride
ethyl chloride and
    dichlorotetrafluoroethane
Fleet® Pain Relief [US-OTC]
Fluoracaine® [US]
Fluro-Ethylv Aerosol [US]
Foille® Medicated First Aid [US-
    OTC]
Foille® Plus [US-OTC]
Foille® [US-OTC]
HDA® Toothache [US-OTC]
hexylresorcinol
Hurricaine® [US]
Isocaine® HCl [US]
Itch-X® [US-OTC]
LidaMantle® [US]
lidocaine
lidocaine and epinephrine
Lidoderm® [US/Can]
L-M-X® 4 [US-OTC]
L-M-X® 5 [US-OTC]
Marcaine® Spinal [US]
Marcaine® [US/Can]
mepivacaine
Mycinettes® [US-OTC]
Naropin™ [US/Can]
Nesacaine®-CE [Can]
Nesacaine®-MPF [US]
Nesacaine® [US]
Novocain® [US/Can]
Nupercainal® [US-OTC]

Ophthetic® [US]
Opticaine® [US]
Orabase®-B [US-OTC]
Orabase® With Benzocaine [US-
    OTC]
Orajel® Baby Nighttime [US-OTC]
Orajel® Baby [US-OTC]
Orajel® Maximum Strength [US-
    OTC]
Orajel® [US-OTC]
Orasol® [US-OTC]
Parcaine® [US]
Phicon® [US-OTC]
Polocaine® MPF [US]
Polocaine® [US/Can]
Pontocaine® [US/Can]
Pontocaine® With Dextrose [US]
PrameGel® [US-OTC]
pramoxine
Prax® [US-OTC]
Premjact® [US-OTC]
prilocaine
procaine
ProctoFoam® NS [US-OTC]
proparacaine
proparacaine and fluorescein
ropivacaine
Sensorcaine®-MPF [US]
Sensorcaine® [US/Can]
Solarcaine® Aloe Extra Burn Relief
    [US-OTC]
Solarcaine® [US-OTC]
Sucrets® Sore Throat [US-OTC]
Sucrets® [US-OTC]
tetracaine
tetracaine and dextrose
Topicaine® [US-OTC]
Trocaine® [US-OTC]
Tronolane® [US-OTC]
Tronothane® [US-OTC]
Xylocaine® MPF [US]
Xylocaine® [US/Can]
Xylocaine® Viscous [US]

Xylocaine® With Epinephrine
  [US/Can]
Xylocard® [Can]
Zilactin® Baby [US/Can]
Zilactin®-B [US/Can]
Zilactin® [Can]
Zilactin-L® [US-OTC]
Local Anesthetic, Amide Derivative
  Chirocaine® [US/Can]
  levobupivacaine
Local Anesthetic, Injectable
  Chirocaine® [US/Can]
  levobupivacaine

ARTHRITIS

Aminoquinoline (Antimalarial)
  Apo®-Hydroxyquine [Can]
  Aralen® Phosphate [US/Can]
  chloroquine phosphate
  hydroxychloroquine
  Plaquenil® [US/Can]
Analgesic, Topical
  Antiphlogistine Rub A-535
    Capsaicin [Can]
  ArthriCare® for Women Extra
    Moisturizing [US-OTC]
  ArthriCare® for Women Silky Dry
    [US-OTC]
  Capsagel® [US-OTC]
  capsaicin
  Capzasin-HP® [US-OTC]
  TheraPatch® Warm [US-OTC]
  Zostrix®-HP [US/Can]
  Zostrix® [US/Can]
Antiinflammatory Agent
  Arava™ [US/Can]
  leflunomide
Antineoplastic Agent
  Apo®-Methotrexate [Can]
  cyclophosphamide
  Cytoxan® [US/Can]
  methotrexate
  Neosar® [US]

Procytox® [Can]
ratio-Methotrexate [Can]
Rheumatrex® [US]
Trexall™ [US]
Antirheumatic, Disease Modifying
  adalimumab
  anakinra
  Enbrel® [US]
  etanercept
  Humira™ [US]
  Kineret™ [US/Can]
Chelating Agent
  Cuprimine® [US/Can]
  Depen® [US/Can]
  penicillamine
Gold Compound
  auranofin
  Aurolate® [US]
  aurothioglucose
  gold sodium thiomalate
  Myochrysine® [Can]
  Ridaura® [US/Can]
  Solganal® [US/Can]
Immunosuppressant Agent
  Alti-Azathioprine [Can]
  Apo®-Azathioprine [Can]
  Apo®-Cyclosporine [Can]
  azathioprine
  cyclosporine
  Gen-Azathioprine [Can]
  Gengraf™ [US]
  Imuran® [US/Can]
  Neoral® [US/Can]
  ratio-Azathioprine [Can]
  Restasis™ [US]
  Rhoxal-cyclosporine [Can]
  Sandimmune® [US/Can]
Monoclonal Antibody
  adalimumab
  Humira™ [US]
Nonsteroidal Antiinflammatory Drug
  (NSAID)
  Advil® Children's [US-OTC]

Advil® Infants' Concentrated Drops [US-OTC]
Advil® Junior [US-OTC]
Advil® Migraine [US-OTC]
Advil® [US/Can]
Albert® Tiafen [Can]
Aleve® [US-OTC]
Amigesic® [US/Can]
Anaprox® DS [US/Can]
Anaprox® [US/Can]
Ansaid® Oral [US/Can]
Apo®-Diclo [Can]
Apo®-Diclo SR [Can]
Apo®-Diflunisal [Can]
Apo®-Flurbiprofen [Can]
Apo®-Ibuprofen [Can]
Apo®-Indomethacin [Can]
Apo®-Keto [Can]
Apo®-Keto-E [Can]
Apo®-Keto SR [Can]
Apo®-Nabumetone [Can]
Apo®-Napro-Na [Can]
Apo®-Napro-Na DS [Can]
Apo®-Naproxen [Can]
Apo®-Naproxen SR [Can]
Apo®-Oxaprozin [Can]
Apo®-Sulin [Can]
Apo®-Tiaprofenic [Can]
Argesic®-SA [US]
Asaphen [Can]
Asaphen E.C. [Can]
Ascriptin® Arthritis Pain [US-OTC]
Ascriptin® Enteric [US-OTC]
Ascriptin® Extra Strength [US-OTC]
Ascriptin® [US-OTC]
Aspercin Extra [US-OTC]
Aspercin [US-OTC]
aspirin
Bayer® Aspirin Extra Strength [US-OTC]
Bayer® Aspirin Regimen Adult Low Strength [US-OTC]
Bayer® Aspirin Regimen Adult Low Strength with Calcium [US-OTC]
Bayer® Aspirin Regimen Children's [US-OTC]
Bayer® Aspirin Regimen Regular Strength [US-OTC]
Bayer® Aspirin [US-OTC]
Bayer® Plus Extra Strength [US-OTC]
Bufferin® Arthritis Strength [US-OTC]
Bufferin® Extra Strength [US-OTC]
Bufferin® [US-OTC]
Cataflam® [US/Can]
choline magnesium trisalicylate
Clinoril® [US]
Daypro™ [US/Can]
diclofenac
diflunisal
Doan's® Original [US-OTC]
Dolobid® [US]
Easprin® [US]
EC-Naprosyn® [US]
Ecotrin® Adult Low Strength [US-OTC]
Ecotrin® Maximum Strength [US-OTC]
Ecotrin® [US-OTC]
Entrophen® [Can]
Extra Strength Doan's® [US-OTC]
Feldene®[US/Can]
fenoprofen
flurbiprofen
Froben® [Can]
Froben-SR® [Can]
Gen-Nabumetone [Can]
Gen-Naproxen EC [Can]
Gen-Piroxicam [Can]
Genpril® [US-OTC]
Halfprin® [US-OTC]
Haltran® [US-OTC]
ibuprofen
Ibu-Tab® [US]
Indocid(R) [Can]

Indocid® P.D.A. [Can]
Indocin® SR [US]
Indocin® [US]
Indo-Lemmon [Can]
indomethacin
I-Prin [US-OTC]
ketoprofen
Keygesic-10® [US]
magnesium salicylate
meclofenamate
Menadol® [US-OTC]
Midol® Maximum Strength Cramp
  Formula [US-OTC]
Momentum® [US-OTC]
Mono-Gesic® [US]
Motrin® Children's [US/Can]
Motrin® IB [US/Can]
Motrin® Infants' [US-OTC]
Motrin® Junior Strength [US-OTC]
Motrin® Migraine Pain [US-OTC]
Motrin® [US/Can]
nabumetone
Nalfon® [US/Can]
Naprelan® [US]
Naprosyn® [US/Can]
naproxen
Naxen® [Can]
Novasen [Can]
Novo-Difenac® [Can]
Novo-Difenac-K [Can]
Novo-Difenac® SR [Can]
Novo-Diflunisal [Can]
Novo-Flurprofen [Can]
Novo-Keto [Can]
Novo-Keto-EC [Can]
Novo-Methacin [Can]
Novo-Naprox [Can]
Novo-Naprox Sodium [Can]
Novo-Naprox Sodium DS [Can]
Novo-Naprox SR [Can]
Novo-Pirocam® [Can]
Novo-Profen® [Can]

Novo-Sundac [Can]
Novo-Tiaprofenic [Can]
Nu-Diclo [Can]
Nu-Diclo-SR [Can]
Nu-Diflunisal [Can]
Nu-Flurprofen [Can]
Nu-Ibuprofen [Can]
Nu-Indo [Can]
Nu-Ketoprofen [Can]
Nu-Ketoprofen-E [Can]
Nu-Naprox [Can]
Nu-Pirox [Can]
Nu-Sundac [Can]
Nu-Tiaprofenic [Can]
Ocufen® Ophthalmic [US/Can]
Orudis® KT [US-OTC]
Orudis® SR [Can]
Oruvail® [US/Can]
oxaprozin
Pennsaid® [Can]
Pexicam® [Can]
piroxicam
PMS-Diclofenac [Can]
PMS-Diclofenac SR [Can]
PMS-Tiaprofenic [Can]
ratio-Flurbiprofen [Can]
ratio-Indomethacin [Can]
Relafen® [US/Can]
Rhodacine® [Can]
Rhodis™ [Can]
Rhodis-EC™ [Can]
Rhodis SR™ [Can]
Rhoxal-nabumetone [Can]
Riva-Diclofenac [Can]
Riva-Diclofenac-K [Can]
Riva-Naproxen [Can]
Salflex® [US/Can]
salsalate
Solaraze™ [US]
St. Joseph® Pain Reliever [US-OTC]
sulindac
Sureprin 81™ [US-OTC]

Surgam® [Can]
Surgam® SR [Can]
tiaprofenic acid (Canada only)
Tolectin® DS [US]
Tolectin® [US/Can]
tolmetin
Tricosal® [US]
Trilisate® [US]
Voltaren Rapide® [Can]
Voltaren® [US/Can]
Voltaren®-XR [US]
Voltare Ophtha(R) [Can]
ZORprin® [US]
Nonsteroidal Antiinflammatory Drug
    (NSAID), COX-2 Selective
    Celebrex® [US/Can]
    celecoxib

ARTHRITIS (RHEUMATOID)

Nonsteroidal Antiinflammatory Drug
    (NSAID), COX-2 Selective
    Bextra™ [US/Can]
    valdecoxib

BACK PAIN (LOW)

Analgesic, Narcotic
    codeine
    Codeine Contin® [Can]
    ratio-Codeine [Can]
Analgesic, Nonnarcotic
    Asaphen [Can]
    Asaphen E.C. [Can]
    Ascriptin® Arthritis Pain [US-OTC]
    Ascriptin® Enteric [US-OTC]
    Ascriptin® Extra Strength [US-OTC]
    Ascriptin® [US-OTC]
    Aspercin Extra [US-OTC]
    Aspercin [US-OTC]
    aspirin
    Bayer® Aspirin Extra Strength [US-
        OTC]
Bayer® Aspirin Regimen Regular
    Strength [US-OTC]
Bayer® Aspirin [US-OTC]
Bayer® Plus Extra Strength [US-
    OTC]
Bufferin® Arthritis Strength [US-
    OTC]
Bufferin® Extra Strength [US-OTC]
Bufferin® [US-OTC]
Easprin® [US]
Ecotrin®Maximum Strength [US-
    OTC]
Ecotrin® [US-OTC]
Entrophen® [Can]
Halfprin® [US-OTC]
Novasen [Can]
St. Joseph® Pain Reliever [US-OTC]
Sureprin 81(TM) [US-OTC]
ZORprin® [US]
Benzodiazepine
    Apo®-Diazepam [Can]
    Diastat® [US/Can]
    Diazemuls® [Can]
    diazepam
    Diazepam Intensol® [US]
    Valium® [US/Can]
Nonsteroidal Antiinflammatory Drug
    (NSAID)
    Doan's®, Original [US-OTC]
    Extra Strength Doan's® [US-OTC]
    Keygesic-10® [US]
    magnesium salicylate
    Momentum® [US-OTC]
Skeletal Muscle Relaxant
    Aspirin® Backache [Can]
    methocarbamol
    methocarbamol and aspirin
    Methoxisal [Can]
    Methoxisal-C [Can]
    Robaxin® [US/Can]

BEHÇET SYNDROME

Immunosuppressant Agent
Alti-Azathioprine [Can]
Apo®Azathioprine [Can]
Apo®-Cyclosporine [Can]
azathioprine
cyclosporine
Gen-Azathioprine [Can]
Gengraf™ [US]
Imuran® [US/Can]
Neoral® [US/Can]
ratio-Azathioprine [Can]
Restasis™ [US]
Rhoxal-cyclosporine [Can]
Sandimmune® [US/Can]

BURSITIS

Nonsteroidal Antiinflammatory Drug
(NSAID)
Advil® Children's [US-OTC]
Advil® [US/Can]
Aleve® [US-OTC]
Anaprox® DS [US/Can]
Anaprox® [US/Can]
Apo®-Ibuprofen [Can]
Apo®-Indomethacin [Can]
Apo®-Napro-Na [Can]
Apo®-Napro-Na DS [Can]
Apo®-Naproxen [Can]
Apo®-Naproxen SR [Can]
Asaphen [Can]
Asaphen E.C. [Can]
Ascriptin® Arthritis Pain [US-OTC]
Ascriptin® Enteric [US-OTC]
Ascriptin® Extra Strength [US-OTC]
Ascriptin® [US-OTC]
Aspercin Extra [US-OTC]
Aspercin [US-OTC]
aspirin
Bayer® Aspirin Extra Strength [US-
OTC]
Bayer® Aspirin Regimen Regular
Strength [US-OTC]
Bayer® Aspirin [US-OTC]
Bayer® Plus Extra Strength [US-
OTC]
Bufferin® Arthritis Strength [US-
OTC]
Bufferin® Extra Strength [US-OTC]
Bufferin® [US-OTC]
choline magnesium trisalicylate
Easprin® [US]
EC-Naprosyn® [US]
Ecotrin® Maximum Strength [US-
OTC]
Ecotrin® [US-OTC]
Entrophen® [Can]
Gen-Naproxen EC [Can]
Genpril® [US-OTC]
Halfprin® [US-OTC]
Haltran® [US-OTC]
ibuprofen
Ibu-Tab® [US]
Indocid® [Can]
Indocid® P.D.A. [Can]
Indocin® SR [US]
Indocin® [US]
Indo-Lemmon [Can]
indomethacin
I-Prin [US-OTC]
Menadol® [US-OTC]
Motrin® IB [US/Can]
Motrin® [US/Can]
Naprelan® [US]
Naprosyn® [US/Can]
naproxen
Naxen® [Can]
Novasen [Can]
Novo-Methacin [Can]
Novo-Naprox [Can]
Novo-Naprox Sodium [Can]
Novo-Naprox Sodium DS [Can]
Novo-Naprox SR [Can]
Novo-Profen® [Can]

Nu-Ibuprofen [Can]
Nu-Indo [Can]
Nu-Naprox [Can]
ratio-Indomethacin [Can]
Rhodacine® [Can]
Riva-Naproxen [Can]
St. Joseph® Pain Reliever [US-OTC]
Sureprin 81™ [US-OTC]
Tricosal® [US]
Trilisate® [US]
ZORprin® [US]

CACHEXIA
Progestin
Apo®-Megestrol [Can]
Lin-Megestrol [Can]
Megace® OS
Megace® [US/Can]
megestrol acetate
Nu-Megestrol [Can]

CLAUDICATION
Blood Viscosity Reducer Agent
Apo®-Pentoxifylline SR [Can]
Nu-Pentoxifylline SR [Can]
pentoxifylline
Pentoxil® [US]
ratio-Pentoxifylline [Can]
Trental® [US/Can]

DEBRIDEMENT OF CALLOUS TISSUE
Keratolytic Agent
trichloroacetic acid
Tri-Chlor® [US]

DEBRIDEMENT OF ESCHAR
Protectant, Topical
Granulex [US]
trypsin, balsam Peru, and castor oil

DECUBITUS ULCER
Enzyme
collagenase
Santyl® [US/Can]
Enzyme, Topical Débridement
Accuzyme™ [US]
papain and urea
Protectant, Topical
Granulex [US]
trypsin, balsam Peru, and castor oil
Topical Skin Product
Accuzyme™ [US]
papain and urea

DEEP VEIN THROMBOSIS (DVT)
Anticoagulant (Other)
Apo®-Warfarin [Can]
Coumadin(R) [US/Can]
dalteparin
danaparoid
enoxaparin
Fragmin® [US/Can]
Gen-Warfarin [Can]
Hepalean® [Can]
Hepalean® Leo [Can]
Hepalean®-LOK [Can]
heparin
Hep-Lock® [US]
Innohep® [US/Can]
Lovenox® [US/Can]
Orgaran® [Can]
Taro-Warfarin [Can]
tinzaparin
warfarin
Factor Xa Inhibitor
Arixtra® [US/Can]
fondaparinux
Low Molecular Weight Heparin
Fraxiparine™ [Can]
Fraxiparine™ Forte [Can]
nadroparin (Canada only)

DWARFISM

Growth Hormone
Genotropin Miniquick® [US]
Genotropin® [US]
human growth hormone
Humatrope® [US/Can]
Norditropin® Cartridges [US]
Norditropin® [US/Can]
Nutropin AQ® [US/Can]
Nutropin Depot® [US]
Nutropin® [US]
Protropin® [US/Can]
Saizen® [US/Can]
Serostim® [US/Can]

EPICONDYLITIS

Nonsteroidal Antiinflammatory Drug
(NSAID)
Advil® [US/Can]
Aleve® [US-OTC]
Anaprox® DS [US/Can]
Anaprox® [US/Can]
Apo®-Ibuprofen [Can]
Apo®-Indomethacin [Can]
Apo®-Napro-Na [Can]
Apo®-Napro-Na DS [Can]
Apo®-Naproxen [Can]
Apo®-Naproxen SR [Can]
EC-Naprosyn® [US]
Gen-Naproxen EC [Can]
Genpril® [US-OTC]
Haltran® [US-OTC]
ibuprofen
Ibu-Tab® [US]
Indocid® [Can]
Indocid® P.D.A. [Can]
Indocin® SR [US]
Indocin® [US]
Indo-Lemmon [Can]
indomethacin
I-Prin [US-OTC]
Menadol® [US-OTC]

Motrin® IB [US/Can]
Motrin® [US/Can]
Naprelan® [US]
Naprosyn® [US/Can]
naproxen
Naxen® [Can]
Novo-Methacin [Can]
Novo-Naprox [Can]
Novo-Naprox Sodium [Can]
Novo-Naprox Sodium DS [Can]
Novo-Naprox SR [Can]
Novo-Profen® [Can]
Nu-Ibuprofen [Can]
Nu-Indo [Can]
Nu-Naprox [Can]
ratio-Indomethacin [Can]
Rhodacine® [Can]
Riva-Naproxen [Can]

FIBROMYOSITIS

Antidepressant, Tricyclic (Tertiary
Amine)
amitriptyline
Apo®-Amitriptyline [Can]
Levate® [Can]
PMS-Amitriptyline [Can]

FUNGUS (DIAGNOSTIC)

Diagnostic Agent
Candida albicans (Monilia)
Candin® [US]
Dermatophytin® [US]
Histolyn-CYL® [US]
histoplasmin
Trichophyton skin test

GOUT

Antigout Agent
colchicine
colchicine and probenecid
ratio-Colchicine [Can]
Nonsteroidal Antiinflammatory Drug
(NSAID)

Drugs by Indication

Advil® [US/Can]
Aleve® [US-OTC]
Anaprox® DS [US/Can]
Anaprox® [US/Can]
Apo®-Diclo [Can]
Apo®-Diclo SR [Can]
Apo®-Ibuprofen [Can]
Apo®-Indomethacin [Can]
Apo®-Napro-Na [Can]
Apo®-Napro-Na DS [Can]
Apo®-Naproxen [Can]
Apo®-Naproxen SR [Can]
Apo®-Sulin [Can]
Cataflam® [US/Can]
Clinoril® [US]
diclofenac
EC-Naprosyn® [US]
Gen-Naproxen EC [Can]
Genpril® [US-OTC]
Haltran® [US-OTC]
ibuprofen
Ibu-Tab® [US]
Indocid® [Can]
Indocid® P.D.A. [Can]
Indocin® SR [US]
Indocin® [US]
Indo-Lemmon [Can]
indomethacin
I-Prin [US-OTC]
Menadol® [US-OTC]
Motrin® IB [US/Can]
Motrin® [US/Can]
Naprelan® [US]
Naprosyn® [US/Can]
naproxen
Naxen® [Can]
Novo-Difenac® [Can]
Novo-Difenac-K [Can]
Novo-Difenac® SR [Can]
Novo-Methacin [Can]
Novo-Naprox [Can]
Novo-Naprox Sodium [Can]
Novo-Naprox Sodium DS [Can]

Novo-Naprox SR [Can]
Novo-Profen® [Can]
Novo-Sundac [Can]
Nu-Diclo [Can]
Nu-Diclo-SR [Can]
Nu-Ibuprofen [Can]
Nu-Indo [Can]
Nu-Naprox [Can]
Nu-Sundac [Can]
PMS-Diclofenac [Can]
PMS-Diclofenac SR [Can]
ratio-Indomethacin [Can]
Rhodacine® [Can]
Riva-Diclofenac [Can]
Riva-Diclofenac-K [Can]
Riva-Naproxen [Can]
sulindac
Voltaren Rapide® [Can]
Voltaren® [US/Can]
Voltaren®-XR [US]
Uricosuric Agent
    Apo®-Sulfinpyrazone [Can]
    Benuryl™ [Can]
    Nu-Sulfinpyrazone [Can]
    probenecid
    sulfinpyrazone
Xanthine Oxidase Inhibitor
    allopurinol
    AloprimTM [US]
    Apo®-Allopurinol [Can]
    Zyloprim® [US/Can]

GRAM-NEGATIVE INFECTION
Aminoglycoside (Antibiotic)
    AKTob® [US]
    Alcomicin® [Can]
    amikacin
    Amikin® [Can]
    Apo®-Tobramycin [Can]
    Diogent® [Can]
    Garamycin® [US/Can]
    Genoptic® [US]

Gentacidin® [US]
Gentak® [US]
gentamicin
kanamycin
Kantrex® [US/Can]
Nebcin® [US/Can]
PMS-Tobramycin [Can]
ratio-Gentamicin [Can]
TOBI® [US/Can]
tobramycin
Tobrex® [US/Can]
Antibiotic, Carbapenem
ertapenem
Invanz™ [US/Can]
Antibiotic, Miscellaneous
Apo®-Nitrofurantoin [Can]
Azactam® [US/Can]
aztreonam
colistimethate
Coly-Mycin® M [US/Can]
Furadantin® [US]
Macrobid® [US/Can]
Macrodantin® [US/Can]
nitrofurantoin
Novo-Furantoin [Can]
Antibiotic, Penicillin
pivampicillin (Canada only)
Pondocillin® [Can]
Antibiotic, Quinolone
gatifloxacin
Levaquin® [US/Can]
levofloxacin
Quixin™ Ophthalmic [US]
Tequin® [US/Can]
Zymar™ [US]
Carbapenem (Antibiotic)
imipenem and cilastatin
meropenem
Merrem® I.V. [US/Can]
Primaxin® [US/Can]
Cephalosporin (First Generation)
Ancef® [US]
Apo®-Cefadroxil [Can]

Apo®-Cephalex [Can]
Biocef® [US]
cefadroxil
cefazolin
cephalexin
cephalothin
cephradine
Ceporacin® [Can]
Duricef® [US/Can]
Keflex® [US]
Keftab® [US/Can]
Novo-Cefadroxil [Can]
Novo-Lexin® [Can]
Nu-Cephalex® [Can]
Velosef® [US]
Cephalosporin (Second Generation)
Apo®-Cefaclor [Can]
Apo®-Cefuroxime [Can]
Ceclor® CD [US]
Ceclor® [US/Can]
cefaclor
Cefotan® [US/Can]
cefotetan
cefoxitin
cefpodoxime
cefprozil
Ceftin® [US/Can]
cefuroxime
Cefzil® [US/Can]
Mefoxin® [US/Can]
Novo-Cefaclor [Can]
Nu-Cefaclor [Can]
PMS-Cefaclor [Can]
ratio-Cefuroxime [Can]
Vantin® [US/Can]
Zinacef® [US/Can]
Cephalosporin (Third Generation)
Cedax® [US]
cefixime
Cefizox® [US/Can]
cefotaxime
ceftazidime
ceftibuten

ceftizoxime
ceftriaxone
Claforan® [US/Can]
Fortaz® [US/Can]
Rocephin® [US/Can]
Suprax® [Can]
Tazicef® [US]
Tazidime® [US/Can]
Cephalosporin (Fourth Generation)
cefepime
Maxipime® [US/Can]
Genitourinary Irrigant
neomycin and polymyxin B
Neosporin® Cream [Can]
Neosporin® G.U. Irrigant [US/Can]
Macrolide (Antibiotic)
Apo®-Erythro Base [Can]
Apo®-Erythro E-C [Can]
Apo®-Erythro-ES [Can]
Apo®-Erythro-S [Can]
azithromycin
Biaxin® [US/Can]
Biaxin® XL [US/Can]
clarithromycin
Diomycin® [Can]
dirithromycin
Dynabac® [US]
E.E.S.® [US/Can]
Erybid™ [Can]
Eryc® [US/Can]
EryPed® [US]
Ery-Tab® [US]
Erythrocin® [US]
erythromycin and sulfisoxazole
erythromycin (systemic)
Eryzole® [US]
Nu-Erythromycin-S [Can]
PCE® [US/Can]
Pediazole® [US/Can]
PMS-Erythromycin [Can]
Tao® [US]
troleandomycin
Zithromax® [US/Can]
Z-PAK® [US/Can]

Penicillin
Alti-Amoxi-Clav® [Can]
amoxicillin
amoxicillin and clavulanate
potassium
Amoxicot® [US]
Amoxil® [US]
ampicillin
ampicillin and sulbactam
Apo®-Amoxi [Can]
Apo®-Amoxi-Clav(R) [Can]
Apo®-Ampi [Can]
Apo®-Pen VK [Can]
Augmentin ES-600™ [US]
Augmentin® [US/Can]
Augmentin XR™ [US]
Bicillin® C-R 900/300 [US]
Bicillin® C-R [US]
Bicillin® L-A [US]
carbenicillin
Clavulin® [Can]
Gen-Amoxicillin [Can]
Geocillin® [US]
Lin-Amox [Can]
Marcillin® [US]
Moxilin® [US]
Nadopen-V® [Can]
Novamoxin® [Can]
Novo-Ampicillin [Can]
Novo-Pen-VK® [Can]
Nu-Amoxi [Can]
Nu-Ampi [Can]
Nu-Pen-VK® [Can]
penicillin G benzathine
penicillin G benzathine and
procaine combined
penicillin G procaine
penicillin V potassium
Permapen® Isoject(R) [US]
piperacillin
piperacillin and tazobactam sodium
Pipracil® [Can]
PMS-Amoxicillin [Can]
Principen® [US]

PVF(R) K [Can]
ratio-AmoxiClav
Suspen® [US]
Tazocin® [Can]
ticarcillin
ticarcillin and clavulanate potassium
Ticar® [US]
Timentin® [US/Can]
Trimox® [US]
Truxcillin® [US]
Unasyn® [US/Can]
Veetids® [US]
Wycillin® [US/Can]
Zosyn® [US]
Quinolone
Apo®-Norflox [Can]
Apo®-Oflox [Can]
Ciloxan® [US/Can]
Cinobac® [US/Can]
cinoxacin
ciprofloxacin
Cipro® [US/Can]
Cipro® XR [US/Can]
Floxin® [US/Can]
lomefloxacin
Maxaquin® [US]
nalidixic acid
NegGram® [US/Can]
norfloxacin
Noroxin® [US/Can]
Novo-Norfloxacin [Can]
Ocuflox® [US/Can]
ofloxacin
PMS-Norfloxacin [Can]
Riva-Norfloxacin [Can]
sparfloxacin
Zagam® [US]
Sulfonamide
Apo®-Sulfatrim [Can]
Bactrim™ DS [US]
Bactrim™ [US]
erythromycin and sulfisoxazole
Eryzole® [US]

Gantrisin® Pediatric Suspension [US]
Novo-Trimel [Can]
Novo-Trimel D.S. [Can]
Nu-Cotrimox® [Can]
Pediazole® [US/Can]
Septra® DS [US/Can]
Septra® [US/Can]
sulfadiazine
sulfamethoxazole and trimethoprim
Sulfatrim® DS [US]
Sulfatrim® [US]
sulfisoxazole
sulfisoxazole and phenazopyridine
Sulfizole® [Can]
Truxazole® [US]
Tetracycline Derivative
Adoxa™ [US]
Alti-Minocycline [Can]
Apo®-Doxy [Can]
Apo®-Doxy Tabs [Can]
Apo®-Minocycline [Can]
Apo®-Tetra [Can]
Brodspec® [US]
Doryx® [US]
Doxy-100® [US]
Doxycin [Can]
doxycycline
Dynacin® [US]
EmTet® [US]
Gen-Minocycline [Can]
Minocin® [US/Can]
minocycline
Monodox® [US]
Novo-Doxylin [Can]
Novo-Minocycline [Can]
Novo-Tetra [Can]
Nu-Doxycycline [Can]
Nu-Tetra [Can]
oxytetracycline
Periostat® [US]
ratio-Doxycycline [Can]
ratio-Minocycline [Can]
Rhoxal-minocycline [Can]

Sumycin® [US]
Terramycin® I.M. [US/Can]
tetracycline
Vibramycin® [US]
Vibra-Tabs® [US/Can]
Wesmycin® [US]

GUILLAIN-BARRÉ SYNDROME

Immune Globulin
Carimune™ [US]
Gamimune® N [US/Can]
Gammagard® S/D [US/Can]
Gammar®-P I.V. [US]
Gamunex® [Can]
immune globulin (intravenous)
Iveegam EN [US]
Iveegam Immuno® [Can]
Panglobulin® [US]
Polygam® S/D [US]
Venoglobulin®-S [US]

INFLAMMATION (NONRHEUMATIC)

Adrenal Corticosteroid
Acthar® [US]
A-HydroCort® [US]
A-methapred® [US]
Apo®-Prednisone [Can]
Aristocort® Forte Injection [US]
Aristocort® Intralesional Injection [US]
Aristocort® Tablet [US/Can]
Aristospan® Intraarticular Injection [US/Can]
Aristospan® Intralesional Injection [US/Can]
Betaject™ [Can]
betamethasone (systemic)
Betnesol® [Can]
Celestone® Phosphate [US]
Celestone® Soluspan(R) [US/Can]
Celestone® [US]
Cel-U-Jec® [US]

Cortef® Tablet [US/Can]
corticotropin
cortisone acetate
Cortone® [Can]
Decadron®-LA [US]
Decadron® [US/Can]
Decaject-LA® [US]
Decaject® [US]
Deltasone® [US]
Depo-Medrol ® [US/Can]
Depopred® [US]
dexamethasone (systemic)
Dexasone® L.A. [US]
Dexasone® [US/Can]
Dexone® LA [US]
Dexone® [US]
Hexadrol® [US/Can]
H.P. Acthar® Gel [US]
hydrocortisone (systemic)
Kenalog® Injection [US/Can]
Medrol® Dosepak™ [US/Can]
Medrol® Tablet [US/Can]
methylprednisolone
Orapred™ [US]
Pediapred® [US/Can]
PMS-Dexamethasone [Can]
Prednicot® [US]
prednisolone (systemic)
Prednisol® TBA [US]
prednisone
Prednisone Intensol™ [US]
Prelone® [US]
ratio-Dexamethasone [Can]
Solu-Cortef® [US/Can]
Solu-Medrol® [US/Can]
Solurex L.A.® [US]
Sterapred® DS [US]
Sterapred® [US]
Tac™-3 Injection [US]
Triam-A® Injection [US]
triamcinolone (systemic)
Triam Forte® Injection [US]
Winpred™ [Can]

INTERMITTENT CLAUDICATION
Platelet Aggregation Inhibitor
  cilostazol
  Pletal® [US/Can]

LEG CRAMP
Blood Viscosity Reducer Agent
  Apo®-Pentoxifylline SR [Can]
  Nu-Pentoxifylline SR [Can]
  pentoxifylline
  Pentoxil® [US]
  ratio-Pentoxifylline [Can]
  Trental® [US/Can]

MARFAN SYNDROME
Rauwolfia Alkaloid
  reserpine

MUSCLE SPASM
Skeletal Muscle Relaxant
  Apo®-Cyclobenzaprine [Can]
  Aspirin® Backache [Can]
  carisoprodol
  carisoprodol and aspirin
  carisoprodol, aspirin, and codeine
  chlorzoxazone
  cyclobenzaprine
  Flexeril® [US/Can]
  Flexitec [Can]
  Gen-Cyclobenzaprine [Can]
  metaxalone
  methocarbamol
  methocarbamol and aspirin
  Methoxisal [Can]
  Methoxisal-C [Can]
  Mivacron® [US/Can]
  mivacurium
  Norflex™ [US/Can]
  Norgesic™ Forte [US/Can]
  Norgesic™ [US/Can]
  Novo-Cycloprine [Can]
  Nu-Cyclobenzaprine [Can]
  Orphenace® [Can]
  orphenadrine
  orphenadrine, aspirin, and caffeine
  Orphengesic Forte [US]
  Orphengesic [US]
  Parafon Forte® [Can]
  Parafon Forte® DSC [US]
  Rhoxal-orphenadrine [Can]
  Robaxin® [US/Can]
  Skelaxin® [US/Can]
  Soma® Compound [US]
  Soma® Compound w/Codeine [US]
  Soma® [US/Can]
  Strifon Forte® [Can]

MYCOSIS (FUNGOIDES)
Psoralen
  methoxsalen
  8-MOP® [US/Can]
  Oxsoralen® Lotion [US/Can]
  Oxsoralen-Ultra® [US/Can]
  Ultramop™ [Can]
  Uvadex® [US/Can]

NERVE BLOCK
Local Anesthetic
  Anestacon® [US]
  Betacaine® [Can]
  bupivacaine
  Carbocaine® [Can]
  chloroprocaine
  Citanest® Forte [Can]
  Citanest® Plain [US/Can]
  Isocaine® HCl [US]
  lidocaine
  lidocaine and epinephrine
  Lidoderm® [US/Can]
  Marcaine® Spinal [US]
  Marcaine® [US/Can]
  mepivacaine
  Nesacaine®-CE [Can]
  Nesacaine®-MPF [US]

Nesacaine® [US]
Novocain® [US/Can]
Polocaine® MPF [US]
Polocaine® [US/Can]
Pontocaine® [US/Can]
Pontocaine® With Dextrose [US]
prilocaine
procaine
Sensorcaine®-MPF [US]
Sensorcaine® [US/Can]
tetracaine
tetracaine and dextrose
Xylocaine® MPF [US]
Xylocaine® [US/Can]
Xylocaine® With Epinephrine
  [US/Can]

NEURALGIA
Analgesic, Topical
  Antiphlogistine Rub A-535
    Capsaicin [Can]
  Antiphlogistine Rub A-535 No
    Odour [Can]
  ArthriCare® for Women Extra
    Moisturizing [US-OTC]
  ArthriCare® for Women Silky Dry
    [US-OTC]
  Capsagel® [US-OTC]
  capsaicin
  Capzasin-HP® [US-OTC]
  Mobisyl® [US-OTC]
  Myoflex® [US/Can]
  Sportscreme® [US-OTC]
  TheraPatch® Warm [US-OTC]
  triethanolamine salicylate
  Zostrix®-HP [US/Can]
  Zostrix(® [US/Can]
Nonsteroidal Antiinflammatory Drug
  (NSAID)
  Asaphen [Can]
  Asaphen E.C. [Can]
  Ascriptin® Arthritis Pain [US-OTC]
  Ascriptin® Enteric [US-OTC]

Ascriptin® Extra Strength [US-OTC]
Ascriptin® [US-OTC]
Aspercin Extra [US-OTC]
Aspercin [US-OTC]
aspirin
Bayer® Aspirin Extra Strength [US-
  OTC]
Bayer® Aspirin Regimen Adult Low
  Strength [US-OTC]
Bayer® Aspirin Regimen Adult Low
  Strength with Calcium [US-OTC]
Bayer® Aspirin Regimen Children's
  [US-OTC]
Bayer® Aspirin Regimen Regular
  Strength [US-OTC]
Bayer® Aspirin [US-OTC]
Bayer® Plus Extra Strength [US-
  OTC]
Bufferin® Arthritis Strength [US-
  OTC]
Bufferin® Extra Strength [US-OTC]
Bufferin® [US-OTC]
Easprin® [US]
Ecotrin® Adult Low Strength [US-
  OTC]
Ecotrin® Maximum Strength [US-
  OTC]
Ecotrin® [US-OTC]
Entrophen® [Can]
Halfprin® [US-OTC]
Novasen [Can]
St. Joseph® Pain Reliever [US-OTC]
Sureprin 81™ [US-OTC]
ZORprin® [US]

ONYCHOMYCOSIS
Antifungal Agent
  Fulvicin® P/G [US]
  Fulvicin-U/F® [US/Can]
  Grifulvin® V Suspension [US]
  griseofulvin
  Gris-PEG® [US]
  Lamisil® Oral [US/Can]
  terbinafine (oral)

OSTEOARTHRITIS

Analgesic, Nonnarcotic
  Arthrotec® [US/Can]
  diclofenac and misoprostol
Analgesic, Topical
  Antiphlogistine Rub A-535
    Capsaicin [Can]
  ArthriCare® for Women Extra
    Moisturizing [US-OTC]
  ArthriCare® for Women Silky Dry
    [US-OTC]
  Capsagel® [US-OTC]
  capsaicin
  Capzasin-HP® [US-OTC]
  TheraPatch® Warm [US-OTC]
  Zostrix®-HP [US/Can]
  Zostrix® [US/Can]
Miscellaneous Product
  sodium hyaluronate/hylan G-F 20
  Synvisc® [US/Can]
Nonsteroidal Antiinflammatory Drug
  (NSAID)
  Advil® Children's [US-OTC]
  Advil(R) Infants' Concentrated
    Drops [US-OTC]
  Advil® Junior [US-OTC]
  Advil® Migraine [US-OTC]
  Advil® [US/Can]
  Albert® Tiafen [Can]
  Aleve® [US-OTC]
  Amigesic® [US/Can]
  Anaprox® DS [US/Can]
  Anaprox® [US/Can]
  Apo®-Diclo [Can]
  Apo®-Diclo SR [Can]
  Apo®-Diflunisal [Can]
  Apo®-Etodolac [Can]
  Apo®-Ibuprofen [Can]
  Apo®-Indomethacin [Can]
  Apo®-Keto [Can]
  Apo®-Keto-E [Can]
  Apo®-Keto SR [Can]
  Apo®-Nabumetone [Can]
  Apo®-Napro-Na [Can]
  Apo®-Napro-Na DS [Can]
  Apo®-Naproxen [Can]
  Apo®-Naproxen SR [Can]
  Apo®-Oxaprozin [Can]
  Apo®-Sulin [Can]
  Apo®-Tiaprofenic [Can]
  Argesic®-SA [US]
  Asaphen [Can]
  Asaphen E.C. [Can]
  Ascriptin® Arthritis Pain [US-OTC]
  Ascriptin® Enteric [US-OTC]
  Ascriptin® Extra Strength [US-
    OTC]
  Ascriptin® [US-OTC]
  Aspercin Extra [US-OTC]
  Aspercin [US-OTC]
  aspirin
  Bayer® Aspirin Extra Strength [US-
    OTC]
  Bayer® Aspirin Regimen Adult Low
    Strength [US-OTC]
  Bayer® Aspirin Regimen Adult Low
    Strength with Calcium [US-OTC]
  Bayer® Aspirin Regimen Children's
    [US-OTC]
  Bayer® Aspirin Regimen Regular
    Strength [US-OTC]
  Bayer® Aspirin [US-OTC]
  Bayer® Plus Extra Strength [US-
    OTC]
  Bufferin® Arthritis Strength [US-
    OTC]
  Bufferin® Extra Strength [US-OTC]
  Bufferin® [US-OTC]
  Cataflam® [US/Can]
  choline magnesium trisalicylate
  Clinoril® [US]
  Daypro™ [US/Can]
  diclofenac
  diflunisal
  Doan's® Original [US-OTC]

Dolobid® [US]
Easprin® [US]
EC-Naprosyn® [US]
Ecotrin® Adult Low Strength [US-OTC]
Ecotrin® Maximum Strength [US-OTC]
Ecotrin® [US-OTC]
Entrophen® [Can]
etodolac
Extra Strength Doan's® [US-OTC]
Feldene® [US/Can]
fenoprofen
Gen-Nabumetone [Can]
Gen-Naproxen EC [Can]
Gen-Piroxicam [Can]
Genpril® [US-OTC]
Halfprin® [US-OTC]
Haltran® [US-OTC]
ibuprofen
Ibu-Tab® [US]
Indocid® [Can]
Indocid® P.D.A. [Can]
Indocin® SR [US]
Indocin® [US]
Indo-Lemmon [Can]
indomethacin
I-Prin [US-OTC]
ketoprofen
Keygesic-10® [US]
Lodine® [US/Can]
Lodine® XL [US]
magnesium salicylate
meclofenamate
meloxicam
Menadol® [US-OTC]
Midol® Maximum Strength Cramp Formula [US-OTC]
Mobicox® [Can]
MOBIC® [US/Can]
Momentum® [US-OTC]
Mono-Gesic® [US]
Motrin® Children's [US/Can]

Motrin® IB [US/Can]
Motrin® Infants' [US-OTC]
Motrin® Junior Strength [US-OTC]
Motrin® Migraine Pain [US-OTC]
Motrin® [US/Can]
nabumetone
Nalfon® [US/Can]
Naprelan® [US]
Naprosyn® [US/Can]
naproxen
Naxen® [Can]
Novasen [Can]
Novo-Difenac® [Can]
Novo-Difenac-K [Can]
Novo-Difenac® SR [Can]
Novo-Diflunisal [Can]
Novo-Keto [Can]
Novo-Keto-EC [Can]
Novo-Methacin [Can]
Novo-Naprox [Can]
Novo-Naprox Sodium [Can]
Novo-Naprox Sodium DS [Can]
Novo-Naprox SR [Can]
Novo-Pirocam® [Can]
Novo-Profen® [Can]
Novo-Sundac [Can]
Novo-Tiaprofenic [Can]
Nu-Diclo [Can]
Nu-Diclo-SR [Can]
Nu-Diflunisal [Can]
Nu-Ibuprofen [Can]
Nu-Indo [Can]
Nu-Ketoprofen [Can]
Nu-Ketoprofen-E [Can]
Nu-Naprox [Can]
Nu-Pirox [Can]
Nu-Sundac [Can]
Nu-Tiaprofenic [Can]
Orudis® KT [US-OTC]
Orudis® SR [Can]
Oruvail® [US/Can]
oxaprozin
Pennsaid® [Can]

Pexicam® [Can]
piroxicam
PMS-Diclofenac [Can]
PMS-Diclofenac SR [Can]
PMS-Tiaprofenic [Can]
ratio-Indomethacin [Can]
Relafen® [US/Can]
Rhodacine® [Can]
Rhodis™ [Can]
Rhodis-EC™ [Can]
Rhodis SR™ [Can]
Rhoxal-nabumetone [Can]
Riva-Diclofenac [Can]
Riva-Diclofenac-K [Can]
Riva-Naproxen [Can]
Salflex® [US/Can]
salsalate
Solaraze™ [US]
St. Joseph® Pain Reliever [US-OTC]
sulindac
Sureprin 81™ [US-OTC]
Surgam® [Can]
Surgam® SR [Can]
tiaprofenic acid (Canada only)
Tolectin® DS [US]
Tolectin® [US/Can]
tolmetin
Tricosal® [US]
Trilisate® [US]
Utradol™ [Can]
Voltaren Rapide® [Can]
Voltaren® [US/Can]
Voltaren®-XR [US]
Voltare Ophtha® [Can]
ZORprin® [US]
Nonsteroidal Antiinflammatory Drug
    (NSAID), COX-2 Selective
    Celebrex® [US/Can]
    celecoxib
    rofecoxib
    Vioxx® [US/Can]
Prostaglandin
    Arthrotec® [US/Can]
    diclofenac and misoprostol

OSTEODYSTROPHY
Vitamin D Analog
    Calciferol™ [US]
    Calcijex™ [US]
    calcitriol
    DHT™ Intensol™ [US]
    DHT™ [US]
    dihydrotachysterol
    Drisdol® [US/Can]
    ergocalciferol
    Hytakerol® [US/Can]
    Ostoforte® [Can]
    Rocaltrol® [US/Can]

OSTEOMALACIA
Vitamin D Analog
    Calciferol™ [US]
    Drisdol® [US/Can]
    ergocalciferol
    Ostoforte® [Can]

OSTEOMYELITIS
Antibiotic, Miscellaneous
    Alti-Clindamycin [Can]
    Apo®-Clindamycin [Can]
    Cleocin HCl® [US]
    Cleocin Pediatric® [US]
    Cleocin Phosphate® [US]
    Cleocin® [US]
    clindamycin
    Dalacin® C [Can]
    Novo-Clindamycin [Can]
    ratio-Clindamycin [Can]
    Vancocin® [US/Can]
    Vancoled® [US]
    vancomycin
Antifungal Agent, Systemic
    Fucidin® [Can]
    Fucithalmic® [Can]
    fusidic acid (Canada only)
Carbapenem (Antibiotic)
    imipenem and cilastatin
    meropenem

Merrem® I.V. [US/Can]
Primaxin® [US/Can]
Cephalosporin (First Generation)
  Ancef® [US]
  cefazolin
  cephalothin
  Ceporacin® [Can]
Cephalosporin (Second Generation)
  Apo®-Cefuroxime [Can]
  Cefotan® [US/Can]
  cefotetan
  cefoxitin
  Ceftin® [US/Can]
  cefuroxime
  Mefoxin® [US/Can]
  ratio-Cefuroxime [Can]
  Zinacef® [US/Can]
Cephalosporin (Third Generation)
  Cefizox® [US/Can]
  cefotaxime
  ceftazidime
  ceftizoxime
  ceftriaxone
  Claforan® [US/Can]
  Fortaz® [US/Can]
  Rocephin®) [US/Can]
  Tazicef® [US]
  Tazidime® [US/Can]
Penicillin
  ampicillin and sulbactam
  dicloxacillin
  nafcillin
  oxacillin
  ticarcillin and clavulanate potassium
  Timentin® [US/Can]
  Unasyn® [US/Can]
Quinolone
  ciprofloxacin
  Cipro® [US/Can]
  Cipro® XR [US/Can]

OSTEOPOROSIS

Bisphosphonate Derivative
  alendronate
  Aredia® [US/Can]
  Didronel® [US/Can]
  etidronate disodium
  Fosamax® [US/Can]
  Gen-Etidronate [Can]
  Novo-Alendronate [Can]
  pamidronate
Electrolyte Supplement, Oral
  Calbon® [US]
  Calcionate® [US-OTC]
  Calciquid® [US-OTC]
  calcium glubionate
  calcium lactate
  calcium phosphate (dibasic)
  Cal-Lac® [US]
  Posture® [US-OTC]
  Ridactate® [US]
Estrogen and Progestin Combination
  estrogens and medroxyprogesterone
  Premphase® [US/Can]
  Prempro™ [US/Can]
Estrogen Derivative
  Alora® [US]
  Cenestin™ [US/Can]
  Climara® [US/Can]
  Congest [Can]
  Delestrogen® [US/Can]
  Depo®-Estradiol [US/Can]
  diethylstilbestrol
  Esclim® [US]
  Estinyl® [US]
  Estrace® [US/Can]
  Estraderm® [US/Can]
  estradiol
  Estring® [US/Can]
  Estrogel® [Can]
  estrogens (conjugated A/synthetic)
  estrogens (conjugated/equine)
  estrogens (esterified)
  ethinyl estradiol

Femring™ [US]
Gynodiol® [US]
Honvol® [Can]
Menest® [US]
Oesclim® [Can]
Premarin® [US/Can]
Vagifem® [US/Can]
Vivelle-Dot® [US]
Vivelle® [US/Can]
Mineral, Oral
ACT® [US-OTC]
Fluor-A-Day® [Can]
fluoride
Fluorigard® [US-OTC]
Fluorinse® [US]
Fluotic® [Can]
Flura-Drops® [US]
Flura-Loz® [US]
Gel-Kam® [US]
Lozi-Flur™ [US]
Luride® Lozi-Tab® [US]
Luride® [US]
NeutraCare® [US]
NeutraGard® [US-OTC]
Pediaflor® [US]
Pharmaflur® [US]
Phos-Flur® [US]
PreviDent® 5000 Plus™ [US]
PreviDent® [US]
Stan-Gard® [US]
Stop® [US-OTC]
Thera-Flur-N® [US]
Polypeptide Hormone
Calcimar® [Can]
calcitonin
Caltine® [Can]
Miacalcin® [US/Can]
Selective Estrogen Receptor Modulator
    (SERM)
Evista® [US/Can]
raloxifene

OSTEOSARCOMA

Antineoplastic Agent
Adriamycin® [Can]
Adriamycin PFS® [US]
Adriamycin RDF® [US]
Apo®-Methotrexate [Can]
Caelyx® [Can]
cisplatin
doxorubicin
methotrexate
Myocet® [Can]
Platinol®-AQ [US]
Platinol® [US]
ratio-Methotrexate [Can]
Rheumatrex® [US]
Rubex® [US]
Trexall™ [US]

PAGET DISEASE OF BONE

Bisphosphonate Derivative
alendronate
Aredia® [US/Can]
Didronel® [US/Can]
etidronate disodium
Fosamax® [US/Can]
Gen-Etidronate [Can]
Novo-Alendronate [Can]
pamidronate
Skelid® [US]
tiludronate
Polypeptide Hormone
Calcimar® [Can]
calcitonin
Caltine® [Can]
Miacalcin® [US/Can]

PAIN

Analgesic, Miscellaneous
acetaminophen and tramadol
Ultracet™ [US]
Analgesic, Narcotic
acetaminophen and codeine

Actiq® [US/Can]
alfentanil
Alfenta® [US/Can]
Anexsia® [US]
Apo®-Butorphanol [Can]
aspirin and codeine
Astramorph/PF™ [US]
Avinza™ [US]
Bancap HC® [US]
belladonna and opium
B&O Supprettes® [US]
Buprenex® [US/Can]
buprenorphine
butalbital compound and codeine
butorphanol
Capital® and Codeine [US]
Ceta-Plus® [US]
codeine
Codeine Contin® [Can]
Co-Gesic® [US]
Coryphen® Codeine [Can]
Damason-P® [US]
Darvocet-N® 50 [US/Can]
Darvocet-N® 100 [US/Can]
Darvon® Compound-65 [US]
Darvon-N® Tablet [US/Can]
Darvon® [US]
Demerol® [US/Can]
dihydrocodeine compound
Dilaudid-5® [US]
Dilaudid-HP-Plus® [Can]
Dilaudid-HP® [US/Can]
Dilaudid® [US/Can]
Dilaudid-XP® [Can]
Dolacet® [US]
Dolophine® [US/Can]
Duragesic® [US/Can]
Duramorph® [US]
Empirin® With Codeine [US]
Endocet® [US/Can]
Endodan® [US/Can]
fentanyl
Fiorinal®-C 1/2 [Can]

Fiorinal®-C 1/4 [Can]
Fiorinal® With Codeine [US]
Hydrocet® [US]
hydrocodone and acetaminophen
hydrocodone and aspirin
hydrocodone and ibuprofen
Hydromorph Contin® [Can]
hydromorphone
Infumorph® [US]
Kadian® [US/Can]
Levo-Dromoran® [US]
levorphanol
Lorcet® 10/650 [US]
Lorcet®-HD [US]
Lorcet® Plus [US]
Lortab® [US]
Margesic® H [US]
Maxidone™ [US]
Mepergan® [US]
meperidine
meperidine and promethazine
Meperitab® [US]
M-Eslon® [Can]
Metadol™ [Can]
methadone
Methadone Intensol™ [US]
Methadose® [US/Can]
Morphine HP® [Can]
morphine sulfate
M.O.S.-Sulfate® [Can]
MS Contin® [US/Can]
MSIR® [US/Can]
nalbuphine
Norco® [US]
Nubain® [US/Can]
Numorphan® [US/Can]
opium tincture
Oramorph SR® [US]
oxycodone
oxycodone and acetaminophen
oxycodone and aspirin
OxyContin® [US/Can]
Oxydose™ [US]

OxyFast® [US]
OxyIR® [US/Can]
oxymorphone
paregoric
PC-Cap® [US]
pentazocine
pentazocine compound
Percocet® [US]
Percodan® [US/Can]
Phenaphen® With Codeine [US]
PMS-Butorphanol [Can]
PMS-Hydromorphone [Can]
PMS-Morphine Sulfate SR [Can]
PMS-Oxycodone-Acetaminophen
  [Can]
Pronap-100® [US]
propoxyphene
propoxyphene and acetaminophen
propoxyphene and aspirin
ratio-Codeine [Can]
ratio-Emtec-30 [Can]
ratio-Lenoltec [Can]
ratio-Morphine [Can]
ratio-Morphine SR [Can]
ratio-Oxycocet [Can]
ratio-Oxycodan® [Can]
ratio-Tecnal C 1/2 [Can]
ratio-Tecnal C 1/4 [Can]
remifentanil
RMS® [US]
Roxanol 100® [US]
Roxanol®-T [US]
Roxanol® [US]
Roxicet® 5/500 [US]
Roxicet™ [US]
Roxicodone™ Intensol™ [US]
Roxicodone™ [US]
Stadol® NS [US/Can]
Stadol® [US]
Stagesic® [US]
Statex® [Can]
Sublimaze® [US]
Subutex® [US]

sufentanil
Sufenta® [US/Can]
Supeudol® [Can]
Synalgos®-DC [US]
642® Tablet [Can]
Talacen® [US]
Talwin® NX [US]
Talwin® [US/Can]
T-Gesic® [US]
Triatec-8 [Can]
Triatec-30 [Can]
Triatec-Strong [Can]
Tylenol® with Codeine [US/Can]
Tylox® [US]
Ultiva™ [US/Can]
Vicodin® ES [US]
Vicodin® HP [US]
Vicodin® [US]
Vicoprofen® [US/Can]
Zydone® [US]

Analgesic, Nonnarcotic
Abenol® [Can]
Acephen® [US-OTC]
acetaminophen
acetaminophen and
  diphenhydramine
acetaminophen and
  phenyltoloxamine
acetaminophen and tramadol
acetaminophen, aspirin, and caffeine
Acular LS™ [US]
Acular® P.F. [US]
Acular® [US/Can]
Advil® Children's [US-OTC]
Advil® Infants' Concentrated Drops
  [US-OTC]
Advil® Junior [US-OTC]
Advil® Migraine [US-OTC]
Advil® [US/Can]
Aleve® [US-OTC]
Amigesic® [US/Can]
Anaprox® DS [US/Can]
Anaprox® [US/Can]

Ansaid® Oral [US/Can]
Apo®-Acetaminophen [Can]
Apo®-Diclo [Can]
Apo®-Diclo SR [Can]
Apo®-Diflunisal [Can]
Apo®-Etodolac [Can]
Apo®-Flurbiprofen [Can]
Apo®-Ibuprofen [Can]
Apo®-Indomethacin [Can]
Apo®-Keto [Can]
Apo®-Keto-E [Can]
Apo®-Ketorolac [Can]
Apo®-Keto SR [Can]
Apo®-Mefenamic [Can]
Apo®-Nabumetone [Can]
Apo®-Napro-Na [Can]
Apo®-Napro-Na DS [Can]
Apo®-Naproxen [Can]
Apo®-Naproxen SR [Can]
Apo®-Oxaprozin [Can]
Apo®-Sulin [Can]
Argesic®-SA [US]
Asaphen [Can]
Asaphen E.C. [Can]
Ascriptin® Arthritis Pain [US-OTC]
Ascriptin® Enteric [US-OTC]
Ascriptin® Extra Strength [US-OTC]
Ascriptin® [US-OTC]
Aspercin Extra [US-OTC]
Aspercin [US-OTC]
aspirin
Atasol® [Can]
Bayer® Aspirin Extra Strength [US-OTC]
Bayer® Aspirin Regimen Adult Low Strength [US-OTC]
Bayer® Aspirin Regimen Adult Low Strength with Calcium [US-OTC]
Bayer® Aspirin Regimen Children's [US-OTC]
Bayer® Aspirin Regimen Regular Strength [US-OTC]
Bayer® Aspirin [US-OTC]

Bayer® Plus Extra Strength [US-OTC]
Brexidol® 20 [Can]
Bufferin® Arthritis Strength [US-OTC]
Bufferin® Extra Strength [US-OTC]
Bufferin® [US-OTC]
Cataflam® [US/Can]
Cetafen Extra® [US-OTC]
Cetafen® [US-OTC]
choline magnesium trisalicylate
Clinoril® [US]
Daypro™ [US/Can]
diclofenac
diflunisal
Dolobid® [US]
Easprin® [US]
EC-Naprosyn® [US]
Ecotrin® Adult Low Strength [US-OTC]
Ecotrin® Maximum Strength [US-OTC]
Ecotrin® [US-OTC]
Entrophen® [Can]
etodolac
Excedrin® Extra Strength [US-OTC]
Excedrin® Migraine [US-OTC]
Excedrin® P.M. [US-OTC]
Feldene® [US/Can]
fenoprofen
Feverall® [US-OTC]
flurbiprofen
Froben® [Can]
Froben-SR® [Can]
Genaced [US-OTC]
Genapap® Children [US-OTC]
Genapap® Extra Strength [US-OTC]
Genapap® Infant [US-OTC]
Genapap® [US-OTC]
Genebs® Extra Strength [US-OTC]
Genebs® [US-OTC]
Genesec® [US-OTC]
Gen-Nabumetone [Can]

Gen-Naproxen EC [Can]
Gen-Piroxicam [Can]
Genpril® [US-OTC]
Goody's® Extra Strength Headache
  Powder [US-OTC]
Goody's PM® Powder [US-OTC]
Halfprin® [US-OTC]
Haltran® [US-OTC]
ibuprofen
Ibu-Tab® [US]
Indocid® [Can]
Indocid® P.D.A. [Can]
Indocin® SR [US]
Indocin® [US]
Indo-Lemmon [Can]
indomethacin
Infantaire [US-OTC]
I-Prin [US-OTC]
ketoprofen
ketorolac
Legatrin PM® [US-OTC]
Liquiprin® for Children [US-OTC]
Lodine® [US/Can]
Lodine® XL [US]
Mapap® Children's [US-OTC]
Mapap® Extra Strength [US-OTC]
Mapap® Infants [US-OTC]
Mapap® [US-OTC]
meclofenamate
mefenamic acid
Menadol® [US-OTC]
Midol® Maximum Strength Cramp
  Formula [US-OTC]
Mono-Gesic® [US]
Motrin® Children's [US/Can]
Motrin® IB [US/Can]
Motrin® Infants' [US-OTC]
Motrin® Junior Strength [US-OTC]
Motrin® Migraine Pain [US-OTC]
Motrin® [US/Can]
nabumetone
Nalfon® [US/Can]
Naprelan® [US]

Naprosyn® [US/Can]
naproxen
Naxen® [Can]
Norgesic™ Forte [US/Can]
Norgesic™ [US/Can]
Novasen [Can]
Novo-Difenac® [Can]
Novo-Difenac-K [Can]
Novo-Difenac® SR [Can]
Novo-Diflunisal [Can]
Novo-Flurprofen [Can]
Novo-Keto [Can]
Novo-Keto-EC [Can]
Novo-Ketorolac [Can]
Novo-Methacin [Can]
Novo-Naprox [Can]
Novo-Naprox Sodium [Can]
Novo-Naprox Sodium DS [Can]
Novo-Naprox SR [Can]
Novo-Pirocam® [Can]
Novo-Profen® [Can]
Novo-Sundac [Can]
Nu-Diclo [Can]
Nu-Diclo-SR [Can]
Nu-Diflunisal [Can]
Nu-Flurprofen [Can]
Nu-Ibuprofen [Can]
Nu-Indo [Can]
Nu-Ketoprofen [Can]
Nu-Ketoprofen-E [Can]
Nu-Mefenamic [Can]
Nu-Naprox [Can]
Nu-Pirox [Can]
Nu-Sundac [Can]
Ocufen® Ophthalmic [US/Can]
orphenadrine, aspirin, and caffeine
Orphengesic Forte [US]
Orphengesic [US]
Orudis® KT [US-OTC]
Orudis® SR [Can]
Oruvail® [US/Can]
oxaprozin
Pediatrix [Can]

Pennsaid® [Can]
Percogesic® Extra Strength [US-OTC]
Percogesic® [US-OTC]
Pexicam® [Can]
Phenylgesic® [US-OTC]
piroxicam
piroxicam and cyclodextrin (Canada only)
PMS-Diclofenac [Can]
PMS-Diclofenac SR [Can]
PMS-Mefenamic Acid [Can]
Ponstan® [Can]
Ponstel® [US/Can]
ratio-Flurbiprofen [Can]
ratio-Indomethacin [Can]
ratio-Ketorolac [Can]
Redutemp® [US-OTC]
Relafen® [US/Can]
Rhodacine® [Can]
Rhodis™ [Can]
Rhodis-EC™ [Can]
Rhodis SR™ [Can]
Rhoxal-nabumetone [Can]
Riva-Diclofenac [Can]
Riva-Diclofenac-K [Can]
Riva-Naproxen [Can]
Salflex® [US/Can]
salsalate
Silapap® Children's [US-OTC]
Silapap® Infants [US-OTC]
sodium salicylate
Solaraze™ [US]
St. Joseph® Pain Reliever [US-OTC]
sulindac
Sureprin 81™ [US-OTC]
Tempra® [Can]
Tolectin® DS [US]
Tolectin® [US/Can]
tolmetin
Toradol® [US/Can]
tramadol
Tricosal® [US]
Trilisate® [US]
Tylenol® Arthritis Pain [US-OTC]
Tylenol® Children's [US-OTC]
Tylenol® Extra Strength [US-OTC]
Tylenol® Infants [US-OTC]
Tylenol® Junior Strength [US-OTC]
Tylenol® PM Extra Strength [US-OTC]
Tylenol® Severe Allergy [US-OTC]
Tylenol® Sore Throat [US-OTC]
Tylenol® [US/Can]
Ultracet™ [US]
Ultram® [US/Can]
Utradol™ [Can]
Valorin Extra [US-OTC]
Valorin [US-OTC]
Vanquish® Extra Strength Pain Reliever [US-OTC]
Voltaren Rapide® [Can]
Voltaren® [US/Can]
Voltaren®-XR [US]
Voltare Ophtha(R) [Can]
ZORprin® [US]

Decongestant/Analgesic
Advil® Cold, Children's [US-OTC]
Advil® Cold & Sinus [US/Can]
Dristan® Sinus Caplets [US]
Dristan® Sinus Tablet [US/Can]
Motrin® Cold and Sinus [US-OTC]
Motrin® Cold, Children's [US-OTC]
pseudoephedrine and ibuprofen

Local Anesthetic
Alcaine® [US/Can]
Diocaine® [Can]
ethyl chloride
ethyl chloride and dichlorotetrafluoroethane
Fluro-Ethyl® Aerosol [US]
Ophthetic® [US]
Parcaine® [US]
proparacaine

Neuroleptic Agent
Apo®-Methoprazine [Can]

methotrimeprazine (Canada only)
Novo-Meprazine [Can]
Nozinan® [Can]
Nonsteroidal Antiinflammatory Drug
   (NSAID)
   Doan's®, Original [US-OTC]
   Extra Strength Doan's® [US-OTC]
   Keygesic-10® [US]
   magnesium salicylate
   Momentum® [US-OTC]
Nonsteroidal Antiinflammatory Drug
   (NSAID), COX-2 Selective
   rofecoxib
   Vioxx® [US/Can]
Nonsteroidal Antiinflammatory Drug
   (NSAID), Oral
   Apo®-Floctafenine [Can]
   floctafenine (Canada only)
   Idarac® [Can]

PAIN (BONE)
Radiopharmaceutical
   Metastron® [US/Can]
   strontium-89

PAIN (LUMBAR PUNCTURE)
Analgesic, Topical
   EMLA® [US/Can]
   lidocaine and prilocaine

PAIN (MUSCLE)
Analgesic, Topical
   dichlorodifluoromethane and
     trichloromonofluoromethane
   Fluori-Methane® [US]

PLANTARIS
Keratolytic Agent
   Duofilm® Solution [US]
   Keralyt® Gel [US-OTC]
   salicylic acid and lactic acid
   salicylic acid and propylene glycol

PLANTAR WART
Keratolytic Agent
   Duofilm® Solution [US]
   salicylic acid and lactic acid
Topical Skin Product
   silver nitrate

POLYMYOSITIS
Antineoplastic Agent
   Apo®-Methotrexate [Can]
   chlorambucil
   cyclophosphamide
   Cytoxan® [US/Can]
   Leukeran® [US/Can]
   methotrexate
   Neosar® [US]
   Procytox® [Can]
   ratio-Methotrexate [Can]
   Rheumatrex® [US]
   Trexall™ [US]
Immunosuppressant Agent
   Alti-Azathioprine [Can]
   Apo®-Azathioprine [Can]
   azathioprine
   Gen-Azathioprine [Can]
   Imuran® [US/Can]
   ratio-Azathioprine [Can]

PSEUDOGOUT
Antigout Agent
   colchicine
   ratio-Colchicine [Can]
Nonsteroidal Antiinflammatory Drug
   (NSAID)
   Apo®-Indomethacin [Can]
   Indocid® [Can]
   Indocid® P.D.A. [Can]
   Indocin® SR [US]
   Indocin® [US]
   Indo-Lemmon [Can]
   indomethacin
   Novo-Methacin [Can]

Nu-Indo [Can]
ratio-Indomethacin [Can]
Rhodacine® [Can]

RHEUMATIC DISORDER
Adrenal Corticosteroid
Acthar® [US]
A-HydroCort® [US]
A-methapred® [US]
Apo®-Prednisone [Can]
Aristocort® Forte Injection [US]
Aristocort® Intralesional Injection [US]
Aristocort® Tablet [US/Can]
Aristospan® Intraarticular Injection [US/Can]
Aristospan® Intralesional Injection [US/Can]
Betaject™ [Can]
betamethasone (systemic)
Betnesol® [Can]
Celestone® Phosphate [US]
Celestone® Soluspan(R) [US/Can]
Celestone® [US]
Cel-U-Jec® [US]
Cortef® Tablet [US/Can]
corticotropin
cortisone acetate
Cortone® [Can]
Decadron®-LA [US]
Decadron® [US/Can]
Decaject-LA® [US]
Decaject® [US]
Deltasone® [US]
Depo-Medrol® [US/Can]
Depopred® [US]
dexamethasone (systemic)
Dexasone® L.A. [US]
Dexasone® [US/Can]
Dexone® LA [US]
Dexone® [US]
Hexadrol® [US/Can]
H.P. Acthar® Gel [US]

hydrocortisone (systemic)
Kenalog® Injection [US/Can]
Medrol® Dosepak(TM) [US/Can]
Medrol® Tablet [US/Can]
methylprednisolone
Orapred™ [US]
Pediapred® [US/Can]
PMS-Dexamethasone [Can]
Prednicot® [US]
prednisolone (systemic)
Prednisol® TBA [US]
prednisone
Prednisone Intensol™ [US]
Prelone® [US]
ratio-Dexamethasone [Can]
Solu-Cortef® [US/Can]
Solu-Medrol® [US/Can]
Solurex L.A.® [US]
Sterapred® DS [US]
Sterapred® [US]
Tac(TM)-3 Injection [US]
Triam-A® Injection [US]
triamcinolone (systemic)
Triam Forte® Injection [US]
Winpred™ [Can]

RHEUMATOID ARTHRITIS
Analgesic, Nonnarcotic
Arthrotec® [US/Can]
diclofenac and misoprostol
Prostaglandin
Arthrotec® [US/Can]
diclofenac and misoprostol

RICKETS
Vitamin D Analog
Calciferol™ [US]
Drisdol® [US/Can]
ergocalciferol
Ostoforte® [Can]

SKIN ULCER
Enzyme
    collagenase
    Santyl®[US/Can]

SPINAL CORD INJURY
Skeletal Muscle Relaxant
    Dantrium® [US/Can]
    dantrolene

SPONDYLITIS (ANKYLOSING)
Nonsteroidal Antiinflammatory Drug (NSAID)
    Apo®-Diclo [Can]
    Apo®-Diclo SR [Can]
    Cataflam® [US/Can]
    diclofenac
    Feldene® [US/Can]
    Gen-Piroxicam [Can]
    Novo-Difenac® [Can]
    Novo-Difenac-K [Can]
    Novo-Difenac® SR [Can]
    Novo-Pirocam® [Can]
    Nu-Diclo [Can]
    Nu-Diclo-SR [Can]
    Nu-Pirox [Can]
    Pennsaid® [Can]
    Pexicam® [Can]
    piroxicam
    PMS-Diclofenac [Can]
    PMS-Diclofenac SR [Can]
    Riva-Diclofenac [Can]
    Riva-Diclofenac-K [Can]
    Solaraze™ [US]
    Voltaren Rapide® [Can]
    Voltaren® [US/Can]
    Voltaren®-XR [US]
    Voltare Ophtha® [Can]

SUDECK ATROPHY
Calcium Channel Blocker
    Adalat® CC [US]
    Adalat® XL(R) [Can]
    Apo®-Nifed [Can]
    Apo®-Nifed PA [Can]
    Nifedical™ XL [US]
    nifedipine
    Novo-Nifedin [Can]
    Nu-Nifed [Can]
    Procardia® [US/Can]
    Procardia XL® [US]

TINEA
Antifungal Agent
    Absorbine Jr.® Antifungal [US-OTC]
    Aftate® Antifungal [US-OTC]
    Aloe Vesta® 2-n-1 Antifungal [US-OTC]
    Apo®-Ketoconazole [Can]
    Baza® Antifungal [US-OTC]
    Blis-To-Sol® [US-OTC]
    butenafine
    Canesten® Topical [Can]
    Canesten® Vaginal [Can]
    carbol-fuchsin solution
    Carrington Antifungal [US-OTC]
    ciclopirox
    Clotrimaderm [Can]
    clotrimazole
    Cruex® [US-OTC]
    Dermasept Antifungal [US-OTC]
    econazole
    Ecostatin® [Can]
    Exelderm® [US/Can]
    Femizol-M™ [US-OTC]
    Fulvicin® P/G [US]
    Fulvicin-U/F® [US/Can]
    Fungi-Guard [US-OTC]
    Fungi-Nail® [US-OTC]
    Fungoid® Tincture [US-OTC]
    Gold Bond® Antifungal [US-OTC]

Grifulvin® V Suspension [US]
griseofulvin
Gris-PEG® [US]
Gyne-Lotrimin® 3 [US-OTC]
Gyne-Lotrimin® [US-OTC]
Gynix® [US-OTC]
ketoconazole
Ketoderm® [Can]
Lamisil® Cream [US]
Loprox® [US/Can]
Lotrimin® AF Athlete's Foot Cream [US-OTC]
Lotrimin® AF Athlete's Foot Solution [US-OTC]
Lotrimin® AF Jock Itch Cream [US-OTC]
Lotrimin® AF Powder/Spray [US-OTC]
Lotrimin® Ultra™ [US-OTC]
Mentax® [US]
Micaderm® [US-OTC]
Micatin® [US/Can]
miconazole
Micozole [Can]
Micro-Guard® [US-OTC]
Mitrazol™ [US-OTC]
Monistat® 1 Combination Pack [US-OTC]
Monistat® 3 [US-OTC]
Monistat® 7 [US-OTC]
Monistat® [Can]
Monistat-Derm® [US]
Mycelex®-7 [US-OTC]
Mycelex® Twin Pack [US-OTC]
Myco-Nail [US-OTC]
naftifine
Naftin® [US]
Nizoral® A-D [US-OTC]
Nizoral® [US/Can]
Novo-Ketoconazole [Can]

oxiconazole
Oxistat® [US/Can]
Penlac™ [US/Can]
Pitrex [CAN]
sodium thiosulfate
Spectazole™ [US/Can]
sulconazole
terbinafine (topical)
Tinactin® Antifungal Jock Itch [US-OTC]
Tinactin® Antifungal [US-OTC]
Tinaderm [US-OTC]
Ting® [US-OTC]
TipTapToe [US-OTC]
tolnaftate
triacetin
Triple Care® Antifungal [OTC]
undecylenic acid and derivatives
Versiclear™ [US]
Zeasorb®-AF [US-OTC]
Antifungal/Corticosteroid
  betamethasone and clotrimazole
  Lotriderm® [Can]
  Lotrisone® [US/Can]
Antiseborrheic Agent, Topical
  Head & Shoulders® Intensive Treatment [US-OTC]
  selenium sulfide
  Selsun Blue® [US-OTC]
  Selsun® [US]
  Versel® [Can]
Disinfectant
  sodium hypochlorite solution

ULCER, DIABETIC FOOT OR LEG

Topical Skin Product
  becaplermin
  Regranex® [US/Can]